British Pharmacopœia 1988

Volume I

British Pharmacopœia 1988

Volume I

Published on the recommendation of the
Medicines Commission
pursuant to the Medicines Act 1968

Effective date: 1 December 1988

London   Her Majesty's Stationery Office

DEPARTMENT OF HEALTH AND SOCIAL SECURITY
SCOTTISH HOME AND HEALTH DEPARTMENT
WELSH OFFICE
MINISTRY OF HEALTH AND SOCIAL SERVICES FOR NORTHERN IRELAND

Office of the British Pharmacopœia Commission:

Market Towers
1 Nine Elms Lane
London SW8 5NQ

Telephone: 01-720 9844
Facsimile: 01-720 5647
Telex: 883669 DHSSHQ G

Laboratory of the British Pharmacopœia Commission:

Government Buildings
Block 2, Honeypot Lane
Stanmore
Middlesex HA7 1AY

Telephone: 01-952 2311
Telex: 94016760

Typography by Her Majesty's Stationery Office

Printed in the United Kingdom
for Her Majesty's Stationery Office

Dd 289915 C250 4/88

ISBN 0 11 320837 5

Contents

Notice

Patents

In this Pharmacopœia certain drugs and preparations have been included notwithstanding the existence of actual or potential patent rights. In so far as such substances are protected by Letters Patent their inclusion in this Pharmacopœia neither conveys, nor implies, licence to manufacture.

Preface

The British Pharmacopœia 1988 is published by Her Majesty's Stationery Office for the Health Ministers on the recommendation of the Medicines Commission in accordance with section 99(6) of the Medicines Act 1968.

The preparation of this edition has made very heavy demands on the members of the British Pharmacopœia Commission, its committees and, in particular, its staff. The Medicines Commission wishes to record appreciation for the services of all who have contributed to this important work. In particular it takes this opportunity to acknowledge the outstanding contribution made by Dr C A Johnson, who retired after exactly twenty-five years of service, of which eight were as Scientific Director and twelve as Secretary and Scientific Director.

British Pharmacopœia Commission

The British Pharmacopœia Commission is appointed by the Secretary of State concerned with health in England, the Secretaries of State respectively concerned with health and with agriculture in Wales and in Scotland, the Minister of Agriculture, Fisheries and Food, the Department of Health and Social Services for Northern Ireland and the Department of Agriculture for Northern Ireland, acting jointly, in exercise of their powers under section 4 of the Medicines Act 1968.

The duties of the British Pharmacopœia Commission are as follows:

(a) the preparation under section 99(1) of the Act of any new edition of the British Pharmacopœia;

(b) the preparation under section 99(1) of the Act, as given effect by section 102(1) thereof, of any amendments of the edition of the British Pharmacopœia published in 1968 or any new edition of it;

(c) the preparation under section 100 of the Act (which provides for the preparation and publication of lists of names to be used as headings to monographs in the British Pharmacopœia) of any list of names and the preparation under that section as given effect by section 102(3) of the Act of any amendments of any published list;

(d) the preparation under section 99(3)(b) of the Act of any compendium or any new edition thereof;

(e) the preparation under section 99(3)(b) of the Act, as given effect by section 102(1) thereof, of any amendments to any such compendium.

Members of the British Pharmacopœia Commission are appointed by Ministers, having regard to recommendations made by the Medicines Commission. Appointments are usually for a (renewable) term of four years.

Membership of the British Pharmacopœia Commission

Chairman

J B Stenlake† CBE DSc PhD FPS CChem FRSC FRSE
Honorary Professor of Pharmacy in the University of Strathclyde

Vice-Chairman

P Turner† MD BSc FRCP HonMPS FIBiol
Professor of Clinical Pharmacology in the University of London

W G Allen† MRCVS
A Veterinary Surgeon

A O Betts★ BSc MA PhD MRCVS
Principal and Dean of The Royal Veterinary College, University of London

D H Calam† MA DPhil CChem FRSC
Head of Antibiotics and Chemistry Division, National Institute for Biological Standards and Control

A C Caws★ BSc CChem MRSC
A Senior Analyst in the Pharmaceutical Industry

J F Chissell★ MSc
A Director of Quality Services in the Pharmaceutical Industry

I Davidson‡ BSc MRCVS
Head of Biological Products and Standards Department, Central Veterinary Laboratory, Weybridge, Ministry of Agriculture, Fisheries and Food

A F Fell★ BPharm PhD MPS CChem FRSC FIQA
Professor of Pharmaceutical Chemistry in the University of Bradford

F Fish★ BPharm PhD FPS
Dean of The School of Pharmacy, University of London

D Ganderton★ BPharm PhD FPS
Professor of Pharmaceutics in the University of London

J A Goldsmith† BSc PhD CChem FRSC FIQA
A Director of Technical Operations in the Pharmaceutical Industry

A Holbrook† MChemA CChem FRSC
A Scientific Adviser in the Pharmaceutical Industry

J A Holgate‡ MB ChB MSc FIBiol
Formerly a Principal Medical Officer in the Department of Health and Social Security

D I Magrath‡ BA PhD
A Member of the Viral Products Division, National Institute for Biological Standards and Control

J M Midgley† BSc MSc PhD FPS CChem MRSC
Professor of Pharmacy and Chairman and Head of the Department of Pharmacy in the University of Strathclyde

G F Phillips† OBE MSc CChem FRSC
Superintendent, Health and Forensic Services Division, Laboratory of the Government Chemist

L E Ramsay* MB ChB FRCP
Consultant Physician, Royal Hallamshire Hospital and Reader in Clinical Pharmacology and Therapeutics, University of Sheffield

J W G Smith§ MD FRCPath FFCM FIBiol DipBact
Lately Director of the National Institute for Biological Standards and Control

W G Thomas§ MSc PhD FPS
Director, Department of Pharmaceutical Sciences, Pharmaceutical Society of Great Britain

B A Wills* BPharm PhD FPS CChem FRSC
Chief Pharmacist, Department of Health and Social Security

Secretary and Scientific Director

C A Johnson CBE DSc(Hon) BPharm BSc FPS CChem FRSC MPhA

*Term of office ends 31 December 1991.
†Term of office ends 31 December 1989.
‡Term of office ended 31 December 1987.
§Term of office ended 31 December 1985.

Membership of Committees and Consultative Groups

The Commission appointed the following Committees and Corresponding Consultative Groups to advise it in carrying out its duties. Membership has changed from time to time; the lists below include all who have served during the period 1984 to 1986.

COMMITTEES

A: Medicinal Chemicals
A C Caws (*Chairman*), J B Stenlake (*Vice-Chairman*), A L Barber, J A Goldsmith, E Mather, N Nix, N Randall, C Ratcliffe, G D Rees, J E Shinner, J Slater

B: Medicinal Chemicals
A Holbrook (*Chairman*), A F Fell (*Vice-Chairman*), F Bailey, J K Bailey, P H Cobb, G Drewery, E J Kempster, M Martin-Smith, R N Thornhill, A A Wagland, D Watt (*Corresponding member* B Warren)

C: General Chemicals
G F Phillips (*Chairman*), A Holbrook (*Vice-Chairman*), G Bratt, D J Brown, A G Davidson, E J Kempster, R E King, G F Lewis, A McCraight, J M Midgley, S U Ruff, D E Simpkins, C H Thorpe

D: Steroids
A Holbrook (*Chairman*), J F Chissell (*Vice-Chairman*), D W Houghton, J P Jefferies, W McMeekin, S Williams

E: Antibiotics
J A Holgate (*Chairman*), J F Chissell (*Vice-Chairman*), E Addison, A E Bird, A K Coulter, P J Duff, J W Lightbown, H C Macfarlane, D Moriau, G F Snook (*Corresponding members* C R Broom, R K Howard, M E Duncan, J Purves, A H Thomas)

F: Pharmacy
D Ganderton (*Chairman*), B A Wills (*Vice-Chairman*), D J G Davies, S S Davis, A L Davison, T Dott, J A Farwell, W L Hooper, T M Jones, J B Kay, A F Lott, W Lund, J M Padfield, W N Pitkethly, G Smith, D F Spooner (*Corresponding members* K A Lees, C J Lewis)

G: Crude Drugs and Galenicals
F Fish (*Chairman*), A C Caws (*Vice-Chairman*), D J Brown, K Helliwell, B P Jackson, N Nix, J D Phillipson, M H Ransom, A R Rixon, A J Woodgate

H: Biological Materials
D H Calam (*Chairman*), D R Bangham (*Vice-Chairman*), D M Benoliel, G W Bisset, A F Bristow, K R Butterworth, J A Holgate, N Randall, G A Sabey, G A Stewart (*Corresponding members* J Tranter, H E Wade)

J: Immunological Products
J W G Smith (Chairman to December 1985), I Davidson (Chairman from January 1986), F W Sheffield (*Vice-Chairman*), I G S Furminger, J R Hepple, P A Knight, A M T Lee, D I Magrath, J Melling, J Prydie, D H Thornton, P W Wells (*Corresponding members* T W F Pay, G C Schild)

K: Blood Products
J A Holgate (*Chairman*), K J Ayling, R S Lane, R J Perry, D S Smith, T Snape, D P Thomas, L Vallet, J G Watt (*Corresponding member* T W Barrowcliffe)

L: Surgical Dressings
F Fish (*Chairman*), T D Turner (*Vice-Chairman*), D T Britton, E H Carus, M G Leakey, K Lunn, D Metcalfe, B W Mitchell, P J Perry, S Thomas (*Corresponding member* R Crabtree)

Membership of the European Pharmacopœia Commission

The membership of the Commission on 30 June 1987 was as follows:

Chairman:	P Arends
Austria (A):	K Pfleger, H Halbich, M Arrouas
Belgium (B):	C L Lapière, P Janssens, H Vanderhaeghe, J Bosly★, P Jacqmain★, R Kinget★
Cyprus (CY):	E Kkolos
Denmark (DK):	P Frandsen, H G Kristensen, P Helboe★, A Sørensen★, M Thomsen★
Finland (SF):	J Halmekoski, L Turakka, A Kaukinen★
France (F):	A Artiges, Y Cohen, M Pesez, J P Billon★, P Delomenie★, F J Pellerin★
Federal Republic of Germany (D):	E Boll, W Hennessen, G Schorn, H D Brede★, K Thoma★
Greece (GR):	S Philianos, G Salem, A Tsoka
Iceland (ISL):	I J Petersen, V G Skulason
Ireland (IRL):	T McGuinn, R F Timoney
Italy (I):	E Cingolani, F Pocchiari, G Vicari, E Ciranni Signoretti★, C Collotti★, M Marchetti★
Luxembourg (L):	J Genoux-Hames, X Perlia, E Duhr★
Netherlands (NL):	A W M Indemans, C A Teijgeler, H L Vos, J van Noordwijk★, H M Smits★
Norway (N):	K Backe-Hansen, K Briseid, H Kristiansen
Spain (E):	A Dominguez-Gil, A Sanchez, A Vardulaki
Sweden (S):	P Lindgren, M B Ohrner, I Sjöholm, L Sjödin★
Switzerland (CH):	G Rotzler, U Salzmann, D Sonanini, P Buri★, I Kapetanidis★
United Kingdom (UK):	J A Holgate, C A Johnson, J B Stenlake, D H Calam★, I Davidson★, B A Wills★
Observers:	
(EEC)	F Sauer
(Portugal)	A Correia Alves, L Nogueira Prista

★Alternates.

Membership of Groups of Experts of the European Pharmacopœia Commission

The membership of the Groups of Experts on 30 June 1987 was as follows:

Group No 1: Biological Methods and Statistical Analysis	J van Noordwijk (*Chairman*), J Dony (*B*), M Gay (*CH*), G Hofrichter (*D*), A German (*F*), R Aureli (*I*), D Fystro (*N*), L Sjödin (*S*), M L Rabouhans (*UK*)
Group No 1CM: Microbiological Contamination	H G Kristensen (*Chairman*), J Dony (*B*), M Gay (*CH*), H Seyfarth (*D*), E A Christensen (*DK*), P Petitjean (*F*), J Lavdiotis (*GR*), R Aureli (*I*), D Fystro (*N*), O Ringertz (*S*), A L Davison (*UK*)
Group No 1L: Limulus Amoebocyte Lysate Test (LAL)	J van Noordwijk (*Chairman*), J Dony (*B*), A Gardi (*CH*), A Krüger (*D*), J Storck (*F*), L Bellentani (*I*), D Fystro (*N*), P Lindgren (*S*), G A Sabey (*UK*)
Group No 1S: Statistics	J van Noordwijk (*Chairman*), H Busse (*D*), J Didry (*F*), G M Leali (*I*), R van Strik (*NL*)
Group No 2: Chemical Methods	M Pesez (*Chairman*), P Dumont (*B*), E Keller (*CH*), E Boll (*D*), P Helboe (*DK*), J P Billon (*F*), G Minola (*I*), X Perlia (*CH*), A Bult (*NL*), G P R Carr (*UK*)
Group No 3: Nomenclature and Drafting	P Jacqmain (*Chairman*), P Braeckman (*B*), L Anker (*CH*), A Erb (*D*), P Delomenie (*F*), E Cingolani (*I*), H L Vos (*NL*), C A Johnson (*UK*)
Group No 4: Physical and Physico-chemical Methods	X Perlia (*Chairman*), L Molle (*B*), E Keller (*CH*), E Boll (*D*), F J Pellerin (*F*), G G Gallo (*I*), A Bult (*NL*), J Vessman (*S*), G P R Carr (*UK*)
Group No 5: Reagents	H L Vos (*Chairman*), A Haemers (*B*), J C Beyer (*CH*), D Giegling (*D*), J L Millet (*F*), A Rossetti (*I*), P W F Brunsmann (*NL*), E J Newman (*UK*)
Group No 6: Biological Substances	J van Noordwijk (*Chairman*), A Lauwers (*B*), E Stürmer (*CH*), A Häussler (*D*), P Frandsen (*DK*), M Percheron (*F*), L Tentori (*I*), F C Arntzen (*N*), F C Hillen (*NL*), L Sjödin (*S*), E Palva (*SF*), A F Bristow (*UK*)
Group No 6B: Human Blood and Blood Products	I Sjöholm (*Chairman*), V Dostal (*A*), C Vermeylen (*B*), N Chariatte (*CH*), G Fürst (*D*), E Sandberg (*DK*), M Netter (*F*), I Liotta (*I*), H Heistø (*N*), H W Krijnen (*NL*), B Karlen (*S*), H Suomela (*SF*), J G Watt (*UK*)
Group No 6I: Insulin Preparations	J van Noordwijk (*Chairman*), E Stürmer (*CH*), H Schöne (*D*), P Frandsen (*DK*), J Macabies (*F*), G W K van Dedem (*NL*), B V Fisher (*UK*)
Group No 7: Antibiotics	H Vanderhaeghe (*Chairman*), J Hoogmartens (*B*), J S Pitton (*CH*), F Sitzius (*D*), A Møller (*DK*), C Pascal (*F*), S Tedeschi (*I*), Ø Karlsson (*N*), C van der Vlies (*NL*), M Fischler (*S*), D H Calam (*UK*)
Group No 8: Dressings and Ligatures	C A Johnson (*Chairman*), Bruyneel (*B*), A Aebi (*CH*), W Triebsch (*D*), J Bilweis (*F*), G Santoni (*I*), G S Groot (*NL*), T D Turner (*UK*)
Group No 8S: Adhesive Dressings	C A Johnson (*Chairman*), Bruyneel (*B*), M Schrenzel (*CH*), D Schulte (*D*)
Group No 9: Inorganic Chemistry	C L Lapière (*Chairman*), Michotte (*B*), J C Beyer (*CH*), D Giegling (*D*), M Mazza (*F*), G Zanni (*I*), S U Ruff (*UK*)
Group No 10A: Organic Chemistry - Synthetic Products	M Pesez (*Chairman*), R Schwarz (*A*), J Bosly (*B*), D Sonanini (*CH*), H Hahn (*D*), M Thomsen (*DK*), J P Billon (*F*), C Loutsidis (*GR*), F La Torre (*I*), X Perlia (*L*), L Borka (*N*), A W M Indemans (*NL*), K G Svensson (*S*), A C Caws (*UK*)

Group No 10B: Organic Chemistry - Synthetic Products	C A Johnson (*Chairman*), R Bouché (*B*), S Weber (*CH*), V Schulze (*D*), A Sørensen (*DK*), F J Pellerin (*F*), E Souli (*GR*), G Cavina (*I*), J L Robert (*L*), A van den Hoek (*NL*), N E Stjernström (*S*), A Kaukinen (*SF*), A Holbrook (*UK*)
Group No 11: Organic Chemistry - Natural Products	G Rotzler (*Chairman*), J De Beer (*B*), H Partenheimer (*CH*), A Müller (*D*), S Kryger (*DK*), J Poisson (*F*), V Hartofylax (*GR*), C Galeffi (*I*), K Øydvin (*N*), H M Smits (*NL*), B Öhrner (*S*), A G Davidson (*UK*)
Group No 11A: Vitamin A	B Borsje (*Chairman*), R Schwob (*CH*), U Thiele (*D*), J Ampilhac (*F*), G Cavina (*I*), G F Phillips (*UK*)
Group No 11C: Cellulose Ethers	W Deckers (*Chairman*), C van Kerchove (*B*), K Münzel (*CH*), L Grosse (*D*), A Reveley (*UK*)
Group No 12: Galenical Products	E Cingolani (*Chairman*), P Braeckman (*B*), K Münzel (*CH*), G Ross (*D*), H G Kristensen (*DK*), P Lotteau (*F*), I Setnikar (*I*), J Karlsen (*N*), H Burger (*NL*), S Wahlgren (*S*), L Turakka (*SF*), D Ganderton (*UK*)
Group No 13: Pharmacognosy	I Kapetanidis (*Chairman*), T Kartnig (*A*), A Vlietinck (*B*), H G Menßen (*D*), R Anton (*F*), S Philianos (*GR*), A Imbesi (*I*), J H Zwaving (*NL*), J D Phillipson (*UK*)
Group No 13H: Fatty Oils	I Kapetanidis (*Chairman*), T Kartnig (*A*), A J Vlietinck (*B*), D Sonanini (*CH*), W Heers (*D*), H G Menßen (*D*), R Anton (*F*), B Entressangles (*F*), A Imbesi (*I*), J H Zwaving (*NL*), J D Phillipson (*UK*)
Group No 14: Radioactive Compounds	K Backe-Hansen (*Chairman*), C Fallais (*B*), P Lerch (*CH*), F Pechtold (*D*), B Pedersen (*DK*), Y Cohen (*F*), R Masi (*I*), P Bremer (*N*), M G Woldring (*NL*), T Bringhammar (*S*), D E Lovett (*UK*)
Group No 15: Sera and Vaccines	W Hennessen (*Chairman*), V Dostal (*A*), P Lemoine (*B*), F Reigel (*CH*), W Schneider (*D*), J Leerhøy (*DK*), A A German (*F*), C Collotti Ferretti (*I*), R Winsnes (*N*), J W Dorpema (*NL*), M Tiru (*S*), T Kuronen (*SF*), D I Magrath (*UK*)
Group No 15V: Veterinary Sera and Vaccines	C Pilet (*Chairman*), H Mathois (*A*), J Leunen (*B*), U Kihm (*CH*), W Schneider (*D*), J Müller (*DK*), J M Person (*F*), C Buonavoglia (*I*), P J O'Connor (*IRL*), H H Lensing (*NL*), K A Karlsson (*S*), I Davidson (*UK*)
Group No 16: Plastic Containers for Pharmaceutical Use	R F Timoney (*Chairman*), W Lhoest (*B*), S Thorens (*CH*), R Rößler (*D*), V Handlos (*DK*), J P Billon (*F*), L Gramiccioni Valsecchi (*I*), J W A Averink (*NL*), A Arbin (*S*), J E Pentelow (*UK*)

Introduction

This edition of the British Pharmacopœia, the fourteenth since the merging of the London, Edinburgh and Dublin Pharmacopœias in 1864, has been prepared by the British Pharmacopœia Commission with the collaboration and support of its advisory committees and other experts. The committees in particular are vital to the healthy growth and maintenance of the Pharmacopœia. For this reason members are selected to provide a wide range of expertise, advice and opinion. In this connection it is of interest to note, and a source of satisfaction to the Commission, that scientists from the National Biological Standards Laboratory in Australia and an officer from the World Health Organization in Geneva have been appointed as corresponding members to three of the committees. The international nature of much pharmaceutical production now demands a more international approach from pharmacopœial authorities. The British Pharmacopœia Commission is very conscious of this and endeavours to foster it by dedicated adherence to the aims of the European Pharmacopœia Commission, by continuing and regular contact with the United States Pharmacopeia Convention and by occasional exchange of views with other pharmacopœial authorities and with the World Health Organization. A further international dimension is brought to the work because of the extensive use made of the British Pharmacopœia in many countries of the world. This is evident from the considerable correspondence received containing comment, question or criticism. In this connection the British Pharmacopœia Commission would like to stress that it relies heavily on dialogue with users of the Pharmacopœia. Constructive comment is welcome from whatever quarter and is vital to the continuing relevance of the Commission's work.

The New Edition

This new edition of the Pharmacopœia contains 2100 monographs for substances and articles used in the practice of medicine. Of these, some 495 are edited versions of monographs now included in the growing European Pharmacopœia (see below). The effective date for this edition is 1 December 1988. From this date this edition supersedes the British Pharmacopœia 1980 as amended by its various addenda. If a monograph that appeared in the earlier edition has not been included in this edition then that monograph remains effective, in accordance with Section 65(4) of the Medicines Act 1968.

There have been some major changes to the Formulated Preparations section which are discussed in greater detail below. These changes have allowed the Pharmacopœia Commission to concentrate its efforts on producing standards that will apply to a range of products of similar type rather than only to a product manufactured to a fixed formulation. They allow greater flexibility in the formulation of many official preparations so that manufacturers may avoid the use of auxiliary ingredients that might from time to time become regarded as undesirable, at least in certain circumstances or conditions. The greater freedom in formulation also allows the development of more stable and possibly more palatable versions of certain products. It has to be borne in mind that many of the fixed formulae included in earlier compendia were designed for extemporaneous dispensing. Over the past two decades or so the practice of manufacturing such preparations in bulk to obviate extemporaneous dispensing has grown and many of the traditional formulae have been shown to be inappropriate for large-scale production and for long-term storage. The greater freedom that is conferred by the new policy allows a manufacturer to modify certain aspects of the formulation to achieve a more commercially acceptable product. This freedom is, however, accompanied by an increased responsibility to ensure the stability and acceptability of the modified preparation.

These changes in the formulary, together with certain other changes of emphasis throughout the Pharmacopœia, have given rise to the need for a substantially revised collection of General Notices. It is stressed that the General Notices are an essential and mandatory part of the Pharmacopœia. Requirements in the monographs must be interpreted in the light of these notices; it follows that the user of the Pharmacopœia must have a ready acquaintance with them. To facilitate this, and to stress their importance, the General Notices have been presented in full on tinted paper at the beginning of both Volumes I and II of this edition.

As in the 1980 edition Volume I contains the monographs for medicinal and auxiliary substances whilst Volume II comprises the formulary (now contained in a section entitled Formulated Preparations), sections dealing with blood products, immunological products, radiopharmaceutical preparations and surgical materials and the extensive appendices. In this edition the necessary infra-red spectra have been incorporated at the end of Volume I.

Some Additions

Monographs included in the Pharmacopœia for the first time are listed at the end of this Introduction. These include aprotinin, a proteolytic enzyme inhibitor, and aprotinin injection; the beta-adrenoceptor antagonist atenolol and atenolol tablets; the oral hypoglycaemic agent glipizide and glipizide tablets; the tranquilliser temazepam; the antispasmodic agent mebeverine hydrochloride and mebeverine tablets and, together with monographs for tablets, the hypotensive agent prazosin hydrochloride and the antacid hydrotalcite.

Also included for the first time is a general monograph for pressurised inhalations which includes a test for deposition of the emitted dose. This general monograph incorporates the requirements of the European Pharmacopœia for Pressurised Pharmaceutical Preparations. With the exception of these European Pharmacopœia requirements, which apply to all pressurised inhalations, the requirements of the general monograph will apply to those pressurised inhalations that are the subject of an individual monograph in the Pharmacopœia. It is hoped to add a monograph for a pressurised inhalation of salbutamol in an addendum to this edition. The test for deposition of the emitted dose uses a simplified cascade impactor. It is an *in vitro* test that is designed to contribute to an assurance of satisfactory aerosol formulation; its role is thus akin to that of the dissolution test for solid oral dosage forms.

The new monographs for atenolol and atenolol tablets referred to above include a high-performance liquid chromatographic test for Related substances that is recognised to provide only partial control of the likely impurities. Other methods are available but none has so far shown itself to be sufficiently robust to serve as a pharmacopœial procedure. The Commission is continuing the development of a more satisfactory test or tests and it is hoped that early improvements to the present requirements will be possible.

Of particular interest is the newly introduced monograph for human insulin. This has been modelled closely on the monograph for insulin and is included as an interim measure whilst work aimed at providing more comprehensive requirements for insulins having the structure of natural human insulin continues in connection with the European Pharmacopœia. The newly introduced monograph defines human insulin as a protein having the normal structure of the natural antidiabetic hormone produced by the human pancreas. Production either by enzymatic modification of insulin obtained from the pancreas of the pig or by a procedure based on recombinant deoxyribonucleic acid (DNA) technology in micro-organisms is recognised. In either case the production must be followed by appropriate purification and, where recombinant DNA technology is used, the production must be based on an approved host-vector system. This interim monograph has been introduced in order that the various monographs for insulin preparations may be modified, where appropriate, to recognise the rapidly growing importance of such preparations made from human insulin.

The Basis of Pharmacopœial Requirements

The basis on which the requirements of the Pharmacopœia are established was discussed in detail in the Introduction to the British Pharmacopœia 1980. Since a proper understanding of the basis is essential to the correct use of the requirements the section is reproduced below in a slightly expanded form.

The Pharmacopœia provides a publicly available statement concerning the quality of a product that is expected to be demonstrable at any time during its accepted shelf-life; it does not provide a collection of minimum standards with which a manufacturer must comply before release of a product. Change may occur during storage and distribution and the pharmacopœial requirements are set to acknowledge acceptable levels of change and to reject materials showing unacceptable levels. It follows that the prudent manufacturer will, where considerations of product stability demand, apply specifications that are more exacting than those laid down in the Pharmacopœia. It also follows that a manufacturer may use any methods of analysis and any general control procedures that are deemed to be appropriate to confirm that the product is acceptable. In so doing the manufacturer must recognise that, at any time during its claimed shelf-life, the product may be challenged independently by the methods of the Pharmacopœia and that compliance with the limits imposed will be required. In the event of any doubt or dispute as to whether or not a material is of pharmacopœial quality, as a General Notice makes clear, the methods of the Pharmacopœia alone are authoritative.

This view of pharmacopœial requirements is also significant when considering the amount of sample to be taken for test. In an overall programme designed to give assurance of quality of a manufactured product the statistical validity of any sampling programme must be beyond doubt. The standards of the Pharmacopœia, on the other hand, are intended to apply to the sample available, perhaps the container of dispensed tablets provided to a patient in accordance with a prescription. The Pharmacopœia requires that twenty of those tablets should meet the test for Uniformity of weight; a manufacturer establishing a sampling and testing protocol designed to ensure ultimate compliance with the pharmacopœial requirements will need to operate at a level designed to show with an acceptable degree of confidence that any twenty tablets, taken at random from a given batch, will meet the requirements.

Pharmacopœial methods and limits are thus set with the intention that they should be used as compliance requirements and not as requirements to guarantee total quality assurance. An article may be said to be of pharmacopœial quality if any sample of the size stipulated in the monograph meets all of the requirements at any time during storage, distribution and use within its accepted shelf-life.

Arising from this it may be useful to underline that compliance of a product with pharmacopœial requirements demands that the product meets *all* aspects of the appropriate monograph and that those requirements shall be interpreted in the light of any relevant General Notices. In certain cases individual requirements of particular tests may seem to be incompatible with those of other tests; where this is apparently the case such requirements have been framed intentionally. Take, for example, the requirements that might be applied to certain tablets. The overall content of active ingredient, as determined on a powdered sample of twenty tablets, might be 90.0 to 110.0 per cent of the prescribed or stated amount. Thus an assay result of 91.0 per cent would indicate compliance. For the Uniformity of content test a further ten tablets might be individually examined, each tablet being required to contain between 85 and 115 per cent of the mean value, with the possibility of a single exception between 80 and 120 per cent. Thus if nine out of ten tablets fall within the range (assuming the mean to be 91.0 per cent) 77.4 and 104.7 per cent and the 10th falls within the range 72.8 to 109.2 per cent then the tablets examined comply with that requirement. For the Dissolution Test each tablet examined might be required to yield at least 70 per cent of the labelled claim into solution within forty-five minutes. It has been suggested that since a single outlier tablet might contain as little as 72.8 per cent of the labelled claim and yet still fall within the acceptance limits for content, the requirements for dissolution should be relaxed to take this into account. In framing requirements, however, the view is taken that it is neither realistic nor profitable to attempt to compound the results of various tests in this way. Each test in a Pharmacopœial monograph and the acceptance limit is therefore framed as an individual entity with requirements based on values encountered in practice; compliance with the monograph requires compliance with each and every test.

The philosophy outlined above has an important bearing on the construction of a monograph for the Pharmacopœia. To achieve maximum benefit from the concept that a product should meet all requirements of the appropriate monograph it follows that, wherever possible, a variety of different approaches to the examination of that product should be employed. The monographs of the British Pharmacopœia are, in general, constructed to use fundamentally different procedures for assay on the one hand and examination for impurities on the other. It has been suggested that liquid chromatography could be employed for identity, impurity control and assay of a medicinal substance thus economising in analytical effort and time. Such a proposal has not commended itself to the British Pharmacopœia Commission. The general approach adopted for a medicinal substance has been to employ chromatographic techniques for control of impurities and to couple them with a precise, even though relatively non-specific, method of assay. In this connection it should be noted that the acceptance limits set down in the opening paragraph of a monograph relate to the method of assay set down under the side heading Assay. Notwithstanding the general approach referred to above there are, of course, exceptions. Moreover, for dosage forms a more specific method of assay, such as liquid chromatography, is being increasingly employed.

Attention is also drawn to the fact that many monographs for preparations in the British Pharmacopœia include tests for impurities, not only those that may result from degradation but also those arising as by-products of the synthetic route used for manufacture of the active ingredient. It has been argued that tests need not be applied for this latter type of impurity since by-products of synthesis will already have been controlled during examination of the substance before formulation. But confirmation of such control will usually be available only to the manufacturer of the finished product who will, of course, know the detailed attributes of the active raw material that has been used. Clearly it would be repetitious and wasteful of resources for tests, often complex in nature, to be repeated simply to demonstrate acceptably low levels of impurities that could only arise during synthesis (as opposed to degradation) of the active ingredient. But for the independent control analyst in a testing laboratory that has access only to the dosage form the profile of synthesis-related impurities offers a valuable indicator as to whether or not the dosage form has been prepared from an active ingredient of pharmacopœial quality. It is primarily for this reason that such tests are included in British Pharmacopœial monographs for dosage forms.

Finally, the key role that is played by the General Notices is stressed since they are all too often overlooked. No requirement of the Pharmacopœia can be taken in isolation; a valid interpretation of any particular requirement depends on it being read in the context of (i) the specified method of analysis (which may include reference to an Appendix), (ii) the monograph as a whole, (iii) where appropriate, the relevant general monograph and (iv) the relevant General Notices. It is clear from queries and comments received from many quarters that appreciation of the above pharmacopœial tenets is commonly lacking.

European Pharmacopœia

As stated above the European Pharmacopœia continues to grow in significance for the United Kingdom and, accordingly, to exercise an increasing influence on the content of and, to some extent, the philosophy that underlies the British Pharmacopœia.

The British Pharmacopœia Commission has, at the request of certain member states party to the Convention on the Elaboration of a European Pharmacopœia, reviewed its policy, introduced in 1980, of reproducing edited versions of almost all of the monographs that currently comprise the European Pharmacopœia. It has decided to maintain this policy, having regard to the many benefits afforded to the user of the British Pharmacopœia, both in the United Kingdom and in many other countries. However, opportunity is again taken to stress that the monographs so presented (distinguished by a five-pointed star against the monograph title) are in an edited and rearranged format designed to effect a style consistent with that used for the national monographs. In the event of doubt of interpretation recourse should be had to the English text published under the direction of the Council of Europe. A General Notice stresses the mandatory nature of this injunction.

The policy of the European Pharmacopœia Commission has been to concentrate effort on the preparation of monographs for medicinal and pharmaceutical substances together with general requirements for dosage forms rather than on the preparation of monographs for specific dosage forms. This policy is reflected in the fact that of the 994 monographs for substances in this edition of the British Pharmacopœia just over 40 per cent now bear the five-pointed star. For the Pharmacopœia as a whole the European contribution now amounts to nearly 25 per cent. The British Pharmacopœia Commission is pleased to acknowledge the significance of this growing presence by listing the names of members of the European Commission and its Groups of Experts who are responsible for preparation of the European Pharmacopœia.

The general monographs for dosage forms developed by the European Pharmacopœia Commission are of special importance. Their provisions apply, not only to those specific preparations of the type described by these general monographs that are themselves the subject of pharmacopœial monographs, but also to all dosage forms of the type described. Thus, any preparation referred to as a tablet, even if it is not included in the Pharmacopœia, must comply with the general requirements of the monograph unless a dispensation has been granted.

The recently introduced European Pharmacopœia general requirements for uniformity of content of unit dosage forms have affected the requirements for a number of individual dosage forms in this edition. For example all tablets containing less than 2 mg or less than 2 per cent of active ingredient are subject to the requirements; as opportunity permits appropriate methods are being developed and included in individual monographs. Even where no test has yet been added, however, the requirements still apply and a preparation would not be of pharmacopœial quality if it could be demonstrated, using a reliable method, that a preparation subject to the requirements fell outside the prescribed limits.

The adoption of a dissolution test method which is closely based on that of the United States Pharmacopeia represents another useful move towards international harmonisation.

Formulated Preparations

As indicated in the opening paragraphs the formulary has undergone far-reaching changes in this edition. The British Pharmacopœia Commission has given consideration to the justification for, and the relevance of, maintaining certain fixed formulations in the British Pharmacopœia. Fixed formulations are those for which a full statement of ingredients and, in some cases, the method of preparation is given in the British Pharmacopœia.

The British Pharmacopœia 1980 contained a greatly increased number of fixed formulations, many of which were established at a time when the preparations concerned were made extemporaneously or in small quantities for short-term storage in the pharmacy. For example, many of the formulations were clearly directed to be 'recently prepared' and it was recognised that such products would not meet the criteria of the test for preservative efficacy. Such formulations are increasingly manufactured on a large scale and have been allocated extended shelf lives. When so prepared they are subject to licensing control under the Medicines Act 1968.

Wide consultations were undertaken with the aim of providing a formulary in which there would be a balance between the needs of extemporaneous preparation and those of modern manufacture. These consultations have resulted in the development of monographs in which the detailed instructions necessary in the former situation are provided in such a way that a certain degree of flexibility of formulation is permitted in the latter. It has been considered appropriate that the manufacturer should be permitted to modify certain of the non-active ingredients or the method of preparation, or both, when manufacturing on a commercial scale with allocation of an extended shelf life. Thus, both freedom and responsibility for formulation have been conferred on the manufacturer who will need to satisfy the appropriate authority that any particular product (including its final container) is acceptable. Monographs constructed in this way have been widely referred to as exhibiting a 'dual format'. While a dual format has been adopted wherever considered appropriate for erstwhile fixed formulation monographs, some fixed formulations have been retained. It has been considered essential, for example, to retain a fixed formula for monographs describing such galenical preparations as Extracts and Tinctures, because of the implications for dispensed medicines if variation in these constituents were to be allowed. For similar reasons a fixed formula has been retained for monographs describing preparations that are used primarily as the basis or vehicle for other preparations, for example, Buffered Cream.

Taking the section on Formulated Preparations as a whole, however, the large majority of monographs are presented as open formulae. This approach, widely used for solid dosage forms in earlier editions, merely defines the preparation in terms of the quality and quantity of the active ingredient. The freedom of formulation is circumscribed only by the obligation to comply with the tests set down in the monograph.

The status and scope of these three categories of Formulary monograph have been clarified by means of appropriate General Notices (see below).

It is recognised that exercise of the greater flexibility in formulation may, in some cases, give rise to problems in applying the analytical methods on which the requirements of monographs depend. Very few problems have so far been encountered but if they are met, users of the Pharmacopœia should report the circumstances in detail to the Secretary and Scientific Director.

As a general observation on auxiliary substances in pharmacopœial preparations opportunity is taken to stress that any preparation described by a name at the head of a monograph in the current edition of the Pharmacopœia, *whether or not it is referred to as BP*, must comply with that monograph. A preparation is not of pharmacopœial quality unless it meets all of the requirements of the monograph when tested by the methods set down.

In this edition a number of statements that related to the presence of auxiliary substances and that were formerly included in the opening paragraphs of specific monographs have been omitted on the grounds that such matters are dealt with in the general monographs pertaining to the product under consideration. For example, statements in specific monographs for injections such as 'the solution may be made isotonic by addition of sodium chloride' or 'the solution may contain suitable buffering and stabilising agents' are now omitted since the points at issue are governed by the general monograph on Parenteral Preparations. The need to consider not only the specific monograph but also the appropriate general monograph is emphasised in this edition by the inclusion of a direct cross-reference.

Provision of apposite General Notices concerning monographs in the section on Formulated Preparations has been crucial to the revision of this part of the Pharmacopœia and opportunity is again taken to stress the key role that General Notices play in interpretation of the Pharmacopœia.

Especial attention should be paid to the General Notices concerning Preparation of Formulated Products. These notices, while incorporating statements in the 1980 Pharmacopœia, have been considerably extended to provide statements covering the different types of monograph (open formula, fixed formula and dual format). In particular, attention is drawn to the statement concerning the criteria to be met by the final product when a dual format formulation is commercially manufactured. These criteria provide the means by which the degree of flexibility of formulation is circumscribed. It is intended to ensure that the essential characteristics of the preparation made strictly according to the extemporaneous formula and instructions are retained.

Declaration of Content

It is evident that some confusion exists with respect to the way in which the content of active substance in a preparation is declared. Opportunity is therefore taken to discuss this subject and also to clarify the method adopted to express the content of the medicinal substances themselves.

The purpose of the assay in monographs for drug substances, taken in conjunction with the tests for impurities, is to determine the purity of the medicinal substance and the limits are therefore usually stated in terms of the molecular entity (salt, ester, etc) and calculated with reference to the anhydrous or dried substance as appropriate (depending on whether the monograph includes a test for water or for loss on drying). One advantage of this form of expression in 'parent' monographs is that it gives an indication 'at a glance' of the purity of the substance. For example (albeit an extreme example) the purity of Amitriptyline Embonate is stated as not less than 98.5 per cent of $(C_{20}H_{23}N)_2,C_{23}H_{16}O_6$ calculated with reference to the anhydrous substance rather than as not less than 57.9 per cent of $C_{20}H_{23}N$ calculated with reference to the anhydrous substance. The mode of expression chosen for the parent monograph in no way circumscribes that which may be used in the monograph for a preparation. There is no reason why the two should be the same and there is frequently good reason why they should be different. In the example of Amitriptyline Embonate the assay limits for the preparation, Amitriptyline Oral Suspension, are stated in terms of amitriptyline, $C_{20}H_{23}N$.

The purpose of the assay in monographs for preparations is to determine whether the content of the active ingredient is within acceptable limits of the labelled claim and the limits are therefore of necessity stated in terms of the moiety declared on the label as established by the manufacturer. Every effort is made in the British Pharmacopœia to achieve internal consistency within monographs, that is, to use the same terms for content statement, assay, label and strengths available. The British Pharmacopœia Commission however has no means of achieving external (inter-monograph) consistency since, unless it perceives there to be a potentially serious risk, it would not seek to obtain a change in a manufacturer's established practice. Problems arise when a manufacturer is not consistent or does not state clearly to what the strength refers and, in particular, when different manufacturers of the same preparation express the content in different terms.

Ideally in many cases where several salts or hydrated forms of the same drug substance are available, the label and dose (and therefore all monograph statements) should be in terms of the anhydrous free base or acid, that is, the active moiety, in order to facilitate comparison and equivalent dosage. Implementation of such a policy would clearly require that each case should be judged on its merits since there would be instances when, for example, a different salt is considered as a different active moiety or where it would be misleading to suggest that two different forms are therapeutically equivalent. Nevertheless it is strongly recommended that as a general rule *for new drug substances*, doses and strengths of preparations should be expressed in terms of the therapeutically active part of the molecule. This recommendation echoes one that was clearly stated in the Introduction to the British Pharmacopœia 1968.

Meanwhile for established materials the Pharmacopœia will continue to reflect current practice. In this respect it should be noted that the labelling requirements of the Pharmacopœia are not comprehensive.

Thus a monograph requirement to state the content of active ingredient in terms of the entire drug substance molecule does not preclude an additional indication of the content expressed in terms of the active moiety where such an indication is considered desirable.

The opportunity afforded by a new edition of the British Pharmacopœia has been taken to clarify the expression of content in monographs for formulated preparations by means of an expanded General Notice on Labelling.

Oral Liquids

As part of the overall review of the formulary a rationalisation of the monographs for Oral Liquids has been undertaken. Because of the difficulties of classification stemming from the changing and imprecise use of terminology there had been a marked blurring of distinction between the categories of oral liquids described in earlier editions.

In this edition there is a single general monograph entitled Oral Liquids that contains sub-sections describing Elixirs, Linctuses, Mixtures, Oral Emulsions, Oral Drops, Oral Solutions and Oral Suspensions. The proposed definitions are not mutually exclusive. For example, a preparation that is a clear solution of an active ingredient dissolved in a flavoured vehicle containing a high proportion of sucrose and ethanol could correctly be called an Oral Solution or an Elixir. Taking this example, for those monographs presented as a fixed formula or in dual format the current title of Elixir has been retained in the title (for example, Phenobarbitone Elixir). For those monographs presented as open formulae the main title is Oral Solution but the subsidiary title Elixir has been retained, at least for this edition. Thus Chlorpheniramine Elixir is now entitled Chlorpheniramine Oral Solution but the older name has been retained as a subsidiary title. Similarly the current titles of Linctus and Mixture have been retained where the monograph in question is presented as a fixed formula or in a dual format but, where an open formula is given, the traditional main titles have given way to Oral Solution or Oral Suspension as appropriate.

Monographs for Syrups have been retained but as a separate part of the section on Formulated Preparations. They are not considered to fall within the scope of the new general monograph for Oral Liquids since they are non-medicated solutions used as vehicle ingredients primarily for their flavouring and sweetening properties rather than as final preparations intended to be administered as such.

As new preparations are added to the Pharmacopœia it is clear that they will be presented as open formulae. It is urged, therefore, that manufacturers in future use the titles Oral Solution or Oral Suspension, as appropriate, rather than the traditional titles such as Elixir or Mixture.

Special consideration has been given to those monographs for which a dual-format approach was earlier planned but that are now presented as open formulae because of the desirability of omiting tartrazine from certain categories of preparation. In these cases the established titles Elixir and Linctus have been retained as the main title.

Powders for Injections

The monographs of the British Pharmacopœia for Powders for Injections have been reviewed with the object of rationalising requirements for compliance with labelled claim and for uniformity of content. In the course of this review it was recognised that the approach adopted in former editions was inconsistent with that adopted for other single-dose preparations such as tablets. The divergence of approach to control of compliance with labelled claim between Powders for Injection and other unit-dose preparations stemmed directly from the practice, common to many monographs for Powders for Injections, of applying the requirements of the monograph for the bulk drug to the contents of the sealed container.

In this edition a new approach has been adopted whereby the assay (commonly carried out on the mixed contents of ten containers) is used to confirm compliance with labelled claim. In general the terms in which the content is declared on the label should be consistent with the approach adopted for other single-dose formulations.

Use of Animals

The British Pharmacopœia Commission is committed to seeking a reduction in animal usage for pharmacopœial testing wherever possible. Removal of an *in vivo* test can be achieved only when such removal is consistent with the provision of satisfactory pharmacopœial standards, that is, when the quality of the material can be controlled adequately by *in vitro* tests. A review of relevant monographs on this basis has enabled a further substantial reduction to be made in this edition. In particular the test for Abnormal toxicity has been deleted from many monographs for antibiotics that are the responsibility of the British rather than the European Pharmacopœia Commission, from all monographs for synthetic peptides and, where appropriate, from monographs for certain materials of biological origin.

In addition biological assays have been omitted from certain preparations where it is now felt that a satisfactory assay can be carried out by physico-chemical methods. For example a colorimetric procedure has replaced the biological assay for Prepared Digitalis and Digitalis Tablets. In addition liquid chromatographic assays have replaced biological assays for Gonadorelin Injection, Tetracosactrin Injection and Tetracosactrin Zinc Injection and have been introduced for Desmopressin Injection and for Desmopressin Intranasal Solution. Further to these, substantial progress has been made towards replacement of biological assays by liquid chromatographic assays for all eight Insulin preparations. This work had not been completed at the time that this edition went to press but promising results had been obtained.

In addition to deletion of the test for prolongation of insulin effect implemented by means of the Addendum 1986 to the British Pharmacopœia 1980 the *in vivo* test for insulin in solution has been omitted from this edition.

Containers

Appendix XIX of the British Pharmacopœia 1980 was confined to the subject of plastic containers. The opportunity has been taken to consolidate this material with other texts concerning containers into a single appendix. The enlarged Appendix XIX so developed and comprises information on both glass and plastic containers together with related topics such as the list of codes for Eye Drops.

In addition to the material contained in Appendix XIX attention is drawn to the section on Plastic Containers included in the European Pharmacopœia. This section, as well as giving general guidance on plastic containers and closures, provides 'type' monographs for materials based on poly(vinyl chloride), low-density polyethylene, high-density polyethylene and polypropylene and specifications for silicones. It is made clear in the general section of the European Pharmacopœia on plastic containers that these monographs are not exclusive and do not restrict the prerogative of a licensing authority to approve materials of different nature, quality or composition from those described, provided it is satisfied in regard to their suitability for the intended purpose. Because these texts are of no more than quasi-official status it has been thought unnecessary to reproduce them, even in summarised form, in the British Pharmacopœia but the attention of those concerned with these materials and containers is drawn to the existence of such sections of the European Pharmacopœia.

Miscellany

The manner of expressing potency requirements for bulk antibiotic substances has been changed in this edition. An individual monograph now states that 'the potency is not less than x Units per mg', but a General Notice makes it clear that this implies that 'the upper fiducial limit of error is not less than x Units per mg', which was the wording previously used in the individual monographs. The prudent manufacturer will wish to be confident that the material supplied will comply with the specification and so will apply the more stringent requirement that the lower fiducial limit of error is not less than x Units per milligram.

Attention is drawn to the fact that when the term Unit is used in official assays and tests it is implied, for the United Kingdom, that the Unit for a particular substance is the specific biological activity contained in that amount of the respective primary standard as the appropriate international or national organisation may from time to time indicate. Where, as in the majority of cases, the primary standard is the respective International Standard, the Unit is the same as the unit, defined by the World Health Organization, which is accepted for international use. Thus, in these circumstances, the term Unit in the British Pharmacopœia, is synonymous with International Unit.

The Action and use statements in this edition of the Pharmacopœia have been simplified and, for medicinal substances, now follow the broad classifications used in the British National Formulary. It is stressed that the indications given have been chosen on the basis of wide acceptance; they do not necessarily reflect all possible uses of the material in question. Dosage statements have been omitted; information regarding dosage is considered to be more satisfactorily provided by other publications.

The second phase of a two-stage change in titles of the monographs for soluble insulin preparations is implemented in this edition, the first phase having been brought into effect by means of Amendments No. 7 to the British Pharmacopœia 1980. The title Insulin Injection and the subsidiary title Soluble Insulin are now used for the clinically-preferred neutral preparation.

In line with the general policy of broadening the scope of certain monographs for formulated products so as to confer greater freedom on their composition and allow wider application, the monograph formerly entitled Compound Sodium Chloride and Glucose Oral Powder has been radically revised. This former monograph, which described a single, fixed, formulation has been replaced by one entitled Oral Rehydration Salts that applies to any products intended for oral rehydration and that contain glucose together with sodium chloride, potassium chloride and either sodium bicarbonate or sodium citrate. This new monograph embraces, amongst other formulations, the two products recommended by the World Health Organization and known as Oral Rehydration Salts—Bicarbonate and Oral Rehydration Salts—Citrate. During the development of this revised monograph the British Pharmacopœia Commission enjoyed considerable co-operation with both the World Health Organization and the United States Pharmacopeial Convention.

The monograph for Dispersible Aspirin Tablets has also been modified to allow greater flexibility in formulation, by making reference to 'a suitable dispersible basis' rather than quoting a specific formula. Coupled with this change a new monograph entitled Soluble Aspirin

Tablets has been introduced. The new monograph makes reference to 'a suitable effervescent basis' and requires that the tablets dissolve to give a clear solution. The free salicylic acid content of Dispersible Aspirin Tablets is required to be less than 0.6 per cent but for the Soluble preparation a more relaxed limit of not more than 3.0 per cent is applied.

The British Pharmacopœia Commission acknowledges difficulty in framing appropriate requirements for modified release tablets that would be equally applicable to all available sources of a given preparation. It is for this reason that the monograph for Slow Lithium Tablets has been withdrawn from this edition until such time as a test can be framed that is equally discriminating and informative for all available brands.

A test, developed by the European Pharmacopœia, to limit the presence of aluminium ions to less than one part per million has been added to monographs for a number of materials that may be used in the preparation of dialysis solutions.

Acknowledgements

The British Pharmacopœia Commission is greatly indebted to the members of its advisory Committees and Consultative Groups without whose dedicated enthusiasm and assistance this edition could not have been prepared.

Close co-operation has continued with many organisations at home and overseas. These include the Department of Pharmaceutical Sciences of the Pharmaceutical Society of Great Britain, the Association of the British Pharmaceutical Industry, the Laboratory of the Government Chemist, the European Pharmacopœia Commission, the National Biological Standards Laboratory (Australia), the Health Protection Branch of the Canadian Department of Health and Welfare, the Committee of Revision of the United States Pharmacopeia, the Pharmaceuticals Unit of the World Health Organization (WHO) and the WHO Collaborating Centre for Chemical Reference Substances.

Special mention must be made of the extensive co-operation that the Commission enjoys with the National Institute for Biological Standards and Control. The support and assistance received from the organisation as a whole and from many individual scientists on its staff is crucial to many aspects of the Commission's task.

The Commission further has pleasure in acknowledging the expert advice provided by a number of individuals who have been consulted on specific topics, notably K Brown, D F Cutler, D T Rossitter, T W Roylance and A Wilson.

Finally, special thanks are due to the staff of Her Majesty's Stationery Office who have given enthusiastic help to the staff of the British Pharmacopœia Commission in the production of this edition. It may seem invidious to single out one member of a team for particular mention but it is felt appropriate, on this occasion, to mention R Marchant who provided so much help and guidance in connection with the transfer of production from traditional methods to computer-based technology.

Additions

The following monographs of the British Pharmacopœia 1988 were not included in the British Pharmacopœia 1980, as amended by the Addendum 1982, the Addendum 1983 and the Addendum 1986.

Medicinal and Pharmaceutical Substances

Aprotinin
Atenolol
Bronopol
Cetyl Alcohol
Desmopressin
Glipizide
Human Insulin
Hydrotalcite
Mebeverine Hydrochloride
Menadiol Sodium Phosphate
Minocycline Hydrochloride
Nicotinyl Alcohol Tartrate
Potassium Hydroxyquinoline Sulphate
Prazosin Hydrochloride
Protamine Sulphate
Temazepam

Formulated Preparations

CAPSULES
Rifampicin Capsules

CREAMS
Clotrimazole Cream
Hydrocortisone and Neomycin Cream
Potassium Hydroxyquinoline Sulphate and Benzoyl Peroxide Cream

EAR DROPS
Hydrocortisone and Neomycin Ear Drops

EYE DROPS
Hydrocortisone and Neomycin Eye Drops

EYE OINTMENTS
Hydrocortisone and Neomycin Eye Ointment

INTRANASAL SOLUTIONS
Desmopressin Intranasal Solution

OINTMENTS
Hydrocortisone Acetate and Neomycin Ointment

ORAL LIQUIDS
Oral Liquids
Diazepam Oral Solution
Naproxen Oral Suspension
Paediatric Codeine Linctus
Paracetamol Oral Suspension
Strong Haloperidol Oral Solution

PARENTERAL PREPARATIONS
Aprotinin Injection
Desmopressin Injection
Biphasic Isophane Insulin Injection

PESSARIES
Clotrimazole Pessaries

PRESSURISED INHALATIONS
Pressurised Inhalations

SUPPOSITORIES
Naproxen Suppositories

TABLETS
Atenolol Tablets
Glipizide Tablets
Hydrotalcite Tablets
Mebeverine Tablets
Menadiol Phosphate Tablets
Minocycline Tablets
Nicotinyl Alcohol Tablets
Prazosin Tablets
Soluble Aspirin Tablets

Blood Products

Hepatitis B Immunoglobulin

Radiopharmaceutical Preparations

Gallium[^{67}Ga] Citrate Injection

Surgical Materials

Long Staple Absorbent Cotton
Sodium Fusidate Gauze Dressing

Omissions

The following monographs of the British Pharmacopœia 1980 as amended by the Addendum 1982, the Addendum 1983 and the Addendum 1986 are not included in the British Pharmacopœia 1988.

Acetarsol
Ajmaline*
Ajmaline Monoethanolate*
Alclofenac
Alphadolone Acetate
Alphaxalone
Alprenolol Hydrochloride
Antimony Sodium Tartrate
Biperiden
Bismuth Subgallate
Brilliant Green
Candicidin
Corticotrophin*

Crystal Violet
Diethyltoluamide
Eugenol
Feprazone
Flufenamic Acid
Glucose for Oral Use
Halquinol
Hydrocortisone Sodium Succinate
Hyoscine Methobromide
Hyoscine Methonitrate*
Lavender Oil
Levallorphan Tartrate
Maize Oil

*Formerly monographs of the European Pharmacopœia

Mastic
Mepacrine Hydrochloride*
Methallenoestril
Methandienone
Methisazone
Methoxyflurane
Nalorphine Hydrobromide
Norethandrolone
Norethynodrel
Nux Vomica
Nystatin (Dermatological)
Oxedrine Tartrate*
Pentetrazol*
Pentolinium Tartrate
Phenformin Hydrochloride
Practolol
Precipitated Sulphur
Prednisolone Pivalate
Prepared Storax
Pumilio Pine Oil
Secbutobarbitone
Serum Gonadotrophin
Siam Benzoin*
Sodium Aminosalicylate*
Stanolone
Sulphamethoxydiazine
Testosterone Phenylpropionate
Thiambutosine
Thiopropazate Hydrochloride
Tolazoline Hydrochloride
Tolu Balsam
Toughened Silver Nitrate
Trichloroacetic Acid*
Trichloroethylene*
Viprynium Embonate
Wild Cherry Bark

Formulary

CAPSULES
Alclofenac Capsules
Amylobarbitone Sodium Capsules
Feprazone Capsules
Flufenamic Acid Capsules
Penicillamine Capsules
Quinalbarbitone Capsules
Troxidone Capsules

CREAMS
Salicylic Acid and Sulphur Cream

EAR DROPS
Hydrogen Peroxide Ear Drops

ELIXIRS
Mepyramine Elixir
Squill Elixir

EMULSIONS
Liquid Paraffin and Phenolphthalein
    Emulsion

EXTRACTS
Cascara Liquid Extract
Nux Vomica Liquid Extract
Senega Liquid Extract

EYE DROPS
Zinc Sulphate and Adrenaline Eye Drops

EYE OINTMENTS
Hyoscine Eye Ointment

IMPLANTS
Deoxycortone Acetate Implants

INFUSIONS
Concentrated Senega Infusion

INHALATIONS
Menthol and Eucalyptus Inhalation

INJECTABLE PREPARATIONS
Alprenolol Injection
Amylobarbitone Injection
Antimony Sodium Tartrate Injection
Biperiden Lactate Injection
Corticotrophin Injection*
Deoxycortone Acetate Injection
Deslanoside Injection
Dipipanone Injection
Levallorphan Injection
Lymecycline and Procaine Injection
Melarsoprol Injection
Mepyramine Injection
Nalorphine Injection
Oxytetracycline Injection
Pentolinium Injection
Practolol Injection
Prednisolone Pivalate Injection
Procaine and Adrenaline Injection
Quinine Dihydrochloride Injection
Serum Gonadotrophin Injection
Testosterone Phenylpropionate Injection
Vasopressin Injection

LOTIONS
Oily Calamine Lotion

LOZENGES
Compound Bismuth Lozenges

MIXTURES
Ipecacuanha and Morphine Mixture
Methisazone Mixture
Paediatric Kaolin Mixture
Viprynium Mixture

OINTMENTS
Ichthammol Ointment
Sulphur Ointment

PAINTS
Brilliant Green and Crystal Violet Paint
Coal Tar Paint
Compound Mastic Paint
Crystal Violet Paint

PASTES
Resorcinol and Sulphur Paste

PASTILLES
Pastille Basis
Opiate Squill Pastilles

PESSARIES
Acetarsol Pessaries
Crystal Violet Pessaries

ORAL POWDERS
Compound Bismuth Oral Powder
Compound Rhubarb Oral Powder
Compound Tragacanth Powder

*Formerly monographs of the European Pharmacopœia

SOLUTIONS
Compound Tartrazine Solution
Green S and Tartrazine Solution

SOLUTION-TABLETS
Mouthwash Solution-tablets

SPRAYS
Compound Adrenaline and Atropine Spray

SUPPOSITORIES
Bismuth Subgallate Suppositories
Compound Bismuth Subgallate
    Suppositories
Phenylbutazone Suppositories

SYRUPS
Wild Cherry Syrup

TABLETS
Alprenolol Tablets
Amylobarbitone Sodium Tablets
Amylobarbitone Tablets
Benzylpenicillin Tablets
Butobarbitone Tablets
Dienoestrol Tablets
Etamiphylline Camsylate Tablets
Ethionamide Tablets
Ethisterone Tablets
Glutethimide Tablets
Hyoscine Methobromide Tablets
Mepacrine Tablets
Meprobamate Tablets
Methallenoestril Tablets
Methandienone Tablets
Methyltestosterone Tablets
Norethandrolone Tablets
Oxyphenbutazone Tablets
Oxytocin Tablets
Paediatric Dispersible Aspirin Tablets
Phenformin Tablets
Phenolphthalein Tablets
Quinalbarbitone Tablets
Reserpine Tablets

Slow Lithium Carbonate Tablets
Slow Orphenadrine Citrate Tablets
Sulphadiazine Tablets
Sulphamethoxydiazine Tablets
Thiambutosine Tablets
Thiopropazate Hydrochloride Tablets
Tolazoline Tablets
Triclofos Tablets
Viprynium Tablets

TINCTURES
Hyoscyamus Tincture
Nux Vomica Tincture
Squill Tincture
Stramonium Tincture

VINEGARS
Squill Vinegar

Blood Products

Antivaccinia Immunoglobulin Injection*
Dried Albumin
Dried Plasma*
Dried Plasma Protein Fraction
Dried Thrombin

Immunological Products

Influenza Vaccine, Live (Intranasal)
Rabies Antiserum*

Radiopharmaceutical Preparations

Iodinated(^{131}I) Albumin Injection
Sodium Iodide(^{131}I) Injection

Surgical Materials

Belladonna Adhesive Plaster
Gauze Pledget
Salicylic Acid Adhesive Plaster
Triangular Calico Bandage

European Pharmacopœia

The following monographs of the European Pharmacopœia are reproduced in edited form in this edition of the British Pharmacopœia. Where a monograph appears in the British Pharmacopœia under a different title, the British Pharmacopœia title is given in parentheses.

Medicinal and Pharmaceutical Substances

Acacia
Acetazolamide
Acetylsalicylic Acid (Aspirin)
Activated Charcoal
Adrenaline Tartrate (Adrenaline Acid
    Tartrate)
Agar
Alexandrian Senna Pods (Alexandrian
    Senna Fruit)
Almond Oil
Alum
Aluminium Sulphate
Amantadine Hydrochloride
Amitriptyline Hydrochloride

Ammonium Chloride
Amobarbital Sodium (Amylobarbitone
    Sodium)
Amoxicillin Trihydrate (Amoxycillin
    Trihydrate)
Amphetamine Sulphate
Ampicillin Trihydrate
Anaesthetic Ether
Anhydrous Ampicillin (Ampicillin)
Anhydrous Chlorobutanol (Anhydrous
    Chlorbutol)
Anhydrous Citric Acid
Anhydrous Dextrose (Anhydrous Glucose)
Anhydrous Ephedrine
Anhydrous Sodium Sulphate
Aniseed
Apomorphine Hydrochloride

*Formerly monographs of the European Pharmacopœia

Arachis Oil
Ascorbic Acid
Atropine Sulphate
Azathioprine
Bacitracin
Bacitracin Zinc
Barbados Aloes (Aloes)
Barbital (Barbitone)*
Barium Sulphate
Belladonna Leaf (Belladonna Herb)
Bendroflumethiazide (Bendrofluazide)
Bentonite
Benzalkonium Chloride
Benzalkonium Chloride Solution
Benzathine Benzylpenicillin (Benzathine
  Penicillin)
Benzocaine
Benzoic Acid
Benzyl Alcohol
Benzylpenicillin Potassium
Benzylpenicillin Sodium
Betamethasone
Betanidine Sulphate (Bethanidine
  Sulphate)
Bismuth Subcarbonate
Borax
Boric Acid
Butobarbital (Butobarbitone)
Caffeine
Caffeine Monohydrate (Caffeine Hydrate)
Calcitonin (Salmon) (Salcatonin)
Calcium Carbonate
Calcium Chloride
Calcium Gluconate
Calcium Hydrogen Phosphate
Calcium Lactate Pentahydrate*
Calcium Lactate Trihydrate
Calcium Pantothenate*
Cape Aloes (Aloes)
Carbon Dioxide
Cascara
Castor Oil
Cefaloridine (Cephaloridine)
Cellulose Acetate Phthalate (Cellacephate)
Cellulose Powder (Powdered Cellulose)
Cetrimide
Cetylpyridinium Chloride
Chloral Hydrate
Chlorambucil
Chloramine
Chloramphenicol
Chloramphenicol Palmitate
Chlordiazepoxide Hydrochloride
Chlorobutanol Hemihydrate (Chlorbutol)
Chlorocresol
Chlorothiazide
Chlorphenamine Maleate
  (Chlorpheniramine Maleate)
Chlorpromazine Hydrochloride
Chlortetracycline Hydrochloride
Cholecalciferol
Cholecalciferol Concentrate (Oily Form)
Cholecalciferol Concentrate (Powder Form)
Chorionic Gonadotrophin
Chymotrypsin
Cinchona Bark

Cinnamon
Citric Acid Monohydrate
Clofibrate
Clonidine Hydrochloride
Clove
Cocaine Hydrochloride
Codeine
Codeine Phosphate Hemihydrate (Codeine
  Phosphate)
Codeine Phosphate Sesquihydrate
Colistimethate Sodium (Colistin
  Sulphomethate Sodium)
Colistin Sulphate
Colloidal Anhydrous Silica
Concentrated Hydrochloric Acid
  (Hydrochloric Acid)
Concentrated Phosphoric Acid (Phosphoric
  Acid)
Cortisone Acetate
Cyanocobalamin
Cyclobarbital Calcium (Cyclobarbitone
  Calcium)
Dapsone
Demeclocycline Hydrochloride
Deoxycortone Acetate
Desipramine Hydrochloride
Deslanoside
Dexamethasone
Dextromethorphan Hydrobromide
Dextromoramide Tartrate
Dextrose Monohydrate (Glucose)
Diazepam
Dienestrol (Dienoestrol)
Diethylcarbamazine Citrate
Diethylstilbestrol (Stilboestrol)
Digitalis Leaf
Digitoxin
Digoxin
Dilute Hydrochloric Acid
Dilute Phosphoric Acid
Dimercaprol
Dimeticone (Dimethicones)
Diphenhydramine Hydrochloride
Diprophylline
Disodium Edetate
Disodium Phosphate Dodecahydrate
  (Sodium Phosphate)
Doxycycline Hyclate (Doxycycline
  Hydrochloride)
Emetine Hydrochloride Heptahydrate
  (Emetine Hydrochloride)
Emetine Hydrochloride Pentahydrate*
Ephedrine Hemihydrate (Ephedrine)
Ephedrine Hydrochloride
Ergocalciferol
Ergometrine Maleate
Ergotamine Tartrate
Erythromycin
Erythromycin Ethylsuccinate
  (Erythromycin Ethyl Succinate)
Erythromycin Stearate
Estradiol Benzoate (Oestradiol Benzoate)
Etacrynic Acid (Ethacrynic Acid)
Ethinylestradiol (Ethinyloestradiol)
Ethionamide
Ethisterone

*Addition to the British Pharmacopœia

Ethylmorphine Hydrochloride
Etofylline
Eucalyptus Oil
Ferrous Gluconate
Ferrous Sulphate
Fluocinolone Acetonide
Folic Acid
Framycetin Sulphate
Frangula Bark
Furosemide (Frusemide)
Gallamine Triethiodide
Gelatin
Gentamicin Sulphate
Gentian Root (Gentian)
Glycerol
Glycerol (85 per cent)
Glyceryl Monostearate 40-50
Griseofulvin
Guanethidine Monosulphate
Halothane
Hard Fat
Heavy Kaolin
Heavy Magnesium Carbonate
Heavy Magnesium Oxide
Heparin Calcium
Heparin Sodium
Hexobarbital (Hexobarbitone)*
Histamine Dihydrochloride
Histamine Phosphate
Homatropine Hydrobromide
Hydrated Aluminium Oxide (Dried
    Aluminium Hydroxide)
Hydrochlorothiazide
Hydrocortisone
Hydrocortisone Acetate
Hydrogen Peroxide Solution (3 Per Cent)
Hydrogen Peroxide Solution (30 Per Cent)
Hydrous Wool Fat
Hydroxyethylcellulose
Hydroxypropylcellulose
Hyoscine Hydrobromide
Hyoscyamine Sulphate
Hyoscyamus Leaf
Imipramine Hydrochloride
Indometacin (Indomethacin)
Insulin
Iodine
Ipecacuanha Root (Ipecacuanha)
Isoniazid
Isoprenaline Sulphate
Kanamycin Acid Sulphate
Kanamycin Monosulphate (Kanamycin
    Sulphate)
Lactic Acid
Lactose
Laevulose (Fructose)
Lanatoside C
Levodopa
Levomepromazine Hydrochloride
    (Methotrimeprazine Hydrochloride)
Levothyroxine Sodium (Thyroxine
    Sodium)
Lidocaine Hydrochloride (Lignocaine
    Hydrochloride)
Light Liquid Paraffin
Light Magnesium Carbonate

Light Magnesium Oxide
Linseed
Liquid Paraffin
Liquorice Root (Liquorice)
Lithium Carbonate
Magnesium Chloride
Magnesium Hydroxide
Magnesium Stearate
Magnesium Sulphate
Magnesium Trisilicate
Maize Starch (Starches)
Maleic Acid
Matricaria Flower (Matricaria Flowers)
Menadione*
Menotrophin
Meprobamate
Mepyramine Maleate
Mercaptopurine
Mestranol
Methadone Hydrochloride
Methaqualone
Methotrexate
Methyl Parahydroxybenzoate (Methyl
    Hydroxybenzoate)
Methyl Salicylate
Methylatropine Bromide (Atropine
    Methobromide)
Methylatropine Nitrate (Atropine
    Methonitrate)
Methylcellulose
Methyldopa
Methylhydroxyethylcellulose
    (Hydroxyethylmethylcellulose)
Methylhydroxypropylcellulose
    (Hypromellose)
Methylhydroxypropylcellulose Phthalate
    (Hypromellose Phthalate)
Methylphenobarbital
    (Methylphenobarbitone)
Methyltestosterone
Miconazole Nitrate
Microcrystalline Cellulose
Morphine Hydrochloride
Naphazoline Nitrate
Neomycin Sulphate
Neostigmine Bromide
Nicotinamide
Nicotinic Acid
Nikethamide
Nitrazepam
Nitrofurantoin
Nitrous Oxide
Noradrenaline Tartrate (Noradrenaline
    Acid Tartrate)
Norethisterone
Noscapine
Noscapine Hydrochloride
Nystatin
Olive Oil
Oxygen
Oxyphenbutazone
Oxytetracycline
Oxytetracycline Hydrochloride
Pancreas Powder (Pancreatic Extract)
Papaverine Hydrochloride
Paracetamol

*Addition to the British Pharmacopœia

Paraldehyde
Pentobarbital (Pentobarbitone)
Pentobarbital Sodium (Pentobarbitone Sodium)
Peppermint Leaf
Peppermint Oil
Pethidine Hydrochloride
Phenazone
Phenobarbital (Phenobarbitone)
Phenolsulfonphthalein (Phenolsulphonphthalein)
Phenoxymethylpenicillin
Phenoxymethylpenicillin Potassium
Phenylbutazone
Phenylmercuric Borate
Phenytoin Sodium
Pholcodine
Phthalylsulfathiazole (Phthalylsulphathiazole)
Physostigmine Salicylate
Pilocarpine Nitrate
Piperazine Adipate
Piperazine Citrate
Piperazine Hydrate
Polymyxin B Sulphate
Polysorbate 20
Polysorbate 60
Polysorbate 80
Potassium Bromide
Potassium Chloride
Potassium Citrate
Potassium Iodide
Potassium Permanganate
Potato Starch (Starches)
Prednisolone
Prednisone
Prepared Belladonna (Prepared Belladonna Herb)
Prepared Hyoscyamus
Prepared Ipecacuanha
Prepared Stramonium
Probenecid
Procaine Benzylpenicillin (Procaine Penicillin)
Procaine Hydrochloride
Prochlorperazine Maleate
Progesterone
Promethazine Hydrochloride
Propyl Parahydroxybenzoate (Propyl Hydroxybenzoate)
Propylene Glycol
Propylthiouracil
Proxyphylline
Purified Water
Pyridoxine Hydrochloride
Pyrimethamine
Quinidine Sulphate
Quinine Hydrochloride
Quinine Sulphate
Reserpine
Resorcinol
Rhatany Root
Rhubarb
Riboflavine
Rice Starch (Starches)
Rifampicin
Rifamycin Sodium
Roman Chamomile Flower (Chamomile Flowers)

Salbutamol
Salicylic Acid
Secobarbital Sodium (Quinalbarbitone Sodium)
Senega Root
Senna Leaf
Sesame Oil
Silver Nitrate
Sodium Acetate
Sodium Benzoate
Sodium Calcium Edetate (Sodium Calciumedetate)
Sodium Carbonate Decahydrate
Sodium Carbonate Monohydrate
Sodium Carboxymethylcellulose (Carmellose Sodium)
Sodium Chloride
Sodium Citrate
Sodium Dihydrogen Phosphate Dihydrate (Sodium Acid Phosphate)
Sodium Fluoride
Sodium Hydrogen Carbonate (Sodium Bicarbonate)
Sodium Iodide
Sodium Lauryl Sulphate
Sodium Salicylate
Sodium Sulphate Decahydrate (Sodium Sulphate)
Sodium Thiosulphate
Sorbitol
Sorbitol 70 Per Cent (Crystallising) [Sorbitol Solution (70 per cent) (Crystallising)]
Sorbitol 70 Per Cent (Non-crystallising) [Sorbitol Solution (70 per cent) (Non-crystallising)]
Spray-dried Acacia
Stramonium Leaf
Streptokinase
Streptomycin Sulphate
Succinylsulfathiazole (Succinylsulphathiazole)
Sucrose
Sulfacetamide Sodium (Sulphacetamide Sodium)
Sulfadiazine (Sulphadiazine)
Sulfadimidine (Sulphadimidine)
Sulfamethoxazole (Sulphamethoxazole)
Suxamethonium Chloride
Synthetic Vitamin A Concentrate (Oily Form)
Synthetic Vitamin A Concentrate (Powder Form)
Synthetic Vitamin A Concentrate (Water-dispersible Form)
Talc (Purified Talc)
Tartaric Acid
Testosterone Propionate
Tetracaine Hydrochloride (Amethocaine Hydrochloride)
Tetracycline
Tetracycline Hydrochloride
Theobromine
Theophylline
Theophylline and Ethylenediamine (Aminophylline)
Theophylline and Ethylenediamine Hydrate (Aminophylline Hydrate)

Theophylline Monohydrate (Theophylline Hydrate)
Thiamine Hydrochloride
Thiamine Nitrate
Thiamphenicol
Thiopental Sodium and Sodium Carbonate (Thiopentone Sodium)
Tinnevelly Senna Pods (Tinnevelly Senna Fruit)
Titanium Dioxide
α-Tocopherol Acetate (Alpha Tocopheryl Acetate)
Tolbutamide
Tragacanth
Triamcinolone Acetonide
Triamterene
Trifluoperazine Hydrochloride
Trimethadione (Troxidone)
Trimethoprim
Trimipramine Maleate
Tubocurarine Chloride
Undecylenic Acid (Undecenoic Acid)
Valerian Root (Valerian)
Water for Injections
Wheat Starch (Starches)
White Beeswax
Wool Fat
Yellow Beeswax
Zinc Chloride
Zinc Oxide
Zinc Stearate
Zinc Sulphate
Zinc Undecylenate (Zinc Undecenoate)

Formulated Preparations

EXTRACTS
Standardised Aloes Dry Extract

PARENTERAL PREPARATIONS
Corticotrophin Zinc Hydroxide Injection (Corticotrophin Zinc Injection)
Lypressin Injection
Oxytocin Injection

SOLUTIONS
Haemodialysis Solutions

Blood Products

Anticoagulant and Preservative Solutions for Human Blood (Anticoagulant and Preservative Solutions for Blood)
Freeze-dried Human Coagulation Factor VIII (Dried Factor VIII Fraction)
Human Albumin Solution (Albumin Solution)
Human Blood (Whole Blood)
Human Measles Immunoglobulin (Measles Immunoglobulin)*
Human Normal Immunoglobulin (Normal Immunoglobulin)
Human Plasma Protein Solution (Plasma Protein Solution)
Human Tetanus Immunoglobulin (Tetanus Immunoglobulin)

Immunological Preparations

ANTISERA
Immunosera for Human Use (Antisera)
Botulinum Antitoxin
Diphtheria Antitoxin
European Viper Venom Antiserum
Gas-gangrene Antitoxin (Novyi)
Gas-gangrene Antitoxin (Perfringens)
Gas-gangrene Antitoxin (Septicum)
Mixed Gas-gangrene Antitoxin
Tetanus Antitoxin for Human Use (Tetanus Antitoxin)

VACCINES
Vaccines for Human Use (Vaccines)
Cholera Vaccine
Diphtheria and Tetanus Vaccine (Adsorbed) (Adsorbed Diphtheria and Tetanus Vaccine)
Diphtheria Vaccine (Adsorbed) (Adsorbed Diphtheria Vaccine)
Diphtheria, Tetanus and Pertussis Vaccine (Adsorbed) (Adsorbed Diphtheria, Tetanus and Pertussis Vaccine)
Freeze-dried BCG Vaccine (Bacillus Calmette-Guérin Vaccine)
Freeze-dried Cholera Vaccine (Cholera Vaccine)
Freeze-dried Smallpox Vaccine (Dermal) (Smallpox Vaccine)
Freeze-dried Typhoid Vaccine (Typhoid Vaccine)
Influenza Vaccine (Inactivated) (Inactivated Influenza Vaccine)
Influenza Vaccine (Split Virion) [Inactivated Influenza Vaccine (Split Virion)]
Measles Vaccine (Live) (Measles Vaccine, Live)
Meningococcal Polysaccharide Vaccine
Mumps Vaccine (Live) (Mumps Vaccine, Live)*
Old Tuberculin for Human Use (Old Tuberculin)
Pertussis Vaccine
Pertussis Vaccine (Adsorbed) (Pertussis Vaccine)
Poliomyelitis Vaccine (Inactivated) (Inactivated Poliomyelitis Vaccine)
Poliomyelitis Vaccine (Oral) (Poliomyelitis Vaccine, Live (Oral))
Rabies Vaccine for Human Use Prepared in Cell Cultures (Rabies Vaccine)
Rubella Vaccine (Live) (Rubella Vaccine, Live)
Tetanus Vaccine (Adsorbed) (Adsorbed Tetanus Vaccine)
Tuberculin Purified Protein Derivative for Human Use (Tuberculin Purified Protein Derivative)
Typhoid Vaccine
Yellow Fever Vaccine (Live) (Yellow Fever Vaccine, Live)

*Addition to the British Pharmacopœia

Radiopharmaceutical Preparations

Radiopharmaceutical Preparations
Chromium[^{51}Cr] Edetate Injection
Colloidal Gold[^{198}Au] Injection
Cyanocobalamin[^{57}Co] Solution
Cyanocobalamin[^{58}Co] Solution
L-Selenomethionine[^{75}Se] Injection
Sodium Chromate[^{51}Cr] Sterile Solution
Sodium Iodide[^{131}I] Solution
Sodium Iodohippurate[^{131}I] Injection
Sodium Pertechnetate[^{99m}Tc] Injection (Fission)
Sodium Pertechnetate[^{99m}Tc] Injection (Non-fission)
Sodium Phosphate[^{32}P] Injection
Technetium[^{99m}Tc] Colloidal Antimony Sulphide Injection
Technetium[^{99m}Tc] Colloidal Sulphur Injection
Technetium[^{99m}Tc] Macrosalb Injection

Technetium[^{99m}Tc] Tin Pyrophosphate Injection
Xenon[^{133}Xe] Injection

Surgical Materials

Absorbent Cotton
Absorbent Cotton and Viscose Ribbon Gauze
Absorbent Cotton Gauze
Absorbent Cotton Ribbon Gauze
Absorbent Viscose Wadding
Self-adhesive Plasters (Adhesive Tapes)
Sterile Braided Silk Suture
Sterile Catgut
Sterile Linen Thread (Sterile Linen Suture)
Sterile Non-absorbable Strands (Sterile Non-absorbable Sutures)
Sterile Polyamide 6 Suture
Sterile Polyamide 6/6 Suture
Sterile Polyester Suture
Sterile Reconstituted Collagen Strands (Sterile Reconstituted Collagen Suture)

The general provisions of the European Pharmacopœia relating to the types of dosage forms listed below are included in edited form in the appropriate general monograph or monographs in that section of the British Pharmacopœia entitled Monographs: Formulated Preparations. (See the General Notice on General Monographs for Formulated Preparations.)

Capsules
Eye-drops
Eye Ointments
Granules
Pessaries
Powders

Preparations for Parenteral Use
Pressurised Pharmaceutical Preparations
Suppositories
Tablets
Topical Semi-solid Preparations

The following materials are the subject of monographs in the European Pharmacopœia but have not been included in the British Pharmacopœia. Nevertheless the standards given in the European Pharmacopœia are those applicable in the United Kingdom.

Medicinal and Pharmaceutical Substances

Mercuric Chloride
Ouabain
Phenacetin
Sodium Bromide

Blood Products

Dried Human Fibrinogen
Human Vaccinia Immunoglobulin

Radiopharmaceutical Preparations

Krypton[^{85}Kr] Injection
Mercuric[^{197}Hg] Chloride Injection

Sodium Iodide [^{125}I] Solution
Technetium [^{99m}Tc] Colloidal Rhenium Sulphide Injection
Tritiated[^{3}H] Water Injection

Surgical Materials

Sterile Absorbent Cotton
Sterile Absorbent Cotton and Viscose Ribbon Gauze
Sterile Absorbent Cotton Gauze
Sterile Absorbent Cotton Ribbon Gauze
Sterile Absorbent Viscose Wadding

The requirements for the above sterile dressings are those of the appropriate non-sterilised dressings with the addition of a requirement for sterility (see Surgical Dressings).

Changes in Title

The following lists give the alterations in the main titles of those monographs of the British Pharmacopœia 1980, as amended by the Addendum 1982, the Addendum 1983 and the Addendum 1986, that have been retained (many with amendments) in the British Pharmacopœia 1988.

BRITISH PHARMACOPŒIA 1980	BRITISH PHARMACOPŒIA 1988
Medicinal and Pharmaceutical Substances	
Oxytetracycline Dihydrate	Oxytetracycline
Powdered Opium	Prepared Opium
Sorbitol Solution (70 per cent)	Sorbitol Solution (70 per cent) (Crystallising)
Formulated Preparations	
Aluminium Hydroxide Mixture	Aluminium Hydroxide Oral Suspension
Aluminium Phosphate Mixture	Aluminium Phosphate Oral Suspension
Aminocaproic Acid Mixture	Aminocaproic Acid Oral Solution
Amiloride Hydrochloride Tablets	Amiloride Tablets
Amitriptyline Embonate Mixture	Amitriptyline Oral Suspension
Amoxycillin Mixture	Amoxycillin Oral Suspension
Ampicillin Mixture	Ampicillin Oral Suspension
Aqueous Iodine Solution	Aqueous Iodine Oral Solution
Atropine Sulphate Injection	Atropine Injection
Atropine Sulphate Tablets	Atropine Tablets
Barium Sulphate Suspension	Barium Sulphate Oral Suspension
Benorylate Mixture	Benorylate Oral Suspension
Bephenium Hydroxynaphthoate Granules	Bephenium Granules
Betamethasone Sodium Phosphate Injection	Betamethasone Injection
Bromhexine Hydrochloride Tablets	Bromhexine Tablets
Bromocriptine Mesylate Capsules	Bromocriptine Capsules
Bromocriptine Mesylate Tablets	Bromocriptine Tablets
Bupivacaine Hydrochloride Injection	Bupivacaine Injection
Calciferol Solution	Calciferol Oral Solution
Cephalexin Mixture	Cephalexin Oral Suspension
Chloramphenicol Palmitate Mixture	Chloramphenicol Oral Suspension
Chlorpheniramine Elixir	Chlorpheniramine Oral Solution
Chlorpromazine Elixir	Chlorpromazine Oral Solution
Chlortetracycline Hydrochloride Eye Ointment	Chlortetracycline Eye Ointment
Clomipramine Hydrochloride Capsules	Clomipramine Capsules
Clonidine Hydrochloride Injection	Clonidine Injection
Clonidine Hydrochloride Tablets	Clonidine Tablets
Cloxacillin Elixir	Cloxacillin Oral Solution
Co-dergocrine Mesylate Tablets	Co-dergocrine Tablets
Co-trimoxazole Mixture	Co-trimoxazole Oral Suspension
Compound Sodium Chloride and Glucose Oral Powder	Oral Rehydration Salts—Formula A
Cyclizine Lactate Injection	Cyclizine Injection
Dextromoramide Tartrate Injection	Dextromoramide Injection
Dichloralphenazone Elixir	Dichloralphenazone Oral Solution
Dicyclomine Elixir	Dicyclomine Oral Solution
Dihydroergotamine Mesylate Injection	Dihydroergotamine Injection
Dihydroergotamine Mesylate Solution	Dihydroergotamine Oral Solution
Dihydroergotamine Mesylate Tablets	Dihydroergotamine Tablets
Diloxanide Furoate Tablets	Diloxanide Tablets
Diphenhydramine Elixir	Diphenhydramine Oral Solution
Dipipanone Hydrochloride and Cyclizine Hydrochloride Tablets	Dipipanone and Cyclizine Tablets
Docusate Sodium Tablets	Docusate Tablets
Dopamine Hydrochloride Intravenous Infusion	Dopamine Intravenous Infusion
Doxapram Hydrochloride Injection	Doxapram Injection
Drostanolone Propionate Injection	Drostanolone Injection
Econazole Nitrate Cream	Econazole Cream

Econazole Nitrate Pessaries	Econazole Pessaries
Ephedrine Hydrochloride Elixir	Ephedrine Elixir
Estramustine Sodium Phosphate Capsules	Estramustine Phosphate Capsules
Etamiphylline Camsylate Injection	Etamiphylline Injection
Etamiphylline Camsylate Suppositories	Etamiphylline Suppositories
Ethamivan Solution	Ethamivan Oral Solution
Ethosuximide Elixir	Ethosuximide Oral Solution
Fenoprofen Calcium Tablets	Fenoprofen Tablets
Fluclorolone Acetonide Ointment	Fluclorolone Ointment
Flucloxacillin Elixir	Flucloxacillin Oral Solution
Flucloxacillin Magnesium Mixture	Flucloxacillin Oral Suspension
Fluocinolone Acetonide Cream	Fluocinolone Cream
Fluocinolone Acetonide Ointment	Fluocinolone Ointment
Fluocortolone Pivalate and Fluocortolone Hexanoate Cream	Fluocortolone Cream
Fluocortolone Pivalate and Fluocortolone Hexanoate Ointment	Fluocortolone Ointment
Fluorescein Sodium Eye Drops	Fluorescein Eye Drops
Fluorescein Sodium Injection	Fluorescein Injection
Flurazepam Monohydrochloride Capsules	Flurazepam Capsules
Fusidic Acid Mixture	Fusidic Acid Oral Suspension
Haloperidol Solution	Haloperidol Oral Solution
High-Strength Calciferol Tablets	Calciferol Tablets
Hydralazine Hydrochloride Injection	Hydralazine Injection
Hydralazine Hydrochloride Tablets	Hydralazine Tablets
Injectable Preparations	Parenteral Preparations
Isoprenaline Hydrochloride Injection	Isoprenaline Injection
Isoxsuprine Hydrochloride Injection	Isoxsuprine Injection
Isoxsuprine Hydrochloride Tablets	Isoxsuprine Tablets
Labetalol Hydrochloride Injection	Labetalol Injection
Labetalol Hydrochloride Tablets	Labetalol Tablets
Lignocaine Hydrochloride and Chlorhexidine Gluconate Gel	Lignocaine and Chlorhexidine Gel
Lignocaine Hydrochloride Gel	Lignocaine Gel
Lignocaine Hydrochloride Injection	Lignocaine Injection
Liquid Paraffin and Magnesium Hydroxide Emulsion	Liquid Paraffin and Magnesium Hydroxide Oral Emulsion
Liquid Paraffin Emulsion	Liquid Paraffin Oral Emulsion
Metaraminol Tartrate Injection	Metaraminol Injection
Mexiletine Hydrochloride Capsules	Mexiletine Capsules
Mexiletine Hydrochloride Injection	Mexiletine Injection
Mianserin Hydrochloride Tablets	Mianserin Tablets
Miconazole Nitrate Cream	Miconazole Cream
Morphine Sulphate Tablets	Morphine Tablets
Nalidixic Acid Mixture	Nalidixic Acid Oral Suspension
Neomycin Sulphate Elixir	Neomycin Oral Solution
Neomycin Sulphate Eye Drops	Neomycin Eye Drops
Neomycin Sulphate Eye Ointment	Neomycin Eye Ointment
Nitrofurantoin Mixture	Nitrofurantoin Oral Suspension
Nystatin Mixture	Nystatin Oral Suspension
Oestradiol Benzoate Injection	Oestradiol Injection
Paediatric Co-trimoxazole Mixture	Paediatric Co-trimoxazole Oral Suspension
Paediatric Digoxin Elixir	Paediatric Digoxin Oral Solution
Paediatric Ferrous Sulphate Mixture	Paediatric Ferrous Sulphate Oral Solution
Paediatric Paracetamol Elixir	Paediatric Paracetamol Oral Solution
Paediatric Sulphadimidine Mixture	Paediatric Sulphadimidine Oral Suspension
Paediatric Trimeprazine Tartrate Elixir	Paediatric Trimeprazine Oral Solution
Pentazocine Lactate Injection	Pentazocine Injection
Phenethicillin Elixir	Phenethicillin Oral Solution
Phenoxymethylpenicillin Mixture	Phenoxymethylpenicillin Oral Suspension
Phenoxymethylpenicillin Potassium Capsules	Phenoxymethylpenicillin Capsules
Phenoxymethylpenicillin Potassium Elixir	Phenoxymethylpenicillin Oral Solution
Phenoxymethylpenicillin Potassium Tablets	Phenoxymethylpenicillin Tablets
Phenylephrine Hydrochloride Injection	Phenylephrine Injection
Phenytoin Mixture	Phenytoin Oral Suspension
Polymyxin B Sulphate and Bacitracin Zinc Eye Ointment	Polymyxin B and Bacitracin Eye Ointment

Prenylamine Lactate Tablets	Prenylamine Tablets
Primidone Mixture	Primidone Oral Suspension
Promethazine Hydrochloride Elixir	Promethazine Oral Solution
Promethazine Hydrochloride Injection	Promethazine Injection
Proxymetacaine Hydrochloride Eye Drops	Proxymetacaine Eye Drops
Pyridoxine Hydrochloride Tablets	Pyridoxine Tablets
Salbutamol Sulphate Injection	Salbutamol Injection
Sodium Valproate Elixir	Sodium Valproate Oral Solution
Spectinomycin Hydrochloride Injection	Spectinomycin Injection
Streptomycin Sulphate Injection	Streptomycin Injection
Strong Paediatric Trimeprazine Tartrate Elixir	Strong Paediatric Trimeprazine Oral Solution
Sulphacetamide Sodium Eye Drops	Sulphacetamide Eye Drops
Sulphacetamide Sodium Eye Ointment	Sulphacetamide Eye Ointment
Tamoxifen Citrate Tablets	Tamoxifen Tablets
Terbutaline Sulphate Tablets	Terbutaline Tablets
Tetracycline Mixture	Tetracycline Oral Suspension
Thiamine Hydrochloride Injection	Thiamine Injection
Thiamine Hydrochloride Tablets	Thiamine Tablets
Timolol Maleate Eye Drops	Timolol Eye Drops
Timolol Maleate Tablets	Timolol Tablets
Triamcinolone Acetonide Cream	Triamcinolone Cream
Triamcinolone Acetonide Dental Paste	Triamcinolone Dental Paste
Triamcinolone Acetonide Ointment	Triamcinolone Ointment
Triclofos Elixir	Triclofos Oral Solution
Trifluoperazine Hydrochloride Tablets	Trifluoperazine Tablets
Triprolidine Hydrochloride Tablets	Triprolidine Tablets
Verapamil Hydrochloride Injection	Verapamil Injection
Verapamil Hydrochloride Tablets	Verapamil Tablets
Xylometazoline Hydrochloride Nasal Drops	Xylometazoline Nasal Drops

Blood Products

Anti-D (Rh$_0$) Immunoglobulin Injection	Anti-D (Rh$_0$) Immunoglobulin
Antirabies Immunoglobulin Injection	Rabies Immunoglobulin
Antitetanus Immunoglobulin Injection	Tetanus Immunoglobulin
Normal Immunoglobulin Injection	Normal Immunoglobulin

Surgical Materials

Adhesive Tapes and Films	Adhesive Tapes
Chlorhexidine Acetate Gauze Dressing	Chlorhexidine Gauze Dressing
Cotton Surgical Tubular Stockinette	Cotton Stockinette
Cotton and Viscose Surgical Tubular Stockinette	Cotton and Viscose Stockinette
Elasticated Surgical Tubular Stockinette	Elasticated Tubular Bandage
Framycetin Sulphate Gauze Dressing	Framycetin Gauze Dressing
Polypropylene Surgical Tubular Stockinette	Polypropylene Stockinette
Ribbed Cotton Surgical Tubular Stockinette	Ribbed Cotton Stockinette
Ribbed Cotton and Viscose Surgical Tubular Stockinette	Ribbed Cotton and Viscose Stockinette
Ribbed Polypropylene Surgical Tubular Stockinette	Ribbed Polypropylene Stockinette
Viscose Surgical Tubular Stockinette	Viscose Stockinette

General Notices

The following general provisions apply to the statements made in the monographs and appendices of the British Pharmacopœia. The word 'official' is used in the Pharmacopœia to signify 'of the Pharmacopœia'. It applies to any title, substance, preparation, method or statement included in the general notices, monographs and appendices of the Pharmacopœia.

European Pharmacopœia

Monographs of the European Pharmacopœia are reproduced in this edition of the British Pharmacopœia in a form designed to effect an editorial style consistent with that of other matter and are included for the convenience of users of the Pharmacopœia. In cases of doubt or dispute reference should be made to the text published under the direction of the Council of Europe (Partial Agreement) in accordance with the Convention on the Elaboration of a European Pharmacopœia (Treaty Series No. 32 (1974) Cmnd 5763). With the exception of general monographs, edited monographs of the European Pharmacopœia are distinguished by a five-pointed star ☆ against the title.

Titles

Where the main title of the monograph for a preparation does not indicate the full nonproprietary name of the active ingredient (for example, Amitriptyline Oral Suspension) a preparation labelled with a title that includes the full name (for example, Amitriptyline Embonate Oral Suspension) must also comply with the requirements of the monograph.

Subsidiary titles, where included, have the same significance as the main titles. An abbreviated title constructed in accordance with the directions given in Appendix XXI has the same significance as the main title.

Titles that are derived by the suitable inversion of words of a main or subsidiary title, with the addition of a preposition if appropriate, are also official titles. Thus, the following are all official titles: Aspirin Tablets, Tablets of Aspirin; Ginger Tincture, Tincture of Ginger; Atropine Injection, Injection of Atropine. The spelling 'cef' may be substituted for 'ceph', 'sulf' may be substituted for 'sulph' and *vice versa* in main and subsidiary titles.

The names of Pharmacopœial substances, preparations and other materials occurring in the text are printed with capital initial letters and these imply that materials of Pharmacopœial quality must be used. Words in the text that name a reagent or other material, a physical characteristic or a process that is described or defined in an appendix are printed in italic type, for example, *ninhydrin reagent, absorbance, gas chromatography*, and these imply compliance with the requirements specified in the appropriate appendix.

Official Standards

The standards of purity and strength stated in the monographs of the Pharmacopœia apply to articles that are intended for medicinal use but not necessarily to articles that may be sold under the same name for other purposes.

A monograph is to be construed in accordance with any general monograph or notice or any appendix, note or other explanatory material that is contained in this edition and that is applicable to that monograph. All statements contained in the monographs, with the exceptions given below, constitute standards for the official substances. A substance is not of Pharmacopœial quality unless it complies with all the requirements stated.

The requirements have been framed to provide appropriate limitation of potential impurities rather than to provide against all possible impurities. It is not to be presumed, for example, that an impurity not precluded by the prescribed tests is tolerated should rational considerations require that it be absent.

The following parts of a monograph do not constitute standards: (a) a chemical formula given at the beginning of a monograph; (b) a Chemical Abstracts Service Registry Number; (c) statements on taste under the side-heading Characteristics; (d) statements given under the side-heading Solubility; (e) information in any annex to a monograph. Monographs may also include non-mandatory advice or information under the side-headings Storage, Action and use and Strengths available.

General Monographs for Formulated Preparations

The general provisions of the European Pharmacopœia relating to different types of dosage form are included in edited form in the appropriate general monograph in that section of the British Pharmacopœia entitled Monographs: Formulated Preparations. These general provisions apply unless otherwise justified and authorised to all dosage forms of the type defined, whether an individual monograph is included in the British Pharmacopœia or not. A statement that is qualified by the phrase 'unless otherwise justified and authorised' implies that the requirement may be modified for application to a particular formulated preparation when modification has been adequately justified to, and authorised by, a competent authority. When the formulated preparation is the subject of a monograph in the British Pharmacopœia any such modification is stated in the monograph. For example, the general monograph for Tablets requires that Uncoated Tablets, except for chewable tablets, disintegrate within 15 minutes; for Calcium Lactate Tablets a time of 30 minutes is permitted.

As with other material edited from the European Pharmacopœia, in cases of doubt or dispute reference should be made to the text published under the direction of the Council of Europe (Partial Agreement) in accordance with the Convention on the Elaboration of a European Pharmacopœia.

Additional statements and requirements applicable to the individual monographs of the British Pharmacopœia are also included in many of the general monographs for formulated preparations. Such statements and requirements apply to all monographs for that dosage form included in the Pharmacopœia unless otherwise indicated in the individual monograph. In those general monographs where the statements and requirements applicable to individual monographs in the British Pharmacopœia are substantial they are provided in a separate section introduced by an italicised statement. Thus, the general monograph for Tablets consists of a preliminary part (an edited version of the European Pharmacopœia monograph for Tablets) that is applicable to all tablets and a supplementary part that relates only to the specific monographs for individual tablets that are contained in the British Pharmacopœia.

Chemical Formulae

When the chemical composition of an official substance is known or generally accepted, the graphic and molecular formula, the molecular weight and the Chemical Abstracts Service Registry Number are normally given at the beginning of the monograph for information. This information refers to the chemically pure substance and is not to be regarded as an indication of the purity of the official material. Elsewhere, in statements of standards of purity and strength and in descriptions of processes of assay, it is evident from the context that the formulae denote the chemically pure substances.

Where the absolute stereochemical configuration is specified the International Union of Pure and Applied Chemistry (IUPAC) *R/S* and

E/Z systems of designation have been used. If the substance is an enantiomer of unknown absolute stereochemistry the sign of the optical rotation, as determined in the solvent and under the conditions specified in the monograph, has been attached to the systematic name. An indication of sign of rotation has also been given where this is incorporated in a trivial name that appears on an IUPAC preferred list.

All amino acids, except glycine, have the L-configuration unless otherwise indicated; the three-letter symbols used for amino acids are those recommended by the Joint Commission on Biochemical Nomenclature of the International Union of Pure and Applied Chemistry and the International Union of Biochemistry.

In the graphic formulae the following abbreviations are used:

Me $-CH_3$	Bu^n $-CH_2 \cdot CH_2 \cdot CH_2 \cdot CH_3$
Et $-CH_2 \cdot CH_3$	Bu^s $-CH(CH_3) \cdot CH_2 \cdot CH_3$
Pr^i $-CH(CH_3)_2$	Bu^t $-C(CH_3)_3$
Pr^n $-CH_2 \cdot CH_2 \cdot CH_3$	Ph $-C_6H_5$
Bu^i $-CH_2 \cdot CH(CH_3)_2$	Ac $-CO \cdot CH_3$

Manufacture of Medicinal and Pharmaceutical Substances

The definitions of certain medicinal and pharmaceutical substances specify a particular method of manufacture although details of the manufacturing processes are not given. A statement that a substance may be prepared by a certain method however indicates that this is one possible method and does not imply that other methods are not permitted.

Manufacture of Formulated Preparations

Attention is drawn to the need to observe adequate hygienic precautions in the preparation and dispensing of pharmaceutical formulations. The principles of good pharmaceutical manufacturing practice should be observed.

Certain pharmaceutical preparations are defined only in terms of the principal ingredients without details of the mode of preparation. Whatever method of preparation is used, the resulting product must conform with the Pharmacopœial requirements and any ingredient, other than those included in the definition, must comply with the general notice on Auxiliary Substances.

Other pharmaceutical preparations are defined by means of a full formula together with, in some cases, directions for their preparation. No deviation from the stated formula and directions is permitted except those allowed by the general notices on Colouring Agents and Antimicrobial Preservatives.

The remaining pharmaceutical preparations are described by means of monographs that include both a definition in terms of the principal ingredients and a full formula together with, in some cases, directions for their preparation. Such full formulae and directions are intended for the *extemporaneous preparation* of relatively small quantities for short-term supply and use. When so prepared, no deviation from the stated formula and directions is permitted.

If, however, such a pharmaceutical preparation is manufactured on a larger scale with the intention that it may be stored, deviations from the stated formula and directions are permitted provided that any ingredient, other than those included in the definition, complies with the general notice on Auxiliary Substances and that the final product meets the following criteria:
(1) accordance with the definition stated in the monograph;
(2) compliance with all the requirements stated in the monograph;

(3) retention of the essential characteristics of the preparation made
strictly in accordance with the formula and directions of the
Pharmacopœia.

In the manufacture of any official preparation on a large scale with the
intention that it should be stored, it is necessary to ascertain that the
product is satisfactory with respect to its physical and chemical stability
and its state of preservation over the claimed shelf-life. This applies
irrespective of whether the formula and instructions of the
Pharmacopœia are followed precisely or modified. Provided that the
preparation has been shown to be stable in other respects, deterioration
due to microbial contamination may be inhibited by the incorporation of
a suitable antimicrobial preservative. In such circumstances the label
states appropriate storage conditions, the date after which the product
should not be used and the identity and concentration of the
antimicrobial preservative.

**Methods of
Sterilisation**

The methods of sterilisation used in preparing the sterile materials
described in the Pharmacopœia are given in Appendix XVIII. For
aqueous preparations, heating in an autoclave is the method of choice
and therefore, wherever it is known to be suitable, this method is
specified in the monographs for such preparations. While the method
specified in any particular monograph is that generally considered to be
the most suitable for the preparation concerned, the use of an alternative
procedure is not precluded provided that it has been validated with
respect to both the assurance of sterility and the integrity of the product
and provided that the final product complies with the requirements of
the monograph.

Water

The term Water used without qualification in formulae means either
potable water freshly drawn direct from the public supply and suitable
for drinking or freshly boiled and cooled Purified Water. The latter
should be used if the public supply is from a local storage tank or if the
potable water is unsuitable for a particular preparation.

Auxiliary Substances

Any substances added in preparing official preparations shall be
innocuous, shall have no adverse influence on the therapeutic efficacy of
the active ingredients and shall not interfere with the assays and tests.
Particular care should be taken to ensure that such substances are free
from harmful organisms.

Colouring Agents

In certain monographs for formulated preparations defined by means of
a full formula a specific colouring agent or agents may be prescribed;
suitable alternatives approved in the country concerned may be
substituted.

**Antimicrobial
Preservatives**

When the term 'suitable antimicrobial preservative' is used it is implied
that the preparation concerned will be effectively preserved according to
the appropriate criteria applied and interpreted as described in the test
for *efficacy of antimicrobial preservatives in pharmaceutical products*
(Appendix XVI C). In certain monographs for formulated preparations
defined by means of a full formula a specific antimicrobial agent or
agents may be prescribed; suitable alternatives may be substituted
provided that their identity and concentration are stated on the label.

**Freshly and Recently
Prepared**

For *extemporaneous preparation*, the direction that a preparation must be
freshly prepared indicates that it must be made not more than twenty-
four hours before it is issued for use. The direction that a preparation

should be recently prepared indicates that deterioration is likely if the preparation is stored for longer than about four weeks at 15° to 25°.

Expression of Standards

Where the standard for a substance described in a monograph is expressed in terms of the chemical formula for that substance an upper limit exceeding 100 per cent may be stated. Such an upper limit applies to the result of the assay calculated in terms of the equivalent content of the specified chemical formula. For example, the statement 'contains not less than 99.0 per cent and not more than 101.0 per cent of $C_{20}H_{24}N_2O_2,HCl$' implies that the result of the assay is not less than 99.0 per cent and not more than 101.0 per cent when calculated in terms of the equivalent content of $C_{20}H_{24}N_2O_2,HCl$.

Where a standard is required to be calculated with reference to the dried substance, the drying conditions prescribed in the test for Loss on drying in the monograph apply. Where the standard is to be calculated with reference to the anhydrous substance, the content of water is determined by the method prescribed in the monograph. Where the standard is to be calculated with reference to the substance free from a specified solvent, the content of that solvent is determined by the method prescribed in the monograph. Where the standard is to be calculated with reference to the peptide content, the content of peptide is determined by the method prescribed in the monograph.

Characteristics

Statements given under the side-heading Characteristics are not to be interpreted in a strict sense and are not to be regarded as analytical requirements. Statements on taste do not form part of the official standards. They are provided only in cases where this property is a guide to the acceptability of the material (for example, a material used primarily for flavouring).

Solubility

Statements given under the side-heading Solubility are intended as information on the approximate solubility at 20°, unless otherwise stated, and are not to be considered as official requirements.

Statements given under side-headings such as Solubility in ethanol express exact requirements and constitute part of the standards for the substances under which they occur.

When the expression parts is used in defining the solubility of a substance, it is to be understood to mean that 1 g of a solid or 1 ml of a liquid is soluble in that number of millilitres of the solvent represented by the stated number of parts.

The following table indicates the meanings of the phrases used in statements of approximate solubilities for which no figures are given:

Descriptive phrase	Approximate quantities of solvent by volume for 1 part of solute by weight
very soluble	less than 1 part
freely soluble	from 1 to 10 parts
soluble	from 10 to 30 parts
sparingly soluble	from 30 to 100 parts
slightly soluble	from 100 to 1000 parts
very slightly soluble	from 1000 to 10,000 parts
practically insoluble	more than 10,000 parts

Identification

The tests described or referred to under the side-heading Identification are not necessarily sufficient to establish absolute proof of identity. They provide a means of verifying that the identity of the material being examined is in accordance with the label on the container. In certain monographs alternative series of identification tests are given; compliance with either one or the other set of tests is adequate to verify the identity of the material.

When tests for infra-red absorption are applied to material extracted from formulated preparations, strict concordance with the specified reference spectrum may not always be possible, but nevertheless a close resemblance between the spectrum of the extracted material and the specified reference spectrum should be achieved.

Assays and Tests

The assays and tests described are the official methods upon which the standards of the Pharmacopœia depend. The analyst is not precluded from employing alternative methods, including methods of micro-analysis, in any assay or test if it is known that the method used will give a result of equivalent accuracy. In the event of doubt or dispute, the methods of analysis of the Pharmacopœia are alone authoritative.

For preparations other than those of fixed strength, the quantity to be taken for an assay or test is usually expressed in terms of the active ingredient. This means that the quantity of the active ingredient expected to be present and the quantity of the preparation to be taken are calculated from the strength stated on the label.

In assays the approximate quantity to be taken for examination is indicated but the quantity actually used must not deviate by more than 10 per cent from that stated. The quantity taken is accurately weighed or measured and the result of the assay is calculated from this exact quantity. Reagents are measured and the procedures are carried out with an accuracy commensurate with the degree of precision implied by the standard stated for the assay.

In tests the stated quantity to be taken for examination must be used unless any divergence can be taken into account in conducting the test and calculating the result. The quantity taken is accurately weighed or measured with the degree of precision implied by the standard or, where the standard is not stated numerically (for example, in tests for Clarity and colour of solution) with the degree of precision implied by the number of significant figures stated. Reagents are measured and the procedures are carried out with an accuracy commensurate with this degree of precision.

At the end of certain tests, the concentration of impurity is given in parentheses in parts per million by weight (ppm) or, when the limit exceeds 500 ppm, as a percentage. These figures are approximations for information only; conformity with the requirements is determined on the basis of compliance or otherwise with the stated test.

Where the solvent used for a solution is not named, the solvent is Purified Water.

The use of a proprietary designation to identify a material used in an assay or test does not imply that another equally suitable material may not be used.

Biological Assays and Tests

Methods of biological (including biochemical and immunochemical) assays and tests are described in Appendix XIV. Where methods of assay are described as Suggested Methods, these are not obligatory, but when another method is used its precision must be not less than that required for the Suggested Method. However, for those substances and preparations that are described in the European Pharmacopœia, in cases of doubt or dispute the methods described in the European Pharmacopœia must be used.

For antibiotics the potency requirement is expressed in the monograph in Units per milligram. The material is not of pharmacopoeial quality if the upper fiducial limit of error is less than the stated potency.

For antibiotics the required precision of the assay is stated in the monograph in terms of the fiducial limits of error about the estimated potency. For other substances and preparations, unless otherwise stated, the precision of the assay is such that the fiducial limits of error, expressed as a percentage of the estimated potency, are within a range not wider than that obtained by multiplying by a factor of ten the square roots of the limits given in the monograph for the fiducial limits of error about the stated potency.

In all cases fiducial limits of error are based on a probability of 95 per cent (P = 0.95).

When the assay is being used to ascertain the purity of the material, the stated potency means the potency stated on the label in terms of Units per gram, Units per milligram or Units per millilitre. When no such statement appears on the label, the stated potency means the fixed or minimum potency required in the monograph. This interpretation of stated potency applies in all cases except where the monograph specifically directs otherwise.

When the assay is being used to determine the total activity in the container, the stated potency means the total number of Units stated on the label or, if no such statement appears, the total activity calculated in accordance with the instructions in the monograph.

When Units are referred to in an assay or test, the Unit for a particular substance or preparation is, for the United Kingdom, the specific biological activity contained in such an amount of the respective primary standard as the appropriate international or national organisation indicates. (The necessary information is provided with the primary standard.)

Wherever possible the primary standard is the respective International Standard or Reference Preparation and the Unit is that defined by the World Health Organization for international use (International Unit).

Unless otherwise directed, animals used in an assay or a test are healthy animals, drawn from a uniform stock, that have not previously been treated with any material that will interfere with the assay or test. Unless otherwise stated, guinea-pigs weigh not less than 250 g or, when used in systemic toxicity tests, not less than 350 g. When used in skin tests they are white or light coloured. Unless otherwise stated, mice weigh not less than 17 g and not more than 22 g.

Certain of the biological assays and tests of the Pharmacopœia are such that in the United Kingdom they may be carried out only in accordance with the Animals (Scientific Procedures) Act 1986. Instructions included in such assays and tests in the Pharmacopœia, with respect to the handling of animals, are therefore confined to those concerned with the accuracy and reproducibility of the assay or test.

Storage   The substances and preparations described in the Pharmacopœia should be stored under conditions that prevent contamination and, as far as possible, deterioration. Precautions that should be taken in relation to the effects of the atmosphere, moisture, heat and light are indicated, where appropriate, in the monographs. Further precautions may be necessary when some materials are stored in tropical climates or under other severe conditions.

Labelling

The labelling requirements of the Pharmacopœia are not comprehensive and laws governing the statements to be declared on labels of official articles should also be met. In the United Kingdom the provisions of regulations issued in accordance with the Medicines Act 1968, together with those of regulations for the labelling of hazardous materials, should be met.

The statements in monographs given under the side-heading Labelling indicate the information required for pharmacopoeial purposes. Such matters as the exact form of wording to be used and whether a particular item of information should appear on the primary label and additionally, or alternatively, on the package or exceptionally in a leaflet are, in general, outside the scope of the Pharmacopœia. When the term 'label' is used in Labelling statements of the Pharmacopœia, decisions as to where the particular statement should appear should therefore be made in accordance with relevant legislation.

The label of every official article states (i) the name at the head of the monograph and (ii) a reference consisting of either figures or letters, or a combination of figures and letters, by which the history of the article may be traced.

The label of every official formulated preparation other than those of fixed strength also states the content of the active ingredient or ingredients expressed in the terms required by the monograph. Where the content of active ingredient is required to be expressed in terms other than the weight of the official medicinal substance used in making the formulation this is specifically stated under the side-heading Labelling. Thus, where no specific requirement is included under the side-heading Labelling, it is implied that the content of active ingredient is expressed in terms of the weight of the official medicinal substance used in making the formulation. For example, for Amodiaquine Tablets, which contain Amodiaquine Hydrochloride but for which the content is expressed in terms of the equivalent amount of amodiaquine base, a specific requirement to this effect is included under the side-heading Labelling. For Amitriptyline Tablets which contain Amitriptyline Hydrochloride and for which the result of the assay is expressed in terms of amitriptyline hydrochloride no specific statement is included under the side-heading Labelling; these Tablets are thus labelled with the nominal weight of Amitriptyline Hydrochloride.

These requirements do not necessarily apply to the labelling of Surgical Dressings, the requirements for which are specified in the section on Surgical Dressings, nor to articles supplied in compliance with a prescription.

Action and Use

The statements given under this side-heading in monographs are intended only as information on the principal pharmacological actions or the uses of the materials in medicine or pharmacy. It should not be assumed that the substance has no other action or use. The statements are not intended to be binding on prescribers or to limit their discretion.

Strengths Available

Statements under the side-headings Strength or Strengths Available are included as a guide and are not necessarily comprehensive. For solid dosage forms such as Capsules and Tablets the strength is given as the amount of active ingredient in each unit. For liquid dosage forms such as Injections and semi-solid dosage forms such as Creams the strength is given as a concentration. For Powders for Injections the strength is given as the amount of active ingredient in each sealed container. Unless otherwise stated the strength is given in terms of the weight or concentration of the official medicinal substance used in making the formulation.

Caution Statements

A number of materials described in the monographs and some of the reagents specified for use in the assays and tests of the Pharmacopœia may be injurious to health unless adequate precautions are taken. The principles of good laboratory practice and the provisions of any appropriate regulations such as those issued in the United Kingdom in accordance with Health and Safety at Work etc. Act (1974) should be observed at all times in carrying out the assays and tests of the Pharmacopœia.

Attention is drawn to particular hazards in certain monographs by means of an italicised statement; the absence of such a statement should not however be taken to mean that no hazard exists.

Atomic Weights

The atomic weights adopted are the values given in the Table of Relative Atomic Weights 1983 published by the International Union of Pure and Applied Chemistry. The values are based on the carbon-12 scale (Appendix XXII).

Temperature

The Celsius thermometric scale is used in expressing temperatures.

Standard Temperature and Pressure

Standard temperature and pressure refers to a temperature of 0° and an atmospheric pressure of 101.3 kPa.

Water-bath

The term water-bath means a bath of boiling water, unless water at some other temperature is indicated in the text. An alternative form of heating may be employed providing that the required temperature is approximately maintained but not exceeded.

Weights and Measures

The metric system of weights and measures is employed; SI Units have generally been adopted. Metric measures are required to have been graduated at 20° and all measurements involved in the analytical operations of the Pharmacopœia are intended, unless otherwise stated, to be made at that temperature. Graduated glass apparatus used in analytical operations should comply with Class A requirements of the appropriate specification issued by the British Standards Institution.

Expression of Concentrations

The expression 'per cent' or the symbol '%' is used, according to circumstances, with one of four different meanings in the expression of concentrations. In order that the meaning to be attached to the expression in each instance is clear, the following notation is used.

Per cent w/w (percentage weight in weight) expresses the number of grams of solute in 100 g of product.

Per cent w/v (percentage weight in volume) expresses the number of grams of solute in 100 ml of product.

Per cent v/v (percentage volume in volume) expresses the number of millilitres of solute in 100 ml of product.

Per cent v/w (percentage volume in weight) expresses the number of millilitres of solute in 100 g of product.

Usually the strength of solutions of solids in liquids is expressed as percentage weight in volume, of liquids in liquids as percentage volume in volume and of gases in liquids as percentage weight in weight. When the concentration of a solution is expressed as parts of dissolved substance in parts of the solution, it is to be understood to mean parts by weight (g) of a solid in parts by volume (ml) of the final solution; or parts by volume (ml) of a liquid in parts by volume (ml) of the final solution; or parts by weight (g) of a gas in parts by weight (g) of the final solution.

When the concentration of a solution is expressed in molarity designated by the symbol M preceded by a number, it denotes the number of moles of the stated solute contained in sufficient Purified Water (unless otherwise stated) to produce 1 litre of solution.

Constant Weight

The term 'constant weight', used in relation to the process of drying, means that two consecutive weighings do not differ by more than 0.5 milligram, the second weighing being made after an additional hour of drying under the specified conditions.

Reagents

The reagents required for the assays and tests of the Pharmacopœia are defined in appendices. The descriptions set out in the appendices do not imply that the materials are suitable for use in medicine.

Indicators

Indicators, the colours of which change over approximately the same range of pH, may be substituted for one another but in the event of doubt or dispute as to the equivalence of indicators for a particular purpose, the indicator specified in the text is alone authoritative.

The quantity of an indicator solution appropriate for use in acid—alkali titrations described in assays or tests is 0.1 ml unless otherwise stated in the text.

Crude Drugs

The macroscopical description of a crude drug includes those features that can be seen by the unaided eye or by the use of a hand lens. The diagnostic characteristics given under a powdered crude drug are to be read in conjunction with the microscopical description given under the whole drug.

Vegetable drugs are required to be free from insects and other animal matter, and from animal excreta. Not more than traces of foreign organic matter may be present in powdered vegetable drugs. Microbial contamination should be minimal.

In determining the Acid-insoluble ash, Ash, Extractive soluble in ethanol, Water-soluble ash and Water-soluble extractive of powdered vegetable drugs, the calculations are made with reference to the drug that has not been specially dried.

In the assays for alkaloids in crude drugs and their preparations, definite quantities of solvents are specified. The quantities are given as being suitable for typical cases; they may, however, be varied where necessary to overcome the difficulties that may be encountered in special instances, provided that the effect of the prescribed directions is ensured.

When it is found necessary to dry a crude drug before it can be reduced to powder for the purpose of assay, a correction is made for the loss on drying and the alkaloidal content is calculated with reference to the undried drug.

Monographs

Medicinal and Pharmaceutical Substances

Acacia ☆

Acacia is the air-hardened, gummy exudate flowing naturally from or obtained by incision of the trunk and branches of *Acacia senegal* L. Willdenow and other species of *Acacia* of African origin.

Characteristics Odourless.

Macroscopical Spheroidal, oval or kidney-shaped pieces (tears), of varying diameter from about 1 to 3 cm, yellowish-white, yellow or pale amber, sometimes with a pinkish tint, friable, opaque, frequently with a cracked surface, easily broken into irregular, whitish or slightly yellowish angular fragments with conchoidal fracture; glassy and transparent appearance. In the centre of unbroken tears there is often a small cavity.

Microscopical The powder presents irregular, colourless, bright fragments. Only traces of starch or vegetable tissue visible. No stratified membrane apparent.

Solubility Almost completely but very slowly soluble in twice its weight of *water*, leaving only a very small residue of vegetable particles; practically insoluble in *ethanol (96%)* and in *ether*.

Identification A. Carry out the method for *thin-layer chromatography*, Appendix III A, using a slurry of *kieselguhr G* in a 1.6% w/v solution of *sodium dihydrogen orthophosphate* to coat the chromatoplate and a mixture of 50 volumes of *acetone*, 40 volumes of *butan-1-ol* and 10 volumes of a 1.6% w/v solution of *sodium dihydrogen orthophosphate* as the mobile phase. Apply separately to the plate 10 µl of each of the following solutions as bands 20 mm long and not more than 3 mm wide. For solution (1) heat 1 g, in powder, with 25 ml of a 4% v/v solution of *sulphuric acid* under a reflux condenser in a water-bath for 90 minutes, neutralise 10 ml of the solution with about 2 g of *barium carbonate*, shake for about 90 minutes, filter, dilute 1 ml of the filtrate with 9 ml of *methanol* and centrifuge. For solution (2) dissolve 10 mg each of D-galactose, D-glucose, L-arabinose and L-rhamnose in 1 ml of *water* and dilute to 10 ml with *methanol*. Develop the plate over a path of 10 cm, remove, dry for a few minutes in a current of warm air and develop over a path of 15 cm using the same mobile phase. After removal of the plate, dry it in an oven at 110° for 10 minutes and spray with *aminohippuric acid reagent*. In the chromatogram obtained with solution (2), four clearly separated bands are obtained which are due to D-galactose (yellowish-brown), D-glucose (yellowish-brown), L-arabinose (reddish-brown) and L-rhamnose (yellow) in order of increasing Rf values. In the chromatogram obtained with solution (1), three bands are present corresponding to D-galactose, L-arabinose and L-rhamnose. The band corresponding to D-glucose is absent and no other bands are visible, particularly in the upper part of the chromatogram.
B. Dissolve 1 g, in powder, in 2 ml of *water* and add 2 ml of *ethanol (96%)*. After shaking, a white gelatinous mucilage is produced which becomes fluid on adding 10 ml of *water*.
C. To 5 ml of a 10% w/v solution add gradually, while shaking, 10 ml of *ethanol (96%)*. The cloudy liquid gives a white precipitate on the addition of 0.5 ml of 5M *acetic acid*. Filter and add to the clear filtrate a few ml of a 4% w/v solution of *ammonium oxalate*; the filtrate becomes cloudy.

D. Dissolve 0.25 g, in powder, in 5 ml of *water*, with shaking, add 0.5 ml of *hydrogen peroxide solution (10 vol)* and 0.5 ml of *guaiacum tincture*. Shake and allow to stand for a few minutes. A deep blue or bluish-green colour is produced.
E. A solution, even of very low concentration (0.01% w/v), gives a precipitate a few minutes after adding *lead subacetate solution*.
F. A 10% w/v solution is laevorotatory.

Agar and sterculia gum To a small quantity, in powder, add freshly prepared *ruthenium red solution* and examine microscopically. The particles are not stained red.

Agar and tragacanth A. To 2 ml of a 10% w/v solution add 8 ml of *water* and 0.2 ml of *lead acetate solution*. No cloudiness is produced on shaking.
B. To 0.1 g, in powder, add 1 ml of 0.01M *iodine*. The mixture does not become crimson or olive green.

Starch and dextrin To 10 ml of a 10% w/v solution, previously boiled and cooled, add 0.1 ml of 0.05M *iodine VS*. No blue or reddish-brown colour is produced.

Sucrose and fructose To 1 ml of a 10% w/v solution add 4 ml of *water*, 0.1 g of *resorcinol* and 2 ml of *hydrochloric acid* and heat on a water-bath. No yellow or pink colour is produced.

Tannins To 10 ml of a 10% w/v solution add 0.1 ml of a 10.5% w/v solution of *iron(III) chloride hexahydrate*. A gelatinous precipitate is produced, but neither the precipitate nor the liquid shows a dark blue colour.

Insoluble matter Not more than 0.5% w/w when determined by the following method. To 5 g, in powder, add 100 ml of *water* and 14 ml of 2M *hydrochloric acid*, boil gently for 15 minutes, shaking frequently, and filter while hot through a sintered-glass filter. Wash the residue with hot *water* and dry at 100° to 105°.

Loss on drying When dried at 100° to 105°, loses not more than 15.0% of its weight. Use 1 g.

Sulphated ash Not more than 5.0%, Appendix IX A, Method II. Use 1 g, in powder.

Microbial contamination 1.0 g is free from *Escherichia coli*, Appendix XVI B1.

Storage Acacia should be kept in a well-closed container.

Action and use Bulk-forming laxative; pharmaceutical aid.

*In certain states party to the Convention on the Elaboration of a European Pharmacopœia, Acacia may be required to comply with a limit for a total viable aerobic count of 10⁴ micro-organisms per gram, determined by plate count, Appendix XVI B2.

Powdered Acacia

Powdered Acacia is Acacia in powder.

Characteristics White or yellowish-white; odourless.

Solubility Almost completely but very slowly soluble in *water*, leaving only a very small residue of vegetable particles; gives a mucilaginous liquid which is colourless or yellowish, dense, viscous, adhesive, translucent and weakly acidic to *litmus paper*; practically insoluble in *ethanol (96%)* and in *ether*.

Identification; Agar and sterculia gum; Agar and tragacanth; Starch and dextrin; Sucrose and fructose;

Tannins; Insoluble matter; Loss on drying; Sulphated ash Complies with the requirements stated under Acacia.

Microbial contamination 1.0 g is free from *Escherichia coli*, Appendix XVI B1.

Storage Powdered Acacia should be kept in a well-closed container.

Action and use Bulk-forming laxative; pharmaceutical aid.

Spray-dried Acacia ☆

Spray-dried Acacia is obtained from a solution of Acacia.

Characteristics White or yellowish-white; odourless.

Microscopical Examined in *ethanol (96%)* the powder consists predominantly of spheroidal particles, 4 to 40 μm in diameter, which show a central cavity containing one or more air bubbles. A few minute flat fragments are present, but no vegetable tissue is visible. Viewed under polarised light, no black cross is seen.

Solubility Completely and rapidly soluble in twice its weight of *water* to produce a mucilaginous liquid which is colourless or yellowish, dense, viscous, adhesive, translucent and weakly acidic to *litmus paper*. Practically insoluble in *ethanol (96%)* and in *ether*.

Identification Complies with tests A, B, C, E and F stated under Acacia.

Agar and sterculia gum; Agar and tragacanth; Starch and dextrin; Sucrose and fructose; Tannins Complies with the requirements stated under Acacia.

Loss on drying When dried at 100° to 105°, loses not more than 10.0% of its weight. Use 1 g.

Sulphated ash Not more than 5.5%, Appendix IX A, Method II. Use 1 g, in powder.

Microbial contamination* 1.0 g is free from *Escherichia coli*, Appendix XVI B1.

Storage Spray-dried Acacia should be kept in an airtight container.

Action and use Pharmaceutical aid.

*In certain states party to the Convention on the Elaboration of a European Pharmacopœia, Spray-dried Acacia may be required to comply with a limit for a total viable aerobic count of 10^4 micro-organisms per gram, determined by plate count, Appendix XVI B2.

Acetazolamide ☆

H₂N·O₂S ⌁ S ⌁ NHAc
(structural formula)

$C_4H_6N_4O_3S_2$ 222.2   59-66-5

Acetazolamide is *N*-(5-sulphamoyl-1,3,4-thia-diazol-2-yl)acetamide. It contains not less than 98.5 per cent and not more than 101.0 per cent of $C_4H_6N_4O_3S_2$, calculated with reference to the dried substance.

Characteristics A white or almost white, crystalline powder; odourless.

Solubility Very slightly soluble in *water*; slightly soluble in *ethanol (96%)* and in *acetone*; practically insoluble in *carbon tetrachloride*, in *chloroform* and in *ether*. It dissolves in dilute solutions of alkali hydroxides.

Identification *Test A may be omitted if tests B, C and D are carried out. Tests C and D may be omitted if tests A and B are carried out.*

A. The *infra-red absorption spectrum*, Appendix II A, is concordant with the spectrum of *acetazolamide EPCRS*. If the spectra are not concordant, dissolve the substances in *ethanol (96%)*, evaporate to dryness and prepare new spectra.

B. The *light absorption*, Appendix II B, in the range 230 to 260 nm of a 0.003% w/v solution in 0.01M *sodium hydroxide* exhibits a maximum at 240 nm; the A(1%, 1 cm) at 240 nm is 162 to 176. The *light absorption* in the range 260 to 350 nm of a 0.00075% w/v solution in 0.01M *sodium hydroxide* exhibits a maximum at 292 nm; the A(1%, 1 cm) at 292 nm is 570 to 620.

C. To 20 mg in a test-tube add 4 ml of 2M *hydrochloric acid* and 0.2 g of *zinc powder* and immediately place a piece of *lead acetate paper* over the mouth of the tube. The paper exhibits a brownish-black colour.

D. Dissolve 25 mg in a mixture of 0.1 ml of 2M *sodium hydroxide* and 5 ml of *water* and add 0.1 ml of *copper sulphate solution*. A greenish-blue precipitate is produced.

Clarity and colour of solution A 10% w/v solution in 1M *sodium hydroxide* is not more opalescent than *reference suspension II*, Appendix IV A, and not more intensely coloured than *reference solution Y_5 or BY_5*, Appendix IV B, Method II.

Heavy metals 1.0 g complies with *limit test C for heavy metals*, Appendix VII (20 ppm). Use 2 ml of *lead standard solution (10 ppm Pb)* to prepare the standard.

Sulphate Dissolve 0.4 g in 20 ml of *water* by heating to boiling. Allow to cool with frequent shaking and filter. 15 ml of the filtrate complies with the *limit test for sulphates*, Appendix VII (500 ppm).

Related substances Carry out the method for *thin-layer chromatography*, Appendix III A, using *silica gel GF254* as the coating substance and a freshly prepared mixture of 50 volumes of *propan-2-ol*, 30 volumes of *ethyl acetate* and 20 volumes of 13.5M *ammonia* as the mobile phase. Use the tank without lining the walls and allow to saturate for 1 hour before development. Apply separately to the chromatoplate 20 μl of each of two solutions of the substance being examined in a mixture of equal volumes of *ethanol (96%)* and *ethyl acetate* containing (1) 0.50% w/v and (2) 0.0050% w/v. After removal of the plate, allow it to dry in air and examine under *ultra-violet light (254 nm)*. Any *secondary spot* in the chromatogram obtained with solution (1) is not more intense than the spot in the chromatogram obtained with solution (2).

Loss on drying When dried to constant weight at 100° to 105°, loses not more than 0.5% of its weight. Use 1 g.

Sulphated ash Not more than 0.1%, Appendix IX A, Method II. Use 1 g.

Assay Dissolve 0.2 g in 25 ml of *dimethylformamide* and titrate with 0.1M *ethanolic sodium hydroxide VS* determining the end-point potentiometrically. Each ml of 0.1M *ethanolic sodium hydroxide VS* is equivalent to 0.02222 g of $C_4H_6N_4O_3S_2$.

Preparation
Acetazolamide Tablets
Action and use Used in treatment of glaucoma.

Glacial Acetic Acid

CH₃·CO₂H

$C_2H_4O_2$ 60.05   *64-19-7*

Glacial Acetic Acid contains not less than 99.0 per cent and not more than 100.5 per cent w/w of $C_2H_4O_2$.

Characteristics A translucent, crystalline mass, or at temperatures above its freezing point, a clear, colourless liquid; odour, pungent.

Solubility Miscible with *water*, with *ethanol (96%)*, with *chloroform* and with most fixed and volatile oils.

Identification A. Strongly acidic, even when diluted freely.
B. When diluted with *water* and neutralised, yields the *reactions* characteristic of acetates, Appendix VI.
C. *Boiling point*, about 117°, Appendix V D.

Freezing point Not lower than 14.8°, Appendix V B.

Weight per ml 1.048 g to 1.051 g, Appendix V G.

Heavy metals Evaporate 3.4 g to dryness and dissolve the residue in 20 ml of *water*. The resulting solution complies with *limit test A for heavy metals*, Appendix VII (6 ppm). Use *lead standard solution (1 ppm Pb)* to prepare the standard.

Chloride Dilute 5.0 ml with sufficient *water* to produce 100 ml. 15 ml of the resulting solution complies with the *limit test for chlorides*, Appendix VII (70 ppm).

Sulphate 12.5 ml of the solution used in the test for Chloride, diluted to 15 ml with *water*, complies with the *limit test for sulphates*, Appendix VII (240 ppm).

Aldehydes Not more than 0.05% w/w, calculated as C_2H_4O, when determined by the following method. To 10 g add 50 ml of *water* and 10 ml of a 1.25% w/v solution of *sodium metabisulphite*, allow to stand for 30 minutes and titrate the excess of sodium metabisulphite with 0.05M *iodine VS*. Repeat the operation without the substance being examined. The difference between the titrations represents the amount of sodium metabisulphite required. Each ml of 0.05M *iodine VS* is equivalent to 0.002203 g of C_2H_4O.

Formic acid and oxidisable impurities Mix 5 ml with 10 ml of *water* and reserve 5.0 ml for the test for Readily oxidisable impurities. To a further 5 ml add 6 ml of *sulphuric acid*, cool, add 2 ml of 0.0167M *potassium dichromate VS*, allow to stand for 1 minute, add 25 ml of *water* and 1 ml of freshly prepared *potassium iodide solution* and titrate the liberated iodine with 0.1M *sodium thiosulphate VS* using *starch mucilage* as indicator. Not less than 1.0 ml of 0.1M *sodium thiosulphate VS* is required.

Readily oxidisable impurities To 5.0 ml of the solution reserved in the test for Formic acid and oxidisable impurities add 20 ml of *water* and 0.2 ml of 0.02M *potassium permanganate VS* and allow to stand for 30 seconds. The colour is not entirely discharged.

Non-volatile matter When evaporated to dryness and dried at 105°, leaves not more than 0.01% w/w of residue.

Assay To 2 g add 50 ml of *water* and titrate with 1M *sodium hydroxide VS* using *phenolphthalein solution* as indicator. Each ml of 1M *sodium hydroxide VS* is equivalent to 0.06005 g of $C_2H_4O_2$.

Storage Glacial Acetic Acid should be kept in a well-closed container.

Acetic Acid (33 per cent)
Acetic Acid

Acetic Acid (33 per cent) contains not less than 32.5 per cent and not more than 33.5 per cent w/w of acetic acid, $C_2H_4O_2$.

Characteristics A clear, colourless liquid; odour, pungent.

Solubility Miscible with *water*, with *ethanol (96%)* and with *glycerol*.

Identification A. Strongly acidic, even when diluted freely.
B. When neutralised, yields the *reactions* characteristic of acetates, Appendix VI.

Weight per ml 1.040 to 1.042 g, Appendix V G.

Heavy metals Evaporate 10.0 ml to dryness and add 20 ml of *water*. 12 ml of the resulting solution complies with *limit test A for heavy metals*, Appendix VII (2 ppm). Use *lead standard solution (1 ppm Pb)* to prepare the standard.

Chloride Dilute 5.0 ml with sufficient *water* to produce 100 ml. 15 ml of the resulting solution complies with the *limit test for chlorides*, Appendix VII (70 ppm).

Sulphate 12.5 ml of the solution used in the test for Chloride, diluted to 15 ml with *water*, complies with the *limit test for sulphates*, Appendix VII (240 ppm).

Aldehydes Distil 15.0 ml. To the first 5 ml of the distillate add 10 ml of a 5% w/v solution of *mercury(II) chloride*, make alkaline with 5M *sodium hydroxide*, allow to stand for 5 minutes and make acidic with 1M *sulphuric acid*. The solution shows not more than a faint turbidity.

Formic acid and oxidisable impurities Mix 5 ml with 6 ml of *sulphuric acid* and cool to 20°. Add 2 ml of 0.0167M *potassium dichromate VS*, allow to stand for 1 minute, add 25 ml of *water* and 1 ml of freshly prepared *potassium iodide solution* and titrate the liberated iodine with 0.1M *sodium thiosulphate VS* using *starch mucilage* as indicator. Not less than 1 ml of 0.1M *sodium thiosulphate VS* is required.

Readily oxidisable impurities To 5.0 ml add 20 ml of *water* and 0.2 ml of 0.02M *potassium permanganate VS* and allow to stand for 1 minute. The pink colour is not entirely discharged.

Non-volatile matter When evaporated to dryness and dried at 105°, leaves not more than 0.01% w/w of residue.

Assay Weigh 5 g into a stoppered flask containing 50 ml of *water* and titrate with 1M *sodium hydroxide VS* using *phenolphthalein solution* as indicator. Each ml of 1M *sodium hydroxide VS* is equivalent to 0.06005 g of $C_2H_4O_2$.

Preparation
Acetic Acid (6 per cent)

Acetic Acid (6 per cent)

Dilute Acetic Acid

Acetic Acid (6 per cent) contains not less than 5.7 per cent and not more than 6.3 per cent w/w of acetic acid, $C_2H_4O_2$. It may be prepared by mixing 182 g of Acetic Acid (33 per cent) with 818 g of Purified Water.

Identification A. Strongly acidic.
B. When neutralised, yields the *reactions* characteristic of acetates, Appendix VI.

Weight per ml About 1.005 g, Appendix V G.

Heavy metals Evaporate 20.0 ml to dryness and add 20 ml of *water*. 12 ml of the resulting solution complies with *limit test A for heavy metals*, Appendix VII (1 ppm). Use *lead standard solution (1 ppm Pb)* to prepare the standard.

Chloride Dilute 5.0 ml with sufficient *water* to produce 100 ml. 15 ml of the resulting solution complies with the *limit test for chlorides*, Appendix VII (70 ppm).

Sulphate 12.5 ml of the solution used in the test for Chloride, diluted to 15 ml with *water*, complies with the *limit test for sulphates*, Appendix VII (240 ppm).

Aldehydes Distil 75 ml. To the first 5 ml of the distillate add 10 ml of a 5% w/v solution of *mercury(II) chloride*, make alkaline with 5M *sodium hydroxide*, allow to stand for 5 minutes and acidify with 1M *sulphuric acid*. The solution shows not more than a faint turbidity.

Formic acid and oxidisable impurities Mix 5 ml with 6 ml of *sulphuric acid* and cool to 20°. Add 0.4 ml of 0.0167M *potassium dichromate VS*, allow to stand for 1 minute, add 25 ml of *water* and 1 ml of freshly prepared *potassium iodide solution* and titrate the liberated iodine with 0.1M *sodium thiosulphate VS* using *starch mucilage* as indicator. Not less than 0.2 ml of 0.1M *sodium thiosulphate VS* is required.

Readily oxidisable impurities To 25.0 ml add 0.2 ml of 0.02M *potassium permanganate VS* and allow to stand for 1 minute. The pink colour is not entirely discharged.

Non-volatile matter When evaporated to dryness and dried at 105°, leaves not more than 0.01% w/w of residue.

Assay Add 30 ml of *water* to 20 g in a stoppered flask and titrate with 1M *sodium hydroxide VS* using *phenolphthalein solution* as indicator. Each ml of 1M *sodium hydroxide VS* is equivalent to 0.06005 g of $C_2H_4O_2$.

Acetohexamide

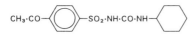

$C_{15}H_{20}N_2O_4S$ 324.4   *968-81-0*

Acetohexamide is 1-(4-acetylbenzenesulphonyl)-3-cyclohexylurea. It contains not less than 98.5 per cent and not more than 101.0 per cent of $C_{15}H_{20}N_2O_4S$, calculated with reference to the dried substance.

Characteristics A white, crystalline powder; odourless or almost odourless.

Solubility Practically insoluble in *water* and in *ether*; slightly soluble in *ethanol (96%)* and in *chloroform*. It dissolves in aqueous solutions of alkali hydroxides.

Identification A. The *infra-red absorption spectrum*, Appendix II A, is concordant with the *reference spectrum* of acetohexamide.
B. The *light absorption*, Appendix II B, in the range 230 to 350 nm of a 0.002% w/v solution in 0.01M *sodium hydroxide* exhibits a maximum at 248 nm. The *absorbance* at 248 nm is about 0.85.

Heavy metals 2.0 g complies with *limit test C for heavy metals*, Appendix VII (20 ppm). Use 2 ml of *lead standard solution (20 ppm Pb)* to prepare the standard.

Cyclohexylamine Prepare a 0.0025% w/v solution of n-*decane* in dichloromethane (solution A). Carry out the method for *gas chromatography*, Appendix III B, using the following solutions. For solution (1) add 50 ml of 0.3M *sodium hydroxide* to 1 ml of a 0.0375% w/v solution of *cyclohexylamine* in 0.5M *hydrochloric acid*, extract with two 5-ml quantities of solution A and combine the extracts. For solution (2) dissolve 3.0 g of the substance being examined in 50 ml of 0.3M *sodium hydroxide*, extract with two 5-ml quantities of *dichloromethane* and combine the extracts. For solution (3) dissolve 3.0 g of the substance being examined in 50 ml of 0.3M *sodium hydroxide*, extract with two 5-ml quantities of solution A and combine the extracts.

The chromatographic procedure may be carried out using a glass column (1.5 m × 4 mm) packed with *acid-washed, silanised diatomaceous support* coated with 10% w/w of Pennwalt 223 and 4% w/w of *potassium hydroxide* and maintained at 120°. In order to ensure a consistent response it may be necessary to saturate the column by making repeated injections of a solution of *cyclohexylamine* in *dichloromethane* before the analysis.

In the chromatogram obtained with solution (3) the ratio of the area of the peak due to cyclohexylamine to that of the internal standard is not greater than the corresponding ratio in the chromatogram obtained with solution (1) (125 ppm).

Dicyclohexylurea Carry out the method for *high-performance liquid chromatography*, Appendix III D, using the following solutions. Solution (1) contains 0.020% w/v of *1,3-dicyclohexylurea* in *methanol*. For solution (2) dissolve 2.0 g of the substance being examined in 50 ml of 0.2M *sodium hydroxide* and extract with three 25-ml quantities of *dichloromethane*, wash the combined extracts with 5 ml of 0.5M *hydrochloric acid*, evaporate to dryness using a rotary evaporator and dissolve the residue in 1 ml of *methanol*.

The chromatographic procedure may be carried out using (a) a stainless steel column (20 cm × 4.6 mm) packed with *stationary phase C* (5 μm) (Spherisorb ODS 1 is suitable), (b) a mixture of 60 volumes of *methanol* and 40 volumes of *water* as the mobile phase with a flow rate of 2 ml per minute and (c) a detection wavelength of 210 nm.

The area of any peak corresponding to 1,3-dicyclohexylurea in the chromatogram obtained with solution (2) is not greater than the area of the peak in the chromatogram obtained with solution (1) (100 ppm).

Related substances Carry out the method for *thin-layer chromatography*, Appendix III A, using *silica gel GF254* as the coating substance and a mixture of 100 volumes of *chloroform*, 50 volumes of *methanol*, 30 volumes of cyclohexane and 11.5 volumes of 13.5M *ammonia* as the mobile phase. Apply separately to the chromatoplate 2 μl of each of three freshly prepared solutions of the substance being examined in *dimethylformamide* containing (1) 5.0% w/v, (2) 0.025% w/v and (3) 0.010% w/v. After removal of the plate, allow it to dry in air and examine under *ultra-violet light (254 nm)*. Any *secondary spot* in the chromatogram obtained with solution (1) is not more intense than the spot in the chromatogram obtained with solution (2) and not more than four such spots are more intense than the spot in the chromatogram obtained with solution (3).

Loss on drying When dried at 105° for 3 hours, loses not more than 1.0% of its weight. Use 1 g.

Sulphated ash Not more than 0.1%, Appendix IX A.

Assay Dissolve 0.6 g in 25 ml of *dimethylformamide* previously neutralised to *thymol blue solution* and titrate with 0.1M *methanolic potassium hydroxide VS* using *thymol blue solution* as indicator. Each ml of 0.1M *methanolic potassium hydroxide VS* is equivalent to 0.03244 g of $C_{15}H_{20}N_2O_4S$.

Preparation

Acetohexamide Tablets

Action and use Hypoglycaemic.

Acetone

CH₃·CO·CH₃

C_3H_6O 58.08   *67-64-1*

Acetone is propan-2-one.

Characteristics A clear, colourless, flammable, mobile, volatile liquid; odour, characteristic.

Solubility Miscible with *water*, with *ethanol (96%)*, with *chloroform* and with *ether*.

Identification A. The *infra-red absorption spectrum*, Appendix II A, is concordant with the *reference spectrum* of acetone.
B. To 1 ml of a 0.5% v/v solution add 1 ml of a 1% w/v solution of *sodium nitroprusside* and 2 ml of 1M *sodium hydroxide*; an orange-red colour is produced. Immediately add a slight excess of 6M *acetic acid*; a purplish-red colour is produced.
C. To 10 ml of a 0.1% v/v solution in *ethanol (50%)* add 1 ml of a 1% w/v solution of *2-nitrobenzaldehyde* in the same solvent followed by 1 ml of 5M *sodium hydroxide*, allow to stand for 2 minutes and acidify with 6M *acetic acid*. A bluish-green colour is produced.

Acidity To 20 ml add 20 ml of *carbon dioxide-free water*, cool and titrate with 0.1M *sodium hydroxide VS* using *phenolphthalein solution* as indicator. Not more than 0.2 ml is required.

Alkalinity Add 10 ml to 10 ml of *carbon dioxide-free water* previously neutralised to 0.05 ml of *methyl red solution*. No change in colour occurs.

Clarity of solution Mix 1.0 ml with 19 ml of *water*. The solution is *clear*, Appendix IV A, Method I.

Distillation range 55.7° to 56.7°, Appendix V C.

Weight per ml 0.789 g to 0.791 g, Appendix V G.

Readily oxidisable substances To 30 ml add 0.1 ml of 0.02M *potassium permanganate VS* and allow to stand protected from light at 15° for 2 hours. The colour is not completely discharged.

Non-volatile matter When evaporated to dryness on a water-bath and dried at 105°, leaves not more than 0.005% w/v of residue.

Storage Acetone should be kept in a well-closed container and stored at a temperature not exceeding 15°.

Acetylcysteine

NHAc
|
HSCH₂---C---CO₂H
|
H

$C_5H_9NO_3S$ 163.2   *616-91-1*

Acetylcysteine is *N*-acetyl-L-cysteine. It contains not less than 98.0 per cent and not more than 102.0 per cent of $C_5H_9NO_3S$, calculated with reference to the dried substance.

Characteristics A white, crystalline powder; odour, faint, of acetic acid.

Solubility Soluble in 8 parts of *water* and in 2 parts of *ethanol (96%)*; practically insoluble in *chloroform* and in *ether*.

Identification A. The *infra-red absorption spectrum*, Appendix II A, is concordant with the *reference spectrum* of acetylcysteine.
B. To 0.5 ml of a 5% w/v solution add 0.05 ml of a 5% w/v solution of *sodium nitroprusside* followed by 0.05 ml of 13.5M *ammonia*. A deep magenta colour is produced.
C. *Melting point*, about 108°, Appendix V A.

Acidity pH of a 1% w/v solution, 2.0 to 2.8, Appendix V L.

Specific optical rotation +21° to +27°, Appendix V F, in a solution prepared by dissolving 1.25 g in a mixture of 1 ml of a 0.1% w/v solution of *disodium edetate*, 7.5 ml of 1M *sodium hydroxide* and sufficient *mixed phosphate buffer pH 7.0* to produce 25 ml.

Non-acetylated amino acids Carry out the method for *thin-layer chromatography*, Appendix III A, using a cellulose precoated chromatoplate (Eastman plates are suitable) and a mixture of 60 volumes of *propan-2-ol*, 25 volumes of 1M *hydrochloric acid* and 15 volumes of *butan-2-one* as the mobile phase but allowing the solvent front to ascend 10 cm above the line of application. Apply separately to the plate 2 μl of each of three solutions containing (1) 5.0% w/v of the substance being examined in *water*, (2) 0.10% w/v of *L-cysteine* in *water* and (3) 5 mg of *L-cystine* dissolved in 0.5 ml of 2M *hydrochloric acid* and diluted to 10 ml with *water*. After removal of the plate, dry it at 105° for 5 minutes, spray with a 0.5% w/v solution of *ninhydrin in butan-1-ol*, heat at 105° for 10 minutes and allow to stand overnight. Any spot corresponding to L-cysteine in the chromatogram obtained with solution (1) is not more intense than the spot in the chromatogram obtained with solution (2) and any other *secondary spot* is not more intense than the spot in the chromatogram obtained with solution (3).

Heavy metals 4.0 g complies with *limit test C for heavy metals*, Appendix VII (10 ppm). Use 4 ml of *lead standard solution (10 ppm Pb)* to prepare the standard.

Iron To 2.0 g in a platinum dish add 0.25 ml of *sulphuric acid*, ignite gently, cool and dissolve the residue in sufficient *water* to produce 30 ml. 10 ml of the resulting solution complies with the *limit test for iron*, Appendix VII (15 ppm).

Zinc Not more than 5 ppm when determined by Method II for *atomic absorption spectrophotometry*, Appendix II D, measuring at 214 nm and using *zinc solution ASp* diluted to contain 1 µg of Zn in 1 ml as the standard solution. To 5-ml quantities of a 10% w/v solution of the substance being examined in 0.001M *hydrochloric acid* add suitable volumes of the prepared standard zinc solution and dilute to 10 ml with *water*.

Loss on drying When dried at 70° at a pressure not exceeding 0.7 kPa for 4 hours, loses not more than 1.0% of its weight. Use 1 g.

Sulphated ash Not more than 0.5%, Appendix IX A.

Assay Dissolve 0.3 g in 30 ml of a 90% v/v solution of *glacial acetic acid* and titrate with 0.05M *iodine VS* until a permanent faint yellow colour is produced. Each ml of 0.05M *iodine VS* is equivalent to 0.01632 g of $C_5H_9NO_3S$.

Storage Acetylcysteine should be kept in a well-closed container, protected from light and stored at a temperature not exceeding 15°.

Action and use Antidote for paracetamol poisoning; mucolytic.

Adrenaline

$C_9H_{13}NO_3$ 183.2   *51-43-4*

Adrenaline is (*R*)-1-(3,4-dihydroxyphenyl)-2-methylaminoethanol and may be prepared by synthesis or isolated from the medulla of the suprarenal glands of certain mammals and substantially freed from noradrenaline. It contains not less than 98.5 per cent and not more than 101.0 per cent of $C_9H_{13}NO_3$, calculated with reference to the dried substance.

Characteristics A white or creamy-white, sphaero-crystalline powder. It darkens in colour on exposure to air and light.

Solubility Sparingly soluble in *water*; practically insoluble in *ethanol (96%)* and in *ether*. It dissolves in solutions of mineral acids, of *sodium hydroxide* and of *potassium hydroxide*, but not in solutions of ammonia or of the alkali carbonates.

It is not stable in neutral or alkaline solutions, which rapidly become red on exposure to air.

Identification A. The *light absorption*, Appendix II B, in the range 230 to 350 nm of a 0.006% w/v solution in

0.01M *hydrochloric acid* exhibits a maximum only at 280 nm. The *absorbance* at 280 nm is about 0.9.

B. To a neutral or faintly acidic solution add a 0.25% w/v solution of *iron(III) chloride hexahydrate*. An emerald-green colour is produced which, on the gradual addition of *sodium hydrogen carbonate solution*, changes first to blue and then to red.

C. *Melting point*, about 212°, with decomposition, the rate of rise of temperature being 10° per minute, Appendix V A.

Specific optical rotation In a freshly prepared 4% w/v solution in 1M *hydrochloric acid*, −50° to −53°, Appendix V F.

Phenones *Absorbance* of a 0.2% w/v solution in 0.1M *hydrochloric acid* at 310 nm, not more than 0.20, Appendix II B.

Noradrenaline Dissolve 5.0 mg in 1 ml of a 0.5% w/v solution of (+)-tartaric acid, add 4 ml of *borate buffer pH 9.6*, mix, add 1 ml of a freshly prepared 0.5% w/v solution of *sodium 1,2-naphthaquinone-4-sulphonate*, mix and allow to stand for 30 minutes. Add 0.2 ml of a 1% v/v solution of *benzalkonium chloride solution*, mix, add 15 ml of *toluene* previously washed with *borate buffer pH 9.6* and filtered through a dry filter paper, shake for 30 minutes and allow to separate, centrifuging if necessary. Any red or purple colour in the toluene layer is not more intense than that produced by treating a solution of 0.40 mg of *noradrenaline acid tartrate* and 9 mg of *noradrenaline-free adrenaline acid tartrate* in 1 ml of *water* in the same manner.

Loss on drying When dried over *phosphorus pentoxide* at a pressure not exceeding 0.7 kPa for 18 hours, loses not more than 1.0% of its weight. Use 1 g.

Sulphated ash Not more than 0.1%, Appendix IX A.

Assay Carry out Method I for *non-aqueous titration*, Appendix VIII A, using 0.3 g and *crystal violet solution* as indicator. Each ml of 0.1M *perchloric acid VS* is equivalent to 0.01832 g of $C_9H_{13}NO_3$.

Storage Adrenaline should be kept in a well-closed container, which is preferably filled with nitrogen, and protected from light.

Action and use Beta-adrenoceptor agonist; used in treatment of glaucoma.

In some countries the material described in this monograph may be known as Epinephrine.

Adrenaline Acid Tartrate ☆

$C_9H_{13}NO_3,C_4H_6O_6$ 333.3   *51-42-3*

Adrenaline Acid Tartrate is (*R*)-1-(3,4-dihydroxyphenyl)-2-methylaminoethanol hydrogen tartrate. It contains not less than 98.5 per cent and not more than 101.0 per cent of $C_9H_{13}NO_3$, $C_4H_6O_6$, calculated with reference to the dried substance.

Characteristics A white to greyish-white, crystalline powder; odourless.

Solubility Freely soluble in *water*; slightly soluble in *ethanol (96%)*; practically insoluble in *chloroform* and in *ether*.

Identification *Test A may be omitted if tests B, C, D, E and F are carried out. Tests B, D and E may be omitted if tests A, C and F are carried out.*

A. Dissolve 2 g in 20 ml of *water* containing 0.1 g of *sodium metabisulphite* and add 10M *ammonia* until an alkaline reaction is obtained. Allow the mixture to stand in ice for 1 hour, filter and retain the filtrate. Wash the precipitate with three 2-ml quantities of *water* followed by 5 ml of *ethanol (96%)* and 5 ml of *ether* and dry the precipitate at a pressure of 1.5 to 2.5 kPa for 3 hours. The *infra-red absorption spectrum* of the residue, Appendix II A, is concordant with the spectrum of adrenaline base prepared by the same method from a suitable quantity of *adrenaline acid tartrate EPCRS*.

B. Dissolve 50 mg in sufficient 0.01M *hydrochloric acid* to produce 100 ml and dilute 10 ml of the solution to 100 ml with the same solvent. The *light absorption* of the resulting solution, Appendix II B, in the range 250 to 300 nm exhibits a maximum only at 279 nm. The A(1%, 1 cm) at 279 nm is 79 to 85.

C. The *specific optical rotation*, determined in a 2% w/v solution of the dried precipitate obtained in test A in 0.5M *hydrochloric acid*, is −50° to −54°, Appendix V F.

D. To 1 ml of a 0.1% w/v solution add 10 ml of *phthalate buffer pH 3.6* and 1 ml of 0.05M *iodine VS*. Allow to stand for 5 minutes and add 2 ml of 0.1M *sodium thiosulphate*. An intense violet-red colour is produced.

E. To 1 ml of a 0.1% w/v solution add 1 ml of a 1.0% v/v solution of *2,5-diethoxytetrahydrofuran* in *glacial acetic acid*. Heat at 80° for 2 minutes, cool in ice and add 3 ml of a 2.0% w/v solution of *4-dimethylaminobenzaldehyde* in a mixture of 1 volume of *hydrochloric acid* and 19 volumes of *glacial acetic acid*. Mix and allow to stand for 2 minutes. The solution shows a yellow colour which is similar to that of a solution prepared in the same manner but omitting the substance being examined.

F. The filtrate obtained in test A yields *reaction B* characteristic of tartrates, Appendix VI.

Clarity and colour of solution A 5.0% w/v solution in *water* examined immediately after preparation is not more opalescent than *reference suspension II*, Appendix IV A, and is not more intensely coloured than *reference solution BY₅*, Appendix IV B, Method II.

Noradrenaline Carry out the method for *thin-layer chromatography*, Appendix III A, using *silica gel G* as the coating substance and a mixture of 100 volumes of *acetone*, 100 volumes of *dichloromethane* and 1 volume of *anhydrous formic acid* as the mobile phase. Apply separately to the chromatoplate, as bands 20 mm × 2 mm, 6 µl of each of solutions (1), (2) and (3) and 12 µl of solution (4). Solutions (1), (2) and (3) are solutions in *water*, prepared immediately before use, containing (1) 2.5% w/v of the substance being examined, (2) 0.125% w/v of *noradrenaline acid tartrate EPCRS* and (3) 0.025% w/v of *noradrenaline acid tartrate EPCRS*. Solution (4) is a mixture of equal volumes of solutions (1) and (3). Allow to dry and spray the bands with a saturated solution of *sodium hydrogen carbonate*; allow the plate to dry in air, spray the bands twice with *acetic anhydride*, drying between the two sprayings and heat the plate at 50° for 90 minutes. After removal of the plate, allow it to dry in air and spray with a freshly prepared mixture of 8 volumes of *methanol*, 2 volumes of *ethylenediamine* and 2 volumes of a 0.5% w/v solution of *potassium hexacyanoferrate(III)*. Dry the plate at 60° for 10 minutes

and examine under *ultra-violet light (254 and 365 nm)*. In the chromatogram obtained with solution (1) any band situated between the two most intense bands is not more intense than the corresponding band in the chromatogram obtained with solution (3). The test is not valid unless the chromatogram obtained with solution (4) shows between the two most intense bands a clearly separated band corresponding to the most intense band in the chromatogram obtained with solution (2).

Phenones *Absorbance* of a 0.2% w/v solution in 0.01M *hydrochloric acid* at 310 nm, not more than 0.10, Appendix II B.

Loss on drying When dried over *phosphorus pentoxide* at a pressure of 1.5 to 2.5 kPa for 18 hours, loses not more than 0.5% of its weight. Use 1 g.

Sulphated ash Not more than 0.1%, Appendix IX A, Method II. Use 1 g.

Assay Dissolve 0.3 g in 50 ml of *anhydrous glacial acetic acid*, heating gently if necessary, and carry out Method I for *non-aqueous titration*, Appendix VIII A, using *crystal violet solution* as indicator. Each ml of 0.1M *perchloric acid VS* is equivalent to 0.03333 g of $C_9H_{13}NO_3,C_4H_6O_6$.

Storage Adrenaline Acid Tartrate should be kept in an airtight container, or preferably in a sealed tube under vacuum or under an inert gas, and protected from light. It darkens in colour on exposure to air and light.

Preparations
Adrenaline Injection
Adrenaline Solution
    Adrenaline Acid Tartrate is an ingredient of:
Bupivacaine and Adrenaline Injection
Lignocaine and Adrenaline Injection

Action and use Beta-adrenoceptor agonist.

The title of the monograph in the European Pharmacopœia is Adrenaline Tartrate. In some countries the material described in this monograph may be known as Epinephrine Bitartrate.

Agar ☆

Agar consists of polysaccharides obtained by extracting various species of Rhodophyceae, mainly those belonging to the genus *Gelidium*, with boiling water, filtering whilst hot and evaporating to dryness.

Characteristics Odourless.

Macroscopical Crumpled strips from 2 to 5 mm wide, sometimes in flakes, colourless to pale yellow, translucent, somewhat tough and difficult to break, becoming more brittle on drying.

Microscopical Examined in 0.005M *iodine VS* appears partly stained brownish-violet. Shows numerous minute, colourless, ovoid or rounded grains on an amorphous background; occasional brown, round or ovoid spores up to 60 µm in size with a reticulate surface may be present.

Identification A. Dissolve 0.1 g in 50 ml of *water* with the aid of heat and allow to cool (solution A). To 1 ml add, without mixing, 3 ml of *water* and 0.1 ml of 0.05M *iodine*. A dark brownish-violet colour is produced at the interface of the two liquids. On mixing, the liquid becomes pale yellow.

B. Heat 5 ml of solution A with 0.5 ml of *hydrochloric acid* for 30 minutes in a water-bath and add 1 ml of a 6.1% w/v solution of *barium chloride*. A white turbidity is produced within 30 minutes.

C. Heat 0.5 g in 50 ml of *water* in a water-bath until a solution is obtained. Only a few fragments remain undissolved and on cooling the solution gels between 35° and 30°. When heated in a water-bath the gel does not liquefy below 80°.

Gelatin Heat 1.00 g in 100 ml of *water* until dissolved and allow to cool to 50°. To 5 ml of the solution add 5 ml of a 1% w/v solution of *2,4,6-trinitrophenol*. The solution does not become turbid within 10 minutes.

Insoluble matter Not more than 0.5% w/w when determined by the following method. To 5 g, in *No. 300 powder*, add 100 ml of *water* and 14 ml of 2M *hydrochloric acid* and boil gently for 15 minutes, stirring frequently. Filter while hot through a sintered-glass filter (BS porosity No. 1 is suitable), wash the residue with hot *water* and dry at 100° to 105°.

Loss on drying When dried at 100° to 105°, loses not more than 20.0% of its weight. Use 1 g, in *No. 300 powder*.

Sulphated ash Not more than 4.5%, Appendix IX A, Method II. Use 1 g, in *No. 300 powder*.

Swelling index Not less than 15, Appendix XI M. Use the substance in *No. 300 powder*.

Microbial contamination⋆ 1.0 g is free from *Escherichia coli*, Appendix XVI B1.

Storage Agar should be kept in a well-closed container.

Action and use Pharmaceutical aid.

⋆In certain states party to the Convention on the Elaboration of a European Pharmacopœia, Agar may be required to comply with a limit for a total viable aerobic count of 10^3 micro-organisms per gram, determined by plate count, Appendix XVI B2.

Powdered Agar

Powdered Agar is Agar in powder.

Characteristics Yellowish-white. Examined under a microscope shows angular fragments with features similar to those seen in the strips or flakes; some fragments are stained brownish-violet with 0.005M *iodine*.

Identification; Gelatin; Insoluble matter; Loss on drying; Sulphated ash; Swelling index Complies with the requirements stated under Agar.

Microbial contamination 1.0 g is free from *Escherichia coli*, Appendix XVI B1.

Storage Powdered Agar should be kept in a well-closed container.

Action and use Pharmaceutical aid.

Allopurinol

$C_5H_4N_4O$ 136.1   1315-30-0

Allopurinol is 1*H*-pyrazolo[3,4-*d*]pyrimidin-4-ol. It contains not less than 98.0 per cent and not more than 101.0 per cent of $C_5H_4N_4O$, calculated with reference to the dried substance.

Characteristics A white or almost white, microcrystalline powder; odourless or almost odourless.

Solubility Very slightly soluble in *water* and in *ethanol* (96%); practically insoluble in *chloroform* and in *ether*. It dissolves in aqueous solutions of alkali hydroxides.

Identification A. The *infra-red absorption spectrum*, Appendix II A, is concordant with the *reference spectrum* of allopurinol.

B. The *light absorption*, Appendix II B, in the range 230 to 350 nm of the solution used in the test for Light absorption exhibits a maximum only at 250 nm. The *absorbance* at 250 nm is about 1.1.

C. Dissolve 50 mg in 5 ml of 1.25M *sodium hydroxide*, add 1 ml of *alkaline potassium mercuri-iodide reagent*, heat to boiling and allow to stand. A flocculent yellow precipitate is produced.

Colour and clarity of solution A 1.0% w/v solution in a 10% w/v solution of *sodium hydroxide* is *clear*, Appendix IV A, and not more intensely coloured than *reference solution* Y_6 or GY_6, Appendix IV B, Method II.

Light absorption Dissolve 0.1 g in 10 ml of 0.1M *sodium hydroxide*, add sufficient 0.1M *hydrochloric acid* to produce 100 ml, dilute 10 ml to 100 ml with 0.1M *hydrochloric acid* and dilute 20 ml of this solution to 100 ml with 0.1M *hydrochloric acid*. The ratio of the *absorbance* of the resulting solution at the minimum at 231 nm to that at the maximum at 250 nm is 0.52 to 0.60, Appendix II B.

Related substances Carry out the method for *thin-layer chromatography*, Appendix III A, using *silica gel GF254* as the coating substance and a mixture of 60 volumes of *butan-2-one*, 20 volumes of *2-methoxyethanol* and 20 volumes of 13.5M *ammonia* as the mobile phase. Apply separately to the chromatoplate 10 μl of each of two solutions in 13.5M *ammonia* containing (1) 2.5% w/v of the substance being examined and (2) 0.0050% w/v of *5-aminopyrazole-4-carboxamide hemisulphate*. After removal of the plate, allow it to dry in a current of air and examine under *ultra-violet light (254 nm)*. Any *secondary spot* in the chromatogram obtained with solution (1) is not more intense than the spot in the chromatogram obtained with solution (2).

Loss on drying When dried to constant weight at 105°, loses not more than 0.5% of its weight. Use 1 g.

Sulphated ash Not more than 0.1%, Appendix IX A.

Assay Dissolve 0.2 g in 50 ml of *dimethylformamide* and carry out Method II for *non-aqueous titration*, Appendix VIII A, using 0.1M *sodium methoxide VS* as titrant and a 0.3% w/v solution of *thymol blue* in *methanol* as indicator. Each ml of 0.1M *sodium methoxide VS* is equivalent to 0.01361 g of $C_5H_4N_4O$.

Preparation
Allopurinol Tablets

Action and use Used in treatment of gout.

Almond Oil ☆

Almond Oil is the fixed oil obtained by cold expression from the ripe seeds of *Prunus dulcis* (Miller) D. A. Webb var. *dulcis* or *Prunus dulcis* (Miller) D. A. Webb var. *amara* (D. C.) Buchheim or a mixture of the two varieties.

Characteristics A pale yellow, clear, transparent oil; odour, slight and characteristic; taste, sweetish and characteristic. It solidifies at about $-18°$.

Solubility Slightly soluble in *ethanol (96%)*; miscible with *chloroform*, with *ether* and with *petroleum spirit (boiling range, 50° to 70°)*.

Identification Carry out the test for *identification of fixed oils by thin-layer chromatography*, Appendix X N. The chromatogram obtained from the oil being examined is concordant with the *typical chromatogram* for almond oil.

Acid value Not more than 1.5, Appendix X B. Use 5 g dissolved in 50 ml of the prescribed mixture of solvents.

Alkaline impurities Complies with the test for *alkaline impurities*, Appendix X N.

Peroxide value Not more than 12, Appendix X F.

Relative density 0.911 to 0.918, Appendix V G.

Unsaponifiable matter Not more than 0.7% w/w, Appendix X H, Method II. Use 5 g.

Apricot-kernel oil and peach-kernel oil Shake 2 ml for 5 minutes with a mixture of 1 ml of *fuming nitric acid* and 1 ml of *water* and allow to separate. No pink or brown colour is produced in either layer.

Foreign fixed oils Carry out the test for *foreign oils by gas chromatography*, Appendix X N. The fatty-acid fraction of the oil has the following composition.

Saturated fatty acids of chain length less than C_{16} Not more than 0.1%.
Palmitic acid 4.0 to 9.0%.
Stearic acid 0.9 to 2.0%.
Oleic acid 67.0 to 86.0%.
Linoleic acid (equivalent chain length on polyethylene glycol adipate 18.9) 7.0 to 25.0%.
Linolenic acid (equivalent chain length on polyethylene glycol adipate 19.7) Not more than 0.1%.
Arachidic acid Not more than 0.1%.
Gadoleic acid (equivalent chain length on polyethylene glycol adipate 20.3) Not more than 0.1%.
Behenic acid Not more than 0.1%.
Erucic acid (equivalent chain length on polyethylene glycol adipate 22.3) Not more than 0.1%.

Sesame oil Shake 10 ml with 5 ml of a mixture of 0.5 volume of a 0.35% v/v solution of *furfuraldehyde* in *acetic anhydride* and 4.5 volumes of *acetic anhydride* for 1 minute, filter through a filter paper impregnated with *acetic anhydride* and add 0.2 ml of *sulphuric acid*. No bluish-green colour is produced.

Storage Almond Oil should be kept in a well-filled, well-closed container and protected from light. Almond Oil intended for use in the manufacture of a parenteral dosage form should be kept in a glass container.

Labelling The label states if the contents of the container are suitable for use in the manufacture of a parenteral dosage form.

Almond Oil intended for use in the manufacture of a parenteral dosage form complies with the above requirements with the following modifications and with the additional test for Water.

Acid value Not more than 0.5, Appendix X B.

Peroxide value Not more than 5.0, Appendix X F.

Water Not more than 0.3%, Appendix IX C. Use 3 g.

Aloes ☆

Aloes consists of the residue obtained by evaporating the juice of the leaves of various species of *Aloe*.

BARBADOS ALOES
Curaçao Aloes

Barbados Aloes consists of the residue obtained by evaporating the juice of the leaves of *Aloe barbadensis* Miller. It contains not less than 28.0 per cent of hydroxyanthracene derivatives, calculated as anhydrous barbaloin.

Characteristics Dark brown masses, slightly shiny or opaque with a conchoidal fracture, or a brown powder; odour, strong and characteristic.

Solubility Soluble in hot *ethanol (96%)*; partly soluble in boiling *water*; practically insoluble in *chloroform* and in *ether*.

Identification A. Carry out the method for *thin-layer chromatography*, Appendix III A, using *silica gel G* as the coating substance and a mixture of 100 volumes of *ethyl acetate*, 17 volumes of *methanol* and 13 volumes of *water* as the mobile phase, but allowing the solvent front to ascend 10 cm above the line of application. Apply separately to the chromatoplate 5 μl of each of the following solutions, as bands 20 mm long and not more than 3 mm wide. For solution (1) heat to boiling in a water-bath 0.5 g, in powder, with 20 ml of *methanol*, shake for a few minutes, decant the supernatant liquid, maintain at 4° and use within 24 hours. For solution (2) dissolve 50 mg of *barbaloin* in 10 ml of *methanol*. After removal of the plate, allow it to dry in air, spray with a 10% w/v solution of *potassium hydroxide* in *methanol* and examine under *ultra-violet light (365 nm)*. The chromatogram obtained with solution (1) shows in the central part a band showing a yellow fluorescence corresponding to that due to barbaloin in the chromatogram obtained with solution (2) and in the lower part a band showing light blue fluorescence corresponding to aloesine. Heat the plate at 110° for 5 minutes. There may also be a band showing violet fluorescence just below the band corresponding to barbaloin.

B. Shake 1 g, in powder, with 100 ml of boiling *water*, cool, add 1 g of *purified talc* and filter. To 10 ml of the filtrate add 0.25 g of *sodium tetraborate*, heat to dissolve and pour 1 to 2 ml of the solution into 20 ml of *water*. A yellowish-green fluorescence is produced which is particularly marked under ultra-violet light (365 nm).

C. Add 5 ml of *bromine water* to 5 ml of the filtrate obtained in test A. A brownish-yellow precipitate is produced and the supernatant liquid is violet.

Loss on drying When dried at 100° to 105°, loses not more than 12.0% of its weight. Use 1 g.

Assay Moisten 0.3 g, in *No. 180 powder*, with 2 ml of *methanol*, add 5 ml of *water* previously warmed to about 60°, mix, add a further 75 ml of *water* at about 60° and shake for 30 minutes. Cool, filter, washing the flask with 20 ml of *water*, and add sufficient *water* to the combined filtrate and washings to produce 1000 ml. Transfer 10 ml of the solution to a flask containing 1 ml of a 60% w/v solution of *iron(III) chloride hexahydrate* and 6 ml of *hydrochloric acid* and heat under a reflux condenser in a water-bath for 4 hours, maintaining the water level above that of the liquid in the flask throughout. Cool and transfer the solution to a separating funnel, rinsing the flask successively with 4 ml of *water*, 4 ml of 1M *sodium hydroxide* and 4 ml of *water* and adding the rinsings to the contents of the separating funnel. Extract with three 20-ml quantities of *carbon tetrachloride* and wash the combined carbon tetrachloride layers with two 10-ml quantities of *water*, discarding the washings. Dilute the organic phase to 100 ml with *carbon tetrachloride*, evaporate 20 ml carefully to dryness on a water-bath and dissolve the residue in 10 ml of a 0.5% w/v solution of *magnesium acetate* in *methanol*. Measure the *absorbance* of the resulting solution at the maximum at 512 nm, Appendix II B, using *methanol* in the reference cell. Calculate the content of hydroxyanthracene derivatives, as anhydrous barbaloin, taking 240 as the value of A(1%, 1 cm) at the maximum at 512 nm.

Action and use Laxative.

CAPE ALOES

Cape Aloes consists of the residue obtained by evaporating the juice of the leaves of various species of *Aloe*, mainly *Aloe ferox* Miller and its hybrids. It contains not less than 18.0 per cent of hydroxyanthracene derivatives, calculated as anhydrous barbaloin.

Characteristics Dark brown masses, tinged with green, with a shiny conchoidal fracture, or a greenish-brown powder; odour, strong and characteristic.

Solubility Soluble in hot *ethanol (96%)*; partly soluble in boiling *water*; practically insoluble in *chloroform* and in *ether*.

Identification A. Carry out test A for Identification described under Barbados Aloes and examine under *ultra-violet light (365 nm)*. The chromatogram obtained with solution (1) shows a yellow band corresponding to that in the chromatogram obtained with solution (2) and in the lower part two yellow bands corresponding to aloinosides A and B as well as a blue fluorescent band corresponding to aloesine. Heat the chromatoplate at 110° for 5 minutes. No violet band appears in the chromatogram obtained with solution (1) just below the yellow band corresponding to barbaloin.

B. Complies with test B for Identification described under Barbados Aloes.

C. To 5 ml of the filtrate obtained in test A add 5 ml of *bromine water*. A yellow precipitate is produced but the supernatant solution is not coloured violet.

Loss on drying When dried at 100° to 105°, loses not more than 10.0% of its weight. Use 1 g.

Assay Carry out the method described under Barbados Aloes, using 0.4 g in *No. 180 powder*.

Action and use Laxative.

Powdered Aloes

Powdered Aloes is either Barbados Aloes in powder or Cape Aloes in powder. It complies with the appropriate requirements for content of anhydrous barbaloin, Identification and Loss on drying stated under Barbados Aloes or Cape Aloes and with the following requirements.

Characteristics Yellowish-brown to dark reddish-brown. When mounted in *lactophenol* and examined under a microscope, it is seen to consist of yellowish- to reddish-brown angular or irregular fragments, which are either amorphous or structureless (Cape Aloes) or composed of masses of small acicular crystals (Barbados Aloes); the powder ultimately dissolves in the mounting liquid.

Solubility in ethanol Almost entirely soluble in *ethanol (60%)*.

Ash Not more than 4.0%, Appendix XI J.

Action and use Laxative.

Labelling The label states whether the Powdered Aloes is made from Barbados Aloes or from Cape Aloes.

Aloin

$C_{21}H_{22}O_9$ 418.4   *5133-19-7*

Aloin is a crystalline substance extracted from Barbados Aloes or, more rarely, Cape Aloes. It contains not less than 70 per cent of anhydrous barbaloin (10-β-D-glucopyranosyl-1,8-dihydroxy-3-hydroxymethylanthracen-9-one), a 10-glucopyranosyl derivative of aloe-emodin-anthrone, calculated with reference to the dried substance.

Characteristics A yellow, crystalline powder; odourless or almost odourless.

Solubility Almost completely soluble in 130 parts of *water*; soluble in *ethanol (96%)* and in *acetone*; very slightly soluble in *chloroform* and in *ether*.

Identification A. Carry out the method for *thin-layer chromatography*, Appendix III A, using *silica gel G* as the coating substance and a mixture of 100 volumes of *ethyl acetate*, 17 volumes of *methanol* and 13 volumes of *water* as the mobile phase, but allowing the solvent front to ascend 10 cm above the line of application. Apply separately to the chromatoplate 5 µl of each of the following solutions, as bands 15 mm long and not more than 5 mm wide. For solution (1) heat 0.5 g to boiling in a water-bath with 20 ml of *methanol*, shake for a few minutes, decant the supernatant liquid, maintain at about 4° and use within 24 hours. For solution (2) dissolve 50 mg of *barbaloin* in 10 ml of *methanol*. After removal of the plate, allow it to dry in air, spray with a 10% w/v solution of *potassium hydroxide* in *methanol* and examine under *ultra-violet light (365 nm)*. The chromatogram obtained with solution (2) shows a yellow band with an Rf value of 0.4 to 0.5. The chromatogram obtained with solution (1) shows a yellow band corresponding to that in the chromatogram obtained with solution (2).

B. Heat 10 ml of a 0.2% w/v solution with 0.1 g of *sodium tetraborate* in a water-bath for 5 minutes. Pour 1 to 2 ml of the resulting solution into 20 ml of *water*. A yellowish-green fluorescence is produced which is particularly marked under ultra-violet light (365 nm).

C. Add 1 ml of *bromine water* to 5 ml of a 0.2% w/v solution. A copious yellow precipitate is produced.

Acidity pH of a 1% w/v suspension, 4.0 to 6.5, Appendix V L.

Light absorption The *light absorption*, Appendix II B, in the range 250 to 370 nm of a freshly prepared 0.0025% w/v solution exhibits maxima at 266, 298 and 354 nm (distinction from amorphous aloin).

Water-insoluble matter Not more than 1.5% when determined by the following method. To 1 g add 120 ml of *water*, shake frequently for 2 hours, maintaining the temperature at 25°, and filter through a sintered-glass filter (BS porosity No. 2). Wash the residue with 25 ml of *water* and dry to constant weight at 70° at a pressure of 2 kPa for 3 hours.

Loss on drying When dried at 70° at a pressure of 2 kPa for 3 hours, loses not more than 5.0% of its weight. Use 1 g.

Ash Not more than 0.5%, Appendix XI J.

Assay Carry out the following procedure protected from light. Dissolve 0.15 g in *water*, with gentle warming if necessary, and add sufficient *water* to produce 100 ml. Dilute 10 ml to 100 ml with *water*. Transfer 10 ml of the resulting solution to a 100-ml round-bottomed flask containing 1 ml of a 60% w/v solution of *iron(III) chloride hexahydrate* and 6 ml of *hydrochloric acid* and heat under a reflux condenser in a water-bath for 4 hours, maintaining the water level above that of the liquid in the flask throughout. Cool and transfer the solution to a separating funnel, rinsing the flask successively with 4 ml of *water*, 4 ml of 1M *sodium hydroxide* and 4 ml of *water* and adding the rinsings to the contents of the separating funnel. Extract with three 20-ml quantities of *carbon tetrachloride* and wash the combined carbon tetrachloride layers with two 10-ml quantities of *water*, discarding the washings. Evaporate the organic phase carefully to dryness on a water-bath, dissolve the residue in a 0.5% w/v solution of *magnesium acetate* in *methanol* and dilute to 50 ml with the same solvent. Measure the *absorbance* of the resulting solution at the maximum at 512 nm, Appendix II B. Calculate the content of anhydrous barbaloin taking 265 as the value of A(1%, 1 cm) at the maximum at 512 nm. The

result of the assay is not valid unless the ratio of the *absorbance* at 512 nm to that at 440 nm is not less than 2.8.

Action and use Stimulant laxative.

Aloxiprin

9014-67-9

Aloxiprin is a polymeric condensation product of aluminium oxide and *O*-acetylsalicylic acid. It contains not less than 7.5 per cent and not more than 8.5 per cent of aluminium, Al, and not less than 79.0 per cent and not more than 87.4 per cent of total salicylates, calculated as *O*-acetylsalicylic acid, $C_9H_8O_4$, both calculated with reference to the dried substance.

Characteristics A fine, white or slightly pink powder; odourless or almost odourless.

Solubility Practically insoluble in *water*, in *ethanol (96%)* and in *ether*; slightly soluble in *chloroform*.

Identification A. Boil 1 g with 20 ml of 2M *hydrochloric acid*, cool, filter and reserve the residue. The filtrate yields the *reactions* characteristic of aluminium, Appendix VI.

B. Dissolve the residue reserved in test A in 10 ml of 0.1M *sodium hydroxide* and neutralise with 1M *acetic acid*. 1 ml of the resulting solution yields *reaction A* characteristic of salicylates, Appendix VI.

Combined salicylate Not more than 9.5%, calculated as salicylic acid, $C_7H_6O_3$, with reference to the content of *O*-acetylsalicylic acid when determined in the following manner. To 0.1 g add 40 ml of a 0.5% w/v solution of *sodium fluoride* in 0.1M *hydrochloric acid* and shake for 5 minutes. Allow the solution to stand for 10 minutes, shaking at frequent intervals. Extract with six 20-ml quantities of *chloroform*, filter the combined extracts through a layer of *anhydrous sodium sulphate*, wash with 30 ml of *chloroform* and dilute the combined filtrate and washings to 200 ml with *chloroform*. Dilute 20 ml of the solution to 50 ml with *chloroform* and measure the *absorbance* of the resulting solution at the maximum at 308 nm, Appendix II B. Calculate the content of $C_7H_6O_3$ taking 293 as the value of A(1%, 1 cm) at the maximum at 308 nm.

Free acetylsalicylic acid To a quantity containing the equivalent of 1.0 g of total salicylates add 50 ml of dry *ether* and shake for 30 minutes. Filter quickly through fluted filter paper, wash the paper with several portions of dry *ether* and dilute the combined filtrate and washings to 100 ml with dry *ether*. The *absorbance* of the solution at the maximum at 278 nm is not more than 0.36, Appendix II B (0.5%, calculated with reference to the content of total salicylates).

Salicylic acid The *absorbance* of the solution used in the test for Free acetylsalicylic acid at the maximum at 308 nm is not more than 0.50, Appendix II B (0.15%, calculated with reference to the content of total salicylates).

Heavy metals Carefully ignite 2.0 g at a low temperature until completely charred, cool, add 2 ml of *nitric acid* and 0.25 ml of *sulphuric acid*, heat cautiously until white fumes are evolved and ignite at 500° to 600°. Cool, add 2 ml of *hydrochloric acid*, evaporate to dryness on a water-bath and carry out the procedure for *limit test C for heavy metals*, Appendix VII, beginning at the words 'Dissolve the residue . . .' (10 ppm). Use 2 ml of *lead standard solution (10 ppm Pb)* to prepare the standard.

Loss on drying When dried to constant weight over *phosphorus pentoxide* at a pressure not exceeding 0.7 kPa, loses not more than 2.0% of its weight. Use 1 g.

Assay *For aluminium* Ignite 2 g in a tared silica crucible, heat gently until the organic matter is destroyed and then ignite to constant weight at 1000°. Each g of residue is equivalent to 0.5292 g of Al.

For total salicylates To 0.25 g add 50 ml of 1M *sodium hydroxide* and boil gently until dissolved. Cool, add 50 ml of *water*, adjust the pH to between 2.40 and 2.50 with 1M *hydrochloric acid* and dilute to 500 ml with *water*. To 5 ml add 4 ml of *iron(III) chloride solution*, allow to stand for 30 minutes, dilute to 50 ml with *water* and measure the *absorbance* of the resulting solution at the maximum at 530 nm, Appendix II B, using in the reference cell a solution prepared by diluting 4 ml of *iron(III) chloride solution* to 50 ml with *water*. Calculate the content of total salicylates as $C_9H_8O_4$ from the *absorbance* obtained by repeating the procedure using 4 ml of a 0.05% w/v solution of *salicylic acid* in place of the solution being examined and beginning at the words 'add 4 ml of *iron(III) chloride solution . . .*'. Each g of salicylic acid is equivalent to 1.305 g of $C_9H_8O_4$.

Storage Aloxiprin should be kept in a well-closed container.

Preparation
Aloxiprin Tablets

Action and use Analgesic; anti-inflammatory.

Alum ☆
Potash Alum; Aluminium Potassium Sulphate

$KAl(SO_4)_2,12H_2O$ 474.4   7784-24-9

Alum contains not less than 99.0 per cent and not more than 100.5 per cent of $KAl(SO_4)_2,12H_2O$.

Characteristics Colourless, transparent crystalline masses or a granular powder; odourless.

Solubility Soluble in 7.5 parts of *water*, in 0.3 part of boiling *water* and in 3 parts of *glycerol*; practically insoluble in *ethanol (96%)*.

Identification A. A 5.0% w/v solution (solution A) yields *reaction A* characteristic of aluminium salts and the *reactions* characteristic of sulphates, Appendix VI.
B. Shake 10 ml of solution A with 0.5 g of *sodium hydrogen carbonate* and filter. The filtrate yields *reaction A* characteristic of potassium salts, Appendix VI.

Clarity and colour of solution Solution A is *clear*, Appendix IV A, and *colourless*, Appendix IV B, Method II.

Acidity pH of a 10% w/v solution, 3.0 to 3.5, Appendix V L.

Ammonium To 1 ml of solution A add 4 ml of *water*. 0.5 ml of the resulting solution, diluted to 14 ml with *water*, complies with the *limit test for ammonium*, Appendix VII (0.2%).

Heavy metals 12 ml of solution A complies with *limit test A for heavy metals*, Appendix VII (20 ppm). Use *lead standard solution (1 ppm Pb)* to prepare the standard.

Iron 2 ml of solution A diluted to 10 ml with *water* complies with the *limit test for iron*, Appendix VII (100 ppm) but using 0.3 ml in place of 0.1 ml of *mercaptoacetic acid*.

Assay Carry out the *complexometric titration of aluminium*, Appendix VIII D, using 0.9 g dissolved in 20 ml of *water*. Each ml of 0.1M *disodium edetate VS* is equivalent to 0.04744 g of $KAl(SO_4)_2,12H_2O$.

Storage Alum should be kept in a well-closed container.

Action and use Astringent.

Aluminium Glycinate

$H_2NCH_2 \cdot CO_2Al(OH)_2, xH_2O$

$C_2H_6AlNO_4$ 135.1   41354-48-7

Aluminium Glycinate is a basic aluminium monoglycinate, partly hydrated. It contains not less than 34.5 per cent and not more than 38.5 per cent of Al_2O_3 and not less than 9.9 per cent and not more than 10.8 per cent of N, both calculated with reference to the dried substance.

Characteristics A white or almost white powder; odourless or almost odourless.

Solubility Practically insoluble in *water* and in organic solvents. It dissolves in dilute mineral acids and in aqueous solutions of the alkali hydroxides.

Identification A. Add 0.1 g to 10 ml of a solution prepared by dissolving 0.84 g of *citric acid* in 8 ml of 1M *sodium hydroxide* and diluting to 20 ml with *water*. Add 0.5 ml of a 0.1% w/v solution of *ninhydrin* in *methanol* and warm. A purple colour is produced.
B. Suspend 1 g in 25 ml of 0.5M *hydrochloric acid* and heat gently until a clear solution is produced. Reserve half of the solution. To 2 ml of the solution add 0.15 ml of *liquefied phenol*, shake and add carefully without shaking 5 ml of *dilute sodium hypochlorite solution*. A blue colour is produced.
C. The solution reserved in test B yields the *reactions* characteristic of aluminium salts, Appendix VI.

Acidity or alkalinity pH of a suspension of 1 g in 25 ml of *carbon dioxide-free water*, 6.5 to 7.5, Appendix V L.

Arsenic Dissolve 2.0 g in 18 ml of *brominated hydrochloric acid* and 32 ml of *water*. 25 ml of the resulting solution complies with the *limit test for arsenic*, Appendix VII (1 ppm).

Heavy metals Dissolve 1.5 g in 20 ml of 2M *hydrochloric acid* and 10 ml of *water*, add 0.5 ml of *nitric acid* and boil for about 30 seconds. Cool, add 2 g of *ammonium chloride* and 2 g of *ammonium thiocyanate* and extract with two 10-ml quantities of a mixture of equal parts of *amyl alcohol* and *ether*. To the aqueous layer add 2 g of *citric acid*. 12 ml of the resulting solution complies with *limit test A for heavy metals*, Appendix VII (20 ppm). Use *lead standard solution (1 ppm Pb)* to prepare the standard.

Mercuric salts Dissolve 2.0 g in 10 ml of 1M *sulphuric acid*, transfer to a separating funnel with the aid of *water*, dilute to about 50 ml with *water* and add 50 ml of 0.5M *sulphuric acid*. Add 100 ml of *water*, 2 g of *hydroxylamine hydrochloride*, 1 ml of 0.05M *disodium edetate* and 1 ml of *glacial acetic acid*. Add 5 ml of *chloroform*, shake, allow to separate and discard the chloroform layer. Titrate the aqueous layer with a 0.0008% w/v solution of *dithizone* in *chloroform* until the chloroform layer remains green. After each addition, shake vigorously, allow the layers to separate and discard the chloroform layer. Repeat the operation using a solution prepared by diluting 1 ml of *mercury standard solution (5 ppm Hg)* to 100 ml with 0.5M *sulphuric acid* and beginning at the words 'Add 100 ml of *water . . .*'. The volume of the dithizone solution required by the substance being examined does not exceed that required by the mercury standard solution.

Chloride Dissolve 1.0 g in 10 ml of 2M *nitric acid* and dilute to 100 ml with *water*. 15 ml of the resulting solution complies with the *limit test for chlorides*, Appendix VII (330 ppm).

Neutralising capacity. Shake 0.2 g vigorously with 25 ml of 0.1M *hydrochloric acid* for 5 minutes and allow to stand for 5 minutes. The pH of the mixture is not more than 3.0, Appendix V L.

Loss on drying When dried to constant weight at 130°, loses not more than 12.0% of its weight. Use 1 g.

Assay *For Al$_2$O$_3$* Carry out Method II for the *complexometric titration of aluminium*, Appendix VIII D, but using 0.25 g dissolved in a mixture of 3 ml of 1M *hydrochloric acid* and 50 ml of *water*. Each ml of 0.05M *disodium edetate VS* is equivalent to 0.002549 g of Al$_2$O$_3$.

For N Carry out Method I for the *determination of nitrogen*, Appendix VIII H, using 0.4 g and 10 ml of *nitrogen-free sulphuric acid*. Each ml of 0.05M *sulphuric acid VS* is equivalent to 0.001401 g of N.

Storage Aluminium Glycinate should be kept in a well-closed container.

Action and use Antacid.

Dried Aluminium Hydroxide ☆

Dried Aluminium Hydroxide Gel

Dried Aluminium Hydroxide contains the equivalent of not less than 47.0 per cent and not more than 60.0 per cent of Al$_2$O$_3$.

Characteristics A white, amorphous powder; odourless.

Solubility Practically insoluble in *water*. It dissolves in dilute mineral acids and in aqueous solutions of alkali hydroxides.

Identification Dissolve 1.25 g in 7.5 ml of *hydrochloric acid* by heating on a water-bath and dilute to 50 ml with *distilled water* (solution A). The solution yields *reaction A* characteristic of aluminium salts, Appendix VI.

Clarity and colour of solution Solution A is not more opalescent than *reference suspension II*, Appendix IV A, and not more intensely coloured than *reference solution GY$_6$*, Appendix IV B, Method II.

Alkalinity Shake 1.0 g with 20 ml of *carbon dioxide-free water* for 1 minute and filter. To 10 ml add 0.1 ml of *phenolphthalein solution*. Any pink colour disappears on the addition of 0.3 ml of 0.1M *hydrochloric acid VS*.

Neutralising capacity Disperse 0.5 g in 100 ml of *water*, heat to 37°, add 100 ml of 0.1M *hydrochloric acid VS* previously heated to 37° and stir continuously, maintaining the temperature at 37°. The pH of the solution at 37° after 10, 15 and 20 minutes is not less than 1.8, 2.3 and 3.0 respectively and at no time is greater than 4.5. Add 10 ml of 0.5M *hydrochloric acid VS* previously heated to 37°, stir continuously for 1 hour maintaining the temperature at 37° and titrate with 0.1M *sodium hydroxide VS* to pH 3.5. Not more than 35.0 ml of 0.1M *sodium hydroxide VS* is required.

Arsenic 10 ml of solution A complies with the *limit test for arsenic*, Appendix VII (4 ppm).

Chloride Dissolve 0.10 g with heating in 10 ml of 2M *nitric acid* and dilute to 100 ml with *water*. 5 ml of the solution diluted to 15 ml with *water* complies with the *limit test for chlorides*, Appendix VII (1%).

Sulphate Dilute 4 ml of solution A to 100 ml with *distilled water*. 15 ml of the solution complies with the *limit test for sulphates*, Appendix VII (1%).

Heavy metals Neutralise 10 ml of solution A with 13.5M *ammonia* using a 0.1% w/v solution of *metanil yellow* in *methanol* as an external indicator. Filter if necessary and dilute to 15 ml with *water*. 12 ml of the solution complies with *limit test A for heavy metals*, Appendix VII (60 ppm). Use 10 ml of *lead standard solution (1 ppm Pb)* to prepare the standard.

Microbial contamination★ 1.0 g is free from *Escherichia coli*, Appendix XVI B1.

Assay Dissolve 0.8 g in 10 ml of 7M *hydrochloric acid* by heating on a water-bath, cool and dilute to 50 ml with *water*. To 10 ml of the solution add 6M *ammonia* until a precipitate begins to appear. Add the minimum quantity of 2M *hydrochloric acid* needed to dissolve the precipitate, dilute to 20 ml with *water* and carry out the *complexometric titration of aluminium*, Appendix VIII D. Each ml of 0.1M *disodium edetate VS* is equivalent to 0.005098 g of Al$_2$O$_3$.

Storage Dried Aluminium Hydroxide Gel should be kept in an airtight container and stored at a temperature not exceeding 30°.

Preparation

Aluminium Hydroxide Tablets

Action and use Antacid.

The title of the monograph in the European Pharmacopœia is Hydrated Aluminium Oxide.

★In certain states party to the Convention on the Elaboration of a European Pharmacopœia, Dried Aluminium Hydroxide Gel may be required to comply either with the test for Enterobacteriaceae and certain other Gram-negative bacteria (1 g), Appendix XVI B1, or with a limit for total viable aerobic count of 10^3 micro-organisms per gram, determined by plate count, Appendix XVI B2, or with both of these tests.

Aluminium Magnesium Silicate

12511-31-8

Aluminium Magnesium Silicate is a native colloidal hydrated aluminium magnesium silicate (saponite) freed from gritty particles.

Characteristics Small creamy-white flakes or a creamy-white powder; odourless or almost odourless. The pH of a

4% dispersion in *water* is about 9 and the viscosity of a 5% dispersion in *water* is about 25 Pa s.

Microscopical A powder or flakes varying in shape and size from about 0.3 × 0.4 mm to 1.0 × 2.0 mm and about 25 to 240 μm thick; many of the flakes are perforated by scattered circular holes about 20 to 120 μm in diameter. Between crossed polars on a dark field innumerable bright specks are observed scattered over the flakes.

Solubility Practically insoluble in *water* but swells to produce a colloidal dispersion; practically insoluble in organic solvents.

Identification A. Fuse 1 g with 2 g of *anhydrous sodium carbonate*, warm the residue with *water*, filter, acidify the filtrate with *hydrochloric acid* and evaporate to dryness on a water-bath. 0.25 g of the residue yields the *reaction* characteristic of silicates, Appendix VI.

B. Dissolve the residue obtained in test A in 5 ml of 2M *hydrochloric acid* and 10 ml of *water*, filter and add *ammonia buffer pH 10.0* to the filtrate; a white, gelatinous precipitate is produced. Centrifuge; the precipitate, when dissolved in 2M *hydrochloric acid*, yields the *reactions* characteristic of aluminium salts, Appendix VI.

C. The supernatant liquid obtained after centrifugation in test B yields the *reactions* characteristic of magnesium salts, Appendix VI.

Alkalinity Disperse 1 g in 50 ml of *carbon dioxide-free water* and titrate with 0.1M *hydrochloric acid VS*. Not more than 10 ml of 0.1M *hydrochloric acid VS* is required to reduce the pH of the suspension to 4.0, Appendix V L.

Loss on drying When dried to constant weight at 105°, loses not more than 10.0% of its weight. Use 1 g.

Loss on ignition When ignited to constant weight at about 800°, loses not more than 17.0% of its weight. Use 1 g.

Action and use Pharmaceutical aid.

Dried Aluminium Phosphate

Dried Aluminium Phosphate Gel

Dried Aluminium Phosphate may be prepared by drying under suitable conditions the product of interaction in aqueous solution of an aluminium salt with an alkali phosphate such as sodium phosphate; it consists mainly of hydrated aluminium orthophosphate. It contains not less than 80.0 per cent of AlPO$_4$.

Characteristics A white powder containing some friable aggregates.

Solubility Practically insoluble in *water* and in *ethanol* (96%); soluble in dilute mineral acids; practically insoluble in solutions of the alkali hydroxides.

Identification A. A solution in 2M *hydrochloric acid* yields the *reactions* characteristic of aluminium salts, Appendix VI.

B. A solution in 2M *nitric acid* yields the *reactions* characteristic of phosphates, Appendix VI.

Alkalinity pH of a 4% w/v suspension in *carbon dioxide-free water*, 5.5 to 6.5, Appendix V L.

Arsenic Dissolve 0.40 g in 18 ml of *brominated hydrochloric acid* and dilute to 50 ml with *water*. 25 ml of the resulting solution complies with the *limit test for arsenic*, Appendix VII (5 ppm).

Heavy metals Dissolve 1.2 g in 20 ml of 1M *hydrochloric acid* and 10 ml of *water*, add 0.5 ml of *nitric acid* and boil for about 30 seconds. Cool, add 2 g of *ammonium chloride* and 2 g of *ammonium thiocyanate* and extract with two 10-ml quantities of a mixture of equal parts of *amyl alcohol* and *ether*. To the aqueous layer add 2 g of *citric acid* and dilute to 40 ml with *water*. 12 ml of the resulting solution complies with *limit test A for heavy metals*, Appendix VII (70 ppm). Use *lead standard solution (2 ppm Pb)* to prepare the standard.

Chloride Dissolve 0.24 g in 10 ml of 2M *nitric acid*, boil, cool, dilute to 1000 ml with *water* and filter. 15 ml of the filtrate complies with the *limit test for chlorides*, Appendix VII (1.4%).

Sulphate Dissolve 0.17 g in 10 ml of 2M *hydrochloric acid*, boil, cool, dilute to 100 ml with *water* and filter. 15 ml of the filtrate, with the addition of 2 ml of 2M *hydrochloric acid*, complies with the *limit test for sulphates*, Appendix VII (0.6%).

Neutralising capacity Pass a sufficient quantity, triturated if necessary, through a sieve of nominal mesh aperture 75 μm, add 0.5 g to 30 ml of 0.1M *hydrochloric acid* previously heated to 37° and maintain at 37° for 30 minutes, stirring continuously. The pH of the mixture at 37° is 2.0 to 2.5, Appendix V L.

Soluble phosphate Not more than 1.0% w/w, calculated as PO$_4$, when determined by the following method. Shake 5.0 g with 150 ml of *water* for 2 hours, filter until the filtrate is clear and wash the filter with 50 ml of *water*. Add to the combined filtrate and washings sufficient *water* to produce 250 ml, mix well and dilute 10 ml to 100 ml with *water*. To 5 ml of the resulting solution add 4 ml of 1M *sulphuric acid*, 1 ml of *ammonium molybdate solution*, 2 ml of *methylaminophenol—sulphite reagent* and 5 ml of *water*. Mix well, allow to stand for 15 minutes and add sufficient *water* to produce 25 ml. Allow to stand for a further 15 minutes and measure the *absorbance* of a 2-cm layer of the resulting solution at 730 nm, Appendix II B. Calculate the content of soluble phosphate from a calibration curve prepared by treating suitable aliquots of a 0.00286% w/v solution of *potassium dihydrogen orthophosphate* in the same manner, beginning at the words 'add 4 ml of 1M *sulphuric acid . . .*'. A 0.00286% w/v solution of *potassium dihydrogen orthophosphate* is equivalent to 0.00100% w/v of PO$_4$.

Assay Dissolve 0.8 g in 15 ml of 2M *hydrochloric acid*, warming if necessary to effect solution, cool and add sufficient 2M *hydrochloric acid* to produce 100 ml. To 10 ml add 25 ml of 0.05M *disodium edetate VS* then add 13.5M *ammonia* dropwise until the solution is just alkaline to *litmus paper*. Boil gently for 5 minutes, cool and add 10 ml of a solution prepared by dissolving 7.7 g of *ammonium acetate* in 50 ml of *water* and adding 6 ml of *glacial acetic acid* and sufficient *water* to produce 100 ml. Adjust the pH to 4.5 with *glacial acetic acid* and add 2 ml of a 0.025% w/v solution of *dithizone* in *ethanol* (96%). Add sufficient *ethanol* (96%) to double the volume of the solution and titrate with 0.05M *zinc chloride VS* until the colour changes to red. Repeat the operation without the substance being examined. The difference between the titrations represents the amount of disodium edetate required. Each ml of 0.05M *disodium edetate VS* is equivalent to 0.006098 g of AlPO$_4$.

Microbial contamination 1 g is free from pseudomonads, Appendix XVI B1.

Storage Dried Aluminium Phosphate should be kept in a well-closed container and stored at a temperature not exceeding 30°.

Preparation
Aluminium Phosphate Tablets

Action and use Antacid.

Aluminium Powder

Al   26.98   *7429-90-5*

Aluminium Powder consists mainly of metallic aluminium in the form of very small flakes, usually with an appreciable proportion of aluminium oxide; it is lubricated with stearic acid to prevent oxidation. It contains not less than 86.0 per cent of Al, calculated with reference to the substance freed from lubricant and volatile matter.

Characteristics A silvery-grey powder; odourless or almost odourless.

Solubility Practically insoluble in *water* and in *ethanol* (96%). It dissolves in dilute acids and in aqueous solutions of alkali hydroxides, with the evolution of hydrogen.

Identification A solution in 2M *hydrochloric acid* yields the *reactions* characteristic of aluminium salts, Appendix VI.

Iron Dissolve 10 mg in 20 ml of 2M *hydrochloric acid* and dilute to 100 ml with *water*. 10 ml of the resulting solution complies with the *limit test for iron*, Appendix VII (1.0%).

Lead Use two solutions prepared as follows. For solution (1) boil 0.40 g with 20 ml of 2M *hydrochloric acid* and 10 ml of *water* until effervescence ceases, add 0.5 ml of *nitric acid*, boil for 30 seconds and cool; add 2 g of *ammonium chloride* and 2 g of *ammonium thiocyanate*, extract with three 10-ml quantities of a mixture of equal volumes of *amyl alcohol* and *ether*, discard the extracts and add 2 g of *citric acid*. For solution (2) dissolve 2 g of *citric acid* in 10 ml of 2M *hydrochloric acid* and add 4 ml of *lead standard solution (10 ppm Pb)*. Make solutions (1) and (2) alkaline with 5M *ammonia* and to each add 1 ml of *potassium cyanide solution PbT*. The solutions should be not more than faintly opalescent. If the colours of the solutions differ, equalise by the addition of about 0.2 ml of a highly diluted solution of burnt sugar or other non-reactive substance. Dilute each solution to 50 ml with *water*, add 0.1 ml of a 10% w/v solution of *sodium sulphide* to each and mix thoroughly. The colour produced in solution (1) is not more intense than that produced in solution (2), when viewed against a white background (100 ppm).

Other metals Dissolve 2 g in 40 ml of 2M *hydrochloric acid*. Dilute 20 ml of the solution to 100 ml with *water*, make alkaline to *litmus paper* by the addition of 5M *ammonia*, boil and filter. Evaporate the filtrate to dryness, add 0.05 ml of *sulphuric acid* and ignite. The residue weighs not more than 2 mg.

Lubricant To 2 g add 100 ml of hot *water*, cover and add, dropwise, sufficient of a mixture of equal volumes of *hydrochloric acid* and *water* to dissolve the metal almost completely. Heat to complete dissolution, cool, filter through a hardened filter paper and wash the vessel and filter paper thoroughly with *water*; dry both the vessel and paper at room temperature. Extract the paper with three 100-ml quantities of boiling, freshly distilled *acetone*, using the original vessel to contain the solvent and then wash the paper with five 10-ml quantities of freshly distilled *acetone*. Evaporate the combined filtrate and washings to dryness using a rotary evaporator. The residue, after drying at 105° for 30 minutes and allowing to cool, weighs 10 to 60 mg.

When the basin containing the residue is floated in a beaker of water suitably stirred and heated, the residue melts between 40° and 60°. The residue is almost completely soluble, with effervescence, in hot *sodium carbonate solution*.

Volatile matter When heated to constant weight at 105°, loses not more than 0.5% of its weight. Use 1 g.

Surface-covering power Not less than 4000 cm^2 per g when determined by the following method. Fill with *water* a shallow trough measuring approximately 60 cm × 12 cm × 1.5 cm, fitted with a movable partition so constructed that it is a sliding fit and can be used to divide the trough into two rectangular areas. Place the movable partition near one end and sprinkle 50 mg of the substance being examined on the surface of the liquid confined in the smaller area. Using a glass rod, spread the powder evenly over the liquid surface until an unbroken film covers the entire surface. Move the partition so as to increase the area confined and again spread the powder to cover the increased surface. Continue this process and determine the maximum unbroken surface area obtained. The surface-covering power is the area covered per g of the powder at the breaking point of the film.

Assay Transfer 0.2 g, previously freed from lubricant by successive washing with *acetone* and drying, to a three-necked 500-ml flask fitted with a 150-ml dropping funnel, an inlet tube connected to a cylinder of *carbon dioxide* and an outlet tube dipping into a water-trap. Add 60 ml of *water* and disperse the substance being examined; replace the air by *carbon dioxide* and add 100 ml of a solution containing 56 g of *ammonium iron(III) sulphate* and 7.5 ml of *sulphuric acid* in *water*. While maintaining an atmosphere of *carbon dioxide* in the flask, heat to boiling, boil for 5 minutes after the sample has dissolved, cool rapidly to 20° and dilute to 250 ml with *water*. To 50 ml add 15 ml of *orthophosphoric acid* and titrate with 0.02M *potassium permanganate VS*. Each ml of 0.02M *potassium permanganate VS* is equivalent to 0.0008994 g of Al.

Storage Aluminium Powder should be kept in a well-closed container.

Preparation
Compound Aluminium Paste

Action and use Topical protective.

Aluminium Sulphate ☆

Al$_2$(SO$_4$)$_3$+aq   342.1 (*anhydrous*)   *17927-65-0*

Aluminium Sulphate contains not less than 51.0 per cent and not more than 59.0 per cent of Al$_2$(SO$_4$)$_3$. It contains a variable quantity of water of crystallisation.

Characteristics Colourless, lustrous crystals or crystalline masses; odourless.

Solubility Soluble in *water*; freely soluble in hot *water*; practically insoluble in *ethanol (96%)*.

Identification A 5.0% w/v solution (solution A) yields *reaction A* characteristic of aluminium salts and the *reactions* characteristic of sulphates, Appendix VI.

Acidity pH of a 2% w/v solution, 2.5 to 4.0, Appendix V L.

Clarity and colour of solution Solution A is not more opalescent than *reference suspension III*, Appendix IV A, and is *colourless*, Appendix IV B, Method II.

Ammonium 0.4 ml of solution A diluted to 14 ml with *water* complies with the *limit test for ammonium*, Appendix VII (0.05%).

Heavy metals Dilute 6 ml of solution A to 15 ml with *water*. 12 ml of the resulting solution complies with *limit test A for heavy metals*, Appendix VII (50 ppm). Use *lead standard solution (1 ppm Pb)* to prepare the standard.

Iron 2 ml of solution A diluted to 10 ml with *water* complies with the *limit test for iron*, Appendix VII (100 ppm) but using 0.3 ml in place of 0.1 ml of *mercaptoacetic acid*.

Alkalis and alkaline-earth metals To 20 ml of solution A add 100 ml of *water*, heat and add 0.1 ml of *methyl red solution*. Add 6M *ammonia* until the colour changes to yellow, dilute to 150 ml with *water*, heat to boiling and filter. Evaporate 75 ml of the filtrate to dryness on a water-bath and ignite. The weight of the residue does not exceed 2 mg.

Assay Carry out the *complexometric titration of aluminium*, Appendix VIII D, using 0.5 g dissolved in 20 ml of *water*. Each ml of 0.1M *disodium edetate VS* is equivalent to 0.01711 g of $Al_2(SO_4)_3$.

Storage Aluminium Sulphate should be kept in an airtight container.

Amantadine Hydrochloride ☆

$C_{10}H_{17}N,HCl$ 187.7   665-67-7

Amantadine Hydrochloride is tricyclo[3.3.1.1³,⁷]-dec-1-ylamine hydrochloride. It contains not less than 98.5 per cent and not more than 101.0 per cent of $C_{10}H_{17}N,HCl$, calculated with reference to the anhydrous substance.

Characteristics A white or almost white crystalline powder. It sublimes when heated.

Solubility Freely soluble in *water* and in *ethanol (96%)*; soluble in *chloroform*; practically insoluble in *ether*.

Identification *Test A may be omitted if tests B, C and D are carried out. Tests B and C may be omitted if tests A and D are carried out.*

A. The *infra-red absorption spectrum*, Appendix II A, is concordant with the spectrum of *amantadine hydrochloride EPCRS*.

B. Dissolve 0.2 g in 1 ml of 0.1M *hydrochloric acid* and add 1 ml of a 50% w/v solution of *sodium nitrite*. A white precipitate is produced.

C. To 0.1 g add 1 ml of *pyridine* and 0.1 ml of *acetic anhydride* and boil for 10 seconds. Pour the hot solution into 10 ml of *hydrochloric acid*, cool to 5° and filter. The *melting point* of the residue, after washing with *water* and drying over *phosphorus pentoxide* at 60° at a pressure of 1.5 to 2.5 kPa for 1 hour, is 147° to 151°, Appendix V A, Method I.

D. 1 ml of a 10% w/v solution in *carbon dioxide-free water* yields *reaction A* characteristic of chlorides, Appendix VI.

Acidity or alkalinity To 10 ml of a 2% w/v solution in *carbon dioxide-free water* add 0.2 ml of 0.01M *sodium hydroxide VS* and 0.1 ml of *methyl red solution*; the solution is yellow. Add 0.4 ml of 0.01M *hydrochloric acid VS*; the solution is red.

Clarity and colour of solution A 10.0% w/v solution in *carbon dioxide-free water* is *clear*, Appendix IV A, and not more intensely coloured than *reference solution Y₇*, Appendix IV B, Method II.

Heavy metals A 10.0% w/v solution in *carbon dioxide-free water* complies with *limit test A for heavy metals*, Appendix VII (20 ppm). Use *lead standard solution (2 ppm Pb)* to prepare the standard.

Related substances Carry out the method for *gas chromatography*, Appendix III B, using 1 μl or other suitable volume of the following solution. Dissolve 0.10 g of the substance being examined in 2 ml of *water*, add 2 ml of a 20% w/v solution of *sodium hydroxide* and 2 ml of *chloroform* and shake for 10 minutes. Separate the chloroform layer, dry over *anhydrous sodium sulphate* and filter.

The chromatographic procedure may be carried out using a glass column (1.8 m × 2 mm) containing a packing material prepared in the following manner. Mix 19.5 g of *silanised diatomaceous support* with 60 ml of a 0.33% w/v solution of *potassium hydroxide* in *methanol* and evaporate the solvent at a pressure of 2 kPa while slowly rotating the mixture. Dissolve 0.4 g of *low-vapour pressure hydrocarbons (type L)* (Apiezon L is suitable) in 60 ml of *toluene* (dissolution requires up to 5 hours), add this solution to the prepared silanised diatomaceous support and evaporate the solvent at a pressure of 2 kPa while slowly rotating the mixture. Programme the temperature of the column to rise from 100° to 200° at a constant rate of 6° per minute and maintain the temperature of the injection port at 220° and that of the detector at 300°. Use 30 ml per minute as the flow rate of the carrier gas. Allow the chromatography to proceed for at least 2.5 times the retention time of the principal peak.

The area of any *secondary peak* is not greater than 0.3% and the sum of the areas of any *secondary peaks* is not greater than 1% by *normalisation*.

Sulphated ash Not more than 0.1%, Appendix IX A, Method II. Use 1 g.

Water Not more than 0.5 per cent, Appendix IX C. Use 2 g.

Assay Dissolve 0.15 g in a mixture of 5 ml of 0.01M *hydrochloric acid VS* and 50 ml of *ethanol (96%)* and titrate with 0.1M *sodium hydroxide VS* determining the end-point potentiometrically. Record the volume added between the two inflections. Each ml of 0.1M *sodium hydroxide VS* is equivalent to 0.01877 g of $C_{10}H_{17}N,HCl$.

Action and use Anticonvulsant; antiviral.

Amethocaine Hydrochloride ☆

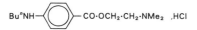

C₁₅H₂₄N₂O₂,HCl   300.8   *136-47-0*

Amethocaine Hydrochloride is 2-dimethyl-aminoethyl 4-butylaminobenzoate hydrochloride. It contains not less than 99.0 per cent and not more than 101.0 per cent of $C_{15}H_{24}N_2O_2,HCl$, calculated with reference to the dried substance.

Characteristics A white, crystalline powder; slightly hygroscopic. It melts at about 148° or may occur in either of two polymorphic modifications which melt at about 134° and 139° respectively. Mixtures of the forms melt within the range 134° to 147°.

Solubility Soluble in 7.5 parts of *water*; soluble in *ethanol (96%)*; sparingly soluble in *chloroform*; practically insoluble in *ether*.

Identification *Test A may be omitted if tests B, C and D are carried out. Test B may be omitted if tests A, C and D are carried out.*
A. The *infra-red absorption spectrum*, Appendix II A, is concordant with the spectrum of *tetracaine hydrochloride EPCRS*.
B. To 5 mg add 0.5 ml of *fuming nitric acid*, evaporate to dryness on a water-bath, cool, dissolve the residue in 5 ml of *acetone* and add 1 ml of *0.1M ethanolic potassium hydroxide*. A violet colour is produced.
C. To 1 ml of a 10% w/v solution add 1 ml of *1M ammonium thiocyanate*. A white, crystalline precipitate is produced which, after recrystallisation from *water* and drying at 80° for 2 hours, has a *melting point* of about 134°, Appendix V A, Method I.
D. Yields *reaction A* characteristic of chlorides, Appendix VI.

Acidity pH of a 1% w/v solution, 4.5 to 5.5, Appendix V L.

Clarity and colour of solution A 10.0% w/v solution is *clear*, Appendix IV A, and *colourless*, Appendix IV B, Method II.

Heavy metals A 10.0% w/v solution complies with *limit test A for heavy metals*, Appendix VII (10 ppm). Use *lead standard solution (1 ppm Pb)* to prepare the standard.

Related substances Carry out the method for *thin-layer chromatography*, Appendix III A, using *silica gel GF254* as the coating substance and a mixture of 80 volumes of *dibutyl ether*, 16 volumes of n-*hexane* and 4 volumes of *glacial acetic acid* as the mobile phase. Place the chromatoplate in the tank so that the plate dips 5 mm beneath the surface of the liquid and allow to stand until the solvent front has ascended about 12 cm, remove the plate and dry it for a few minutes in a current of warm air. Allow to cool and apply separately 5 μl of each of two solutions in *water* containing (1) 10.0% w/v of the substance being examined and (2) 0.0050% w/v of *4-aminobenzoic acid*. Allow the solvent front to ascend 10 cm above the line of application. After removal of the plate, dry it at 100° to 105° for 10 minutes and examine under *ultra-violet light (254 nm)*. Any *secondary spot* in the chromatogram obtained with solution (1) is not more intense than the spot in the chromatogram obtained with

solution (2). The principal spot remains on the line of application.

Loss on drying When dried to constant weight at 100° to 105°, loses not more than 1.0% of its weight. Use 1 g.

Sulphated ash Not more than 0.1%, Appendix IX A, Method II. Use 1 g.

Assay Dissolve 0.25 g in a mixture of 5 ml of *acetic anhydride* and 25 ml of *anhydrous glacial acetic acid*, heat under a reflux condenser for 2 minutes, add 6 ml of *mercury(II) acetate solution* and carry out Method I for *non-aqueous titration*, Appendix VIII A, using 0.05 ml of *crystal violet solution* as indicator. Each ml of 0.1M *perchloric acid VS* is equivalent to 0.03008 g of C₁₅H₂₄N₂O₂,HCl.

Storage Amethocaine Hydrochloride should be kept in a well-closed container and protected from light.

Preparation
Amethocaine Eye Drops

Action and use Local anaesthetic.

The title of the monograph in the European Pharmacopœia is Tetracaine Hydrochloride.

Amiloride Hydrochloride

C₆H₈ClN₇O,HCl,2H₂O   302.1   *17440-83-4*

Amiloride Hydrochloride is *N*-amidino-3,5-diamino-6-chloropyrazine-2-carboxamide hydrochloride dihydrate. It contains not less than 98.0 per cent and not more than 101.0 per cent of $C_6H_8ClN_7O,HCl$, calculated with reference to the dried substance.

Characteristics A pale yellow to greenish-yellow powder; odourless or almost odourless.

Solubility Slightly soluble in *water* and in *ethanol (96%)*; practically insoluble in *chloroform* and in *ether*.

Identification A. The *infra-red absorption spectrum*, Appendix II A, is concordant with the *reference spectrum* of amiloride hydrochloride.
B. The *light absorption*, Appendix II B, in the range 230 to 380 nm of a 0.001% w/v solution in 0.1M *hydrochloric acid* exhibits two maxima, at 285 nm and 361 nm. The *absorbance* at 285 nm is about 0.55 and at 361 nm is about 0.61.
C. Yields *reaction A* characteristic of chlorides, Appendix VI.

Acidity pH of a 0.5% w/v solution, 3.8 to 5.2, Appendix V L.

Related substances Carry out the method for *thin-layer chromatography*, Appendix III A, using a silica gel precoated chromatoplate (Merck silica gel 60 plates are suitable) and a freshly prepared mixture of 90 volumes of *1,4-dioxan* and 12 volumes of *3M ammonia* as the mobile phase. Apply separately to the plate 5 μl of each of three solutions in *methanol* containing (1) 0.40% w/v of the substance being examined, (2) 0.0020% w/v of *methyl 3,5-diamino-6-chloropyrazine-2-carboxylate BPCRS* and (3)

0.00080% w/v of *methyl 3,5-diamino-6-chloropyrazine-2-carboxylate BPCRS*. After removal of the plate, allow it to dry in air and examine under *ultra-violet light (365 nm)*. Any spot corresponding to methyl 3,5-diamino-6-chloro-pyrazine-2-carboxylate in the chromatogram obtained with solution (1) is not more intense than the spot in the chromatogram obtained with solution (2). Any other *secondary spot* in the chromatogram obtained with solution (1) is not more intense than the spot in the chromatogram obtained with solution (2) and not more than one such spot is more intense than the spot in the chromatogram obtained with solution (3).

Loss on drying When dried to constant weight at 100° at a pressure not exceeding 0.7 kPa, loses 11.0% to 13.0% of its weight. Use 1 g.

Sulphated ash Not more than 0.1%, Appendix IX A.

Assay Dissolve 0.45 g in a mixture of 100 ml of *anhydrous glacial acetic acid*, 15 ml of *1,4-dioxan* and 10 ml of *mercury(II) acetate solution* and carry out Method I for *non-aqueous titration*, Appendix VIII A, determining the end-point potentiometrically. Each ml of 0.1M *perchloric acid VS* is equivalent to 0.02661 g of $C_6H_8ClN_7O,HCl$.

Storage Amiloride Hydrochloride should be kept in a well-closed container and protected from light.

Preparation
Amiloride Tablets

Action and use Diuretic.

Aminobenzoic Acid

$H_2N—\langle\bigcirc\rangle—CO_2H$

$C_7H_7NO_2$ 137.1   *150-13-0*

Aminobenzoic Acid is 4-aminobenzoic acid. It contains not less than 98.5 per cent and not more than 100.5 per cent of $C_7H_7NO_2$, calculated with reference to the dried substance.

Characteristics White or slightly yellow crystals or crystalline powder, gradually darkening on exposure to air and light; odourless or almost odourless.

Solubility Slightly soluble in *water*; soluble in 8 parts of *ethanol (96%)*. It dissolves in solutions of alkali hydroxides and carbonates.

Identification A. The *infra-red absorption spectrum*, Appendix II A, is concordant with the *reference spectrum* of aminobenzoic acid.
B. The *light absorption*, Appendix II B, in the range 230 to 350 nm of a 0.005% w/v solution in *ethanol (96%)* exhibits a maximum at 280 nm; the *absorbance* at 280 nm is about 0.48. A 0.005% w/v solution in 0.1M *sodium hydroxide* exhibits a maximum at 265 nm; the *absorbance* at 265 nm is about 0.53.
C. Dissolve 0.1 g in 2 ml of 2M *hydrochloric acid*, heating if necessary. Cool in ice, add 4 ml of a freshly prepared 1% w/v solution of *sodium nitrite* and pour the mixture into 2 ml of *2-naphthol solution* containing 1 g of *sodium acetate*. A bright red precipitate is produced.

Melting point 186° to 189°, Appendix V A.

Aromatic amines Carry out the method for *thin-layer chromatography*, Appendix III A, using *silica gel G* as the coating substance and a mixture of 90 volumes of *toluene*, 5 volumes of *ethyl acetate* and 5 volumes of *glacial acetic acid* as the mobile phase. Apply separately to the chromatoplate 10 μl of each of the following solutions. For solution (1) dissolve 2.0 g of the substance being examined in 10 ml of 2M *sodium hydroxide* and extract with two 10-ml quantities of *1,2-dichloroethane*. Wash the combined dichloroethane extracts with 5 ml of 2M *sodium hydroxide* followed by 5 ml of *water*, shake with anhydrous *sodium sulphate* and filter. Evaporate to a low volume using a rotary evaporator and dilute to 2 ml with *1,2-dichloroethane*. Solution (2) contains 0.0020% w/v of *aniline* in *1,2-dichloroethane*. Solution (3) contains 0.0020% w/v of *ethyl 4-aminobenzoate* in *1,2-dichloroethane*. After removal of the plate, dry it in a current of warm air and spray with *dimethylaminobenzaldehyde solution*. Any spots corresponding to aniline and ethyl 4-aminobenzoate in the chromatogram obtained with solution (1) are not more intense than the spots in the chromatograms obtained with solutions (2) and (3) respectively.

Iron Ignite 0.25 g with 0.25 g of *anhydrous sodium carbonate*, dissolve the residue in 4 ml of 2M *hydrochloric acid* and dilute to 10 ml with *water*. The solution complies with the *limit test for iron*, Appendix VII (40 ppm).

4-Nitrobenzoic acid Carry out the method for *thin-layer chromatography*, Appendix III A, using *cellulose F254* as the coating substance and the upper layer obtained by mixing 70 volumes of *2-methylpropan-1-ol*, 30 volumes of *water* and 15 volumes of 5M *ammonia* as the mobile phase. Apply separately to the chromatoplate 5 μl of each of two solutions in *ethanol (96%)* containing (1) 10% w/v of the substance being examined and (2) 0.020% w/v of *4-nitrobenzoic acid*. After removal of the plate, allow it to dry in a current of air and examine under *ultra-violet light (254 nm)*. Any spot corresponding to 4-nitrobenzoic acid in the chromatogram obtained with solution (1) is not more intense than the spot in the chromatogram obtained with solution (2).

Loss on drying When dried to constant weight at 60° at a pressure not exceeding 0.7 kPa, loses not more than 0.5% of its weight. Use 1 g.

Sulphated ash Not more than 0.2%, Appendix IX A.

Assay Dissolve 0.3 g in 60 ml of *ethanol (50%)* and titrate with 0.1M *sodium hydroxide VS* using *phenolphthalein solution* as indicator. Each ml of 0.1M *sodium hydroxide VS* is equivalent to 0.01371 g of $C_7H_7NO_2$.

Storage Aminobenzoic Acid should be kept in a well-closed container and protected from light.

Preparation
Aminobenzoic Acid Lotion

Action and use Skin protective.

Aminocaproic Acid

$H_2N\cdot(CH_2)_5\cdot CO_2H$

$C_6H_{13}NO_2$ 131.2   *60-32-2*

Aminocaproic Acid is 6-aminohexanoic acid. It contains not less than 98.5 per cent and not more than 101.0 per cent of $C_6H_{13}NO_2$, calculated with reference to the dried substance.

Characteristics Colourless crystals or a white, crystalline powder; odourless or almost odourless.

Solubility Soluble in 1.5 parts of *water*.

Identification A. The *infra-red absorption spectrum*, Appendix II A, is concordant with the *reference spectrum* of aminocaproic acid.

B. Carry out the method for *thin-layer chromatography*, Appendix III A, using *silica gel G* as the coating substance and a mixture of 100 volumes of *ethanol (96%)*, 16 volumes of 13.5M *ammonia* and 12 volumes of *water* as the mobile phase. Apply separately to the chromatoplate 2 µl of each of two solutions in *water* containing (1) 0.25% w/v of the substance being examined and (2) 0.25% w/v of *aminocaproic acid BPCRS*. After removal of the plate, spray it with a 0.25% w/v solution of *ninhydrin* in a mixture of equal volumes of *methanol* and *pyridine* and heat at 105° for 2 minutes. The principal spot in the chromatogram obtained with solution (1) corresponds to that in the chromatogram obtained with solution (2).

C. *Melting point*, about 204°, with decomposition, Appendix V A.

Alkalinity pH of a 20% w/v solution, 7.5 to 8.0, Appendix V L.

Clarity and colour of solution A 20% w/v solution remains *clear* for 24 hours, Appendix IV A, and is *colourless*, Appendix IV B, Method II.

Stability A. The *absorbance* of a 20% w/v solution at 287 nm is not more than 0.10 and at 450 nm is not more than 0.03, Appendix II B.

B. Place 20.0 g in an even layer in a shallow dish 9 cm in diameter, cover and allow to stand at 98° to 102° for 72 hours. Dissolve in sufficient *water* to produce 100 ml and measure the *absorbance* of the resulting solution at 287 nm and at 450 nm, Appendix II B. The absorbance at 287 nm is not more than 0.15 and at 450 nm is not more than 0.03.

Heavy metals Dissolve 3.0 g in 15 ml of *water*. 12 ml of the resulting solution complies with *limit test A for heavy metals*, Appendix VII (10 ppm). Use *lead standard solution (2 ppm Pb)* to prepare the standard.

Loss on drying When dried to constant weight at 105°, loses not more than 0.5% of its weight. Use 1 g.

Sulphated ash Not more than 0.1%, Appendix IX A.

Assay Dissolve 0.15 g in 20 ml of *anhydrous glacial acetic acid* and carry out Method I for *non-aqueous titration*, Appendix VIII A, using *crystal violet solution* as indicator. Each ml of 0.1M *perchloric acid VS* is equivalent to 0.01312 g of $C_6H_{13}NO_2$.

Preparations
Aminocaproic Acid Oral Solution
Aminocaproic Acid Effervescent Oral Powder

Action and use Antifibrinolytic; haemostatic.

Aminophylline ☆

$(C_7H_8N_4O_2)_2, C_2H_8N_2$ 420.4   *317-34-0*

Aminophylline is a stable mixture or combination of theophylline and ethylene-diamine. It contains the equivalent of not less than 84.0 per cent and not more than 87.4 per cent of theophylline, $C_7H_8N_4O_2$, and the equivalent of not less than 13.5 per cent and not more than 15.0 per cent of ethylene-diamine, $C_2H_8N_2$, both calculated with reference to the anhydrous substance.

Characteristics A white or slightly yellowish powder or granular powder; odourless or with a slight ammoniacal odour.

Solubility Soluble in 5 parts of *water* (the solution may become cloudy in the presence of carbon dioxide); practically insoluble in *absolute ethanol* and in *ether*.

Identification *Test A may be omitted if tests B, C, D, E and F are carried out. Tests B, D and F may be omitted if tests A, C and E are carried out.*

A. Dissolve 1 g in 10 ml of *water* and add 2 ml of 2M *hydrochloric acid* dropwise, with shaking. Filter the precipitate and reserve the filtrate for test E. The *infra-red absorption spectrum*, Appendix II A, of the precipitate, after washing with *water* and drying at 100° to 105°, is concordant with the spectrum of *theophylline EPCRS*.

B. Dissolve 10 mg of the precipitate obtained in test A in 10 ml of *water*, add 0.5 ml of a 5% w/v solution of *mercury(II) acetate* and allow to stand. A white, crystalline precipitate is produced.

C. Complies with the test for Water.

D. The *melting point* of the precipitate obtained in test A, after washing with *water* and drying at 100° to 105°, is 270° to 274°, Appendix V A, Method I.

E. To the filtrate obtained in test A add 0.2 ml of *benzoyl chloride*, make alkaline with 2M *sodium hydroxide* and shake vigorously. Filter, wash the precipitate with 10 ml of *water*, dissolve in 5 ml of hot *ethanol (96%)* and add 5 ml of *water*. The *melting point* of the precipitate, after washing and drying at 100° to 105°, is 248° to 252°, Appendix V A, Method I.

F. The precipitate obtained in test A yields the *reaction* characteristic of xanthines, Appendix VI.

Clarity and colour of solution Dissolve 0.5 g in 10 ml of *carbon dioxide-free water* with the aid of gentle heat. The solution is not more opalescent than *reference suspension II*, Appendix IV A, and not more intensely coloured than *reference solution GY₆*, Appendix IV B, Method II.

Heavy metals 1.0 g complies with *limit test C for heavy metals*, Appendix VII (20 ppm). Use 2 ml of *lead standard solution (10 ppm Pb)* to prepare the standard.

Related substances Carry out the method for *thin-layer chromatography*, Appendix III A, using *silica gel GF254* as the coating substance and a mixture of 40 volumes of *butan-1-ol*, 30 volumes of *acetone*, 30 volumes of *chloroform* and 10 volumes of 13.5M *ammonia* as the mobile phase. Apply separately to the chromatoplate 10 µl of each of the following solutions. For solution (1) dissolve 0.2 g of the substance being examined in 2 ml of *water* with the aid of heat and dilute to 10 ml with *methanol*. For solution (2) dilute 1 volume of solution (1) to 200 volumes with *methanol*. After removal of the plate, allow it to dry in air and examine under *ultra-violet light (254 nm)*. Any *secondary spot* in the chromatogram obtained with solution (1) is not more intense than the spot in the chromatogram obtained with solution (2).

Sulphated ash Not more than 0.1%, Appendix IX A, Method II. Use 1 g.

Water Not more than 1.5% w/w, Appendix IX C. Use 2 g dissolved in 20 ml of *pyridine*.

Assay *For ethylenediamine* Dissolve 0.25 g in 30 ml of *water* and titrate with 0.1M *hydrochloric acid VS*, using *bromocresol green solution* as indicator, until a green colour is produced. Each ml of 0.1M *hydrochloric acid VS* is equivalent to 0.003005 g of $C_2H_8N_2$.

For theophylline Dry 0.2 g to constant weight at 135°. Dissolve the residue in 100 ml of *water* with the aid of heat, allow to cool, add 20 ml of 0.1M *silver nitrate VS* and titrate with 0.1M *sodium hydroxide VS*, using 1 ml of *aqueous bromothymol blue solution* as indicator, until a blue colour is produced. Each ml of 0.1M *sodium hydroxide VS* is equivalent to 0.01802 g of $C_7H_8N_4O_2$.

Storage Aminophylline should be kept in a well-filled, airtight container and protected from light.

Preparations
Aminophylline Injection
Aminophylline Suppositories
Aminophylline Tablets

Action and use Xanthine bronchodilator.

The title of the monograph in the European Pharmacopœia is Theophylline and Ethylenediamine.

Aminophylline Hydrate ☆

5877-66-5

Aminophylline Hydrate is a stable mixture or combination of theophylline and ethylene-diamine containing water of hydration. It contains the equivalent of not less than 84.0 per cent and not more than 87.4 per cent of theophylline, $C_7H_8N_4O_2$, and the equivalent of not less than 13.5 per cent and not more than 15.0 per cent of ethylenediamine, $C_2H_8N_2$, both calculated with reference to the anhydrous substance.

Characteristics A white or slightly yellowish powder or granular powder; odourless or with a slight ammoniacal odour.

Solubility Soluble in 5 parts of *water* (the solution may become cloudy in the presence of carbon dioxide); practically insoluble in *absolute ethanol* and in *ether*.

Identification; Clarity and colour of solution; Heavy metals; Related substances; Sulphated ash Complies with the requirements stated under Aminophylline.

Water 3.0 to 8.0% w/w, Appendix IX C. Use 0.5 g dissolved in 20 ml of *pyridine*.

Assay Carry out the Assays for ethylenediamine and for theophylline described under Aminophylline. Each ml of 0.1M *hydrochloric acid VS* is equivalent to 0.003005 g of $C_2H_8N_2$ and to 0.01802 g of $C_7H_8N_4O_2$.

Storage Aminophylline Hydrate should be kept in a well-filled, airtight container and protected from light.

Preparation
Aminophylline Injection

Action and use Xanthine bronchodilator.

The title of the monograph in the European Pharmacopœia is Theophylline and Ethylenediamine Hydrate.

Amitriptyline Embonate

$(C_{20}H_{23}N)_2,C_{23}H_{16}O_6$ 943.2   *17086-03-2*

Amitriptyline Embonate is 3-(10,11-dihydro-5*H*-dibenzo[*a,d*]cyclohept-5-ylidene)propyl-dimethylamine 4,4′-methylenebis(3-hydroxy-2-naphthoate). It contains not less than 98.5 per cent and not more than 101.0 per cent of $C_{40}H_{46}N_2,C_{23}H_{16}O_6$, calculated with reference to the anhydrous substance.

Characteristics A pale yellow to brownish-yellow powder; odourless or almost odourless.

Solubility Practically insoluble in *water*; slightly soluble in *ethanol (96%)*; soluble in 8 parts of *chloroform*.

Identification A. Dissolve 40 mg in 100 ml of *methanol*. To 1 ml of the solution add 1 ml of a 2.5% w/v solution of *sodium hydrogen carbonate*, 1 ml of a 2.0% w/v solution of *sodium metaperiodate* and 1 ml of a 0.3% w/v solution of *potassium permanganate*, shake and allow to stand for 15 minutes. Acidify with 1M *sulphuric acid*, extract with 10 ml of *2,2,4-trimethylpentane* and filter. The *light absorption* of the filtrate, Appendix II B, in the range 230 to 350 nm exhibits a maximum only at 265 nm.
B. Dissolve 0.2 g in 10 ml of *dichloromethane*, add 5 ml of 1.25M *sodium hydroxide* and shake. The aqueous layer exhibits a green fluorescence when examined under ultra-violet light (365 nm).

Chloride Not more than 0.2% when determined by the following method. Dissolve 1 g in a mixture of 50 ml of *acetone* and 50 ml of *water*, add 2 ml of *nitric acid* and 75 ml of *acetate buffer pH 5.0* and titrate with 0.01M *silver nitrate VS* determining the end-point potentiometrically. Each ml of 0.01M *silver nitrate VS* is equivalent to 0.0003545 g of Cl.

Dibenzosuberone Carry out the method for *thin-layer chromatography*, Appendix III A, using *silica gel G* as the coating substance and a mixture of 70 volumes of *toluene* and 30 volumes of *carbon tetrachloride* as the mobile phase but allowing the solvent front to ascend 12 cm above the line of application. Apply separately to the chromatoplate 5 μl of each of two solutions in *ethanol (96%)* containing (1) 2.0% w/v of the substance being examined and (2) 0.0010% w/v of *dibenzosuberone*. After removal of the plate, allow it to dry in air until the odour of solvent is no longer detectable, spray with *sulphuric acid* containing 4% v/v of *formaldehyde solution* and examine immediately under *ultra-violet light (365 nm)*. Any spot corresponding to dibenzosuberone in the chromatogram obtained with solution (1) is not more intense than the spot in the chromatogram obtained with solution (2).

Sulphated ash Not more than 0.2%, Appendix IX A.

Water Not more than 5.0% w/w, Appendix IX. Use 0.5 g.

Assay Dissolve 0.6 g in 50 ml of *acetic anhydride* and carry out Method I for *non-aqueous titration*, Appendix VIII A, using *1-naphtholbenzein solution* as indicator. Each ml of 0.1M *perchloric acid VS* is equivalent to 0.04716 g of $(C_{20}H_{23}N_2)_2,C_{23}H_{16}O_6$.

Storage Amitriptyline Embonate should be protected from light.

Preparation
Amitriptyline Oral Suspension

Action and use Antidepressant.

Amitriptyline Hydrochloride ☆

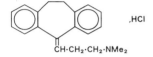

$C_{20}H_{23}N,HCl$ 313.9   *549-18-8*

Amitriptyline Hydrochloride is 3-(10,11-dihydro-5*H*-dibenzo[*a,d*]cyclohept-5-ylidene)-propyldimethylamine hydrochloride. It contains not less than 99.0 per cent and not more than 101.0 per cent of $C_{20}H_{23}N,HCl$, calculated with reference to the dried substance.

Characteristics Colourless crystals or a white or almost white powder; odourless or almost odourless.

Solubility Soluble in 1 part of *water*, in 1.5 parts of *ethanol (96%)*, in 1 part of *methanol* and in 1.2 parts of *chloroform*; practically insoluble in *ether*.

Identification *Test A may be omitted if tests B, C, D and E are carried out. Tests B and C may be omitted if tests A, D and E are carried out.*
A. The *infra-red absorption spectrum*, Appendix II A, is concordant with the spectrum of *amitriptyline hydrochloride EPCRS*.
B. The *light absorption*, Appendix II B, in the range 230 to 350 nm of a 0.00125% w/v solution in *methanol* exhibits a maximum only at 239 nm. The A(1%, 1 cm) at 239 nm is 435 to 475.
C. Dissolve 0.1 g in 10 ml of 1M *sulphuric acid* and add 2 ml of a saturated solution of *potassium permanganate*; the violet colour quickly disappears. Heat in a water-bath until the brown precipitate is almost completely dissolved, cool, shake with 15 ml of *ether* to remove the white turbidity and discard the ether layer. Add to the aqueous layer 5 ml of *ammonia*, shake for 2 minutes, add 3 ml of *chloroform* and shake. The chloroform layer is violet-red.
D. 50 mg yields *reaction A* characteristic of chlorides, Appendix VI.
E. *Melting point*, 195° to 199°, Appendix V A, Method I.

Acidity or alkalinity Dissolve 0.2 g in sufficient *carbon dioxide-free water* to produce 10 ml and add 0.1 ml of *methyl red solution* and 0.2 ml of 0.01M *sodium hydroxide*

VS; the solution is yellow. Add 0.4 ml of 0.01M *hydrochloric acid VS*; the solution is red.

Clarity and colour of solution Dissolve 1.25 g in sufficient *water* to produce 25 ml. The solution is *clear*, Appendix IV A, and not more intensely coloured than *reference solution B_7*, Appendix IV B, Method II.

Heavy metals 1.0 g complies with *limit test C for heavy metals*, Appendix VII (20 ppm). Use 2 ml of *lead standard solution (10 ppm)* to prepare the standard.

Related substances Carry out the method for *thin-layer chromatography*, Appendix III A, using *silica gel G* as the coating substance and a mixture of 85 volumes of *cyclohexane*, 15 volumes of *ethyl acetate* and 3 volumes of *diethylamine* as the mobile phase, but allowing the solvent front to ascend 14 cm above the line of application in an unlined tank. Apply separately to the chromatoplate 10 μl of each of three solutions in *chloroform* containing (1) 2.0% w/v of the substance being examined, (2) 0.001% w/v of *dibenzosuberone EPCRS* and (3) 0.004% w/v of *cyclobenzaprine hydrochloride EPCRS*. After removal of the plate, allow it to dry in air, spray with a freshly prepared mixture of 4 volumes of *formaldehyde* and 96 volumes of *sulphuric acid*, heat at 100° to 105° for 10 minutes and examine under *ultra-violet light (254 nm)*. In the chromatogram obtained with solution (1) any spots corresponding to dibenzosuberone and cyclobenzaprine are not more intense than the spots in the chromatograms obtained with solutions (2) and (3) respectively and any other *secondary spot* is not more intense than the spot in the chromatogram obtained with solution (3).

Loss on drying When dried at 100° to 105° for 2 hours, loses not more than 0.5% of its weight. Use 1 g.

Sulphated ash Not more than 0.1%, Appendix IX A, Method II. Use 1 g.

Assay Dissolve 0.25 g in 30 ml of *ethanol (96%)* and titrate with 0.1M *sodium hydroxide VS* determining the end-point potentiometrically. Each ml of 0.1M *sodium hydroxide VS* is equivalent to 0.03139 g of $C_{20}H_{23}N,HCl$.

Storage Amitriptyline Hydrochloride should be kept in a well-closed container.

Preparation
Amitriptyline Tablets

Action and use Antidepressant.

Strong Ammonia Solution

Content of ammonia, NH_3 27.0 to 30.0% w/w.

Characteristics A clear, colourless liquid; odour, strongly pungent and characteristic.

Identification A. Strongly alkaline, even when freely diluted with *water*.
B. When the vapour is brought into contact with gaseous hydrochloric acid, dense white fumes are produced.

Weight per ml 0.892 to 0.901 g, Appendix V G.

Arsenic Evaporate 10 g on a water-bath until reduced to 2 ml, add 40 ml of *water* and 7 ml of *brominated hydrochloric acid* and dilute to 100 ml with *water*. 25 ml of the resulting solution complies with the *limit test for arsenic*, Appendix VII (0.4 ppm).

Heavy metals Dilute 10 g to 20 ml with *water*. 12 ml of the resulting solution complies with *limit test A for heavy* *metals*, Appendix VII (2 ppm). Use *lead standard solution (1 ppm Pb)* to prepare the standard.

Tarry matter Dilute 5 ml to 10 ml with *water* and dissolve 6 g of powdered *citric acid* in the resulting solution. No tarry or unpleasant odour is produced.

Pyridine and homologues *Absorbance* at the maximum at 252 nm, not more than 0.045, Appendix II B.

Non-volatile matter 100 ml, when evaporated on a water-bath and dried to constant weight at 105°, leaves not more than 10 mg of residue.

Assay To 50 ml of 1M *hydrochloric acid VS* add 2 g, taking precautions during the addition to avoid loss of ammonia, and titrate the excess of acid with 1M *sodium hydroxide VS* using *methyl red solution* as indicator. Each ml of 1M *hydrochloric acid VS* is equivalent to 0.01703 g of NH_3.

Storage Strong Ammonia Solution should be kept in a well-closed container and stored at a temperature not exceeding 20°.

Preparation
Dilute Ammonia Solution

Ammonium Bicarbonate

NH_4HCO_3 79.06   *1066-33-7*

Ammonium Bicarbonate is ammonium hydrogen carbonate. It contains not less than 98.0 per cent and not more than 101.0 per cent of NH_4HCO_3.

Characteristics White crystals, a white, fine crystalline powder or a colourless, glassy solid; odour, slightly ammoniacal; slightly hygroscopic. It volatilises rapidly at 60°, with dissociation into ammonia, carbon dioxide and water; the volatilisation takes place slowly at ambient temperatures if the substance is slightly moist.

Solubility Soluble in 5 parts of *water*; practically insoluble in *ethanol (96%)*.

Identification Yields the *reactions* characteristic of ammonium salts and of bicarbonates, Appendix VI.

Arsenic Boil 0.50 g with 25 ml of *water* until most of the ammonia is volatilised. The resulting solution complies with the *limit test for arsenic*, Appendix VII (2 ppm).

Iron Dissolve 0.50 g in 20 ml of *water*, boil to remove the ammonia and restore to the original volume. 10 ml of the resulting solution complies with the *limit test for iron*, Appendix VII (40 ppm).

Heavy metals Dissolve 2.5 g in 25 ml of 1M *hydrochloric acid*. 12 ml of the resulting solution complies with *limit test A for heavy metals*, Appendix VII (10 ppm). Use *lead standard solution (1 ppm Pb)* to prepare the standard.

Chloride Dissolve 1.4 g in 30 ml of *water*, boil to remove the ammonia and restore to the original volume. 15 ml of the resulting solution complies with the *limit test for chlorides*, Appendix VII (70 ppm).

Sulphate Dissolve 3.5 g in 25 ml of *water*, boil to remove the ammonia and restore to the original volume. 15 ml of the resulting solution complies with the *limit test for sulphates*, Appendix VII (70 ppm).

Sulphide Dissolve 5.0 g in 50 ml of *carbon dioxide-free water* and add 2 ml of a solution containing 1.7% w/v of *lead(II) acetate*, 3.4% w/v of *potassium citrate* and 50% w/v

of *potassium hydroxide*. No darkening in colour is produced.

Tarry matter Mix 5.0 g with 15 ml of *water* and 5 g of *citric acid*. No tarry odour is detectable.

Non-volatile matter When heated to constant weight at 300°, leaves not more than 0.01% of residue.

Assay Dissolve 2 g in 40 ml of 1M *hydrochloric acid VS* diluted with 50 ml of *water*, boil, cool and titrate the excess of acid with 1M *sodium hydroxide VS* using *methyl red solution* as indicator. Each ml of 1M *hydrochloric acid VS* is equivalent to 0.07906 g of NH_4HCO_3.

Storage Ammonium Bicarbonate should be kept in a well-closed container and at a temperature not exceeding 15°.

Preparations
Ammonia and Ipecacuanha Mixture
Ammonium Chloride and Morphine Mixture
Aromatic Ammonia Solution
Strong Ammonium Acetate Solution
Aromatic Ammonia Spirit

Action and use Expectorant.

When Ammonium Carbonate is prescribed or demanded, Ammonium Bicarbonate shall be dispensed or supplied.

Ammonium Chloride ☆

NH_4Cl 53.49   *12125-02-9*

Ammonium Chloride contains not less than 99.0 per cent and not more than 100.5 per cent of NH_4Cl, calculated with reference to the dried substance.

Characteristics Colourless crystals or a white, crystalline powder; odourless.

Solubility Soluble in 2.7 parts of *water*.

Identification Yields the *reactions* characteristic of ammonium salts and of chlorides, Appendix VI.

Acidity or alkalinity To 10 ml of a 10.0% w/v solution in *distilled water* (solution A) add 0.05 ml of *methyl red solution*. Not more than 0.5 ml of either 0.01M *hydrochloric acid VS* or 0.01M *sodium hydroxide VS* is required to change the colour of the solution.

Clarity and colour of solution Solution A is *clear*, Appendix IV A, and *colourless*, Appendix IV B, Method II.

Calcium 5 ml of solution A diluted to 15 ml with *distilled water* complies with the *limit test for calcium*, Appendix VII (200 ppm).

Heavy metals 12 ml of solution A complies with *limit test A for heavy metals*, Appendix VII (10 ppm). Use *lead standard solution (1 ppm Pb)* to prepare the standard.

Iron 5 ml of solution A diluted to 10 ml with *water* complies with the *limit test for iron*, Appendix VII (20 ppm).

Bromide and iodide To 10 ml of solution A add 0.1 ml of 2M *hydrochloric acid* and 0.05 ml of a 2% w/v solution of *chloramine T*; after 1 minute add 2 ml of *chloroform* and shake vigorously. The chloroform layer remains *colourless*, Appendix IV B, Method I.

Sulphate 10 ml of solution A diluted to 15 ml with *distilled water* complies with the *limit test for sulphates*, Appendix VII (150 ppm).

Loss on drying When dried at 100° to 105° for 2 hours, loses not more than 1.0% of its weight. Use 1 g.

Sulphated ash Not more than 0.1%, Appendix IX A, Method II. Use 2 g.

Assay Dissolve 1 g in 20 ml of *water* and add a mixture of 5 ml of *formaldehyde solution* previously neutralised to *dilute phenolphthalein solution* and 20 ml of *water*. Allow to stand for 1 to 2 minutes and then titrate slowly with 1M *sodium hydroxide VS* using a further 0.2 ml of *dilute phenolphthalein solution* as indicator. Each ml of 1M *sodium hydroxide VS* is equivalent to 0.05349 g of NH_4Cl.

Preparations

Ammonium Chloride Mixture

Ammonium Chloride and Morphine Mixture

Action and use Used for the acidification of urine and to correct metabolic alkalosis.

Amodiaquine Hydrochloride

$C_{20}H_{22}ClN_3O,2HCl,2H_2O$ 464.8   *6398-98-7*

Amodiaquine Hydrochloride is 4-(7-chloro-4-quinolylamino)-2-(diethylaminomethyl)phenol dihydrochloride dihydrate. It contains not less than 98.0 per cent and not more than 101.5 per cent of $C_{20}H_{22}ClN_3O,2HCl$, calculated with reference to the anhydrous substance.

Characteristics A yellow, crystalline powder; odourless or almost odourless.

Solubility Soluble in 22 parts of *water* and in 70 parts of *ethanol (96%)*; practically insoluble in *chloroform* and in *ether*.

Identification A. Dissolve 0.1 g in 10 ml of *water* and add 2 ml of 2M *sodium hydroxide*. Extract with two 20-ml quantities of *chloroform*, wash the combined chloroform extracts with 5 ml of *water*, dry with *anhydrous sodium sulphate* and evaporate to dryness. Dissolve the residue in 2 ml of *chloroform*. The *infra-red absorption spectrum* of the resulting solution, Appendix II A, is concordant with the *reference spectrum* of amodiaquine.

B. The *light absorption*, Appendix II B, in the range 240 to 360 nm of a 0.003% w/v solution in 0.1M *hydrochloric acid* exhibits a maximum only at 343 nm. The *absorbance* at 343 nm is about 1.1.

C. To 1 ml of a 2% w/v solution add 0.5 ml of *cobalt thiocyanate reagent*. A green precipitate is produced.

D. Yields the *reactions* characteristic of chlorides, Appendix VI.

E. *Melting point* of the undried substance, about 158°, Appendix V A.

Acidity pH of a 2.0% w/v solution, 3.6 to 4.6, Appendix V L.

4-(7-Chloro-4-quinolylamino)phenol hydrochloride Carry out the method for *thin-layer chromatography*, Appendix III A, using *silica gel G* as the coating substance, spread in a layer about 0.5 mm thick, and a mixture of 50 volumes of *chloroform*, 40 volumes of *butan-2-one* and 10 volumes of *diethylamine* as the mobile phase. Apply separately to the chromatoplate 5 μl of each of two solutions in *methanol* containing (1) 10.0% w/v of the substance being examined and (2) 10.0% w/v of *amodiaquine hydrochloride BPCRS* and 0.020% w/v of *4-(7-chloro-4-quinolylamino)phenol hydrochloride BPCRS*. After removal of the plate, heat it at 105° for 10 minutes, spray with a freshly prepared mixture of equal volumes of a 10% w/v solution of *iron(III) chloride* and a 1% w/v solution of *potassium hexacyanoferrate(III)* and examine immediately. Any spot corresponding to 4-(7-chloro-4-quinolylamino)phenol in the chromatogram obtained with solution (1) is not more intense than the spot with lower Rf value in the chromatogram obtained with solution (2).

Sulphated ash Not more than 0.1%, Appendix IX A.

Water 6.0 to 10.0% w/w, Appendix IX C. Use 0.5 g.

Assay Carry out Method I for *non-aqueous titration*, Appendix VIII A, using 0.2 g, 7 ml of *mercury(II) acetate solution* and *1-naphtholbenzein solution* as indicator. Each ml of 0.1M *perchloric acid VS* is equivalent to 0.02144 g of $C_{20}H_{22}ClN_3O,2HCl$.

Preparation

Amodiaquine Tablets

Action and use Antimalarial.

Amoxycillin Trihydrate ☆

$C_{16}H_{19}N_3O_5S,3H_2O$ 419.5   *61336-70-7*

Amoxycillin Trihydrate is (6R)-6-(α-D-p-hydroxyphenylglycylamino)penicillanic acid trihydrate. It contains not less than 95.0 per cent and not more than 100.5 per cent of $C_{16}H_{19}N_3O_5S$, calculated with reference to the anhydrous substance.

Characteristics A white or almost white, crystalline powder.

Solubility Slightly soluble in *water* and in *ethanol (96%)*; practically insoluble in *chloroform*, in *ether* and in fixed oils. It dissolves in dilute solutions of acids and of alkali hydroxides.

Identification *Test A may be omitted if tests B, C, D and E are carried out. Tests B, C and E may be omitted if tests A and D are carried out.*

A. The *infra-red absorption spectrum*, Appendix II A, is concordant with the spectrum of *amoxicillin trihydrate EPCRS*.

B. Prepare a 0.01% w/v solution in *0.0067M mixed phosphate buffer pH 7.0* (solution A). To 10 ml of solution A add 0.5 ml of *dilute penicillinase solution* and allow to stand for 10 minutes at 30° (solution B). To 5 ml of solution A and to 5 ml of solution B, in separate test-tubes, add 10 ml of *acetate buffer pH 4.6* and 5 ml of 0.0005M *iodine VS*. Mix the contents of each tube and add, to each, 0.1 ml of *starch solution*. The mixture produced with solution A is blue; the mixture produced with solution B remains colourless.

C. Suspend 10 mg in 1 ml of *water* and add 2 ml of a mixture of 2 volumes of *modified potassium cupri-tartrate solution* and 6 volumes of *water*. A violet colour is produced.

D. Dissolve 10 mg in 2 ml of *water*. Heat on a water-bath for 2 minutes and while heating add 0.5 ml of *mercury—nitric acid solution*. The solution becomes red and a red precipitate is produced.

E. Yields the *reaction* characteristic of penicillins and cephalosporins, Appendix VI.

Acidity pH of a 0.2% w/v solution, prepared by mixing in an ultrasonic bath or by gentle heating, 3.5 to 5.5, Appendix V L.

Clarity of solution Dissolve 1.0 g in 10 ml of 0.5M *hydrochloric acid*. Separately dissolve 1.0 g in 10 ml of 2M *ammonia*. The solutions, examined immediately after dissolution, are not more opalescent than *reference suspension II*, Appendix IV A.

Specific optical rotation In a 0.2% w/v solution in *carbon dioxide-free water*, prepared with the aid of ultrasound or gentle heating, +290° to +315°, Appendix V F.

Heavy metals 1.0 g complies with *limit test C for heavy metals*, Appendix VII (20 ppm). Use 2 ml of *lead standard solution (10 ppm Pb)* to prepare the standard.

N,N-Dimethylaniline Not more than 20 ppm when determined by the following method. Prepare a 0.005% w/v solution of *naphthalene* (internal standard) in *cyclohexane* (solution A). Mix 50 mg of N,N-*dimethylaniline* with 2 ml of *hydrochloric acid* and 20 ml of *water*, shake to dissolve, add sufficient *water* to produce 50 ml and dilute 5 ml of the resulting solution to 250 ml with *water* (solution B). Carry out the method for *gas chromatography*, Appendix III B, injecting 1 μl of each of the following solutions. For solution (1) add 5 ml of 1M *sodium hydroxide* and 1 ml of solution A to 1 ml of solution B, shake vigorously for 1 minute, centrifuge if necessary and use the clear, upper layer. For solution (2) dissolve 1.00 g of the substance being examined in 5 ml of 1M *sodium hydroxide*, add 1 ml of *cyclohexane*, shake vigorously for 1 minute, centrifuge if necessary and use the clear, upper layer. Prepare solution (3) in the same manner as solution (2) but adding 1 ml of solution A in place of the *cyclohexane*.

The chromatographic procedure may be carried out using a glass column (2 m × 2 mm) packed with *acid-washed, silanised diatomaceous support* (Gas Chrom Q is suitable) coated with 3% w/w of phenyl methyl silicone fluid (50% phenyl) (OV-17 is suitable) and maintained at 120° with both the inlet port temperature and the detector temperature at 150° and using 30 ml per minute as the flow rate of the carrier gas.

Sulphated ash Not more than 1.0%, Appendix IX A, Method II. Use 1 g.

Water 11.5 to 14.5% w/w, Appendix IX C. Use 0.1 g.

Assay Dissolve 50 mg in 10 ml of *boric buffer pH 9.0* and 0.2 ml of *acetic anhydride* and stir for 3 minutes. Add 10 ml of 1M *sodium hydroxide* and allow to stand for 15 minutes. Add 10 ml of 1M *nitric acid* and 20 ml of *acetate buffer pH 4.6* and immediately titrate with 0.02M *mercury(II) nitrate VS*. Titrate slowly so that the titration takes about 15 minutes. Determine the end-point potentiometrically using a platinum or mercury indicator

electrode and a mercury—mercury(I) sulphate reference electrode. Ignore any preliminary inflection on the titration curve. Each ml of 0.02M *mercury(II) nitrate VS* is equivalent to 0.007308 g of total penicillins, calculated as $C_{16}H_{19}N_3O_5S$.

To a further 0.25 g add 25 ml of *boric buffer pH 9.0* and 0.5 ml of *acetic anhydride*, stir for 3 minutes, add 10 ml of *acetate buffer pH 4.6* and immediately titrate with 0.02M *mercury(II) nitrate VS*. Determine the end-point potentiometrically using a platinum or mercury indicator electrode and a mercury—mercury(I) sulphate reference electrode. Each ml of 0.02M *mercury(II) nitrate VS* is equivalent to 0.007308 g of degradation products, calculated as $C_{16}H_{19}N_3O_5S$.

Calculate the percentage content of total penicillins and the percentage content of degradation products. The content of amoxycillin, $C_{16}H_{19}N_3O_5S$, is the difference between the two percentages.

Storage Amoxycillin Trihydrate should be kept in an airtight container and stored at a temperature not exceeding 30°.

Labelling The label states (1) the date after which the material is not intended to be used; (2) the conditions under which it should be stored.

Preparations
Amoxycillin Capsules
Amoxycillin Oral Suspension

Action and use Antibacterial.

The title of the monograph in the European Pharmacopœia is Amoxicillin Trihydrate.

Amphetamine Sulphate ☆

$(C_9H_{13}N)_2,H_2SO_4$ 368.5   *300-62-9*

Amphetamine Sulphate is α-methylphenethylamine sulphate. It contains not less than 99.0 per cent and not more than 100.5 per cent of $(C_9H_{13}N)_2,H_2SO_4$, calculated with reference to the dried substance.

Characteristics A white powder.

Solubility Soluble in 9 parts of *water*; slightly soluble in *ethanol (96%)*; practically insoluble in *ether*.

Identification *Test A may be omitted if tests B, C, D and E are carried out. Tests C and D may be omitted if tests A, B and E are carried out.*

A. The *infra-red absorption spectrum*, Appendix II A, is concordant with the European Pharmacopœia reference spectrum of amphetamine sulphate. Examine the substance as a dispersion in *liquid paraffin*.

B. The *optical rotation* of a 2% w/v solution in *carbon dioxide-free water* is −0.04° to +0.04°, Appendix V F. Use a 2-dm tube.

C. Dissolve 1 g in 50 ml of *water*, add 5 ml of 10M *sodium hydroxide* and 0.5 ml of *benzoyl chloride* and shake. Continue adding *benzoyl chloride* in 0.5-ml quantities until no further precipitate is produced. Collect the precipitate on a filter, wash with *water* and recrystallise twice from a mixture of equal volumes of *ethanol (96%)* and *water*. The *melting point* of the crystals, after drying at 100° to 105°, is 131° to 135°, Appendix V A, Method I.

D. To 2 mg add 1 ml of *sulphuric acid—formaldehyde reagent*. An orange colour is produced which rapidly changes to dark brown.

E. A 2% w/v solution yields the *reactions* characteristic of sulphates, Appendix VI.

Acidity or alkalinity To 25 ml of a 2% w/v solution add 0.1 ml of *methyl red solution*. Not more than 0.1 ml of 0.01M *hydrochloric acid VS* or 0.01M *sodium hydroxide VS* is required to change the colour of the solution.

Clarity and colour of solution A 2.0% w/v solution in *carbon dioxide-free water* is *clear*, Appendix IV A, and *colourless*, Appendix IV B, Method II.

Loss on drying When dried to constant weight at 100° to 105°, loses not more than 1.0% of its weight. Use 1 g.

Sulphated ash Not more than 0.1%, Appendix IX A, Method II. Use 1 g.

Assay Dissolve 0.3 g in 30 ml of *anhydrous glacial acetic acid* and carry out Method II for *non-aqueous titration*, Appendix VIII A, using 0.1M *perchloric acid VS* as titrant and determining the end-point potentiometrically. Each of 0.1M *perchloric acid VS* is equivalent to 0.03685 g of $(C_9H_{13}N)_2,H_2SO_4$.

Action and use Central nervous system stimulant.

Amphotericin

$C_{47}H_{73}NO_{17}$ 924.1   *1397-89-3*

Amphotericin is a mixture of antifungal polyenes produced by the growth of certain strains of *Streptomyces nodosus* or by any other means. It consists largely of amphotericin B which is (3*R*,5*R*,8*R*,9*R*,11*S*,13*R*,15*S*,16*R*, 17*S*,19*R*,34*S*,35*R*,36*R*,37*S*)-19-(3-amino-3,6-dideoxy-β-D-mannopyranosyloxy)-16-carboxy-3,5,8,9,11,13,15,35-octahydroxy-34,36-dimethyl-13,17-epoxyoctatriaconta-20,22,24,26,28,30,32-heptaen-37-olide. The potency is not less than 750 Units per mg, calculated with reference to the dried substance.

Characteristics A yellow to orange powder.

Solubility Practically insoluble in *water*, in *ethanol (96%)* and in *ether*; soluble in *dimethyl sulphoxide* and in *propane-1,2-diol*; slightly soluble in *dimethylformamide* and in *methanol*.

Identification A. The *infra-red absorption spectrum*, Appendix II A, is concordant with the *reference spectrum* of

amphotericin. If the spectra are not concordant, dry a sufficient quantity at 60° at a pressure not exceeding 0.7 kPa for 1 hour and prepare a new spectrum.

B. Dissolve 25 mg in 5 ml of *dimethyl sulphoxide*, add sufficient *methanol* to produce 50 ml and dilute 2 ml to 200 ml with *methanol*. The *light absorption* of the resulting solution, Appendix II B, in the range 300 to 450 nm exhibits three maxima, at 362, 381 and 405 nm. The ratio of the *absorbance* at the maximum at 362 nm to that at the maximum at 381 nm is 0.5 to 0.6. The ratio of the *absorbance* at the maximum at 381 nm to that at the maximum at 405 nm is about 0.9.

C. To 1 ml of a 0.05% w/v solution in *dimethyl sulphoxide* add 5 ml of *orthophosphoric acid* to form a lower layer; a blue ring is immediately produced at the junction of the liquids. Mix; an intense blue colour is produced. Add 15 ml of *water* and mix; the solution becomes pale straw coloured.

Content of tetraenes Not more than 10.0% when determined by the following method. For solution (1) dissolve 50 mg in 5 ml of *dimethyl sulphoxide*, add sufficient *methanol* to produce 50 ml and dilute 4 ml to 50 ml with *methanol*. Prepare solution (2) in the same manner but using 50 mg of *amphotericin B BPCRS* in place of the substance being examined. For solution (3) dissolve 25 mg of *nystatin BPCRS* in 25 ml of *dimethyl sulphoxide*, dilute to 250 ml with *methanol* and dilute 4 ml to 50 ml with *methanol*. Measure the *absorbances* of solutions (1) and (2) at the maximum at 282 nm and that of solution (3) at the same wavelength, Appendix II B, using a 0.8% v/v solution of *dimethyl sulphoxide* in *methanol* in the reference cell. Then measure the *absorbance* of solution (3) at the maximum at 304 nm and those of solution (1) and (2) at the same wavelength. Calculate the A(1%, 1 cm) (specific absorbance) of the substance being examined, of *nystatin BPCRS* and of *amphotericin B BPCRS* at both wavelengths and calculate the content of tetraenes from the expression

$$F + 100(B_1S_2 - B_2S_1)/(N_2B_1 - N_1B_2)$$

where S_1 and S_2 are the specific absorbances of the substance being examined at 282 nm and 304 nm respectively, N_1 and N_2 are the specific absorbances of *nystatin BPCRS* at 282 nm and 304 nm respectively, B_1 and B_2 are the specific absorbances of *amphotericin B BPCRS* at 282 and 304 nm respectively and F is the declared content of tetraenes in *amphotericin B BPCRS*.

Loss on drying When dried to constant weight at 60° at a pressure not exceeding 0.7 kPa, loses not more than 5.0% of its weight. Use 1 g.

Sulphated ash Not more than 3.0%, Appendix IX A.

Assay Triturate 60 mg with *dimethylformamide* and add, with shaking, sufficient *dimethylformamide* to produce 100 ml. Dilute 10 ml to 100 ml with *dimethylformamide*. Carry out the *biological assay of antibiotics*, Appendix XIV A. The precision of the assay is such that the fiducial limits of error are not less than 95% and not more than 105% of the estimated potency.

Storage Amphotericin should be kept in a well-closed container, protected from light and stored at a temperature of 2° to 8°. Amphotericin is sensitive to light in dilute solutions and is inactivated at low pH values.

Labelling The label states (1) the number of Units per mg; (2) the date after which the material is not intended to be used; (3) the conditions under which it should be stored.

Preparation
Amphotericin Lozenges
Action and use Antifungal.

Ampicillin ☆

C$_{16}$H$_{19}$N$_3$O$_4$S   349.4   *69-53-4*

Ampicillin is (6*R*)-6-(α-D-phenylglycylamino)-
penicillanic acid. It contains not less than 96.0
per cent and not more than 100.5 per cent of
C$_{16}$H$_{19}$N$_3$O$_4$S, calculated with reference to the
anhydrous substance.

Characteristics A white, crystalline powder; odourless or
almost odourless.

Solubility Sparingly soluble in *water*; practically insoluble
in *ethanol (96%)*, in *acetone*, in *chloroform*, in *ether* and in
fixed oils. It dissolves in dilute solutions of acids and of
alkali hydroxides.

Identification *Test A may be omitted if tests B, C, D and E
are carried out. Tests B, C, D and E may be omitted if test A
is carried out.*
A. The *infra-red absorption spectrum*, Appendix II A, is
concordant with the spectrum of *anhydrous ampicillin
EPCRS*.
B. Prepare a 0.01% w/v solution in *0.0067M mixed
phosphate buffer pH 7.0* (solution A). To 10 ml of solution
A add 0.5 ml of *dilute penicillinase solution* and allow to
stand for 10 minutes at 30° (solution B). To 5 ml of
solution A and to 5 ml of solution B, in separate test-
tubes, add 10 ml of *acetate buffer pH 4.6* and 5 ml of
0.0005M iodine VS. Mix the contents of each tube and
add, to each, 0.1 ml of *starch solution*. The mixture
obtained with solution A is blue; the mixture obtained
with solution B remains colourless.
C. Suspend 10 mg in 1 ml of *water* and add 2 ml of a
mixture of 2 volumes of *modified potassium cupri-tartrate
solution* and 6 volumes of *water*. A violet colour is
produced immediately.
D. Dissolve 10 mg in 2 ml of *water*. Heat on a water-bath
for 2 minutes and while heating add 0.5 ml of *mercury—
nitric acid solution*. A white precipitate is produced and the
supernatant liquid is yellow.
E. Yields the *reaction* characteristic of penicillins and
cephalosporins, Appendix VI.

Acidity pH of a 0.25% w/v solution, 3.5 to 5.5, Appendix
V L.

Clarity of solution Dissolve 1.0 g in 10 ml of *1M
hydrochloric acid*. Separately dissolve 1.0 g in 10 ml of *2M
ammonia*. The solutions, examined immediately after
dissolution, are not more opalescent than *reference
suspension II*, Appendix IV A.

Specific optical rotation In a 0.25% w/v solution, +280°
to +305°, Appendix V F.

Heavy metals 1.0 g complies with *limit test C for heavy
metals*, Appendix VII (20 ppm). Use 2 ml of *lead standard
solution (10 ppm Pb)* to prepare the standard.

N,N-Dimethylaniline Not more than 20 ppm when
determined by the following method. Prepare a
0.005% w/v solution of *naphthalene* (internal standard) in
cyclohexane (solution A). Dissolve 50 mg of N,N-
dimethylaniline in a mixture of 2 ml of *hydrochloric acid*
and 20 ml of *water* with shaking, add sufficient *water* to
produce 50 ml and dilute 5 ml of the resulting solution to
250 ml with *water* (solution B). Carry out the method for
gas chromatography, Appendix III B, using the following
solutions. For solution (1) add 5 ml of 1M *sodium
hydroxide* and 1 ml of solution A to 1 ml of solution B,
shake vigorously for 1 minute, centrifuge if necessary and
use the clear, upper layer. For solution (2) dissolve 1.00 g
of the substance being examined in 5 ml of 1M *sodium
hydroxide*, add 1 ml of *cyclohexane*, shake vigorously for 1
minute, centrifuge if necessary and use the clear, upper
layer. Prepare solution (3) in the same manner as solution
(2) but using 1 ml of solution A in place of the
cyclohexane.

The chromatographic procedure may be carried out
using a glass column (2 m × 2 mm) packed with *acid-
washed, silanised diatomaceous support* (Gas Chrom Q or
Chromosorb W/AW/DMCS is suitable) coated with
3% w/w of phenyl methyl silicone fluid (50% phenyl)
(OV-17 or XE-60 is suitable) and maintained at 120° with
both the inlet port temperature and the detector
temperature at 150°.

Sulphated ash Not more than 0.5%, Appendix IX A,
Method II. Use 1 g.

Water Not more than 2.0% w/w, Appendix IX C. Use
0.3 g.

Assay Dissolve 50 mg in 10 ml of *boric buffer pH 9.0* and
0.2 ml of *acetic anhydride* and stir for 3 minutes. Add
10 ml of 1M *sodium hydroxide* and allow to stand for 15
minutes. Add 10 ml of 1M *nitric acid* and 20 ml of *acetate
buffer pH 4.6* and titrate immediately with *0.02M
mercury(II) nitrate VS*. Titrate slowly so that the titration
takes about 15 minutes. Determine the end-point
potentiometrically using a platinum or mercury indicator
electrode and a mercury—mercury(I) sulphate reference
electrode. Disregard any preliminary inflection on the
titration curve. Each ml of 0.02M *mercury(II) nitrate VS* is
equivalent to 0.006988 g of total penicillins, calculated as
C$_{16}$H$_{19}$N$_3$O$_4$S.

To a further 0.25 g add 25 ml of *boric buffer pH 9.0* and
0.5 ml of *acetic anhydride*, stir for 3 minutes, add 10 ml of
acetate buffer pH 4.6 and titrate immediately with *0.02M
mercury(II) nitrate VS*. Determine the end-point
potentiometrically using a platinum or mercury indicator
electrode and a mercury—mercury(I) sulphate reference
electrode. Each ml of 0.02M *mercury(II) nitrate VS* is
equivalent to 0.006988 g of degradation products,
calculated as C$_{16}$H$_{19}$N$_3$O$_4$S.

Calculate the percentage content of total penicillins and
the percentage content of degradation products. The
content of ampicillin, C$_{16}$H$_{19}$N$_3$O$_4$S, is the difference
between the two percentages.

Storage Ampicillin should be kept in an airtight container
and stored at a temperature not exceeding 30°.

Labelling The label states (1) the date after which the
material is not intended to be used; (2) the conditions
under which it should be stored.

Preparations
Ampicillin Capsules
Ampicillin Oral Solution

Paediatric Ampicillin Tablets

Action and use Antibacterial.

The title of the monograph in the European Pharmacopœia is Anhydrous Ampicillin.

Ampicillin Sodium

$C_{16}H_{18}N_3NaO_4S$ 371.4   69-53-4

Ampicillin Sodium is sodium (6R)-6-(α-D-phenylglycylamino)penicillanate. It contains not less than 92.5 per cent and not more than 101.0 per cent of ampicillin, $C_{16}H_{18}N_3NaO_4S$, calculated with reference to the anhydrous substance.

Characteristics A white, crystalline or amorphous powder; hygroscopic.

Solubility Soluble in 2 parts of *water* and in 50 parts of *acetone*; slightly soluble in *chloroform*; practically insoluble in *ether*, in *liquid paraffin* and in *fixed oils*.

Identification A. The *infra-red absorption spectrum*, Appendix II A, is concordant with the *reference spectrum* of ampicillin sodium.
B. Place 0.1 ml of a 0.1% w/v solution of *ninhydrin* on a filter paper, dry at 105°, superimpose 0.1 ml of a 0.1% w/v solution of the substance being examined, heat for 5 minutes at 105° and allow to cool. A mauve colour is produced.
C. Suspend 10 mg in 1 ml of *water* and add 2 ml of a mixture of 2 ml of *potassium cupri-tartrate solution* and 6 ml of *water*. A magenta-violet colour is produced immediately.
D. Yields the *reactions* characteristic of sodium salts, Appendix VI.

Alkalinity pH of a 10% w/v solution, 8.0 to 10.0, Appendix V L, measured within 10 minutes of preparing the solution.

Clarity of solution A. To 1.0 g in a conical flask add slowly 10 ml of 1M *hydrochloric acid*, swirling continuously. Separately dissolve 1.0 g in 10 ml of *water*. Both solutions are not more opalescent than *reference solution II*, Appendix IV A, when examined immediately after preparation.
B. The *absorbance* of a 10% w/v solution at 430 nm is not more than 0.15, Appendix II B.

Specific optical rotation In a 0.25% w/v solution in a 0.02M solution of *potassium hydrogen phthalate*, +258° to +287°, Appendix V F.

Heavy metals 1.0 g complies with *limit test C for heavy metals*, Appendix VII (20 ppm). Use 2 ml of *lead standard solution (10 ppm Pb)* to prepare the standard.

Dichloromethane Not more than 0.2% cent w/w when determined by the method for *gas chromatography*, Appendix III B, using solutions in *water* containing (1) 0.020% v/v of *dichloromethane* and 0.020% v/v of *1,2-dichloroethane* (internal standard), (2) 10.0% w/v of the substance being examined and (3) 10.0% w/v of the substance being examined and 0.020% v/v of the internal standard.

The chromatographic procedure may be carried out using a glass column (1.5 m × 4 mm) packed with *acid-washed, silanised diatomaceous support* (100 to 120 mesh) coated with 10% w/w of polyethylene glycol 1000 and maintained at 60°.

Calculate the percentage w/w of dichloromethane, taking its weight per ml at 20° to be 1.325 g.

***N,N*-Dimethylaniline** Dissolve 75 mg of N,N-*diethyl-aniline* (internal standard) in a mixture of 2 ml of *hydrochloric acid* and 20 ml of *water* and add sufficient *water* to produce 50 ml. Dilute 2 ml of the resulting solution to 100 ml with *water* (solution A). Prepare a further solution in exactly the same manner as solution A but using 50 mg of N,N-*dimethylaniline* in place of the 75 mg of internal standard (solution B). Examine by the method for *gas chromatography*, Appendix III B, using the following solutions. For solution (1) add 1 ml of solution A to 1 ml of solution B, 1 ml of 1.25M *sodium hydroxide* and 1 ml of *cyclohexane*, shake vigorously for 1 minute, centrifuge if necessary and use the clear upper layer. For solution (2) dissolve 1.0 g of the substance being examined in 3 ml of 1.25M *sodium hydroxide*, add 1 ml of *cyclohexane*, shake vigorously for 1 minute, centrifuge if necessary and use the clear upper layer. Prepare solution (3) in exactly the same manner as solution (2) but using a mixture of 1 ml of solution A and 2 ml of 1.25M *sodium hydroxide* in place of the 3 ml of 1.25M *sodium hydroxide*.

The chromatographic procedure may be carried out using a glass column (1.5 m × 4 mm) packed with *acid-washed, silanised diatomaceous support* (80 to 100 mesh) coated with 3% w/w of phenyl methyl silicone fluid (50% phenyl) (OV-17 is suitable) and maintained at 80°.

In the chromatogram obtained with solution (3) the ratio of the area of any peak due to *N,N*-dimethylaniline to the area of the peak due to the internal standard is not greater than the corresponding ratio in the chromatogram obtained with solution (1).

Iodine-absorbing substances Dissolve 0.25 g in sufficient *water* to produce 100 ml. To 10 ml add 0.5 ml of 1M *hydrochloric acid* and 10 ml of 0.01M *iodine VS* and titrate immediately with 0.02M *sodium thiosulphate VS* using *starch mucilage*, added towards the end of the titration, as indicator. Repeat the operation without the substance being examined. The difference between the titrations represents the amount of iodine-absorbing substances present. Each ml of 0.02M *sodium thiosulphate VS* is equivalent to 0.0007392 g of iodine-absorbing substances. Calculate the percentage of iodine-absorbing substances in the substance being examined. The sum of the percentage of iodine-absorbing substances and that of $C_{16}H_{19}N_3O_4S$ as determined by the Assay, both calculated with reference to the anhydrous substance, is not less than 92.0%.

Related substances Carry out the method for *agarose—starch gel electrophoresis*, Appendix III F, using the following solutions in *phosphate buffer pH 7.0*. Solution (1) contains 0.00020% w/v of *benzylpenicillin sodium EPCRS*. Solution (2) is a solution of the substance being examined containing the equivalent of 0.020% w/v of ampicillin, $C_6H_{19}N_3O_4S$. The diameter of the zone of inhibition produced by solution (1) is greater than that of any corresponding zone of inhibition produced by solution (2).

Water Not more than 2.0% w/w, Appendix IX C. Use 0.3 g.

Assay Dissolve 0.17 g in sufficient *water* to produce 500 ml. Transfer 10 ml of the resulting solution to a 100-ml graduated flask, add 10 ml of *boric buffer pH 9.0* followed by 1 ml of *acetic anhydride—dioxan solution*, allow to stand for 5 minutes and add sufficient *water* to produce

100 ml. Place two 2-ml aliquots of this solution in separate stoppered tubes. To one tube add 10 ml of *imidazole—mercury reagent*, mix, stopper the tube and immerse in a water-bath at 60° for exactly 25 minutes, swirling occasionally. Remove from the water-bath and cool rapidly to 20° (solution A). To the second tube add 10 ml of *water* and mix (solution B). Without delay measure the *absorbances* of solutions A and B at the maximum at 325 nm, Appendix II B, using in the reference cell a mixture of 2 ml of *water* and 10 ml of *imidazole—mercury reagent* for solution A and *water* for solution B. Calculate the content of $C_{16}H_{18}N_3NaO_4S$ from the difference between the absorbances of solutions A and B, from the difference obtained by repeating the operation using 0.17 g of *ampicillin trihydrate BPCRS* in place of the substance being examined and from the declared equivalent content of $C_{16}H_{18}N_3NaO_4S$ in *ampicillin trihydrate BPCRS*.

Storage Ampicillin Sodium should be kept in a well-closed container and stored at a temperature not exceeding 25°. If it is intended for use in the manufacture of a parenteral dosage form, the container should be sterile and sealed so as to exclude micro-organisms.

Labelling The label states (1) the date after which the material is not intended to be used; (2) the conditions under which it should be stored; (3) whether or not it is intended for use in the manufacture of a parenteral dosage form.

Preparation
Ampicillin Injection

Action and use Antibacterial.

Ampicillin Sodium intended for use in the manufacture of a parenteral dosage form complies with the following additional requirements.

Pyrogens Complies with the *test for pyrogens*, Appendix XIV K. Use per kg of the rabbit's weight 1 ml of a solution in *water for injections* containing 6 mg per ml.

Sterility When intended for use in the manufacture of a parenteral dosage form without further sterilisation, complies with the *test for sterility*, Appendix XVI A.

Ampicillin Trihydrate ☆

$C_{16}H_{19}N_3O_4S,3H_2O$ 403.5   *7177-48-2*

Ampicillin Trihydrate is (6*R*)-6-(α-D-phenyl-glycylamino)penicillanic acid trihydrate. It contains not less than 96.0 per cent and not more than 100.5 per cent of $C_{16}H_{19}N_3O_4S$, calculated with reference to the anhydrous substance.

Characteristics A white, crystalline powder; odourless or almost odourless.

Solubility Slightly soluble in *water*; practically insoluble in *ethanol (96%)*, in *chloroform*, in *ether* and in fixed oils. It dissolves in dilute solutions of acids and of alkali hydroxides.

Identification *Test A may be omitted if tests B, C, D and E are carried out. Tests B, C, D and E may be omitted if test A is carried out.*

A. The *infra-red absorption spectrum*, Appendix II A, is concordant with the spectrum of *ampicillin trihydrate EPCRS*.

B. Prepare a 0.01% w/v solution in *0.0067M mixed phosphate buffer pH 7.0* (solution A). To 10 ml of solution A add 0.5 ml of *dilute penicillinase solution* and allow to stand for 10 minutes at 30° (solution B). To 5 ml of solution A and to 5 ml of solution B, in separate test-tubes, add 10 ml of *acetate buffer pH 4.6* and 5 ml of *0.0005M iodine VS*. Mix the contents of each tube and add, to each, 0.1 ml of *starch solution*. The mixture obtained with solution A is blue; the mixture obtained with solution B remains colourless.

C. Suspend 10 mg in 1 ml of *water* and add 2 ml of a mixture of 2 ml of *modified potassium cupri-tartrate solution* and 6 ml of *water*. A violet colour is produced immediately.

D. Dissolve 10 mg in 2 ml of *water*. Heat in a water-bath for 2 minutes and while heating add 0.5 ml of *mercury—nitric acid solution*. A white precipitate is produced and the supernatant liquid is yellow.

E. Yields the *reaction* characteristic of penicillins and cephalosporins, Appendix VI.

Acidity; Clarity of solution; Specific optical rotation; Heavy metals; *N,N*-Dimethylaniline; Sulphated ash Complies with the requirements stated under Ampicillin.

Water 12.0 to 15.0% w/w, Appendix IX C. Use 0.3 g.

Assay Carry out the Assay described under Ampicillin.

Storage Ampicillin Trihydrate should be kept in an airtight container and stored at a temperature not exceeding 30°.

Labelling The label states (1) the date after which the material is not intended to be used; (2) the conditions under which it should be stored.

Preparations
Ampicillin Capsules
Ampicillin Oral Suspension
Paediatric Ampicillin Tablets

Action and use Antibacterial.

Amylmetacresol

OH
C₅H₁₁
Me

$C_{12}H_{18}O$ 178.3   *1300-94-3*

Amylmetacresol is 5-methyl-2-pentylphenol. It contains not less than 96.0 per cent and not more than 104.0 per cent of $C_{12}H_{18}O$.

Characteristics A clear or almost clear liquid or a solid crystalline mass, colourless or slightly yellow when freshly prepared, which darkens on keeping; odour, characteristic.

Solubility Practically insoluble in *water*; soluble in *ethanol (96%)*, in *ether* and in fixed and volatile oils.

Identification A. The *infra-red absorption spectrum*, Appendix II A, is concordant with the *reference spectrum* of amylmetacresol.

B. The *light absorption*, Appendix II B, in the range 230 to 350 nm of a 0.004% w/v solution in *absolute ethanol* containing 2% v/v of 0.1M *hydrochloric acid* exhibits a maximum at 278 nm and a less well-defined maximum at 286 nm. The *absorbance* at 278 nm is about 0.53.

C. To 5 ml of a 0.5% v/v solution in *methanol* add 5 ml of *bromine water*. A yellow precipitate is produced.

D. *Freezing point*, about 22°, Appendix V B.

Weight per ml 0.947 to 0.953 g, Appendix V G.

Related substances Carry out the method for *gas chromatography*, Appendix III B, using the following solutions. Solution (1) contains 1% w/v of the substance being examined in *chloroform* and solution (2) is the substance being examined.

The chromatographic procedure may be carried out using a glass column (1.8 m × 3 mm) packed with *acid-washed, silanised diatomaceous support* (80 to 100 mesh) coated with 10% w/w of silicone grease (Apiezon L is suitable) and maintained at 180°.

In the chromatogram obtained with solution (2) the area of any *secondary peak* is not greater than 2% and the sum of the areas of any *secondary peaks* is not greater than 3% by *normalisation*.

Sulphated ash Not more than 0.1%, Appendix IX A.

Assay Dissolve 0.2 g in *absolute ethanol* containing 2% v/v of 0.1M *hydrochloric acid* and dilute to 100 ml with the same solvent. Dilute 2 ml of the solution to 100 ml with the same solvent and measure the *absorbance* of the resulting solution at the maximum at 278 nm, Appendix II B. Calculate the content of $C_{12}H_{18}O$ taking 132 as the value of A(1%, 1 cm) at the maximum at 278 nm.

Storage Amylmetacresol should be kept in a well-closed container and protected from light.

Action and use Antiseptic.

Amylobarbitone

$C_{11}H_{18}N_2O_3$ 226.3   *57-43-2*

Amylobarbitone is 5-ethyl-5-isopentylbarbituric acid.

Characteristics A white, crystalline powder; odourless or almost odourless.

Solubility Very slightly soluble in *water*; soluble in 5 parts of *ethanol (96%)*, in 20 parts of *chloroform* and in 6 parts of *ether*. It dissolves in aqueous solutions of alkali hydroxides and carbonates.

Identification A. The *infra-red absorption spectrum*, Appendix II A, is concordant with the *reference spectrum* of amylobarbitone. If the spectra are not concordant, dissolve a sufficient quantity in the minimum volume of *ethanol (25%)*, evaporate to dryness, dry the residue at 105° and prepare a new spectrum.

B. Dissolve 50 mg in 2 ml of a 0.2% w/v solution of *cobalt(II) acetate* in *methanol*, warm, add 50 mg of

powdered *sodium tetraborate* and heat to boiling. A bluish-violet colour is produced.

C. Triturate 0.6 g with 0.15 g of *anhydrous sodium carbonate* and 5 ml of *water*, add a solution of 0.45 g of *4-nitrobenzyl chloride* in 10 ml of *ethanol (96%)* and warm on a water-bath for 30 minutes. Cool, allow to stand for 1 hour, filter and wash the residue with 10 ml of 1M *sodium hydroxide* and then with *water*. The melting point of the residue, after recrystallisation from *ethanol (96%)*, is about 150° or about 168°, Appendix V A.

D. A saturated solution is acidic to *litmus solution*.

Melting point 155° to 158°, Appendix V A.

Neutral and basic substances Dissolve 1.0 g in a mixture of 2 ml of 5M *sodium hydroxide* and 13 ml of *water* and shake for 1 minute with 25 ml of *ether*. Wash the ether layer with three 5-ml quantities of *water*, evaporate the ether and dry the residue at 105° for 1 hour. The residue weighs not more than 3 mg.

Loss on drying When dried to constant weight at 105°, loses not more than 0.5% of its weight. Use 1 g.

Sulphated ash Not more than 0.1%, Appendix IX A.

Action and use Sedative and hypnotic.

In some countries the material described in this monograph may be known as Amobarbital.

Amylobarbitone Sodium ☆

$C_{11}H_{17}N_2NaO_3$ 248.3   *64-43-7*

Amylobarbitone Sodium is sodium 5-ethyl-5-isopentylbarbiturate. It contains not less than 98.5 per cent and not more than 102.0 per cent of $C_{11}H_{17}N_2NaO_3$, calculated with reference to the dried substance.

Characteristics A white, granular powder; odourless; hygroscopic.

Solubility Very soluble in *carbon dioxide-free water*, sometimes leaving a small insoluble residue; freely soluble in *ethanol (96%)*; practically insoluble in *chloroform* and in *ether*.

Identification *Test A may be omitted if tests B, C, D and E are carried out. Tests B and D may be omitted if tests A, C and E are carried out.*

A. Acidify 10 ml of a 10% w/v solution in *ethanol (50%)* with 2M *hydrochloric acid* and shake with 20 ml of *ether*. Separate the ether layer, wash with 10 ml of *water*, dry over *anhydrous sodium sulphate* and filter. Evaporate the filtrate to dryness and dry the residue at 100° to 105°. The *infra-red absorption spectrum* of the residue, Appendix II A, is concordant with the spectrum obtained using the residue similarly prepared from 0.1 g of *amobarbital sodium EPCRS*.

B. Complies with the test for *identification of barbiturates*, Appendix III A.

C. Determine the *melting point*, Appendix V A, Method I, of the residue obtained in test A (about 157°). Mix equal parts of the residue with the residue obtained from *amobarbital sodium EPCRS* and determine the *melting point* of the mixture. The difference between the melting points is not greater than 2°.

D. Yields the *reaction* characteristic of non-nitrogen substituted barbiturates, Appendix VI.

E. Yields *reaction A* characteristic of sodium salts, Appendix VI.

Alkalinity pH of a 10% w/v solution, ignoring any slight residue, not more than 11.0, Appendix V L.

Clarity and colour of solution A 10.0% w/v solution in *ethanol (50%)* is *clear*, Appendix IV A, and not more intensely coloured than *reference solution Y₇*, Appendix IV B, Method II.

Related substances Complies with the test for *related substances in barbiturates*, Appendix III A.

Loss on drying When dried to constant weight at 130°, loses not more than 3.0% of its weight. Use 0.5 g.

Assay Dissolve 0.2 g in 5 ml of *absolute ethanol*, add 10 ml of *silver nitrate—pyridine reagent* and titrate with 0.1M *ethanolic sodium hydroxide VS*, using 0.5 ml of *thymolphthalein solution* as indicator, until a pure blue colour is obtained. Repeat the operation without the substance being examined. The difference between the titrations represents the amount of sodium hydroxide required. Each ml of 0.1M *ethanolic sodium hydroxide VS* is equivalent to 0.02483 g of $C_{11}H_{17}N_2NaO_3$.

Storage Amylobarbitone Sodium should be kept in an airtight container.

Action and use Sedative and hypnotic.

The title of the monograph in the European Pharmacopœia is Amobarbital Sodium.

Anise Oil
Aniseed Oil

Anise Oil is obtained by distillation from the dried fruits of the star anise, *Illicium verum* Hook. f., or from the dried ripe fruits of *Pimpinella anisum* L.

Characteristics A clear, colourless or pale yellow liquid, visibly free from water; odour, that of the crushed fruit; taste, sweet and aromatic. Crystallises on cooling.

Freezing point Not below 15°, Appendix V B.

Optical rotation −2° to +1°, Appendix V F.

Refractive index 1.55 to 1.560, Appendix V E.

Solubility in ethanol Soluble, at 20°, in 3 volumes of *ethanol (90%)*; the solution may show an opalescence not greater than that produced on adding 0.5 ml of 0.1M *silver nitrate* to a mixture of 0.5 ml of 0.02M *sodium chloride* and 50 ml of *water*.

Weight per ml 0.978 to 0.992 g, Appendix V G.

Storage Anise Oil should be kept in a well-filled, well-closed container, protected from light and stored at a temperature not exceeding 25°. If the oil has crystallised, it should be melted and mixed before use.

Preparation
Concentrated Anise Water

Action and use Flavour.

Aniseed ☆
Anise

Aniseed is the dried fruit of *Pimpinella anisum* L.

Characteristics Odour, reminiscent of that of anethole.

Macroscopical Fruit generally whole (cremocarp) with a small fragment of the thin, rigid, slightly curved pedicel frequently attached; cremocarps ovoid or pyriform, slightly compressed laterally, yellowish-green or greenish-grey, 3 to 5 mm long, up to 3 mm wide; stylopod with two short reflexed stylar points. Mericarps attached by their tops to the carpophore with a plane commissural surface and convex dorsal surface, the latter covered with short warty trichomes visible using a lens; with five primary ridges, running longitudinally, comprising three dorsal ridges and two lateral ridges, non-prominent and lighter in colour.

Microscopical Transverse section of the mericarp showing an epicarp with numerous short covering trichomes, usually unicellular and conical, with thick walls and warty cuticle. On the dorsal side the mesocarp shows an almost continuous layer of vittae. Ridges containing a narrow bundle of fibro-vascular tissue. In the commissural zone narrow sclereids, longitudinally elongated with numerous pits. Endosperm, non-invaginated, made up of colourless, thick-walled polygonal cells containing many droplets of fatty oil, aleurone grains and micro-rosettes of calcium oxalate.

Identification Carry out the method for *thin-layer chromatography*, Appendix III A, using *silica gel GF254* as the coating substance and *toluene* as the mobile phase, but allowing the solvent front to ascend 10 cm above the line of application. Apply separately to the chromatoplate, at 2-cm intervals, 2 µl and 3 µl of solution (1) and 1 µl, 2 µl and 3 µl of solution (2). For solution (1) stir 0.1 g, in powder, with 2 ml of *dichloromethane* for 15 minutes, filter, evaporate the filtrate on a water-bath at about 60° and dissolve the residue in 0.5 ml of *toluene*. For solution (2) dissolve 3 µl of *anethole* and 40 µl of *olive oil* in 1 ml of *toluene*. After removal of the plate, allow it to dry in air and examine under *ultra-violet light (254 nm)*.

Dark spots corresponding to anethole are seen in the central part of the chromatogram. Spray the plate with a freshly prepared 20% w/v solution of *phosphomolybdic acid* in *ethanol (96%)*, using about 10 ml for a 200 mm × 200 mm plate, and heat at 120° for 5 minutes. The chromatogram obtained with 2 µl of solution (1) exhibits a blue spot due to anethole against a yellow background; the spot is intermediate in size between the corresponding spots obtained with 1 µl and 3 µl of solution (2). A blue spot due to triglycerides appears in the lower third of the chromatogram obtained with solution (1) corresponding in position to the blue spot due to triglycerides of olive oil in the chromatogram obtained with solution (2).

Foreign matter Not more than 2%, Appendix XI D, Test B.

Acid-insoluble ash Not more than 2.5%, Appendix XI K, Method II.

Sulphated ash Not more than 12.0%, Appendix IX A, Method II. Use 2 g, in powder.

Volatile oil Not less than 2.0% v/w when determined by the method for the *determination of essential oils in vegetable drugs*, Appendix XI E. Use 100 ml of *water* as the distillation liquid in a 250-ml round-bottomed flask and use 0.5 ml of *xylene* in the graduated tube. Use 10 g of the substance being examined in *coarse powder* immediately after grinding and distil for 2 hours.

Water Not more than 7.0% w/w, Appendix IX C, Method II. Use 20 g, in powder.

Storage Aniseed should be protected from light and moisture.

Action and use Carminative.

Powdered Aniseed

Powdered Aniseed is Aniseed in powder.

Characteristics Greenish-yellow or brownish-green. Diagnostic structures, whole or broken trichomes, mostly unicellular, sometimes curved, with blunt apex and warty cuticle; fragments of epidermis with striated cuticle, occasional *anomocytic* stomata, fragments of numerous narrow, branched vittae, fragments of endosperm containing aleurone grains and micro-rosettes of calcium oxalate; oblong sclereids from the commissural zone and bundles of sclerenchymatous fibres from the carpophore and the pedicel. Starch absent.

Identification Complies with the test described under Aniseed.

Acid-insoluble ash; Sulphated ash; Water Complies with the requirements stated under Aniseed.

Storage Powdered Aniseed should be protected from light and moisture.

Action and use Carminative.

Apomorphine Hydrochloride ☆

$C_{17}H_{17}NO_2,HCl,\frac{1}{2}H_2O$ 312.8   *41372-20-7*

Apomorphine Hydrochloride is (*R*)-10,11-dihydroxy-6a-aporphine hydrochloride hemihydrate. It contains not less than 98.0 per cent and not more than 101.0 per cent of $C_{17}H_{17}NO_2,HCl$, calculated with reference to the dried substance.

Characteristics White or faintly yellow to green-tinged greyish crystals or crystalline powder; on exposure to air and light the green tinge becomes more pronounced.

Solubility Soluble in 50 parts of *water* and in 50 parts of *ethanol (96%)*; practically insoluble in *chloroform*; very slightly soluble in *ether*.

Identification A. The *light absorption*, Appendix II B, in the range 230 to 350 nm of a 0.001% w/v solution in 0.1M *hydrochloric acid* exhibits a maximum at 273 nm and a shoulder at 300 to 310 nm. The A(1%, 1 cm) at 273 nm is 530 to 570.

B. To 5 ml of a 1% w/v solution add *sodium hydrogen carbonate solution* until a permanent, white precipitate is obtained; the precipitate slowly becomes greenish. Add 0.25 ml of 0.05M *iodine VS* and shake; the precipitate becomes greyish-green. The precipitate is soluble in *ether* giving a purple solution, in *chloroform* giving a violet-blue solution and in *ethanol (96%)* giving a blue solution.

C. Mix 2 ml of a 1% w/v solution with 0.1 ml of 2M *nitric acid* and filter. The filtrate yields *reaction A* characteristic of chlorides, Appendix VI.

Acidity pH of a 1% w/v solution, prepared without heating, 4.0 to 5.0, Appendix V L.

Clarity and colour of solution 10 ml of a 1.0% w/v solution, prepared without heating, is *clear*, Appendix IV A, and not more intensely coloured than a reference solution prepared in the following manner. Dissolve 5 mg in 100 ml of *water*, transfer 1 ml to a test-tube, add 6 ml of *water*, 1 ml of *sodium hydrogen carbonate solution* and 0.5 ml of 0.05M *iodine VS*, allow to stand for 30 seconds, add 0.6 ml of 0.1M *sodium thiosulphate* and dilute to 10 ml with *water*.

Specific optical rotation In a 1% w/v solution in 0.02M *hydrochloric acid*, −48° to −52°, Appendix V F.

Morphine Carry out the method for *thin-layer chromatography*, Appendix III A, using *silica gel G* as the coating substance and a mixture of 30 volumes of *acetonitrile*, 30 volumes of *dichloromethane*, 30 volumes of *ethyl acetate*, 5 volumes of *anhydrous formic acid* and 5 volumes of *water* as the mobile phase. Apply separately to the chromatoplate 5 μl of each of two solutions of the substance being examined in *methanol* containing (1) 0.20% w/v and (2) 0.004% w/v. After removal of the plate, dry it in a current of cold air until all traces of solvent have disappeared and spray with a 3% w/v solution of *sodium nitrite*. Expose the plate to ammonia vapour for a few minutes and allow to stand in daylight for 1 hour. In the chromatogram obtained with solution (1), there is no reddish-orange spot with an Rf value of 0.3 to 0.5 relative to the principal spot (about 2% of morphine). The test is not valid unless there is a clearly visible spot in the chromatogram obtained with solution (2).

Loss on drying When dried to constant weight at 100° to 105°, loses 2.5 to 4.2% of its weight. Use 0.5 g.

Sulphated ash Not more than 0.1%, Appendix IX A, Method II. Use 0.5 g.

Assay Dissolve 0.25 g in 5 ml of *anhydrous formic acid*. Add 30 ml of *anhydrous glacial acetic acid* and 5 ml of *mercury(II) acetate solution* and carry out Method I for *non-aqueous titration*, Appendix VIII A, determining the end-point potentiometrically. Each ml of 0.1M *perchloric acid VS* is equivalent to 0.03038 g of $C_{17}H_{17}NO_2,HCl$.

Storage Apomorphine Hydrochloride should be kept in an airtight container and protected from light.

Action and use Emetic.

Aprotinin

Aprotinin is a polypeptide consisting of fifty-eight amino acids that inhibits stoichiometrically the activity of certain proteolytic enzymes such as chymotrypsin, kallikrein, plasmin and trypsin. It is obtained by extraction from bovine tissues and purified by a suitable process such as gel filtration. It is prepared in conditions designed to minimise the risk of microbial contamination.

Aprotinin is presented either as a liquid or as a solid. When presented as a liquid, it contains not less than 3.0 Units per mg calculated with reference to the dry residue and not less than 15.0 Units per ml. When presented as a solid, it contains not less than 3.0 Units per mg calculated with reference to the dried substance.

Characteristics When presented as a liquid, a clear, colourless solution. When presented as a solid, an almost white powder; hygroscopic.

Solubility When presented as a solid, soluble in *water* and in solutions isotonic with blood; practically insoluble in organic solvents.

Identification A. Carry out the method for *thin-layer chromatography*, Appendix III A, using *silica gel G* as the coating substance but allowing the solvent front to ascend 12 cm above the line of application. Use a 10% w/v solution of *sodium acetate* in a mixture of 50 volumes of *glacial acetic acid* and 40 volumes of *water* as the mobile phase. Apply separately to the chromatoplate 10 μl of each of the following solutions. For solution (1) prepare a dilution of the liquid or a solution of the solid being examined containing 15 Units per ml. For solution (2) use *aprotinin solution BPCRS*. After removal of the plate, allow it to dry in air and spray with a solution containing 0.1 g of *ninhydrin* in a mixture of 70 ml of *absolute ethanol*, 21 ml of *glacial acetic acid* and 6 ml of a 1% w/v solution of *copper(II) chloride*. Dry the plate at 60°. The principal spot in the chromatogram obtained with solution (1) corresponds in position, colour and size to that in the chromatogram obtained with solution (2).
B. Dilute 1 ml of solution (1) from test A to 50 ml with *phosphate buffer pH 7.2*. Mix 1 ml of the resulting solution with 1 ml of a solution containing 0.01% of *trypsin EPCRS* in 0.002M *hydrochloric acid* and allow to stand for 10 minutes. Add 1 ml of a 0.2% solution of *casein* in *phosphate buffer pH 7.2* and incubate at 35° for 30 minutes. Cool in ice and add 0.5 ml of a mixture of 50 volumes of *absolute ethanol*, 49 volumes of *water* and 1 volume of *glacial acetic acid*. Shake and allow to stand at room temperature for 15 minutes; the solution becomes cloudy. Repeat the operation using *phosphate buffer pH 7.2* in place of the solution being examined; the solution remains clear.

Clarity of solution Prepare a dilution of the liquid or a solution of the solid being examined containing 15 Units per ml (solution A). The solution is *clear*, Appendix IV A.

Light absorption The *light absorption* of solution A diluted to contain 3 Units per ml, Appendix II B, exhibits a maximum at 277 nm. The *absorbance* at 277 nm is not more than 0.80.

Proteins of higher molecular weight Carry out the method for *size-exclusion chromatography*, Appendix III C, equilibrating the column with 2M *acetic acid*. When presented as a liquid, freeze dry a volume containing 300 Units at −30° at a pressure of 2.7 Pa; the procedure, including a period of drying at 15° to 25°, should take 6 to 12 hours. Dissolve the dry residue thus obtained in 1 ml

of 2M *acetic acid* and apply to the top of the column. When presented as a solid, dissolve a quantity containing 300 Units in 1 ml of 2M *acetic acid* and apply to the top of the column.

The chromatographic procedure may be carried out using (a) a column (80 to 100 cm × 25 mm) packed with a cross-linked dextran suitable for fractionation of proteins in the range of molecular weights from 1,500 to 30,000 (Sephadex G-50-SF is suitable), (b) 2M *acetic acid* as the mobile phase and (c) a detection wavelength of 277 nm.

Collect the eluate in 2-ml fractions. No peak is eluted in advance of the principal peak.

Dry residue When presented as a liquid evaporate 25 ml to dryness, dry the residue at 110° for 15 hours and weigh. Calculate the number of Units per mg of dry residue from the weight thus obtained and the activity determined in the Assay.

Loss on drying Aprotinin presented as a solid when dried to constant weight over *phosphorus pentoxide* at a pressure of 1.5 to 2.5 kPa, loses not more than 6.0% of its weight. Use 0.1 g.

Assay Carry out the *assay of aprotinin*, Appendix XIV E6. The estimated activity is not less than 90% and not more than 110% of the stated activity.

Storage Aprotinin should be kept in an airtight, tamper-evident container.

Labelling The label states (1) the number of Units in the container; (2) the date after which the material is not intended to be used; (3) the conditions under which it should be stored.

When presented as a liquid, the label also states the number of Units per ml and the number of Units per mg of the dry residue.

When presented as a solid, the label also states the number of Units per mg.

Action and Use Proteolytic enzyme inhibitor.

Preparation
Aprotinin Injection

Aprotinin intended for use in the manufacture of a parenteral dosage form complies with the following additional requirement.

Histamine Not more than 0.2 μg of histamine per 3 Units when determined by the *test for histamine*, Appendix XIV N.

Aprotinin intended for use in the manufacture of a parenteral dosage form without further appropriate procedure for the removal of pyrogens complies with the following additional requirement.

Pyrogens Complies with the *test for pyrogens*, Appendix XIV K. Use per kg of the rabbit's weight 1 ml of a solution containing 15 Units per ml. When presented as a liquid, dilute if necessary with a sufficient volume of *water for injections*. When presented as a solid, dissolve in a sufficient volume of *water for injections*.

Aprotinin intended for use in the manufacture of a parenteral dosage form without further appropriate procedure of sterilisation complies with the following additional requirement.

Sterility Complies with the *test for sterility*, Appendix XVI A.

Arachis Oil ☆

Ground-nut Oil; Peanut Oil

Arachis Oil is the fixed oil obtained from the shelled seeds of *Arachis hypogaea* L. and refined.

Characteristics A clear, yellowish, viscous oil; odourless. It solidifies at about 2°.

Solubility Very slightly soluble in *ethanol (96%)*; miscible with *chloroform*, with *ether* and with *petroleum spirit (boiling range, 40° to 60°)*.

Identification Carry out the test for *identification of fixed oils by thin-layer chromatography*, Appendix X N. The chromatogram obtained from the oil being examined is concordant with the *typical chromatogram* for arachis oil.

Acid value Not more than 0.6, Appendix X B.

Alkaline impurities Complies with the test for *alkaline impurities*, Appendix X N.

Peroxide value Not more than 5.0, Appendix X F.

Relative density 0.912 to 0.918, Appendix V G.

Unsaponifiable matter Not more than 1.0% w/w, Appendix X H, Method II. Use 5 g.

Foreign fixed oils Carry out the test for *foreign oils by gas chromatography*, Appendix X N. The fatty-acid fraction of the oil has the following composition.

Saturated fatty acids of chain length less than C_{16} Not more than 0.4%.
Palmitic acid 7.0 to 16.0%.
Stearic acid 1.3 to 6.5%.
Oleic acid 35.0 to 72.0%.
Linoleic acid (equivalent chain length on polyethylene glycol adipate 18.9) 13.0 to 43.0%.
Linolenic acid (equivalent chain length on polyethylene glycol adipate 19.7) Not more than 0.6%.
Arachidic acid 1.0 to 3.0%.
Gadoleic acid (equivalent chain length on polyethylene glycol adipate 20.3) 0.5 to 2.1%.
Behenic acid 1.0 to 5.0%.
Erucic acid (equivalent chain length on polyethylene glycol adipate 22.3) Not more than 0.5%.
Lignoceric acid 0.5 to 3.0%.

The ratio of linoleic acid to behenic acid is not more than 13.

Semi-drying oils To 1.0 g of the oil being examined add 5 ml of a mixture of 3 volumes of *2M ethanolic potassium hydroxide* and 1 volume of *ethanol (96%)*, boil under a reflux condenser for 5 minutes, add 1.5 ml of *5.4M acetic acid* and 50 ml of *ethanol (70%)* and heat until the solution is clear. Cool very slowly with a thermometer in the liquid. The temperature at which the liquid becomes cloudy is not less than 36°.

Sesame oil Shake 10 ml with 5 ml of a mixture of 0.5 volume of a 0.35% v/v solution of *furfuraldehyde* in *acetic anhydride* and 4.5 volumes of *acetic anhydride* for 1 minute, filter the solution through a filter paper impregnated with *acetic anhydride* and add 0.2 ml of *sulphuric acid*. No bluish-green colour is produced.

Storage Arachis Oil should be kept in a well-filled, well-closed container and protected from light. Arachis Oil intended for use in the manufacture of a parenteral dosage form should be kept in a glass container.

Labelling The label states if the contents of the container are suitable for use in the manufacture of a parenteral dosage form.

Arachis Oil intended for use in the manufacture of a parenteral dosage form complies with the above requirements with the following modification and with the additional test for Water.

Acid value Not more than 0.5, Appendix X B.

Water Not more than 0.3%, Appendix IX C. Use 3 g.

Ascorbic Acid ☆

Vitamin C

$C_6H_8O_6$ 176.1 *50-81-7*

Ascorbic Acid is L-ascorbic acid. It contains not less than 99.0 per cent and not more than 100.5 per cent of $C_6H_8O_6$.

Characteristics Colourless crystals or a white or almost white, crystalline powder which discolours on exposure to air and moisture; odourless or almost odourless. It melts at about 190°, with decomposition.

Solubility Soluble in 3.5 parts of *water* and in 25 parts of *ethanol (96%)*; practically insoluble in *chloroform*, in *ether* and in *petroleum spirit (boiling range, 40° to 60°)*.

Identification *Test A may be omitted if tests B, C and D are carried out. Tests B and C may be omitted if tests A and D are carried out.*
A. The *infra-red absorption spectrum*, Appendix II A, is concordant with the spectrum of *ascorbic acid EPCRS*. Examine as discs containing 1 mg.
B. Dissolve 0.1 g in sufficient *water* to produce 100 ml and dilute 1 ml to 100 ml with *0.01M hydrochloric acid*. The *light absorption* of the resulting solution, Appendix II B, when examined immediately, exhibits a maximum only at 243 nm. The A(1%, 1 cm) at 243 nm is 545 to 585.
C. To 1 ml of a 5% w/v solution add about 0.2 ml of *2M nitric acid* and 0.2 ml of *0.1M silver nitrate*. A grey precipitate is produced.
D. pH of a 5% w/v solution, 2.1 to 2.6, Appendix V L.

Clarity and colour of solution A 5.0% w/v solution in *carbon dioxide-free water* is *clear*, Appendix IV A, and not more intensely coloured than *reference solution BY_7*, Appendix IV B, Method II.

Specific optical rotation In a 10% w/v solution, +20.5° to +21.5°, Appendix V F.

Copper Not more than 5 ppm of Cu when determined by *atomic absorption spectrophotometry*, Appendix II D, using a solution prepared by dissolving 2 g of the substance being examined in 25 ml of *0.1M nitric acid* and measuring at 324.8 nm. Use *copper solution ASp*, diluted if necessary with *0.1M nitric acid*, to prepare the standard.

Heavy metals 2.0 g complies with *limit test D for heavy metals*, Appendix VII (10 ppm). Use 2 ml of *lead standard solution (10 ppm Pb)* to prepare the standard.

Iron Not more than 2 ppm of Fe when determined by *atomic absorption spectrophotometry*, Appendix II D, using a 20% w/v solution in *0.1M nitric acid* and measuring at

248.3 nm. Use *iron solution ASp*, diluted if necessary with 0.1M *nitric acid*, to prepare the standard.

Oxalic acid Dissolve 0.25 g in 5 ml of *water* and neutralise to *litmus paper* using 2M *sodium hydroxide*. Add 1 ml of 2M *acetic acid* and 0.5 ml of 0.5M *calcium chloride*. After allowing to stand for 60 minutes any opalescence in the test solution is not more intense than that in a solution prepared at the same time and in the following manner. Dissolve 70 mg of *oxalic acid* in 500 ml of *water* and to 5 ml of the resulting solution add 1 ml of 2M *acetic acid* and 0.5 ml of 0.5M *calcium chloride* (0.2%).

Sulphated ash Not more than 0.1%, Appendix IX A, Method II. Use 1 g.

Assay Dissolve 0.15 g in a mixture of 80 ml of *carbon dioxide-free water* and 10 ml of 1M *sulphuric acid*. Titrate with 0.05M *iodine VS*, using 1 ml of *starch solution* as indicator, until a persistent violet-blue colour is obtained. Each ml of 0.05M *iodine VS* is equivalent to 0.008805 g of $C_6H_8O_6$.

Storage Ascorbic Acid should be kept in a well-closed container, free from contact with metal and protected from light. Solutions of Ascorbic Acid deteriorate rapidly in contact with air.

Preparation
Ascorbic Acid Tablets

Aspirin ☆
Acetylsalicylic Acid

Note The name Aspirin may be used freely in many countries including the United Kingdom. In countries where exclusive proprietary rights in this name are claimed, the official title is Acetylsalicylic Acid.

$C_9H_8O_4$ 180.2   *50-78-2*

Aspirin is *O*-acetylsalicylic acid. It contains not less than 99.5 per cent and not more than 101.0 per cent of $C_9H_8O_4$, calculated with reference to the dried substance.

Characteristics Colourless crystals or a white, crystalline powder; odourless or almost odourless. It melts at about 143°, Appendix V A, Method VI.

Solubility Slightly soluble in *water*; soluble in 7 parts of *ethanol (96%)*, in 17 parts of *chloroform* and in 20 parts of *ether*.

Identification *Test A may be omitted if tests B, C and D are carried out. Tests C and D may be omitted if tests A and B are carried out.*
A. The *infra-red absorption spectrum*, Appendix II A, is concordant with the spectrum of *acetylsalicylic acid EPCRS*.
B. Heat 0.2 g to boiling for 3 minutes with 4 ml of 2M *sodium hydroxide*, cool, add 5 ml of 1M *sulphuric acid* and filter. The *melting point* of the precipitate, after washing and drying at 100° to 105°, is 156° to 161°, Appendix V A, Method I.

C. Mix 0.1 g with 0.5 g of *calcium hydroxide* and heat; the fumes produced turn *nitrobenzaldehyde paper* yellowish-green or bluish-green. Moisten the paper with 2M *hydrochloric acid*; the colour changes to blue.
D. Heat 20 mg of the precipitate obtained in test B with 10 ml of *water* and cool. The resulting solution yields *reaction A* characteristic of salicylates, Appendix VI.

Clarity and colour of solution A solution of 1.0 g in 9 ml of *ethanol (96%)* is *clear*, Appendix IV A, and *colourless*, Appendix IV B, Method II.

Heavy metals Dissolve 0.75 g in 9 ml of *acetone* and dilute to 15 ml with *water*. 12 ml of the solution complies with *limit test B for heavy metals*, Appendix VII (20 ppm). Use a solution prepared by diluting *lead standard solution (100 ppm Pb)* with a mixture of 9 volumes of *acetone* and 6 volumes of *water* to contain 1 µg of Pb per ml as the standard.

Salicylic acid Dissolve 0.1 g in 5 ml of *ethanol (96%)* and 15 ml of iced *water* and add 0.05 ml of a 0.5% w/v solution of *iron(III) chloride*. After 1 minute the colour of the solution is not more intense than that of a solution prepared at the same time by adding a mixture of 4 ml of *ethanol (96%)*, 0.1 ml of 5M *acetic acid*, 15 ml of *water* and 0.5 ml of a 0.5% w/v solution of *iron(III) chloride* to 1 ml of a 0.005% w/v solution of *salicyclic acid* in *ethanol (96%)*.

Related substances Dissolve 0.15 g in 10 ml of 0.1M *tetrabutylammonium hydroxide* in *propan-2-ol* and allow to stand for 10 minutes. Add 8 ml of 0.1M *hydrochloric acid* and 20 ml of a 1.9% w/v solution of *sodium tetraborate* and mix. Add with constant swirling 2 ml of a 1% w/v solution of *dimethylaminoantipyrine* and 2 ml of *potassium hexacyanoferrate(III) solution*. After 2 minutes dilute to 100 ml with *water* and allow to stand for 20 minutes. The *absorbance* at 505 nm of a 2-cm layer of the resulting solution is not more than 0.25, Appendix II B.

Loss on drying When dried to constant weight over *phosphorus pentoxide* at a pressure of 1.5 to 2.5 kPa, loses not more than 0.5% of its weight. Use 1 g.

Sulphated ash Not more than 0.1%, Appendix IX A, Method II. Use 1 g.

Assay Dissolve 1 g in 10 ml of *ethanol (96%)*, add 50 ml of 0.5M *sodium hydroxide VS*, stopper the flask and allow to stand for 1 hour. Add 0.2 ml of *dilute phenolphthalein solution* and titrate with 0.5M *hydrochloric acid VS*. Repeat the operation without the substance being examined. The difference between the titrations represents the amount of sodium hydroxide required. Each ml of 0.5M *sodium hydroxide VS* is equivalent to 0.04504 g of $C_9H_8O_4$.

Storage Aspirin should be kept in an airtight container. It is stable in dry air but in contact with moisture it is gradually hydrolysed to acetic and salicylic acids.

Preparations
Aspirin Tablets
Dispersible Aspirin Tablets
Soluble Aspirin Tablets
Aspirin and Caffeine Tablets
Co-codaprin Tablets
Dispersible Co-codaprin Tablets

Action and use Analgesic; antipyretic.

The title of the monograph in the European Pharmacopœia is Acetylsalicylic Acid.

Atenolol

OH
|
O·CH₂·CH·CH₂·NHPrⁱ

CH₂·CONH₂

C₁₄H₂₂N₂O₃   266.3   29122-68-7

Atenolol is 4-(2-hydroxy-3-isopropylamino-propoxy)phenylacetamide. It contains not less than 99.0 per cent and not more than 101.0 per cent of C₁₄H₂₂N₂O₃, calculated with reference to the dried substance.

Characteristics A white or almost white powder; odourless or almost odourless.

Solubility Sparingly soluble in *water*; soluble in *absolute ethanol*; practically insoluble in *ether*.

Identification A. The *infra-red absorption spectrum*, Appendix II A, is concordant with the *reference spectrum* of atenolol.
B. The *light absorption*, Appendix II B, in the range 230 to 350 nm of a 0.01% w/v solution in *methanol* exhibits maxima at 275 nm and 282 nm. The *absorbance* at 275 nm is about 0.54 and at 282 nm is about 0.46.

Melting point 152° to 155°, Appendix V A.

Chloride Dissolve 50 mg in 15 ml of *water*. The resulting solution complies with the *limit test for chlorides*, Appendix VII (0.1%).

Related substances Carry out the method for *high-performance liquid chromatography*, Appendix III D, using the following solutions. For solution (1) dilute 1 volume of solution (2) to 200 volumes with *methanol (40%)*. For solution (2) dissolve 0.1 g of the substance being examined in sufficient *methanol (40%)* to produce 10 ml. Solution (3) contains 1% w/v of *atenolol impurity standard BPCRS* in *methanol (40%)*.

The chromatographic procedure may be carried out using (a) a stainless steel column (20 cm × 5 mm) packed with *stationary phase C* (5 μm) (Hypersil ODS is suitable), (b) as the mobile phase with a flow rate of 1 ml per minute a mixture of 600 volumes of a 0.166% w/v solution of *sodium octyl sulphate*, 10 volumes of *sulphuric acid (10%)* and sufficient *methanol* to produce a chromatogram with solution (3) closely resembling that of the reference chromatogram supplied with the impurity standard (400 volumes of *methanol* is usually suitable) and that complies with the system validity test and (c) a detection wavelength of 226 nm.

In the chromatogram obtained with solution (2) any *secondary peak* with a retention time greater than that of the peak due to 4-hydroxyphenylacetamide and *p*-2,3-di-hydroxypropoxyphenylacetamide (diol) in the chromatogram obtained with solution (3) is not greater than the area of the peak in the chromatogram obtained with solution (1) and the sum of the areas of any such secondary peaks is not greater than 1.5 times the area of the peak in the chromatogram obtained with solution (1).

The test is not valid unless in the chromatogram obtained with solution (3) a peak due to 4-hydroxyphenyl-acetamide and *p*-2,3-dihydroxypropoxyphenylacetamide elutes within 5 minutes of injection and peaks due to *p,p'*-

[*N*-isopropyl-3,3'-iminobis(2-hydroxypropoxy)]bis(phenyl-acetamide) (tertiary amine) and 4-(2-hydroxy-3-isopropylaminopropoxy)phenylacetic acid (blocker acid) elute after the principal peak. Adjust the setting of the amplifier so that the peak due to tertiary amine in the chromatogram obtained with solution (3) is between 30 and 80% of full-scale deflection on the chart paper. Measure the height (*a*) of the peak due to tertiary amine and the height (*b*) of the lowest part of the curve separating this peak from the principal peak. The test is not valid unless *a* is greater than 3*b*.

Loss on drying When dried to constant weight at 105°, loses not more than 0.5% of its weight. Use 1 g.

Sulphated ash Not more than 0.2%, Appendix IX A.

Assay Carry out Method I for *non-aqueous titration*, Appendix VIII A, using 0.6 g and *1-naphtholbenzein solution* as indicator. Each ml of 0.1M *perchloric acid VS* is equivalent to 0.02663 g of C₁₄H₂₂N₂O₃.

Preparation
Atenolol Tablets

Action and use Beta-adrenoceptor antagonist.

Atropine Methobromide ☆

Me   Me
N⁺

H   Br⁻

OCO·CH·CH₂OH
|
Ph

C₁₈H₂₆BrNO₃   384.3   2870-71-5

Atropine Methobromide is (1*R*,3*r*,5*S*)-8-methyl-3-tropoyloxytropanium bromide. It contains not less than 99.0 per cent and not more than 101.0 per cent of C₁₈H₂₆BrNO₃, calculated with reference to the dried substance.

Characteristics Colourless crystals or a white, crystalline powder. It melts at about 219°, with decomposition.

Solubility Freely soluble in *water*; sparingly soluble in *ethanol (96%)*; practically insoluble in *ether*.

Identification *Test A may be omitted if tests B, C, D and E are carried out. Tests B, C and D may be omitted if tests A and E are carried out.*
A. The *infra-red absorption spectrum*, Appendix II A, is concordant with the spectrum of *methylatropine bromide EPCRS*.
B. Complies with the test for Optical rotation.
C. To 1 mg add 0.2 ml of *fuming nitric acid* and evaporate to dryness on a water-bath. Dissolve the residue in 2 ml of *acetone* and add 0.1 ml of a 3% w/v solution of *potassium hydroxide* in *methanol*. A violet colour is produced.
D. To 5 ml of a 5% w/v solution add 2 ml of 2M *sodium hydroxide*. No precipitate is produced.
E. Yields *reaction A* characteristic of bromides, Appendix VI.

Acidity or alkalinity To 10 ml of a 5.0% w/v solution in *carbon dioxide-free water* add 0.1 ml of *dilute phenolphthalein solution*; the solution is colourless. Add 0.5 ml of 0.01M *sodium hydroxide*; the solution is red.

Clarity and colour of solution A 5.0% w/v solution in *carbon dioxide-free water* is *clear*, Appendix IV A, and not more intensely coloured than *reference solution B₉*, Appendix IV B, Method II.

Optical rotation In a 10% w/v solution, −0.25° to +0.05°, Appendix V F, determined using a 2-dm tube.

Apomethylatropine Determine the *absorbance*, Appendix II B, of a 0.1% w/v solution in 0.01M *hydrochloric acid* at the maxima at 252 nm and 257 nm. The ratio of the absorbance at 257 nm to that at 252 nm is not less than 1.19.

Related substances Carry out the method for *thin-layer chromatography*, Appendix III A, using *silica gel G* as the coating substance and a mixture of 60 volumes of *ethyl acetate*, 15 volumes of *anhydrous formic acid*, 15 volumes of *water* and 10 volumes of *methanol* as the mobile phase. Apply separately to the chromatoplate 5 µl of each of two solutions of the substance being examined in *methanol (90%)* containing (1) 4.0% w/v and (2) 0.020% w/v. After removal of the plate, dry it at 100° to 105° until the odour of the solvent is no longer detectable, allow to cool and spray with *dilute potassium iodobismuthate solution* until spots appear. Any *secondary spot* in the chromatogram obtained with solution (1) is not more intense than the spot in the chromatogram obtained with solution (2).

Loss on drying When dried to constant weight at 100° to 105°, loses not more than 0.5% of its weight. Use 0.5 g.

Sulphated ash Not more than 0.1%, Appendix IX A, Method II. Use the residue from the test for Loss on drying.

Assay Dissolve 0.3 g in 50 ml of *anhydrous glacial acetic acid*, warming slightly if necessary, add 5 ml of *mercury(II) acetate solution* and carry out Method I for *non-aqueous titration*, Appendix VIII A, determining the end-point potentiometrically. Each ml of 0.1M *perchloric acid VS* is equivalent to 0.03843 g of $C_{18}H_{26}BrNO_3$.

Storage Atropine Methobromide should be kept in a well-closed container and protected from light.

Action and use Antispasmodic.

The title of the monograph in the European Pharmacopœia is Methylatropine Bromide.

Atropine Methonitrate ☆

$C_{18}H_{26}N_2O_6$ 366.4   *52-88-0*

Atropine Methonitrate is (1*R*,3*r*,5*S*)-8-methyl-3-tropoyloxytropanium nitrate. It contains not less than 99.0 per cent and not more than 101.0 per cent of $C_{18}H_{26}N_2O_6$, calculated with reference to the dried substance.

Characteristics Colourless crystals or a white, crystalline powder. It melts at about 167°.

Solubility Freely soluble in *water*; soluble in 13 parts of *ethanol (96%)*; practically insoluble in *chloroform* and in *ether*.

Identification *Test A may be omitted if tests B, C, D and E are carried out. Tests B, C and D may be omitted if tests A and E are carried out.*

A. The *infra-red absorption spectrum*, Appendix II A, is concordant with the spectrum of *methylatropine nitrate EPCRS*.

B. Complies with the test for Optical rotation.

C. To 1 mg add 0.2 ml of *fuming nitric acid* and evaporate to dryness on a water-bath. Dissolve the residue in 2 ml of *acetone* and add 0.25 ml of a 3% w/v solution of *potassium hydroxide* in *methanol*. A violet colour is produced.

D. To 5 ml of a 2.5% w/v solution add 2 ml of 2M *sodium hydroxide*. No precipitate is produced.

E. To 0.05 ml of *diphenylamine solution* add 0.05 ml of a 0.5% w/v solution of the substance being examined. An intense blue colour is produced.

Acidity or alkalinity To 10 ml of a 5.00% w/v solution in *carbon dioxide-free water* (solution A) add 0.1 ml of *dilute phenolphthalein solution*; the solution is colourless. Add 0.5 ml of 0.01M *sodium hydroxide*; the solution is red.

Clarity and colour of solution Solution A is *clear*, Appendix IV A, and not more intensely coloured than *reference solution B₉*, Appendix IV B, Method II.

Optical rotation In a 10.0% w/v solution, −0.25° to +0.05°, Appendix V F, determined using a 2-dm tube.

Silver To 10 ml of a 10% w/v solution add 0.1 ml of *sodium sulphide solution* and allow to stand for 2 minutes. The solution is not more intensely coloured than *reference solution B₈*, Appendix IV B, Method II (10 ppm).

Halides 15 ml of solution A complies with the *limit test for chlorides*, Appendix VII (10 ppm). Use 1.5 ml of *chloride standard solution (5 ppm Cl)* to prepare the standard.

Apomethylatropine Ratio of the *absorbance* of a 0.1% w/v solution in 0.01M *hydrochloric acid* at the maximum at 257 nm to that at the maximum at 252 nm, not less than 1.17, Appendix II B.

Related substances Carry out the method for *thin-layer chromatography*, Appendix III A, using *silica gel G* as the coating substance and a mixture of 60 volumes of *ethyl acetate*, 15 volumes of *anhydrous formic acid*, 15 volumes of *water* and 10 volumes of *methanol* as the mobile phase. Apply separately to the chromatoplate 5 µl of each of two solutions of the substance being examined in *methanol (90%)* containing (1) 4% w/v and (2) 0.020% w/v. After removal of the plate, dry it at 100° to 105° until the odour of the solvent is no longer detectable, allow to cool and spray with *dilute potassium iodobismuthate solution* until spots appear. Any *secondary spot* in the chromatogram obtained with solution (1) is not more intense than the spot in the chromatogram obtained with solution (2).

Loss on drying When dried to constant weight at 100° to 105°, loses not more than 0.5% of its weight. Use 0.5 g.

Sulphated ash Not more than 0.1% when determined on the residue obtained in the test for Loss on drying, Appendix IX A, Method II.

Assay Dissolve 0.3 g in 50 ml of *anhydrous glacial acetic acid* and carry out Method I for *non-aqueous titration*, Appendix VIII A, determining the end-point potentiometrically. Each ml of 0.1M *perchloric acid VS* is equivalent to 0.03664 g of $C_{18}H_{26}N_2O_6$.

Storage Atropine Methonitrate should be kept in a well-closed container and protected from light.

Action and use Antispasmodic.

The title of the monograph in the European Pharmacopœia is Methylatropine Nitrate.

Atropine Sulphate ☆

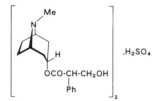

(C₁₇H₂₃NO₃)₂,H₂SO₄,H₂O   694.8   5908-89-6

Atropine Sulphate is (1*R*,3*r*,5*S*)-tropan-3-yl (±)-tropate sulphate monohydrate. It contains not less than 99.0 per cent and not more than 101.0 per cent of (C₁₇H₂₃NO₃)₂,H₂SO₄, calculated with reference to the anhydrous substance.

Characteristics Colourless crystals or a white, crystalline powder; odourless. It melts at about 190°, with decomposition, after drying at 135° for 15 minutes.

Solubility Very soluble in *water*; freely soluble in *ethanol* (96%); practically insoluble in *chloroform* and in *ether*.

Identification *Tests A and B may be omitted if tests C, D, E and F are carried out. Tests C, D and E may be omitted if tests A, B and F are carried out.*
A. The *infra-red absorption spectrum*, Appendix II A, is concordant with the spectrum of *atropine sulphate EPCRS*.
B. An aqueous solution shows almost no optical rotation.
C. To 5 ml of a 1% w/v solution add 5 ml of a 1% w/v solution of *2,4,6-trinitrophenol*. The *melting point* of the precipitate, after washing and drying at 100° to 105° for 2 hours, is 174° to 179°, Appendix V A, Method I.
D. To 1 mg add 0.2 ml of *fuming nitric acid* and evaporate to dryness in a water-bath. Dissolve the residue in 2 ml of *acetone* and add 0.1 ml of a 3% w/v solution of *potassium hydroxide* in *methanol*. A violet colour is produced.
E. Yields the *reaction* characteristic of alkaloids, Appendix VI.
F. Yields the *reactions* characteristic of sulphates, Appendix VI.

Acidity pH of a 2% w/v solution, 4.5 to 6.2, Appendix V L.

Specific optical rotation In a 10% w/v solution, −0.50° to +0.05°, Appendix V F, determined using a 2-dm tube.

Related substances and decomposition products Carry out the method for *thin-layer chromatography*, Appendix III A, using *silica gel G* as the coating substance and a mixture of 90 volumes of *acetone*, 7 volumes of *water* and 3 volumes of 13.5M *ammonia* as the mobile phase, but allowing the solvent front to ascend 10 cm above the line of application. Apply separately to the chromatoplate 10 μl of each of three solutions of the substance being examined in *methanol* containing (1) 2% w/v, (2) 0.020% w/v and (3) 0.010% w/v. After removal of the plate, dry it at 100° to 105° for 15 minutes, allow to cool and spray with *dilute potassium iodobismuthate solution* until spots appear. Any *secondary spot* in the chromatogram obtained with solution (1) is not more intense than the spot in the chromatogram obtained with solution (2) and not more than one such spot is more intense than the spot in the chromatogram obtained with solution (3).

Apoatropine The A(1%, 1 cm) in a 0.1% w/v solution in 0.01M *hydrochloric acid* at 245 nm is not more than 4.0, Appendix II B (about 0.5%).

Water 2.0 to 4.0% w/w, Appendix IX C. Use 0.5 g.

Sulphated ash Not more than 0.1%, Appendix IX A, Method II. Use 1 g.

Assay Dissolve 0.5 g in 30 ml of *anhydrous glacial acetic acid*, warming if necessary. Cool the solution and carry out Method I for *non-aqueous titration*, Appendix VIII A, determining the end-point potentiometrically. Each ml of 0.1M *perchloric acid VS* is equivalent to 0.06768 g of (C₁₇H₂₃NO₃)₂,H₂SO₄.

Storage Atropine Sulphate should be kept in a well-closed container and protected from light.

Preparations
Atropine Eye Drops
Atropine Eye Ointment
Atropine Injection
Atropine Tablets
Morphine and Atropine Injection

Action and use Antispasmodic.

Attapulgite

Attapulgite is a purified native hydrated magnesium aluminium silicate essentially consisting of the clay mineral palygorskite.

Characteristics A light, cream or buff, very fine powder, free or almost free from gritty particles.

Identification A. Ignite 0.5 g with 2 g of *anhydrous sodium carbonate* for 20 minutes, cool and extract with 25 ml of boiling *water*. Cool, filter, wash the residue with *water* and add the washings to the filtrate. Reserve the residue for test B. Cautiously acidify the combined filtrate and washings with *hydrochloric acid*, evaporate to dryness, moisten the residue with 0.2 ml of *hydrochloric acid*, add 10 ml of *water* and stir. A white, gelatinous precipitate is produced.
B. Wash again the residue reserved in test A with *water* and dissolve in 10 ml of 2M *hydrochloric acid*. To 2 ml of the solution add a 10% w/v solution of *ammonium thiocyanate*. An intense red colour is produced.
C. To 2 ml of the solution obtained in test B add 5M *ammonia* until a faint precipitate is produced, add 0.25 ml of a freshly prepared 0.05% w/v solution of *quinalizarin* in a 1% w/v solution of *sodium hydroxide*, heat to boiling, cool and acidify with 6M *acetic acid*. A reddish-violet colour is produced.
D. To 2 ml of the solution obtained in test B add *ammonium chloride* and an excess of 13.5M *ammonia* and filter. To the filtrate add 0.15 ml of *magneson reagent* and an excess of 5M *sodium hydroxide*. A blue precipitate is produced.
E. *Moisture adsorption*, 5 to 14%, Appendix IX F.

Acidity or alkalinity pH of a 5% w/v suspension in *carbon dioxide-free water* after shaking for 5 minutes, 7.0 to 9.5, Appendix V L.

Arsenic To 0.13 g add 5 ml of *water*, 2 ml of *sulphuric acid* and 10 ml of *sulphurous acid* and evaporate on a water-bath until the sulphurous acid is removed and the volume reduced to about 2 ml. Transfer the solution to the generator flask with the aid of 5 ml of *water*. The resulting solution complies with the *limit test for arsenic*, Appendix VII (8 ppm).

Heavy metals A. Not more than 20 ppm when determined by the following method. Shake 6.0 g with 40 ml of 0.5M *hydrochloric acid* at 37° for 30 minutes, cool and filter. Wash the residue with *water* and dilute the combined filtrate and washings to 50 ml with *water*. To 20 ml add 2 g each of *ammonium chloride* and *ammonium thiocyanate* and dissolve. Shake the solution with 80 ml of a mixture of equal volumes of *ether* and *amyl alcohol* and separate, retaining the aqueous layer. Extract with a further 80 ml of the mixture. To the aqueous layer add 2 g of *citric acid*, neutralise with 13.5M *ammonia* and dilute to 25 ml with *water*. 12 ml of the resulting solution complies with *limit test A for heavy metals*, Appendix VII. Use *lead standard solution (2 ppm Pb)* to prepare the standard.
B. Not more than 10 ppm when determined by the following method. Shake 6.0 g with 40 ml of 0.5M *sodium hydroxide* at 37° for 30 minutes, cool and filter. Wash the residue with *water* and dilute the combined filtrate and washings to 50 ml with *water*. Neutralise 20 ml of the solution with *hydrochloric acid* and dilute to 25 ml with *water*. 12 ml of the resulting solution complies with *limit test A for heavy metals*, Appendix VII. Use *lead standard solution (1 ppm Pb)* to prepare the standard.

Acid-soluble matter Boil 2 g with 100 ml of 0.2M *hydrochloric acid* under a reflux condenser for 5 minutes, cool and filter. Evaporate 50 ml of the filtrate to dryness. The residue, after ignition at about 600° for 30 minutes, weighs not more than 0.25 g.

Water-soluble matter Boil 10 g with 100 ml of *water* under a reflux condenser for 5 minutes, cool and filter. Evaporate 50 ml of the filtrate to dryness. The residue, after ignition at 600° for 30 minutes, weighs not more than 50 mg.

Loss on drying When dried to constant weight at 105°, loses not more than 17.0% of its weight. Use 1 g.

Loss on ignition When ignited at 600°, loses 15.0 to 27.0% of its weight. Use 1 g.

Action and use Pharmaceutical aid.

Activated Attapulgite

Activated Attapulgite is a purified native hydrated magnesium aluminium silicate essentially consisting of the clay mineral palygorskite that has been carefully heated to increase its adsorptive capacity.

Characteristics A light, cream or buff, very fine powder, free or almost free from gritty particles.

Identification Complies with tests A to D for Identification stated under Attapulgite and with the test for Adsorptive capacity.

Adsorptive capacity In a stoppered bottle shake 1.0 g, in *very fine powder*, with 50 ml of a 0.12% w/v solution of *methylene blue* for 5 minutes, allow to settle and centrifuge. The colour of the clear supernatant solution is not more intense than that of a 0.0012% w/v solution of *methylene blue*.

Acidity or alkalinity; Arsenic; Heavy metals; Acid-soluble matter; Water-soluble matter Complies with the requirements stated under Attapulgite.

Loss on drying When dried to constant weight at 105°, loses not more than 4.0% of its weight. Use 1 g.

Loss on ignition When ignited at 600°, loses not more than 9.0% of its weight. Use 1 g.

Action and use Antidiarrhoeal.

Azathioprine ☆

$C_9H_7N_7O_2S$ 277.3   446-86-6

Azathioprine is 6-(1-methyl-4-nitroimidazol-5-ylthio)purine. It contains not less than 98.5 per cent and not more than 101.0 per cent of $C_9H_7N_7O_2S$, calculated with reference to the dried substance.

Characteristics A pale yellow powder.

Solubility Practically insoluble in *water*, in *ethanol (96%)* and in *chloroform*; sparingly soluble in dilute mineral acids. It dissolves in dilute solutions of alkali hydroxides.

Identification A. The *infra-red absorption spectrum*, Appendix II A, is concordant with the spectrum of *azathioprine EPCRS*.
B. Dissolve 0.15 g in 30 ml of *dimethyl sulphoxide* and dilute to 500 ml with 0.1M *hydrochloric acid*. Dilute 25 ml of this solution to 1000 ml with 0.1M *hydrochloric acid*. The *light absorption* of the resulting solution, Appendix II B, in the range 230 to 350 nm exhibits a maximum at 280 nm. The A(1%, 1 cm) at 280 nm is 600 to 660.
C. Heat 20 mg with 100 ml of *water* and filter. To 5 ml of the filtrate add 1 ml of *hydrochloric acid* and 10 mg of *zinc powder* and allow to stand for 5 minutes; the solution becomes yellow. Filter, cool in ice, add 0.1 ml of *sodium nitrite solution* and 0.1 g of *sulphamic acid* and shake until the bubbles disappear. Add 1 ml of *2-naphthol solution*; a pale pink precipitate is produced.

Acidity or alkalinity Shake 0.5 g with 25 ml of *carbon dioxide-free water* for 15 minutes and filter. To 20 ml of the filtrate add 0.1 ml of *methyl red solution*. Not more than 0.2 ml of 0.01M *hydrochloric acid VS* or 0.2 ml of 0.01M *sodium hydroxide VS* is required to change the colour of the solution.

5-Chloro-1-methyl-4-nitroimidazole and 6-mercapto-purine Carry out the method for *thin-layer chromatography*, Appendix III A, using *cellulose F254* as the coating substance and *butan-1-ol* saturated with 6M *ammonia* as the mobile phase. Apply separately to the chromatoplate 5 μl of each of three solutions prepared immediately before use in 6M *ammonia* containing (1) 2.0% w/v of the substance being examined, (2) 0.020% w/v of *chloromethylnitro-imidazole EPCRS* and (3) 0.020% w/v of *6-mercaptopurine*. After removal of the plate, dry it at 50° and examine under *ultra-violet light (254 nm)*. Any spots corresponding to 5-chloro-1-methyl-4-nitroimidazole and 6-mercaptopurine in the chromatogram obtained with solution (1) are not more intense than the spots in the chromatograms obtained with solutions (2) and (3) respectively.

Loss on drying When dried to constant weight at 100° to 105°, loses not more than 1.0% of its weight. Use 0.5 g.

Sulphated ash Not more than 0.1%, Appendix IX A, Method II. Use 1 g.

Assay Dissolve 0.25 g in 25 ml of *dimethylformamide* and carry out Method II for *non-aqueous titration*, Appendix VIII A, using 0.1M *tetrabutylammonium hydroxide VS* as titrant and determining the end-point potentiometrically. Each ml of 0.1M *tetrabutylammonium hydroxide VS* is equivalent to 0.02773 g of $C_9H_7N_7O_2S$.

Storage Azathioprine should be kept in a well-closed container and protected from light.

Preparation
Azathioprine Tablets

Action and use Immunosuppressant.

Bacitracin ☆

1405-87-4

Bacitracin consists of one or more of the antimicrobial polypeptides produced by certain strains of *Bacillus licheniformis* and by *B. subtilis* var. *Tracy* and yields on hydrolysis the amino-acids L-cysteine, D-glutamic acid, L-histidine, L-isoleucine, L-leucine, L-lysine, D-ornithine, D-phenylalanine and DL-aspartic acid. The potency is not less than 60 Units per mg, calculated with reference to the dried substance.

Characteristics A white or almost white powder; hygroscopic.

Solubility Freely soluble in *water* and in *ethanol* (96%); practically insoluble in *chloroform* and in *ether*.

Identification A. Carry out the method for *thin-layer chromatography*, Appendix III A, protected from light, using *silica gel G* as the coating substance and a mixture of 75 parts of *phenol* and 25 parts of *water* as the mobile phase but allowing the solvent front to ascend 12 cm above the line of application. Apply separately to the chromatoplate 5 μl of each of the following solutions as bands 10 mm wide. For solution (1) dissolve 5 mg of the substance being examined in a mixture of 0.5 ml of *hydrochloric acid* and 0.5 ml of *water*, heat in a sealed tube at 135° for 5 hours, evaporate to dryness on a water-bath, continue to heat until the odour of hydrogen chloride is no longer detectable and dissolve the residue in 0.5 ml of *water*. Prepare solution (2) in the same manner, but using *bacitracin zinc EPCRS* in place of the substance being examined. Place the plate in the tank so that it is not in contact with the mobile phase and allow to stand for at least 12 hours before development. After removal of the plate, allow it to dry at 100° to 105°, spray with *ethanolic ninhydrin solution* and heat at 110° for 5 minutes. The bands in the chromatogram obtained with solution (1) correspond to those in the chromatogram obtained with solution (2).
B. Dissolve 5 mg in 3 ml of *water* and add 3 ml of 2M *sodium hydroxide*. Shake and add 0.5 ml of a 1% w/v solution of *copper(II) sulphate*. A violet colour is produced.

C. Ignite 0.2 g; an insignificant residue remains which is not yellow at high temperatures. Allow to cool, dissolve in 0.1 ml of 2M *hydrochloric acid* and add 5 ml of *water* and 0.2 ml of 10M *sodium hydroxide*; no white precipitate is produced.

Acidity or alkalinity pH of a 1% w/v solution, 6.0 to 7.0, Appendix V L.

Clarity and colour of solution A 1.0% w/v solution in *carbon dioxide-free water* is *clear*, Appendix IV A, and not more intensely coloured than *reference solution BY₅*, Appendix IV B, Method II.

Bacitracin F and related substances The ratio of the *absorbance* at 290 nm to that at 252 nm of a 0.03% w/v solution in 0.05M *sulphuric acid* is not more than 0.20, Appendix II B.

Loss on drying When dried over *phosphorus pentoxide* at 60° at a pressure not exceeding 0.1 kPa for 3 hours, loses not more than 5.0% of its weight. Use 1 g.

Sulphated ash Not more than 3.0%, Appendix IX A, Method II. Use 1 g.

Assay Carry out the *biological assay of antibiotics*, Appendix XIV A. The precision of the assay is such that the fiducial limits of error are not less than 95% and not more than 105% of the estimated potency.

Storage Bacitracin should be kept in an airtight container and stored at a temperature of 8° to 15°. If it is intended for the preparation of eye drops, the container should be sterile, tamper-evident and sealed so as to exclude micro-organisms.

Labelling The label states (1) the number of Units per mg; (2) the date after which the material is not intended to be used; (3) the conditions under which it should be stored; (4) whether or not it is intended for the preparation of eye drops.

Action and use Antibacterial.

Bacitracin intended for the preparation of eye drops without further treatment complies with the following additional requirement.

Sterility Complies with the *test for sterility*, Appendix XVI A.

Bacitracin Zinc ☆

1405-89-6

Bacitracin Zinc is the zinc complex of bacitracin, which consists of one or more of the antimicrobial polypeptides produced by certain strains of *Bacillus licheniformis* and by *B. subtilis* var. *Tracy* and which yields on hydrolysis the amino-acids L-cysteine, D-glutamic acid, L-histidine, L-isoleucine, L-leucine, L-lysine, D-ornithine, D-phenylalanine and DL-aspartic acid. The potency is not less than 60 Units per mg, calculated with reference to the dried substance.

Characteristics A white or light yellowish-grey powder; hygroscopic.

Solubility Slightly soluble in *water* and in *ethanol* (96%); practically insoluble in *chloroform*; very slightly soluble in *ether*.

Identification A. Carry out the method for *thin-layer chromatography*, Appendix III A, protected from light, using *silica gel G* as the coating substance and a mixture of 75 parts of *phenol* and 25 parts of *water* as the mobile phase but allowing the solvent front to ascend 12 cm above the line of application. Apply separately to the chromatoplate 5 µl of each of the following solutions as bands 10 mm wide. For solution (1) dissolve 5 mg of the substance being examined in a mixture of 0.5 ml of *hydrochloric acid* and 0.5 ml of *water*, heat in a sealed tube at 135° for 5 hours, evaporate to dryness on a water-bath, continue to heat until the odour of hydrogen chloride is no longer detectable and dissolve the residue in 0.5 ml of *water*. Prepare solution (2) in the same manner but using *bacitracin zinc EPCRS* in place of the substance being examined. Place the plate in the tank so that it is not in contact with the mobile phase and allow to stand for at least 12 hours before development. After removal of the plate, allow it to dry at 100° to 105°, spray with *ethanolic ninhydrin solution* and heat at 110° for 5 minutes. The bands in the chromatogram obtained with solution (1) correspond to those in the chromatogram obtained with solution (2).

B. Dissolve 5 mg in 3 ml of *water* and add 3 ml of 2M *sodium hydroxide*. Shake well and add 0.5 ml of a 1% w/v solution of *copper(II) sulphate*. A violet colour is produced.

C. Ignite 0.15 g, allow to cool, dissolve the residue in 1 ml of 2M *hydrochloric acid* and add 4 ml of *water*. The solution yields the *reaction* characteristic of zinc salts, Appendix VI.

Acidity or alkalinity Shake 1 g with 10 ml of *carbon dioxide-free water* for 1 minute and filter. The pH of the filtrate is 6.0 to 7.5, Appendix V L.

Bacitracin F and related substances The ratio of the *absorbance* at 290 nm to that at 252 nm of a 0.03% w/v solution in 0.05M *sulphuric acid* is not more than 0.15, Appendix II B.

Zinc 4.0 to 6.0%, calculated with reference to the dried substance, when determined by the following method. Dissolve 0.2 g in a mixture of 2.5 ml of 2M *acetic acid* and 2.5 ml of *water* and add 50 ml of *water*, 50 mg of *xylenol orange mixture* and sufficient *hexamine* to produce a red solution. Add 2 g of *hexamine* in excess and titrate with 0.01M *disodium edetate VS* until the colour changes to yellow. Each ml of 0.01M *disodium edetate VS* is equivalent to 0.000654 g of Zn.

Loss on drying When dried over *phosphorus pentoxide* at 60° at a pressure not exceeding 0.1 kPa for 3 hours, loses not more than 5.0% of its weight. Use 1 g.

Assay Suspend 50 mg in 5 ml of *water*, add 0.5 ml of 2M *hydrochloric acid* and dilute to 100 ml with *water*. Allow to stand for 30 minutes and carry out the *biological assay of antibiotics*, Appendix XIV A. The precision of the assay is such that the fiducial limits of error are not less than 95% and not more than 105% of the estimated potency.

Storage Bacitracin Zinc should be kept in an airtight container. If it is intended for administration by spraying into internal body cavities, the container should be sterile, tamper-evident and sealed so as to exclude micro-organisms.

Labelling The label states (1) the number of Units per mg; (2) the date after which the material is not intended to be used; (3) the conditions under which it should be stored; (4) whether or not it is intended for administration by spraying into internal body cavities.

Action and use Antibacterial.

Bacitracin Zinc intended for administration by spraying into internal body cavities complies with the following additional requirements.

Abnormal toxicity Complies with the *test for abnormal toxicity*, Appendix XIV L. Use 0.5 mg suspended in 0.5 ml of *saline solution* and inject the suspension intraperitoneally; a suitable suspending agent may be used in the suspension.

Pyrogens Complies with the *test for pyrogens*, Appendix XIV K. Use per kg of the rabbit's weight 1 ml of the supernatant liquid obtained by centrifuging a 1.1% w/v suspension in *saline solution*.

Sterility Complies with the *test for sterility*, Appendix XVI A.

Baclofen

H₂NCH₂·CH·CH₂·CO₂H

$C_{10}H_{12}ClNO_2$ 213.7   *1134-47-0*

Baclofen is 4-amino-3-(4-chlorophenyl)butyric acid. It contains not less than 99.0 per cent and not more than 101.0 per cent of $C_{10}H_{12}ClNO_2$, calculated with reference to the anhydrous substance.

Characteristics A white or creamy-white powder.

Solubility Slightly soluble in *water*; practically insoluble in organic solvents. It dissolves in dilute mineral acids and alkali hydroxides.

Identification A. The *infra-red absorption spectrum*, Appendix II A, is concordant with the *reference spectrum* of baclofen.

B. In the test for Related substances, the principal spot in the chromatogram obtained with solution (2) corresponds to that in the chromatogram obtained with solution (5).

Clarity and colour of solution A 2.0% w/v solution in 1M *sodium hydroxide* is *clear*, Appendix IV A, and not more intensely coloured than *reference solution BY₅*, Appendix IV B, Method I.

Related substances Carry out the method for *thin-layer chromatography*, Appendix III A, using *silica gel G* as the coating substance and a mixture of 40 volumes of *ethyl acetate*, 30 volumes of *chloroform*, 20 volumes of *methanol*, 5 volumes of *anhydrous formic acid* and 5 volumes of *water* as the mobile phase. Apply separately to the chromato-plate 5 µl of each of the following solutions in the mobile phase. Solutions (1) to (4) contain (1) 1.0% w/v, (2) 0.10% w/v, (3) 0.010% w/v and (4) 0.0050% w/v respectively of the substance being examined. Solution (5) contains 0.10% w/v of *baclofen BPCRS*. After removal of the plate, allow the solvent to evaporate and place in a closed tank containing chlorine gas, produced by mixing equal volumes of a 1.5% w/v solution of *potassium permanganate* and 3M *hydrochloric acid* in a container placed at the bottom of the tank, and allow to stand for 15 minutes. Remove the plate from the tank and remove the chlorine in a current of cold air until an area below the line of application does not produce a blue colour on the addition of 0.05 ml of *starch—iodide solution*. Spray the plate with *starch—iodide solution*. Any *secondary spot* in the chromatogram obtained with solution (1) is not more intense than the spot in the chromatogram obtained with solution (3) and not more than one such spot is more intense than the spot in the chromatogram obtained with solution (4).

Sulphated ash Not more than 0.1%, Appendix IX A.

Water Not more than 1.0% w/w, Appendix IX C. Use 1 g.

Assay Carry out Method I for *non-aqueous titration*, Appendix VIII A, using 0.5 g and *1-naphtholbenzein solution* as indicator. Each ml of 0.1M *perchloric acid VS* is equivalent to 0.02137 g of $C_{10}H_{12}ClNO_2$.

Preparation

Baclofen Tablets

Action and use Skeletal muscle relaxant.

Barbitone ☆

O
H
N
O
Et
NH
Et
O

$C_8H_{12}N_2O_3$ 184.2   *57-44-3*

Barbitone is 5,5-diethylbarbituric acid. It contains not less than 99.0 per cent and not more than 101.0 per cent of $C_8H_{12}N_2O_3$, calculated with reference to the dried substance.

Characteristics A white, crystalline powder or colourless crystals; odourless.

Solubility Slightly soluble in *water* and in *chloroform*; soluble in boiling *water*, in *ethanol (96%)* and in *ether*. It dissolves in aqueous solutions of alkali hydroxides and carbonates and in aqueous ammonia.

Identification *Test A may be omitted if tests B, C and D are carried out. Tests B and C may be omitted if tests A and D are carried out.*

A. The *infra-red absorption spectrum*, Appendix II A, is concordant with the spectrum of *barbital EPCRS*.

B. Complies with the test for *identification of barbiturates*, Appendix III A, but applying separately to the chromatoplate 10 µl of each of two solutions in *ethanol (96%)* containing (1) 0.30% w/v of the substance being examined and (2) 0.30% w/v of *barbital EPCRS*.

C. Yields the *reaction* characteristic of non-nitrogen substituted barbiturates, Appendix VI.

D. Determine the *melting point*, Appendix V A, Method I, of the substance being examined (about 190°). Mix equal parts of the substance being examined and *barbital EPCRS* and determine the *melting point* of the mixture. The difference between the melting points is not greater than 2°.

Acidity Boil 1 g with 50 ml of *water* for 2 minutes, allow to cool and filter. To 10 ml of the filtrate add 0.15 ml of *methyl red solution*. The solution is orange-yellow and not

more than 0.1 ml of 0.1M *sodium hydroxide VS* is required to produce a pure yellow colour.

Clarity and colour of solution A solution containing 1.0 g in a mixture of 4 ml of 2M *sodium hydroxide* and 6 ml of *carbon dioxide-free water* is clear, Appendix IV A, and not more intensely coloured than *reference solution Y_6*, Appendix IV B, Method II.

Related substances Complies with the test for *related substances in barbiturates*, Appendix III A.

Loss on drying When dried to constant weight at 100° to 105°, loses not more than 0.5% of its weight. Use 1 g.

Sulphated ash Not more than 0.1%, Appendix IX A, Method II. Use 1 g.

Assay Dissolve 85 mg in 5 ml of *pyridine*, add 10 ml of *silver nitrate—pyridine reagent* and titrate with 0.1M *ethanolic sodium hydroxide VS*, using 0.5 ml of *thymolphthalein solution* as indicator, until a pure blue colour is produced. Repeat the operation without the substance being examined. The difference between the titrations represents the amount of sodium hydroxide required. Each ml of 0.1M *ethanolic sodium hydroxide VS* is equivalent to 0.00921 g of $C_8H_{12}N_2O_3$.

The title of the monograph in the European Pharmacopœia is Barbital.

Barium Sulphate ☆

$BaSO_4$ 233.4   *7727-43-7*

Characteristics A fine, heavy, white powder, free from grittiness; odourless.

Solubility Practically insoluble in *water* and in organic solvents; very slightly soluble in acids and in alkali hydroxides.

Identification A. Boil 0.2 g with 5 ml of a 50% w/v solution of *sodium carbonate* for 5 minutes, add 10 ml of *water* and filter. Reserve the filtrate for test B. Wash the residue with three successive small quantities of *water*. To the residue add 5 ml of 2M *hydrochloric acid*, filter and to the filtrate add 0.3 ml of 1M *sulphuric acid*. A white precipitate is produced which is insoluble in 2M *sodium hydroxide*.

B. Acidify a portion of the filtrate obtained in test A with 2M *hydrochloric acid*. The solution yields the *reactions* characteristic of sulphates, Appendix VI.

Acidity or alkalinity Heat 5 g with 20 ml of *carbon dioxide-free water* for 5 minutes on a water-bath and filter. To 10 ml of the filtrate add 0.05 ml of *bromothymol blue solution*. Not more than 0.5 ml of either 0.01M *hydrochloric acid VS* or 0.01M *sodium hydroxide VS* is required to change the colour of the solution.

Arsenic In a long-necked combustion flask shake 0.50 g with 2 ml of *nitric acid* and 30 ml of *water*, insert a small funnel into the neck of the flask, heat in an inclined position on a water-bath for 2 hours, allow to cool, adjust to the original volume with *water* and filter. Wash the residue by decantation with three 5-ml quantities of *water*, combine the filtrate and washings, add 1 ml of *sulphuric acid*, evaporate on a water-bath and heat until white fumes are evolved. Dissolve the residue in 10 ml of 1M *sulphuric acid* and add 10 ml of *water*. The resulting solution complies with the *limit test for arsenic*, Appendix VII (2 ppm).

Soluble barium salts Boil 20 g with a mixture of 40 ml of *water* and 60 ml of 2M *acetic acid* for 5 minutes, filter, allow to cool and dilute to 100 ml with *water* (solution A). To 10 ml of solution A add 1 ml of 1M *sulphuric acid*. After 1 hour any opalescence in the solution is not more intense than that in a mixture of 10 ml of solution A and 1 ml of *water*.

Heavy metals Dilute 7.5 ml of solution A to 15 ml with *water*. 12 ml of the resulting solution complies with *limit test A for heavy metals*, Appendix VII (10 ppm). Use *lead standard solution (1 ppm Pb)* to prepare the standard.

Oxidisable sulphur compounds Shake 1.0 g with 5 ml of *water* for 30 seconds and filter. To the filtrate add 0.1 ml of *starch solution*, dissolve 0.1 g of *potassium iodide* in the mixture, add 1 ml of a freshly prepared 0.00036% w/v solution of *potassium iodate* and 1 ml of 1M *hydrochloric acid* and shake well. The colour produced is more intense than that of a solution prepared at the same time and in the same manner, but omitting the potassium iodate solution.

Phosphate To 1.0 g add a mixture of 3 ml of 2M *nitric acid* and 7 ml of *water*, heat on a water-bath for 5 minutes, filter, dilute the filtrate to 10 ml with *water*, add 5 ml of *molybdovanadic reagent* and allow to stand for 5 minutes. Any yellow colour produced is not more intense than that of a standard prepared at the same time and in the same manner using 10 ml of *phosphate standard solution (5 ppm PO₄)* (50 ppm).

Acid-soluble substances Evaporate 25 ml of solution A to dryness on a water-bath. The residue, when dried to constant weight at 100° to 105°, weighs not more than 15 mg.

Sedimentation Place 5.0 g in a 50-ml glass-stoppered graduated cylinder with the 50-ml graduation mark 14 cm from the base. Add sufficient *water* to produce 50 ml, shake for 5 minutes and allow to stand for 15 minutes. The barium sulphate does not settle below the 15-ml graduation mark.

Loss on ignition When ignited at 600°, loses not more than 2.0% of its weight. Use 1 g.

Action and use Radio-opaque substance used in the investigation of the gastro-intestinal tract.

Barium Sulphate for Suspension

Barium Sulphate for Suspension is a dry mixture of Barium Sulphate with suitable flavours, antimicrobial preservatives and a suitable dispersing agent. It contains not less than 85.0 per cent w/w of barium sulphate, BaSO₄.

Characteristics A fine, white or creamy-white powder.

Identification A. Ignite 1 g to constant weight. To 0.2 g of the residue add 5 ml of a 50% w/v solution of *sodium carbonate* and boil for 5 minutes. Add 10.0 ml of *water* and filter. Reserve the filtrate for test B. Wash the residue with *water*, add 5 ml of 2M *hydrochloric acid*, mix well and filter. Add 0.3 ml of 1M *sulphuric acid* to the filtrate. A white precipitate is produced which is insoluble in 2M *hydrochloric acid*.

B. Acidify a portion of the filtrate obtained in test A with 2M *hydrochloric acid*. The solution yields the *reactions* characteristic of sulphates, Appendix VI.

Acidity or alkalinity pH of an aqueous suspension containing 75% w/v of Barium Sulphate, 4.5 to 7.0, Appendix V L.

Soluble barium compounds To 10 g of an aqueous suspension containing 75% w/v of Barium Sulphate add 10 ml of 2M *hydrochloric acid* and 90 ml of *water*. Boil for 10 minutes, cool and filter. Wash the residue with *water* and dilute the combined filtrate and washings to 100 ml with *water*. Carefully evaporate 50 ml of the resulting solution to avoid charring, add 0.1 ml of 2M *hydrochloric acid* and 10 ml of hot *water* to the residue and filter. To the clear filtrate add 0.5 ml of 1M *sulphuric acid* and allow to stand for 30 minutes. The solution is *clear*, Appendix IV A.

Loss on drying When dried at 105° for 4 hours, loses not more than 1.0% of its weight. Use 1 g.

Assay To 0.75 g contained in a platinum dish add 5 g of *sodium carbonate* and 5 g of *potassium carbonate* and mix. Heat to 1000° and maintain at this temperature for 15 minutes. Allow to cool and suspend the residue in 150 ml of *water*. Wash the dish with 2 ml of 6M *acetic acid* and add the washings to the suspension. Cool in ice and decant the supernatant liquid, transferring as little of the solid matter as possible to the filter. Wash the residue with successive quantities of a 2% w/v solution of *sodium carbonate* until the washings are free from sulphate and discard the washings. Add 5 ml of 2M *hydrochloric acid* to the filter, wash through into the vessel containing the bulk of the solid matter with *water*, add 5 ml of *hydrochloric acid* and dilute to 100 ml with *water*. Add 10 ml of a 40% w/v solution of *ammonium acetate*, 25 ml of a 10% w/v solution of *potassium dichromate* and 10 g of *urea*. Cover and digest in a hot-air oven at 80° to 85° for 16 hours. Filter whilst still hot through a sintered-glass filter (BS porosity No. 4), washing the precipitate initially with a 0.5% w/v solution of *potassium dichromate* and finally with 2 ml of *water*. Dry to constant weight at 105°. Each g of the residue is equivalent to 0.9213 g of barium sulphate, BaSO₄.

Preparation

Barium Sulphate Oral Suspension

Action and use Radio-opaque preparation used in the investigation of the gastro-intestinal tract.

Beclamide

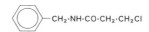

C₁₀H₁₂ClNO   197.7   *501-68-8*

Beclamide is *N*-benzyl-3-chloropropionamide. It contains not less than 99.0 per cent and not more than 101.0 per cent of C₁₀H₁₂ClNO, calculated with reference to the dried substance.

Characteristics A white, crystalline powder.

Solubility Sparingly soluble in *water*; soluble in *ethanol (96%)*; freely soluble in *chloroform*.

Identification A. The *infra-red absorption spectrum*, Appendix II A, is concordant with the *reference spectrum* of beclamide.

B. Carry out the method for *thin-layer chromatography*, Appendix III A, using *silica gel GF254* as the coating substance and a mixture of 90 volumes of *chloroform* and 10 volumes of *ethanol (96%)* as the mobile phase. Apply separately to the chromatoplate 10 µl of each of two solutions in *absolute ethanol* containing (1) 0.5% w/v of the substance being examined and (2) 0.5% w/v of *beclamide BPCRS*. After removal of the plate, allow it to dry in air and examine under *ultra-violet light (254 nm)*. The principal spot in the chromatogram obtained with solution (1) corresponds to that in the chromatogram obtained with solution (2).

Melting point 91° to 94°, Appendix V A.

Benzylamine and *N*-benzylacrylamide Carry out the method for *high-performance liquid chromatography*, Appendix III D, using the following solutions. Solution (1) contains 0.0025% w/v of N-*benzylacrylamide BPCRS* in *methanol (40%)*. Solution (2) contains 0.0050% w/v of *benzylamine* in *methanol (40%)*. For solution (3) dissolve 0.10 g of the substance being examined in 8 ml of *methanol* and dilute to 20 ml with *water*. For solution (4) dissolve 1.0 g of the substance being examined in 5 ml of *chloroform*, shake with 2 ml of 0.1M *hydrochloric acid* and centrifuge. Use 1 ml of the upper layer in which 15 mg of *sodium acetate* has been dissolved.

The chromatographic procedure may be carried out using (a) a stainless steel column (20 cm × 4 mm) packed with *stationary phase C* (10 µm) (Nucleosil C18 is suitable), (b) a mixture of 3 volumes of 0.008M *sodium hexanesulphonate* and 2 volumes of *methanol*, the pH of which has been adjusted to 3.5 with *glacial acetic acid*, as the mobile phase and (c) a detection wavelength of 215 nm.

In the chromatogram obtained with solution (3) the area of any peak corresponding to *N*-benzylacrylamide is not greater than the area of the principal peak in the chromatogram obtained with solution (1). In the chromatogram obtained with solution (4) the area of any peak corresponding to benzylamine is not greater than the area of the peak in the chromatogram obtained with solution (2).

Loss on drying When dried to constant weight at 60° at a pressure not exceeding 0.7 kPa, loses not more than 0.5% of its weight. Use 1 g.

Sulphated ash Not more than 0.1%, Appendix IX A.

Assay To 0.4 g add 20 ml of 0.5M *ethanolic potassium hydroxide*, heat under a reflux condenser for 1 hour, cool, add 20 ml of 1M *nitric acid* and 25 ml of 0.1M *silver nitrate VS*, mix and titrate the excess silver nitrate with 0.1M *ammonium thiocyanate VS* using 5 ml of *ammonium iron(III) sulphate solution* as indicator. Each ml of 0.1M *silver nitrate VS* is equivalent to 0.01977 g of $C_{10}H_{12}ClNO$.

Storage Beclamide should be kept in a well-closed container.

Preparation
Beclamide Tablets

Action and use Anticonvulsant.

Beclomethasone Dipropionate

$C_{28}H_{37}ClO_7$ 521.0   *5534-09-8*

Beclomethasone Dipropionate is 9α-chloro-11β,17α,21-trihydroxy-16β-methylpregna-1,4-diene-3,20-dione 17,21-dipropionate. It contains not less than 96.0 per cent and not more than 104.0 per cent of $C_{28}H_{37}ClO_7$, calculated with reference to the dried substance.

Characteristics A white to creamy-white powder; odourless or almost odourless.

Solubility Practically insoluble in *water*; soluble in 60 parts of *ethanol (96%)* and in 8 parts of *chloroform*.

Identification A. The *infra-red absorption spectrum*, Appendix II A, is concordant with the *reference spectrum* of beclomethasone dipropionate.
B. Complies with the test for *identification of steroids*, Appendix III A, using *impregnating solvent II* and *mobile phase D*.
C. Burn 25 mg by the method for *oxygen-flask combustion*, Appendix VIII C, using a mixture of 20 ml of *water* and 1 ml of 1M *sodium hydroxide* as the absorbing liquid. The liquid yields *reaction A* characteristic of chlorides, Appendix VI.
D. Carry out the *reaction* for acetyl groups, Appendix VI. A blue colour slowly appears at the junction of the two liquids.
E. *Melting point*, about 212°, with decomposition, Appendix V A.

Light absorption *Absorbance* of a 0.0020% w/v solution in *absolute ethanol* at the maximum at 238 nm, 0.57 to 0.60, Appendix II B. The ratio of the absorbance at the maximum at 238 nm to that at 263 nm is 2.25 to 2.45.

Specific optical rotation In a 1% w/v solution in *1,4-dioxan*, +88° to +94°, Appendix V F.

Related foreign steroids Carry out Method B for *related foreign steroids*, Appendix III A, using for solution (3) a solution containing 0.030% w/v each of *beclomethasone 17-propionate BPCRS* and *beclomethasone 21-propionate BPCRS* in a mixture of 9 volumes of *chloroform* and 1 volume of *methanol*. Any *secondary spot* in the chromatogram obtained with solution (1) is not more intense than the proximate spot in the chromatogram obtained with solution (3). The test is not valid unless the principal spot in the chromatogram obtained with solution (1) corresponds in Rf value, colour and intensity to the principal spot in the chromatogram obtained with solution (2).

Loss on drying When dried to constant weight at 105°, loses not more than 0.5% of its weight. Use 1 g.

Sulphated ash Not more than 0.1%, Appendix IX A.

Assay Carry out the *tetrazolium assay of steroids*, Appendix VIII P, allowing the reaction to proceed at 35° for 2 hours, and calculate the content of $C_{28}H_{37}ClO_7$ from the *absorbance* obtained by repeating the operation using *beclomethasone dipropionate BPCRS* in place of the substance being examined.

Storage Beclomethasone Dipropionate should be protected from light.

Preparations
Beclomethasone Cream
Beclomethasone Ointment

Action and use Corticosteroid.

White Beeswax ☆

White Beeswax is obtained by bleaching Yellow Beeswax.

Characteristics White or yellowish-white pieces or plates, translucent when thin, with a fine-grained, matt, non-crystalline fracture; becomes soft and pliable when warmed by hand. Odour, similar to that of yellow beeswax, though fainter, never rancid. It is tasteless and does not stick to the teeth. Relative density, about 0.96.

Solubility Practically insoluble in *water*; partially soluble in *ethanol (90%)* and in *ether*; completely soluble in volatile and fixed oils.

Melting point 61° to 65°, Appendix V A, Method III, Test B. Melt the substance by heating on a water-bath, pour onto a glass plate and allow to cool to a semi-solid mass. Fill the metal cup by inserting the wider end into the wax and repeating the procedure until the wax is extruded from the narrow opening. Remove the excess with a spatula and insert the thermometer immediately. Remove the wax displaced and allow to stand at ambient temperature for at least 12 hours before determining the melting point.

Acid value 17 to 24 when determined by the following method. To 2 g in a 250-ml conical flask fitted with a reflux condenser add 40 ml of *xylene* and a few glass beads, heat until dissolved, add 20 ml of *ethanol (96%)* and 0.5 ml of a 1% w/v solution of *phenolphthalein* in *ethanol (70%)* and titrate the hot solution with 0.5M *ethanolic potassium hydroxide VS* until a red colour persists for at least 10 seconds (n_1 ml). Repeat the procedure omitting the substance being examined (n_2 ml). Calculate the Acid value from the expression $28.05(n_1 - n_2)/w$, where w is the weight, in g, of substance taken.

Ester value 70 to 80, determined by subtracting the Acid value from the Saponification value.

Ratio number The Ester value divided by the Acid value, determined by the method described above, is 3.3 to 4.3.

Saponification value 87 to 104 when determined by the following method. To 2 g in a 250-ml conical flask add 30 ml of a mixture of equal volumes of *xylene* and *ethanol (96%)* and a few glass beads, heat until dissolved, add 25 ml of 0.5M *ethanolic potassium hydroxide VS* and heat under a reflux condenser for 3 hours. Titrate the hot solution immediately with 0.5M *hydrochloric acid VS* using *dilute phenolphthalein solution* as indicator, bringing the solution back to the boil several times during the titration (n_1 ml). Repeat the procedure omitting the substance being examined (n_2 ml). Calculate the Saponification value from the expression $28.05(n_2 - n_1)/w$, where w is the weight, in g, of substance taken.

Ceresin, paraffin and certain other waxes To 3.0 g in a 100-ml round-bottomed flask add 30 ml of a 4% w/v solution of *potassium hydroxide* in *aldehyde-free ethanol (96%)* and boil gently under a reflux condenser for 2 hours. Remove the condenser and immediately insert a thermometer, place the flask in a water-bath at 80° and allow to cool with continuous swirling. The solution may be opalescent, but no precipitate is formed before the temperature reaches 65°.

Glycerol and other polyhydric alcohols Not more than 0.5% w/w, calculated as glycerol, when determined by the following method. To 0.2 g add 10 ml of *ethanolic potassium hydroxide solution*, heat under a reflux condenser on a water-bath for 30 minutes, add 50 ml of 1M *sulphuric acid*, cool and filter. Rinse the flask and filter with 1M *sulphuric acid*, combine the filtrate and washings and dilute to 100 ml with 1M *sulphuric acid* (solution A). Into two matched test-tubes introduce, respectively, 1 ml of solution A and 1 ml of a 0.001% w/v solution of glycerol in 1M *sulphuric acid* (solution B). Add 0.5 ml of 0.05M *sodium metaperiodate* to each tube, allow to stand for 5 minutes, add to each tube 1 ml of *decolorised magenta solution* and mix. Any precipitate disappears. Place the tubes in a beaker containing water at about 40° and observe for 10 to 15 minutes during cooling. Any bluish-violet colour in the tube containing solution A is not more intense than that in the tube containing solution B.

Action and use Pharmaceutical aid.

Yellow Beeswax ☆

Yellow Beeswax is the wax obtained by melting the walls of the honeycomb of the bee, *Apis mellifera* L. with hot water and removing the foreign matter.

Characteristics Yellow or light brown pieces or plates, with a fine-grained, matt, non-crystalline fracture; becomes soft and pliable when warmed by hand. Odour, faint and characteristic of honey. Relative density, about 0.96.

Solubility Practically insoluble in *water*; partially soluble in *ethanol (90%)* and in *ether*; completely soluble in volatile and fixed oils.

Melting point Complies with the requirement stated under White Beeswax.

Acid value 17 to 22 when determined by the method described under White Beeswax.

Ester value 70 to 80, determined by subtracting the Acid value from the Saponification value.

Ratio number The Ester value divided by the Acid value, determined by the method described under White Beeswax, is 3.3 to 4.3.

Saponification value 87 to 102 when determined by the method described under White Beeswax.

Ceresin, paraffin and certain other waxes Complies with the requirement stated under White Beeswax.

Glycerol and other polyhydric alcohols Not more than 0.5% w/w, calculated as glycerol, when determined by the method described under White Beeswax.

Action and use Pharmaceutical aid.

Belladonna Herb ☆

Belladonna Herb consists of the dried leaf or the dried leaf, flowering tops and occasionally fruits of *Atropa belladonna* L. It contains not less than 0.30 per cent of total alkaloids, calculated as hyoscyamine with reference to the material dried at 100° to 105°. The alkaloids consist mainly of those of the hyoscyamine—atropine group together with small quantities of hyoscine.

Characteristics Odour, slightly nauseous.

Macroscopical Leaves green to greenish-brown, slightly darker on the upper surface, often crumpled or rolled and partly matted together. When whole, lamina 5 to 25 cm long, 3 to 12 cm wide, elliptical to broadly ovate, acuminate at the apex, narrowing at the acute and decurrent base; margin entire. Petiole 0.5 to 4 cm in length. Young leaves pubescent, older leaves only slightly pubescent, mainly along the veins. Pinnate venation with secondary veins leaving the midrib at about 60° and anastomosing near the margin. Under a hand lens, crystal idioblasts visible between veins as dark points by transmitted light or bright points by reflected light. In flowering tops, stems hollow and flattened, bearing at each node a pair of leaves of unequal size, in the axils of which are single flowers or fruits. Flowers with gamosepalous calyx having five triangular lobes and campanulate corolla, purple to yellowish-brown, with five short lobes. Fruits, subspherical berries, green to violet-black, surrounded by the persistent calyx with widely separated lobes; when mature, they contain numerous brown seeds.

Microscopical Epidermal cells with slightly sinuous anticlinal walls and a frequently striated cuticle. Covering and glandular trichomes infrequent, but more numerous on the young leaves and on the veins; covering trichomes multicellular, uniseriate, with thin, smooth walls; glandular trichomes short and clavate or, less frequently, long with uniseriate stalks and ovoid unicellular heads. Stomata *anisocytic*, more frequent on the lower epidermis. Midrib characterised by an open arc of vascular bundles with isolated groups of intraxylary phloem. Throughout the mesophyll and particularly just below the palisade layer are cells containing microsphenoidal crystals of calcium oxalate or, very rarely, prisms or cluster crystals. Stems show epidermis with few trichomes, pericyclic fibres, intraxylary phloem and xylem with wide reticulately-thickened vessels; cortical parenchymatous cells and pith cells containing microsphenoidal crystals of calcium oxalate. Inner epidermis of corolla papillose on upper part, bearing numerous covering trichomes on basal part; outer epidermis has wavy anticlinal walls and numerous glandular trichomes.

Identification A. Carry out the method for *thin-layer chromatography*, Appendix III A, using *silica gel G* as the coating substance and a mixture of 90 volumes of *acetone*, 7 volumes of *water* and 3 volumes of 13.5M *ammonia* as the mobile phase but allowing the solvent front to ascend 10 cm above the line of application. Apply separately to a 200 mm × 200 mm chromatoplate, as bands 20 mm × 3 mm, 1 cm apart, 10 μl and 20 μl of each of the following solutions. For solution (1) add 15 ml of 0.05M *sulphuric acid* to 0.6 g of the material being examined, in *fine powder*, shake for 15 minutes, filter and wash the filter with 0.05M *sulphuric acid* until 20 ml of filtrate is obtained; add 1 ml of 13.5M *ammonia* to the filtrate, extract with two 10-ml quantities of *peroxide-free ether*, separate the ether layer, by centrifugation if necessary, dry the combined ether extracts over *anhydrous sodium sulphate*, filter, evaporate to dryness on a water-bath and dissolve the residue in 0.5 ml of *methanol*. For solution (2) dissolve 50 mg of *hyoscyamine sulphate* in 9 ml of *methanol* (solution A) and dissolve 15 mg of *hyoscine hydrobromide* in 10 ml of *methanol* (solution B); mix 8.0 ml of solution A with 1.8 ml of solution B.

After removal of the plate, dry it at 100° to 105° for 15 minutes, allow to cool and spray with 10 ml of *modified potassium iodobismuthate solution* until the bands become visible as orange or brown on a yellow background. The bands in the chromatograms obtained with solution (1) have similar Rf values to those in the chromatograms obtained with solution (2) (hyoscyamine in the lower third of the chromatogram; hyoscine in the upper third) and are similar in colour and at least equal in size. Faint secondary bands may appear, particularly in the middle of the chromatogram obtained with 20 μl of solution (1) or near the line of application in the chromatogram obtained with 10 μl of solution (1). Spray the plate with a freshly prepared 10% w/v solution of *sodium nitrite* until transparent and examine after 15 minutes. The colours due to hyoscyamine in the chromatograms change from brown to reddish-brown but not to greyish-blue (atropine); any secondary bands are no longer visible.
B. Shake 1 g, in powder, with 10 ml of 0.05M *sulphuric acid* for 2 minutes, filter, add 1 ml of 13.5M *ammonia* and 5 ml of *water* to the filtrate, extract cautiously with 15 ml of *chloroform* to avoid the formation of an emulsion, dry the chloroform layer over *anhydrous sodium sulphate* and filter. Evaporate the chloroform in a porcelain dish, add 0.5 ml of *fuming nitric acid* and evaporate to dryness on a water-bath. Add 10 ml of *acetone* and, dropwise, a 3% w/v solution of *potassium hydroxide* in *ethanol* (96%). A deep violet colour is produced.

Foreign matter Not more than 3% of stem with a diameter exceeding 5 mm, Appendix XI D, Test B.

Acid-insoluble ash Not more than 4.0%, Appendix XI K, Method II.

Assay Reduce 50 g, selected from a well-mixed sample, to *No. 180 powder* and determine the moisture content of 2 g by drying to constant weight at 100° to 105°. Moisten 10 g of the powdered herb with a mixture of 5 ml of 10M *ammonia*, 10 ml of *ethanol* (96%) and 30 ml of *peroxide-free ether* and mix thoroughly. Transfer the mixture to a small percolator with the aid of the extracting mixture if necessary, allow to macerate for 4 hours and then percolate with a mixture of 1 volume of *chloroform* and 3 volumes of *peroxide-free ether* until *complete extraction* of the alkaloids is effected. Concentrate the percolate to about 50 ml by distillation on a water-bath and transfer to a separating funnel using *peroxide-free ether*. Add a quantity of *peroxide-free ether* at least 2.1 times the volume of the percolate to produce a liquid considerably less dense than water. Extract the solution with not less than three 20-ml quantities of 0.25M *sulphuric acid*, separating the layers by centrifugation if necessary, and transfer each acid extract to a second separating funnel. Make the combined acid extracts alkaline with 10M *ammonia* and extract with three 30-ml quantities of *chloroform*. Combine the chloroform extracts, add 4 g of *anhydrous sodium* *sulphate* and allow to stand for 30 minutes, shaking occasionally. Decant the chloroform and wash the sodium sulphate with three 10-ml quantities of *chloroform*. Evaporate the combined chloroform extracts and washings to dryness on a water-bath and heat the residue at 100° to 105° for 15 minutes. Dissolve the residue in several ml of *chloroform*, add 20 ml of 0.01M *sulphuric acid VS*, remove the chloroform by evaporation on a water-bath and titrate the excess acid with 0.02M *sodium hydroxide VS* using *methyl red solution* as indicator. Each ml of 0.01M *sulphuric acid VS* is equivalent to 0.005788 g of total alkaloids calculated as hyoscyamine.

Storage Belladonna Herb should be kept in an airtight container and protected from light.

Preparations
Prepared Belladonna Herb
Belladonna Dry Extract
Belladonna Tincture

Action and use Antispasmodic.

The title of the monograph in the European Pharmacopœia is Belladonna Leaf.

When Belladonna Herb or Belladonna Leaf is prescribed, Prepared Belladonna Herb shall be dispensed.

Powdered Belladonna Herb

Powdered Belladonna Herb is Belladonna Herb in powder. It contains not less than 0.30 per cent of total alkaloids, calculated as hyoscyamine with reference to the powder dried at 100° to 105°. The alkaloids consist mainly of those of the hyoscyamine—atropine group together with small quantities of hyoscine.

Characteristics Dark green; odour, that of the unground drug. Diagnostic structures: fragments of leaf lamina showing sinuous-walled epidermal cells with sinuous striated cuticle and numerous *anisocytic* stomata. Few covering and glandular trichomes; fragments of parenchyma with covering trichomes and cells containing microsphenoidal crystals of calcium oxalate. Occasional fibres and reticulately-thickened vessels from the stem. Subspherical pollen grains, 40 to 50 μm in diameter. Numerous isolated microsphenoidal crystals of calcium oxalate measuring from 0.5 to several μm; occasional prisms.

Identification Complies with the tests for Identification described under Belladonna Herb.

Acid-insoluble ash Not more than 4.0%, Appendix XI K.

Assay Carry out the Assay described under Belladonna Herb.

Storage Powdered Belladonna Herb should be kept in an airtight container and protected from light.

Action and use Antispasmodic.

When Powdered Belladonna Herb is prescribed, Prepared Belladonna Herb shall be dispensed.

Prepared Belladonna Herb ☆

Prepared Belladonna Herb is Belladonna Herb in *No. 180 powder* adjusted, if necessary, by the addition of Lactose or of belladonna leaf powder of lower alkaloidal content to contain 0.28 to 0.32 per cent of total alkaloids, calculated as hyoscyamine with reference to the material dried at 100° to 105°.

Characteristics Greyish-green powder; odour, slightly nauseous. Diagnostic structures, as described under Powdered Belladonna Herb; additionally, when mounted in *glycerol (85%)*, crystals of lactose may be seen.

Identification Complies with the tests for Identification described under Belladonna Herb.

Acid-insoluble ash Not more than 4.0%, Appendix XI K, Method II.

Loss on drying When dried to constant weight at 100° to 105°, loses not more than 5.0% of its weight. Use 1 g.

Assay Carry out the Assay described under Belladonna Herb.

Storage Prepared Belladonna Herb should be kept in an airtight container and protected from light.

The title of the monograph in the European Pharmacopœia is Prepared Belladonna.

Bendrofluazide ☆

$C_{15}H_{14}F_3N_3O_4S_2$ 421.4   *73-48-3*

Bendrofluazide is 3-benzyl-3,4-dihydro-6-trifluoromethyl-2*H*-1,2,4-benzothiadiazine-7-sulphonamide 1,1-dioxide. It contains not less than 98.0 per cent and not more than 102.0 per cent of $C_{15}H_{14}F_3N_3O_4S_2$, calculated with reference to the dried substance.

Characteristics A white or almost white, crystalline powder; odourless or almost odourless.

Solubility Practically insoluble in *water* and in *chloroform*; soluble in 17 parts of *ethanol (96%)* and in 1.5 parts of *acetone*; slightly soluble in *ether*.

Identification *Test A may be omitted if tests B, C and D are carried out. Tests B, C and D may be omitted if test A is carried out.*

A. The *infra-red absorption spectrum*, Appendix II A, is concordant with the spectrum of *bendroflumethiazide EPCRS*.

B. In the test for Related substances, the principal spot in the chromatogram obtained with 4 μl of solution (1) is similar in position, colour and size to the principal spot in the chromatogram obtained with solution (2).

C. Heat 0.5 ml of *chromic—sulphuric acid mixture* in a small test-tube in a naked flame until white fumes are produced in the upper part of the tube; the solution wets the sides of the tube and there is no greasiness. Add 2 mg

Free acid Not more than 1.0% w/v, calculated as benzoic acid, $C_7H_6O_2$, when determined by the following method. To 10 ml add 20 ml of *ethanol (96%)* previously neutralised to *phenolphthalein solution* and titrate with 0.1M *sodium hydroxide VS* using *phenolphthalein solution* as indicator. Each ml of 0.1M *sodium hydroxide VS* is equivalent to 0.01221 g of $C_7H_6O_2$.

Chlorinated compounds Not more than 0.05% w/v, calculated as Cl, when determined by the following method. To 5 ml add 50 ml of *amyl alcohol* and 3 g of *sodium* and boil under a reflux condenser for 1 hour. Cool, add 50 ml of *water* and 15 ml of *nitric acid*, cool, add 5 ml of 0.1M *silver nitrate VS*, shake and titrate the excess silver nitrate with 0.1M *ammonium thiocyanate VS* using *ammonium iron(III) sulphate solution* as indicator. Repeat the procedure without the substance being examined. The difference between the titrations represents the amount of silver nitrate required. Each ml of 0.1M *silver nitrate VS* is equivalent to 0.003545 g of Cl.

Assay Carry out the method for *determination of aldehydes*, Appendix X K, using 0.5 g. Each ml of 0.5M *potassium hydroxide in ethanol (60%) VS* is equivalent to 0.05348 g of C_7H_6O.

Storage Benzaldehyde should be kept in a well-filled, well-closed container, protected from light and stored at a temperature not exceeding 15°.

Preparation
Benzaldehyde Spirit

Action and use Flavour.

Benzalkonium Chloride ☆

8001-54-5

Benzalkonium Chloride is a mixture of alkylbenzyldimethylammonium chlorides, the alkyl groups having chain lengths of C_8 to C_{18}. It contains not less than 95.0 per cent and not more than 104.0 per cent of alkylbenzyldimethylammonium chlorides, calculated as $C_{22}H_{40}ClN$ (354.0) with reference to the anhydrous substance.

Characteristics A white or yellowish-white powder or gelatinous, yellowish-white fragments; hygroscopic; unctuous. It forms a clear molten mass on heating.

Solubility Very soluble in *water*, foaming strongly on shaking, and in *ethanol (96%)*.

Identification A. Dissolve 80 mg in sufficient *water* to produce 100 ml. The *light absorption* of the resulting solution, Appendix II B, in the range 220 to 350 nm exhibits three maxima, at 257, 263 and 269 nm and a shoulder at 250 nm.

B. To 5 ml of 2M *sodium hydroxide* add 0.1 ml of *aqueous bromophenol blue solution* and 5 ml of *chloroform* and shake; the chloroform layer is colourless. Add 0.1 ml of a 1.0% w/v solution in *carbon dioxide-free water* (solution A) and shake; the chloroform layer becomes blue.

C. To 2 ml of solution A add 0.1 ml of *glacial acetic acid* and, dropwise, 1 ml of a 1.0% w/v solution of *sodium tetraphenylborate*; a white precipitate is produced. Filter and dissolve the precipitate in a mixture of 5 ml of *ethanol (96%)* and 1 ml of *acetone*, heating to a temperature not exceeding 70°. To the warm solution add *water*, dropwise, until a slight opalescence is produced, heat gently until the solution becomes clear and allow to cool; white crystals are produced. Filter, wash with three 10-ml quantities of *water* and dry over *phosphorus pentoxide* or *self-indicating silica gel* at a temperature not exceeding 50° and at a pressure of 1.5 to 2.5 kPa. The *melting point* of the crystals is 127° to 133°, Appendix V A.

D. To 2 ml of solution A add 1 ml of 2M *nitric acid*. A white precipitate is produced which dissolves on the addition of 5 ml of *ethanol (96%)*. The resulting solution yields *reaction A* characteristic of chlorides, Appendix VI.

Acidity or alkalinity To 50 ml of solution A add 0.1 ml of *bromocresol purple solution*. Not more than 0.1 ml of 0.1M *hydrochloric acid VS* or 0.1M *sodium hydroxide VS* is required to change the colour of the solution.

Clarity and colour of solution Solution A is *clear*, Appendix IV A, and not more intensely coloured than *reference solution Y_6*, Appendix IV B, Method II.

Non-quaternised amines Dissolve 5 g with heating in 20 ml of a mixture of 3 volumes of 1M *hydrochloric acid* and 97 volumes of *methanol* and add 100 ml of *propan-2-ol*. Pass a stream of *nitrogen* slowly through the solution and titrate potentiometrically with 0.1M *tetrabutyl-ammonium hydroxide VS* until a total of 12.0 ml has been added. If two inflections are observed the volume of titrant added between the two points is not greater than 5.0 ml. If no inflection is observed the substance being examined does not comply with the test. If only one inflection is observed repeat the procedure but add 3.0 ml of a 2.5% w/v solution of N,N-*dimethyltetradecylamine* in *propan-2-ol* before the titration. If the titration curve shows only one inflection after the addition of 12.0 ml of the titrant the substance being examined does not comply with the test.

Sulphated ash Not more than 0.1% w/w, Appendix IX A, Method II. Use 1 g.

Water Not more than 10.0% w/w, Appendix IX C. Use 0.3 g.

Assay Dissolve 2 g in sufficient *water* to produce 100 ml. Transfer 25 ml of the solution to a separating funnel, add 25 ml of *chloroform*, 10 ml of 0.1M *sodium hydroxide* and 10.0 ml of a freshly prepared 5.0% w/v solution of *potassium iodide*. Shake well, allow to separate and discard the chloroform layer. Wash the aqueous layer with three 10-ml quantities of *chloroform* and discard the washings. Add 40 ml of *hydrochloric acid*, allow to cool and titrate with 0.05M *potassium iodate VS* until the deep brown colour is almost discharged. Add 2 ml of *chloroform* and continue the titration, shaking vigorously, until the chloroform layer no longer changes colour. Carry out a blank titration on a mixture of 10.0 ml of the freshly prepared potassium iodide solution, 20 ml of *water* and 40 ml of *hydrochloric acid*. The difference between the titrations represents the amount of potassium iodate required. Each ml of 0.05M *potassium iodate VS* is equivalent to 0.0354 g of $C_{22}H_{40}ClN$.

Action and use Antiseptic detergent.

Benzalkonium Chloride Solution ☆

Benzalkonium Chloride Solution is a solution of a mixture of alkylbenzyldimethylammonium chlorides, the alkyl groups having chain lengths of C_8 to C_{18}; it may contain Ethanol (96 per cent). It contains not less than 47.5 per cent w/v and not more than 52.5 per cent w/v of alkylbenzyldimethylammonium chlorides, calculated as $C_{22}H_{40}ClN$.

In making Benzalkonium Chloride Solution, the Ethanol (96 per cent) may be replaced by Industrial Methylated Spirit, diluted so as to be of equivalent alcoholic strength, provided that the law and statutory regulations governing the use of Industrial Methylated Spirit are observed.

Characteristics A clear, colourless or slightly yellowish liquid. It foams strongly on shaking.

Solubility Miscible with *water* and with *ethanol (96%)*.

Identification A. Dilute 0.3 ml to 100 ml with *water*. The *light absorption*, Appendix II B, in the range 220 to 350 nm exhibits three maxima, at 257, 263 and 269 nm, and a shoulder at 250 nm.

B. To 5 ml of 2M *sodium hydroxide* add 0.1 ml of *aqueous bromophenol blue solution* and 5 ml of *chloroform* and shake; the chloroform layer is colourless. Add 0.05 ml of the solution being examined and shake; the chloroform layer becomes blue.

C. To 0.05 ml add 2 ml of *water*, 0.1 ml of *glacial acetic acid* and, dropwise, 1 ml of a 1% w/v solution of *sodium tetraphenylborate*; a white precipitate is produced. Filter and dissolve the precipitate in a mixture of 5 ml of *ethanol (96%)* and 1 ml of *acetone*, heating to a temperature not exceeding 70°. To the warm solution add *water*, dropwise, until a slight opalescence is produced, heat gently until the solution becomes clear and allow to cool; white crystals are produced. Filter, wash with three 10-ml quantities of *water* and dry over *phosphorus pentoxide* or *self-indicating silica gel* at a temperature not exceeding 50° and at a pressure of 1.5 to 2.5 kPa. The *melting point* of the crystals is 127° to 133°, Appendix V A.

D. To 0.05 ml add 1 ml of 2M *nitric acid*. A white precipitate is produced which dissolves on the addition of 5 ml of *ethanol (96%)*. The resulting solution yields *reaction A* characteristic of chlorides, Appendix VI.

Acidity or alkalinity Dilute 2.0 g to 100 ml with *carbon dioxide-free water* (solution A). Add 0.1 ml of *bromocresol purple solution* to 50 ml of solution A. Not more than 0.1 ml of 0.1M *hydrochloric acid VS* or 0.1M *sodium hydroxide VS* is required to change the colour of the solution.

Clarity and colour of solution Solution A is *clear*, Appendix IV A, and not more intensely coloured than *reference solution Y_6*, Appendix IV B, Method II.

Non-quaternised amines Mix 10.0 g, while heating, with 20 ml of a mixture of 3 volumes of 1M *hydrochloric acid* and 97 volumes of *methanol* and add 100 ml of *propan-2-ol*. Pass a stream of *nitrogen* slowly through the solution and titrate potentiometrically with 0.1M *tetrabutylammonium hydroxide VS* until a total of 12.0 ml has been added. If two inflections are observed the volume of titrant added between the two points is not greater than 5.0 ml. If no inflection is observed the substance being examined does not comply with the test. If only one inflection is observed repeat the procedure but add 3.0 ml of a 2.5% w/v solution of N,N-*dimethyltetradecylamine* in *propan-2-ol* before the titration. If the titration curve shows only one inflection after the addition of 12.0 ml of the titrant the substance being examined does not comply with the test.

Sulphated ash Not more than 0.1%, Appendix IX A, Method II. Use 1 g.

Assay Dilute 4 g to 100 ml with *water*. Transfer 25 ml of the solution to a separating funnel, add 25 ml of *chloroform*, 10 ml of 0.1M *sodium hydroxide* and 10.0 ml of a freshly prepared 5.0% w/v solution of *potassium iodide*. Shake well, allow to separate and discard the chloroform layer. Wash the aqueous layer with three 10-ml quantities of *chloroform*, discarding the chloroform layers. Add 40 ml of *hydrochloric acid*, allow to cool and titrate with 0.05M *potassium iodate VS* until the deep brown colour is almost discharged. Add 2 ml of *chloroform* and continue the titration, shaking vigorously, until the chloroform layer no longer changes colour. Carry out a blank titration on a mixture of 10.0 ml of the freshly prepared of *potassium iodide solution*, 20 ml of *water* and 40 ml of *hydrochloric acid*. The difference between the titrations represents the amount of potassium iodate required. Each ml of 0.05M *potassium iodate VS* is equivalent to 0.0354 g of $C_{22}H_{40}ClN$. Determine the *weight per ml* of the solution being examined, Appendix V G, and calculate the percentage content of $C_{22}H_{40}ClN$, weight in volume.

Labelling The label states, where appropriate, the content of Ethanol (96 per cent).

Action and use Antiseptic detergent.

Benzathine Penicillin ☆

$CH_2 \cdot NH \cdot CH_2Ph$
$CH_2 \cdot NH \cdot CH_2Ph$ · [PhCH₂·CO·NH ... S Me ... Me ... CO_2H]₂

$C_{16}H_{20}N_2,(C_{16}H_{18}N_2O_4S)_2$ 909.1   *1538-09-6*

Benzathine Penicillin is N,N'-dibenzylethylenediammonium bis[$(6R)$-6-(2-phenylacetamido)-penicillanate] containing a variable amount of water. It contains not less than 96.0 per cent and not more than 100.5 per cent of penicillins calculated as $C_{16}H_{20}N_2,(C_{16}H_{18}N_2O_4S)_2$ and not less than 24.0 per cent and not more than 27.0 per cent of N,N'-dibenzylethylenediamine, $C_{16}H_{20}N_2$, both calculated with reference to the anhydrous substance.

Characteristics A white powder.

Solubility Very slightly soluble in *water* and in *chloroform*; slightly soluble in *ethanol (96%)*; soluble in 7 parts of *dimethylformamide* and in 10 parts of *formamide*; practically insoluble in *ether*.

Identification *Test A may be omitted if tests B, C and D are carried out. Tests B, C and D may omitted if test A is carried out.*

A. The *infra-red absorption spectrum*, Appendix II A, is concordant with the spectrum of *benzathine benzylpenicillin EPCRS*.

B. Use a 1% w/v solution in *dimethylformamide* to prepare a 0.01% w/v solution in *0.0067M mixed phosphate buffer pH 7.0* (solution A). To 10 ml of solution A add 0.5 ml of *dilute penicillinase solution* and allow to stand at 30° for 10 minutes (solution B). To 5 ml of solution A and 5 ml of solution B, in separate test-tubes, add 10 ml of *acetate buffer pH 4.6* and 5 ml of 0.0005M *iodine VS*. Mix the contents of each tube and add, to each, 0.1 ml of *starch solution*. The mixture obtained with solution A is blue; the mixture obtained with solution B remains colourless.

C. Shake 0.1 g with 2 ml of 1M *sodium hydroxide* for 2 minutes, extract the mixture with two 3-ml quantities of *ether*, evaporate the combined extracts and dissolve the residue in 1 ml of *ethanol (50%)*. Add 5 ml of a 1% w/v solution of *2,4,6-trinitrophenol*, heat at 90° for 5 minutes and allow to cool slowly. The *melting point* of the precipitate, after recrystallisation from hot *ethanol (25%)* containing 1% w/v of *2,4,6-trinitrophenol*, is about 214°, Appendix V A, Method I.

D. Yields the *reaction* characteristic of penicillins and cephalosporins, Appendix VI.

Acidity or alkalinity To 0.5 g add 100 ml of *carbon dioxide-free water*, shake for 5 minutes and filter through sintered glass. To 20 ml of the filtrate add 0.1 ml of *bromothymol blue solution*. The solution is green or yellow and not more than 0.2 ml of 0.02M *sodium hydroxide VS* is required to change the colour of the solution to blue.

Water 5.0 to 8.0% w/w, Appendix IX C. Use 0.3 g.

Assay *For penicillins* Dissolve 70 mg in 20 ml of *methanol*. Add 5 ml of *water* and 5 ml of 1M *sodium hydroxide* and allow to stand for 15 minutes. Add 5 ml of 1M *nitric acid*, 20 ml of *acetate buffer pH 4.6* and 20 ml of *water* and titrate at 35° to 40° with 0.02M *mercury(II) nitrate VS*. Titrate slowly so that the titration takes about 15 minutes. Determine the end-point potentiometrically using a platinum or mercury indicator electrode and a mercury—mercury(I) sulphate reference electrode. Disregard any preliminary inflection on the titration curve. Each ml of 0.02M *mercury(II) nitrate VS* is equivalent to 0.00909 g of total penicillins, calculated as $C_{48}H_{56}N_6O_8S_2$.

To a further 0.25 g dissolved in 50 ml of *methanol* add 25 ml of *acetate buffer pH 4.6* and titrate immediately at room temperature with 0.02M *mercury(II) nitrate VS*. Determine the end-point potentiometrically using a platinum or mercury indicator electrode and a mercury—mercury(I) sulphate reference electrode. Each ml of 0.02M *mercury(II) nitrate VS* is equivalent to 0.00909 g of degradation products, calculated as $C_{48}H_{56}N_6O_8S_2$.

Calculate the percentage content of total penicillins and the percentage content of degradation products. The difference between the two percentages is the content of penicillins.

For N,N'-dibenzylethylenediamine To 1 g add 30 ml of a saturated solution of *sodium chloride* and 10 ml of 5M *sodium hydroxide* and shake with four 50-ml quantities of *ether*. Wash the combined extracts with three 10-ml quantities of *water*, extract the combined washings with 25 ml of *ether* and add the extract to the main ether solution. Evaporate the ether solution to a small volume, add 2 ml of *absolute ethanol* and evaporate to dryness. Dissolve the residue in 50 ml of *glacial acetic acid* and titrate with 0.1M *perchloric acid VS* using 1 ml of *1-naphtholbenzein solution* as indicator. Repeat the operation without the substance being examined. The difference between the titrations represents the amount of perchloric acid required to neutralise the liberated base. Each ml of 0.1M *perchloric acid VS* is equivalent to 0.01202 g of $C_{16}H_{20}N_2$.

Storage Benzathine Penicillin should be kept in an airtight container and stored at a temperature not exceeding 30°. If it is intended for use in the manufacture of a parenteral dosage form, the container should be sterile, tamper-evident and sealed so as to exclude micro-organisms.

Labelling The label states (1) the date after which the material is not intended to be used; (2) the conditions under which it should be stored; (3) whether or not it is intended for use in the manufacture of a parenteral dosage form.

Action and use Antibacterial.

Benzathine Penicillin intended for use in the manufacture of a parenteral dosage form complies with the following additional requirements.

Pyrogens Complies with the *test for pyrogens*, Appendix XIV K. Use per kg of the rabbit's weight 1 ml of the supernatant liquid obtained by suspending 40 mg in 20 ml of *water for injections*, shaking thoroughly and centrifuging.

Sterility Complies with the *test for sterility*, Appendix XVI A.

The title of the monograph in the European Pharmacopœia is Benzathine Benzylpenicillin.

Benzhexol Hydrochloride

$C_{20}H_{31}NO,HCl$ 337.9   *52-49-3*

Benzhexol Hydrochloride is 1-cyclohexyl-1-phenyl-3-piperidin-1-ol hydrochloride. It contains not less than 98.0 per cent and not more than 101.0 per cent of $C_{20}H_{31}NO,HCl$, calculated with reference to the dried substance.

Characteristics A white or creamy-white, crystalline powder; odourless or almost odourless.

Solubility Slightly soluble in *water*; soluble in 22 parts of *ethanol (96%)*, in 10 parts of *methanol* and in 15 parts of *chloroform*.

Identification A. The *infra-red absorption spectrum*, Appendix II A, is concordant with the *reference spectrum* of benzhexol hydrochloride.

B. Dissolve 0.5 g in 5 ml of warm *methanol* and make just alkaline to *litmus paper* with 5M *sodium hydroxide*. A precipitate is produced, which, after recrystallisation from *methanol*, has a *melting point* of about 114°, Appendix V A.

C. Yields the *reactions* characteristic of chlorides, Appendix VI.

Acidity Dissolve 1 g in 50 ml of *carbon dioxide-free water* with the aid of heat. Cool to room temperature and dilute to 100 ml with the same solvent. The pH of the resulting solution is 5.2 to 6.2, Appendix V L.

Piperidylpropiophenone Dissolve 0.1 g in a mixture of 40 ml of *water* and 1 ml of 1M *hydrochloric acid* using heat, cool and add sufficient *water* to produce 100 ml. The *absorbance* of the resulting solution at 247 nm is not more than 0.5, Appendix II B.

Loss on drying When dried to constant weight at 105°, loses not more than 0.5% of its weight. Use 1 g.

Sulphated ash Not more than 0.1%, Appendix IX A.

Assay Carry out Method I for *non-aqueous titration*, Appendix VIII A, using 0.7 g and *1-naphtholbenzein solution* as indicator. Each ml of 0.1M *perchloric acid VS* is equivalent to 0.03379 g of $C_{20}H_{31}NO,HCl$.

Preparation

Benzhexol Tablets

Action and use Used in treatment of Parkinson's disease.

In some countries the material described in this monograph may be known as Trihexyphenidyl Hydrochloride.

Benzocaine ☆

$C_9H_{11}NO_2$ 165.2   *94-09-7*

Benzocaine is ethyl 4-aminobenzoate. It contains not less than 99.0 per cent and not more than 101.0 per cent of $C_9H_{11}NO_2$, calculated with reference to the dried substance.

Characteristics Colourless crystals or a white, crystalline powder.

Solubility Very slightly soluble in *water*; soluble in 8 parts of *ethanol (96%)*, in 2 parts of *chloroform*, in 4 parts of *ether* and in 50 parts of fixed oils.

Identification *Test A may be omitted if tests B, C and D are carried out. Tests B and C may be omitted if tests A and D are carried out.*

A. The *infra-red absorption spectrum*, Appendix II A, is concordant with the spectrum of *benzocaine EPCRS*.

B. Place 50 mg in a test-tube, add 0.2 ml of a 50% w/v solution of *chromium trioxide*, cover the mouth of the tube with a piece of filter paper moistened with a freshly prepared solution consisting of equal volumes of a 5% w/v solution of *sodium nitroprusside* and a 20% w/v solution of *piperazine hydrate* and boil gently for at least 30 seconds. A blue colour is produced on the filter paper.

C. 2 ml of a 0.05% w/v solution in *ethanol (96%)* yields the *reaction* characteristic of primary aromatic amines, Appendix VI.

D. *Melting point*, 89° to 92°, Appendix V A, Method I.

Acidity or alkalinity Dissolve 0.5 g in 10 ml of *ethanol (96%)* previously neutralised to 0.05 ml of *dilute phenolphthalein solution* and add 10 ml of *carbon dioxide-free water*. The solution remains colourless and not more than 0.5 ml of 0.01M *sodium hydroxide VS* is required to change the colour of the solution.

Clarity and colour of solution A 5.0% w/v solution in *ethanol (96%)* is *clear*, Appendix IV A, and *colourless*, Appendix IV B, Method II.

Loss on drying When dried to constant weight over *phosphorus pentoxide* at a pressure of 1.5 to 2.5 kPa, loses not more than 0.5% of its weight. Use 1 g.

Sulphated ash Not more than 0.1%, Appendix IX A, Method II. Use 1 g.

Assay Dissolve 0.4 g in a mixture of 25 ml of *hydrochloric acid* and 50 ml of *water* and add 3 g of *potassium bromide*. Cool, if necessary, in ice and carry out the method for

amperometric titration, Appendix VIII B. Each ml of 0.1M *sodium nitrite VS* is equivalent to 0.01652 g of $C_9H_{11}NO_2$.

Storage Benzocaine should be protected from light.

Action and use Local anaesthetic.

Benzoic Acid ☆

$C_7H_6O_2$ 122.1   *65-85-0*

Benzoic Acid contains not less than 99.0 per cent and not more than 100.5 per cent of $C_7H_6O_2$.

Characteristics Colourless crystals or a white, crystalline powder; odourless or with a very slight, characteristic odour.

Solubility Slightly soluble in *water*; soluble in *boiling water*; freely soluble in *ethanol (96%)*, in *chloroform*, in *ether* and in fixed oils.

Identification A. A 5% w/v solution in *ethanol (96%)* yields *reaction A* characteristic of benzoates, Appendix VI.

B. *Melting point*, 121° to 124°, Appendix V A, Method I.

Clarity and colour of solution A 5.0% w/v solution in *ethanol (96%)* is *clear*, Appendix IV A, and *colourless*, Appendix IV B, Method II.

Carbonisable substances Dissolve 0.5 g, with shaking, in 5 ml of *sulphuric acid (96% w/w)* and allow to stand for 5 minutes. Any colour produced in the solution is not more intense than that of *reference solution Y_5*, Appendix IV B, Method I.

Oxidisable substances Dissolve 0.2 g in 10 ml of boiling *water*, cool, shake and filter. To the filtrate add 1 ml of 1M *sulphuric acid* and 0.2 ml of 0.02M *potassium permanganate* and allow to stand for 5 minutes. The solution remains pink.

Heavy metals 12 ml of a 5.0% w/v solution in *ethanol (96%)* complies with *limit test B for heavy metals*, Appendix VII (10 ppm). Use a mixture of 5 ml of *lead standard solution (1 ppm Pb)* and 5 ml of *ethanol (96%)* to prepare the standard.

Halogenated compounds and halides For solution (1) dissolve 6.7 g in 40 ml of 1M *sodium hydroxide* and 50 ml of *ethanol (96%)* and dilute to 100 ml with *water*. To 10 ml of the solution add 7.5 ml of 2M *sodium hydroxide* and 0.125 g of *Raney nickel catalyst* and heat on a water-bath for 10 minutes. Allow to cool, filter and wash with three 2-ml quantities of *ethanol (96%)*. Dilute the filtrate and washings to 25 ml with *water*. Prepare solution (2) in the same manner but omitting the substance being examined. Solution (3) is a solution of 30 g of *ammonium iron(III) sulphate* in 40 ml of *nitric acid* diluted to 100 ml with *water*, filtered if necessary and stored protected from light.

To four 25-ml graduated flasks labelled A, B, C and D transfer respectively 10 ml each of solution (1), solution (2), *chloride standard solution (8 ppm Cl)* and *water*. To each flask add 5 ml of solution (3), mix and add dropwise with swirling 2 ml of *nitric acid* and 5 ml of a recently prepared 0.3% w/v solution of *mercury(II) thiocyanate* in absolute ethanol. Shake, dilute the resulting solutions to 25 ml with *water* and allow to stand in a water-bath at 20° for 15 minutes. Measure the *absorbance* at 460 nm of solution A using solution B in the reference cell and that of solution C using solution D in the reference cell, Appendix II B. The absorbance of solution A is not more than that of solution C (300 ppm).

Sulphated ash Not more than 0.1%, Appendix IX A, Method II. Use 1 g.

Assay Dissolve 0.2 g in 20 ml of *ethanol (96%)* and titrate with 0.1M *sodium hydroxide VS*, using *phenol red solution* as indicator, until the colour changes from yellow to violet-red. Each ml of 0.1M *sodium hydroxide VS* is equivalent to 0.01221 g of $C_7H_6O_2$.

Preparations
Benzoic Acid Solution
Compound Benzoic Acid Ointment

Action and use Antimicrobial preservative.

Sumatra Benzoin

Benzoin

Sumatra Benzoin is the balsamic resin obtained from the incised stem of *Styrax benzoin* Dryand. and of *S. paralleloneurus* Perkins. It contains not less than 25 per cent of total balsamic acids, calculated as cinnamic acid, $C_9H_8O_2$, with reference to the dried material.

Characteristics Hard, brittle masses consisting of whitish tears embedded in a greyish-brown to reddish-brown translucent matrix, known in commerce as block benzoin. It also occurs in the form of tears with cream-coloured surfaces and, when broken, exhibiting surfaces having a milky-white colour. Odour, agreeable and balsamic.

Identification A. Heat 0.5 g gently in a dry test-tube. It melts and white fumes are evolved which form a white, crystalline sublimate.
B. Warm gently 1 g, in powder, with 5 ml of *potassium permanganate solution*. A distinct odour of benzaldehyde is produced.
C. Triturate 0.1 g, in powder, with 5 ml of *ethanol (96%)*, filter and add 0.5 ml of a 5% w/v solution of *iron(III) chloride* in *ethanol (96%)*. No bright green colour is produced.

Matter insoluble in ethanol (90%) Not more than 20.0% when determined by the following method. Warm 2 g, in *coarse powder*, with 25 ml of *ethanol (90%)*, filter, wash the residue with hot *ethanol (90%)* until extraction is complete and dry to constant weight at 100°.

Loss on drying Not more than 10.0% when determined by the following method. Spread evenly 2 g, in *coarse powder*, in a flat-bottomed dish (9 cm × 1.5 cm) and dry over *phosphorus pentoxide* at a pressure not exceeding 2.7 kPa for 4 hours.

Ash Not more than 2.0%, Appendix XI J.

Assay Boil 1.25 g with 25 ml of *ethanolic potassium hydroxide solution* under a reflux condenser for 1 hour. Evaporate the ethanol, disperse the residue in 50 ml of hot *water*, cool, add 80 ml of *water* and 1.5 g of *magnesium sulphate* dissolved in 50 ml of *water*. Mix thoroughly and allow to stand for 10 minutes. Filter, wash the residue on

the filter with 20 ml of *water*, acidify the combined filtrate and washings with *hydrochloric acid* and extract with four 40-ml quantities of *ether*. Discard the aqueous solution, combine the ether extracts and extract with successive quantities of 20, 20, 10, 10 and 10 ml of *sodium hydrogen carbonate solution*, washing each aqueous extract with the same 20 ml of *ether*. Discard the ether layers, carefully acidify the combined aqueous extracts with *hydrochloric acid* and extract with successive quantities of 30, 20, 20 and 10 ml of *chloroform*, filtering each extract through *anhydrous sodium sulphate* supported on absorbent cotton. Distil the chloroform from the combined filtrates until 10 ml remains and remove the remainder in a current of air. Dissolve the residue, with the aid of gentle heat, in 10 ml of *ethanol (96%)*, previously neutralised to *phenol red solution*, cool and titrate with 0.1M *sodium hydroxide VS* using *phenol red solution* as indicator. Each ml of 0.1M *sodium hydroxide VS* is equivalent to 0.01482 g of total balsamic acids, calculated as cinnamic acid, $C_9H_8O_2$.

Storage Sumatra Benzoin should be kept in a well-closed container, protected from light and stored at a temperature not exceeding 25°.

Preparations
Benzoin Inhalation
Compound Benzoin Tincture

Hydrous Benzoyl Peroxide

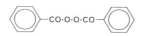

$C_{14}H_{10}O_4$ 242.2   *94-36-0*

Hydrous Benzoyl Peroxide contains not less than 95.0 per cent and not more than 105.0 per cent of the declared content of $C_{14}H_{10}O_4$. It contains not less than 23 per cent of water to ensure safety in transit and handling.

CAUTION Hydrous Benzoyl Peroxide may explode at temperatures higher than 60° or cause fires in the presence of reducing substances. Anhydrous benzoyl peroxide may be exploded by percussion or excessive heat.

Characteristics A white, amorphous or granular powder or paste that has been moistened with water.

Solubility Sparingly soluble in *water* and in *absolute ethanol*; soluble in *acetone*; soluble in *chloroform* and in *ether* with the separation of water.

Mix the entire sample thoroughly before carrying out the following tests.

Identification A. Shake a quantity containing the equivalent of 0.5 g of anhydrous benzoyl peroxide with 10 ml of *chloroform IR* and filter through *anhydrous sodium sulphate*. The *infra-red absorption spectrum* of the filtrate, Appendix II A, is concordant with the *reference spectrum* of benzoyl peroxide.
B. The *light absorption*, Appendix II B, in the range 220 to 350 nm of a solution containing the equivalent of 0.0008% w/v of anhydrous benzoyl peroxide in *absolute ethanol* exhibits a maximum at 235 nm. The *absorbance* at 235 nm is about 1.05.

Acidity Dissolve a quantity containing the equivalent of 2.0 g of anhydrous benzoyl peroxide in 10 ml of *acetone* by heating in a water-bath maintained at 50°, add 25 ml of *water* and filter. Wash the residue with three 10-ml quantities of *water*. Titrate the combined filtrate and washings with 0.1M *sodium hydroxide VS* using *phenolphthalein solution* as indicator. Not more than 2.5 ml is required.

Chloride Dissolve a quantity containing the equivalent of 0.5 g of anhydrous benzoyl peroxide in 10 ml of *acetone*, add, while stirring, 25 ml of 0.05M *nitric acid* and filter. Wash the residue with 10 ml of 0.05M *nitric acid*, combine the washings and filtrate and dilute to 50 ml with 0.05M *nitric acid*. To 10 ml of the resulting solution add 0.1 ml of *silver nitrate solution*. The solution is not more opalescent than a standard prepared by adding 0.1 ml of *silver nitrate solution* to 10 ml of a 0.0038% w/v solution of *sodium chloride* in 0.05M *nitric acid*.

Related substances Carry out the method for *high-performance liquid chromatography*, Appendix III D, using the following solutions in the mobile phase. For solution (1) dilute 1 volume of solution (2) to 100 volumes with the mobile phase. Solution (2) is a solution of the substance being examined containing the equivalent of 0.20% w/v of anhydrous benzoyl peroxide. Solutions (3) to (5) contain (3) 0.0030% w/v of *benzoic acid*, (4) 0.0020% w/v of *ethyl benzoate* and (5) 0.0020% w/v of *benzaldehyde*.

The chromatographic procedure may be carried out using (a) a stainless steel column (20 cm × 4.6 mm) packed with *stationary phase C* (10 μm) (Spherisorb ODS 1 is suitable), (b) a mixture of 500 volumes of *acetonitrile*, 500 volumes of *water* and 1 volume of *glacial acetic acid* as the mobile phase with a flow rate of 1 ml per minute and (c) a detection wavelength of 235 nm.

In the chromatogram obtained with solution (2) the areas of any peaks corresponding to benzoic acid, ethyl benzoate and benzaldehyde are not greater than the areas of the principal peaks in the chromatograms obtained with solutions (3), (4) and (5) respectively and the area of any other *secondary peak* is not greater than the area of the principal peak in the chromatogram obtained with solution (1). The sum of the areas of the *secondary peaks* is not greater than three times the area of the principal peak in the chromatogram obtained with solution (1).

Water Not less than 23.0%, Appendix IX C. Dissolve a quantity expected to contain about 0.25 g of water in sufficient *anhydrous methanol* to produce 250 ml and use 25 ml of the resulting solution.

Assay Dissolve a quantity containing the equivalent of 3 g of anhydrous benzoyl peroxide in sufficient *acetone* to produce 200 ml. To 20 ml of the solution add 3 ml of a 50% w/v solution of *potassium iodide* and titrate with 0.1M *sodium thiosulphate VS* using *starch mucilage*, added towards the end of the titration, as indicator. Repeat the operation without the substance being examined. The difference between the titrations represents the amount of sodium thiosulphate required. Each ml of 0.1M *sodium thiosulphate VS* is equivalent to 0.01211 g of $C_{14}H_{10}O_4$.

Storage Hydrous Benzoyl Peroxide should be kept in the original container which has been treated to reduce static discharge. Unused material must not be returned to the original container but destroyed by treating with a 10% w/v solution of sodium hydroxide until addition of a crystal of potassium iodide does not liberate free iodine.

Labelling The label states the percentage content of anhydrous benzoyl peroxide.

Preparations
Benzoyl Peroxide Cream
Benzoyl Peroxide Gel
Benzoyl Peroxide Lotion
Potassium Hydroxyquinoline Sulphate and Benzoyl Peroxide Cream

Action and use Used topically in treatment of acne.

Benztropine Mesylate

$C_{21}H_{25}NO,CH_4O_3S$ 403.5   *132-17-2*

Benztropine Mesylate is (1*R*,3*r*,5*S*)-3-benz-hydryloxytropane methanesulphonate. It contains not less than 98.0 per cent and not more than 100.5 per cent of $C_{21}H_{25}NO,CH_4O_3S$, calculated with reference to the dried substance.

Characteristics A white, crystalline powder; odourless or almost odourless.

Solubility Soluble in 0.7 part of *water* and in 1.5 parts of *ethanol (96%)*; practically insoluble in *ether*.

Identification A. The *infra-red absorption spectrum*, Appendix II A, is concordant with the *reference spectrum* of benztropine mesylate.
B. The *light absorption*, Appendix II B, in the range 230 to 350 nm of a 0.01% w/v solution in 2M *hydrochloric acid* exhibits two maxima, at 253 and 258 nm. The *absorbance* at 253 nm is about 0.96 and at 258 nm is about 1.1.
C. Add 1 mg to 0.2 ml of *fuming nitric acid*; a reddish colour is produced. Evaporate to dryness; a brownish-yellow, oily residue is obtained which becomes yellow on the addition of 2 ml of *acetone* and gives a brownish-red precipitate on the addition of 0.2 ml of a 3% w/v solution of *potassium hydroxide* in *methanol*.
D. Dissolve 10 mg in 10 ml of *sulphuric acid*; an orange solution is produced. To 5 ml of the solution add 0.2 ml of *potassium dichromate solution*, warm and allow to stand; the colour of the solution slowly changes from red to brown. Pour the remainder of the solution into about 10 ml of *water*; a colourless, opalescent solution is produced.
E. Dissolve 10 mg in 2 ml of *water*, pour into 5 ml of hot *trinitrophenol solution* and allow to cool. The *melting point* of the precipitate, after drying at 105°, is about 185°, Appendix V A.

Melting point 142° to 144°, Appendix V A.

Tropine Carry out the method for *thin-layer chromatography*, Appendix III A, using *silica gel G* as the coating substance and a mixture of 75 volumes of *ethanol (96%)* and 15 volumes of 13.5M *ammonia* as the mobile phase. Apply separately to the chromatoplate 10 μl of each of two solutions in *acetone* containing (1) 4.0% w/v of the substance being examined and (2) 0.020% w/v of *tropine*. After removal of the plate, allow it to dry in air and spray

with *sodium iodobismuthate solution* and then with a
0.4% w/v solution of *sulphuric acid*. Any spot
corresponding to tropine in the chromatogram obtained
with solution (1) is not more intense than the spot in the
chromatogram obtained with solution (2).

Loss on drying When dried to constant weight at 105°,
loses not more than 5.0% of its weight. Use 1 g.

Sulphated ash Not more than 0.1%, Appendix IX A.

Assay Dissolve 0.6 g in 25 ml of *water*, add 5 ml of
sodium carbonate solution and extract with four 10-ml
quantities of *chloroform*. Wash the combined extracts with
10 ml of *water*, extract the washings with 5 ml of
chloroform and add the chloroform to the combined
extracts. Filter and wash the filter with 5 ml of *chloroform*.
To the combined filtrate and washings add 25 ml of
1,4-dioxan and titrate with 0.1M *perchloric acid VS* using
0.15 ml of a 0.1% w/v solution of *methyl red* in *methanol* as
indicator. Each ml of 0.1M *perchloric acid VS* is equivalent
to 0.04035 g of $C_{21}H_{25}NO,CH_4O_3S$.

Storage Benztropine Mesylate should be kept in a well-
closed container.

Preparations
Benztropine Injection
Benztropine Tablets

Action and use Used in treatment of Parkinson's disease.

In some countries the material described in this
monograph may be known as Benzatropine Mesylate.

Benzyl Alcohol ☆

C_7H_8O 108.1   *100-51-6*

Benzyl Alcohol contains not less than 97.0 per
cent and not more than 100.5 per cent of
C_7H_8O.

Characteristics A clear, colourless, refringent, oily liquid;
odour, slightly aromatic.

Solubility Soluble in 25 parts of *water*; miscible with
ethanol (96%), with *chloroform*, with *ether* and with fixed
and volatile oils.

Identification Add 0.1 ml to 5 ml of a 3.0% w/v solution
of *potassium permanganate* acidified with 1 ml of 1M
sulphuric acid. Benzaldehyde, recognisable by its odour, is
produced.

Acidity To 10 ml add 10 ml of *ethanol (96%)* and 1 ml of
dilute phenolphthalein solution. Not more than 1 ml of 0.1M
sodium hydroxide VS is required to change the colour of
the solution.

Clarity of solution Shake 2.0 ml with 60 ml of *water*. The
resulting solution is *clear*, Appendix IV A.

Peroxide value Not more than 5, Appendix X F.

Refractive index 1.538 to 1.541, Appendix V E.

Relative density 1.043 to 1.049, Appendix V G.

Benzaldehyde and other related substances Carry out
the method for *gas chromatography*, Appendix III B, using
as solution (1) the substance being examined containing

0.1% w/v of *dibutyl phthalate* and 0.1% w/v of *benzaldehyde*
and as solution (2) the substance being examined.

The chromatographic procedure may be carried out
using a glass column (2 m × 3 mm) packed with *acid-
washed, silanised diatomaceous support* (Chromosorb W/HP
is suitable) coated with 3% w/w of phenyl methyl silicone
fluid (50% phenyl) (OV-17 is suitable) with the
temperature rising at a rate of 10° per minute from 85° to
290°, an inlet port temperature of 210° and a detector
temperature of 275° and using 20 ml per minute as the
flow rate of the carrier gas. Inject 1 μl of each solution
using on-column injection or a glass-lined injector.

In the chromatogram obtained with solution (2) the area
of any peak corresponding to benzaldehyde is not greater
than 1.5 times the area of the peak due to dibutyl
phthalate in the chromatogram obtained with solution (1)
(0.15%); the sum of the areas of any other *secondary peaks*
is not greater than twice the area of the peak due to
dibutyl phthalate in the chromatogram obtained with
solution (1) (0.2%).

*Benzyl Alcohol intended for use in the manufacture of a
parenteral dosage form contains not more than 0.05% of
benzaldehyde and not more than 0.1% of other related
substances.*

Halogenated compounds and halides All glassware must
be chloride-free and may be prepared by soaking
overnight in a 50% v/v solution of *nitric acid*, rinsing with
water and storing full of *water*. Dissolve 6.7 g in 50 ml of
ethanol (96%) and dilute to 100 ml with *water*. To 10 ml
of the resulting solution add 7.5 ml of 2M *sodium hydroxide*
and 0.125 g of *Raney nickel* and heat on a water-bath for
10 minutes. Cool to room temperature, filter, wash the
filter with three 2-ml quantities of *ethanol (96%)* and
dilute to 25 ml with *water*. Prepare a blank solution using
10 ml of a mixture of equal volumes of *ethanol (96%)* and
water and beginning at the words 'add 7.5 ml of . . .'. To
four 25-ml graduated flasks labelled A, B, C and D
transfer respectively 10 ml each of the test solution, the
blank solution, *chloride standard solution (8 ppm Cl)* and
water. To each flask add 5 ml of *ammonium iron(III)
sulphate—nitric acid solution* and 5 ml of a 0.3% w/v
solution of *mercury(II) thiocyanate* in *ethanol (96%)*. Shake,
dilute the contents of each flask to 25 ml with *water* and
allow the solutions to stand in a water-bath at 20° for 15
minutes. Measure the *absorbance* at 460 nm, Appendix
II B, of solution (A) using solution (B) in the reference
cell and of solution (C) using solution (D) in the reference
cell. The absorbance of solution (A) is not more than that
of solution (C) (300 ppm).

Non-volatile matter Evaporate 2 g to dryness on a water-
bath, dry at 100° to 105° for 1 hour and cool in a
desiccator. The residue weighs not more than 1 mg
(0.05%).

Assay To 0.9 g add 15 ml of a mixture of 7 volumes of
pyridine and 1 volume of *acetic anhydride* and heat under a
reflux condenser on a water-bath for 30 minutes. Cool,
add 25 ml of *water* and titrate with 1M *sodium hydroxide
VS* using 0.25 ml of *dilute phenolphthalein solution* as
indicator. Repeat the operation without the substance
being examined. The difference between the titrations
represents the amount of sodium hydroxide required.
Each ml of 1M *sodium hydroxide VS* is equivalent to
0.1081 g of C_7H_8O.

Storage Benzyl Alcohol should be kept in a completely
filled and well-closed container and protected from light.

Action and use Local anaesthetic; disinfectant.

Benzyl Benzoate

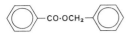

C$_{14}$H$_{12}$O$_2$ 212.3   *120-51-4*

Benzyl Benzoate contains not less than 99.0 per cent and not more than 100.5 per cent w/w of C$_{14}$H$_{12}$O$_2$.

Characteristics Colourless crystals or a colourless, oily liquid; odour, faintly aromatic.

Solubility Practically insoluble in *water*; miscible with *ethanol (96%)*, with *chloroform* and with *ether*; practically insoluble in *glycerol*.

Identification A. Boil 2 g with 25 ml of *ethanolic potassium hydroxide solution* under a reflux condenser for 2 hours. Remove the ethanol on a water-bath, add 50 ml of *water* and distil until the liquid distilling is no longer turbid. The liquid remaining in the flask, after acidification with 2M *hydrochloric acid*, yields a white crystalline precipitate of benzoic acid.

B. To the distillate obtained in test A add 2.5 g of *potassium permanganate* and 2 ml of 5M *sodium hydroxide*, boil under a reflux condenser for 15 minutes, cool and filter. The filtrate, after acidification with 2M *hydrochloric acid*, yields a white crystalline precipitate of benzoic acid.

C. *Boiling point*, about 320°, Appendix V D.

Freezing point Not below 17.0°, Appendix V B.

Refractive index 1.568 to 1.570, Appendix V E.

Weight per ml 1.116 to 1.120 g, Appendix V G.

Sulphated ash Not more than 0.1%, Appendix IX A.

Assay Carry out the method for the *determination of esters*, Appendix VIII L, using 40 ml of 0.5M *ethanolic potassium hydroxide VS*. Each ml of 0.5M *ethanolic potassium hydroxide VS* is equivalent to 0.1061 g of C$_{14}$H$_{12}$O$_2$.

Preparation

Benzyl Benzoate Application

Action and use Used topically in the treatment of scabies.

Benzyl Hydroxybenzoate

Benzylparaben

HO—⟨◯⟩—CO·O·CH$_2$—⟨◯⟩

C$_{14}$H$_{12}$O$_3$ 228.3   *94-18-8*

Benzyl Hydroxybenzoate is benzyl 4-hydroxy-benzoate. It contains not less than 99.0 per cent and not more than 101.0 per cent of C$_{14}$H$_{12}$O$_3$.

Characteristics A white to creamy-white, crystalline powder; odourless or almost odourless.

Solubility Practically insoluble in *water*; soluble in 2.5 parts of *ethanol (96%)* and in 6 parts of *ether*. It dissolves in solutions of alkali hydroxides.

Identification A. The *infra-red absorption spectrum*, Appendix II A, is concordant with the *reference spectrum* of benzyl hydroxybenzoate.

B. The *light absorption*, Appendix II B, in the range 230 to 350 nm of a 0.001% w/v solution in *ethanol (96%)* exhibits a maximum only at 260 nm. The *absorbance* at 260 nm is about 0.76.

C. Dissolve 0.1 g in 2 ml of *ethanol (96%)*, boil and add 0.5 ml of *mercury—nitric acid solution*. A precipitate is produced slowly and the supernatant liquid becomes red.

D. *Melting point*, about 112°, Appendix V A.

Acidity Dissolve 0.2 g in 10 ml of *ethanol (50%)* previously neutralised to *methyl red solution* and titrate with 0.1M *sodium hydroxide VS* using *methyl red solution* as indicator. Not more than 0.1 ml of 0.1M *sodium hydroxide VS* is required to change the colour of the solution.

Related substances Carry out the method for *thin-layer chromatography*, Appendix III A, using a chromatoplate precoated with silica gel F254 the surface of which has been modified with chemically-bonded octadecylsilyl groups (Whatman KC18F plates are suitable) and a mixture of 70 volumes of *methanol*, 30 volumes of *water* and 1 volume of *glacial acetic acid* as the mobile phase. Apply separately to the plate 2 μl of each of two solutions of the substance being examined in *acetone* containing (1) 1.0% w/v and (2) 0.010% w/v. After removal of the plate, allow it to dry in air and examine under *ultra-violet light (254 nm)*. Any *secondary spot* in the chromatogram obtained with solution (1) is not more intense than the spot in the chromatogram obtained with solution (2).

Sulphated ash Not more than 0.1%, Appendix IX A.

Assay Gently boil 0.12 g under a reflux condenser with 20 ml of 2M *sodium hydroxide* for 30 minutes. Cool and extract with three 20-ml quantities of *1,2-dichloroethane*. Wash the combined extracts with 20 ml of 0.1M *sodium hydroxide* and add the washings to the main aqueous phase, discarding the organic layer. To the aqueous solution add 25 ml of 0.0333M *potassium bromate VS*, 5 ml of a 12.5% w/v solution of *potassium bromide* and 10 ml of *hydrochloric acid* and immediately stopper the flask. Shake for 15 minutes and allow to stand for 15 minutes. Add 25 ml of *potassium iodide solution* and shake vigorously. Titrate the liberated iodine with 0.1M *sodium thiosulphate VS* using *starch mucilage*, added towards the end of the titration, as indicator. The volume of 0.0333M *potassium bromate VS* used is equivalent to half of the volume of 0.1M *sodium thiosulphate VS* required for the titration. Each ml of 0.0333M *potassium bromate VS* is equivalent to 0.007608 g of C$_{14}$H$_{12}$O$_3$.

Action and use Antimicrobial preservative.

Benzylpenicillin Potassium ☆
Penicillin G Potassium

PhCH₂·CO·NH— ... structure ...

$C_{16}H_{17}KN_2O_4S$ 372.5   113-98-4

Benzylpenicillin Potassium is potassium (6R)-6-(2-phenylacetamido)penicillanate, produced by the growth of certain strains of *Penicillium notatum* or related organisms, or obtained by any other means. It contains not less than 96.0 per cent and not more than 100.5 per cent of penicillins, calculated as $C_{16}H_{17}KN_2O_4S$ with reference to the dried substance.

Characteristics A white or almost white, crystalline powder with a faint characteristic odour.

Solubility Very soluble in *water*; practically insoluble in *chloroform*, in *ether*, in fixed oils and in *liquid paraffin*.

Identification *Test A may be omitted if tests B, C and D are carried out. Tests B and C may be omitted if tests A and D are carried out.*
A. The *infra-red absorption spectrum*, Appendix II A, is concordant with the spectrum of *benzylpenicillin potassium EPCRS*.
B. To 10 ml of a 0.01% w/v solution in *0.0067M mixed phosphate buffer pH 7.0* (solution A) add 0.5 ml of a solution prepared by diluting 1 ml of *penicillinase solution* to 10 ml with *water* and allow to stand at 30° for 10 minutes (solution B). To 5 ml of solution A and to 5 ml of solution B, in separate test-tubes, add 10 ml of *acetate buffer pH 4.6* and 5 ml of 0.0005M *iodine VS*. Mix the contents of each tube and add to each 0.1 ml of *starch solution*. The mixture obtained with solution A is blue; the mixture obtained with solution B remains colourless.
C. Yields the *reaction* characteristic of penicillins and cephalosporins, Appendix VI.
D. Yields *reaction A* characteristic of potassium salts, Appendix VI.

Acidity or alkalinity pH of a 10% w/v solution, 5.5 to 7.5, Appendix V L.

Light absorption Dissolve 94 mg in sufficient *water* to produce 50 ml. Measure the *absorbances* at 325 nm, at 280 nm and at the maximum at 264 nm, Appendix II B, diluting the solution, if necessary, for the measurement at 264 nm. The absorbances at 325 and 280 nm are not more than 0.10 and that at the maximum at 264 nm, calculated on the basis of the undiluted solution (0.188% w/v), is 0.80 to 0.88.
Determine the *resolution power* of the spectrophotometer, Appendix II B. The test is not valid unless the ratio of the absorbances is not less than 1.7.

Specific optical rotation In a 2% w/v solution in *carbon dioxide-free water*, +270° to +300°, Appendix V F.

Loss on drying When dried to constant weight at 100° to 105°, loses not more than 1.0% of its weight. Use 1 g.

Assay Dissolve 50 mg in 5 ml of *water*, add 5 ml of 1M *sodium hydroxide* and allow to stand for 15 minutes. Add 5 ml of 1M *nitric acid*, 20 ml of *acetate buffer pH 4.6* and 20 ml of *water* and titrate at 35° to 40° with 0.02M *mercury(II) nitrate VS*. Titrate slowly so that the titration takes about 15 minutes. Determine the end-point potentiometrically using a platinum or mercury indicator electrode and a mercury—mercury(I) sulphate reference electrode. Disregard any preliminary inflection on the titration curve. Each ml of 0.02M *mercury(II) nitrate VS* is equivalent to 0.007450 g of total penicillins, calculated as $C_{16}H_{17}KN_2O_4S$.
To a further 0.25 g add 25 ml of *water* and 25 ml of *acetate buffer pH 4.6* and shake until solution is complete. Titrate immediately at room temperature with 0.02M *mercury(II) nitrate VS* determining the end-point as above. Each ml of 0.02M *mercury(II) nitrate VS* is equivalent to 0.007450 g of degradation products, calculated as $C_{16}H_{17}KN_2O_4S$.
Calculate the percentage content of total penicillins and the percentage content of degradation products. The difference between the two percentages is the content of penicillins.

Storage Benzylpenicillin Potassium should be kept in a well-closed container, protected from moisture and stored at a temperature not exceeding 30°. If the contents are intended for use in the manufacture of a parenteral dosage form, the container should be sterile, tamper-evident and sealed so as to exclude micro-organisms.

Labelling The label states (1) the date after which the material is not intended to be used; (2) the conditions under which it should be stored; (3) whether or not it is intended for use in the manufacture of a parenteral dosage form.

Preparations
Benzylpenicillin Injection
Fortified Procaine Penicillin Injection

Action and use Antibacterial.

Benzylpenicillin Potassium intended for use in the manufacture of a parenteral dosage form complies with the following additional requirements.

Pyrogens Complies with the *test for pyrogens*, Appendix XIV K. Use per kg of the rabbit's weight 1 ml of a solution containing 1.5 mg per ml of the substance being examined in *water for injections*.

Sterility Complies with the *test for sterility*, Appendix XVI A.

Benzylpenicillin Sodium ☆
Penicillin G Sodium

$C_{16}H_{17}N_2NaO_4S$ 356.4   69-57-8

Benzylpenicillin Sodium is sodium (6R)-6-(2-phenylacetamido)penicillanate, produced by the growth of certain strains of *Penicillium notatum* or related organisms, or obtained by any other means. It contains not less than 96.0 per cent and not more than 100.5 per cent of penicillins, calculated as $C_{16}H_{17}N_2NaO_4S$ with reference to the dried substance.

Characteristics A white or almost white, crystalline powder with a faint characteristic odour.

Solubility Very soluble in *water*; practically insoluble in *chloroform*, in *ether*, in fixed oils and in *liquid paraffin*.

Identification *Test A may be omitted if tests B, C and D are carried out. Tests B and C may be omitted if tests A and D are carried out.*

A. The *infra-red absorption spectrum*, Appendix II A, is concordant with the spectrum of *benzylpenicillin sodium EPCRS*.

B. To 10 ml of a 0.01% w/v solution in *0.0067M mixed phosphate buffer pH 7.0* (solution A) add 0.5 ml of a solution prepared by diluting 1 ml of *penicillinase solution* to 10 ml with *water* and allow to stand at 30° for 10 minutes (solution B). To 5 ml of solution A and to 5 ml of solution B, in separate test-tubes, add 10 ml of *acetate buffer pH 4.6* and 5 ml of 0.0005M *iodine VS*. Mix the contents of each tube and add to each 0.1 ml of *starch solution*. The mixture obtained with solution A is blue; the mixture obtained with solution B remains colourless.

C. Yields the *reaction* characteristic of penicillins and cephalosporins, Appendix VI.

D. Yields *reaction A* characteristic of sodium salts, Appendix VI.

Acidity or alkalinity pH of a 10% w/v solution, 5.5 to 7.5, Appendix V L.

Light absorption Dissolve 90 mg in sufficient *water* to produce 50 ml. Measure the *absorbances* at 325 nm, at 280 nm and at the maximum at 264 nm, Appendix II B, diluting the solution, if necessary, for the measurement at 264 nm. The absorbances at 325 and 280 nm are not more than 0.10 and that at the maximum at 264 nm, calculated on the basis of the undiluted solution (0.180% w/v), is 0.80 to 0.88.

Determine the *resolution power* of the spectrophotometer, Appendix II B. The test is not valid unless the ratio of absorbances is not less than 1.7.

Specific optical rotation In a 2% w/v solution in *carbon dioxide-free water*, +285° to +310°, Appendix V F.

Loss on drying When dried to constant weight at 100° to 105°, loses not more than 1.0% of its weight. Use 1 g.

Assay Carry out the Assay described under Benzylpenicillin Potassium. Each ml of 0.02M *mercury(II) nitrate VS* is equivalent to 0.007128 g of total penicillins, calculated as $C_{16}H_{17}N_2NaO_4S$, and is also equivalent to 0.007128 g of degradation products, calculated as $C_{16}H_{17}N_2NaO_4S$. Calculate the percentage content of total penicillins and the percentage content of degradation products. The difference between the two percentages is the content of penicillins.

Storage Benzylpenicillin Sodium should be kept in a well-closed container, protected from moisture and stored at a temperature not exceeding 30°. If the contents are intended for use in the manufacture of a parenteral dosage form, the container should be sterile, tamper-evident and sealed so as to exclude micro-organisms.

Labelling The label states (1) the date after which the material is not intended to be used; (2) the conditions under which it should be stored; (3) whether or not it is intended for use in the manufacture of a parenteral dosage form.

Preparations

Benzylpenicillin Injection
Fortified Procaine Penicillin Injection

Action and use Antibacterial.

Benzylpenicillin Sodium intended for use in the manufacture of a parenteral dosage form complies with the following additional requirements.

Pyrogens Complies with the *test for pyrogens*, Appendix XIV K. Use per kg of the rabbit's weight 1 ml of a solution containing 1.5 mg per ml of the substance being examined in *water for injections*.

Sterility Complies with the *test for sterility*, Appendix XVI A.

Bephenium Hydroxynaphthoate

$C_{28}H_{29}NO_4$ 443.5   *3818-50-6*

Bephenium Hydroxynaphthoate is benzyl-dimethyl-2-phenoxyethylammonium 3-hydroxy-2-naphthoate. It contains not less than 99.0 per cent and not more than 101.0 per cent of $C_{28}H_{29}NO_4$, calculated with reference to the dried substance.

Characteristics A yellow, crystalline powder; odourless or almost odourless.

Solubility Practically insoluble in *water*; soluble in 50 parts of *ethanol (96%)*.

Identification A. The *infra-red absorption spectrum*, Appendix II A, is concordant with the *reference spectrum* of bephenium hydroxynaphthoate.

B. Examine under ultra-violet light. A green fluorescence is produced.

C. Dissolve 0.2 g in 10 ml of warm *absolute ethanol*, add 15 ml of *trinitrophenol solution* and allow to stand. The *melting point* of the precipitate, after washing with *ethanol (96%)* and then with *water* and drying at 105°, is about 134°, with decomposition, Appendix V A.

D. *Melting point*, about 170°, with decomposition, Appendix V A.

Specific surface area Not less than 7000 cm² per g when determined using an air-permeability specific surface area measuring equipment (a Fisher Sub-sieve Sizer is suitable), operated in accordance with the manufacturer's instructions. Prepare a compact of suitable size in the sample tube. Measure the permeability of the compact using a manometer and a defined flow rate. Calculate the specific surface area assuming the true powder density to be 1.298 g per cm³.

Chloride Boil 0.7 g with 50 ml of *water*, cool in ice and filter. To 5 ml of the filtrate add 10 ml of 2M *nitric acid*, shake and filter. The filtrate complies with the *limit test for chlorides*, Appendix VII (0.07%).

Related substances Carry out the method for *thin-layer chromatography*, Appendix III A, using *silica gel GF254* as the coating substance and a mixture of 75 volumes of *butan-1-ol*, 30 volumes of *water* and 15 volumes of *glacial acetic acid* as the mobile phase. Apply separately to the chromatoplate 5 µl of each of two solutions of the substance being examined in *methanol* containing (1) 4.0% w/v and (2) 0.040% w/v. After removal of the plate, allow it to dry in air and examine under *ultra-violet light (254 and 365 nm)*. In each of the chromatograms obtained two principal spots are revealed under ultra-violet light (254 nm); the spot of higher Rf value exhibits fluorescence under ultra-violet light (365 nm). Any *secondary spot* which absorbs at 254 nm but does not fluoresce at 365 nm in the chromatogram obtained with solution (1) is not more intense than the principal spot of lower Rf value in the chromatogram obtained with solution (2).

Spray the plate with *sodium molybdotungstophosphate solution* and then with a 20% w/v solution of *sodium carbonate*. In each of the chromatograms obtained two principal spots are revealed. Any *secondary spot* in the chromatogram obtained with solution (1), other than any absorbing spot that has been assessed under ultra-violet light, is not more intense than the principal spot of higher Rf value in the chromatogram obtained with solution (2).

Loss on drying When dried to constant weight at 105°, loses not more than 1.0% of its weight. Use 1 g.

Assay Carry out Method I for *non-aqueous titration*, Appendix VIII A, using 1 g and determining the end-point potentiometrically. Each ml of 0.1M *perchloric acid VS* is equivalent to 0.04435 g of $C_{28}H_{29}NO_4$.

Preparation
Bephenium Granules

Action and use Anthelmintic.

Betamethasone ☆

CH$_2$OH
CO
HO   Me   --OH
Me   H
F   H   Me
O

$C_{22}H_{29}FO_5$ 392.5   *378-44-9*

Betamethasone is 9α-fluoro-11β,17α,21-trihydr-oxy-16β-methylpregna-1,4-diene-3,20-dione. It contains not less than 96.0 per cent and not more than 104.0 per cent of $C_{22}H_{29}FO_5$, calculated with reference to the dried substance.

Characteristics A white or almost white, crystalline powder. It melts at about 240° with decomposition.

Solubility Practically insoluble in *water*; soluble in 75 parts of *ethanol (96%)*; very slightly soluble in *chloroform*.

Identification *Test A may be omitted if tests B, C, D and E are carried out. Tests C, D and E may be omitted if tests A and B are carried out.*
A. The *infra-red absorption spectrum*, Appendix II A, is concordant with the spectrum of *betamethasone EPCRS*. If the spectra obtained are not concordant, dissolve the substances separately in the minimum volume of *chloroform IR*, evaporate to dryness on a water-bath and prepare new spectra of the residues either as halide discs or as dispersions in *liquid paraffin*.
B. To 2 ml of a 0.01% w/v solution in *absolute ethanol* in a stoppered tube add 10 ml of *phenylhydrazine sulphate solution*, mix, place in a water-bath at 60° for 20 minutes and cool immediately. The *absorbance* of the resulting solution at the maximum at 450 nm is not more than 0.25, Appendix II B.
C. Carry out the method for *thin-layer chromatography*, Appendix III A, using the coating substance prescribed in

the test for Related substances, and a mixture of 85 volumes of *ether*, 10 volumes of *toluene* and 5 volumes of *butan-1-ol* saturated with *water* as the mobile phase. Apply separately to the chromatoplate 2 μl of each of the following solutions in a mixture of 9 volumes of *chloroform* and 1 volume of *methanol*. Solution (1) contains 0.25% w/v of the substance being examined. Solution (2) contains 0.25% w/v of *betamethasone EPCRS*. Solution (3) contains 0.125% w/v each of the substance being examined and *betamethasone EPCRS*. Solution (4) contains 0.125% w/v each of the substance being examined and *dexamethasone EPCRS*. After removal of the plate, allow it to dry in air and spray with *ethanolic sulphuric acid (20%)*. Heat at 120° for 10 minutes or until spots are produced, allow to cool and examine in daylight and under *ultra-violet light (365 nm)*. The principal spot in the chromatogram obtained with solution (1) is similar in colour in daylight, fluorescence under ultra-violet light (365 nm), position and size to the principal spot in the chromatogram obtained with solution (2). The test is not valid unless the chromatogram obtained with solution (3) shows only one spot and the chromatogram obtained with solution (4) shows two principal spots that are close to one another but separated.
D. Heat 0.5 ml of *chromic—sulphuric acid mixture* in a small test-tube in a naked flame until white fumes appear in the upper part of the tube; the solution wets the sides of the tube readily and there is no greasiness. Add 2 mg of the substance being examined and again heat in a naked flame until white fumes appear; the solution does not wet the sides of the tube.
E. Add 2 mg to 2 ml of *sulphuric acid* and shake to dissolve; a faint reddish-brown colour is produced within 5 minutes. Add the solution to *water* and mix; the colour disappears.

Light absorption Dissolve 50 mg in sufficient *ethanol (96%)* to produce 100 ml and dilute 1 ml to 50 ml with the same solvent. The A(1%, 1 cm) of the resulting solution at the maximum at 240 nm is 370 to 400, Appendix II B.

Specific optical rotation In a 0.5% w/v solution in *1,4-dioxan*, +114° to +122°, Appendix V F.

Related substances Carry out the method for *thin-layer chromatography*, Appendix III A, using as the coating substance a suitable silica gel containing a fluorescent indicator with an optimal intensity at 254 nm (Merck silica gel 60 F254 is suitable) and a mixture of 77 volumes of *dichloromethane*, 15 volumes of *ether*, 8 volumes of *methanol* and 1.2 volumes of *water* as the mobile phase. Apply separately to the chromatoplate 5 μl of each of the following solutions in a mixture of 9 volumes of *chloroform* and 1 volume of *methanol*. Solutions (1), (2) and (3) contain 1.0% w/v, 0.020% w/v and 0.010% w/v respectively of the substance being examined. Solution (4) contains 0.10% w/v each of the substance being examined and *prednisone EPCRS*. After removal of the plate, allow it to dry in air and examine under *ultra-violet light (254 nm)*. Any *secondary spot* in the chromatogram obtained with solution (1) is not more intense than the spot in the chromatogram obtained with solution (2) and not more than one such spot is more intense than the spot in the chromatogram obtained with solution (3). The test is not valid unless the chromatogram obtained with solution (4) shows two clearly separated principal spots.

Loss on drying When dried at 100° to 105° at a pressure not exceeding 0.7 kPa for 3 hours, loses not more than 0.5% of its weight. Use 0.5 g.

Assay Carry out the *tetrazolium assay of steroids*, Appendix VIII P, and calculate the content of $C_{22}H_{29}FO_5$ from the *absorbance* obtained by repeating the operation using *betamethasone EPCRS* in place of the substance being examined.

Storage Betamethasone should be kept in a well-closed container and protected from light.

Preparation
Betamethasone Tablets

Action and use Corticosteroid.

Betamethasone Sodium Phosphate

$C_{22}H_{28}FNa_2O_8P$ 516.4   *151-73-5*

Betamethasone Sodium Phosphate is disodium 9α-fluoro-11β,17α-dihydroxy-16β-methyl-3,20-dioxopregna-1,4-dien-21-yl orthophosphate. It contains not less than 96.0 per cent and not more than 103.0 per cent of $C_{22}H_{28}FNa_2O_8P$, calculated with reference to the anhydrous substance.

Characteristics A white or almost white powder or lumpy powder; odourless or almost odourless; hygroscopic.

Solubility Soluble in 2 parts of *water*; slightly soluble in *absolute ethanol*; practically insoluble in *chloroform*.

Identification *Test A may be omitted if tests B, C, D, E and F are carried out. Tests B, C, D and E may be omitted if tests A and F are carried out.*
A. Dissolve 50 mg in 1 ml of *deuterium oxide* containing 0.1% w/v of *sodium 3-trimethylsilylpropanesulphonate*. The *nuclear magnetic resonance spectrum*, Appendix II C, is concordant with that of a similar solution of *betamethasone sodium phosphate BPCRS*.
B. Carry out the method for *thin-layer chromatography*, Appendix III A, using *silica gel G* as the coating substance and a freshly prepared mixture of 60 volumes of *butan-1-ol*, 20 volumes of *acetic anhydride* and 20 volumes of *water* as the mobile phase. Apply separately to the chromatoplate 2 μl of each of the following solutions in *methanol*. Solution (1) contains 0.25% w/v of the substance being examined. Solution (2) contains 0.25% w/v of *betamethasone sodium phosphate BPCRS*. Solution (3) is a mixture of equal volumes of solutions (1) and (2). Solution (4) is a mixture of equal volumes of solution (1) and a 0.25% w/v solution of *prednisolone sodium phosphate BPCRS* in *methanol*. After removal of the plate, allow it to dry in air, spray with *ethanolic sulphuric acid (20%)*, heat at 120° for 10 minutes, allow to cool and examine under *ultra-violet light (365 nm)*. The principal spot in the chromatogram obtained with solution (1) corresponds to that in the chromatogram obtained with solution (2). The principal spot in the chromatogram obtained with solution

(3) appears as a single, compact spot and the chromatogram obtained with solution (4) shows two principal spots with almost identical Rf values.
C. To 2 ml of a 0.013% w/v solution in *ethanol (96%)* in a stoppered tube add 10 ml of *phenylhydrazine sulphate solution*, mix, place in a water-bath at 60° for 20 minutes and cool immediately. The *absorbance* of the resulting solution at the maximum at 450 nm is not more than 0.13, Appendix II B.
D. Dissolve 2 mg in 2 ml of *sulphuric acid* and allow to stand for 2 minutes. No red colour or yellowish-green fluorescence is produced (distinction from prednisolone sodium phosphate and hydrocortisone sodium phosphate).
E. Heat 0.5 ml of *chromic—sulphuric acid mixture* in a small test-tube in a naked flame until white fumes appear in the upper part of the tube; the solution wets the sides of the tube readily and there is no greasiness. Add 2 or 3 mg of the substance being examined and again heat in a naked flame until white fumes appear; the solution does not wet the sides of the tube and does not pour easily from the tube.
F. Heat gently 40 mg with 2 ml of *sulphuric acid* until white fumes are evolved, add *nitric acid* dropwise until oxidation is complete and cool. Add 2 ml of *water*, heat until white fumes are evolved again, cool, add 10 ml of *water* and neutralise to *litmus paper* with 5M *ammonia*. The solution yields *reaction A* characteristic of sodium salts and *reaction B* characteristic of phosphates, Appendix VI.

Alkalinity pH of a 0.5% w/v solution, 7.5 to 9.0, Appendix V L.

Specific optical rotation In a 1% w/v solution, +98° to +104°, Appendix V F.

Inorganic phosphate Dissolve 25 mg in 10 ml of *water*, add 4 ml of 1M *sulphuric acid*, 1 ml of a 10% w/v solution of *ammonium molybdate* and 2 ml of *methylaminophenol—sulphite reagent* and allow to stand for 15 minutes. Add sufficient *water* to produce 25 ml and allow to stand for a further 15 minutes. The *absorbance* of a 4-cm layer of the resulting solution, Appendix II B, at 730 nm is not more than the absorbance of a 4-cm layer of a solution prepared by treating 10 ml of a 0.0036% w/v solution of *potassium dihydrogen orthophosphate* in the same manner, beginning at the words 'add 4 ml . . .'.

Free betamethasone and other derivatives Carry out the method for *thin-layer chromatography*, Appendix III A, using *silica gel GF254* as the coating substance and *methanol* as the mobile phase. Apply separately to the chromatoplate 2 μl of each of three solutions in *methanol* containing (1) 1.0% w/v of the substance being examined, (2) 1.0% w/v of *betamethasone sodium phosphate BPCRS* and (3) 0.020% w/v of *betamethasone EPCRS*. After removal of the plate, allow it to dry in air for 5 minutes and examine under *ultra-violet light (254 nm)*. Any *secondary spot* in the chromatogram obtained with solution (1) is not more intense than the spot in the chromatogram obtained with solution (3).

Water Not more than 8.0% w/w, Appendix IX C. Use 0.5 g.

Assay Dissolve 0.2 g in sufficient *water* to produce 200 ml. Dilute 10 ml to 250 ml with *water* and measure the *absorbance* of the resulting solution at the maximum at 241 nm, Appendix II B. Calculate the content of $C_{22}H_{28}FNa_2O_8P$ taking 297 as the value of A(1%, 1 cm) at the maximum at 241 nm.

Storage Betamethasone Sodium Phosphate should be kept in a well-closed container and protected from light.

Preparations
Betamethasone Injection
Betamethasone Sodium Phosphate Tablets

Action and use Corticosteroid.

Betamethasone Valerate

$C_{17}H_{37}FO_6$ 476.6   *2152-44-5*

Betamethasone Valerate is 9α-fluoro-11β,17α,21-trihydroxy-16β-methylpregna-1,4-diene-3,20-dione 17-valerate (9α-fluoro-16β-methylprednisolone 17-valerate). It contains not less than 96.0 per cent and not more than 102.0 per cent of $C_{17}H_{37}FO_6$, calculated with reference to the dried substance.

Characteristics A white to creamy-white powder.

Solubility Practically insoluble in *water*; soluble in 12 parts of *ethanol (96%)* and in 2 parts of *chloroform*.

Identification A. The *infra-red absorption spectrum*, Appendix II A, is concordant with the *reference spectrum* of betamethasone valerate.

B. Complies with the test for *identification of steroids*, Appendix III A, using *impregnating solvent I* and *mobile phase B* and applying to the chromatoplate 1 μl of each of the solutions.

C. In the Assay, the chromatogram obtained with solution (2) shows a peak having the same retention time as the peak due to betamethasone valerate in the chromatogram obtained with solution (1).

Light absorption *Absorbance* of a 0.0020% w/v solution in *absolute ethanol* at the maximum at 240 nm, 0.63 to 0.67, Appendix II B.

Specific optical rotation In a 1% w/v solution in *1,4-dioxan*, +75° to +81°, Appendix V F.

Related foreign steroids Carry out *Method B* for *related foreign steroids*, Appendix III A, using for solution (3) a solution containing 0.030% w/v each of *betamethasone EPCRS* and *betamethasone 21-valerate BPCRS*. The principal spot in the chromatogram obtained with solution (1) corresponds in position, colour and intensity to the principal spot in the chromatogram obtained with solution (2). Any *secondary spot* in the chromatogram obtained with solution (1) is not more intense than the proximate spot in the chromatogram obtained with solution (3).

Loss on drying When dried to constant weight at 105°, loses not more than 0.5% of its weight. Use 1 g.

Sulphated ash Not more than 0.1%, Appendix IX A.

Assay Carry out the method for *high-performance liquid chromatography*, Appendix III D, using the following solutions. For solution (1) mix 10 ml of a solution in *absolute ethanol* containing 0.05% w/v of *betamethasone valerate BPCRS* and 0.0025% w/v of *betamethasone 21-valerate BPCRS* with 5 ml of a 0.15% w/v solution of *beclomethasone dipropionate BPCRS* (internal standard) in *absolute ethanol* and 10 ml of *water*. For solution (2) mix 10 ml of a solution in *absolute ethanol* containing 0.05% w/v of the substance being examined with 5 ml of *absolute ethanol* and 10 ml of *water*. For solution (3) mix 10 ml of a 0.05% w/v solution of the substance being examined in *absolute ethanol* with 5 ml of a 0.15% w/v solution of the internal standard in *absolute ethanol* and 10 ml of *water*.

The chromatographic procedure may be carried out using (a) a stainless steel column (10 cm × 5 mm) packed with *stationary phase C* (5 μm) (Spherisorb ODS 1 is suitable) and maintained at 60°, (b) as the mobile phase with a flow rate of 2 ml per minute a mixture of *absolute ethanol* and *water* adjusted so that baseline separation is obtained between betamethasone valerate (retention time about 5 minutes) and betamethasone 21-valerate (retention time about 7 minutes) and between betamethasone 21-valerate and beclomethasone dipropionate (retention time about 8 minutes) (a mixture of 42 volumes of *absolute ethanol* and 58 volumes of *water* is usually suitable) and (c) a detection wavelength of 238 nm.

Calculate the content of $C_{17}H_{37}FO_6$ using the declared content of $C_{17}H_{37}FO_6$ in *betamethasone valerate BPCRS*.

Storage Betamethasone Valerate should be protected from light.

Preparations
Betamethasone Valerate Scalp Application
Betamethasone Valerate Cream
Betamethasone Valerate Lotion
Betamethasone Valerate Ointment

Action and use Corticosteroid.

Bethanidine Sulphate ☆

$C_{20}H_{30}N_6,H_2SO_4$ 452.6   *114-85-2*

Bethanidine Sulphate is 2-benzyl-1,3-dimethyl-guanidine sulphate. It contains not less than 98.0 per cent and not more than 101.0 per cent of $C_{20}H_{30}N_6,H_2SO_4$, calculated with reference to the dried substance.

Characteristics A white powder; odourless.

Solubility Freely soluble in *water*; sparingly soluble in *ethanol (96%)*; practically insoluble in *ether*.

Identification *Test A may be omitted if tests B, C, D and E are carried out. Tests B, C and D may be omitted if tests A and E are carried out.*

A. The *infra-red absorption spectrum*, Appendix II A, is concordant with the spectrum of *betanidine sulphate EPCRS*.

B. The *light absorption*, Appendix II B, in the range 230 to 350 nm of a 0.05% w/v solution exhibits three maxima, at 251, 257 and 263 nm. The *absorbance* at 257 nm is more than the *absorbances* at 251 nm and 263 nm.

C. Dissolve 25 mg in 5 ml of *water*, add 1 ml of 10M *sodium hydroxide*, 1 ml of *dilute 1-naphthol solution* and, dropwise with shaking, 1 ml of *sodium hypochlorite solution*. A bright pink precipitate is produced which becomes violet-red on standing.

D. Dissolve 0.1 g in 10 ml of *water* and add 20 ml of a 1.0% w/v solution of *2,4,6-trinitrophenol*. The *melting point* of the precipitate, after washing with *water* and drying at 80° for 30 minutes, is 147° to 152°, Appendix V A, Method I.

E. A 1% w/v solution yields *reaction A* characteristic of sulphates, Appendix VI.

Acidity or alkalinity Dissolve 0.2 g in sufficient *carbon dioxide-free water* to produce 10 ml and add 0.1 ml of *dilute phenolphthalein solution*; the solution is colourless. Add 0.2 ml of 0.01M *sodium hydroxide VS*; the solution is red. Add 0.4 ml of 0.01M *hydrochloric acid VS* and 0.25 ml of *methyl red solution*; the solution is red or orange.

Heavy metals A 10.0% w/v solution complies with *limit test A for heavy metals*, Appendix VII (20 ppm). Use *lead standard solution (2 ppm Pb)* to prepare the standard.

Trimethylguanidine Carry out the method for *thin-layer chromatography*, Appendix III A, using *silica gel G* as the coating substance and a mixture of 50 volumes of *ethyl acetate*, 24 volumes of *glacial acetic acid*, 16 volumes of *water* and 10 volumes of *ethanol (96%)* as the mobile phase. Apply separately to the chromatoplate 10 μl of each of two solutions in *methanol* containing (1) 4.0% w/v of the substance being examined and (2) 4.0% w/v of *betanidine sulphate EPCRS* and 0.03% of *trimethylguanidine sulphate EPCRS*. After removal of the plate, allow it to dry in air and spray with *acetic potassium iodobismuthate solution*. Any spot corresponding to trimethylguanidine in the chromatogram obtained with solution (1) is not more intense than the smaller spot in the chromatogram obtained with solution (2).

Loss on drying When dried to constant weight at 100° to 105°, loses not more than 1.0% of its weight. Use 1 g.

Sulphated ash Not more than 0.1%, Appendix IX A, Method II. Use 1 g.

Assay Carry out Method I for *non-aqueous titration*, Appendix VIII A, using 0.4 g dissolved in 30 ml of *anhydrous glacial acetic acid* and determining the end-point potentiometrically. Each ml of 0.1M *perchloric acid VS* is equivalent to 0.04526 g of $C_{20}H_{30}N_6,H_2SO_4$.

Preparation
Bethanidine Tablets

Action and use Antihypertensive.

The title of the monograph in the European Pharmacopœia is Betanidine Sulphate.

Bisacodyl

$C_{22}H_{19}NO_4$ 361.4   *603-50-9*

Bisacodyl is 4,4′-(2-pyridylmethylene)di(phenyl acetate). It contains not less than 98.0 per cent and not more than 101.0 per cent of $C_{22}H_{19}NO_4$, calculated with reference to the dried substance.

Characteristics A white or almost white, crystalline powder; odourless or almost odourless.

Solubility Practically insoluble in *water*; slightly soluble in *ethanol (96%)* and in *ether*; soluble in 35 parts of *chloroform*.

Identification A. The *light absorption*, Appendix II B, in the range 230 to 350 nm of a 0.002% w/v solution in 0.1M *methanolic potassium hydroxide* exhibits a maximum only at 248 nm. The *absorbance* at 248 nm is about 1.3.

B. Carry out the method described under Related substances applying to the chromatoplate 5 μl of each of two solutions in *acetone* containing (1) 0.5% w/v of the substance being examined and (2) 0.5% w/v of *bisacodyl BPCRS*. The principal spot in the chromatogram obtained with solution (1) corresponds to that in the chromatogram obtained with solution (2).

Acidity or alkalinity Boil 1.0 g with 20 ml of *carbon dioxide-free water* and cool rapidly. Add 0.1 ml of *bromocresol purple solution*. A grey colour is produced or the colour becomes grey on the addition of 0.05 ml of either 0.01M *sodium hydroxide VS* or 0.01M *hydrochloric acid VS*.

Melting point 133° to 135°, Appendix V A.

Related substances Carry out the method for *thin-layer chromatography*, Appendix III A, using *silica gel GF254* as the coating substance and a mixture of equal volumes of *butan-2-one* and *xylene* as the mobile phase. Apply separately to the chromatoplate 10 μl of each of two solutions of the substance being examined in *acetone* containing (1) 2.0% w/v and (2) 0.020% w/v. After removal of the plate, allow it to dry in air and examine under *ultra-violet light (254 nm)*. Any *secondary spot* in the chromatogram obtained with solution (1) is not more intense than the spot in the chromatogram obtained with solution (2).

Loss on drying When dried to constant weight at 105°, loses not more than 1.0% of its weight. Use 1 g.

Sulphated ash Not more than 0.1%, Appendix IX A.

Assay Carry out Method I for *non-aqueous titration*, Appendix VIII A, using 0.5 g and *1-naphtholbenzein solution* as indicator. Each ml of 0.1M *perchloric acid VS* is equivalent to 0.03614 g of $C_{22}H_{19}NO_4$.

Storage Bisacodyl should be kept in a well-closed container and protected from light.

Preparations
Bisacodyl Suppositories
Bisacodyl Tablets

Action and use Stimulant laxative.

Bismuth Subcarbonate ☆
Bismuth Carbonate

5892-10-4

Bismuth Subcarbonate contains not less than 80.0 per cent and not more than 82.5 per cent of Bi, calculated with reference to the dried substance.

Characteristics A white or almost white powder; odourless.

Solubility Practically insoluble in *water*, in *ethanol (96%)* and in *ether*; soluble with effervescence in mineral acids.

Identification Yields the *reactions* characteristic of bismuth compounds and *reaction A* characteristic of carbonates, Appendix VI.

Clarity and colour of solution Shake 5.0 g with 10 ml of *water* and add 20 ml of *nitric acid*. Heat to dissolve, cool and dilute to 100 ml with *water* (solution A). Solution A is not more opalescent than *reference suspension II*, Appendix IV A, and is *colourless*, Appendix IV B, Method II.

Alkalis and alkaline earths To 1 g add 10 ml of *water* and 10 ml of 5M *acetic acid*, boil for 2 minutes, cool, filter and wash the residue with 20 ml of *water*. To the combined filtrate and washings add 2 ml of 2M *hydrochloric acid* and 20 ml of *water*. Boil, pass *hydrogen sulphide* through the boiling solution until no further precipitate is produced, filter and wash the residue with *water*. Evaporate the combined filtrate and washings to dryness, add 0.5 ml of *sulphuric acid*, ignite gently and allow to cool. The residue weighs not more than 10 mg (1.0%).

Arsenic To 0.5 g in a distillation flask add 5 ml of *water* and 7 ml of *sulphuric acid*, cool and add 5 g of a mixture prepared by grinding together, in the following order, 20 mg of *potassium bromide*, 0.5 g of *hydrazine sulphate* and 5 g of *sodium chloride*. Add 10 ml of *hydrochloric acid*, connect the flask to an air-condenser, heat gradually to boiling during 15 to 30 minutes and continue heating at such a rate that the distillation proceeds steadily and until the volume in the flask is reduced by half, or until 5 minutes after the condenser has become full of steam. Distillation should be discontinued before fumes of sulphur trioxide are evolved. Collect the distillate in a tube containing 15 ml of *water* cooled in ice. Wash the condenser with *water* and dilute the combined distillate and washings to 25 ml with *water*. The resulting solution complies with the *limit test for arsenic*, Appendix VII (5 ppm). Use 2.5 ml of *arsenic standard solution (1 ppm As)*, diluted to 25 ml with *water*, to prepare the standard.

Copper To 5 ml of solution A add 2 ml of 10M *ammonia*, dilute to 50 ml with *water* and filter. To 10 ml of the filtrate add 1 ml of a 0.1% w/v solution of *sodium diethyldithiocarbamate*. The colour produced is not more intense than that produced by treating in the same manner a solution containing 0.25 ml of *copper standard solution (10 ppm Cu)* diluted to 10 ml with *water* (50 ppm).

Lead Not more than 20 ppm when determined by the following method. Dissolve 12.5 g in 75 ml of a mixture of equal volumes of *nitric acid* and *water*, boil for 1 minute, cool and dilute to 100 ml with *water*. Determine by *atomic absorption spectrophotometry*, Appendix II D, Method II, measuring at either 217.0 nm or 283.3 nm, depending on the apparatus used, and using an air—acetylene flame. Use *lead solution ASp*, suitably diluted with a 37% v/v solution of *nitric acid*, to prepare the standard solutions.

Silver To 2.0 g add 1 ml of *water* and 4 ml of *nitric acid*. Heat slightly to dissolve and dilute to 11 ml with *water*. Cool, add 2 ml of 1M *hydrochloric acid* and allow to stand for 5 minutes protected from light. Any opalescence produced is not more intense than that produced by treating in the same manner and at the same time a solution containing 10 ml of *silver standard solution (5 ppm Ag)*, 2 ml of 1M *hydrochloric acid* and 1 ml of *nitric acid* (25 ppm).

Chloride To 6.6 ml of solution A add 4 ml of *nitric acid* and dilute to 50 ml with *water*. 15 ml of the resulting solution complies with the *limit test for chlorides*, Appendix VII (500 ppm).

Nitrate To 0.25 g add 20 ml of *water*, 0.05 ml of *indigo carmine VS* and then, as a single addition but with caution, 30 ml of *sulphuric acid*. Titrate immediately with *indigo carmine VS* until a stable blue colour is produced. The volume of *indigo carmine VS* required is not more than that equivalent to 1 mg of NO_3 (0.4%).

Loss on drying When dried to constant weight at 100° to 105°, loses not more than 1.0% of its weight. Use 1 g.

Assay Dissolve 0.5 g in 3 ml of *nitric acid*, dilute to 250 ml with *water* and carry out the *complexometric titration of bismuth*, Appendix VIII D. Each ml of 0.1M *disodium edetate VS* is equivalent to 0.02090 g of Bi.

Storage Bismuth Subcarbonate should be protected from light.

Action and use Antacid.

Black Currant
Ribes Nigrum

Black Currant consists of the fresh ripe fruits of *Ribes nigrum* L., together with their pedicels and rachides.

Characteristics Odour, strong and characteristic; taste, pleasantly acidic.

Macroscopical Berries: globose, ranging in diameter from about 7 to 15 mm, occurring in pendulous racemes; epicarp shiny black externally, enclosing a yellowish-green translucent pulp containing numerous flattened ovoid seeds, about 2.5 mm long, 1.25 mm wide and 1 mm thick; berry crowned with withered remains of five-cleft calyx; pedicels thin, up to about 10 mm long, attached to a rachis of varying length.

Microscopical Epicarp: glands yellow, disc-shaped, roughly circular or broadly elliptical, varying in diameter from about 140 to 240 μm, each consisting of a single layer of cells attached in the centre to the epicarp by means of a short, multiseriate stalk. Calyx: trichomes unicellular, blunt-ended with thin, crooked walls, about 10 to 14 μm wide and averaging about 350 μm in length. Seed: testa with pigment layer composed of small cells with horseshoe-shaped wall thickenings as seen in cross section, each cell containing one or two prismatic crystals of calcium oxalate; endosperm cells with irregularly thickened walls.

Preparation
Black Currant Syrup

Action and use Flavour; source of vitamin C.

Borax ☆

Sodium Borate; Sodium Tetraborate

$Na_2B_4O_7,10H_2O$ 381.4   *1303-96-4*

Borax is sodium tetraborate decahydrate. It contains not less than 99.0 per cent and not more than 103.0 per cent of $Na_2B_4O_7,10H_2O$.

Characteristics Colourless crystals or crystalline masses or a white, crystalline powder; odourless; efflorescent.

Solubility Soluble in 20 parts of *water*, in 0.6 part of boiling *water* and in 1 part of *glycerol*.

Identification A. To a mixture of 1 ml of a 4.0% w/v solution in *carbon dioxide-free water* prepared from *distilled water* (solution A) and 0.1 ml of *sulphuric acid* add 5 ml of *methanol* and ignite. It burns with a flame tinged with green.
B. To 5 ml of solution A add 0.1 ml of *dilute phenolphthalein solution*. A red colour is produced which disappears on the addition of 5 ml of *glycerol*.
C. Solution A yields *reactions A* and *B* characteristic of sodium salts, Appendix VI.

Alkalinity pH of solution A, 9.0 to 9.6, Appendix V L.

Clarity and colour of solution Solution A is *clear*, Appendix IV A, and *colourless*, Appendix IV B, Method II.

Ammonium 6 ml of solution A diluted to 14 ml with *water* complies with the *limit test for ammonium*, Appendix VII (10 ppm). Use a mixture of 2.5 ml of *ammonium standard solution (1 ppm NH₄)* and 7.5 ml of *water* to prepare the standard.

Arsenic 5 ml of solution A complies with the *limit test for arsenic*, Appendix VII (5 ppm).

Calcium 15 ml of solution A complies with the *limit test for calcium*, Appendix VII (100 ppm). Use a mixture of 6 ml of *calcium standard solution (10 ppm Ca)* and 9 ml of *distilled water* to prepare the standard.

Heavy metals 12 ml of solution A complies with *limit test A for heavy metals*, Appendix VII (25 ppm). Use *lead standard solution (1 ppm Pb)* to prepare the standard.

Sulphate 15 ml of solution A complies with the *limit test for sulphates*, Appendix VII (50 ppm). Use a mixture of 3 ml of *sulphate standard solution (10 ppm SO₄)* and 12 ml of *distilled water* to prepare the standard.

Assay Dissolve 20 g of *mannitol* in 100 ml of *water*, heating if necessary. Cool, add 0.5 ml of *dilute phenolphthalein solution* and neutralise with 0.1M *sodium hydroxide VS* until the colour of the solution changes to pink. Add 3 g of the substance being examined, heat to dissolve, cool and titrate with 1M *sodium hydroxide VS* until the colour of the solution again becomes pink. Each ml of 1M *sodium hydroxide VS* is equivalent to 0.1907 g of $Na_2B_4O_7,10H_2O$.

Storage Borax should be kept in a well-closed container.

Boric Acid ☆

H_3BO_3 61.83   *10043-35-3*

Boric Acid is orthoboric acid. It contains not less than 99.0 per cent and not more than 100.5 per cent of H_3BO_3.

Characteristics Colourless brilliant plates, white crystals or a white crystalline powder; unctuous to the touch; odourless.

Solubility Soluble in 20 parts of *water*, in 3.6 parts of boiling *water*, in 16 parts of *ethanol (96%)* and in 4 parts of *glycerol (85%)*.

Identification A. Dissolve 0.1 g by heating in a mixture of 5 ml of *methanol* and 0.1 ml of *sulphuric acid* and ignite. The flame is tinged with green.
B. Dissolve 3.3 g in 80 ml of boiling *water*, cool and dilute to 100 ml with *carbon dioxide-free water* (solution A). The solution is acidic.

Acidity pH of solution A, 3.8 to 4.8, Appendix V L.

Clarity and colour of solution Solution A is *clear*, Appendix IV A, and *colourless*, Appendix IV B, Method II.

Solubility in ethanol Dissolve 1.0 g in 10 ml of boiling *ethanol (96%)*. The solution is not more opalescent than *reference suspension II*, Appendix IV A, and is *colourless*, Appendix IV B, Method II.

Heavy metals 12 ml of solution A complies with *limit test A for heavy metals*, Appendix VII (15 ppm). Use a mixture of 2.5 ml of *lead standard solution (2 ppm Pb)* and 7.5 ml of *water* to prepare the standard.

Sulphate 10 ml of solution A diluted to 15 ml with *water* complies with the *limit test for sulphates*, Appendix VII (450 ppm).

Carbonisable substances Heat progressively to dull redness. No darkening is produced.

Assay Dissolve a mixture of 1 g and 15 g of *mannitol* in 100 ml of *water* with heating and titrate with 1M *sodium hydroxide VS* using 0.5 ml of *dilute phenolphthalein solution* as indicator. Each ml of 1M *sodium hydroxide VS* is equivalent to 0.06183 g of H_3BO_3.

Preparation
Chlorinated Lime and Boric Acid Solution

Bromhexine Hydrochloride

$C_{14}H_{20}Br_2N_2,HCl$ 412.6   *611-75-6*

Bromhexine Hydrochloride is 2-amino-3,5-dibromobenzyl(cyclohexyl)methylamine hydrochloride. It contains not less than 98.5 per cent and not more than 101.5 per cent of $C_{14}H_{20}Br_2N_2,HCl$, calculated with reference to the dried substance.

Characteristics A white or almost white, crystalline powder; odourless or almost odourless.

Solubility Practically insoluble in *water*; sparingly soluble in *ethanol (96%)* and in *methanol*; slightly soluble in *chloroform*.

Identification A. The *infra-red absorption spectrum*, Appendix II A, is concordant with the *reference spectrum* of bromhexine hydrochloride.

B. The *light absorption*, Appendix II B, in the range 280 to 350 nm of a 0.01% w/v solution in 0.1M *methanolic hydrochloric acid* exhibits a maximum only at 317 nm. The *absorbance* at 317 nm is about 0.86.

C. Yields *reaction A* characteristic of chlorides, Appendix VI.

Related substances Carry out the method for *thin-layer chromatography*, Appendix III A, using *silica gel G* as the coating substance and a mixture of 90 volumes of *heptane* and 10 volumes of *absolute ethanol* as the mobile phase. Apply separately to the chromatoplate 10 µl of each of two solutions of the substance being examined in *methanol* containing (1) 2.0% w/v and (2) 0.0050% w/v. Treat each application with 10 µl of 13.5M *ammonia*. After removal of the plate, dry it in a current of warm air, place in a tank containing a freshly prepared mixture of 1 g of *sodium nitrite* and 10 ml of 5M *hydrochloric acid* and allow to stand for 1 minute. Remove the plate and immediately spray with a 0.5% w/v solution of N-(*1-naphthyl*)*ethylenediamine dihydrochloride* in *methanol*. Any *secondary spot* in the chromatogram obtained with solution (1) is not more intense than the spot in the chromatogram obtained with solution (2).

Loss on drying When dried at 105° for 2 hours, loses not more than 1.0% of its weight. Use 1 g.

Sulphated ash Not more than 0.1%, Appendix IX A.

Assay Dissolve 0.4 g in a mixture of 80 ml of *anhydrous glacial acetic acid* and 10 ml of *acetic anhydride*, add 7 ml of *mercury(II) acetate solution* and carry out Method I for *non-aqueous titration*, Appendix VIII A, determining the end-point potentiometrically. Each ml of 0.1M *perchloric acid VS* is equivalent to 0.04126 g of $C_{14}H_{20}Br_2N_2,HCl$.

Storage Bromhexine Hydrochloride should be protected from light.

Preparation
Bromhexine Tablets

Action and use Expectorant.

Bromocriptine Mesylate

$C_{32}H_{40}BrN_5O_5,CH_4O_3S$ 750.7   *22260-51-1*

Bromocriptine Mesylate is (5'S)-2-bromo-12'-hydroxy-2'-(1-methylethyl)-5'-(2-methylpropyl)-ergotaman-3',6',18-trione methanesulphonate. It contains not less than 98.0 per cent and not more than 102.0 per cent of $C_{32}H_{40}BrN_5O_5$,

CH_4O_3S, calculated with reference to the dried substance.

Characteristics A white or greyish-white to pale yellow, crystalline powder; odourless or almost odourless.

Solubility Practically insoluble in *water*; sparingly soluble in *absolute ethanol*; soluble in *ethanol (96%)*; freely soluble in *methanol*; very slightly soluble in *chloroform*.

Identification A. The *infra-red absorption spectrum*, Appendix II A, is concordant with the *reference spectrum* of bromocriptine mesylate.

B. The *light absorption*, Appendix II B, in the range 230 to 380 nm of a 0.005% w/v solution in 0.1M *methanesulphonic acid* in *methanol* exhibits a maximum only at 305 nm. The *absorbance* at 305 nm is about 0.66.

C. In the test for Related substances the principal spot in the chromatogram obtained with solution (2) corresponds to that in the chromatogram obtained with solution (3).

Clarity and colour of solution A 1.0% w/v solution in *methanol* is clear, Appendix IV A, and not more intensely coloured than *reference solution B_4, Y_4 or BY_4*, Appendix IV B, Method II.

Specific optical rotation In a 1% w/v solution in a mixture of equal volumes of *methanol* and *dichloromethane*, +95° to +105°, Appendix V F. Prepare the solution in subdued light and carry out the test as rapidly as possible.

Acidity pH of a 1% w/v solution in *methanol (20%)*, 3.0 to 4.0, Appendix V L.

Heavy metals To the cooled residue obtained in the test for Sulphated ash add 2 ml of *hydrochloric acid*, evaporate to dryness on a water-bath, add 0.05 ml of *hydrochloric acid* and 10 ml of *water* and heat on a water-bath for 2 minutes. Add 2M *ammonia* dropwise to the cooled solution until it is alkaline to *litmus paper*, acidify with 2M *acetic acid* and add 1 ml of the acetic acid in excess, filter if necessary and dilute to 20 ml with *water*. 12 ml of the resulting solution complies with *limit test A for heavy metals*, Appendix VII (20 ppm). Use *lead standard solution (1 ppm Pb)* to prepare the standard.

Related substances Carry out in subdued light the method for *thin-layer chromatography*, Appendix III A, using a silica gel F254 precoated chromatoplate (Merck silica gel 60 F254 plates are suitable) and a mixture of 180 volumes of *dichloromethane*, 15 volumes of *1,4-dioxan*, 5 volumes of *ethanol (96%)* and 0.1 volume of 13.5M *ammonia* as the mobile phase. Apply separately to the plate 10 µl of each of the following six freshly prepared solutions in a mixture of equal volumes of *methanol* and *chloroform*. Solutions (1) and (2) contain 1.0 and 0.1% w/v respectively of the substance being examined. Solutions (3), (4), (5) and (6) contain 0.1, 0.010, 0.0050 and 0.0025% w/v respectively of *bromocriptine mesylate BPCRS*. After removal of the plate, allow it to dry at a pressure of 2 kPa for 15 minutes and spray with *dilute potassium iodobismuthate solution* followed by *hydrogen peroxide solution (30 vol)*. Any *secondary spot* in the chromatogram obtained with solution (1) is not more intense than the spot in the chromatogram obtained with solution (4). Not more than one such spot is more intense than the spot in the chromatogram obtained with solution (5) and not more than a further two such spots are more intense than the spot in the chromatogram obtained with solution (6).

Loss on drying When dried to constant weight at 80° at a pressure not exceeding 13 Pa, loses not more than 6.0% of its weight. Use 0.5 g.

Sulphated ash Not more than 0.1%, Appendix IX A. Use 1.0 g.

Assay Dissolve 30 mg in a sufficient quantity of 0.1M *methanesulphonic acid* in *methanol* to produce 50 ml. Dilute 5 ml to 100 ml with the same solvent and compare the *absorbance* of the resulting solution at the maximum at 305 nm, Appendix II B, with that of a solution prepared in the same manner but using 30 mg of *bromocriptine mesylate BPCRS* in place of the substance being examined. Calculate the content of $C_{32}H_{40}BrN_5O_5,CH_4O_3S$ using the declared content of $C_{32}H_{40}BrN_5O_5,CH_4O_3S$ in *bromocriptine mesylate BPCRS*.

Storage Bromocriptine Mesylate should be kept in an airtight container, protected from light and stored at a temperature not exceeding $-18°$.

Preparations
Bromocriptine Capsules
Bromocriptine Tablets

Action and use Dopamine agonist.

Bronopol

$$HOCH_2 \cdot \overset{\overset{\displaystyle Br}{|}}{\underset{\underset{\displaystyle NO_-}{|}}{C}} CH_2OH$$

$C_3H_6BrNO_4$ 200.0   *52-51-7*

Bronopol is 2-bromo-2-nitropropane-1,3-diol. It contains not less than 99.0 per cent and not more than 101.0 per cent of $C_3H_6BrNO_4$, calculated with reference to the anhydrous substance.

Characteristics White or almost white crystals or crystalline powder; odourless or almost odourless.

Solubility Soluble in 4 parts of *water* and in 2 parts of *ethanol (96%)*; slightly soluble in *glycerol* and in *liquid paraffin*.

Identification A. The *infra-red absorption spectrum*, Appendix II A, is concordant with the *reference spectrum* of bronopol.
B. Dissolve 0.1 g in 10 ml of *water*, add 10 ml of 7.5M *sodium hydroxide* and, carefully with constant stirring and cooling, 0.5 g of *Raney nickel catalyst*. Allow the reaction to subside, filter and carefully neutralise with *nitric acid*. The resulting solution yields *reaction A* characteristic of bromides, Appendix VI.
C. *Melting point*, after drying over *phosphorus pentoxide* at a pressure not exceeding 0.7 kPa, about 130°, Appendix V A.

Acidity or alkalinity pH of a 1% w/v solution, 5.0 to 7.0, Appendix V L.

Related substances Prepare a 0.05% w/v solution of *biphenyl* (internal standard) in *pyridine* (solution A) and a mixture of 9 volumes of *bis(trimethylsilyl)trifluoroacetamide* and 1 volume of *trimethylchlorosilane* (solution B). Carry out the method for *gas chromatography*, Appendix III B, using the following solutions. For solution (1) add 1 ml of solution A and 1 ml of solution B to 1 ml of a 0.05% w/v solution of the substance being examined in *pyridine*, mix and heat at 70° for 20 minutes. For solution (2) add 2 ml of *pyridine* to 0.1 g of the substance being examined,

shake to dissolve, add 1 ml of solution B, mix and heat at 70° for 20 minutes. For solution (3) add 1 ml of solution A and 1 ml of *pyridine* to 0.1 g of the substance being examined, shake to dissolve, add 1 ml of solution B, mix and heat at 70° for 20 minutes.

The chromatographic procedure may be carried out using a glass column (1.5 m × 4 mm) packed with *acid-washed, silanised diatomaceous support* (80 to 100 mesh) coated with 3% w/w of phenyl methyl silicone fluid (50% phenyl) (OV-17 is suitable) and maintained at 115°.

In the chromatogram obtained with solution (3) the ratio of the area of any *secondary peak* to the area of the peak due to the internal standard is not greater than the ratio of the area of the peak corresponding to bronopol to the area of the peak due to the internal standard in the chromatogram obtained with solution (1). In the chromatogram obtained with solution (3) the ratio of the sum of the areas of any *secondary peaks* to the area of the peak due to the internal standard is not greater than twice the ratio of the area of the peak corresponding to bronopol to the area of the peak due to the internal standard in the chromatogram obtained with solution (1).

Sulphated ash Not more than 0.1%, Appendix IX A.

Water Not more than 0.5% w/w, Appendix IX C, Method I B. Use 5 g.

Assay In a flask fitted with a reflux condenser dissolve 0.4 g in 15 ml of *water* and add 15 ml of 7.5M *sodium hydroxide*. Slowly, with caution, add 2 g of *Raney nickel catalyst* through the reflux condenser, agitating the flask whilst cooling under running water. Allow the mixture to stand for 10 minutes and boil for 1 hour. Cool and filter under reduced pressure, washing the condenser, flask and residue with 150 ml of *water*. Combine the filtrate and washings, add 25 ml of *nitric acid* and 40 ml of 0.1M *silver nitrate VS*, shake vigorously and titrate with 0.1M *ammonium thiocyanate VS* using *ammonium iron(III) sulphate solution* as indicator. Repeat the operation without the substance being examined. The difference between the titrations represents the amount of silver nitrate required. Each ml of 0.1M *silver nitrate VS* is equivalent to 0.02000 g of $C_3H_6BrNO_4$.

Storage Bronopol should be kept in a well-closed container and protected from light.

Action and use Preservative; mild antiseptic.

Bupivacaine Hydrochloride

$C_{18}H_{28}N_2O,HCl,H_2O$ 342.9   *14252-80-3*

Bupivacaine Hydrochloride is 1-butyl-2-piperidylformo-2′,6′-xylidide hydrochloride monohydrate. It contains not less than 98.5 per cent and not more than 101.0 per cent of $C_{18}H_{28}N_2O,HCl$, calculated with reference to the dried substance.

Characteristics A white, crystalline powder; odourless or almost odourless.

Solubility Soluble in 25 parts of *water* and in 8 parts of *ethanol (96%)*; slightly soluble in *chloroform* and in *ether*.

Identification A. Dissolve 0.1 g in 5 ml of *water*, add 2 ml of 5M *ammonia* and filter. Wash the precipitate with *water* and dry at 60° at a pressure not exceeding 0.7 kPa. The *infra-red absorption spectrum* of the residue, Appendix II A, is concordant with the *reference spectrum* of bupivacaine.
B. The *light absorption*, Appendix II B, in the range 230 to 350 nm of a 0.08% w/v solution in 0.01M *hydrochloric acid* exhibits two maxima, at 263 and 271 nm. The *absorbance* at 263 nm is about 1.1 and at 271 nm is about 0.90.
C. Dissolve 0.15 g in 10 ml of *water* and add 15 ml of *trinitrophenol solution*. The *melting point* of the precipitate, after rapid washing with a small quantity of *water*, with successive 2-ml quantities of *methanol* and with *ether*, is about 194°, Appendix V A.
D. Yields *reaction A* characteristic of chlorides, Appendix VI.
E. *Melting point*, about 250°, Appendix V A.

Acidity pH of a 1% w/v solution, 4.5 to 6.0, Appendix V L.

Light absorption *Absorbance* of a 0.04% w/v solution in 0.01M *hydrochloric acid* at 263 nm, 0.53 to 0.58 and at 271 nm, 0.43 to 0.48, Appendix II B.

Copper To 0.25 g dissolved in 10 ml of *water* add 0.25 ml of 0.05M *disodium edetate*, allow to stand for 2 minutes, add 0.2 g of *citric acid*, 1 ml of 5M *ammonia* and 1 ml of *sodium diethyldithiocarbamate solution* and shake with 10 ml of *carbon tetrachloride* for 2 minutes. The colour of the carbon tetrachloride extract is not more intense than that produced when 10 ml of a mixture of 3 volumes of *copper standard solution (10 ppm Cu)* and 397 volumes of *water* is treated in the same manner (3 ppm).

Iron Ignite 1.0 g with 1 g of *anhydrous sodium carbonate*, cool and dissolve the residue in sufficient of a mixture of 1 volume of 2M *hydrochloric acid* and 2 volumes of *water* to produce 10 ml. The resulting solution complies with the *limit test for iron*, Appendix VII (10 ppm).

Dimethylaniline To 2 ml of a 2.5% w/v solution of the substance being examined in *methanol* (solution A) add 1 ml of a 1% w/v solution of *4-dimethylaminobenzaldehyde* in *methanol* and 2 ml of *glacial acetic acid* and allow to stand for 10 minutes at room temperature. The yellow colour produced is not more intense than that obtained by repeating the operation using 2 ml of a solution in *methanol* containing 2.5 µg of *2,6-dimethylaniline* per ml in place of solution A (100 ppm).

Related bases Carry out the method for *thin-layer chromatography*, Appendix III A, using *silica gel G* as the coating substance and *ethanol (96%)* as the mobile phase. Apply separately to the chromatoplate 2 µl of each of two solutions of the substance being examined in *methanol* containing (1) 5.0% w/v and (2) 0.050% w/v. After removal of the plate, allow it to dry in air and spray with *dilute potassium iodobismuthate solution*. Any *secondary spot* in the chromatogram obtained with solution (1) is not more intense than the spot in the chromatogram obtained with solution (2).

Loss on drying When dried to constant weight at 105°, loses 4.5% to 6.0% of its weight. Use 1 g.

Sulphated ash Not more than 0.1%, Appendix IX A.

Assay Carry out Method I for *non-aqueous titration*, Appendix VIII A, using 0.6 g and *crystal violet solution* as

indicator. Each ml of 0.1M *perchloric acid VS* is equivalent to 0.03249 g of $C_{18}H_{28}N_2O,HCl$.

Preparations
Bupivacaine Injection
Bupivacaine and Adrenaline Injection

Action and use Local anaesthetic.

Busulphan

$$CH_3 \cdot SO_2 \cdot O \cdot (CH_2)_4 \cdot OSO_2CH_3$$

$C_6H_{14}O_6S_2$ 246.3   *55-98-1*

Busulphan is tetramethylene di(methanesulphonate). It contains not less than 98.5 per cent and not more than 100.5 per cent of $C_6H_{14}O_6S_2$, calculated with reference to the dried substance.

Characteristics A white, crystalline powder.

Solubility Slightly soluble in *water* and in *ethanol (96%)*; soluble in 25 parts of *acetone*.

Identification A. The *infra-red absorption spectrum*, Appendix II A, is concordant with the *reference spectrum* of busulphan.
B. Fuse 0.1 g with 0.1 g of *potassium nitrate* and 0.25 g of *potassium hydroxide*, cool, dissolve the residue in *water*, acidify with 2M *hydrochloric acid* and add 2 ml of 0.25M *barium chloride*. A white precipitate is produced.
C. Heat 0.1 g with 15 ml of *water* and 1 ml of 5M *sodium hydroxide* until solution is effected. An intense, characteristic odour of methanesulphonic acid is produced. Cool the solution. To one half add 0.05 ml of *potassium permanganate solution*; the purple colour changes to violet, then to blue and finally to emerald-green. Acidify the remainder with 1M *sulphuric acid* and add 0.05 ml of *potassium permanganate solution*; the colour of the permanganate is not discharged.

Acidity Dissolve 0.2 g in 50 ml of warm *ethanol (70%)* previously neutralised to *methyl red solution* and titrate with 0.1M *sodium hydroxide VS* using *methyl red solution* as indicator. Not more than 0.05 ml is required to change the colour of the solution.

Melting point 115° to 118°, Appendix V A.

Loss on drying When dried to constant weight at 60° at a pressure not exceeding 0.7 kPa, loses not more than 2.0% of its weight. Use 1 g.

Sulphated ash Not more than 0.1%, Appendix IX A.

Assay To 0.25 g add 25 ml of *water* and boil gently under a reflux condenser for 30 minutes. Wash the condenser with a small quantity of *water*, cool and titrate with 0.1M *sodium hydroxide VS* using *phenolphthalein solution* as indicator. Each ml of 0.1M *sodium hydroxide VS* is equivalent to 0.01232 g of $C_6H_{14}O_6S_2$.

Storage Busulphan should be kept in a well-closed container and protected from light.

Preparation
Busulphan Tablets

Action and use Cytotoxic.

Butobarbitone ☆

$C_{10}H_{16}N_2O_3$ 212.2   77-28-1

Butobarbitone is 5-butyl-5-ethylbarbituric acid. It contains not less than 99.0 per cent and not more than 101.0 per cent of $C_{10}H_{16}N_2O_3$, calculated with reference to the dried substance.

Characteristics Colourless crystals or a white, crystalline powder; practically odourless.

Solubility Slightly soluble in *water*; freely soluble in *ethanol (96%)* and in *chloroform*; soluble in *ether*. It dissolves in aqueous solutions of alkali hydroxides and carbonates and in aqueous ammonia.

Identification *Test A may be omitted if tests B, C and D are carried out. Tests B and D may be omitted if tests A and C are carried out.*
A. The *infra-red absorption spectrum*, Appendix II A, is concordant with the spectrum of *butobarbital EPCRS*.
B. Complies with the test for *identification of barbiturates*, Appendix III A.
C. Determine the *melting point*, Appendix V A, Method I, of the substance being examined (about 124°). Mix equal quantities of the substance being examined and *butobarbital EPCRS* and determine the *melting point* of the mixture. The difference between the melting points is not greater than 2°.
D. Yields the *reaction* characteristic of non-nitrogen substituted barbiturates, Appendix VI.

Acidity Boil 1 g with 50 ml of *water* for 2 minutes, allow to cool and filter. To 10 ml of the filtrate add 0.15 ml of *methyl red solution*. The solution is orange-yellow and not more than 0.1 ml of 0.1M *sodium hydroxide VS* is required to change the colour of the solution to a pure yellow.

Clarity and colour of solution Dissolve 1.0 g in a mixture of 4 ml of 2M *sodium hydroxide* and 6 ml of *water*. The solution is *clear*, Appendix IV A, and not more intensely coloured than *reference solution Y_6*, Appendix IV B, Method II.

Related substances Carry out the test for *related substances in barbiturates*, Appendix III A, but use as solution (2) a 0.020% w/v solution of the substance being examined in *ethanol (96%)*, applying separately to the chromatoplate 20 μl and 5 μl. Any *secondary spot* in the chromatogram obtained with solution (1) is not more intense than the spot in the chromatogram obtained with 20 μl of solution (2) and not more than one such spot is more intense than the spot in the chromatogram obtained with 5 μl of solution (2).

Loss on drying When dried to constant weight at 100° to 105°, loses not more than 0.5% of its weight. Use 1 g.

Sulphated ash Not more than 0.1%, Appendix IX A, Method II. Use 1 g.

Assay Dissolve 0.1 g in 5 ml of *pyridine*, add 10 ml of *silver nitrate—pyridine reagent* and titrate with 0.1M *ethanolic sodium hydroxide VS*, using 0.5 ml of *thymolphthalein solution* as indicator, until a pure blue colour is obtained. Repeat the operation without the substance being examined. The difference between the titrations represents the amount of sodium hydroxide required. Each ml of 0.1M *ethanolic sodium hydroxide VS* is equivalent to 0.01061 g of $C_{10}H_{16}N_2O_3$.

Action and use Sedative and hypnotic.

The title of the monograph in the European Pharmacopœia is Butobarbital.

Butyl Hydroxybenzoate
Butylparaben

$C_{11}H_{14}O_3$ 194.2   94-26-8

Butyl Hydroxybenzoate is butyl 4-hydroxybenzoate. It contains not less than 99.0 per cent and not more than 101.0 per cent of $C_{11}H_{14}O_3$.

Characteristics A white, crystalline powder; odourless or almost odourless.

Solubility Very slightly soluble in *water*; soluble in 1 part of *ethanol (96%)*; slightly soluble in *glycerol*. It dissolves in solutions of alkali hydroxides.

Identification The *infra-red absorption spectrum*, Appendix II A, is concordant with the *reference spectrum* of butyl hydroxybenzoate.
B. The *light absorption*, Appendix II B, in the range 230 to 350 nm of a 0.001% w/v solution in *ethanol (96%)* exhibits a maximum only at 259 nm. The *absorbance* at 259 nm is about 0.84.
C. Dissolve 0.1 g in 2 ml of *ethanol (50%)*, boil and add 0.5 ml of *mercury—nitric acid solution*. A precipitate is produced slowly and the supernatant liquid becomes red.
D. *Melting point*, about 69°, Appendix V A.

Acidity Dissolve 0.2 g in 10 ml of *ethanol (50%)* previously neutralised to *methyl red solution* and titrate with 0.1M *sodium hydroxide VS* using *methyl red solution* as indicator. Not more than 0.1 ml of 0.1M *sodium hydroxide VS* is required to change the colour of the solution.

Related substances Carry out the method for *thin-layer chromatography*, Appendix III A, using a chromatoplate precoated with silica gel F254 the surface of which has been modified with chemically-bonded octadecylsilyl groups (Whatman KC18F plates are suitable) and a mixture of 70 volumes of *methanol*, 30 volumes of *water* and 1 volume of *glacial acetic acid* as the mobile phase. Apply separately to the plate 2 μl of each of two solutions of the substance being examined in *acetone* containing (1) 1.0% w/v and (2) 0.010% w/v. After removal of the plate, allow it to dry in air and examine under *ultra-violet light (254 nm)*. Any *secondary spot* in the chromatogram obtained with solution (1) is not more intense than the spot in the chromatogram obtained with solution (2).

Sulphated ash Not more than 0.1%, Appendix IX A.

Assay Gently boil 0.1 g under a reflux condenser with 20 ml of 2M *sodium hydroxide* for 30 minutes. Allow to cool, add 25 ml of 0.0333M *potassium bromate VS*, 5 ml of a 12.5% w/v solution of *potassium bromide* and 10 ml of *hydrochloric acid* and immediately stopper the flask. Shake for 15 minutes and allow to stand for 15 minutes. Add 25 ml of *potassium iodide solution* and shake vigorously. Titrate the liberated iodine with 0.1M *sodium thiosulphate VS* using *starch mucilage*, added towards the end of the titration, as indicator. The volume of 0.0333M *potassium bromate VS* used is equivalent to half of the volume of 0.1M *sodium thiosulphate VS* required for the titration. Each ml of 0.0333M *potassium bromate VS* is equivalent to 0.006474 g of $C_{11}H_{14}O_3$.

Action and use Antimicrobial preservative.

Butylated Hydroxyanisole

$C_{11}H_{16}O_2$ 180.2   *25013-16-5*

Butylated Hydroxyanisole is 2-*tert*-butyl-4-methoxyphenol containing a variable amount of 3-*tert*-butyl-4-methoxyphenol.

Characteristics A white or almost white, crystalline powder or a yellowish-white, waxy solid; odour, aromatic.

Solubility Practically insoluble in *water*; soluble in *ethanol (96%)*, in *propane-1,2-diol* and in *arachis oil*. It dissolves in solutions of alkali hydroxides.

Identification A. Dissolve 0.1 g in 10 ml of *ethanol (96%)* and add 2 ml of a 2% w/v solution of *sodium tetraborate* and a few crystals of *dichloroquinonechloroimine*. A blue colour is produced (distinction from butylated hydroxytoluene).

B. Dissolve 10 mg in 10 ml of *ethanol (96%)* and add 0.5 ml of a 0.2% w/v solution of *potassium hexacyanoferrate(III)* and 0.5 ml of a 0.5% w/v solution of *ammonium iron(III) sulphate* in 0.5M *sulphuric acid*. A green to blue colour is produced.

Hydroquinone Carry out the method for *thin-layer chromatography*, Appendix III A, using *silica gel G* as the coating substance and a mixture of 80 volumes of *chloroform* and 20 volumes of *ethyl acetate* as the mobile phase. Apply separately to the chromatoplate 3 μl of each of two solutions in *ether* containing (1) 5.0% w/v of the substance being examined and (2) 0.010% w/v of *hydroquinone*. After removal of the plate, allow it to dry in air for a few minutes and spray with a 5% w/v solution of *phosphomolybdic acid* in *absolute ethanol*. While still damp expose it to ammonia vapour and examine immediately the yellow background has disappeared. Any spot corresponding to hydroquinone in the chromatogram obtained with solution (1) is not more intense than the spot in the chromatogram obtained with solution (2).

Related substances Carry out the method for *high-performance liquid chromatography*, Appendix III D, using four solutions in the mobile phase containing (1) 0.10% w/v of *4-chlorophenol* (internal standard) and 0.050% w/v of 3-tert-*butyl-4-methoxyphenol BPCRS*, (2) 5.0% w/v of the substance being examined, (3) 5.0% w/v of the substance being examined and 0.10% w/v of the internal standard and (4) 0.050% w/v of the substance being examined.

The chromatographic procedure may be carried out using (a) a stainless steel column (30 cm × 4 mm) packed with *stationary phase A* (10 μm) (μPorasil is suitable), (b) a mixture of 50 volumes of *ethanol-free chloroform*, 50 volumes of n-*hexane* and 0.1 volume of *glacial acetic acid* as the mobile phase with a flow rate of 2 ml per minute and (c) a detection wavelength of 290 nm.

In the chromatogram obtained with solution (1) the peak due to 3-*tert*-butyl-4-methoxyphenol is eluted before the peak due to the internal standard. In the chromatogram obtained with solution (3) the ratio of the sum of the areas of all of the *secondary peaks* with a retention time of up to twice that of the internal standard, other than the peak corresponding to 3-*tert*-butyl-4-methoxyphenol, to the area of the internal standard peak is not greater than the ratio of the area of the peak corresponding to 3-*tert*-butyl-4-methoxyphenol to that of the internal standard peak in the chromatogram obtained with solution (1). In the chromatogram obtained with solution (4) the area of the peak corresponding to 3-*tert*-butyl-4-methoxyphenol is not greater than 15% by *normalisation*.

Sulphated ash Not more than 0.05%, Appendix IX A. Use 2 g.

Storage Butylated Hydroxyanisole should be protected from light.

Action and use Antioxidant.

Butylated Hydroxytoluene

$C_{15}H_{24}O$ 220.4   *128-37-0*

Butylated Hydroxytoluene is 2,6-di-*tert*-butyl-*p*-cresol.

Characteristics Colourless crystals or a white, crystalline powder; odourless or almost odourless.

Solubility Practically insoluble in *water*, in *glycerol* and in *propane-1,2-diol*; soluble in 4 parts of *ethanol (96%)*, in 0.5 part of *ether*, in 5 parts of *liquid paraffin* and in 3 parts of fixed oils; practically insoluble in solutions of the alkali hydroxides.

Identification A. The *light absorption*, Appendix II B, in the range 230 to 350 nm of a 0.010% w/v solution in *absolute ethanol* exhibits a maximum only at 278 nm. The *absorbance* at 278 nm is about 0.85.

B. Dissolve 0.1 g in 10 ml of *ethanol (96%)*, add 2 ml of a 2.0% w/v solution of *sodium tetraborate* and a few crystals of *dichloroquinonechloroimine*. Not more than a faint blue colour is produced (distinction from butylated hydroxyanisole).

C. Dissolve a few crystals in 10 ml of *ethanol (96%)* and add 0.5 ml of a 0.2% w/v solution of *potassium hexacyanoferrate(III)* and 0.5 ml of a 0.5% w/v solution of *ammonium iron(III) sulphate* in 0.5M *sulphuric acid*. A green to blue colour is produced.

Acid value Not more than 0.05, Appendix X B.

Freezing point Not lower than 69.2°, Appendix V B, with the following modifications. After determining the approximate freezing point and remelting the crystals, insert the inner tube into the jacket with the temperature of the cooling bath between 6° and 8° below the expected freezing point. Measure the temperature at intervals of 30 seconds, with continuous and gentle stirring, so that a seed crystal is present as the temperature of the butylated hydroxytoluene falls to that at which crystallisation commences. The freezing point corresponds to the first five consecutive readings during which the temperature remains constant within 0.05°. If super-cooling occurs, the constant temperature may be observed immediately after the temperature rise, provided that the rise does not exceed 1°. If a constant temperature is not obtained over the first five readings after the rise in temperature, take six readings commencing with the point at which the maximum temperature is first attained. Plot the readings against time and draw a straight line to lie evenly between the first and second and between the fifth and sixth of the six points. Extrapolate this line until it intersects the portion of the curve before the temperature rise. Take the point of intersection as the freezing point.

Sulphated ash Not more than 0.1%, Appendix IX A.

Action and use Antioxidant.

Caffeine ☆

Anhydrous Caffeine

$C_8H_{10}N_4O_2$ 194.2   58-08-2

Caffeine is 1,3,7-trimethylpurine-2,6(3H,1H)-dione. It contains not less than 98.5 per cent and not more than 101.5 per cent of $C_8H_{10}N_4O_2$, calculated with reference to the dried substance.

Characteristics Silky, white crystals or a white, crystalline powder. It sublimes readily.

Solubility Soluble in 60 parts of *water*; freely soluble in boiling *water* and in *chloroform*; slightly soluble in *ethanol* (96%) and in *ether*. It dissolves in concentrated solutions of alkali benzoates or salicylates.

Identification *Test A may be omitted if tests B, C, D, E and F are carried out. Tests B, C and E may be omitted if tests A, D and F are carried out.*

A. The *infra-red absorption spectrum*, Appendix II A, is concordant with the spectrum of *caffeine EPCRS*.

B. To 2 ml of a saturated solution add 0.05 ml of *iodine solution*; the solution remains clear. Add 0.1 ml of 2M *hydrochloric acid*; a brown precipitate is produced which dissolves on neutralisation with 2M *sodium hydroxide*.

C. Dissolve 10 mg in 0.25 ml of a mixture of 0.5 ml of *acetylacetone* and 5 ml of 2M *sodium hydroxide*. Heat in a stoppered test-tube on a water-bath at 80° for 7 minutes, allow to cool and add 0.5 ml of a solution prepared immediately before use by dissolving, without heating,

0.2 g of *4-dimethylaminobenzaldehyde* in a mixture of 5.5 ml of *hydrochloric acid* and 4.5 ml of *water*. Heat on a water-bath at 80° for a further 7 minutes, allow to cool and add 10 ml of *water*. An intense blue colour is produced.

D. Complies with the test for Loss on drying.

E. Yields the *reaction* characteristic of xanthines, Appendix VI.

F. *Melting point*, 234° to 239°, Appendix V A, Method I.

Acidity or alkalinity Dissolve 0.5 g in 50 ml of *carbon dioxide-free water* with the aid of heat and cool (solution A). To 10 ml add 0.05 ml of *bromothymol blue solution*. The solution is green or yellow and not more than 0.2 ml of 0.01M *sodium hydroxide VS* is required to change the colour of the solution to blue.

Clarity and colour of solution Solution A is *clear*, Appendix IV A, and *colourless*, Appendix IV B, Method II.

Heavy metals 1.0 g complies with *limit test C for heavy metals*, Appendix VII (20 ppm). Use 2 ml of *lead standard solution (10 ppm Pb)* to prepare the standard.

Sulphate Solution A complies with the *limit test for sulphates*, Appendix VII (500 ppm). Use a mixture of 7.5 ml of *sulphate standard solution (10 ppm SO₄)* and 7.5 ml of *water* to prepare the standard.

Related substances Carry out the method for *thin-layer chromatography*, Appendix III A, using *silica gel GF254* as the coating substance and a mixture of 40 volumes of *butan-1-ol*, 30 volumes of *acetone*, 30 volumes of *chloroform* and 10 volumes of 13.5M *ammonia* as the mobile phase. Apply separately to the chromatoplate 10 μl of each of two solutions of the substance being examined in a mixture of 3 volumes of *chloroform* and 2 volumes of *methanol* containing (1) 2% w/v and (2) 0.010% w/v. After removal of the plate, allow it to dry in air and examine under *ultra-violet light (254 nm)*. Any *secondary spot* in the chromatogram obtained with solution (1) is not more intense than the spot in the chromatogram obtained with solution (2).

Loss on drying When dried at 100° to 105° for 1 hour, loses not more than 0.5% of its weight. Use 1 g.

Sulphated ash Not more than 0.1%, Appendix IX A, Method II. Use 1 g.

Assay Dissolve 0.17 g in 5 ml of *anhydrous glacial acetic acid* with the aid of heat. Allow to cool, add 10 ml of *acetic anhydride* and 20 ml of *toluene* and carry out Method I for *non-aqueous titration*, Appendix VIII A, determining the end-point potentiometrically. Each ml of 0.1M *perchloric acid VS* is equivalent to 0.01942 g of $C_8H_{10}N_4O_2$.

Storage Caffeine should be kept in a well-closed container.

Preparation

Aspirin and Caffeine Tablets

Action and use Central nervous stimulant.

Caffeine Hydrate ☆

$C_8H_{10}N_4O_2,H_2O$ 212.2   5743-12-4

Caffeine Hydrate is 1,3,7-trimethylpurine-2,6(3H,1H)-dione monohydrate. It contains not less than 98.5 per cent and not more than 101.5 per cent of $C_8H_{10}N_4O_2$, calculated with reference to the dried substance.

Characteristics Silky, white crystals or a white, crystalline powder. It sublimes readily.

Solubility Soluble in 60 parts of *water*; freely soluble in boiling *water* and in *chloroform*; slightly soluble in *ethanol (96%)* and in *ether*. It dissolves in concentrated solutions of alkali benzoates or salicylates.

Identification Complies with the tests described under Caffeine but dry the substance being examined at 100° to 105° before carrying out tests A and F.

Acidity or alkalinity; Clarity and colour of solution; Heavy metals; Sulphate; Related substances; Sulphated ash Complies with the tests described under Caffeine.

Loss on drying When dried at 100° to 105° for 1 hour, loses 5.0 to 9.0% of its weight. Use 1 g.

Assay Dissolve 0.17 g, previously dried at 100° to 105°, in 5 ml of *anhydrous glacial acetic acid* with heating. Allow to cool, add 10 ml of *acetic anhydride* and 20 ml of *toluene* and carry out Method I for *non-aqueous titration*, Appendix VIII A, determining the end-point potentiometrically. Each ml of 0.1M *perchloric acid VS* is equivalent to 0.01942 g of $C_8H_{10}N_4O_2$.

Storage Caffeine Hydrate should be kept in a well-closed container.

Action and use Central nervous stimulant.

The title of the monograph in the European Pharmacopœia is Caffeine Monohydrate.

Calamine

Prepared Calamine

Calamine is a basic zinc carbonate suitably coloured with iron(III) oxide.

Characteristics An amorphous, impalpable, pink or reddish-brown powder, the colour depending on the variety and amount of iron(III) oxide present and the process by which it is incorporated.

Solubility Practically insoluble in *water*. It dissolves with effervescence in *hydrochloric acid*.

Identification A. Yields the *reactions* characteristic of carbonates, Appendix VI.
B. A solution in *hydrochloric acid*, after neutralisation, yields *reactions* B and C characteristic of iron salts and the *reactions* characteristic of zinc salts, Appendix VI.

Calcium Dissolve 0.50 g in a mixture of 10 ml of *water* and 2.5 ml of *glacial acetic acid* and filter. To 0.5 ml of the filtrate add 15 ml of 5M *ammonia* and 2 ml of a 2.5% w/v solution of *ammonium oxalate* and allow to stand for 2 minutes. The solution remains clear.

Soluble barium salts To the remainder of the filtrate obtained in the test for Calcium add 2 ml of 1M *sulphuric acid* and allow to stand for 5 minutes. The solution remains clear.

Lead Dissolve 2.0 g in a mixture of 20 ml of *water* and 5 ml of *glacial acetic acid*, filter and add 0.25 ml of *potassium chromate solution*. The solution remains clear for 5 minutes.

Chloride Dissolve 0.15 g in *water* with the addition of 1 ml of *nitric acid*, filter and dilute to 30 ml with *water*. The resulting solution complies with the *limit test for chlorides*, Appendix VII (0.07%).

Sulphate Dissolve 0.1 g in *water* with the addition of 3 ml of 2M *hydrochloric acid*, filter and dilute to 60 ml with *water*. The resulting solution complies with the *limit test for sulphates*, Appendix VII (0.6%).

Ethanol-soluble dyes Shake 1.0 g with 10 ml of *ethanol (90%)* and filter. The filtrate is *colourless*, Appendix IV B, Method II.

Matter insoluble in hydrochloric acid Dissolve 1 g in 20 ml of warm 2M *hydrochloric acid* and filter. The residue, when washed with *water* and dried to constant weight at 105°, weighs not more than 10 mg.

Water-soluble dyes Shake 1.0 g with 10 ml of *water* and filter. The filtrate is *colourless*, Appendix IV B, Method II.

Residue on ignition 68.0 to 74.0%, when ignited at a temperature not lower than 900° until, after further ignition, two successive weighings do not differ by more than 0.2% of the weight of the residue.

Preparations
Aqueous Calamine Cream
Calamine and Coal Tar Ointment
Calamine Lotion
Calamine Ointment

Calcitonin (Pork)

12321-44-7

Calcitonin (Pork) is a polypeptide hormone of ultimobranchial origin, obtained from pork thyroid, that lowers the calcium concentration in plasma of mammals by diminishing the rate of bone resorption. It contains not less than 60 Units per mg calculated with reference to the dried substance.

Calcitonin (Pork) may be prepared from dried pork thyroid by extraction with dilute acid or organic solvents and purified by precipitation. It is prepared in conditions designed to minimise microbial contamination.

Characteristics A white or almost white powder.

Solubility Soluble in *water*; practically insoluble in *ethanol (96%)*, in *acetone*, in *chloroform* and in *ether*; sparingly soluble in solutions of mineral acids. It dissolves in solutions of alkali hydroxides.

Identification Carry out the method for *thin-layer chromatography*, Appendix III A, using *microcrystalline cellulose* as the coating substance and a mixture of 30 volumes of *butan-1-ol*, 24 volumes of *water*, 20 volumes of *pyridine* and 6 volumes of *glacial acetic acid* as the mobile phase. Apply separately to the chromatoplate 1 µl of each of two freshly prepared solutions in 0.1M *acetic acid* containing (1) 0.25% w/v of the substance being examined and (2) 0.25% w/v of *calcitonin (pork) BPCRS*. After removal of the plate, allow it to dry in air for 1 hour, heat at 110° for 10 minutes and spray the hot plate with a solution prepared immediately before use by diluting *sodium hypochlorite solution* with *water* to contain 0.5% w/v of available chlorine. Dry in a current of cold air until a sprayed area of the plate below the line of application gives at most a very faint blue colour with 0.05 ml of *potassium iodide and starch solution*; avoid prolonged exposure to cold air. Spray the plate with *potassium iodide and starch solution*. The spots in the chromatogram obtained with solution (1) correspond to those in the chromatogram obtained with solution (2) and no additional spots are present.

Clarity of solution A 0.10% w/v solution in 0.01M *hydrochloric acid* is not more opalescent than *reference suspension II*, Appendix IV A.

Light absorption *Absorbance* of a 0.025% w/v solution in 0.01M *hydrochloric acid* at the maximum at 278 nm, 0.30 to 0.50, Appendix II B.

Uniformity of molecular size Carry out the method for *size-exclusion chromatography*, Appendix III C, applying about 0.5 ml of a solution in 0.045M *formic acid* containing 0.1% w/v of *bovine serum albumin* (retention volume V_0), 0.025% w/v of L-*tyrosine* (V_T) and 0.2% w/v of the substance being examined (V_R).

The chromatographic procedure may be carried out at 20° to 25° using (a) a column (100 cm × 9 to 10 mm) packed with a gel of a cross-linked dextran suitable for fractionation of proteins in the range of molecular weights from 1000 to 6000 (Sephadex G 50, Fine grade is suitable), (b) 0.045M *formic acid* that has been freed from oxygen by slow passage of *oxygen-free nitrogen* just before use as the mobile phase with a flow rate not exceeding 30 ml per hour and (c) a detection wavelength of 280 nm.

The substance being examined gives one principal peak with a *distribution coefficient* of 0.58 to 0.68.

Liothyronine and thyroxine Not more than 20 ng of liothyronine and not more than 50 ng of thyroxine per Unit of calcitonin when determined by the following method. Carry out the method for *high-performance liquid chromatography*, Appendix III D, using 0.1 ml of each of the following solutions. Dissolve 10 mg of *liothyronine EPCRS* and 25 mg of *thyroxine sodium EPCRS* in 50 ml of a mixture of 19 volumes of *methanol* and 1 volume of 13.5M *ammonia* and add sufficient of the same solvent to produce 100 ml (solution A). For solution (1) transfer 0.1 ml of solution A to a test-tube, add 1.2 ml of 0.0083M *hydrochloric acid* and then add 3 ml of a solution in *tris— chloride buffer pH 8.6* containing 20 mg of a suitable broad-spectrum bacterial protease and mix. Stopper the tube and incubate at 37° for 24 hours. Extract the resulting mixture with two 6-ml quantities of *butan-1-ol* saturated with 0.1M *sodium thiosulphate*. (To ensure saturation add the 0.1M *sodium thiosulphate*, in small quantities, to the *butan-1-ol*, shaking vigorously after each addition, until two liquid layers are obtained.) Centrifuge after each extraction, combine the upper layers and evaporate to dryness on a water-bath in a current of nitrogen. Dissolve the cold residue in 1.0 ml of *fluorenone solution* (internal standard) shaking to assist solution. For solution (2) add 1.2 ml of 0.0083M *hydrochloric acid* to a quantity of the substance being examined containing 1500 Units (approximately 25 mg), mixing during the addition, and continue as described for solution (1), beginning at the words 'add 3 ml . . .'. Prepare solution (3) in the same manner as solution (2) but using *methanol* in place of *fluorenone solution* to dissolve the cold residue.

The chromatographic procedure may be carried out using (a) a stainless steel column (25 cm × 4.6 mm) packed with *stationary phase C* (10 μm) (Spherisorb ODS 1 is suitable), (b) a solution prepared as described below as the mobile phase with a flow rate of 1 ml per minute and (c) a detection wavelength of 230 nm. To prepare the mobile phase dissolve 13.6 g of *sodium acetate* and 46 g of *sodium dihydrogen orthophosphate* in 500 ml of *water*, adjust the pH to 4.0 with a 10% v/v solution of *orthophosphoric acid* and dilute to 1000 ml with *water*. Add sufficient *methanol* to 105 ml of the resulting solution to produce a volume of 300 ml after shaking.

In the chromatogram obtained with solution (1) the peaks appear in the order liothyronine, thyroxine and fluorenone. Calculate the content of liothyronine and thyroxine in nanograms per Unit of calcitonin.

Loss on drying When dried over *phosphorus pentoxide* at a pressure not exceeding 0.7 kPa for 24 hours, loses not more than 6.0% of its weight. Use 0.25 g.

Pyrogens Complies with the *test for pyrogens*, Appendix XIV K. Use a quantity containing 10 Units per kg of the rabbit's weight dissolved in not more than 5 ml of *albumin solution*.

Assay Carry out the *biological assay of calcitonin (pork)*, Appendix XIV C1. The estimated potency is not less than 80% and not more than 125% of the stated potency. The fiducial limits of error are not less than 64% and not more than 156% of the stated potency.

Storage Calcitonin should be kept in a well-closed container, protected from light and stored at a temperature not exceeding 25°. Under these conditions it may be expected to retain its potency for not less than 2 years.

Labelling The label states (1) the number of Units in the container; (2) the number of Units per mg; (3) the date after which the material is not intended to be used; (4) the conditions under which it should be stored.

Preparation
Calcitonin (Pork) Injection

Action and use Hypocalcaemic hormone.

Calcium Acetate

$C_4H_6CaO_4$ 158.2   62-54-4

Calcium Acetate contains not less than 98.0 per cent and not more than 100.5 per cent of $C_4H_6CaO_4$, calculated with reference to the anhydrous substance.

Characteristics A white powder; odourless or almost odourless; hygroscopic.

Solubility Soluble in 3 parts of *water*; slightly soluble in *ethanol (96%)*.

Identification Yields the *reactions* characteristic of calcium salts and of acetates, Appendix VI.

Alkalinity pH of a 5% w/v solution, 7.2 to 8.2, Appendix V L.

Aluminium Dissolve 4.0 g in 100 ml of *water* and add 10 ml of *acetate buffer pH 6.0*. The resulting solution complies with the *limit test for aluminium*, Appendix VII (1 ppm).

Arsenic 0.50 g dissolved in 25 ml of *water* complies with the *limit test for arsenic*, Appendix VII (2 ppm).

Barium Not more than 50 ppm of Ba when determined by *atomic emission spectrophotometry*, Appendix II D, Method II, using a 5.0% w/v solution and measuring at 455.5 nm with a nitrous oxide—acetylene flame. Use *barium solution*

ASp, suitably diluted with *water*, for the standard solution.

Heavy metals Dissolve 2.0 g in 20 ml of *water*. 12 ml of the resulting solution complies with *limit test A for heavy metals*, Appendix VII (20 ppm). Use *lead standard solution (2 ppm Pb)* to prepare the standard.

Magnesium Not more than 500 ppm of Mg when determined by *atomic absorption spectrophotometry*, Appendix II D, Method II, using a 0.20% w/v solution and measuring at 285.2 nm. Use *magnesium solution ASp*, suitably diluted with *water*, for the standard solution.

Potassium Not more than 0.1% of K when determined by *atomic emission spectrophotometry*, Appendix II D, Method II, using a 1.25% w/v solution and measuring at 766.7 nm. Use *potassium solution ASp*, suitably diluted with *water*, for the standard solution.

Sodium Not more than 0.5% of Na when determined by *atomic emission spectrophotometry*, Appendix II D, Method II, using a 1.0% w/v solution and measuring at 589.0 nm. Use *sodium solution ASp*, suitably diluted with *water*, for the standard solution.

Strontium Not more than 500 ppm of Sr when determined by *atomic absorption spectrophotometry*, Appendix II D, Method II, using a 2.0% w/v solution and measuring at 460.7 nm. Use *strontium solution ASp*, suitably diluted with *water*, for the standard solution.

Chloride 0.15 g complies with the *limit test for chlorides*, Appendix VII (330 ppm).

Nitrate Dissolve 1.0 g in 10 ml of *water*, add 5 mg of *sodium chloride*, 0.05 ml of *indigo carmine solution* and, with stirring, 10 ml of *nitrogen-free sulphuric acid*. The blue colour remains for at least 10 minutes.

Sulphate 0.25 g complies with the *limit test for sulphates*, Appendix VII (600 ppm).

Readily oxidisable substances Dissolve 2.0 g in 100 ml of boiling *water*, add a few anti-bumping granules, 6 ml of 5M *sulphuric acid* and 0.3 ml of 0.02M *potassium permanganate*, mix, boil gently for 5 minutes and allow the precipitate to settle. The pink colour in the supernatant liquid is not completely discharged.

Water Not more than 7.0% w/w, Appendix IX C. Use 0.7 g and add 20 ml of *anhydrous glacial acetic acid* to the titration vessel in addition to the methanol.

Assay Dissolve 0.6 g in 15 ml of *water*, add 5 ml of *diethylamine* and titrate with 0.1M *disodium edetate VS* using *methyl thymol blue mixture* as indicator. Each ml of 0.1M *disodium edetate VS* is equivalent to 0.01582 g of $C_4H_6CaO_4$.

Storage Calcium Acetate should be kept in a well-closed container.

Action and use Used in solutions for haemodialysis and peritoneal dialysis.

Calcium Carbonate ☆

CaCO₃   100.1   *471-34-1*

Calcium Carbonate contains not less than 98.5 per cent and not more than 100.5 per cent of $CaCO_3$, calculated with reference to the dried substance.

Characteristics A white powder; odourless.

Solubility Practically insoluble in *water*.

Identification A. Dissolve 5.0 g in 80 ml of 2M *acetic acid*. When effervescence ceases, boil the solution for 2 minutes, allow to cool, dilute to 100 ml with 2M *acetic acid* and filter, if necessary, through a sintered-glass filter, reserving any residue for the test for Substances insoluble in acetic acid. The resulting solution (solution A) yields *reactions A* and *B* characteristic of calcium salts, Appendix VI.

B. Yields *reaction A* characteristic of carbonates, Appendix VI.

Substances insoluble in acetic acid Wash any residue produced in the preparation of solution A with four successive 5-ml quantities of hot *water* and dry at 100° to 105° for 1 hour. The residue weighs not more than 10 mg (0.2%).

Arsenic 5 ml of solution A complies with the *limit test for arsenic*, Appendix VII (4 ppm).

Barium To 10 ml of solution A add 10 ml of *calcium sulphate solution*. After 15 minutes the solution is not more opalescent than a mixture of 10 ml of solution A and 10 ml of *distilled water*.

Heavy metals 12 ml of solution A complies with *limit test A for heavy metals*, Appendix VII (20 ppm). Use *lead standard solution (1 ppm Pb)* to prepare the standard.

Iron 50 mg dissolved in 5 ml of 2M *hydrochloric acid* and diluted to 10 ml with *water* complies with the *limit test for iron*, Appendix VII (200 ppm).

Magnesium and alkali metals Dissolve 1.0 g in 10 ml of 2M *hydrochloric acid*, boil for 2 minutes and add 20 ml of *water*, 1 g of *ammonium chloride* and 0.1 ml of *methyl red solution*. Add 6M *ammonia* until the solution changes colour and add a further 2 ml. Heat to boiling and add 50 ml of a hot 4% w/v solution of *ammonium oxalate*. Allow to stand for 4 hours, dilute to 100 ml with *water* and filter. To 50 ml of the filtrate add 0.25 ml of *sulphuric acid* and evaporate to dryness on a water-bath. The residue, when ignited to constant weight at 600°, weighs not more than 5 mg (1.0%).

Chloride 3 ml of solution A diluted to 15 ml with *water* complies with the *limit test for chlorides*, Appendix VII (330 ppm).

Sulphate 1.2 ml of solution A diluted to 15 ml with *distilled water* complies with the *limit test for sulphates*, Appendix VII (0.25%).

Loss on drying When dried to constant weight at 200°, loses not more than 2.0% of its weight. Use 1 g.

Assay Dissolve 0.15 g in a mixture of 3 ml of 2M *hydrochloric acid* and 20 ml of *water*, boil for 2 minutes, allow to cool, dilute to 50 ml with *water* and carry out the *complexometric titration of calcium*, Appendix VIII D. Each ml of 0.1M *disodium edetate VS* is equivalent to 0.01001 g of $CaCO_3$.

Action and use Antacid.

Calcium Chloride ☆

Calcium Chloride Dihydrate

$CaCl_2,2H_2O$ 147.0   *10035-04-8*

Calcium Chloride contains not less than 97.0 per cent and not more than 103.0 per cent of $CaCl_2,2H_2O$.

Characteristics A white, crystalline powder; odourless; hygroscopic.

Solubility Soluble in 1.2 parts of *water* and in 4 parts of *ethanol* (96%).

Identification A. Yields *reactions A* and *B* characteristic of calcium salts, Appendix VI.
B. A 10.0% w/v solution in *carbon dioxide-free water* prepared from *distilled water* (solution A) yields *reaction A* characteristic of chlorides, Appendix VI.

Acidity or alkalinity To 10 ml of solution A add 0.1 ml of *dilute phenolphthalein solution*. Not more than 0.2 ml of either 0.01M *hydrochloric acid VS* or 0.01M *sodium hydroxide VS* is required to change the colour of the solution.

Clarity and colour of solution Solution A is *clear*, Appendix IV A, and not more intensely coloured than *reference solution Y_6*, Appendix IV B, Method II.

Aluminium To 10 ml of solution A add 2 ml of 2M *ammonium chloride* and 1 ml of 6M *ammonia* and boil. No turbidity or precipitate is produced.

Barium To 10 ml of solution A add 1 ml of *calcium sulphate solution*. After 15 minutes the solution is not more opalescent than a mixture of 10 ml of solution A and 1 ml of *distilled water*.

Heavy metals 12 ml of solution A complies with *limit test A for heavy metals*, Appendix VII (20 ppm). Use *lead standard solution (2 ppm Pb)* to prepare the standard.

Iron 10 ml of solution A complies with the *limit test for iron*, Appendix VII (10 ppm).

Magnesium and alkali metals To a mixture of 20 ml of solution A and 80 ml of *water* add 2 g of *ammonium chloride* and 2 ml of 6M *ammonia*. Heat to boiling and add a hot solution of 5 g of *ammonium oxalate* in 75 ml of *water*. Allow to stand for 4 hours, dilute to 200 ml with *water* and filter. To 100 ml of the filtrate add 0.5 ml of *sulphuric acid*, evaporate to dryness on a water-bath and ignite to constant weight at 600°. The residue weighs not more than 5 mg (0.5%).

Sulphate 5 ml of solution A diluted to 15 ml with *distilled water* complies with the *limit test for sulphates*, Appendix VII (300 ppm).

Assay Carry out the *complexometric titration of calcium*, Appendix VIII D, using 0.28 g dissolved in 100 ml of *water*. Each ml of 0.1M *disodium edetate VS* is equivalent to 0.01470 g of $CaCl_2,2H_2O$.

Storage Calcium Chloride should be kept in a well-closed container.

Calcium Gluconate ☆

$C_{12}H_{22}CaO_{14},H_2O$ 448.4   *18016-24-5*

Calcium Gluconate★ is calcium D-gluconate monohydrate. It contains not less than 98.5 per cent and not more than 102.0 per cent of $C_{12}H_{22}CaO_{14}$, calculated with reference to the dried substance.

Characteristics A white, crystalline or granular powder; odourless.

Solubility Soluble in 30 parts of *water* and in 5 parts of boiling *water*.

Identification A. Carry out the method for *thin-layer chromatography*, Appendix III A, using *silica gel G* as the coating substance and a mixture of 50 volumes of *ethanol* (96%), 30 volumes of *water*, 10 volumes of 13.5M *ammonia* and 10 volumes of *ethyl acetate* as the mobile phase, but allowing the solvent front to ascend 10 cm above the line of application. Apply separately to the chromatoplate 5 μl of each of two solutions in *water* containing (1) 2.0% w/v of the substance being examined and (2) 2.0% w/v of *calcium gluconate EPCRS*, heating, if necessary, to 60° on a water-bath to effect dissolution. After removal of the plate, dry it at 100° for 20 minutes, cool and spray with a 5% w/v solution of *potassium dichromate* in a 40% w/w solution of *sulphuric acid*. After 5 minutes the principal spot in the chromatogram obtained with solution (1) is similar in position, colour and size to that in the chromatogram obtained with solution (2).
B. A 2% w/v solution yields the *reactions A* and *B* characteristic of calcium salts, Appendix VI.

Colour and clarity of solution A 2.0% w/v solution at 60° is not more intensely coloured than *reference solution Y_6*, Appendix IV B, Method II. On cooling to room temperature the solution is not more opalescent than *reference suspension II*, Appendix IV A.

Heavy metals 2.0 g complies with *limit test D for heavy metals*, Appendix VII (10 ppm). Heat gradually and with care until the substance being examined is almost completely transformed into a white mass and then ignite. Use 2 ml of *lead standard solution (10 ppm Pb)* to prepare the standard.

Magnesium and alkali metals Dissolve 1 g in 100 ml of boiling *water*, add 10 ml of 2M *ammonium chloride*, 1 ml of 10M *ammonia* and, dropwise, 50 ml of a hot 4% w/v solution of *ammonium oxalate*. Allow to stand for 4 hours, dilute to 200 ml with *water* and filter. Evaporate 100 ml of the filtrate to dryness and ignite. The residue weighs not more than 2 mg (0.4%).

Chloride 12.5 ml of a 2.0% w/v solution diluted to 15 ml with *water* complies with the *limit test for chlorides*, Appendix VII (200 ppm).

Sulphate Dissolve 10.0 g in a mixture of 10 ml of 5M *acetic acid* and 90 ml of *water* by heating. 15 ml of the resulting solution complies with the *limit test for sulphates*, Appendix VII (100 ppm).

Readily carbonisable substances and boric acid Mix 0.5 g with 2 ml of cooled *sulphuric acid (96% w/w)* in a porcelain dish previously rinsed with the same reagent and placed in ice; no yellow or brown colour is produced. Add 1 ml of *chromotrope 2B solution* and mix; a violet colour is produced which does not become dark blue. Compare the colour obtained with that of a mixture of 1 ml of *chromotrope 2B solution* and 2 ml of cooled *sulphuric acid (96% w/w)*.

Sucrose and reducing sugars Dissolve 0.5 g in a mixture of 10 ml of *water* and 2 ml of *7M hydrochloric acid*, boil for 5 minutes, cool, add 10 ml of *sodium carbonate solution* and allow to stand. Dilute to 25 ml with *water*, filter and to 5 ml of the filtrate add 2 ml of *potassium cupri-tartrate solution* and boil for 1 minute. No red precipitate is produced.

Loss on drying When dried to constant weight at 110° at a pressure not exceeding 13 Pa, loses 3.5 to 6.5% of its weight. Use 0.5 g, finely powdered.

Assay Dissolve 0.8 g in 20 ml of hot *water*, allow to cool, dilute to 50 ml and carry out Method I for the *complexometric titration of calcium*, Appendix VIII D. Each ml of *0.1M disodium edetate VS* is equivalent to 0.04304 g of $C_{12}H_{22}CaO_{14}$.

Preparations
Calcium Gluconate Injection
Calcium Gluconate Tablets
Effervescent Calcium Gluconate Tablets

Action and use Used in treatment of calcium deficiency.

*In certain states party to the Convention on the Elaboration of a European Pharmacopœia, Calcium Gluconate may be required to comply with a limit for a total viable aerobic count of 10^3 micro-organisms per gram, determined by plate count, Appendix XVI B2.

Calcium Hydrogen Phosphate ☆
Dibasic Calcium Phosphate

$CaHPO_4,2H_2O$ 172.1   7789-77-7

Calcium Hydrogen Phosphate contains not less than 98.0 per cent and not more than 105.0 per cent of $CaHPO_4,2H_2O$.

Characteristics A white, crystalline powder; odourless.

Solubility Practically insoluble in cold *water* and in *ethanol (96%)*. It dissolves in dilute acids.

Identification A. Yields *reaction B* characteristic of calcium salts, Appendix VI.
B. Dissolve 0.1 g in a mixture of 5 ml of *2M nitric acid* and 5 ml of *water*. The solution yields *reaction B* characteristic of phosphates, Appendix VI.

Arsenic Dissolve 2.5 g in 20 ml of *2M hydrochloric acid*, filter if necessary, add *5M ammonia* until a precipitate begins to form, then add just sufficient *2M hydrochloric acid* to dissolve the precipitate and dilute to 50 ml with *distilled water* (solution A). 2 ml of the solution complies with the *limit test for arsenic*, Appendix VII (10 ppm).

Barium To 10 ml of solution A add 0.5 ml of *1M sulphuric acid*. After 15 minutes the solution is not more opalescent than a mixture of 10 ml of solution A and 0.5 ml of *distilled water*.

Heavy metals Dilute 7.5 ml of solution A to 15 ml with *water*. 12 ml of the resulting solution complies with *limit test A for heavy metals*, Appendix VII (40 ppm). Use *lead standard solution (1 ppm Pb)* to prepare the standard.

Iron 0.5 ml of solution A diluted to 10 ml with *water* complies with the *limit test for iron*, Appendix VII (400 ppm).

Carbonate Mix 0.5 g with 5 ml of *carbon dioxide-free water* and add 1 ml of *hydrochloric acid*. No effervescence is produced.

Chloride Dissolve 0.5 g in a mixture of 10 ml of *water* and 1 ml of *nitric acid* and dilute to 50 ml with *water*. 15 ml of the resulting solution complies with the *limit test for chlorides*, Appendix VII (330 ppm).

Fluoride 0.5 g complies with *limit test B for fluorides*, Appendix VII (100 ppm).

Sulphate Dilute 1 ml of solution A to 25 ml with *distilled water*. 15 ml of the resulting solution complies with the *limit test for sulphates*, Appendix VII (0.5%).

Monocalcium and tricalcium phosphates Dissolve 2 g in 30 ml of *1M hydrochloric acid VS*, add 20 ml of *water* and 0.05 ml of *methyl orange solution* and titrate the excess of acid with *1M sodium hydroxide VS*. Not less than 11.0 ml and not more than 12.5 ml of *1M hydrochloric acid VS* is required.

Assay Dissolve 0.3 g in a mixture of 5 ml of *water* and 1 ml of *7M hydrochloric acid*, add 25 ml of *0.1M disodium edetate VS* and dilute to 200 ml with *water*. Neutralise with *13.5M ammonia*, add 10 ml of *ammonia buffer pH 10* and 50 mg of *mordant black 11 mixture* and titrate the excess of disodium edetate with *0.1M zinc sulphate VS*. Each ml of *0.1M disodium edetate VS* is equivalent to 0.01721 g of $CaHPO_4,2H_2O$.

Storage Calcium Hydrogen Phosphate should be kept in a well-closed container.

Calcium Hydroxide

$Ca(OH)_2$ 74.09   1305-62-0

Calcium Hydroxide contains not less than 90.0 per cent of $Ca(OH)_2$.

Characteristics A soft, white powder.

Solubility Almost entirely soluble in 600 parts of *water*; soluble in aqueous solutions of *glycerol* and of sugars.

Identification A solution in *6M acetic acid* yields *reactions B* and *C* characteristic of calcium salts, Appendix VI.

Alkalinity A solution is alkaline to *phenolphthalein solution*.

Aluminium, iron, phosphate and matter insoluble in hydrochloric acid Dissolve 2 g in a mixture of 10 ml of *hydrochloric acid* and 75 ml of *water*, boil to remove carbon dioxide and make alkaline with *5M ammonia* using *methyl red solution* as indicator. Boil for 1 minute, filter and wash the precipitate with a hot 2% w/v solution of *ammonium chloride*. Dissolve the precipitate as completely as possible by passing 20 ml of hot *2M hydrochloric acid* through the filter and wash the filter with sufficient hot *water* to adjust the volume of the solution to 50 ml. Boil the solution and make alkaline with *5M ammonia* using *methyl red solution* as indicator. Boil for 1 minute, filter through the same filter, wash the precipitate with a hot 2% w/v solution of *ammonium nitrate*, dry and ignite at a temperature not lower than 1000°. The residue weighs not more than 20 mg.

Arsenic Dissolve 0.50 g in 5 ml of *brominated hydrochloric acid* and dilute to 50 ml with *water*. 25 ml of the resulting solution complies with the *limit test for arsenic*, Appendix VII (4 ppm).

Heavy metals Dissolve 3.0 g in 30 ml of 1M *hydrochloric acid*, add 0.5 ml of *nitric acid* and boil to remove any carbon dioxide. Cool, add 20 ml of a 0.01% w/v solution of *iron(III) chloride*, make alkaline with 5M *ammonia*, filter and wash the precipitate with *water*. Pass 20 ml of hot 1M *hydrochloric acid* through the filter, cool the filtrate, add 2 g of *ammonium thiocyanate* and extract with two successive 10-ml quantities of a mixture of equal volumes of *amyl alcohol* and *ether*. Dilute the aqueous solution to 60 ml with *water* and add 2 g of *citric acid*. 12 ml of the resulting solution complies with *limit test A for heavy metals*, Appendix VII (20 ppm). Use *lead standard solution (1 ppm Pb)* to prepare the standard.

Chloride Dissolve 0.30 g in *water* with the addition of 2 ml of *nitric acid* and dilute to 30 ml with *water*. 15 ml of the resulting solution complies with the *limit test for chlorides*, Appendix VII (330 ppm).

Sulphate Dissolve 0.15 g in *water* with the addition of 1 ml of 1M *hydrochloric acid* and dilute to 60 ml with *water*. 15 ml of the resulting solution complies with the *limit test for sulphates*, Appendix VII (0.4%).

Assay To 1.5 g add 5 ml of *ethanol (96%)* previously neutralised to *phenolphthalein solution*, shake gently and add 250 ml of a 10% w/v solution of *sucrose* previously neutralised to *phenolphthalein solution*. Shake vigorously for 5 minutes and then at frequent intervals during 4 hours. Add sufficient of the neutralised sucrose solution to produce 500 ml, filter and titrate 250 ml of the filtrate with 1M *hydrochloric acid VS* using *phenolphthalein solution* as indicator. Each ml of 1M *hydrochloric acid VS* is equivalent to 0.03705 g of $Ca(OH)_2$.

Storage Calcium Hydroxide should be kept in a well-closed container.

Preparation
Calcium Hydroxide Solution

Calcium Lactate Pentahydrate ☆
Calcium Lactate

$$\left[\begin{array}{c} CH_3 \cdot CH \cdot CO_2 - \\ | \\ OH \end{array} \right]_2 Ca$$

$C_6H_{10}CaO_6,5H_2O$ *(approx)*   218.2 *(anhydrous)*
814-80-2 *(anhydrous)*

Calcium Lactate Pentahydrate is hydrated calcium (*RS*)-2-hydroxypropionate or mixtures of calcium (*R*)-, (*S*)- and (*RS*)-2-hydroxypropionate. It contains not less than 98.0 per cent and not more than 102.0 per cent of $C_6H_{10}CaO_6$, calculated with reference to the dried substance. It contains not less than 22.0

per cent and not more than 27.0 per cent of water.

Characteristics A white or almost white, crystalline or granular powder; slightly efflorescent.

Solubility Soluble in *water*; freely soluble in boiling *water*; very slightly soluble in *ethanol (96%)*.

Identification A. Yields *reaction B* characteristic of calcium salts, Appendix VI.
B. Yields *reaction A* characteristic of lactates, Appendix VI.
C. Complies with the test for Loss on drying.

Acidity or alkalinity To 10 ml of a 5.0% w/v solution in *carbon dioxide-free water* prepared from *distilled water* (solution A) add 0.1 ml of *dilute phenolphthalein solution* and 0.5 ml of 0.01M *hydrochloric acid VS*. The solution is colourless and not more than 2.0 ml of 0.01M *sodium hydroxide VS* is required to change the colour of the solution to pink.

Clarity and colour of solution Solution A is not more opalescent than *reference suspension II*, Appendix IV A, and not more intensely coloured than *reference solution BY₆*, Appendix IV B, Method II.

Barium To 10 ml of solution A add 1 ml of *calcium sulphate solution* and allow to stand for 15 minutes. The mixture is not more opalescent than a mixture of 10 ml of solution A and 1 ml of *distilled water*.

Heavy metals 12 ml of solution A complies with *limit test A for heavy metals*, Appendix VII (20 ppm). Use *lead standard solution (1 ppm Pb)* to prepare the standard.

Iron 4 ml of solution A diluted to 10 ml with *water* complies with the *limit test for iron*, Appendix VII (50 ppm).

Magnesium and alkali salts To 20 ml of solution A add 20 ml of *water*, 2 g of *ammonium chloride* and 2 ml of 6M *ammonia*, heat to boiling and add rapidly 40 ml of a hot 4% w/v solution of *ammonium oxalate*. Allow to stand for 4 hours, dilute to 100 ml with *water* and filter. To 50 ml of the filtrate add 0.5 ml of *sulphuric acid*, evaporate to dryness and ignite to constant weight at 600°. The residue weighs not more than 5 mg (1%).

Chloride 5 ml of solution A diluted to 15 ml with *water* complies with the *limit test for chlorides*, Appendix VII (200 ppm).

Sulphate 7.5 ml of solution A diluted to 15 ml with *distilled water* complies with the *limit test for sulphates*, Appendix VII (400 ppm).

Volatile acids Mix 0.5 g with 1 ml of *orthophosphoric acid* in a 100-ml ground-glass stoppered flask and heat cautiously at 50° for 10 minutes. No odour of volatile fatty acids is detectable immediately after opening the flask.

Loss on drying When dried to constant weight at 125°, loses 22.0 to 27.0% of its weight. Use 0.5 g.

Assay Dissolve 0.2 g in sufficient *water* to produce 300 ml and carry out the method for the *complexometric titration of calcium*, Appendix VIII D. Each ml of 0.1M *disodium edetate VS* is equivalent to 0.02182 g of $C_6H_{10}CaO_6$.

Storage Calcium Lactate Pentahydrate should be kept in a well-closed container.

Preparation
Calcium Lactate Tablets

Action and use Used in treatment of calcium deficiency.

Calcium Lactate Trihydrate ☆

$C_6H_{10}CaO_6,3H_2O$ (approx)   218.2 (anhydrous)
814-80-2 (anhydrous)

Calcium Lactate Trihydrate is hydrated calcium (RS)-2-hydroxypropionate or mixtures of calcium (R)-, (S)- and (RS)-2-hydroxypropionate. It contains not less than 98.0 per cent and not more than 102.0 per cent of $C_6H_{10}CaO_6$, calculated with reference to the dried substance. It contains not less than 15.0 per cent and not more than 20.0 per cent of water.

Characteristics A white or almost white, crystalline or granular powder.

Solubility Soluble in water; freely soluble in boiling water; very slightly soluble in ethanol (96%).

Identification A. Complies with tests A and B for Identification described under Calcium Lactate Pentahydrate.
B. Complies with the test for Loss on drying.

Acidity or alkalinity; Clarity and colour of solution; Barium; Heavy metals; Iron; Magnesium and alkali salts; Chloride; Sulphate; Volatile acids Complies with the tests described under Calcium Lactate Pentahydrate.

Loss on drying When dried to constant weight at 125°, loses 15.0 to 20.0% of its weight. Use 0.5 g.

Assay Dissolve 0.2 g in sufficient water to produce 300 ml and carry out the method for the complexometric titration of calcium, Appendix VIII D. Each ml of 0.1M disodium edetate VS is equivalent to 0.02182 g of $C_6H_{10}CaO_6$.

Storage Calcium Lactate Trihydrate should be kept in a well-closed container.

Preparation
Calcium Lactate Tablets.

Action and use Used in treatment of calcium deficiency.

Calcium Pantothenate ☆

$$\left[HOCH_2 \cdot CMe_2 - \overset{\overset{\displaystyle OH}{|}}{\underset{\underset{\displaystyle H}{|}}{C}} - CO \cdot NH \cdot CH_2 \cdot CH_2 \cdot CO_2 - \right]_2 Ca$$

$C_{18}H_{32}CaN_2O_{10}$ 476.5   137-08-6

Calcium Pantothenate is calcium bis[(R)-N-(2,4-dihydroxy-3,3-dimethylbutyryl)-β-alaninate]. It contains not less than 98.0 per cent and not more than 101.0 per cent of $C_{18}H_{32}CaN_2O_{10}$, calculated with reference to the dried substance.

Characteristics A white powder; slightly hygroscopic.

Solubility Freely soluble in water; slightly soluble in ethanol (96%); practically insoluble in ether.

Identification A. In the test for β-Alanine, the principal spot in the chromatogram obtained with solution (2) is similar in colour, position and size to that in the chromatogram obtained with solution (3).
B. Complies with the test for Specific optical rotation.
C. To 1 ml of a 5.0% w/v solution in carbon dioxide-free water (solution A) add 1 ml of 2M sodium hydroxide and 0.1 ml of a 12.5% w/v solution of copper(II) sulphate. A blue colour is produced.
D. Yields reaction A characteristic of calcium salts, Appendix VI.

Acidity or alkalinity pH of solution A, 6.8 to 8.0, Appendix V L.

Clarity and colour of solution Solution A is clear, Appendix IV A, and colourless, Appendix IV B, Method II.

Specific optical rotation In solution A, +25.5° to +27.5°, Appendix V F.

β-Alanine Carry out the method for thin-layer chromatography, Appendix III A, using silica gel G as the coating substance and a mixture of 65 volumes of absolute ethanol and 35 volumes of water as the mobile phase but allowing the solvent front to ascend 12 cm above the line of application. Apply separately to the chromatoplate 5 μl of each of four solutions in water containing (1) 4.0% w/v of the substance being examined, (2) 0.4% w/v of the substance being examined, (3) 0.4% w/v of calcium pantothenate EPCRS and (4) 0.02% w/v of β-alanine. After removal of the plate, dry it in a current of air, spray with ethanolic ninhydrin solution and heat at 110° for 10 minutes. Any spot corresponding to β-alanine in the chromatogram obtained with solution (1) is not more intense than the spot in the chromatogram obtained with solution (4).

Chloride Dilute 5 ml of solution A to 15 ml. The resulting solution complies with the limit test for chlorides, Appendix VII (200 ppm).

Heavy metals 12 ml of solution A complies with limit test A for heavy metals, Appendix VII (20 ppm). Use lead standard solution (1 ppm Pb) to prepare the standard.

Loss on drying When dried to constant weight at 100° to 105°, loses not more than 3.0% of its weight. Use 1 g.

Assay Dissolve 0.18 g in 50 ml of glacial acetic acid and carry out Method I for non-aqueous titration, Appendix VIII A, determining the end-point potentiometrically. Each ml of 0.1M perchloric acid VS is equivalent to 0.02383 g of $C_{18}H_{32}CaN_2O_{10}$.

Storage Calcium Pantothenate should be kept in an airtight container.

Action and use Component of vitamin B.

Calcium Phosphate
Tribasic Calcium Phosphate

7758-23-8

Calcium Phosphate consists mainly of tricalcium diorthophosphate, $Ca_3(PO_4)_2$, together with calcium phosphates of more acidic or basic character. It contains not less than 90.0 per cent of calcium phosphates, calculated as $Ca_3(PO_4)_2$.

Characteristics A white, amorphous powder; odourless or almost odourless. At relative humidities between about 15 and 65%, the equilibrium moisture content at 25° is about 2%, but at relative humidities above about 75% it absorbs small additional amounts of moisture.

Solubility Practically insoluble in water. It dissolves in dilute mineral acids.

Identification Yields the *reactions* characteristic of calcium salts and of phosphates, Appendix VI.

Arsenic 0.25 g complies with the *limit test for arsenic*, Appendix VII (4 ppm).

Heavy metals Dissolve 2.5 g in 20 ml of 1M *hydrochloric acid*, filter if necessary, add 5M *ammonia* until a precipitate just begins to form, add just sufficient 2M *hydrochloric acid* to redissolve the precipitate and dilute to 50 ml with *water*. Dilute 10 ml of this solution to 15 ml with *water*. 12 ml of the resulting solution complies with *limit test A for heavy metals*, Appendix VII (30 ppm). Use *lead standard solution (1 ppm Pb)* to prepare the standard.

Iron Dissolve 0.25 g in a mixture of 50 ml of *water* and 5 ml of *hydrochloric acid* and dilute to 100 ml with *water*. 10 ml of the resulting solution complies with the *limit test for iron*, Appendix VII (400 ppm).

Carbonate 5.0 g suspended in 30 ml of *carbon dioxide-free water* dissolves with not more than a slight effervescence on the addition of 10 ml of *hydrochloric acid*.

Chloride Dissolve 0.10 g in *water* with the addition of 1 ml of *nitric acid* and dilute to 100 ml with *water*. 15 ml of the resulting solution complies with the *limit test for chlorides*, Appendix VII (0.35%).

Fluoride 4.0 g complies with the *limit test for fluorides*, Appendix VII (50 ppm).

Sulphate Dissolve 0.10 g in *water* with the addition of 3 ml of 1M *hydrochloric acid* and dilute to 60 ml with *water*. 15 ml of the resulting solution complies with the *limit test for sulphates*, Appendix VII (0.6%).

Acid-insoluble matter Dissolve 5.0 g in 30 ml of *water* and 10 ml of *hydrochloric acid*, filter, wash the residue with *water* and dry to constant weight at 105°. The residue weighs not more than 0.3% of the weight taken.

Water Not more than 2.5% w/w, Appendix IX C. Use 1 g.

Assay Dissolve 1 g in 10 ml of *hydrochloric acid* by heating on a water-bath, add 50 ml of *water*, cool and dilute to 250 ml with *water*. To 25 ml of the resulting solution add 30 ml of 0.05M *disodium edetate VS*, 10 ml of *ammonia buffer pH 10.9* and 100 ml of *water* and titrate the excess of disodium edetate with 0.05M *zinc chloride VS* using *mordant black 11 solution* as indicator. Each ml of 0.05M *disodium edetate VS* is equivalent to 0.005170 g of $Ca_3(PO_4)_2$.

Action and use Pharmaceutical aid.

Calcium Sodium Lactate

$2C_3H_5NaO_3,(C_3H_5O_3)_2Ca,4H_2O$ 514.4

Calcium Sodium Lactate contains not less than 7.5 per cent w/w and not more than 8.5 per cent w/w of calcium, Ca, and not less than 8.5 per cent w/w and not more than 10.0 per cent w/w of sodium, Na.

Characteristics A white powder or granules; odour, slight and characteristic; deliquescent.

Solubility Soluble in 14 parts of *water* and in 25 parts of boiling *ethanol (96%)*; practically insoluble in *ether*.

Identification A. Heat 1 g gently with 10 ml of 1M *sulphuric acid* and 0.1 g of *potassium permanganate*. The odour of acetaldehyde is produced.

B. Yields the *reactions* characteristic of calcium salts and of sodium salts, Appendix VI.

Acidity or alkalinity Dissolve 5 g in 100 ml of hot *carbon dioxide-free water*. The solution is not alkaline to *phenolphthalein solution* and requires not more than 2.5 ml of 0.1M *sodium hydroxide VS* to change the colour of the solution to pink.

Heavy metals A 10.0% w/v solution complies with *limit test A for heavy metals*, Appendix VII (10 ppm). Use *lead standard solution (1 ppm Pb)* to prepare the standard.

Chloride Dissolve 0.50 g in 100 ml of *water* containing 1.5 ml of *nitric acid*. 15 ml of the resulting solution complies with the *limit test for chlorides*, Appendix VII (700 ppm).

Sulphate Dissolve 0.25 g in 60 ml of *water* containing 3 ml of 2M *hydrochloric acid*. 15 ml of the resulting solution complies with the *limit test for sulphates*, Appendix VII (0.24%).

Reducing sugars 1.0 g dissolved in 10 ml of *water* and boiled with 5 ml of *potassium cupri-tartrate solution* yields not more than the slightest trace of a red precipitate.

Assay *For calcium* Carry out Method II for the *complexometric titration of calcium*, Appendix VIII D, using 0.5 g. Each ml of 0.05M *disodium edetate VS* is equivalent to 0.002004 g of Ca.

For sodium Ignite 2 g gently until carbonised, cool, boil the residue with 50 ml of *water* and 50 ml of 0.5M *hydrochloric acid VS* and filter. Wash the residue with *water* and titrate the excess of acid in the combined filtrate and washings with 0.5M *sodium hydroxide VS* using *methyl orange solution* as indicator. Each ml of 0.5M *hydrochloric acid VS*, after the subtraction of one-fifth of the volume of 0.05M *disodium edetate VS* that would be required by the calcium in the weight of sample taken, is equivalent to 0.01149 g of Na.

Storage Calcium Sodium Lactate should be kept in a well-closed container.

Action and use Used in treatment of calcium deficiency.

Dried Calcium Sulphate

Exsiccated Calcium Sulphate; Plaster of Paris

$CaSO_4,\frac{1}{2}H_2O$ 145.1   *26499-65-0*

Dried Calcium Sulphate is prepared by heating powdered gypsum, $CaSO_4,2H_2O$, at about 150° in a controlled manner such that it is substantially converted into the hemihydrate, $CaSO_4,\frac{1}{2}H_2O$, with minimum production of the anhydrous phases of calcium sulphate. It may contain suitable setting accelerators or decelerators.

Characteristics A white or almost white powder; odourless or almost odourless; hygroscopic.

Solubility Slightly soluble in *water*; more soluble in dilute mineral acids; practically insoluble in *ethanol (96%)*.

Identification Yields the *reactions* characteristic of calcium salts and of sulphates, Appendix VI.

Setting properties 20 g mixed with 10 ml of *water* at 15° to 20° in a cylindrical mould about 2.4 cm in diameter sets in 4 to 11 minutes. The mass thus produced, after standing for 3 hours, possesses sufficient hardness to resist pressure of the fingers at the edges, which retain their sharpness of outline and do not crumble.

Loss on ignition When ignited to constant weight at red heat, loses 4.5% to 8.0% of its weight.

Storage Dried Calcium Sulphate should be kept in a well-closed container.

Camphor

$C_{10}H_{16}O$ 152.2   77-22-2

Camphor is obtained from *Cinnamomum camphora* (L.) Nees and Eberm. and purified by sublimation (natural camphor) or it may be prepared synthetically (synthetic camphor).

Characteristics Colourless, transparent crystals, crystalline masses, blocks of tough consistence or crumbly masses known as 'flowers of camphor'; odour, penetrating and characteristic. Readily pulverisable in the presence of a little *ethanol (96%)*, *ether* or *chloroform*.

Solubility Slightly soluble in *water*; soluble in in 1 part of *ethanol (96%)* and in 0.25 part of *chloroform*; very soluble in *ether*; freely soluble in fixed oils.

Identification A. Burns readily with a bright smoky flame and slowly volatilises at 20°.

B. The *light absorption*, Appendix II B, in the range 230 to 350 nm of a 0.5% w/v solution in *ethanol (96%)* exhibits a maximum only at 289 nm. The *absorbance* at 289 nm is about 1.04.

Melting point 174° to 181°, Appendix V A, but using a capillary tube with an internal diameter not greater than 2 mm.

Specific optical rotation In a 10% w/v solution in *ethanol (96%)*, natural camphor, +40° to +43°; synthetic camphor, −1.5° to +1.5°, Appendix V F.

Water 1.0 g forms a clear solution with 10 ml of *petroleum spirit (boiling range, 40° to 60°)*.

Non-volatile matter When volatilised at 105°, leaves not more than 0.1% of residue. Use 5 g.

Storage Camphor should be kept in a well-closed container and stored at a temperature not exceeding 25°.

Preparations
Camphorated Opium Tincture
Concentrated Camphorated Opium Tincture
Concentrated Camphor Water

Action and use Counter-irritant.

Capreomycin Sulphate

1405-37-4

Capreomycin Sulphate is a mixture of the sulphates of the antimicrobial substances produced by certain strains of *Streptomyces capreolus*. The potency is not less than 700 Units per mg.

Characteristics A white, or almost white, solid.

Solubility Soluble in 1 part of *water*; practically insoluble in *ethanol (96%)*, in *chloroform* and in *ether*.

Identification A. The *light absorption*, Appendix II B, in the range 230 to 350 nm of a 0.004% w/v solution in 0.1M *hydrochloric acid* exhibits a maximum only at 268 nm. The *absorbance* at 268 nm is about 1.2.

B. The *light absorption*, Appendix II B, in the range 230 to 350 nm of a 0.004% w/v solution in 0.1M *sodium hydroxide* exhibits a maximum only at 287 nm. The *absorbance* at 287 nm is about 0.8.

C. Carry out the method for *thin-layer chromatography*, Appendix III A, using *microcrystalline cellulose* as the coating substance and a mixture of 60 volumes of *propan-2-ol*, 25 volumes of 1M *hydrochloric acid* and 15 volumes of *butan-2-one* as the mobile phase. Apply separately to the chromatoplate 5 µl of each of the following solutions. For solution (1) dissolve 5 mg of the substance being examined in a mixture of 0.5 ml of *hydrochloric acid* and 0.5 ml of *water*, heat in a sealed tube at 100° for 16 hours, evaporate to dryness on a water-bath, continue to heat until the odour of hydrogen chloride is no longer detectable and dissolve the residue in 1 ml of *water*. Prepare solution (2) in the same manner, but using *capreomycin sulphate BPCRS* in place of the substance being examined. After removal of the plate, dry it in a stream of cold air for 15 minutes and then at 100° for 15 minutes. Allow to cool, spray with *cadmium and ninhydrin solution* and heat at 100° for 30 minutes. The spots in the chromatogram obtained with solution (1) correspond to those in the chromatogram obtained with solution (2).

D. A solution is laevorotatory.

E. Yields the *reactions* characteristic of sulphates, Appendix VI.

Acidity or alkalinity pH of a 3% w/v solution, 4.5 to 7.5, Appendix V L.

Capreomycin I Not less than 90% when determined by the following method. Carry out the method for *descending paper chromatography*, Appendix III E, using a mixture of 70 volumes of *propan-1-ol* and 30 volumes of *water* as the saturating solvent and allowing to stand for 48 hours at 20° to 25°. Use three strips of paper, 50 cm × 20 cm in size. Apply to one of the strips, evenly across the paper, 0.1 ml of a freshly prepared 2.0% w/v solution of the substance being examined (solution A; this solution must be kept at 2° to 8° before use) and dry in a current of warm air. Place this strip, and a second unspotted strip, in the tank and allow chromatography to proceed for 16 hours using a mixture of 75 volumes of *propan-1-ol*, 33 volumes of *water*, 8 volumes of *glacial acetic acid* and 8 volumes of *triethylamine* as the mobile phase.

Remove the strips from the tank, allow to dry in air for 1 hour, examine the first strip under *ultra-violet light (254 nm)* and mark the main band (capreomycin I). (A subsidiary band preceding the main band may appear; this is due to capreomycin II.) Cut out the capreomycin I band and the corresponding portion from the second (unspotted) strip and treat each in the following manner. Cut into small pieces, place in a 50-ml glass-stoppered flask and add 30 ml of a citrate buffer solution prepared by dissolving 21.0 g of *citric acid* in 1000 ml of *water* and adjusting the pH to 6.2 with a 50% w/v solution of *sodium hydroxide*. Shake for 1 hour, filter and dilute 10 ml of the filtrate to 50 ml with *water*. Apply evenly across the third strip of paper 100 µl of solution A, allow to dry in a current of warm air, cut out the area containing the streak and a similarly sized area from an unused portion of the strip and treat each as described above beginning at the words 'Cut into small pieces . . .'. Measure the *absorbance* of each solution, Appendix II B, at the maximum at 268 nm using *water* in the reference cell. Subtract the absorbance of the solution obtained from the second strip of paper from that of the solution obtained from the first strip. The difference is not less than 90% of the difference obtained by subtracting the absorbance of the solution obtained from the unused area of the third strip from that of the solution obtained from the area of the third strip containing the streak.

Loss on drying When dried at 100° at a pressure not exceeding 0.7 kPa for 4 hours, loses not more than 10.0% of its weight. Use 1 g.

Sulphated ash Not more than 3.0%, Appendix IX A.

Assay Carry out the *biological assay of antibiotics*, Appendix XIV A. The precision of the assay is such that the fiducial limits of error are not less than 95% and not more than 105% of the estimated potency.

Storage Capreomycin Sulphate should be kept in a well-closed container and stored at a temperature not exceeding 15°. If it is intended for use in the manufacture of a parenteral dosage form, the container should be sterile and sealed so as to exclude micro-organisms.

Labelling The label states (1) the number of Units per mg; (2) the date after which the material is not intended to be used; (3) the conditions under which it should be stored; (4) whether or not it is intended for use in the manufacture of a parenteral dosage form.

Preparation
Capreomycin Injection

Action and use Antituberculous.

Capreomycin Sulphate intended for use in the manufacture of a parenteral dosage form complies with the following additional requirements.

Pyrogens Complies with the *test for pyrogens*, Appendix XIV K. Use per kg of the rabbit's weight 1 ml of a solution in *water for injections* containing 7000 Units per ml.

Sterility When intended for use in the manufacture of a parenteral dosage form without further sterilisation, complies with the *test for sterility*, Appendix XVI A.

Caraway

Caraway consists of the dried ripe fruits of *Carum carvi* L.

Characteristics Odour of the crushed fruit, aromatic and characteristic; taste, aromatic and characteristic.

Macroscopical Cremocarp oblong, ellipsoidal, laterally compressed. Mericarps glabrous, brown, free from the pedicel and carpophores; up to about 7 mm long and 2 mm broad, tapered to curved ends; five narrow, slightly yellow primary ridges. Pericarp thin, endosperm oily, without a ventral groove.

Microscopical Trichomes absent. Pericarp: cells of outer epidermis polygonal in surface view, with striated cuticle and occasional stomata, tabular. Inner epidermal cells thin-walled, subrectangular and elongated tangentially, each about 10 to 20 µm wide and 40 to 100 µm long, appearing parallel with each other in surface view and showing no parquetry arrangement. Vittae: four dorsal, two commissural; epithelium brown-celled; cavity containing oil. Mericarp with five ribs each containing a vascular strand supported by a cap of finely pitted sclerenchyma. Mesocarp parenchymatous without reticulate thickening. A single, small secretory canal at the outer margin of each vascular bundle. Endosperm parenchymatous with thick cellulose walls, containing much oil and numerous small aleurone grains up to 10 µm in diameter and each usually with one or more microrosettes of calcium oxalate.

Acid-insoluble ash Not more than 1.5%, Appendix XI K.

Foreign matter Not more than 2.0%, Appendix XI D.

Volatile oil Not less than 3.5% v/w, Appendix XI E, Method I. Use 20 g, unground, and distil for 4 hours.

Storage Caraway should be stored at a temperature not exceeding 25°.

Action and use Flavour.

Powdered Caraway

Powdered Caraway is Caraway in powder.

Characteristics Fawn to brown. Diagnostic structures: epidermal cells of pericarp with striated cuticle; fragments of brown epithelium of vittae; parenchymatous cells of the mesocarp without reticulate thickening; rectangular sclereids of the mesocarp; parenchymatous cells of the endosperm containing much oil and numerous aleurone grains containing calcium oxalate; no parquetry arrangement of endocarp cells; trichomes and starch absent.

Acid-insoluble ash Not more than 1.5%, Appendix XI K.

Volatile oil Not less than 2.5% v/w, Appendix XI E, Method I. Use 20 g and distil for 4 hours.

Storage Powdered Caraway should be kept in a well-closed container that prevents the loss of volatile oil and stored at a temperature not exceeding 25°.

Action and use Flavour.

Caraway Oil

Caraway Oil is obtained by distillation from Caraway.

Characteristics A clear, colourless or pale yellow liquid, visibly free from water; odour, that of caraway.

Optical rotation +74° to +80°, Appendix V F.

Refractive index 1.485 to 1.492, Appendix V E.

Solubility in ethanol Soluble, at 20°, in 7 volumes of *ethanol (80%)*, Appendix X M.

Weight per ml 0.902 to 0.912 g, Appendix V G.

Content of ketones 53.0 to 63.0% w/w, calculated as carvone, $C_{10}H_{14}O$, Appendix X L. Each ml of 1M *potassium hydroxide in ethanol (90%) VS* is equivalent to 0.1514 g of $C_{10}H_{14}O$.

Storage Caraway Oil should be kept in a well-filled, well-closed container, protected from light and stored at a temperature not exceeding 25°.

Action and use Carminative and flavour.

Carbamazepine

$C_{15}H_{12}N_2O$ 236.3   *298-46-4*

Carbamazepine is 5*H*-dibenz[*b,f*]azepine-5-carboxamide. It contains not less than 97.0 per cent and not more than 103.0 per cent of $C_{15}H_{12}N_2O$, calculated with reference to the dried substance.

Characteristics A white or almost white, crystalline powder.

Solubility Practically insoluble in *water* and in *ether*; sparingly soluble in *ethanol (96%)*; soluble in 10 parts of *chloroform*.

Identification A. The *light absorption*, Appendix II B, in the range 230 to 300 nm of a 0.002% w/v solution in *ethanol (96%)* exhibits maxima at 238 and 285 nm. The *absorbance* at 285 nm is about 0.98.
B. Exhibits an intense blue fluorescence in ultra-violet light (365 nm).
C. Heat 0.1 g with 2 ml of *nitric acid* in a water-bath for 3 minutes. An orange-red colour is produced.

Acidity or alkalinity Stir 1 g with 20 ml of *water* for 15 minutes and filter. Titrate 10 ml of the filtrate with 0.01M *sodium hydroxide VS* using 0.05 ml of *phenolphthalein solution* as indicator; not more than 0.5 ml is required. Add 0.15 ml of a 0.05% w/v solution of *methyl red* and titrate with 0.01M *hydrochloric acid VS* until the colour changes to red; not more than 1.0 ml is required.

Melting point 189° to 193°, Appendix V A.

Chloride 0.30 g complies with the *limit test for chlorides*, Appendix VII (170 ppm).

Related substances Carry out the method for *thin-layer chromatography*, Appendix III A, using *silica gel G* as the coating substance and a mixture of 95 volumes of *toluene* and 5 volumes of *methanol* as the mobile phase. Apply separately to the chromatoplate 10 μl of each of two solutions containing (1) 2.50% w/v of the substance being examined in *chloroform* and (2) 0.0050% w/v of *iminodibenzyl* in *methanol*. After removal of the plate, allow it to dry in air for 15 minutes and spray with a 0.5% w/v solution of *potassium dichromate* in *sulphuric acid (20%)*. Any *secondary spot* in the chromatogram obtained with solution (1) is not more intense than the spot in the chromatogram obtained with solution (2).

Loss on drying When dried at 105° for 2 hours, loses not more than 0.5% of its weight. Use 1 g.

Sulphated ash Not more than 0.1%, Appendix IX A.

Assay Dissolve 0.1 g in sufficient *ethanol (96%)* to produce 100 ml. Dilute 10 ml to 100 ml with *ethanol (96%)* and dilute 10 ml of the dilution to 100 ml with *ethanol (96%)*. Measure the *absorbance* of the resulting solution at the maximum at 285 nm, Appendix II B. Calculate the content of $C_{15}H_{12}N_2O$ taking 490 as the value of A(1%, 1 cm) at the maximum at 285 nm.

Preparation
Carbamazepine Tablets

Action and use Anticonvulsant.

Carbenicillin Sodium

$C_{17}H_{16}N_2Na_2O_6S$ 422.4   *4800-94-6*

Carbenicillin Sodium is disodium (6*R*)-6-[2-carboxy-2-phenylacetamido]penicillanate. It contains not less than 89.0 per cent and not more than 100.5 per cent of $C_{17}H_{16}N_2Na_2O_6S$, calculated with reference to the anhydrous substance.

Characteristics A white or almost white powder; hygroscopic.

Solubility Soluble in 1.2 parts of *water* and in 25 parts of *ethanol (96%)*; practically insoluble in *chloroform* and in *ether*.

Identification A. The *infra-red absorption spectrum*, Appendix II A, is concordant with the *reference spectrum* of carbenicillin sodium.
B. Heat 0.5 g in a small sealed container on a water-bath for 3 minutes, remove the seal and immediately replace by a cork fitted with a platinum loop carrying a drop of a solution freshly prepared by mixing 1 ml of a 0.5% w/v solution of *sodium carbonate*, 1 ml of *phenolphthalein solution* and 10 ml of *water*. The reagent is decolorised within 2 minutes.
C. Yields the *reactions* characteristic of sodium salts, Appendix VI.

Acidity or alkalinity pH of a 10% w/v solution, 6.0 to 8.0, Appendix V L.

Specific optical rotation In a 1% w/v solution, +182° to +196°, Appendix V F.

Palladium Not more than 25 ppm when determined by the following method. Moisten 1 g in a silica crucible with 2 ml of *sulphuric acid*. Heat, gently at first, then more strongly until all carbon is removed and a white ash is obtained. Allow to cool, add 5 ml of a mixture of 3 volumes of *nitric acid* and 4 volumes of *hydrochloric acid* and evaporate to dryness on a water-bath. Add 3 ml of *hydrochloric acid*, warm to dissolve and add sufficient *water* to produce 25 ml. Determine the palladium by Method II for *atomic absorption spectrophotometry*, Appendix II D, measuring at 248 nm and using *palladium solution ASp* suitably diluted with *water* as the standard solution.

Total carbenicillin sodium, benzylpenicillin sodium, iodine-absorbing substances and water 96.0 to 102.0%

when determined by adding together the percentages of carbenicillin sodium (corrected for benzylpenicillin sodium), benzylpenicillin sodium, iodine-absorbing substances (all calculated with reference to the undried substance) and water found by the methods described below.

Benzylpenicillin sodium Not more than 5.0%, calculated with reference to the anhydrous substance, when determined by Method I for *agar-gel electrophoresis*, Appendix III F, using the following solutions. Solution (1) contains 0.00080% w/v of *benzylpenicillin sodium BPCRS* in *mixed phosphate buffer pH 6.5*. Solution (2) is a mixture of 1 volume of solution (1) and 3 volumes of *mixed phosphate buffer pH 6.5*. For solution (3) dissolve a sufficient quantity of the substance being examined in *mixed phosphate buffer pH 6.5* to produce a solution containing 0.00080% w/v of benzylpenicillin sodium (determine the approximate content of benzylpenicillin sodium by a preliminary test). Solution (4) is a mixture of 1 volume of solution (3) and 3 volumes of *mixed phosphate buffer pH 6.5*.

Iodine-absorbing substances Not more than 8.0%, calculated with reference to the anhydrous substance, when determined by the following method. Dissolve 0.125 g in sufficient *mixed phosphate buffer pH 7.0* to produce 25 ml. To 10 ml add 10 ml of *mixed phosphate buffer pH 4.0* and 10 ml of 0.01M *iodine VS* and titrate immediately with 0.01M *sodium thiosulphate VS* using *starch mucilage*, added towards the end of the titration, as indicator. Repeat the operation without the substance being examined. The difference between the titrations represents the amount of iodine-absorbing substances present. Each ml of 0.01M *sodium thiosulphate VS* is equivalent to 0.000489 g of iodine-absorbing substances.

Related substances Carry out the method for *thin-layer chromatography*, Appendix III A, using a silanised silica gel precoated chromatoplate (Merck silica gel 60 silanised plates are suitable), allowing the plate to dry at 110° for 1 hour before use and using as the mobile phase a mixture of 70 volumes of a 2.0% w/v solution of *sodium acetate*, previously adjusted to pH 7.0 with 1M *acetic acid*, and 30 volumes of *acetone*. Apply separately to the plate 5 μl of each of three solutions in the mobile phase containing (1) 10.0% w/v of the substance being examined, (2) 0.20% w/v of *benzylpenicillin sodium BPCRS* and (3) 0.050% w/v of *sodium α-benzyloxycarbonylbenzylpenicillin BPCRS* and develop immediately, without allowing the spots to dry. After removal of the plate, dry it at 60° for 10 minutes and spray with a freshly prepared solution containing 10% w/v of *hydroxylamine hydrochloride* and 5% w/v of *sodium hydroxide*, adjusted to pH 7.0 with either 0.1M *sodium hydroxide* or 0.1M *hydrochloric acid*, followed by a freshly prepared 20% w/v solution of *ammonium iron(III) sulphate* in a 12.4% w/v solution of *sulphuric acid*. In the chromatogram obtained with solution (1) any *secondary spot* with an Rf value higher than that of the principal spot is not more intense than the spot in the chromatogram obtained with solution (2) and any spot corresponding to α-benzyloxycarbonylbenzylpenicillin is not more intense than the spot in the chromatogram obtained with solution (3). Disregard any spot in the chromatogram obtained with solution (1) that corresponds to the spot in the chromatogram obtained with solution (2).

Water Not more than 5.5% w/w, Appendix IX C. Use 0.3 g.

Assay Dissolve 0.25 g (W_1) in sufficient *water* to produce 500 ml and dilute 10 ml to 100 ml with *water*. Place two 2-ml quantities of the resulting solution in separate stoppered tubes. To one tube add 10 ml of *imidazole—mercury reagent*, mix, stopper the tube and immerse in a water-bath at 60° for exactly 25 minutes, swirling occasionally. Remove from the water-bath and cool rapidly to 20° (solution A). To the second tube add 10 ml of *water* and mix (solution B). Without delay measure the *absorbances* of solutions A and B at the maximum at 325 nm, Appendix II B, using in the reference cell a mixture of 2 volumes of *water* and 10 volumes of *imidazole—mercury reagent* for solution A and *water* for solution B. Calculate the difference (S_1) between the absorbances of solutions A and B.

Repeat the procedure using 0.21 g (W_2) of *benzylpenicillin sodium BPCRS* in place of the substance being examined. Calculate the difference (S_2) between the absorbances of solutions A and B.

Calculate the percentage of total penicillins from the expression $1.185 S_1 W_2 F / S_2 W_1$, where F is the declared content of $C_{16}H_{17}N_2NaO_4S$ in *benzylpenicillin sodium BPCRS*. Subtract the percentage of benzylpenicillin sodium, determined in the test for Benzylpenicillin sodium, multiplied by 1.185. The difference is the content of carbenicillin sodium, $C_{17}H_{16}N_2Na_2O_6S$.

Storage Carbenicillin Sodium should be kept in a well-closed container and stored at a temperature not exceeding 5°. If it is intended for use in the manufacture of a parenteral dosage form the container should be sterile and sealed so as to exclude micro-organisms.

Labelling The label on the container states (1) the date after which the material is not intended to be used; (2) the conditions under which it should be stored; (3) whether or not it is intended for use in the manufacture of a parenteral dosage form.

Preparation
Carbenicillin Injection

Action and use Antibacterial.

Carbenicillin Sodium intended for use in the manufacture of a parenteral dosage form complies with the following additional requirements.

Pyrogens Complies with the *test for pyrogens*, Appendix XIV K. Use per kg of the rabbit's weight 1 ml of *water for injections* containing 6 mg per ml.

Sterility When intended for use in the manufacture of a parenteral dosage form without further sterilisation complies with the *test for sterility*, Appendix XVI A.

Carbenoxolone Sodium

$C_{34}H_{48}Na_2O_7$ 614.7   7421-40-1

Carbenoxolone Sodium is disodium 3β-(3-carboxylatopropionyloxy)-11-oxo-olean-12-en-30-oate. It contains not less than 97.0 per cent and not more than 103.0 per cent of $C_{34}H_{48}Na_2O_7$, calculated with reference to the anhydrous substance.

Characteristics A white or pale cream powder; hygroscopic. The powder is irritant to nasal membranes.

Solubility Soluble in 6 parts of *water* and in 30 parts of *ethanol (96%)*; practically insoluble in *chloroform* and in *ether*.

Identification A. Dissolve 0.1 g in 5 ml of *water* and make just acid with 2M *hydrochloric acid*, stir well and filter. Wash the residue with *water* until the washings are no longer acidic and dry to constant weight at 105°. The *infra-red absorption spectrum* of the residue, Appendix II A, is concordant with the *reference spectrum* of carbenoxolone.
B. The *light absorption*, Appendix II B, in the range 230 to 350 nm of a 0.0050% w/v solution in a mixture of equal volumes of *methanol* and 0.02M *sodium carbonate* exhibits a maximum only at 256 nm. The *absorbance* at 256 nm is about 1.0.
C. Mix 5 mg with 50 mg of *resorcinol* and 2 ml of *sulphuric acid (80%)*. Heat at 200° for 10 minutes, cool, pour into 200 ml of *water* and add sufficient 5M *sodium hydroxide* to make the mixture just alkaline. An intense green fluorescence is produced.
D. Yields the *reactions* characteristic of sodium salts, Appendix VI.

Alkalinity pH of a 10% w/v solution, 8.0 to 9.2, Appendix V L.

Specific optical rotation In a 1% w/v solution in a mixture of equal volumes of *methanol* and 0.02M *sodium carbonate*, +132° to +140°, Appendix V F.

Related substances Carry out the method for *thin-layer chromatography*, Appendix III A, using a silica gel F254 precoated chromatoplate (Merck silica gel 60 F254 plates are suitable) and a mixture of 60 volumes of *ethyl acetate*, 20 volumes of *methanol*, 11 volumes of *water* and 1 volume of 13.5M *ammonia* as the mobile phase. Apply separately to the chromatoplate 5 μl of each of two solutions of the substance being examined in *methanol* containing (1) 1.50% w/v and (2) 0.030% w/v. After removal of the plate, allow it to dry in air and examine under *ultra-violet light (254 nm)*. Spray with a 1.5% w/v solution of *vanillin* in *sulphuric acid (60%)* and heat at 105° for 10 to 15 minutes. By both methods of visualisation, any *secondary spot* in the chromatogram obtained with solution (1) is not more intense than the spot in the chromatogram obtained with solution (2).

Water Not more than 4.0% w/w, Appendix IX C. Use 0.6 g.

Assay Dissolve 1 g in 30 ml of *water*, add 30 ml of *chloroform* and 15 ml of a mixture of 1 volume of 2M *hydrochloric acid* and 9 volumes of *water*, shake and allow to separate. Add the chloroform layer to 40 ml of a 20% w/v solution of *sodium chloride*, shake and allow to separate. Repeat the extraction with four 15-ml quantities of *chloroform*, combine the chloroform extracts and add sufficient *chloroform* to produce 100 ml. Evaporate 25 ml, dry the residue at 100° at a pressure of 2 kPa, dissolve in 10 ml of *dimethylformamide* and carry out Method I for *non-aqueous titration*, Appendix VIII A, using 0.1M *tetrabutylammonium hydroxide VS* as titrant and *thymol blue solution* as indicator. Each ml of 0.1M *tetrabutylammonium hydroxide VS* is equivalent to 0.03073 g of $C_{34}H_{48}Na_2O_7$.

Storage Carbenoxolone Sodium should be kept in a well-closed container.

Preparation Carbenoxolone Tablets

Action and use Used in treatment of gastric ulcer.

Carbidopa

$C_{10}H_{14}N_2O_4,H_2O$ 244.2   38821-49-7

Carbidopa is (S)-2-(3,4-dihydroxybenzyl)-2-hydrazinopropionic acid monohydrate. It contains not less than 99.0 per cent and not more than 101.0 per cent of $C_{10}H_{14}N_2O_4$, calculated with reference to the anhydrous substance.

Characteristics A white or creamy-white powder; odourless or almost odourless.

Solubility Slightly soluble in *water*; very slightly soluble in *ethanol (96%)*; practically insoluble in *chloroform* and in *ether*.

Identification A. The *infra-red absorption spectrum*, Appendix II A, is concordant with the *reference spectrum* of carbidopa.
B. The *light absorption*, Appendix II B, in the range 230 to 350 nm of a 0.01% w/v solution in 0.1M *methanolic hydrochloric acid* exhibits a maximum only at 282 nm. The *absorbance* at 282 nm is about 1.30.
C. In the test for Methyldopa and 3-O-methylcarbidopa, the chromatogram obtained with solution (5) shows a peak with the same retention time as the principal peak in the chromatogram obtained with solution (4).

Acidity pH of a suspension prepared by shaking 0.1 g with 10 ml of *water* for 15 minutes, 4.0 to 6.0, Appendix V L.

Colour of solution A 1.0% w/v solution in 1M *hydrochloric acid* is not more intensely coloured than *reference solution* BY_6 or B_6, Appendix IV B, Method II.

Specific optical rotation In a 1% w/v solution in *aluminium chloride solution*, −22.5° to −26.5°, Appendix V F.

Heavy metals 1.0 g complies with *limit test C for heavy metals*, Appendix VII (20 ppm). Use 2 ml of *lead standard solution (10 ppm Pb)* to prepare the standard.

Methyldopa and 3-*O*-methylcarbidopa Carry out the method for *high-performance liquid chromatography*, Appendix III D, using five solutions in 0.1M *hydrochloric acid* containing (1) 0.0050% w/v of *methyldopa BPCRS*, 0.0050% w/v of *3-O-methylcarbidopa BPCRS* and 0.010% w/v of *3-O-methylmethyldopa BPCRS* (internal standard), (2) 1.00% w/v of the substance being examined, (3) 1.00% w/v of the substance being examined and 0.010% w/v of the internal standard, (4) 0.010% w/v of *carbidopa BPCRS* and (5) 0.010% w/v of the substance being examined.

The chromatographic procedure may be carried out using (a) a stainless steel column (20 cm × 4 mm) packed with *stationary phase B* (10 µm) (Lichrosorb RP-8 is suitable), (b) a mixture of 98 volumes of 0.1M *potassium dihydrogen orthophosphate* and 2 volumes of *methanol* as the mobile phase with a flow rate of 1.5 ml per minute and (c) a detection wavelength of 282 nm.

In the chromatogram obtained with solution (1) the peaks other than any solvent peak appear in the order methyldopa, 3-*O*-methylmethyldopa and 3-*O*-methylcarbidopa. In the chromatogram obtained with solution (1) the ratios of the areas of the peaks due to methyldopa and 3-*O*-methylcarbidopa to the area of the internal standard peak are greater than the corresponding ratios in the chromatogram obtained with solution (3).

Sulphated ash Not more than 0.1%, Appendix IX A.

Water 6.9 to 7.9% w/w, Appendix IX C. Use 0.5 g.

Assay To 0.3 g add 25 ml of 0.1M *perchloric acid VS*, swirl and warm gently to dissolve using the minimum of heat. Titrate the excess perchloric acid with 0.1M *sodium acetate in glacial acetic acid VS* determining the end-point potentiometrically. Each ml of 0.1M *perchloric acid VS* is equivalent to 0.02262 g of $C_{10}H_{14}N_2O_4$.

Preparation
Levodopa and Carbidopa Tablets

Action and use Used in treatment of Parkinson's disease.

Carbimazole

$C_7H_{10}N_2O_2S$ 186.2   *22232-54-8*

Carbimazole is ethyl 3-methyl-2-thioxo-4-imidazoline-1-carboxylate. It contains not less than 98.5 per cent and not more than 100.5 per cent of $C_7H_{10}N_2O_2S$, calculated with reference to the dried substance.

Characteristics A white or creamy-white, crystalline powder; odour, characteristic.

Solubility Slightly soluble in *water* and in *ether*; soluble in 50 parts of *ethanol (96%)*, in 17 parts of *acetone* and in 3 parts of *chloroform*.

Identification A. The *infra-red absorption spectrum*, Appendix II A, is concordant with the *reference spectrum* of carbimazole.
B. Heat 0.2 g with 5 ml of 0.1M *sodium hydroxide* on a water-bath for 1 hour. Cool, acidify with 2M *hydrochloric acid* and extract with three 5-ml quantities of *chloroform*.

Wash the combined chloroform extracts with 0.5 ml of *water*, filter through a dry filter paper and evaporate the chloroform. The *melting point* of the residue, after recrystallisation from *ethanol (96%)*, is about 140°, Appendix V A.
C. To a few mg add 0.05 ml of *dilute potassium iodobismuthate solution*. A scarlet colour is produced.

Melting point 122° to 125°, Appendix V A.

Methimazole Carry out the method for *thin-layer chromatography*, Appendix III A, using *silica gel G* as the coating substance and a mixture of 80 volumes of *chloroform* and 20 volumes of *acetone* as the mobile phase. Apply separately to the chromatoplate 10 µl of each of two solutions in *chloroform* containing (1) 1.0% w/v of the substance being examined and (2) 0.0050% w/v of *methimazole* and develop immediately. After removal of the plate, allow it to dry in air and spray with *dilute potassium iodobismuthate solution*. Any spot corresponding to methimazole in the chromatogram obtained with solution (1) is not more intense than the spot in the chromatogram obtained with solution (2).

Loss on drying When dried over *phosphorus pentoxide* at a pressure not exceeding 0.7 kPa for 24 hours, loses not more than 0.5% of its weight. Use 1 g.

Sulphated ash Not more than 0.1%, Appendix IX A.

Assay Dissolve 50 mg in sufficient *water* to produce 500 ml. To 10 ml of the solution, add 10 ml of 1M *hydrochloric acid* and sufficient *water* to produce 100 ml and measure the *absorbance* of the resulting solution at the maximum at 291 nm, Appendix II B. Calculate the content of $C_7H_{10}N_2O_2S$ taking 557 as the value of A(1%, 1 cm) at the maximum at 291 nm.

Storage Carbimazole should be kept in a well-closed container.

Preparation
Carbimazole Tablets

Action and use Antithyroid.

Carbomer

Carbomer is a synthetic high molecular weight polymer of acrylic acid cross-linked with allylsucrose. It contains not less than 56.0 per cent and not more than 68.0 per cent of carboxylic acid (-COOH) groups, calculated with reference to the dried substance.

Characteristics A white, fluffy powder; odour, slight and characteristic; hygroscopic.

Solubility After neutralisation with alkali hydroxides or amines, soluble in *water*, in *ethanol (96%)* and in *glycerol*.

Identification A. A 1% w/v dispersion is orange with *thymol blue solution* and yellow with *cresol red solution*.
B. Adjust a 1% w/v dispersion to about pH 7.5 with 1M *sodium hydroxide*. A very viscous gel is produced.

Yield value Mean zone diameter, 2.0 to 2.2 cm, using a gel prepared in the following manner. Add carefully 2.5 g to 500 ml of *water* containing 0.25 g of *sodium chloride* in a 1000-ml beaker, while stirring continuously at 990 to 1010 revolutions per minute with the stirrer shaft set at an angle of 60° from the vertical and to one side of the beaker and with the stirrer set near the bottom of the beaker.

Allow 45 to 90 seconds for addition of the substance being examined at a uniform rate, ensuring that any loose aggregates of powder are broken up, and continue stirring at 990 to 1010 revolutions per minute for 15 minutes. Remove the stirrer and allow the beaker containing the dispersion to stand in a water-bath maintained at 24.8° to 25.2° for 30 minutes. Insert the stirrer to a depth such that air is not drawn into the dispersion and, while stirring at 290 to 310 revolutions per minute, add 0.2 ml of *phenolphthalein solution* and 1.5 ml of *bromothymol blue solution*. Add rapidly about 5 ml of 5M *sodium hydroxide* below the surface and stir for 2 to 3 minutes until neutralisation, indicated by a uniform light blue colour, is complete. The pH, determined potentiometrically using glass and calomel electrodes should be between 7.3 and 7.8, Appendix V L. If it is below 7.3 add more 5M *sodium hydroxide* and mix; if the pH is above 7.8, discard the mucilage and prepare another using a smaller amount of sodium hydroxide for neutralisation. Return the neutralised mucilage to the water-bath and maintain at 25° for 1 hour.

The apparatus consists of two clear soda-glass plates, 100 mm × 100 mm × 3 mm. Give two opposing faces of the plates an even matt surface by rubbing together by hand with fine carborundum paste. Mark the plates with a diamond marker to show centre and corner alignment and four sample location points equidistant from the plate centre and the four corners.

Equilibrate the plates in a water-bath at 24.8° to 25.2° and dry rapidly before use. Apply 0.1 g of the dispersion of the gel to each of the sample location points on the matt surface of one of the plates. Align the second plate and lower it carefully, matt-side downwards, onto the lower plate. Add a suitable weight so that the combined weight of the top plate and applied weight equals 100 g. Allow the apparatus to stand for 10 minutes and determine the average zone diameter of the four samples using a strip of paper calibrated in mm.

Loss on drying When dried at 80° for 1 hour, loses not more than 2.0% of its weight. Use 1 g.

Sulphated ash Not more than 0.1%, Appendix IX A.

Assay Slowly add 0.4 g, previously dried for 1 hour at 80°, to 400 ml of *water* stirred continuously with a magnetic stirrer and continue stirring until solution is complete. Reduce the stirring speed and titrate with 0.2M *sodium hydroxide VS* determining the end-point potentiometrically using glass and calomel electrodes. Stir for 1 minute after each addition of 0.2M *sodium hydroxide VS* before recording the pH. Each ml of 0.2M *sodium hydroxide VS* is equivalent to 0.009004 g of carboxylic acid (-COOH) groups.

Storage Carbomer should be kept in a well-closed container.

Action and use Pharmaceutical aid.

Carbon Dioxide ☆

CO₂   44.01   *124-38-9*

Carbon Dioxide contains not less than 99.0 per cent v/v of CO_2.

Store the cylinder of the gas being examined at room temperature for not less than 6 hours before carrying out the following tests. For each test keep the cylinder in a vertical position with the outlet valve uppermost and deliver the gas at a steady rate of 4 litres per hour unless otherwise stated.

Characteristics A colourless gas; odourless.

Solubility At 20° and at a pressure of 101.3 kPa, soluble in about 1 volume of *water*.

Identification A. Extinguishes a flame.
B. Pass through a 5% w/v solution of *barium hydroxide*. A white precipitate is produced which dissolves, with effervescence, in 2M *acetic acid*.

Acidity Use a hermetically closed, flat-bottomed, glass cylinder with dimensions such that 50 ml of liquid reaches a height of 12 to 14 cm, fitted with an outlet tube and with an inlet tube with an orifice of internal diameter 1 mm reaching to within 2 mm of the bottom of the cylinder.

For solution (1) pass 5.0 litres of the gas being examined through a mixture of 0.1 ml of *hydrogen peroxide solution (10 vol)* diluted to contain 1% w/v of H_2O_2 and 50 ml of *carbon dioxide-free water*. Pass 5 litres of *nitrogen* at a rate of 15 to 20 litres per hour. For solution (2) add 0.1 ml of the hydrogen peroxide solution and 0.5 ml of 0.01M *hydrochloric acid* to 50 ml of *carbon dioxide-free water* in an identical cylinder. To each solution add 0.1 ml of *methyl orange—bromocresol green solution*. Any orange-yellow colour in solution (1) is not more intense than that in solution (2) (20 ppm v/v, calculated as HCl).

Phosphoric hydrides, hydrogen sulphide and organic reducing substances Use the apparatus described in the test for Acidity. Pass 1.0 litre of the gas being examined through a mixture of 20 ml of *ammoniacal silver nitrate solution*, 15 ml of *water* and 5 ml of 13.5M *ammonia*. The solution is not darker than a reference solution prepared at the same time and in the same manner but through which the gas has not been passed.

Carbon monoxide Carry out the *limit test for carbon monoxide in medicinal gases*, Appendix IX E, using 5 litres mixed with an equal volume of *argon*. Repeat the operation using 10 litres of *argon*. The difference between the titrations is not more than 0.5 ml (10 ppm v/v).

Assay Carry out Method I for the *assay of medicinal gases*, Appendix VIII J, using a 40% w/v solution of *potassium hydroxide* as the absorbent solution.

Storage Carbon Dioxide should be kept liquefied under pressure in approved metal cylinders.

Labelling The metal cylinder should be painted grey and carry a label stating 'Carbon Dioxide'. In addition, 'Carbon Dioxide' or the symbol 'CO₂' should be stencilled in paint on the shoulder of the cylinder.

Carbromal

Br
|
Et₂CCO·NH·CO·NH₂

$C_7H_{13}BrN_2O_2$ 237.1   *77-65-6*

Carbromal is (2-bromo-2-ethylbutyryl)urea. It contains not less than 98.0 per cent and not more than 101.0 per cent of $C_7H_{13}BrN_2O_2$.

Characteristics A white, crystalline powder; odourless or almost odourless.

Solubility Slightly soluble in *water*; soluble in 18 parts of *ethanol (96%)*, in 2 parts of *chloroform* and in 25 parts of *ether*.

Identification A. The *infra-red absorption spectrum*, Appendix II A, is concordant with the *reference spectrum* of carbromal.

B. Heat 0.2 g with 5 ml of 1M *sodium hydroxide*. Ammonia is evolved and the resulting solution yields the *reactions* characteristic of bromides, Appendix VI.

Clarity of solution A 20.0% w/v solution in *chloroform* is *clear*, Appendix IV A.

Melting point 117° to 120°, Appendix V A.

Halide ions Shake 0.70 g with 100 ml of *water* and filter. 5 ml of the filtrate complies with the *limit test for chlorides*, Appendix VII (0.14%).

Sulphate Shake 0.60 g with 100 ml of *water* and filter. 5 ml of the filtrate complies with the *limit test for sulphates*, Appendix VII (0.48%).

α-Ethylcrotonoylurea Carry out the method for *thin-layer chromatography*, Appendix III A, using *silica gel GF254* as the coating substance and a mixture of 75 volumes of *chloroform* and 25 volumes of *ether* as the mobile phase. Apply separately to the chromatoplate 10 μl of each of two solutions in *chloroform* containing (1) 2.0% w/v of the substance being examined and (2) 0.020% w/v of *α-ethylcrotonoylurea BPCRS*. After removal of the plate, allow it to dry in air and examine under *ultra-violet light (254 nm)*. Any spot corresponding to α-ethylcrotonoylurea in the chromatogram obtained with solution (1) is not more intense than the spot in the chromatogram obtained with solution (2).

Sulphated ash Not more than 0.1%, Appendix IX A.

Assay Dissolve 0.3 g in 20 ml of 2M *sodium hydroxide* and boil under a reflux condenser for 15 minutes. Cool, add 100 ml of *water* followed by 5 ml of *nitric acid* and boil for 5 minutes. Cool again, add 20 ml of 0.1M *silver nitrate VS*, shake vigorously and titrate with 0.1M *ammonium thiocyanate VS* using *ammonium iron(III) sulphate solution* as indicator. Each ml of 0.1M *silver nitrate VS* is equivalent to 0.02371 g of $C_7H_{13}BrN_2O_2$.

Action and use Hypnotic.

Cardamom Fruit

Cardamom Fruit consists of the dried, nearly ripe fruit of *Elettaria cardamomum* Maton var. *minuscula* Burkill.

Characteristics Odour and taste of the seeds, strongly aromatic.

Macroscopical Fruit: a trilocular inferior capsule, up to about 2 cm long, ovoid or oblong, dull green to pale buff, plump or slightly shrunken, obtusely triangular in cross-section, nearly smooth or longitudinally striated. Seeds in each loculus in two rows, forming an adherent mass attached to the axile placenta. Seed: pale to dark reddish-brown, about 4 mm long and 3 mm broad, irregularly angular, marked with six to eight transverse wrinkles, with a longitudinal channel containing the raphe, each seed enveloped by a colourless, membranous aril. Transversely cut surface of seed showing a brown testa, white starchy perisperm, grooved on one side, yellowish endosperm and a paler embryo.

Microscopical Seed: aril composed of flattened, thin-walled, parenchymatous cells. Testa composed of the following layers: (i) outer epidermis of thick-walled, narrow, axially elongated cells; (ii) a layer of collapsed parenchyma subjacent to the outer epidermis; (iii) a single layer (two or three layers near the raphe) of large, thin-walled, rectangular cells containing volatile oil; (iv) two or three layers of parenchyma; (v) layers of thin-walled, flattened cells; (vi) distinctive sclerenchymatous layer of closely-packed brown, thick-walled cells, each with a bowl-shaped cavity in the upper part containing a warty silica body; (vii) inner layer consisting of flattened cells. Perisperm: cells thin-walled, packed with numerous starch granules up to 6 μm in diameter and, in a small cavity, one to seven prisms of calcium oxalate about 10 to 30 μm long. Endosperm parenchymatous, thin-walled, with a granular hyaline mass of protein in each cell. Embryo: cells small, containing aleurone grains.

Acid-insoluble ash Of the seeds, not more than 3.5%, Appendix XI K.

Ash Of the seeds, not more than 6.0%, Appendix XI J.

Foreign matter Of the fruit, not more than 1.0%; of the separated seeds, not more than 3.0%, Appendix XI D.

Volatile oil In the seeds, not less than 4.0% v/w, Appendix XI, Method I. Use 20 g of the unground seeds and distil for 5 hours.

Action and use Flavour.

In making preparations of Cardamom, only the seed is used. The seed is removed from the fruit, immediately powdered or bruised and used immediately in making the preparation. Cardamom seed, after removal from the fruit, should not be stored.

Cardamom Oil

Cardamom Oil is obtained by distillation from crushed Cardamom Fruit.

Characteristics A clear, colourless or pale yellow liquid, visibly free from water; odour, that of Cardamom Fruit.

Optical rotation +20° to +40°, Appendix V F.

Refractive index 1.461 to 1.467, Appendix V E.

Solubility in ethanol Soluble, at 20°, in 6 volumes of *ethanol (70%)*, Appendix X M.

Weight per ml 0.917 to 0.940 g, Appendix V G.

Ester value 90 to 156, Appendix X C.

Storage Cardamom Oil should be kept in a well-filled, well-closed container, protected from light and stored at a temperature not exceeding 25°.

Preparations
Aromatic Cardamom Tincture
Compound Cardamom Tincture

Action and use Carminative and flavour.

Carmellose Sodium ☆

9004-32-4

Carmellose Sodium is the sodium salt of a partially-substituted poly(carboxymethyl) ether of cellulose. It contains not less than 6.5 per cent and not more than 10.8 per cent of sodium, Na, calculated with reference to the dried substance.

Characteristics A white or almost white, granular powder; odourless; hygroscopic after drying.

Solubility Practically insoluble in *absolute ethanol*, in *acetone*, in *ether* and in *toluene*. It is easily dispersed in *water* forming colloidal solutions.

Identification A. Sprinkle a quantity containing the equivalent of 1.0 g of the dried substance on to 90 ml of *carbon dioxide-free water* at 40° to 50°, stir vigorously until a colloidal solution is produced, cool and dilute to 100 ml with *carbon dioxide-free water* (solution A). To 10 ml of solution A add 1 ml of *copper sulphate solution*. A blue, cotton-like precipitate is produced.
B. Boil 5 ml of solution A for a few minutes. No precipitate is produced.
C. The solution obtained in the test for Heavy metals yields the *reactions* characteristic of sodium salts, Appendix VI.

Acidity or alkalinity pH of solution A, 6.0 to 8.0, Appendix V L.

Clarity and colour of solution Solution A is not more opalescent than *reference suspension III*, Appendix IV A, and not more intensely coloured than *reference solution Y$_6$*, Appendix IV B, Method II.

Apparent viscosity 75 to 140% of the declared value when determined by the following method. To 50 ml of *water* heated to 90° add, with stirring, a quantity containing the equivalent of 2 g of the dried substance or, for a product of low viscosity, use the quantity required to give the concentration on the label. Allow to cool, dilute to 100 ml with *water* and continue stirring until solution is complete. Determine the *viscosity*, Appendix V H, Method IV, at 20° using a shear rate of 10 s^{-1}. If necessary, use rates slightly below and slightly above 10 s^{-1} and interpolate.

Heavy metals To the residue obtained in the test for Sulphated ash add 1 ml of *hydrochloric acid*, evaporate to dryness on a water-bath and dissolve the residue in 20 ml of *water*. 12 ml of the resulting solution complies with *limit test A for heavy metals*, Appendix VII (20 ppm). Use *lead standard solution (1 ppm Pb)* to prepare the standard.

Chloride 2 ml of solution A diluted to 15 ml with *water* complies with the *limit test for chlorides*, Appendix VII (0.25%).

Sodium glycollate To a quantity containing the equivalent of 0.5 g of the dried substance add 5 ml of 5.4M *acetic acid* and 5 ml of *water* and stir until dissolution is complete (about 30 minutes). Add 80 ml of *acetone* and 2 g of *sodium chloride*, filter through a fast filter paper moistened with *acetone*, rinse the flask and filter paper with *acetone*, dilute to 100 ml with *acetone* and allow to stand for 24 hours without shaking. Place 2 ml of the clear supernatant liquid in a graduated flask, heat on a water-bath to remove the acetone, cool to room temperature, add 5 ml of *naphthalenediol reagent*, shake and add a further 15 ml of *naphthalenediol reagent*. Close

the flask with aluminium foil and heat on a water-bath for 20 minutes. Cool under running water, dilute to 25 ml with *sulphuric acid* and transfer 10 ml to a flat-bottomed tube within 10 minutes. When viewed vertically, the colour of the solution is not more intense than that of a standard solution prepared at the same time in the following manner. Dissolve 0.310 g of *glycollic acid*, previously dried over *phosphorus pentoxide* at a pressure of 1.5 to 2.5 kPa, in sufficient *water* to produce 1000 ml. To 5 ml of this solution add 5 ml of 5.4M *acetic acid*, allow to stand for 30 minutes, add 80 ml of *acetone* and 2 g of *sodium chloride* and dilute to 100 ml with *acetone*. Place 2 ml of the solution in a graduated flask and continue as described above beginning at the words 'heat on a water-bath to remove the acetone . . .' (0.4%).

Loss on drying When dried to constant weight at 100° to 105°, loses not more than 10.0% of its weight. Use 1 g.

Sulphated ash 20.0 to 33.3%, calculated with reference to the dried substance, Appendix IX A, Method II. Use 1 g and a mixture of equal volumes of *sulphuric acid* and *water*. The limits correspond to a content of 6.5 to 10.8% of Na.

Storage Carmellose Sodium should be kept in a well-closed container.

Labelling The label states (1) the apparent viscosity in millipascal seconds of a 2% w/v solution or, for a product of low viscosity, the concentration of the solution to be used and the apparent viscosity in millipascal seconds; (2) that the contents are not intended for use in the manufacture of a parenteral dosage form.

Action and use Pharmaceutical aid.

The title of the monograph in the European Pharmacopœia is Sodium Carboxymethylcellulose.

Carnauba Wax

Carnauba Wax is obtained from the leaves of *Copernicia cerifera* (Mart.) and purified to remove foreign matter.

Characteristics Light brown to pale yellow, moderately coarse powder, or flakes or irregular lumps of hard, brittle wax; odour, characteristic and free from rancidity.

Solubility Practically insoluble in *water*; slightly soluble in boiling *ethanol (96%)*; soluble in warm *chloroform* and in warm *toluene*.

Melting point 78° to 85°, Appendix V A, Method V.

Acid value Not more than 12.0, Appendix X B.

Iodine value 7 to 14 (*iodine monochloride method*), Appendix X E.

Saponification value 75 to 95, Appendix X G.

Storage Carnauba Wax should be kept in a well-closed container.

Action and use Pharmaceutical aid.

Cascara ☆

Cascara consists of the dried bark of *Rhamnus purshianus* DC [*Frangula purshiana* (DC) A Gray ex J C Cooper]. It contains not less than 8 per cent of hydroxyanthracene glycosides of which not less than 60 per cent consists of cascarosides, both calculated as cascaroside A.

Characteristics Odour, characteristic but not powerful.

Macroscopical Quilled, channelled or nearly flat pieces, 1 to 5 mm thick, varying greatly in length and width; sometimes broken into small, nearly flat, uniform fragments. Outer surface nearly smooth, cork dark purplish-brown with scattered lenticels and sometimes more or less completely covered by a whitish coat of lichen, epiphytic moss and foliaceous liverwort. Inner surface yellow to reddish-brown or almost black, with longitudinal striations and faint, transverse corrugations. Fracture short and granular in the outer part, somewhat fibrous in the inner part.

Microscopical Cork composed of a few layers of flattened thin-walled, prismatic cells containing yellowish-brown amorphous masses. Cortex, narrow and consisting of a few outer layers of collenchymatous cells and an inner parenchymatous region; cortex and, less frequently, phloem containing ovoid or irregular groups consisting of few to numerous sclereids. Phloem, wide and composed of tangential bands of sieve tissue, alternating with zones of parenchyma, each enclosing a band or smaller group of up to 30 phloem fibres, individual fibres about 8 to 15 μm wide. Medullary rays multiseriate. Parenchymatous sheaths surrounding the groups of sclereids and phloem fibres with prisms of calcium oxalate in many of the cells; numerous cells of the remaining parenchyma containing cluster crystals of calcium oxalate up to about 10 to 25 μm, rarely up to 45 μm, in diameter, others containing starch granules about 6 μm in diameter and yellow colouring matter, changed to dark red when treated with a 0.5% w/v solution of *sodium hydroxide*. In young bark, a persistent epidermis with mostly unicellular, conical trichomes up to 200 μm long.

Identification A. Heat 0.1 g, in powder, with 50 ml of *water* on a water-bath for 15 minutes, cool and filter. To 10 ml of the filtrate add 20 ml of 7M *hydrochloric acid* and heat on a water-bath for 15 minutes, cool, transfer to a separating funnel and extract with three 20-ml quantities of *ether*. Reserve the aqueous layer, combine the ether extracts and shake with 10 ml of 2M *ammonia*. The aqueous layer becomes reddish-purple (hydroxyanthracene O-glycosides).

B. Add 5 g of *iron(III) chloride hexahydrate* to the aqueous layer reserved in test A, heat on a water-bath for 30 minutes, cool, transfer to a separating funnel and extract with 15 ml of *chloroform*. Wash the chloroform layer with 10 ml of *water* and shake with 5 ml of 2M *ammonia*. The aqueous layer becomes red (hydroxyanthracene C-glycosides).

C. Carry out the method for *thin-layer chromatography*, Appendix III A, using *silica gel G* as the coating substance and a mixture of 100 volumes of *ethyl acetate*, 17 volumes of *methanol* and 13 volumes of *water* as the mobile phase, but allowing the solvent front to ascend 10 cm above the line of application. Apply separately to the chromatoplate 10 μl of each of the following solutions as bands 20 mm long and not more than 3 mm wide. For solution (1) heat to boiling 0.5 g, in *fine powder*, with 5 ml of *ethanol (70%)*, cool, centrifuge and immediately decant the supernatant liquid and use within 30 minutes. For solution (2) dissolve 20 mg of *barbaloin* in sufficient *ethanol (70%)* to produce 10 ml. After removal of the plate, allow the solvent to evaporate for 5 minutes and immediately spray with a freshly prepared 0.1% w/v solution of N,N-*dimethyl-p-nitrosoaniline* in *pyridine*, using

about 10 ml for a plate 200 mm × 200 mm in size, and examine without delay. No grey bands appear (anthrones). Then spray with a 5% w/v solution of *potassium hydroxide* in *ethanol (50%)*, heat for 15 minutes at 100° to 105° and examine the plate immediately.

In the chromatogram obtained with solution (2) a reddish-brown band is present with an Rf value of 0.4 to 0.5 (barbaloin). The chromatogram obtained with solution (1) shows several reddish-brown bands with different intensities, of which three faint bands are at about the mid-point of the chromatogram, one strong band in the upper third and one faint band in the lower third. Examine under *ultra-violet light (365 nm)*. The band corresponding to barbaloin exhibits an intense yellowish-brown fluorescence. In the chromatogram obtained with solution (1) several bands are visible with the same yellowish-brown fluorescence, situated above and, particularly, below that due to barbaloin (cascarosides). No bands exhibit a blue fluorescence (absence of other species of *Rhamnus*); no reddish-orange fluorescent band is present between the zones due to barbaloin and cascarosides (absence of *Rhamnus frangula*).

Foreign matter Not more than 1%, Appendix XI D.

Sulphated ash Not more than 6.0%, Appendix IX A, Method II. Use 1 g, in powder.

Assay Stir 1 g, in *No. 180 powder*, into 100 ml of boiling *water*, continue boiling and stirring for 5 minutes, cool, dilute to 100 ml with *water*, shake well and filter. Transfer 10 ml of the filtrate to a separating funnel, add 0.1 ml of 1M *hydrochloric acid* and shake with two 20-ml quantities of *carbon tetrachloride*. Wash the combined carbon tetrachloride layers with 5 ml of *water* and add the washings to the aqueous solution. Extract the aqueous solution with four 30-ml quantities of water-saturated ethyl acetate freshly prepared by shaking 150 ml of *ethyl acetate* with 15 ml of *water* for 3 minutes and allowing to separate. Use the combined ethyl acetate extracts for the determination of hydroxyanthracene glycosides other than cascarosides and the aqueous solution for the determination of cascarosides.

For hydroxyanthracene glycosides other than cascarosides Remove the solvent from the combined ethyl acetate extracts and evaporate almost to dryness, dissolve the residue in 0.3 to 0.5 ml of *methanol*, transfer to a flask with the aid of warm *water*, cool and add sufficient *water* to produce 50 ml. Add 20 ml of the solution to a mixture of 2 g of *iron(III) chloride hexahydrate* and 12 ml of *hydrochloric acid* and heat under a reflux condenser in a water-bath for 4 hours, maintaining the level of the water above that of the liquid in the flask. Allow to cool, transfer to a separating funnel and wash the flask successively with 3 to 4 ml of 1M *sodium hydroxide* and with 3 to 4 ml of *water*, adding the washings to the separating funnel. Extract with three 30-ml quantities of *carbon tetrachloride*, washing the combined carbon tetrachloride layers with two 10-ml quantities of *water*, discard the washings and add sufficient *carbon tetrachloride* to produce 100 ml. Evaporate 20 ml carefully to dryness on a water-bath, dissolve the residue in 10 ml of a 0.5% w/v solution of *magnesium acetate* in *methanol* and measure the *absorbance* at 515 nm and at 440 nm, Appendix II B, using *methanol* in the reference cell. Calculate the content of hydroxyanthracene glycosides other than cascarosides, as cascaroside A, from the absorbance at 515 nm taking 169 as the value of A(1%,

1 cm). The result of the assay is not valid unless the ratio of the *absorbance* at 515 nm to that at 440 nm is not less than 2.6.

For cascarosides To the aqueous layer reserved from the preliminary extraction add sufficient *water* to produce 50 ml and carry out the Assay for hydroxyanthracene glycosides other than cascarosides, beginning at the words 'Add 20 ml . . .'. Calculate the content of cascarosides, as cascaroside A, from the *absorbance* at 515 nm, Appendix II B, taking 169 as the value of A(1%, 1 cm). The result of the assay is not valid unless the ratio of the absorbance at 515 nm to that at 440 nm is not less than 2.7.

Storage Cascara should be kept in a well-closed container and protected from light.

Preparations

Cascara Dry Extract

Cascara Elixir

Action and use Stimulant laxative.

Powdered Cascara

Powdered Cascara is Cascara in powder. It contains not less than 8 per cent of hydroxy-anthracene glycosides of which not less than 60 per cent consists of carcarosides, both calculated as cascaroside A.

Characteristics Light yellowish-brown to brownish-green; odour, that of the unground drug. Diagnostic structures: bundles of slender lignified phloem fibres, accompanied by crystal sheaths containing prisms of calcium oxalate; groups of sclereids accompanied by crystal sheaths; cluster crystals of calcium oxalate. Cork cells and, occasionally, epiphytes, which may be liverworts, entire or in fragments, having a lamina one cell thick without a midrib and composed of isodiametric cells, or leaves of mosses, having a lamina one cell thick composed of elongated cells and possessing a midrib several cells thick. Some parenchymatous cells contain a yellow substance that is coloured deep red when treated with a 0.5% w/v solution of *sodium hydroxide*.

Identification Complies with the tests stated under Cascara.

Sulphated ash Not more than 6.0%, Appendix IX A, Method II. Use 1 g.

Assay Carry out the Assay described under Cascara.

Storage Powdered Cascara should be kept in a well-closed container and protected from light.

Action and use Stimulant laxative.

Castor Oil ☆

Castor Oil is the fixed oil obtained by cold expression from the seeds of *Ricinus communis* L.

Characteristics A clear, almost colourless or slightly yellow, viscid liquid; odour, very slight and characteristic; taste at first bland, but afterwards slightly acrid.

Solubility Soluble in 2.5 parts of *ethanol (96%)*; soluble in *chloroform* and in *ether*; slightly soluble in *petroleum spirit*;

miscible in all proportions with *absolute ethanol* and with *glacial acetic acid*.

Optical rotation +3.5° to +6.0°, Appendix V F.

Acid value Not more than 2.0, Appendix X B. Dissolve 5 g in 25 ml of the prescribed mixture of solvents.

Hydroxyl value Not less than 150, Appendix X D, Method II.

Iodine value 82 to 90 (*iodine bromide method*), Appendix X E.

Peroxide value Not more than 5.0, Appendix X F.

Refractive index 1.477 to 1.481, Appendix V E.

Relative density 0.952 to 0.965, Appendix V G.

Saponification value 176 to 187, Appendix X G, Method II.

Unsaponifiable matter Not more than 0.8% w/w, Appendix X H, Method II.

Foreign fatty substances A. A mixture of 2 ml of the oil and 8 ml of *ethanol (96%)* is *clear*, Appendix IV A. B. Shake 10.0 ml with 20.0 ml of *petroleum spirit (boiling range 60° to 80°)* and allow to separate. The volume of the lower layer is not less than 16.0 ml.

Light absorption *Absorbance* of a 1% w/v solution in *ethanol (96%)* at the maximum at 269 nm, not more than 1.0, Appendix II B.

Storage Castor Oil should be kept in a well-filled, well-closed container, protected from light and stored at a temperature not exceeding 15°. Castor Oil intended for use in the manufacture of a parenteral dosage form should be kept in a glass container.

Labelling The label states (1) the name and quantity of any added antioxidant; (2) if the contents of the container are suitable for use in the manufacture of a parenteral dosage form.

Preparation

Zinc and Castor Oil Ointment

Action and use Stimulant laxative; emollient.

Castor Oil intended for use in the manufacture of a parenteral dosage form does not contain any added antioxidant. It complies with the above requirements and with the following additional test for Water.

Water Not more than 0.3% w/w, Appendix IX C. Use 3 g.

Catechu

Pale Catechu

Catechu is a dried aqueous extract prepared from the leaves and young shoots of *Uncaria gambier* (Hunter) Roxb.

Characteristics Odourless or almost odourless.

Macroscopical Catechu usually occurs as cubes, which are sometimes more or less agglutinated and mixed with fragments of broken cubes; the cubes are friable and porous and measure about 2.5 cm in each direction; larger cubes and brick-shaped pieces, up to 4 cm long, also occur and are sometimes broken. Their colour is dull, pale greyish-brown to dark reddish-brown externally and pale brown internally.

Microscopical The diagnostic characters are: the abundant yellowish-brown masses of acicular catechin crystals, soluble in hot *water*; varying amounts of fragments from the leaves and flowering shoots of the plant including: unicellular covering trichomes, 250 to 540 μm long with lignified walls, pitted at the base, some with one or two thin transverse septa; fewer smaller trichomes, 25 to 45 μm long, conical, with warty, unlignified walls, epidermal cells of the leaves thin-walled with a finely striated cuticle and *paracytic* stomata on the lower epidermis only; reddish-brown corolla segments with numerous covering trichomes and characteristic pitted and lignified cicatrices in the epidermis; parenchymatous cells containing calcium oxalate as cluster crystals and crystal sand; subspherical pollen grains, 11 to 18 μm in diameter with three pores, three furrows and a minutely pitted exine; occasional fragments of cork.

Identification Warm 0.3 g with 2 ml of *ethanol (96%)*, cool and filter. Add 2 ml of 5M *sodium hydroxide* to the filtrate, shake, add 2 ml of *petroleum spirit (boiling range, 40° to 60°)*, shake and allow to separate. A brilliant greenish fluorescence is produced in the upper layer.

Matter insoluble in ethanol (96%) Not more than 34.0%, calculated with reference to the dried material, when determined by the following method. Macerate 5 g, in *coarse powder*, with 100 ml of *ethanol (96%)*, allow to stand for 6 hours shaking frequently and allow to stand for a further 18 hours. Filter, wash the residue with *ethanol (96%)* and dry to constant weight at 100°.

Starch The residue obtained in the test for Matter insoluble in ethanol (96%) contains not more than an occasional starch granule.

Water-insoluble matter Not more than 33.0%, calculated with reference to the dried material, when determined by the method for Matter insoluble in ethanol (96%), but using *water* in place of the *ethanol (96%)*.

Loss on drying When dried to constant weight at 105°, loses not more than 15.0% of its weight. Use 1 g.

Ash Not more than 8.0%, Appendix XI J.

Preparation
Catechu Tincture

Action and use Intestinal astringent.

Powdered Catechu

Powdered Catechu is Catechu in powder.

Characteristics Pale brown. Diagnostic structures: yellowish-brown acicular catechin crystals; unicellular covering trichomes, pitted at the base, some with one or two thin transverse septa; epidermal cells with a finely striated cuticle, *paracytic* stomata, characteristic pitted and lignified cicatrices; pollen grains; occasional fragments of cork.

Identification; Matter insoluble in ethanol (96%); Starch; Water-insoluble mater; Loss on drying Complies with the requirements stated under Catechu.

Action and use Intestinal astringent.

Cellacephate ☆

9004-38-0

Cellacephate is a cellulose, some of the hydroxyl groups of which are esterified by hydrogen phthaloyl groups and others by acetyl groups. It contains not less than 30.0 per cent and not more than 40.0 per cent of hydrogen phthaloyl groups and not less than 17.0 per cent and not more than 26.0 per cent of acetyl groups, both calculated with reference to the anhydrous substance.

Characteristics A white, free-flowing powder or colourless flakes; odourless, or with a faint odour of acetic acid; hygroscopic.

Solubility Practically insoluble in *water*, in *ethanol (96%)* and in chlorinated and non-chlorinated aliphatic hydrocarbons; freely soluble in *acetone*; soluble in *diethylene glycol* and in *1,4-dioxan*. It dissolves in dilute solutions of alkalis.

Identification A. Mix thoroughly 1 g with 2 g of finely powdered *manganese(II) sulphate* in a test-tube about 16 cm long. Impregnate a strip of filter paper with a freshly prepared mixture of 11 volumes of a 5% w/v solution of *sodium nitroprusside* and 1 volume of a 20% v/v solution of *diethanolamine*, adjusted to pH 9.8 with 1M *hydrochloric acid*. Insert the strip to a depth of 2 cm into the upper part of the tube, immerse the tube to a depth of 8 cm in a silicone oil-bath and heat at 190° to 200°. The filter paper does not become blue within 10 minutes. Carry out a blank test.
B. Without heating, completely dissolve 0.2 g in 15 ml of a 70% w/w solution of *sulphuric acid*, pour the solution, with stirring, into 100 ml of iced *water* and dilute to 250 ml with iced *water*. In a test-tube kept in ice, mix thoroughly 1 ml of the solution with 8 ml of *sulphuric acid*, added dropwise. Heat on a water-bath for exactly 3 minutes and cool immediately in ice. When the mixture is cool, add carefully 0.6 ml of a solution of 3 g of *ninhydrin* in 100 ml of a 4.55% w/v solution of *sodium metabisulphite*, mix well and allow to stand at 25°. A pink colour is produced immediately which does not become violet within 100 minutes.
C. Gently boil 0.5 g with 5 ml of 2M *sodium hydroxide* and 50 ml of *water* for 15 minutes, cool and filter. To the filtrate add 5 ml of 2M *hydrochloric acid*, evaporate the solution on a water-bath and dry the residue at 100° to 105°. To 0.1 g of the residue in a dry boiling-tube add 0.1 g of *resorcinol* and 3 ml of *sulphuric acid* and heat gently (below 180°) over a small flame until the liquid becomes dark brown. Cool, pour the mixture into 150 ml of *water* and make strongly alkaline by adding 20 ml of 10M *sodium hydroxide*. A yellow colour with an intense green fluorescence is produced.

Clarity and colour of solution Dissolve 15.0 g in 85 g of *acetone* with a water content of 0.35 to 0.45% w/w (solution A). Solution A is not more opalescent than *reference suspension III*, Appendix IV A, and not more intensely coloured than *reference solution Y₆*, Appendix IV B, Method II.

Appearance of a film Allow 1 ml of solution A to flow over a glass plate and dry. A thin, colourless, transparent and glossy film is produced.

Solubility of a film Immerse a glass tube (15 cm ×
1.5 cm) to a depth of not less than 3 cm in a mixture of
50 ml of solution A and 1.5 ml of *glycerol triacetate*, the
immersed end being covered by a piece of absorbent
gauze held in position by adhesive tape. Remove the tube,
fix in a vertical position and allow the mixture to drain.
Allow the resulting film to dry at 20° in an atmosphere
with a relative humidity not exceeding 60%. Carry out
this procedure twice more. Pour 2 ml of a 0.15% w/v
solution of *methylene blue* into the tube and immerse the
closed end of the tube in 0.1M *hydrochloric acid* to a depth
of 1 cm at 37° for 3 hours; the acid solution is not blue.
Remove the tube, rinse the outside with *water* and
immerse it in *citro-phosphate buffer pH 6.8* at 37° for 20
minutes; the buffer solution is blue.

Free acid Not more than 3.0%, calculated as phthalic
acid, $C_8H_6O_4$, with reference to the anhydrous substance.
Shake 1 g, in fine powder, for 5 minutes with 100 ml of
carbon dioxide-free water and filter. Wash the flask and the
filter with two 10-ml quantities of *carbon dioxide-free
water*. Titrate the combined filtrate and washings with
0.1M *sodium hydroxide VS*, using *dilute phenolphthalein
solution* as indicator, until a faint pink colour is obtained.
Repeat the operation without the substance being
examined. The difference between the titrations represents
the amount of sodium hydroxide required. Each ml of
0.1M *sodium hydroxide VS* is equivalent to 0.0083 g of
$C_8H_6O_4$.

Heavy metals 2.0 g complies with *limit test C for heavy
metals*, Appendix VII (10 ppm). Use 2 ml of *lead standard
solution (10 ppm)* to prepare the standard.

Sulphated ash Not more than 0.1%, Appendix IX A.

Water Not more than 5.0%, Appendix IX C. Use 0.5 g
dissolved in 20 ml of a mixture of equal volumes of
anhydrous methanol and *chloroform*.

Assay *For hydrogen phthaloyl groups* Without heating,
dissolve 0.4 g (x g, calculated with reference to the
anhydrous substance) in 20 ml of *2-methoxyethanol*
previously neutralised to 0.1 ml of *dilute phenolphthalein
solution*. Titrate with 0.1M *sodium hydroxide VS* until a
faint pink colour is obtained (b ml). Calculate the
percentage content of hydrogen phthaloyl groups, $C_8H_5O_3$,
from the expression

$$(1.49b/x) - 1.795S$$

where S is the percentage content of free acid.

For acetyl groups Heat 0.1 g (y g, calculated with
reference to the anhydrous substance) with 25 ml of 0.1M
sodium hydroxide VS under a reflux condenser on a water-
bath for 30 minutes. Cool and titrate with 0.1M
hydrochloric acid VS, using *dilute phenolphthalein solution* as
indicator, until the colour is discharged (d ml). Repeat the
operation without the substance being examined (c ml).
Calculate the percentage content of acetyl groups, C_2H_3O,
from the expression

$$[0.43(c - d)/y] - (0.578P + 0.518S)$$

where P is the percentage content of hydrogen phthaloyl
groups and S is the percentage content of free acid.

Storage Cellacephate should be kept in an airtight
container and stored at a temperature of 8° to 15°.

Action and use Pharmaceutical aid.

The title of the monograph in the European
Pharmacopœia is Cellulose Acetate Phthalate. In some
countries the material described in this monograph may
be known as Cellacefate.

Dispersible Cellulose

Dispersible Cellulose is a colloid-forming,
attrited mixture of Microcrystalline Cellulose
and Carmellose Sodium.

Content of carmellose sodium 75.0 to 125.0% w/w of the
stated amount.

Characteristics A white or off-white, coarse or fine
powder; odourless or almost odourless.

Solubility Disperses in *water* producing a white, opaque
dispersion or gel; practically insoluble in organic solvents
and in dilute acids.

Identification A. Mix 6 g with 300 ml of *water* stirring at
18,000 revolutions per minute for 5 minutes. A white,
opaque, bubble-free dispersion is obtained which does not
produce a supernatant liquid.
B. Add several drops of the dispersion obtained in test A
to a 10% w/v solution of *aluminium chloride hexahydrate*.
Each drop forms a white, opaque globule which does not
disperse on standing.
C. Add 2 ml of *iodine solution* to the dispersion obtained
in test A. No blue or purplish colour is produced.
D. The solution obtained in the test for Heavy metals
yields the *reactions* characteristic of sodium salts,
Appendix VI.

Acidity or alkalinity pH of the dispersion obtained in the
test for Apparent viscosity, 6.0 to 8.0, Appendix V L.

Clarity of solution Dissolve 50 mg in 10 ml of *copper
tetrammine hydroxide solution*. The solution is *clear*,
Appendix IV A.

Apparent viscosity 60 to 140% of the declared value when
determined by the following method. Calculate the
quantity (x g) needed to prepare exactly 600 g of a
dispersion of the stated percentage w/w, with reference to
the dried substance. To (600 − x) g of *water* at 23° to 25°
contained in a 1000-ml high-speed blender bowl add x g
of the substance being examined, stirring at reduced
speed, taking care to avoid contacting the sides of the
bowl with the powder. Continue stirring at low speed for
15 seconds after the addition and then stir at 18,000
revolutions per minute for exactly 2 minutes. Immerse the
appropriate spindle of a rotational viscometer, switch on
after 30 seconds and after a further 30 seconds determine
the *viscosity*, Appendix V H, Method IV, using a speed of
20 revolutions per minute (2.09 radians per second).

Heavy metals To the residue obtained in the test for
Sulphated ash add 1 ml of *hydrochloric acid*, evaporate to
dryness on a water-bath and dissolve the residue in 20 ml
of *water*. 12 ml of the resulting solution complies with
limit test A for heavy metals, Appendix VII (10 ppm). Use
lead standard solution (1 ppm Pb) to prepare the standard.

Loss on drying When dried to constant weight at 105°,
loses not more than 8.0% of its weight. Use 1 g.

Sulphated ash Not more than 5.0%, Appendix IX A. Use
2.0 g.

Assay Heat 2 g with 75 ml of *anhydrous glacial acetic acid*
under a reflux condenser for 2 hours, cool and carry out
Method I for *non-aqueous titration*, Appendix VIII A,
determining the end-point potentiometrically. Each ml of
0.1M *perchloric acid VS* is equivalent to 0.0296 g of
carmellose sodium.

Storage Dispersible Cellulose should be kept in a well-
closed container and stored at a temperature of 8° to 15°.

Labelling The label states (1) the percentage w/w of Carmellose Sodium; (2) the viscosity of a dispersion in water of a stated percentage w/w of Carmellose Sodium.

Action and use Pharmaceutical aid.

Microcrystalline Cellulose ☆

9004-34-6

Microcrystalline Cellulose is partially depolymerised cellulose and is prepared from alpha-cellulose. According to its use, it is defined by its particle size which ranges from 20 to 150 µm.

Characteristics A fine or granular, white or almost white powder; odourless.

Solubility Practically insoluble in *water*, in *absolute ethanol*, in *acetone* and in *toluene*.

Identification A. Place 10 mg on a watch-glass and disperse in 2 ml of *iodinated zinc chloride solution*. The powder becomes violet-blue.

B. Sieve 20 g for 5 minutes on an air-jet sieve equipped with a screen with a nominal mesh aperture of 38 µm. If more than 5% is retained on the screen, mix 30 g with 270 ml of *water*; otherwise, mix 45 g with 255 ml of *water*. Mix at 18,000 revolutions per minute for 5 minutes. Transfer 100 ml of the mixture to a 100-ml graduated cylinder and allow to stand for 3 hours. A white, opaque, bubble-free dispersion is obtained that does not produce a supernatant liquid.

Acidity or alkalinity Shake 2 g with 100 ml of *carbon dioxide-free water* for 5 minutes. The pH of the supernatant liquid is 5.0 to 7.5, Appendix V L.

Solubility in copper tetrammine hydroxide Dissolve 50 mg in 10 ml of *copper tetrammine hydroxide solution*. It dissolves completely without leaving any residue.

Ether-soluble substances Place 10 g in a column 20 mm in internal diameter. Pass 50 ml of *peroxide-free ether* through the column and evaporate the eluate to dryness. The residue weighs not more than 5 mg (0.05%).

Water-soluble substances Shake 5 g with 80 ml of *water* for 10 minutes, filter and evaporate the filtrate to dryness on a water-bath. The residue, after drying at 100° to 105° for 1 hour, weighs not more than 10 mg (0.2%).

Starch and dextrins Shake 0.1 g with 5 ml of *water* and add 0.2 ml of *iodine solution*. No blue or reddish-brown colour is produced.

Heavy metals 2.0 g complies with *limit test C for heavy metals*, Appendix VII (10 ppm). Use 2 ml of *lead standard solution (10 ppm Pb)* to prepare the standard.

Organic impurities Place 10 mg on a watch-glass and add 0.05 ml of a solution prepared immediately before use by dissolving 0.1 g of *phloroglucinol* in 5 ml of *hydrochloric acid*. No red colour is produced.

Loss on drying When dried at 100° to 105° for 5 hours, loses not more than 6.0% of its weight. Use 1 g.

Sulphated ash Not more than 0.1%, Appendix IX A, Method II. Use 1 g.

Action and use Pharmaceutical aid.

Powdered Cellulose ☆

$(C_6H_{10}O_5)_n$

Powdered Cellulose is a purified and mechanically powdered cellulose prepared from alpha-cellulose.

Characteristics A white or almost white, fine or granular powder; odourless.

Solubility Practically insoluble in *water*, in *absolute ethanol*, in *acetone*, in *toluene*, in dilute acids and in most organic solvents.

Identification A. Place 10 mg on a watch-glass and disperse in 2 ml of *iodinated zinc chloride solution*. The powder becomes violet-blue.

B. Mix 30 g with 270 ml of *water* at 18,000 revolutions per minute for 5 minutes. Transfer 100 ml of the mixture to a 100-ml graduated cylinder and allow to stand for 3 hours. A white, opaque, bubble-free dispersion with a supernatant liquid is produced.

Acidity or alkalinity Shake 2 g with 100 ml of *carbon dioxide-free water* for 5 minutes. The pH of the supernatant liquid is 5.0 to 7.5, Appendix V L.

Solubility in copper tetrammine hydroxide Dissolve 50 mg in 10 ml of *copper tetrammine hydroxide solution*. It dissolves completely without leaving any residue.

Ether-soluble substances Place 10 g in a column 20 mm in internal diameter. Pass 50 ml of *peroxide-free ether* through the column and evaporate the eluate to dryness. The residue weighs not more than 15 mg (0.15%).

Water-soluble substances Shake 5 g with 80 ml of *water* for 10 minutes, filter and evaporate the filtrate to dryness on a water-bath. The residue, after drying at 100° to 105° for 1 hour, weighs not more than 50 mg (1.0%).

Starch and dextrins Shake 0.1 g with 5 ml of *water* and add 0.2 ml of *iodine solution*. No blue or brownish-red colour is produced.

Heavy metals 2.0 g complies with *limit test C for heavy metals*, Appendix VII (10 ppm). Use 2 ml of *lead standard solution (10 ppm Pb)* to prepare the standard.

Organic impurities Place 10 mg on a watch-glass and add 0.05 ml of a solution prepared immediately before use by dissolving 0.1 g of *phloroglucinol* in 5 ml of *hydrochloric acid*. No red colour is produced.

Loss on drying When dried at 100° to 105° for 2 hours, loses not more than 6.0% of its weight. Use 1 g.

Sulphated ash Not more than 0.3%, Appendix IX A, Method II. Use 1 g.

Action and use Pharmaceutical aid.

The title of the monograph in the European Pharmacopœia is Cellulose Powder.

Cephalexin

$C_{16}H_{17}N_3O_4S,H_2O$ 365.4   23325-78-2

Cephalexin is 7-α-D-phenylglycylamino-3-methyl-3-cephem-4-carboxylic acid monohydrate. It contains not less than 95.0 per cent and not more than 103.0 per cent of $C_{16}H_{17}N_3O_4S$, calculated with reference to the anhydrous substance.

Characteristics A white to cream, crystalline powder; odour, characteristic.

Solubility Slightly soluble in *water*; practically insoluble in *ethanol (96%)*, in *chloroform* and in *ether*.

Identification A. The *infra-red absorption spectrum*, Appendix II A, is concordant with the *reference spectrum* of cephalexin.
B. In the test for Related substances, the principal spot in the chromatogram obtained with solution (2) corresponds to that in the chromatogram obtained with solution (4).
C. Mix 20 mg with 0.25 ml of a 1% v/v solution of *glacial acetic acid* and add 0.1 ml of a 1% w/v solution of *copper(II) sulphate* and 0.05 ml of 2M *sodium hydroxide*. An olive-green colour is produced.

Acidity pH of a 0.5% w/v solution, 3.5 to 5.5, Appendix V L.

Light absorption *Absorbance* of a 0.002% w/v solution at the maximum at 260 nm, 0.44 to 0.49, Appendix II B.

Specific optical rotation In a 0.5% w/v solution in *phthalate buffer pH 4.4*, +149° to +158°, Appendix V F.

Related substances Carry out the method for *thin-layer chromatography*, Appendix III A, using a silica gel G precoated chromatoplate (Analtech plates are suitable) and a mixture of 120 volumes of 0.1M *citric acid*, 80 volumes of 0.2M *disodium hydrogen orthophosphate* and 3 volumes of *acetone* as the mobile phase. Impregnate the plate by placing it in a tank containing a shallow layer of a 5% w/v solution of n-*tetradecane* in n-*hexane*, allowing the impregnating solvent to ascend to the top, removing the plate from the tank and allowing the solvent to evaporate; use with the flow of the mobile phase in the direction in which impregnation was carried out. Apply separately to the plate 2 μl of each of five freshly prepared solutions in 0.5M *hydrochloric acid* containing (1) 5.0% w/v of the substance being examined, (2) 0.2% w/v of the substance being examined, (3) 0.050% w/v of the substance being examined, (4) 0.2% w/v of *cephalexin BPCRS* and (5) 0.050% w/v of α-*phenylglycine BPCRS* and 0.050% w/v of 7-*aminodesacetoxycephalosporanic acid BPCRS*. After removal of the plate, heat it at 90° for 2 to 3 minutes and spray the hot plate with a 0.1% w/v solution of *ninhydrin* in the mobile phase. Heat at 90° for 15 minutes and allow to cool. In the chromatogram obtained with solution (1) any spots corresponding to α-phenylglycine and 7-amino-desacetoxycephalosporanic acid are not more intense than the spots in the chromatogram obtained with solution (5) and any other *secondary spot* in the chromatogram obtained with solution (1) is not more intense than the spot in the chromatogram obtained with solution (3).

Sulphated ash Not more than 0.2%, Appendix IX A.
Water 4.0 to 8.0% w/w, Appendix IX C. Use 0.3 g.

Assay Dissolve 0.1 g in sufficient *water* to produce 100 ml. Transfer 10 ml to a stoppered flask, add 5 ml of 1M *sodium hydroxide* and allow to stand for 20 minutes. Add 20 ml of a freshly prepared buffer solution containing 5.44% w/v of *sodium acetate* and 2.40% w/v of *glacial acetic acid*. Add 5 ml of 1M *hydrochloric acid* and 25 ml of 0.01M *iodine VS*, close the flask with a wet stopper and allow to stand for 20 minutes, protected from light. Titrate the excess of iodine with 0.02M *sodium thiosulphate VS* using *starch mucilage*, added towards the end of the titration, as indicator. To a further 10 ml of the solution add 20 ml of the buffer solution and 25 ml of 0.01M *iodine VS*, allow to stand for 20 minutes and titrate with 0.02M *sodium thiosulphate VS* using *starch mucilage*, added towards the end of the titration, as indicator. The difference between the titrations represents the amount of iodine equivalent to the cephalexin present.

Calculate the content of $C_{16}H_{17}N_3O_4S$ from the difference obtained by carrying out the assay at the same time using *cephalexin BPCRS* in place of the substance being examined and from the declared content of $C_{16}H_{17}N_3O_4S$ in *cephalexin BPCRS*.

Storage Cephalexin should be kept in a well-closed container, protected from light and stored at a temperature not exceeding 30°.

Labelling The label states (1) the date after which the material is not intended to be used; (2) the conditions under which it should be stored.

Preparations
Cephalexin Capsules
Cephalexin Oral Suspension
Cephalexin Tablets

Action and use Antibacterial.

Cephaloridine ☆

$C_{19}H_{17}N_3O_4S_2$ 415.5   50-59-9

Cephaloridine is (7R)-3-(1-pyridiniomethyl)-7-[(2-thienyl)acetamido]ceph-3-em-4-carboxylate (α-form or δ-form) and is derived from cephalosporin C produced by the growth of certain strains of various species of *Cephalosporium* in a suitable medium or obtained by other means. It contains not less than 96.0 per cent and not more than 102.0 per cent of $C_{19}H_{17}N_3O_4S_2$, calculated with reference to the anhydrous substance.

Characteristics A white or almost white, crystalline powder.

Solubility Soluble in *water*; slightly soluble in *ethanol (96%)*; practically insoluble in *chloroform* and in *ether*.

Identification A. The *infra-red absorption spectrum*, Appendix II A, is concordant with the spectrum of either *cefaloridine (α-form) EPCRS* or *cefaloridine (δ-form) EPCRS*.

B. To 20 mg add 0.25 ml of a mixture of 1 volume of *nitric acid*, 20 volumes of *water* and 80 volumes of *sulphuric acid*. A bluish-green colour is produced.

C. Yields the *reaction* characteristic of penicillins and cephalosporins, Appendix VI.

Acidity Dissolve 1 g in *carbon dioxide-free water* at 30°, cool to 20° and dilute to 10 ml with the same solvent. The pH of the resulting solution is 4.0 to 6.0, Appendix V L.

Light absorption Dissolve 12 mg in sufficient *water* to produce 100 ml. Dilute 10 ml to 100 ml with *water*. The *absorbance* of the resulting solution at the maximum at 240 nm is 0.43 to 0.48, Appendix II B. The ratio of the absorbance at the maximum at 240 nm to that at 255 nm is not more 1.10.

Specific optical rotation In a 1% w/v solution, +46° to +50°, Appendix V F.

Pyridine Dissolve 25 mg in 10 ml of *water* and add 2.5 ml of a solution prepared by adjusting a 5% w/v solution of *anhydrous disodium hydrogen orthophosphate* to pH 6.0 with *orthophosphoric acid* and adding 1% v/v of *aniline*. Add 1.25 ml of a solution prepared by decolorising a 0.5% v/v solution of *bromine* with *potassium cyanide solution*. Shake, allow to stand for 2 minutes, dilute to 25 ml with *water* and allow to stand for 25 minutes. Measure the *absorbance* of the resulting solution, Appendix II B, at the maximum at 462 nm, using in the reference cell a solution prepared in the same manner but omitting the substance being examined. The absorbance is not more than that of a solution prepared by treating in the same manner 2.5 ml of a 0.005% w/v solution of *pyridine* diluted to 10 ml with *water*, beginning at the words 'add 2.5 ml of a solution . . .'.

Related substances Carry out the method for *paper electrophoresis*, Appendix III F, using to fill the trough a buffer solution containing 188 volumes of *water*, 6 volumes of *acetone*, 5 volumes of *glacial acetic acid* and 1 volume of *anhydrous formic acid*. Elute the paper* with a mixture of 2 volumes of *acetone* and 1 volume of *water* for 16 hours, allow to dry and cut into strips, 230 mm × 170 mm.

Apply separately to the paper 5 μl of solution (1) containing 0.10% w/v of *cyanocobalamin*, 2 μl of solution (2) containing 0.10% w/v of *crystal violet*, 10 μl of solution (3) containing 0.20% w/v of *cefaloridine (δ-form) EPCRS*, 10 μl of solution (4) containing 20% w/v of the substance being examined, 10 μl of solution (5) containing 0.020% w/v of *cefaloridine (δ-form) EPCRS*, 5 μl of solution (1) and 2 μl of solution (2). Solutions (1) and (2) may be superimposed.

Allow electrophoresis to proceed protected from light until the crystal violet band has moved 6 cm from the line of application. Calculate the movement of the bands on the assumption that the cyanocobalamin spots indicate the true line of application. Any *secondary band* in the electrophoretogram obtained with solution (4) is not more intense than the principal band in the electrophoretogram obtained with solution (3). Any band in the electrophoretogram obtained with solution (4) that has moved between 1.2 and 1.6 times the distance moved by the principal band in the electrophoretogram obtained with solution (2) is not more intense than the principal band in the electrophoretogram obtained with solution (5). The test is not valid if the cyanocobalamin bands have moved more than 1.2 cm from the line of application. Spray the paper evenly on both sides with freshly prepared *iodoplatinate reagent* and apply the same criteria to the resulting bands.

Residual solvents Carry out the method for *gas chromatography*, Appendix III B, using solutions in *water* containing (1) 0.25% w/v of *butan-2-one* (internal standard) and 0.375% w/v of *dimethylformamide* (internal standard), (2) 25% w/v of the substance being examined, (3) 25% w/v of the substance being examined, 0.25% w/v of *butan-2-one* and 0.375% w/v of *dimethylformamide* and (4) 4.5% w/v of *pyridine*.

The chromatographic procedure may be carried out using a column (1.5 m × 5 mm) packed with *diatomaceous support* (100 to 120 mesh) coated with 10% w/w of *polyethylene glycol 1000* and maintained at 120° with an inlet port temperature of 230°. Continue the chromatography for five times the retention time of dimethylformamide (the retention time of dimethylformamide is about 9 minutes).

In the chromatogram obtained with solution (3) the height or area of the butan-2-one peak is greater than the sum of the heights or areas of any other peaks with a retention time less than that of pyridine and the height or area of the dimethylformamide peak is greater than the sum of the heights or areas of any other peaks with a retention time greater than that of pyridine.

Water Not more than 0.5% w/w for the α-form and not more than 3.0% w/w for the δ-form, Appendix IX C, Method I B. Use 0.25 g and, as the solvent, a mixture of equal volumes of *anhydrous methanol* and *anhydrous pyridine*.

Assay Dissolve 60 mg in sufficient *water* to produce 50 ml. Transfer 10 ml to a stoppered flask, add 5 ml of 1M *sodium hydroxide*, allow to stand for 20 minutes and add 20 ml of a buffer solution containing 35.0% w/v of *sodium acetate* and 42.4% v/v of *glacial acetic acid*. Add 5 ml of 1M *hydrochloric acid* and 25 ml of 0.01M *iodine VS*, close the flask with a wet stopper and allow to stand in a water-bath at 30° for 3 hours, protected from light. Titrate the excess of iodine with 0.02M *sodium thiosulphate VS* using 1 ml of *starch solution*, added towards the end of the titration, as indicator. To a further 10 ml of the solution add 20 ml of the buffer solution and 25 ml of 0.01M *iodine VS*, allow to stand in a water-bath at 30° for 3 hours protected from light and titrate with 0.02M *sodium thiosulphate VS* using 1 ml of *starch solution*, added towards the end of the titration, as indicator. The difference between the titrations represents the amount of iodine equivalent to the cephaloridine present. Calculate the content of $C_{19}H_{17}N_3O_4S_2$ from the difference obtained by carrying out the assay at the same time using *cefaloridine (δ-form) EPCRS* in place of the substance being examined and the declared content of $C_{19}H_{17}N_3O_4S_2$ in *cefaloridine (δ-form) EPCRS*.

Storage Cephaloridine should be kept in an airtight container, protected from light and stored at a temperature of 8° to 15°. If it is intended for use in the manufacture of a parenteral dosage form, the container should be sterile, tamper-evident and sealed so as to exclude micro-organisms.

Labelling The label states (1) whether the material is Cephaloridine (α-form) or Cephaloridine (δ-form); (2) the date after which it is not intended to be used; (3) the conditions under which it should be stored; (4) whether or not it is intended for use in the manufacture of a parenteral dosage form.

Preparation
Cephaloridine Injection

Action and use Antibacterial.

Cephaloridine intended for use in the manufacture of a parenteral dosage form complies with the following additional requirements.

Pyrogens Complies with the *test for pyrogens*, Appendix XIV K. Use per kg of the rabbit's weight 1 ml of a solution in *water for injections* containing 50 mg per ml.

Sterility Complies with the *test for sterility*, Appendix XVI A.

*A paper with a weight per unit area of 185 g m⁻², thickness of 0.33 mm and a capillary rise for water of 130 mm in 30 minutes can be used (Whatman 3MM is suitable).

Cephalothin Sodium

$C_{16}H_{15}N_2NaO_6S_2$ 418.4   *58-71-9*

Cephalothin Sodium is sodium 7-(2-thienyl-acetamido)cephalosporanate. It contains not less than 95.0 per cent and not more than 101.0 per cent of $C_{16}H_{15}N_2NaO_6S_2$, calculated with reference to the dried substance.

Characteristics A white or almost white, crystalline powder.

Solubility Soluble in 3.5 parts of *water*; slightly soluble in *ethanol (96%)*; practically insoluble in *chloroform* and in *ether*.

Identification A. The *infra-red absorption spectrum*, Appendix II A, is concordant with the *reference spectrum* of cephalothin sodium.
B. Mix 20 mg with 0.2 ml of *sulphuric acid (80%)* containing 1% v/v of *nitric acid*. An olive-green colour is produced which changes to reddish-brown.
C. Yields the *reactions* characteristic of sodium salts, Appendix VI.

Acidity or alkalinity pH of a 10% w/v solution, 4.5 to 7.0, Appendix V L.

Light absorption *Absorbance* of a 0.002% w/v solution at the maximum at 237 nm, 0.65 to 0.72, Appendix II B.

Specific optical rotation In a 5% w/v solution, +124° to +134°, Appendix V F.

Loss on drying When dried at 60° at a pressure not exceeding 0.7 kPa for 3 hours, loses not more than 1.5% of its weight. Use 1 g.

Assay Dissolve 0.2 g in sufficient *water* to produce 100 ml. Transfer 10 ml to a stoppered flask, add 5 ml of 1M *sodium hydroxide* and allow to stand for 20 minutes. Add 20 ml of a freshly prepared buffer solution containing 5.44% w/v of *sodium acetate* and 2.40% w/v of *glacial acetic acid*, 5 ml of 1M *hydrochloric acid* and 25 ml of 0.01M

iodine VS, close the flask with a wet stopper and allow to stand for 20 minutes, protected from light. Titrate the excess of iodine with 0.02M *sodium thiosulphate VS* using *starch mucilage*, added towards the end of the titration, as indicator. To a further 10 ml of the solution add 20 ml of the buffer solution and 25 ml of 0.01M *iodine VS*, allow to stand for 20 minutes and titrate with 0.02M *sodium thiosulphate VS* using *starch mucilage*, added towards the end of the titration, as indicator. The difference between the titrations represents the amount of iodine equivalent to the cephalothin present.

Calculate the content of $C_{16}H_{15}N_2NaO_6S_2$ from the difference obtained by carrying out the procedure at the same time using *cephalothin sodium BPCRS* in place of the substance being examined and using the declared content of $C_{16}H_{15}N_2NaO_6S_2$ in *cephalothin sodium BPCRS*.

Storage Cephalothin Sodium should be kept in a well-closed container and stored at a temperature not exceeding 25°. If it is intended for use in the manufacture of a parenteral dosage form, the container should be sterile and sealed so as to exclude micro-organisms.

Labelling The label states (1) the date after which the material is not intended to be used; (2) the conditions under which it should be stored; (3) whether or not it is intended for use in the manufacture of a parenteral dosage form.

Preparation
Cephalothin Injection

Action and use Antibacterial.

Cephalothin Sodium intended for use in the manufacture of a parenteral dosage form complies with the following additional requirements.

Pyrogens Complies with the *test for pyrogens*, Appendix XIV K. Use per kg of the rabbit's weight 1 ml of a solution in *water for injections* containing 50 mg per ml.

Sterility When intended for use in the manufacture of a parenteral dosage form without further sterilisation, complies with the *test for sterility*, Appendix XVI A.

Cephradine

$C_{16}H_{19}N_3O_4S$ 349.4   *38821-53-3*

Cephradine is 7-[α-D-(cyclohexa-1,4-dienyl)-glycylamino]-3-methyl-3-cephem-4-carboxylic acid. It contains not less than 95.0 per cent and not more than 100.5 per cent of $C_{16}H_{19}N_3O_4S$, calculated with reference to the anhydrous substance.

Characteristics A white to cream, crystalline powder.

Solubility Slightly soluble in *water*; insoluble in *ethanol (96%)*, in *chloroform* and in *ether*; soluble in 70 parts of *methanol*; freely soluble in *propane-1,2-diol*.

Identification A. The *infra-red absorption spectrum*, Appendix II A, is concordant with the *reference spectrum* of cephradine. If the spectra are not concordant, dissolve

30 mg in 10 ml of *methanol*, evaporate to dryness at 40° at a pressure of 2 kPa and prepare a new spectrum of the residue.

B. Carry out the method described under Related substances applying to the chromatoplate 5 µl of each of two solutions in 0.01M *ammonia* containing (1) 0.04% w/v of the substance being examined and (2) 0.04% w/v of *cephradine BPCRS*. The principal spot in the chromatogram obtained with solution (1) corresponds to that in the chromatogram obtained with solution (2).

Acidity pH of a 1% w/v solution, 3.5 to 6.0, Appendix V L.

Specific optical rotation Prepare an acetate buffer by dissolving 1.36 g of *sodium acetate* in 50 ml of *water*, adjusting to pH 4.6 with *glacial acetic acid* and adding sufficient *water* to produce 100 ml. The *specific optical rotation* in a 1% w/v solution in the acetate buffer is +80° to +90°, Appendix V F.

Related substances Carry out the method for *thin-layer chromatography*, Appendix III A, using a silica gel G precoated chromatoplate (Analtech plates are suitable) and a mixture of 120 volumes of 0.1M *citric acid*, 80 volumes of 0.2M *anhydrous disodium hydrogen orthophosphate* and 3 volumes of *acetone* as the mobile phase. Impregnate the plate by placing it in a tank containing a shallow layer of a 5% w/v solution of n-*tetradecane* in n-*hexane*, allowing the impregnating solvent to ascend to the top, removing the plate from the tank and allowing the solvent to evaporate; use with the flow of the mobile phase in the direction in which impregnation was carried out. Apply separately to the plate, as bands about 3 cm wide, 40 µl of each of three freshly prepared solutions in 0.01M *ammonia* containing (1) 0.40% w/v of the substance being examined, (2) 0.0020% w/v of the substance being examined and (3) 0.020% w/v of *cephalexin BPCRS*, 0.0040% w/v of *cyclohexa-1,4-dienylglycine BPCRS* and 0.0040% w/v of *7-aminodesacetoxycephalosporanic acid BPCRS*. After removal of the plate, heat it at 90° for 2 to 3 minutes and spray the hot plate with a 0.1% w/v solution of *ninhydrin* in the mobile phase. Heat at 90° for 15 minutes in a circulating air oven with the plates parallel to the airflow, cool for 15 minutes protected from light and examine in daylight. The bands in the chromatogram obtained with solution (3) are more intense than any corresponding bands in the chromatogram obtained with solution (1). Any other *secondary band* in the chromatogram obtained with solution (1) is not more intense than the band in the chromatogram obtained with solution (2).

Sulphated ash Not more than 0.2%, Appendix IX A.

Water Not more than 6.0%, Appendix IX C. Use 0.5 g.

Assay Dissolve 90 mg in sufficient *0.1M mixed phosphate buffer pH 7.0* to produce 100 ml and transfer 5 ml to a stoppered flask. Add 4 ml of *cephalosporinase solution*, close the flask with a wet stopper and gently swirl the contents to mix. Allow to stand for 30 minutes at 23° to 25°. Add 20 ml of *phthalate buffer pH 4.5* and 20 ml of *0.005M iodine VS*, close the flask with a wet stopper and allow to stand for 30 minutes protected from light. Titrate the excess of iodine with 0.01M *sodium thiosulphate VS* using *starch mucilage*, added towards the end of the titration, as indicator. To a further 5 ml of the solution add 4 ml of *0.1M mixed phosphate buffer pH 8.0*, close the flask with a wet stopper, gently swirl the contents to mix and repeat the procedure beginning at the words 'Allow to

stand for 30 minutes . . .'. The difference between the titrations represents the amount of iodine equivalent to the cephradine present. Calculate the content of $C_{16}H_{19}N_3O_4S$ from the difference obtained by carrying out the assay at the same time using *cephadrine BPCRS* in place of the substance being examined and from the declared content of $C_{16}H_{19}N_3O_4S$ in *cephradine BPCRS*.

Storage Cephradine should be kept in a well-closed container, protected from light and stored at a temperature not exceeding 30°.

Labelling The label states (1) the date after which the material is not intended to be used; (2) the conditions under which it should be stored.

Preparation
Cephradine Capsules

Action and use Antibacterial.

Cetomacrogol 1000

Cetomacrogol 1000 may be prepared by condensing cetyl or cetostearyl alcohol with ethylene oxide under controlled conditions. It is represented by the formula $CH_3 \cdot (CH_2)_m \cdot (O \cdot CH_2 \cdot CH_2)_n \cdot OH$, where *m* is 15 or 17 and *n* is 20 to 24.

Characteristics A cream-coloured, waxy, unctuous mass, pellets or flakes melting, when heated, to a clear brownish-yellow liquid; odourless or almost odourless.

Solubility Soluble in *water*, in *ethanol (96%)* and in *acetone*; insoluble in petroleum spirit.

Identification A. Dissolve 0.1 g in 5 ml of *water*, add 10 ml of 2M *hydrochloric acid*, 10 ml of *barium chloride solution* and 10 ml of a 10% w/v solution of *phosphomolybdic acid*. A greenish-yellow precipitate is produced.
B. Dissolve 0.1 g in 5 ml of *water* and add gradually a 10% w/v solution of *tannic acid*. The precipitate produced initially dissolves and is reprecipitated on further addition of the tannic acid solution.

Acid value Not more than 0.5, Appendix X B.

Alkalinity Dissolve 2 g in 20 ml of hot *water*. Not more than 0.5 ml of 0.1M *hydrochloric acid VS* is required for neutralisation using *phenolphthalein solution* as indicator.

Hydroxyl value 40.0 to 52.5, Appendix X D. Use 10 g.

Melting point Not lower than 38°, Appendix V A, Method IV, but allowing an air-pocket between the column of the substance and the lower end of the capillary tube.

Refractive index At 60°, 1.448 to 1.452, Appendix V E.

Saponification value Not more than 1.0, Appendix X G. Use 10 g.

Water Not more than 1.0% w/w, Appendix IX C. Use 2.5 g.

Preparation
Cetomacrogol Emulsifying Wax

Action and use Pharmaceutical aid.

Cetostearyl Alcohol

Cetostearyl Alcohol is a mixture of solid aliphatic alcohols consisting chiefly of stearyl and cetyl alcohols. It may be obtained by reduction of the appropriate fatty acids.

Characteristics A white or cream, unctuous mass or almost white flakes or granules; odour, faint and characteristic. When heated it melts to a clear, colourless or pale yellow liquid free from cloudiness or suspended matter.

Solubility Practically insoluble in *water*; soluble in *ether*; less soluble in *ethanol (96%)* and in *petroleum spirit (boiling range, 40° to 60°)*.

Acidity To 20 g add a mixture of 40 ml of *ether* and 75 ml of *ethanol (96%)* previously neutralised to *phenolphthalein solution* and warm gently until solution is effected. Titrate with 0.1M *sodium hydroxide VS*, using *phenolphthalein solution* as indicator, until a pink colour is produced which persists for at least 15 seconds. Not more than 1.0 ml of 0.1M *sodium hydroxide VS* is required.

Iodine value Not more than 3.0 (*iodine monochloride method*), Appendix X E.

Saponification value Not more than 2.0, Appendix X G. Use 20 g.

Solidifying point 45° to 53°, Appendix V B, with the following modifications. Place in the inner test-tube sufficient of the melted substance to fill the tube to a depth of 5 cm. Stir the substance gently and steadily, without scraping the wall of the tube, while the tube and its contents are allowed to cool. The temperature at which the level of the mercury in the thermometer remains stationary for a short time is regarded as the solidifying point.

Alcohols To 3.5 g add 12 g of *stearic anhydride* and 10 ml of *xylene* and heat gently under a reflux condenser for 30 minutes. Cool, add a mixture of 40 ml of *pyridine* and 4 ml of *water*, reflux for a further 30 minutes and titrate the hot solution with 1M *sodium hydroxide VS* using *phenolphthalein solution* as indicator. Repeat the operation without the substance being examined. The difference between the titrations is 12.8 ml to 14.2 ml.

Hydrocarbons Dissolve 2 g in 100 ml of *petroleum spirit (boiling range, 40° to 60°)*, warming slightly if necessary, and transfer the solution to a column (25 cm × 1 cm) of *anhydrous aluminium oxide* that has been slurried with *petroleum spirit (boiling range, 40° to 60°)*. Elute with two 50-ml quantities of *petroleum spirit (boiling range, 40° to 60°)*, filter into a flask, remove the petroleum spirit and dry at 80°. The residue weighs not more than 30 mg.

Cetrimide ☆

505-86-2

Cetrimide consists of trimethyltetradecyl-ammonium bromide and may contain smaller amounts of dodecyl- and hexadecyltrimethyl-ammonium bromides. It contains not less than 96.0 per cent and not more than 101.0 per cent of alkyltrimethylammonium bromides,

calculated as $C_{17}H_{38}BrN$ (336.4) with reference to the dried substance.

Characteristics A white or almost white, voluminous, free-flowing powder; odour, slight and characteristic.

Solubility Soluble in 2 parts of *water*; freely soluble in *ethanol (96%)* and in *chloroform*; practically insoluble in *ether*.

Identification A. Dissolve 0.25 g in sufficient *ethanol (96%)* to produce 25 ml. The *absorbance* of the solution, Appendix II B, in the range 260 to 280 nm is not more than 0.05.
B. Dissolve 5 mg in 5 ml of *phosphate buffer pH 8* and add a strip of *methyl green—iodomercurate paper*. After 5 minutes the greenish-blue colour of the solution is more intense than that of a solution prepared at the same time and in the same manner but omitting the substance being examined.
C. Yields *reaction A* characteristic of bromides, Appendix VI.
D. A 2.0% w/v solution in *carbon dioxide-free water* (solution A) foams strongly on shaking.

Acidity or alkalinity To 50 ml of solution A add 0.1 ml of *bromocresol purple solution*. Not more than 0.1 ml of either 0.1M *hydrochloric acid VS* or 0.1M *sodium hydroxide VS* is required to change the colour of the solution.

Clarity and colour of solution Solution A is *clear*, Appendix IV A, and *colourless*, Appendix IV B, Method II.

Non-quaternised amines Dissolve 5 g in 30 ml of a mixture of 99 volumes of *methanol* and 1 volume of 1M *hydrochloric acid* and add 100 ml of *propan-2-ol*. Pass a stream of *nitrogen* slowly through the solution and titrate potentiometrically with 0.1M *tetrabutylammonium hydroxide VS* until a total of 15.0 ml has been added. If two inflections are observed the volume of titrant added between the two points is not greater than 2.0 ml.

Loss on drying When dried at 100° to 105° for 2 hours, loses not more than 2.0% of its weight. Use 1 g.

Sulphated ash Not more than 0.5%, Appendix IX A, Method II. Use 1 g.

Assay Dissolve 2 g in sufficient *water* to produce 100 ml. Transfer 25 ml of the solution to a separating funnel, add 25 ml of *chloroform*, 10 ml of 0.1M *sodium hydroxide* and 10.0 ml of a freshly prepared 5.0% w/v solution of *potassium iodide*. Shake well, allow to separate and discard the chloroform layer. Wash the aqueous layer with three 10-ml quantities of *chloroform* and discard the washings. Add 40 ml of *hydrochloric acid*, cool and titrate with 0.05M *potassium iodate VS* until the deep brown colour is almost discharged. Add 2 ml of *chloroform* and continue the titration, with shaking, until the chloroform layer no longer changes colour. Carry out a blank titration on a mixture of 10.0 ml of the freshly prepared potassium iodide solution, 20 ml of *water* and 40 ml of *hydrochloric acid*. The difference between the titrations represents the amount of potassium iodate required. Each ml of 0.05M *potassium iodate VS* is equivalent to 0.03364 g of $C_{17}H_{38}BrN$.

Preparations
Cetrimide Cream
Cetrimide Emulsifying Ointment

Action and use Antiseptic detergent.

Strong Cetrimide Solution

Strong Cetrimide Solution is an aqueous solution of cetrimide. It contains 20 to 40 per cent w/v of cetrimide, calculated as $C_{17}H_{38}BrN$. It contains Ethanol (96 per cent) or Isopropyl Alcohol or both. It may be perfumed and may contain colouring matter.

In making Strong Cetrimide Solution, Ethanol (96 per cent) may be replaced by Industrial Methylated Spirit, provided that the law and the statutory regulations governing the use of Industrial Methylated Spirit are observed.

Content of cetrimide, $C_{17}H_{38}BrN$ 95.0 to 105.0% of the prescribed or stated amount.

Identification A. Dilute a volume of the solution containing 0.1 g of cetrimide to 5 ml with *water* and add 2 ml of a 5% w/v solution of *potassium hexacyanoferrate(III)*. A yellow precipitate is produced.
B. Shake together 5 ml of *water*, 1 ml of 2M *sulphuric acid*, 2 ml of *chloroform* and 0.05 ml of *methyl orange solution*; the chloroform layer is colourless. Add 0.1 ml of the solution being examined and shake; a yellow colour is produced slowly in the chloroform layer.
C. Yields the *reactions* characteristic of bromides, Appendix VI.

Acidity or alkalinity Dilute a volume of the solution containing 10 g of cetrimide to 100 ml and add 0.1 ml of *bromocresol purple solution*. Not more than 1.0 ml of either 0.1M *hydrochloric acid VS* or 0.1M *sodium hydroxide VS* is required to change the colour of the solution.

Miscibility with ethanol Mix a volume of the solution containing 1.6 g of cetrimide with a mixture of 2 ml of *water* and 16 ml of *ethanol (96%)*. The solution remains *clear*, Appendix IV A.

Neutral substances To a volume of the solution containing 10 g of cetrimide add 25 ml of *ethanol (50%)*. Acidify to *bromophenol blue solution* by the dropwise addition of *hydrochloric acid* and add 0.05 ml in excess. Transfer quantitatively to the extraction compartment of an apparatus designed for continuous liquid—liquid extraction by fluids of a lesser density than water, washing out the beaker with 10 ml of *ethanol (50%)* and adding the washings to the bulk of the solution in the extractor. Add sufficient *ethanol (50%)*, if necessary, to half-fill the extraction chamber to the level of the overflow limb. Add sufficient *purified hexane* to fill the extraction chamber, secure an overflow volume of about 30 ml in the ebullition flask and heat using an electrically heated mantle. Ensure that a continuous flow of hexane through the aqueous ethanol layer is observed and continue the extraction for 16 hours. Transfer the hexane extract to a separating funnel, washing out the flask with 10 ml of *purified hexane*. Shake the combined extract and washings with 25 ml of *ethanol (50%)* and discard the aqueous ethanol layer. Filter the hexane layer through a dry filter paper (Whatman No. 1 is suitable) into a tared flask and remove the solvent using a rotary evaporator at 40° and then at room temperature at a pressure not exceeding 0.7 kPa for 2 hours. The residue weighs not more than 0.4 g.

Non-quaternised amines To a volume of the solution containing 10 g of cetrimide add a mixture of 100 ml of *propan-2-ol*, 0.1 ml of *hydrochloric acid* and 20 ml of

methanol. Titrate with 0.1M *tetrabutylammonium hydroxide VS* passing a slow stream of *nitrogen* through the solution and determining the end-point potentiometrically using a platinum—glass electrode system. Inflections in the titration curve indicate (A) neutralisation of excess hydrochloric acid and (B) neutralisation of non-quaternised amine salts. The difference between the volumes corresponding to A and B is not more than 10 ml (2.4%, calculated as $C_{16}H_{35}N$).

Ethanol; Isopropyl alcohol Carry out one or both of the following methods according to the declared alcohol content of the solution being examined.
ETHANOL Not more than 10.0% v/v, by the method for the *determination of ethanol*, Appendix VIII F. Use on-column injection and do not heat the injection port.
ISOPROPYL ALCOHOL Not more than 10.0% v/v, by the method for the *determination of ethanol*, Appendix VIII F, with the following modifications. For solution (1) use a solution containing 5.0% v/v of *propan-2-ol* and 5.0% v/v of *propan-1-ol* (internal standard). For solution (2) use the solution being examined, diluted with *water*, if necessary, to contain about 5.0% v/v of isopropyl alcohol. Maintain the column temperature at 170°, use on-column injection and do not heat the injection port.

Assay Dilute a volume containing 4 g of cetrimide with sufficient *water* to produce 100 ml. Transfer 25 ml of the solution to a separating funnel and add 25 ml of *chloroform*, 10 ml of 0.1M *sodium hydroxide* and 10.0 ml of a freshly prepared 8.0% w/v solution of *potassium iodide*. Shake well, allow to separate and discard the chloroform layer. Wash the aqueous layer with three 10-ml quantities of *chloroform* and discard the washings. Add 40 ml of *hydrochloric acid*, cool and titrate with 0.05M *potassium iodate VS* until the deep brown colour is almost discharged. Add 2 ml of *chloroform* and continue the titration, with shaking, until the chloroform layer becomes colourless. Carry out a blank titration on a mixture of 10.0 ml of the freshly prepared 8.0% w/v potassium iodide solution, 20 ml of *water* and 40 ml of *hydrochloric acid*. The difference between the titrations represents the amount of potassium iodate required. Each ml of 0.05M *potassium iodate VS* is equivalent to 0.03364 g of $C_{17}H_{38}BrN$. Determine the *weight per ml* of the solution, Appendix V G, and calculate the percentage content of $C_{17}H_{38}BrN$, weight in volume.

Storage Strong Cetrimide Solution should be kept in a well-closed container and stored at a temperature above 15°.

Labelling The label states whether Ethanol, Isopropyl Alcohol or both are present and the percentage of cetrimide, weight in volume.

Preparation
Cetrimide Solution

Action and use Antiseptic detergent.

Cetyl Alcohol

36653-82-4

Cetyl Alcohol is a mixture of solid alcohols consisting mainly of hexadecan-1-ol, $C_{16}H_{34}O$.

Characteristics A white, unctuous mass, powder, flakes or granules; odour, slight.

Solubility Practically insoluble in *water*; freely to sparingly soluble in *ethanol (96%)*; freely soluble in *ether*. When melted it is miscible with *liquid paraffin*, with animal oils, with vegetable oils and with melted wool fat.

Identification A. *Hydroxyl value*, 218 to 238, Appendix X D, Method II.

B. *Melting point*, 46° to 52°, Appendix V A, Method I.

Acid value Not more than 1.0, Appendix X A.

Clarity and colour of solution Dissolve 0.5 g in boiling *ethanol (96%)*, cool and dilute to 20 ml with the same solvent. The resulting solution is *clear*, Appendix IV A, and not more intensely coloured than *reference solution B₆*, Appendix IV B, Method II.

Iodine value Not more than 2.0 (*iodine bromide method*), Appendix X E. Use 2 g dissolved in 25 ml of *chloroform*.

Saponification value Not more than 2.0, Appendix X G, Method II. Use 2 g.

Storage Cetyl Alcohol should be kept in a well-closed container.

Cetylpyridinium Chloride ☆

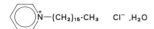

$C_{21}H_{38}ClN,H_2O$ 358.0   6004-24-6

Cetylpyridinium Chloride is 1-hexadecyl-pyridinium chloride monohydrate. It contains not less than 96.0 per cent and not more than 101.0 per cent of $C_{21}H_{38}ClN$, calculated with reference to the anhydrous substance.

Characteristics A white, unctuous powder.

Solubility Soluble in 20 parts of *water*, foaming strongly on shaking, in *ethanol (96%)* and in *chloroform*; very slightly soluble in *ether*.

Identification *Test A may be omitted if tests B, C and D are carried out. Tests B and C may be omitted if tests A and D are carried out.*
A. The *infra-red absorption spectrum*, Appendix II A, is concordant with the spectrum of *cetylpyridinium chloride EPCRS*.
B. Dissolve 0.1 g in sufficient *water* to produce 100 ml and dilute 5 ml to 100 ml with *water*. The *light absorption* of the resulting solution, Appendix II B, in the range 240 to 300 nm exhibits a maximum at 259 nm and two shoulders, at 254 nm and 265 nm. The A(1%, 1 cm) at the maximum is 126 to 134.
C. To 5 ml of 2M *sodium hydroxide* add 0.1 ml of *aqueous bromophenol blue solution* and 5 ml of *chloroform* and shake; the chloroform layer is colourless. Add 0.1 ml of a solution prepared by dissolving 1.0 g in sufficient *carbon dioxide-free water* to produce 100 ml (solution A) and shake; the chloroform layer becomes blue.
D. Solution A yields *reaction A* characteristic of chlorides, Appendix VI.

Acidity To 50 ml of solution A add 0.1 ml of *dilute phenolphthalein solution*. Not more than 2.5 ml of 0.02M *sodium hydroxide VS* is required to change the colour of the solution.

Clarity and colour of solution Solution A is not more opalescent than *reference suspension II*, Appendix IV A, and is *colourless*, Appendix IV B, Method II.

Non-quaternised amines Dissolve 5 g with heating in 20 ml of a mixture of 97 volumes of *methanol* and 3 volumes of 1M *hydrochloric acid* and add 100 ml of *propan-2-ol*. Pass a stream of *nitrogen* slowly through the solution and titrate potentiometrically with 0.1M *tetrabutyl-ammonium hydroxide VS* until a total of 12.0 ml has been added. If two inflections are observed the volume of titrant added between the two points is not greater than 5.0 ml. If no inflection is observed the substance being examined does not comply with the test. If only one inflection is observed repeat the procedure but add 3.0 ml of a 2.5% w/v solution of N,N-*dimethyltetradecylamine* in *propan-2-ol* before the titration. If the titration curve shows only one inflection after the addition of 12.0 ml of the titrant the substance being examined does not comply with the test.

Sulphated ash Not more than 0.2%, Appendix IX A, Method II. Use 1 g.

Water 4.5 to 5.5% w/w, Appendix IX C. Use 0.3 g.

Assay Dissolve 2 g in sufficient *water* to produce 100 ml. Transfer 25 ml to a separating funnel and add 25 ml of *chloroform*, 10 ml of 0.1M *sodium hydroxide* and 10.0 ml of a freshly prepared 5.0% w/v solution of *potassium iodide*. Shake well, allow to separate and discard the chloroform layer. Wash the aqueous layer with three 10-ml quantities of *chloroform* and discard the washings. Add 40 ml of *hydrochloric acid*, allow to cool and titrate with 0.05M *potassium iodate VS* until the deep brown colour is almost discharged. Add 2 ml of *chloroform* and continue the titration, shaking vigorously, until the chloroform layer no longer changes colour. Carry out a blank titration on a mixture of 10.0 ml of the freshly prepared potassium iodide solution, 20 ml of *water* and 40 ml of *hydrochloric acid*. The difference between the titrations represents the amount of potassium iodate required. Each ml of 0.05M *potassium iodate VS* is equivalent to 0.03400 g of $C_{21}H_{38}ClN$.

Action and use Antiseptic detergent.

Chalk

Prepared Chalk

$CaCO_3$ 100.1

Chalk is a native form of calcium carbonate freed from most of its impurities by elutriation and dried. It contains not less than 97.0 per cent and not more than 100.5 per cent of $CaCO_3$, calculated with reference to the dried substance.

Characteristics Odourless or almost odourless. It absorbs water readily.

Macroscopical White or greyish-white, small friable masses, usually conical in form, or in powder; amorphous; earthy; soft to the touch.

Microscopical Consists of the calcareous shells and detritus of various foraminifera; the calcareous shells vary from about 35 to 100 μm in breadth and from about 50 to 180 μm in length; among the detritus are numerous small rings and discs about 5 to 10 μm in diameter.

Solubility Practically insoluble in *water*; slightly soluble in *water* containing carbon dioxide.

Identification A. A solution in 6M *acetic acid* yields *reaction C* characteristic of calcium salts, Appendix VI. B. Yields *reaction A* characteristic of carbonates, Appendix VI.

Acidity or alkalinity 1 g, boiled with 50 ml of *water* and filtered, yields a filtrate which is neutral to *bromothymol blue solution* or requires not more than 0.05 ml of 0.1M *hydrochloric acid VS* to make it so.

Aluminium, iron, phosphate and matter insoluble in hydrochloric acid Dissolve 2 g in a mixture of 5 ml of *hydrochloric acid* and 75 ml of *water*, boil to remove carbon dioxide and make alkaline with 5M *ammonia* using *methyl red solution* as indicator. Boil for 1 minute, filter and wash the precipitate with a hot 2% w/v solution of *ammonium chloride*. Dissolve the precipitate as completely as possible by passing 20 ml of hot 2M *hydrochloric acid* through the filter and wash the filter with sufficient hot *water* to adjust the volume of the solution to 50 ml. Boil the solution and make alkaline with 5M *ammonia* using *methyl red solution* as indicator. Boil for 1 minute, filter through the same filter, wash the precipitate with a hot 2% w/v solution of *ammonium nitrate*, dry and ignite at a temperature not lower than 1000°. The residue weighs not more than 40 mg.

Arsenic Dissolve 0.5 g in 5 ml of *brominated hydrochloric acid* and dilute to 50 ml with *water*. 25 ml of the resulting solution complies with the *limit test for arsenic*, Appendix VII (4 ppm).

Heavy metals Dissolve 1.0 g in 10 ml of 2M *hydrochloric acid*, add 0.1 ml of *nitric acid* and boil to remove carbon dioxide. Cool, make alkaline with 5M *ammonia*, filter and wash the precipitate with *water*. Pass 5 ml of hot 2M *hydrochloric acid* through the filter, cool the filtrate, add 0.5 g of *ammonium thiocyanate* and extract with two successive 5-ml quantities of a mixture of equal volumes of *amyl alcohol* and *ether*. To the aqueous layer add 0.5 g of *citric acid* and dilute to 20 ml with *water*. 12 ml of the resulting solution complies with *limit test A for heavy metals*, Appendix VII (40 ppm). Use *lead standard solution (2 ppm Pb)* to prepare the standard.

Chloride Dissolve 0.3 g in 2 ml of *nitric acid* and 10 ml of *water*, filter and dilute the filtrate to 30 ml with *water*. 15 ml of the resulting solution complies with the *limit test for chlorides*, Appendix VII (330 ppm).

Sulphate Dissolve 0.25 g in 5.5 ml of 2M *hydrochloric acid*, dilute to 30 ml with *water* and filter. 15 ml of the resulting solution complies with the *limit test for sulphates*, Appendix VII (0.12%).

Loss on drying When dried to constant weight at 105°, loses not more than 1.0% of its weight. Use 1 g.

Assay To 2 g in 100 ml of *water* add 50 ml of 1M *hydrochloric acid VS*, boil to remove carbon dioxide, cool and titrate the excess of acid with 1M *sodium hydroxide VS* using *methyl orange solution* as indicator. Each ml of 1M *hydrochloric acid VS* is equivalent to 0.05004 g of $CaCO_3$.

Preparations
Paediatric Chalk Mixture
Aromatic Chalk with Opium Mixture

Action and use Antacid.

Chamomile Flowers ☆

Chamomile Flowers consist of the dried flower heads of the cultivated double variety of *Anthemis nobilis* L. (*Chamaemelum nobile* L.)

Characteristics Odour, strong, pleasant, characteristic; taste, bitter and aromatic. Flower heads white to yellowish-grey consisting of solitary, hemispherical capitula, 8 to 20 mm in diameter, each composed of a solid conical receptacle bearing florets each subtended by a transparent palea. Receptacle base surrounded by an involucre consisting of two or three rows of compact, imbricated bracts with scarious margins. Florets usually ligulate, white, dull, lanceolate and reflexed with a dark brown, inferior ovary, filiform style and bifid stigma; occasional pale yellow, tubular florets in the central region with a five-toothed corolla tube, five syngenesious, epipetalous stamens, gynoecium as in ligulate florets.

Identification Carry out the method for *thin-layer chromatography*, Appendix III A, using *silica gel G* as the coating substance and a mixture of 66 volumes of *butan-1-ol*, 17 volumes of *glacial acetic acid* and 17 volumes of *water* as the mobile phase, but allowing the solvent front to ascend 10 cm above the line of application. Apply separately to the chromatoplate, as bands 20 mm × 3 mm, 10 μl each of the following solutions. For solution (1) shake 0.5 g, in *No. 710 powder*, with 10 ml of *methanol* in a water-bath at 60° for 5 minutes, cool and filter. For solution (2) dissolve 1 mg of *caffeic acid* and 2.5 mg of *rutin* in 10 ml of *methanol* and use immediately. After removal of the plate, dry it at 80° to 100° for 5 minutes and spray with a 1% w/v solution of *diphenylboric acid—ethanolamine reagent* in *methanol*, using about 10 ml for a 200 mm × 200 mm plate. Spray the plate with the same volume of a 5% w/v solution of *polyethylene glycol 400* in *methanol*, allow to stand for 30 minutes and examine under *ultra-violet light (365 nm)*.

The chromatogram obtained with solution (2) shows a band with bright blue fluorescence in the upper part and a band with brownish-yellow fluorescence in the middle part due to caffeic acid and rutin respectively. In the chromatogram obtained with solution (1) the band with the highest Rf value shows a yellowish-green fluorescence (apigenin) and at a lower Rf value there is a faint band with bright blue fluorescence corresponding in position and fluorescence to the band due to caffeic acid in the chromatogram obtained with solution (2). At an Rf value slightly lower than the band corresponding to caffeic acid there is a band showing brownish fluorescence (ruteolin). There is also a band showing light brown fluorescence with an Rf value slightly higher than that of rutin in the chromatogram obtained with solution (2) (apiin). At Rf values slightly higher and lower than the apiin band are bands with yellowish fluorescence (apigenin-7-glucoside) and strong, bright blue fluorescence, respectively. There is also a band with bright blue fluorescence with an Rf value lower than that of rutin and other faint bands showing bluish fluorescence may be present.

Small or blemished flowers Not more than 3% of flower heads with a diameter of less than 8 mm; brown or darkened flower heads absent.

Sulphated ash Not more than 12.0%, Appendix IX A, Method II. Use 1 g.

Volatile oil Not less than 0.7% v/w, Appendix XI E. Use a 500-ml round-bottomed flask, 250 ml of *water* as the distillation liquid and 0.50 ml of *xylene* in the graduated tube. Use 20 g and distil at a rate of 3 to 3.5 ml per minute for 3 hours.

Water Not more than 10.0%, Appendix IX C, Method II. Use 20 g.

Storage Chamomile Flowers should be kept in a well-closed container and protected from light.

The title of the monograph in the European Pharmacopœia is Roman Chamomile Flower.

Activated Charcoal ☆
Decolorising Charcoal

16291-96-6

Activated Charcoal* is obtained from vegetable matter by suitable carbonisation processes intended to confer a high adsorbing power.

Characteristics A light, black powder, free from grittiness; odourless.

Solubility Practically insoluble in all usual solvents.

Identification A. When heated to redness, burns slowly without flame.

B. Complies with the test for Adsorbing power.

Acidity or alkalinity Boil 2.0 g in 40 ml of *water* for 5 minutes. Cool, restore to the original weight with *carbon dioxide-free water* and filter, discarding the first 20 ml of filtrate. To 10 ml of the filtrate add 0.25 ml of *bromothymol blue solution* and 0.25 ml of 0.02M *sodium hydroxide VS*. The solution is blue and not more than 0.75 ml of 0.02M *hydrochloric acid VS* is required to change the colour to yellow.

Acid-soluble substances To 1 g add 25 ml of 2M *nitric acid* and boil for 5 minutes. Filter whilst hot through a sintered-glass filter (BS porosity No. 4) and wash with 10 ml of hot *water*. Evaporate the combined filtrate and washings on a water-bath, add to the residue 1 ml of *hydrochloric acid* and evaporate again. The residue after drying to constant weight at 100° to 105°, weighs not more than 30 mg.

Alkali-soluble coloured matter To 0.25 g add 10 ml of 2M *sodium hydroxide*, boil for 1 minute, cool and filter. The filtrate, when diluted to 10 ml with *water*, is not more intensely coloured than *reference solution GY₄*, Appendix IV B, Method II.

Ethanol-soluble substances To 2 g add 50 ml of *ethanol (96%)* and boil under a reflux condenser for 10 minutes. Filter immediately, cool and adjust the volume to 50 ml with *ethanol (96%)*. The filtrate is not more intensely coloured than *reference solution BY₆* or *Y₆*, Appendix IV B, Method II. Evaporate 40 ml of the filtrate to dryness. The residue, after drying to constant weight at 100° to 105°, weighs not more than 8 mg (0.5%).

Fluorescent substances Extract 10 g with 100 ml of *cyclohexane FT* for 2 hours using a Soxhlet apparatus. Adjust the volume of the extract to 100 ml and examine under ultra-violet light (365 nm). The fluorescence of the solution is not more intense than that of a solution containing 83 μg of *quinine* in 1000 ml of 0.005M *sulphuric acid*.

Copper Not more than 25 ppm of Cu when determined by *atomic absorption spectrophotometry*, Appendix II D, measuring at 325 nm using an air—acetylene flame and a solution prepared in the following manner. Boil 2 g of the substance being examined with 50 ml of 2M *hydrochloric acid* under a reflux condenser for 1 hour. Filter, wash the filtrate with 2M *hydrochloric acid* and evaporate the combined filtrate and washings to dryness in a water-bath. Dissolve the residue in sufficient 0.1M *hydrochloric acid* to produce 50 ml (solution A). Use *copper solution ASp*, suitably diluted with 0.1M *hydrochloric acid*, for the standard solution.

Lead Not more than 10 ppm of Pb when determined by *atomic absorption spectrophotometry*, Appendix II D, measuring at 283.3 nm or 217 nm and using an air—acetylene flame. Use solution A as the test solution and *lead standard solution ASp*, suitably diluted with 0.1M *hydrochloric acid*, for the standard solution.

Zinc Not more than 25 ppm of Zn when determined by *atomic absorption spectrophotometry*, Appendix II D, measuring at 214 nm and using an air—acetylene flame. Use solution A as the test solution and *zinc standard solution ASp*, suitably diluted with 0.1M *hydrochloric acid*, for the standard solution.

Sulphide To 1.0 g add 20 ml of *water* and 5 ml of 7M *hydrochloric acid* and heat to boiling. The fumes evolved do not turn *lead acetate paper* brown.

Loss on drying When heated at 120° for 4 hours, loses not more than 15% of its weight. Use 1 g.

Sulphated ash Not more than 5.0%, Appendix IX A, Method II. Use 1 g.

Adsorbing power Not less than 40% of its own weight of *phenazone*, calculated with reference to the dried substance, when determined by the following method. To 0.3 g add 25 ml of a freshly prepared 1% w/v solution of *phenazone*, shake thoroughly for 15 minutes, filter and discard the first 5 ml of filtrate. To 10 ml of the filtrate add 1.0 g of *potassium bromide* and 20 ml of 2M *hydrochloric acid* and titrate with 0.0167M *potassium bromate VS*, using 0.1 ml of *ethoxychrysoidine hydrochloride solution* as indicator, until the colour changes from reddish-pink to yellowish-pink, and titrating at the rate of 0.05 ml every 15 seconds towards the end of the titration (*b* ml). Repeat the titration using 10 ml of the phenazone solution and beginning at the words 'add 1.0 g . . .' (*a* ml). Calculate the percentage of phenazone adsorbed with reference to the dried substance using the expression $2.353(a - b)/w$ where w is the weight, in g, of the substance being examined.

Storage Activated Charcoal should be kept in an airtight container.

Action and use Adsorbent.

*In certain states party to the Convention on the Elaboration of a European Pharmacopœia, Activated Charcoal may be required to comply with a limit for a total viable aerobic count of 10^2 micro-organisms per gram, determined by plate count, Appendix XVI B2.

Chloral Hydrate ☆

CCl₃·CH(OH)₂

$C_2H_3Cl_3O_2$ 165.4   *302-17-0*

Chloral Hydrate is 2,2,2-trichloroethane-1,1-diol. It contains not less than 98.5 per cent and not more than 101.0 per cent of $C_2H_3Cl_3O_2$.

Characteristics Colourless, transparent crystals; odour, pungent.

Solubility Soluble in 0.3 part of *water*, in 0.2 part of *ethanol (96%)* and in 3 parts of *chloroform*; freely soluble in *ether*.

Identification A. To 10 ml of a 10.0% w/v solution in *carbon dioxide-free water* (solution A) add 2 ml of *2M sodium hydroxide*. The mixture becomes cloudy and when heated evolves an odour of chloroform.
B. To 1 ml of solution A add 2 ml of *sodium sulphide solution*. A yellow colour is produced which quickly becomes reddish-brown. On standing, a red precipitate may be produced.

Acidity pH of solution A, 3.5 to 5.5, Appendix V L.

Clarity and colour of solution Solution A is *clear*, Appendix IV A, and *colourless*, Appendix IV B, Method I.

Chloral alcoholate Dissolve 1.0 g in 10 ml of *2M sodium hydroxide* with gentle heating, filter the upper layer and add 0.05M *iodine* dropwise until a yellow colour is obtained. No precipitate is produced within 1 hour.

Heavy metals 7.5 ml of solution A diluted to 15 ml with *water* complies with *limit test A for heavy metals*, Appendix VII (20 ppm). Use *lead standard solution (1 ppm Pb)* to prepare the standard.

Chloride 5 ml of solution A diluted to 15 ml with *water* complies with the *limit test for chlorides*, Appendix VII (100 ppm).

Non-volatile residue Evaporate 2 g on a water-bath. The residue weighs not more than 2 mg (0.1%).

Assay Dissolve 4 g in 10 ml of *water* and add 40 ml of 1M *sodium hydroxide VS*. Allow to stand for exactly 2 minutes and titrate with 0.5M *sulphuric acid VS* using *dilute phenolphthalein solution* as indicator. Titrate the neutralised solution with 0.1M *silver nitrate VS* using 0.2 ml of *potassium chromate solution* as indicator. Calculate the number of ml of 1M sodium hydroxide used in the reaction by adding to the volume of 0.5M sulphuric acid used in the first titration two-fifteenths of the volume of 0.1M silver nitrate used in the second titration and subtracting the figure so obtained from the volume of 1M sodium hydroxide added. Each ml of 1M *sodium hydroxide VS* is equivalent to 0.1654 g of $C_2H_3Cl_3O_2$.

Storage Chloral Hydrate should be kept in an airtight container.

Preparations
Chloral Mixture
Paediatric Chloral Elixir

Action and use Hypnotic.

Chlorambucil ☆

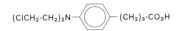
(ClCH₂·CH₂)₂N—⟨○⟩—(CH₂)₃·CO₂H

$C_{14}H_{19}Cl_2NO_2$ 304.2   *305-03-3*

Chlorambucil is 4-[4-bis(2-chloroethyl)amino-phenyl]butyric acid. It contains not less than 98.5 per cent and not more than 101.0 per cent of $C_{14}H_{19}Cl_2NO_2$, calculated with reference to the anhydrous substance.

Characteristics A white, crystalline powder.

Solubility Practically insoluble in *water*; soluble in 1.5 parts of *ethanol (96%)*, in 2 parts of *acetone* and in 2.5 parts of *chloroform*.

Identification *Test A may be omitted if tests B, C and D are carried out. Tests B and C may be omitted if tests A and D are carried out.*
A. The *infra-red absorption spectrum*, Appendix II A, is concordant with the spectrum of *chlorambucil EPCRS*.
B. Mix 0.4 g with 10 ml of *2M hydrochloric acid* and allow to stand for 30 minutes, shaking occasionally. Filter, wash the residue with two 10-ml quantities of *water* and add 0.5 ml of *potassium mercuri-iodide solution* to 10 ml of the mixed filtrate and washings; a buff precipitate is produced. To a further 10 ml add 0.5 ml of *potassium permanganate solution*; the purple colour is immediately discharged.
C. Dissolve 50 mg in 5 ml of *acetone* and dilute to 10 ml with *water*. Add 0.05 ml of *2M nitric acid* and 0.2 ml of *dilute silver nitrate solution*; no opalescence is produced immediately. Heat on a water-bath; an opalescence is produced.
D. *Melting point*, 64° to 67°, Appendix V A, Method I.

Related substances Carry out the method for *thin-layer chromatography*, Appendix III A, using *silica gel GF254* as the coating substance and a mixture of 40 volumes of *toluene*, 25 volumes of *methanol*, 20 volumes of *butan-2-one* and 20 volumes of n-*heptane* as the mobile phase, but allowing the solvent front to ascend 10 cm above the line of application. Apply separately to the chromatoplate 5 μl of each of three solutions of the substance being examined in *acetone* containing (1) 2.0% w/v, (2) 0.040% w/v and (3) 0.010% w/v. After removal of the plate, allow it to dry in air and examine under *ultra-violet light (254 nm)*. Any *secondary spot* in the chromatogram obtained with solution (1) is not more intense than the spot in the chromatogram obtained with solution (2) and not more than one such spot is more intense than the spot in the chromatogram obtained with solution (3).

Sulphated ash Not more than 0.1%, Appendix IX A, Method II. Use 1 g.

Water Not more than 0.5% w/w, Appendix IX C. Use 1 g.

Assay Dissolve 0.2 g in 10 ml of *acetone*, add 10 ml of *water* and titrate with 0.1M *sodium hydroxide VS* using *dilute phenolphthalein solution* as indicator. Each ml of 0.1M *sodium hydroxide VS* is equivalent to 0.03042 g of $C_{14}H_{19}Cl_2NO_2$.

Storage Chlorambucil should be kept in a well-closed container and protected from light.

Preparation
Chlorambucil Tablets

Action and use Cytotoxic.

Chloramine ☆

Chloramine T

$C_7H_7ClNNaO_2S,3H_2O$ 281.7   *127-65-1*

Chloramine is sodium *N*-chlorotoluene-*p*-sulphonimidate trihydrate. It contains not less than 98.0 per cent and not more than 103.0 per cent of $C_7H_7ClNNaO_2S,3H_2O$.

Characteristics A white or slightly yellow, crystalline powder.

Solubility Freely soluble in *water*; soluble in *ethanol (96%)*; practically insoluble in *chloroform* and in *ether*.

Identification A. A 5.0% w/v solution in *carbon dioxide-free water* (solution A) first turns *litmus paper* blue and then bleaches it.
B. To 10 ml of solution A add 10 ml of *hydrogen peroxide solution (10 vol)*; a white precipitate is produced which dissolves on heating. Filter the hot solution and allow to cool; white crystals are produced. The *melting point* of the crystals, after washing with *water* and drying at 100° to 105°, is 137° to 140°, Appendix V A, Method I.
C. Cautiously ignite 1 g and dissolve the residue in 10 ml of *water*. The solution yields *reaction B* characteristic of sodium salts, *reaction A* characteristic of chlorides and *reaction A* characteristic of sulphates, Appendix VI.

Alkalinity pH of solution A, 8.0 to 10.0, Appendix V L.

Clarity and colour of solution Solution A is not more opalescent than *reference suspension II*, Appendix IV A, and is *colourless*, Appendix IV B, Method II.

Ethanol-insoluble matter Shake 1 g for 30 minutes with 20 ml of *ethanol (96%)* and filter on a tared filter. Any residue, when washed with 5 ml of *ethanol (96%)* and dried at 100° to 105°, weighs not more than 20 mg (2.0%).

Ortho compound To 2 g add 10 ml of *water*, mix, add 1 g of *sodium metabisulphite* and heat to boiling. Cool to 0°, filter rapidly and wash with three 5-ml quantities of iced *water*. The *melting point* of the precipitate, after drying over *phosphorus pentoxide* at a pressure not exceeding 0.6 kPa, is not less than 134°, Appendix V A, Method I.

Assay Dissolve 0.125 g in 100 ml of *water* in a stoppered flask. Add 1 g of *potassium iodide* and 5 ml of 1M *sulphuric acid*, allow to stand for 3 minutes and titrate the liberated iodine with 0.1M *sodium thiosulphate VS* using 1 ml of *starch solution* as indicator. Each ml of 0.1M *sodium thiosulphate VS* is equivalent to 0.01408 g of $C_7H_7ClNNaO_2S,3H_2O$.

Storage Chloramine should be kept in an airtight container, protected from light and stored at a temperature of 8° to 15°.

Action and use Antiseptic; disinfectant.

Chloramphenicol ☆

$C_{11}H_{12}Cl_2N_2O_5$ 323.1   *56-75-7*

Chloramphenicol is 2,2-dichloro-*N*-[($\alpha R,\beta R$)-β-hydroxy-α-hydroxymethyl-4-nitrophenethyl]-acetamide. It is produced by the growth of certain strains of *Streptomyces venezuelae* in a suitable medium, but is normally prepared by synthesis. It contains not less than 98.0 per cent and not more than 102.0 per cent of $C_{11}H_{12}Cl_2N_2O_5$, calculated with reference to the dried substance.

Characteristics A white to greyish-white or yellowish-white, fine crystalline powder or fine crystals, needles or elongated plates. A solution in *ethyl acetate* is laevo-rotatory; a solution in *absolute ethanol* is dextrorotatory.

Solubility Slightly soluble in *water* and in *ether*; soluble in 2.5 parts of *ethanol (96%)* and in 7 parts of *propane-1,2-diol*.

Identification *Test A may be omitted if tests B, C, D and E are carried out. Tests B, C and D may be omitted if tests A and E are carried out.*
A. The *infra-red absorption spectrum*, Appendix II A, is concordant with the spectrum of *chloramphenicol EPCRS*.
B. In the test for Related substances the principal spot in the chromatogram obtained with 1 µl of solution (1) is similar in position and size to the spot in the chromatogram obtained with solution (2).
C. Dissolve 10 mg in 1 ml of *ethanol (50%)*, add 3 ml of a 1% w/v solution of *calcium chloride* and 50 mg of *zinc powder* and heat on a water-bath for 10 minutes. Filter the hot solution, allow the filtrate to cool, add 0.1 ml of *benzoyl chloride* and shake for 1 minute. Add 0.5 ml of a 10.5% w/v solution of *iron(III) chloride hexahydrate* and 2 ml of *chloroform* and shake. The aqueous layer is light violet-red to purple.
D. To 50 mg in a porcelain crucible add 0.5 g of *anhydrous sodium carbonate*, heat over an open flame for 10 minutes and allow to cool. Extract the residue with 5 ml of 2M *nitric acid*, filter and to 1 ml of the filtrate add 1 ml of *water*. The solution yields *reaction A* characteristic of chlorides, Appendix VI.
E. *Melting point*, 149° to 153°, Appendix V A, Method I.

Acidity or alkalinity Shake 0.1 g with 20 ml of *carbon dioxide-free water* and add 0.1 ml of *bromothymol blue solution*. Not more than 0.1 ml of either 0.02M *hydrochloric acid VS* or 0.02M *sodium hydroxide VS* is required to change the colour of the solution.

Specific optical rotation In a 6% w/v solution in *absolute ethanol*, +18.5° to +20.5°, Appendix V F.

Chloride Shake 0.25 g with 50 ml of *water*, filter and to 20 ml of the filtrate add 1 ml of 2M *nitric acid* and 0.3 ml of *silver nitrate solution*. Any opalescence produced is not more intense than that produced in a mixture of 20 ml of the filtrate, 1 ml of 2M *nitric acid* and 0.3 ml of *water*.

Related substances Carry out the method for *thin-layer chromatography*, Appendix III A, using *silica gel GF254* as the coating substance and a mixture of 90 volumes of *chloroform*, 10 volumes of *methanol* and 1 volume of *water* as the mobile phase. Apply separately to the chromato-plate 1 μl and 20 μl of solution (1), 1 μl of solution (2) and 20 μl of solution (3). Solution (1) contains 1% w/v of the substance being examined in *acetone*. Solution (2) contains 1% w/v of *chloramphenicol EPCRS* in *acetone*. For solution (3) dilute 0.5 ml of solution (2) to 100 ml with *acetone*. After removal of the plate, allow it to dry in air and examine under *ultra-violet light (254 nm)*. Any *secondary spot* in the chromatogram obtained with 20 μl of solution (1) is not more intense than the spot in the chromatogram obtained with solution (3).

Loss on drying When dried to constant weight at 100° to 105°, loses not more than 0.5% of its weight. Use 1 g.

Sulphated ash Not more than 0.1%, Appendix IX A, Method II. Use 2 g.

Assay Dissolve 0.1 g in sufficient *water* to produce 500 ml. Dilute 10 ml to 100 ml with *water* and measure the *absorbance* of the resulting solution at the maximum at 278 nm, Appendix II B. Calculate the content of $C_{11}H_{12}Cl_2N_2O_5$ taking 297 as the value of A(1%, 1 cm) at the maximum at 278 nm.

Storage Chloramphenicol should be protected from light. If the material is intended for use in the manufacture of a parenteral dosage form the container should be sterile and sealed so as to exclude micro-organisms.

Labelling The label states (1) the date after which the material is not intended to be used; (2) the conditions under which it should be stored; (3) whether or not it is intended for use in the manufacture of a parenteral dosage form.

Preparations
Chloramphenicol Capsules
Chloramphenicol Ear Drops
Chloramphenicol Eye Drops
Chloramphenicol Eye Ointment

Action and use Antibacterial.

Chloramphenicol intended for use in the manufacture of a parenteral dosage form complies with the following additional requirements.

Abnormal toxicity Complies with the *test for abnormal toxicity*, Appendix XIV L. Use 0.5 ml of a solution containing 2 mg per ml.

Pyrogens Complies with the *test for pyrogens*, Appendix XIV K. Use per kg of the rabbit's weight 2.5 ml of a solution in *water for injections* containing 2 mg per ml.

Sterility Complies with the *test for sterility*, Appendix XVI A.

Chloramphenicol Palmitate ☆

$O_2N \!-\! \langle \text{ring} \rangle \!-\! \overset{\overset{HO}{|}}{\underset{\underset{H}{|}}{C}} \!-\! \overset{\overset{H}{|}}{\underset{\underset{NH\cdot CO\cdot CHCl_2}{|}}{C}} \!-\! CH_2\cdot OCO\cdot(CH_2)_{14}\cdot CH_3$

$C_{27}H_{42}Cl_2N_2O_6$ 561.6   *530-43-8*

Chloramphenicol Palmitate is (2*R*,3*R*)-2-(2,2-dichloroacetamido)-3-hydroxy-3-(4-nitro-phenyl)propyl palmitate. It contains not less than 98.0 per cent and not more than 102.0 per cent of $C_{27}H_{42}Cl_2N_2O_6$, calculated with reference to the dried substance.

Characteristics A fine, white or almost white, unctuous powder. It melts at 87° to 95°. It is polymorphic and the thermodynamically stable form has low bioavailability following oral administration.

Solubility Practically insoluble in *water*; soluble in 45 parts of *ethanol (96%)*, in 6 parts of *chloroform* and in 14 parts of *ether*; freely soluble in *acetone*; very slightly soluble in *hexane*.

Identification A. Carry out the method for *thin-layer chromatography*, Appendix III A, using *silanised silica gel H* as the coating substance and a mixture of 70 volumes of *ethanol (96%)* and 30 volumes of a 10% w/v solution of *ammonium acetate* as the mobile phase. Apply separately to the chromatoplate 4 μl of each of the following solutions. For solution (1) dissolve 50 mg of the substance being examined in a mixture of 1 ml of 1M *sodium hydroxide* and 5 ml of *acetone*, allow to stand for 30 minutes and add 1.1 ml of 1M *hydrochloric acid* and 3 ml of *acetone*. Solution (2) contains 0.2% w/v of *chloramphenicol EPCRS* in *acetone*. Solution (3) contains 0.2% w/v of *palmitic acid* in *acetone*. Solution (4) contains 0.2% w/v of the substance being examined in *acetone*. After removal of the plate, allow it to dry in air and spray with a solution containing 0.02% w/v of *2,7-dichlorofluorescein* and 0.01% w/v of *rhodamine B* in *ethanol (96%)*. Allow the plate to dry in air and examine under *ultra-violet light (254 nm)*. The chromatogram obtained with solution (1) shows three spots corresponding in position to the principal spots in the chromatograms obtained with solutions (2), (3) and (4).

B. Dissolve 0.2 g in 2 ml of *pyridine*, add 2 ml of a 10% w/v solution of *potassium hydroxide* and heat on a water-bath. A red colour is produced.

C. Dissolve 10 mg in 5 ml of *ethanol (96%)*, add 4.5 ml of 1M *sulphuric acid* and 50 mg of *zinc powder* and allow to stand for 10 minutes. Decant the supernatant liquid or filter if necessary. Cool the resulting solution in ice and add 0.5 ml of *sodium nitrite solution*. Allow to stand for 2 minutes and add 1 g of *urea* followed by 1 ml of *2-naphthol solution* and 2 ml of 10M *sodium hydroxide*. A red colour is produced.

Acidity Dissolve 1 g by warming to 35° with 5 ml of a mixture of equal volumes of *ethanol (96%)* and *ether* and add 0.2 ml of *phenolphthalein solution*. Not more than 0.4 ml of 0.1M *sodium hydroxide VS* is required to produce a pink colour that persists for 30 seconds.

Specific optical rotation In a 5% w/v solution in *absolute ethanol*, +22.5° to +25.5°, Appendix V F.

Free chloramphenicol Not more than 450 ppm when determined by the following method. Dissolve 1.0 g in 80 ml of *xylene* with the aid of gentle heat, cool and extract with three 15-ml quantities of *water*. Discard the xylene and dilute the combined aqueous extracts to 50 ml with *water*. Shake the solution with 10 ml of *carbon tetrachloride*, allow to separate, discard the carbon tetrachloride and centrifuge a portion of the aqueous solution. Measure the *absorbance* of the clear supernatant liquid, Appendix II B, at the maximum at 278 nm, using in the reference cell a solution obtained by repeating the procedure without the substance being examined. The *absorbance* of the reference solution must be not more than 0.05. Calculate the content of free chloramphenicol taking 298 as the value of A(1%, 1 cm) at the maximum at 278 nm.

Related substances Carry out the method for *thin-layer chromatography*, Appendix III A, using *silica gel GF254* as the coating substance and a mixture of 50 volumes of *cyclohexane*, 40 volumes of *chloroform* and 10 volumes of *methanol* as the mobile phase. Apply separately to the chromatoplate 10 µl of each of four solutions in *acetone* containing (1) 1.0% w/v of the substance being examined, (2) 0.020% w/v of *chloramphenicol palmitate isomer EPCRS*, (3) 0.020% w/v of *chloramphenicol dipalmitate EPCRS* and (4) 0.0050% w/v of *chloramphenicol EPCRS*. After removal of the plate, allow it to dry in air and examine under *ultra-violet light (254 nm)*. In the chromatogram obtained with solution (1) any spots corresponding to chloramphenicol palmitate isomer and chloramphenicol dipalmitate are not more intense than the spots in the chromatograms obtained with solutions (2) and (3) respectively and any other *secondary spot* is not more intense than the spot in the chromatogram obtained with solution (4).

Loss on drying When dried over *phosphorus pentoxide* at 80° at a pressure not exceeding 0.1 kPa for 3 hours, loses not more than 0.5% of its weight. Use 1 g.

Sulphated ash Not more than 0.1%, Appendix IX A, Method II. Use 1 g.

Assay Dissolve 90 mg in sufficient *ethanol (96%)* to produce 100 ml. Dilute 10 ml of this solution to 250 ml with *ethanol (96%)* and measure the *absorbance* at the maximum at 271 nm, Appendix II B. Calculate the content of $C_{27}H_{42}Cl_2N_2O_6$ taking 178 as the value of A(1%, 1 cm) at the maximum at 271 nm.

Storage Chloramphenicol Palmitate should be protected from light.

Labelling The label states (1) the date after which the material is not intended to be used; (2) the conditions under which it should be stored.

Preparation
Chloramphenicol Oral Suspension

Action and use Antibacterial.

Chloramphenicol Sodium Succinate

O_2N—⟨benzene ring⟩—$\overset{\overset{HO}{|}}{\underset{\underset{H}{|}}{C}}$—$\overset{\overset{H}{|}}{\underset{\underset{NH \cdot CO \cdot CHCl_2}{|}}{C}}$—$CH_2 \cdot OCO \cdot CH_2 \cdot CH_2 \cdot CO_2Na$

$C_{15}H_{15}Cl_2N_2NaO_8$ 445.2   *982-57-0*

Chloramphenicol Sodium Succinate is sodium (2R,3R)-2-(2,2-dichloroacetamido)-3-hydroxy-3-(4-nitrophenyl)propyl succinate. It contains not less than 98.0 per cent and not more than 102.0 per cent of $C_{15}H_{15}Cl_2N_2NaO_8$, calculated with reference to the anhydrous substance.

Characteristics A white or yellowish-white powder; hygroscopic.

Solubility Soluble in less than 1 part of *water* and in 1 part of *ethanol (96%)*; practically insoluble in *chloroform* and in *ether*.

Identification A. The *light absorption*, Appendix II B, in the range 230 to 350 nm of a 0.004% w/v solution exhibits a maximum only at 276 nm. The *absorbance* at 276 nm is about 0.86.

B. Dissolve 10 mg in 2 ml of *ethanol (50%)*, add 4.5 ml of 1M *sulphuric acid* and 50 mg of *zinc powder*, allow to stand for 10 minutes and decant the supernatant liquid or filter if necessary. Cool the resulting solution in ice and add 0.5 ml of *sodium nitrite solution* and, after 2 minutes, 1 g of *urea* followed by 1 ml of *2-naphthol solution* and 2 ml of 10M *sodium hydroxide*; a red colour is produced. Repeat the test omitting the *zinc powder*; no red colour is produced.

C. To 5 ml of a 0.1% w/v solution add 0.2 ml of 0.1M *silver nitrate*; no precipitate is produced. Heat 50 mg with 2 ml of *ethanolic potassium hydroxide solution* on a water-bath for 15 minutes, add 15 mg of *decolorising charcoal*, shake and filter. The filtrate, when treated with 0.1M *silver nitrate*, yields a curdy precipitate which is insoluble in *nitric acid* but soluble, after being well washed with *water*, in 5M *ammonia* from which it is reprecipitated on the addition of *nitric acid*.

D. Yields the *reactions* characteristic of sodium salts, Appendix VI.

Acidity or alkalinity pH of a 25% w/v solution, 6.0 to 7.0, Appendix V L.

Specific optical rotation In a 5% w/v solution, +5.0° to +8.0°, Appendix V F.

Chloramphenicol Carry out the method for *thin-layer chromatography*, Appendix III A, using *silica gel GF254* as the coating substance and a mixture of 90 volumes of *chloroform*, 10 volumes of *methanol* and 1 volume of *water* as the mobile phase. Apply separately to the chromatoplate 10 µl of each of two solutions in *acetone* containing (1) 1.0% w/v of the substance being examined and (2) 0.020% w/v of *chloramphenicol EPCRS*. After removal of the plate, allow it to dry in air and examine under *ultra-violet light (254 nm)*. Any spot corresponding to chloramphenicol in the chromatogram obtained with solution (1) is not more intense than the spot in the chromatogram obtained with solution (2).

Water Not more than 2.0% w/w, Appendix IX C. Use 1.25 g.

Assay Dissolve 0.2 g in *water* and add sufficient *water* to produce 500 ml. Dilute 5 ml to 100 ml with *water* and measure the *absorbance* of the resulting solution at the maximum at 276 nm, Appendix II B. Calculate the content of $C_{15}H_{15}Cl_2N_2NaO_8$ taking 216 as the value of A(1%, 1 cm) at the maximum at 276 nm.

Storage Chloramphenicol Sodium Succinate should be kept in an airtight container and protected from light. If it is intended for use in the manufacture of a parenteral dosage form, the container should be sterile and sealed so as to exclude micro-organisms.

Labelling The label states (1) the date after which the material is not intended to be used; (2) the conditions under which it should be stored; (3) whether or not it is intended for use in the manufacture of a parenteral dosage form.

Preparation
Chloramphenicol Sodium Succinate Injection

Action and use Antibacterial.

Chloramphenicol Sodium Succinate intended for use in the manufacture of a parenteral dosage form complies with the following additional requirements.

Pyrogens Complies with the *test for pyrogens*, Appendix XIV K. Use, per kg of the rabbit's weight 2 ml of a solution in *water for injections* containing the equivalent of 2.5 mg of chloramphenicol per ml.

Sterility When intended for use in the manufacture of a parenteral dosage form without further sterilisation, complies with the *test for sterility*, Appendix XVI A.

Chlorbutol ☆

$CCl_3 \cdot CMe_2OH, \frac{1}{2}H_2O$

$C_4H_7Cl_3O, \frac{1}{2}H_2O$ 186.5   *6001-64-5*

Chlorbutol is 1,1,1-trichloro-2-methylpropan-2-ol hemihydrate. It contains not less than 98.0 per cent and not more than 101.0 per cent of $C_4H_7Cl_3O$, calculated with reference to the anhydrous substance.

Characteristics A white crystalline powder or colourless crystals; sublimes readily. It melts at about 78°, determined without previous drying.

Solubility Slightly soluble in *water*; soluble in 0.6 part of *ethanol (96%)*; freely soluble in *chloroform*; very soluble in *ether*; soluble in *glycerol (85%)*.

Identification A. Heat 20 mg with 2 ml of 10M *sodium hydroxide* and 1 ml of *pyridine* on a water-bath and shake. The separated pyridine layer becomes red.
B. Warm 20 mg with 5 ml of *ammoniacal silver nitrate solution*. A black precipitate is produced.
C. Shake 20 mg with 3 ml of 1M *sodium hydroxide* until dissolved, add 5 ml of *water* and then, slowly, 2 ml of *iodine solution*. The odour of iodoform is detectable and a yellowish precipitate is produced.
D. Complies with the test for Water.

Acidity To 4 ml of a 50.0% w/v solution in *ethanol (96%)* (solution A) add 15 ml of *ethanol (96%)* and 0.1 ml of *bromothymol blue solution*. Not more than 0.1 ml of 0.1M *sodium hydroxide VS* is required to change the colour of the solution.

Clarity and colour of solution Solution A is not more opalescent than *reference suspension II*, Appendix IV A, and not more intensely coloured than *reference solution BY₅*, Appendix IV B, Method II.

Chloride To 1 ml of solution A add 4 ml of *ethanol (96%)* and dilute to 15 ml with *water*. The resulting solution complies with the *limit test for chlorides*, Appendix VII (100 ppm). Use 5 ml of *ethanol (96%)* in place of the 5 ml of water to prepare the standard.

Sulphated ash Not more than 0.1%, Appendix IX A, Method II. Use 1 g.

Water 4.5 to 5.5%, Appendix IX C. Use 0.3 g.

Assay Dissolve 0.1 g in 20 ml of *ethanol (96%)*, add 10 ml of 2M *sodium hydroxide* and heat on a water-bath for 5 minutes. Cool, add 20 ml of 2M *nitric acid* and 25 ml of 0.1M *silver nitrate VS*, shake vigorously with 2 ml of *dibutyl phthalate*, add 2 ml of a 10% w/v solution of *ammonium iron(III) sulphate* and titrate the excess of silver nitrate with 0.1M *ammonium thiocyanate VS*. Each ml of 0.1M *silver nitrate VS* is equivalent to 0.00592 g of $C_4H_7Cl_3O$.

Storage Chlorbutol should be kept in an airtight container and stored at a temperature of 8° to 15°.

Action and use Antimicrobial preservative.

The title of the monograph in the European Pharmacopœia is Chlorobutanol Hemihydrate.

Anhydrous Chlorbutol ☆

$C_4H_7Cl_3O$ 177.5   *57-15-8*

Anhydrous Chlorbutol is 1,1,1-trichloro-2-methylpropan-2-ol. It contains not less than 98.0 per cent and not more than 101.0 per cent of $C_4H_7Cl_3O$, calculated with reference to the anhydrous substance.

Characteristics A white crystalline powder or colourless crystals; sublimes readily. It melts at about 95°, determined without previous drying.

Solubility Slightly soluble in *water*; soluble in 0.6 part of *ethanol (96%)*; freely soluble in *chloroform*; very soluble in *ether*; soluble in *glycerol (85%)*.

Identification Complies with tests A, B and C for Identification described under Chlorbutol.
D. Complies with the test for Water.

Acidity; Clarity and colour of solution; Sulphated ash Complies with the tests described under Chlorbutol.

Chloride Dissolve 0.17 g in 5 ml of *ethanol (96%)* and dilute to 15 ml with *water*. The resulting solution complies with the *limit test for chlorides*, Appendix VII (300 ppm). Use 5 ml of *ethanol (96%)* in place of the 5 ml of water to prepare the standard.

Water Not more than 1.0% w/w, Appendix IX C. Use 2 g.

Assay Carry out the Assay described under Chlorbutol. Each ml of 0.1M *silver nitrate VS* is equivalent to 0.00592 g of $C_4H_7Cl_3O$.

Storage Anhydrous Chlorbutol should be kept in an airtight container and stored at a temperature of 8° to 15°.

Action and use Antimicrobial preservative.

The title of the monograph in the European Pharmacopœia is Anhydrous Chlorobutanol.

Chlorcyclizine Hydrochloride

$C_{18}H_{21}ClN_2, HCl$ 337.3   *1620-21-9*

Chlorcyclizine Hydrochloride is 1-(4-chloro-benzhydryl)-4-methylpiperazine hydrochloride. It contains not less than 98.0 per cent and not more than 101.0 per cent of $C_{18}H_{21}ClN_2, HCl$, calculated with reference to the dried substance.

Characteristics A white, crystalline powder; odourless or almost odourless.

Solubility Soluble in 2 parts of *water*, in 11 parts of *ethanol (96%)* and in 4 parts of *chloroform*; practically insoluble in *ether*.

Identification A. The *infra-red absorption spectrum*, Appendix II A, is concordant with the *reference spectrum* of chlorcyclizine hydrochloride.

B. The *light absorption*, Appendix II B, in the range 225 to 350 nm of a 0.002% w/v solution in 0.05M *sulphuric acid* exhibits a maximum only at 231 nm. The *absorbance* at 231 nm is about 1.0.

C. Yields the *reactions* characteristic of chlorides, Appendix VI.

N-Methylpiperazine Carry out the method for *thin-layer chromatography*, Appendix III A, using *silica gel G* as the coating substance and a mixture of 90 volumes of *chloroform*, 8 volumes of *methanol* and 2 volumes of 13.5M *ammonia* as the mobile phase. Apply separately to the chromatoplate 20 µl of each of two freshly prepared solutions in *methanol* containing (1) 1.0% w/v of the substance being examined and (2) 0.0050% w/v of N-*methylpiperazine*. After removal of the plate, allow it to dry in air and expose to iodine vapour for 10 minutes. Any spot corresponding to N-methylpiperazine in the chromatogram obtained with solution (1) is not more intense than the spot in the chromatogram obtained with solution (2).

Loss on drying When dried at 120° for 3 hours, loses not more than 2.5% of its weight. Use 1 g.

Sulphated ash Not more than 0.1%, Appendix IX A.

Assay Carry out Method I for *non-aqueous titration*, Appendix VIII A, using 0.5 g, adding 20 ml of *mercury (II) acetate solution* and determining the end-point potentiometrically. Each ml of 0.1M *perchloric acid VS* is equivalent to 0.01686 g of $C_{18}H_{21}ClN_2,HCl$.

Action and use Antiemetic.

Chlordiazepoxide

$C_{16}H_{14}ClN_3O$ 299.8   *58-25-3*

Chlordiazepoxide is 7-chloro-2-methylamino-5-phenyl-3*H*-1,4-benzodiazepine-4-oxide. It contains not less than 99.0 per cent and not more than 101.0 per cent of $C_{16}H_{14}ClN_3O$, calculated with reference to the dried substance.

Characteristics A yellow, crystalline powder; odourless or almost odourless.

Solubility Practically insoluble in *water*; sparingly soluble in *ethanol (96%)* and in *chloroform*.

Identification A. The *infra-red absorption spectrum*, Appendix II A, is concordant with the *reference spectrum* of chlordiazepoxide.

B. The *light absorption*, Appendix II B, in the range 230 to 350 nm of a 0.001% w/v solution in 0.1M *hydrochloric acid* exhibits two maxima, at 246 nm and 308 nm. The *absorbance* at 246 nm is about 1.1 and at 308 nm is about 0.33.

C. Dissolve 0.2 g in 4 ml of hot 2M *hydrochloric acid*, heat at 100° for 10 minutes, cool and filter. 2 ml of the filtrate yields the *reaction* characteristic of primary aromatic amines, Appendix VI, producing a bright pinkish-red precipitate.

D. Carry out the method for *reaction B* characteristic of chlorides, Appendix VI. The paper does not turn violet-red.

Heavy metals To the residue obtained in the test for Sulphated ash add 2 ml of *hydrochloric acid* and evaporate slowly to dryness on a water-bath. Moisten the residue with 0.05 ml of *hydrochloric acid*, add 10 ml of boiling *water* and heat for 10 minutes on a water-bath. Cool, filter if necessary and adjust the volume of the filtrate and washings to 20 ml with *water*. 12 ml of the resulting solution complies with *limit test A for heavy metals*, Appendix VII (20 ppm). Use *lead standard solution (1 ppm Pb)* to prepare the standard.

Related substances and decomposition products Carry out in subdued light the method for *thin-layer chromatography*, Appendix III A, using *silica gel HF254* as the coating substance and a mixture of 95 volumes of *ethyl acetate* and 5 volumes of *absolute ethanol* as the mobile phase, but allowing the solvent front to ascend 12 cm above the line of application. Prepare the following solutions immediately before use. Solution (1) contains 2.0% w/v of the substance being examined in a mixture of 97 volumes of *methanol* and 3 volumes of 6M *ammonia*. Solution (2) contains 0.0050% w/v of *2-amino-5-chloro-benzophenone* in *methanol*. Solution (3) contains 0.010% w/v of the substance being examined in a mixture of 97 volumes of *methanol* and 3 volumes of 6M *ammonia*. Apply separately to the chromatoplate 25 µl of solution (1) as five 5-µl quantities at one point, allowing the solvent to evaporate between applications, and 5 µl of each of solutions (2) and (3). After removal of the plate, allow the solvent to evaporate and examine under *ultra-violet light (254 nm)*. Any *secondary spot* in the chromatogram obtained with solution (1) is not more intense than the spot in the chromatogram obtained with solution (3). Spray the plate with a freshly prepared 1% w/v solution of *sodium nitrite* in 1M *hydrochloric acid* and, after 1 minute, with a 0.4% w/v solution of N-*(1-naphthyl)ethylenediamine dihydrochloride* in *methanol*. Any violet spot in the chromatogram obtained with solution (1) is not more intense than the spot in the chromatogram obtained with solution (2).

Loss on drying When dried at 60° at a pressure not exceeding 0.7 kPa for 4 hours, loses not more than 0.5% of its weight. Use 1 g.

Sulphated ash Not more than 0.1%, Appendix IX A, Method II. Use 1.0 g.

Assay Carry out Method I for *non-aqueous titration*, Appendix VIII A, using 0.6 g and determining the end-point potentiometrically. Each ml of 0.1M *perchloric acid VS* is equivalent to 0.02998 g of $C_{16}H_{14}ClN_3O$.

Storage Chlordiazepoxide should be kept in a well-closed container and protected from light.

Preparation
Chlordiazepoxide Tablets

Action and use Anxiolytic.

Chlordiazepoxide Hydrochloride ☆

$C_{16}H_{14}ClN_3O,HCl$ 336.2   *438-41-5*

Chlordiazepoxide Hydrochloride is 7-chloro-2-methylamino-5-phenyl-3*H*-1,4-benzodiazepine-4-oxide hydrochloride. It contains not less than 99.0 per cent and not more than 101.0 per cent of $C_{16}H_{14}ClN_3O,HCl$, calculated with reference to the dried substance.

Characteristics A white or slightly yellow, crystalline powder. It melts at about 216°, with decomposition.

Solubility Soluble in 10 parts of *water* and in 40 parts of *ethanol (96%)*; practically insoluble in *chloroform* and in *ether*.

Identification *Test A may be omitted if tests B, C, D and E are carried out. Tests B, C and D may be omitted if tests A and E are carried out.*
A. The *infra-red absorption spectrum*, Appendix II A, is concordant with the spectrum of *chlordiazepoxide hydrochloride EPCRS*.
B. Carry out the test in subdued light and prepare the solutions immediately before use. The *light absorption*, Appendix II B, in the range 230 to 320 nm of a 0.0005% w/v solution in 0.1M *hydrochloric acid* exhibits two maxima, at 246 nm and 309 nm. The A(1%, 1 cm) at the maximum at 246 nm is 996 to 1058 and the A(1%, 1 cm) at the maximum at 309 nm is 280 to 298.
C. Examine the chromatograms obtained in the test for Related substances under *ultra-violet light (254 nm)*. The principal spot in the chromatogram obtained with solution (2) is similar in position and size to that in the chromatogram obtained with solution (4).
D. Dissolve 20 mg in a mixture of 5 ml of *hydrochloric acid* and 10 ml of *water*. Boil for 5 minutes, cool and add 2 ml of a 0.1% w/v solution of *sodium nitrite*. Allow to stand for 1 minute, add 1 ml of a 0.5% w/v solution of *sulphamic acid*, mix, allow to stand for 1 minute and add 1 ml of a 0.1% w/v solution of N-*(1-naphthyl)ethylene-diamine dihydrochloride*. A violet-red colour is produced.
E. Dissolve 50 mg in 5 ml of *water*, add 1 ml of 6M *ammonia*, mix, allow to stand for 5 minutes and filter. The filtrate, after acidifying with 2M *nitric acid*, yields *reaction A* characteristic of chlorides, Appendix VI.

Clarity and colour of solution A 10.0% w/v solution in *carbon dioxide-free water* is clear, Appendix IV A, and not more intensely coloured that *reference solution GY₆*, Appendix IV B, Method II.

Heavy metals 1.0 g complies with *limit test C for heavy metals*, Appendix VII (20 ppm). Use 2 ml of *lead standard solution (10 ppm Pb)* to prepare the standard.

Related substances Carry out in subdued light the method for *thin-layer chromatography*, Appendix III A, using *silica gel GF254* as the coating substance and a mixture of 85 volumes of *chloroform*, 14 volumes of *methanol* and 1 volume of 13.5M *ammonia* as the mobile phase. Prepare the following solutions immediately before use. Solution (1) contains 2% w/v of the substance being examined in a mixture of 3 volumes of 6M *ammonia* and 97 volumes of *methanol*. For solution (2) dilute 1 volume of solution (1) to 10 volumes with *methanol*. Solution (3) contains 0.010% w/v of *2-amino-5-chlorobenzophenone* in *methanol*. Solution (4) contains 0.20% w/v of *chlordiazepoxide hydrochloride EPCRS* in a mixture of 3

volumes of 6M *ammonia* and 97 volumes of *methanol*. For solution (5) dilute 1 volume of solution (1) to 200 volumes with *methanol*. Apply separately to the chromatoplate 25 µl of solution (1) as five 5-µl quantities at one point, allowing the solvent to evaporate between applications, and 5 µl of each of solutions (2), (3), (4) and (5). After removal of the plate, allow it to dry in air and examine under *ultra-violet light (254 nm)*. Any *secondary spot* in the chromatogram obtained with solution (1) is not more intense than the spot in the chromatogram obtained with solution (5). Spray the plate with about 10 ml of a freshly prepared 1% w/v solution of *sodium nitrite* in 1M *hydrochloric acid*, dry it in a current of cold air and spray with a 0.4% w/v solution of N-*(1-naphthyl)ethylene-1,2-diamine dihydrochloride* in *ethanol (96%)*. Any *violet spot* corresponding to 2-amino-5-chlorobenzophenone in the chromatogram obtained with solution (1) is not more intense than the spot in the chromatogram obtained with solution (3).

Loss on drying When dried over *phosphorus pentoxide* at 60° at a pressure of 1.5 to 2.5 kPa for 4 hours, loses not more than 0.5% of its weight. Use 1 g.

Sulphated ash Not more than 0.1%, Appendix IX A, Method II. Use 1 g.

Assay Dissolve 0.25 g in 80 ml of *anhydrous glacial acetic acid*, heating if necessary, cool and add 10 ml of *mercury(II) acetate solution*. Carry out Method I for *non-aqueous titration*, Appendix VIII A, determining the end-point potentiometrically. Each ml of 0.1M *perchloric acid VS* is equivalent to 0.03362 g of $C_{16}H_{14}ClN_3O,HCl$.

Storage Chlordiazepoxide Hydrochloride should be kept in a well-closed container and protected from light.

Preparations
Chlordiazepoxide Capsules
Chlordiazepoxide Hydrochloride Tablets

Action and use Sedative.

Chlorhexidine Acetate

$C_{22}H_{30}Cl_2N_{10},2C_2H_4O_2$ 625.6   *56-95-1*

Chlorhexidine Acetate is 1,1'-hexamethylenebis-[5-(4-chlorophenyl)biguanide] diacetate. It contains not less than 97.5 per cent and not more than 101.0 per cent of $C_{22}H_{30}Cl_2N_{10}$, $2C_2H_4O_2$, calculated with reference to the dried substance.

Characteristics A white to pale cream, microcrystalline powder; odourless or almost odourless.

Solubility Soluble in 55 parts of *water* and in 15 parts of *ethanol (96%)*; very slightly soluble in *glycerol* and in *propane-1,2-diol*.

Identification A. The *infra-red absorption spectrum*, Appendix II A, is concordant with the *reference spectrum* of chlorhexidine acetate.

B. Dissolve 0.1 g in 5 ml of a warm 20% w/v solution of *cetrimide* and add 1 ml of 5M *sodium hydroxide* and 1 ml of *bromine water*. A deep red colour is produced.

C. Dissolve 0.1 g in 10 ml of *water* and add, with shaking, 0.15 ml of *ammoniacal copper chloride solution*. A purple precipitate is produced immediately which changes to blue on the addition of a further 0.5 ml of *ammoniacal copper chloride solution*.

D. Yields the *reactions* characteristic of acetates, Appendix VI.

4-Chloroaniline Dissolve 0.20 g in 30 ml of *water* and add in rapid succession, with mixing between each addition, 5 ml of 1M *hydrochloric acid*, 1 ml of 0.5M *sodium nitrite* and 2 ml of a 5% w/v solution of *ammonium sulphamate*. Add 5 ml of a 0.1% w/v solution of N-(*1-naphthyl*)ethylene-diamine dihydrochloride, 1 ml of *ethanol (96%)* and sufficient *water* to produce 50 ml and allow to stand for 30 minutes. Any magenta colour produced is not more intense than that produced by treating in the same manner and at the same time 10 ml of a 0.0010% w/v solution of *4-chloroaniline* diluted to 30 ml with *water* slightly acidified with *hydrochloric acid*.

Related substances Carry out the method for *high-performance liquid chromatography*, Appendix III D, using the following solutions. For solution (1) dilute 2 volumes of solution (2) to 100 volumes with the mobile phase. Solution (2) contains 0.20% w/v of the substance being examined in the mobile phase. Solution (3) contains 0.10% w/v of *chlorhexidine impurity standard BPCRS* in the mobile phase.

The chromatographic procedure may be carried out using (a) a stainless steel column (20 cm × 4 mm) packed with *stationary phase C* (10 μm) (Nucleosil ODS is suitable), (b) as the mobile phase with a flow rate of 1.5 ml per minute 0.01M *sodium octanesulphonate* in a mixture of 73 volumes of *methanol*, 27 volumes of *water* and sufficient *glacial acetic acid* (12 volumes may be suitable) to produce with solution (3) a chromatogram resembling the reference chromatogram and (c) a detection wavelength of 254 nm. Pass the mobile phase through the column for at least 1 hour before starting the analysis.

In the chromatogram obtained with solution (2) the sum of the areas of the *secondary peaks* is not greater than 1.5 times the area of the principal peak in the chromatogram obtained with solution (1). After use, the apparatus should be thoroughly flushed with *methanol*.

The test is not valid unless the chromatogram obtained with solution (3) closely resembles the reference chromatogram in that the retention time of the principal peak is 5.5 to 8.0 minutes, the retention time of peak D is 20 to 25 minutes, the height of peak B is at least 75% of full-scale deflection on the chart paper and peaks B and C are at least partially resolved. Increasing the concentration of glacial acetic acid in the mobile phase reduces the retention times and reducing the concentration of glacial acetic acid in the mobile phase increases the retention times. If peaks B and C are not resolved when satisfactory retention times have been obtained for the principal peak and peak D the column should be equilibrated for a further 12 hours and if still unsatisfactory conditioned by the injection of ten 20-μl quantities of solution (3) in quick succession. If after this treatment a chromatogram resembling the reference chromatogram cannot be obtained the column should be repacked.

Loss on drying When dried to constant weight at 105°, loses not more than 3.5% of its weight. Use 1 g.

Sulphated ash Not more than 0.2%, Appendix IX A.

Assay Carry out Method I for *non-aqueous titration*, Appendix VIII A, using 0.45 g and *1-naphtholbenzein solution* as indicator. Each ml of 0.1M *perchloric acid VS* is equivalent to 0.01564 g of $C_{22}H_{30}Cl_2N_{10},2C_2H_4O_2$.

Storage Chlorhexidine Acetate should be kept in a well-closed container and protected from light.

Action and use Disinfectant.

Chlorhexidine Gluconate Solution

Chlorhexidine Gluconate Solution is an aqueous solution of 1,1'-hexamethylenebis[5-(4-chloro-phenyl)biguanide] digluconate. It contains not less than 19.0 per cent w/v and not more than 21.0 per cent w/v of $C_{22}H_{30}Cl_2N_{10},2C_6H_{12}O_7$.

Characteristics An almost colourless to pale straw-coloured, clear or not more than slightly opalescent liquid; odourless or almost odourless.

Solubility Miscible with *water*, with not more than 5 parts of *ethanol (96%)* and with not more than 3 parts of *acetone*.

Identification A. To 1 ml add 40 ml of *water*, cool in ice, add 5M *sodium hydroxide* dropwise with stirring until the solution is slightly alkaline to *titan yellow paper* and add 1 ml in excess. Filter, wash the precipitate with *water* until the washings are no longer alkaline to *titan yellow paper*, recrystallise from *ethanol (70%)* and dry at 105°. The *infra-red absorption spectrum* of the residue, Appendix II A, is concordant with the *reference spectrum* of chlorhexidine.

B. To 0.5 ml add 10 ml of *water* and 0.5 ml of *copper sulphate solution*. A white precipitate is produced which on boiling flocculates and becomes lilac.

C. To 0.05 ml add 5 ml of a warm 1% w/v solution of *cetrimide*, 1 ml of 5M *sodium hydroxide* and 1 ml of *bromine water*. A deep red colour is produced.

D. *Melting point* of the residue obtained in test A, about 132°, Appendix V A.

Acidity or alkalinity pH of a solution containing 5% v/v of the solution being examined, 5.5 to 7.0, Appendix V L.

Weight per ml 1.06 to 1.07 g, Appendix V G.

4-Chloroaniline Dilute 2.0 ml to 100 ml with *water*. To 10 ml of the resulting solution add 20 ml of *water* and, in rapid succession with mixing between each addition, 5 ml of 1M *hydrochloric acid*, 1 ml of 0.5M *sodium nitrite* and 2 ml of a 5% w/v solution of *ammonium sulphamate*. Add 5 ml of a 0.1% w/v solution of N-(*1-naphthyl*)ethylene-diamine dihydrochloride, 1 ml of *ethanol (96%)* and sufficient *water* to produce 50 ml and allow to stand for 30 minutes. Any magenta colour produced is not more intense than that produced by treating in the same manner and at the same time 10 ml of a 0.0010% w/v solution of *4-chloroaniline* in *water* slightly acidified with *hydrochloric acid*, beginning at the words 'add 20 ml of *water* . . .'.

Related substances Complies with the test described under Chlorhexidine Acetate but using as solution (2) a solution prepared by diluting 1 ml of the solution being examined to 100 ml with the mobile phase.

Sulphated ash Not more than 0.1% w/v, Appendix IX A.

Assay Carry out Method I for *non-aqueous titration*, Appendix VIII A, using 5 g evaporated to low volume and determining the end-point potentiometrically. Each ml of 0.1M *perchloric acid VS* is equivalent to 0.02244 g of $C_{22}H_{30}Cl_2N_{10},2C_6H_{12}O_7$. Using the weight per ml, calculate the percentage of $C_{22}H_{30}Cl_2N_{10},2C_6H_{12}O_7$ weight in volume.

Storage Chlorhexidine Gluconate Solution should be protected from light and stored at a temperature not exceeding 25°.

Preparations
Chlorhexidine Cream
Lignocaine and Chlorhexidine Gel.

Action and use Disinfectant.

Chlorhexidine Hydrochloride

$C_{22}H_{30}Cl_2N_{10},2HCl$ 578.4   *3697-42-5*

Chlorhexidine Hydrochloride is 1,1′-hexamethylenebis[5-(4-chlorophenyl)biguanide] dihydrochloride. It contains not less than 98.0 per cent and not more than 101.0 per cent of $C_{22}H_{30}Cl_2N_{10},2HCl$, calculated with reference to the dried substance.

Characteristics A white or almost white, crystalline powder; odourless or almost odourless.

Solubility Sparingly soluble in *water*; very slightly soluble in *ethanol (96%)*; soluble in 50 parts of *propane-1,2-diol*.

Identification A. The *infra-red absorption spectrum*, Appendix II A, is concordant with the *reference spectrum* of chlorhexidine hydrochloride.
B. Dissolve 5 mg in 5 ml of a warm 1% w/v solution of *cetrimide* and add 1 ml of 5M *sodium hydroxide* and 1 ml of *bromine water*. A deep red colour is produced.
C. Dissolve 0.3 g in 10 ml of a mixture of equal parts of *hydrochloric acid* and *water*, add 40 ml of *water*, filter, cool the filtrate in ice, add 5M *sodium hydroxide* dropwise with stirring until the solution is slightly alkaline to *titan yellow paper* and add 1 ml in excess. Filter, wash the precipitate with *water* until the washings are no longer alkaline to *titan yellow paper*, recrystallise from *ethanol (70%)* and dry at 105°. The *melting point* of the residue is about 132°, Appendix V A.
D. Yields *reaction B* characteristic of chlorides, Appendix VI.

4-Chloroaniline To 0.20 g add 1 ml of *hydrochloric acid*, shake until the solution is clear and immediately add sufficient *water* to produce 10 ml. Add 20 ml of *water* and, in rapid succession with mixing between each addition, 5 ml of 1M *hydrochloric acid*, 1 ml of 0.5M *sodium nitrite* and 2 ml of a 5% w/v solution of *ammonium sulphamate*. Add 5 ml of a 0.1% w/v solution of N-*(1-naphthyl)ethylenediamine dihydrochloride*, 1 ml of *ethanol (96%)* and sufficient *water* to produce 50 ml and allow to stand for 30 minutes. Any magenta colour produced is not more intense than that produced by treating in the same manner and at the same time 10 ml of a 0.0010% w/v solution of *4-chloroaniline* in *water* slightly acidified with *hydrochloric acid*, beginning at the words 'Add 20 ml of water . . .'.

Related substances Complies with the test described under Chlorhexidine Acetate.

Loss on drying When dried to constant weight at 130°, loses not more than 2.0% of its weight. Use 1 g.

Sulphated ash Not more than 0.1%, Appendix IX A.

Assay Carry out Method I for *non-aqueous titration*, Appendix VIII A, using 0.4 g and 10 ml of mercury *(II)* acetate solution and determining the end-point potentiometrically. Each ml of 0.1M *perchloric acid VS* is equivalent to 0.01446 g of $C_{22}H_{30}Cl_2N_{10},2HCl$.

Storage Chlorhexidine Hydrochloride should be protected from light.

Preparation
Chlorhexidine Dusting Powder

Action and use Disinfectant.

Chlorinated Lime

Chlorinated Lime contains not less than 30.0 per cent w/w of available chlorine, Cl.

Characteristics A dull white powder; odour, characteristic.

Solubility Partly soluble in *water* and in *ethanol (96%)*.

Identification A. Evolves chlorine copiously on the addition of 2M *hydrochloric acid*.
B. When shaken with *water* and filtered, the filtrate yields *reaction C* characteristic of calcium salts and *reaction A* characteristic of chlorides, Appendix VI.

Assay Triturate 4 g with successive small quantities of *water*, dilute to 1000 ml with *water* and shake thoroughly. Mix 100 ml of the resulting suspension with a solution containing 3 g of *potassium iodide* in 100 ml of *water*, acidify with 5 ml of 6M *acetic acid* and titrate the liberated iodine with 0.1M *sodium thiosulphate VS*. Each ml of 0.1M *sodium thiosulphate VS* is equivalent to 0.003545 g of available chlorine, Cl.

Storage Chlorinated Lime should be kept in a well-closed container. On exposure to air it becomes moist and gradually decomposes, carbon dioxide being absorbed and chlorine evolved.

Preparation
Chlorinated Lime and Boric Acid Solution

Action and use Disinfectant.

Chlormethiazole

ClCH₂·CH₂ — S / Me — N (structure)

C_6H_8ClNS 161.6   *533-45-9*

Chlormethiazole is 5-(2-chloroethyl)-4-methylthiazole. It contains not less than 98.0 per cent and not more than 101.0 per cent of C_6H_8ClNS.

Characteristics A colourless to slightly yellowish-brown liquid; odour, characteristic.

Solubility Slightly soluble in *water*; miscible with *ethanol (96%)*, with *chloroform* and with *ether*.

Identification A. The *infra-red absorption spectrum*, Appendix II A, is concordant with the *reference spectrum* of chlormethiazole.

B. The *light absorption*, Appendix II B, in the range 230 to 350 nm of a 0.004% w/v solution in 0.1M *hydrochloric acid* exhibits a maximum only at 257 nm. The *absorbance* at 257 nm is about 1.1.

C. Mix 0.1 g with 0.2 g of powdered *sodium hydroxide*, heat to fusion and continue heating for a further few seconds. Cool, add 0.5 ml of *water* and a slight excess of 2M *hydrochloric acid* and warm. Any fumes evolved do not turn moistened *starch—iodate paper* blue (distinction from chlormethiazole edisylate).

Acidity or alkalinity pH of a 0.5% w/v solution, 5.5 to 7.0, Appendix V L.

Heavy metals Moisten the residue obtained in the test for Sulphated ash with 2 ml of *hydrochloric acid* and evaporate to dryness. Dissolve the residue in *water* and add sufficient *water* to produce 20 ml. 12 ml of the resulting solution complies with *limit test A for heavy metals*, Appendix VII (20 ppm). Use *lead standard solution (1 ppm Pb)* to prepare the standard.

Related substances Carry out the method for *gas chromatography*, Appendix III B, using solutions in *chloroform* containing (1) 0.030% w/v of the substance being examined and 0.015% w/v of *dibenzyl* (internal standard), (2) 6.0% w/v of the substance being examined and (3) 6.0% w/v of the substance being examined and 0.015% w/v of the internal standard.

The chromatographic procedure may be carried out using a glass column (1.5 m × 4 mm) packed with *acid-washed, silanised diatomaceous support* (80 to 100 mesh) (Gas Chrom Q is suitable) coated with 8% of butane-1,4-diol succinate polyester and maintained at 170°.

In the chromatogram obtained with solution (3), the ratio of the sum of the areas of any *secondary peaks* to the area of the peak due to the internal standard is not greater than the ratio of the area of the peak due to chlormethiazole to that of the peak due to the internal standard in the chromatogram obtained with solution (1)

Sulphated ash Not more than 0.1%, Appendix IX A. Use 1.0 g.

Assay Carry out Method I for *non-aqueous titration*, Appendix VIII A, using 0.3 g and determining the end-point potentiometrically. Each ml of 0.1M *perchloric acid VS* is equivalent to 0.01616 g of C_6H_8ClNS.

Storage Chlormethiazole should be kept in a well-closed container and stored at a temperature of 2° to 8°.

Preparation
Chlormethiazole Capsules

Action and use Hypnotic; sedative; anticonvulsant.

In some countries the material described in this monograph may be known as Clomethiazole.

Chlormethiazole Edisylate

$$\left[\begin{array}{c} ClCH_2\cdot CH_2 \quad S \\ \diagdown \diagdown \\ Me \quad N \end{array} \right]_2 \cdot \begin{array}{c} CH_2\cdot SO_3H \\ CH_2\cdot SO_3H \end{array}$$

$(C_6H_8ClNS)_2,C_2H_6O_6S_2$ 513.5   *1867-58-9*

Chlormethiazole Edisylate is 5-(2-chloroethyl)-4-methylthiazole ethanedisulphonate. It contains not less than 99.0 per cent and not more than 101.0 per cent of $(C_6H_8ClNS)_2$, $C_2H_6O_6S_2$, calculated with reference to the dried substance.

Characteristics A white, crystalline powder; odour, characteristic.

Solubility Freely soluble in *water*; soluble in *ethanol* (96%); practically insoluble in *ether*.

Identification A. The *infra-red absorption spectrum*, Appendix II A, is concordant with the *reference spectrum* of chlormethiazole edisylate.

B. The *light absorption*, Appendix II B, in the range 230 to 350 nm of a 0.005% w/v solution in 0.1M *hydrochloric acid* exhibits a maximum only at 257 nm. The *absorbance* at 257 nm is about 0.92.

C. Mix 0.1 g with 0.2 g of powdered *sodium hydroxide*, heat to fusion and continue heating for a further few seconds. Cool, add 0.5 ml of *water* and a slight excess of 2M *hydrochloric acid* and warm. Fumes are evolved which turn moistened *starch—iodate paper* blue (distinction from chlormethiazole).

D. *Melting point*, about 128°, Appendix V A.

Calcium 10 ml of a 10.0% w/v solution diluted to 15 ml with *water* complies with the *limit test for calcium*, Appendix VII (100 ppm).

Heavy metals Moisten the residue obtained in the test for Sulphated ash with 2 ml of *hydrochloric acid* and evaporate to dryness. Dissolve the residue in *water* and add sufficient *water* to produce 20 ml. 12 ml of the resulting solution complies with *limit test A for heavy metals*, Appendix VII (20 ppm). Use *lead standard solution (1 ppm Pb)* to prepare the standard.

Chloride 10 ml of a 10% w/v solution diluted to 15 ml with *water* complies with the *limit test for chlorides*, Appendix VII (50 ppm).

Sulphate 10 ml of a 1.0% w/v solution diluted to 15 ml with *water* complies with the *limit test for sulphates*, Appendix VII (0.15%).

Related substances Carry out the method for *gas chromatography*, Appendix III B, using the following solutions. For solution (1) dilute 1 volume of solution (2) to 100 volumes with *chloroform*. To 25 volumes of this solution add 10 volumes of a 0.075% w/v solution of *dibenzyl* (internal standard) in *chloroform* and dilute to 50 volumes with *chloroform*. For solution (2) dissolve 0.5 g of the substance being examined in 10 ml of *water* and add 2 ml of 1M *sodium hydroxide*. Extract with two 10-ml quantities of *chloroform*, evaporate the combined extracts to a volume of about 2 ml and dilute to 5 ml with *chloroform*. Prepare solution (3) in the same manner as solution (2) but adding 1 ml of the internal standard solution before the final dilution.

The chromatographic procedure may be carried out using a glass column (1.5 m × 4 mm) packed with *acid-washed, silanised diatomaceous support* (80 to 100 mesh)

(Gas Chrom Q is suitable) coated with 8% of butane-1,4-diol succinate polyester and maintained at 170°.

The ratio of the sum of the areas of any *secondary peaks* to the area of the peak due to the internal standard in the chromatogram obtained with solution (3) is not greater than the ratio of the area of the peak due to chlormethiazole to that of the peak due to the internal standard in the chromatogram obtained with solution (1).

Loss on drying When dried at 50° at a pressure not exceeding 0.7 kPa for 6 hours, loses not more than 0.5% of its weight. Use 1 g.

Sulphated ash Not more than 0.3%, Appendix IX A. Use 1.0 g.

Assay Dissolve 0.4 g in 50 ml of *water* and titrate with 0.1M *sodium hydroxide VS* using *phenolphthalein solution* as indicator. Each ml of 0.1M *sodium hydroxide VS* is equivalent to 0.02567 g of $(C_6H_8ClNS)_2,C_2H_6O_6S_2$.

Storage Chlormethiazole Edisylate should be kept in a well-closed container.

Action and use Hypnotic; sedative; anticonvulsant.

In some countries the material described in this monograph may be known as Clomethiazole Edisilate.

Chlorocresol ☆

C$_7$H$_7$ClO   142.6   *59-50-7*

Chlorocresol is 4-chloro-3-methylphenol and contains not less than 98.0 per cent and not more than 101.0 per cent of C_7H_7ClO.

Characteristics Colourless or almost colourless crystals or a white, crystalline powder; odour, characteristic.

Solubility Slightly soluble in *water*; very soluble in *ethanol (96%)*; freely soluble in *ether* and in fatty oils. It dissolves in aqueous solutions of alkali hydroxides.

Identification A. To 3.0 g, finely powdered, add 60 ml of *carbon dioxide-free water*, shake for 2 minutes and filter (solution A). To 5 ml of solution A add 0.1 ml of *iron(III) chloride test-solution*. A bluish colour is produced.
B. To 0.1 g add 0.2 ml of *benzoyl chloride* and 0.5 ml of 2M *sodium hydroxide*. Shake vigorously until a white precipitate is produced, add 5 ml of *water* and filter. The *melting point* of the residue, after recrystallisation from *methanol* and drying at 70°, is 85° to 88°, Appendix V A, Method I.
C. *Melting point*, 64° to 67°, Appendix V A, Method I.

Acidity or alkalinity To 10 ml of solution A add 0.1 ml of *methyl red solution*. The solution is orange or red and not more than 0.2 ml of 0.01M *sodium hydroxide* is required to change the colour of the solution to yellow.

Clarity and colour of solution Dissolve 1.25 g in sufficient *ethanol (96%)* to produce 25 ml. The solution is *clear*, Appendix IV A, and not more intensely coloured than *reference solution BY₆*, Appendix IV B, Method II.

Related substances Carry out the method for *gas chromatography*, Appendix III B, using a 1.0% w/v solution of the substance being examined in *acetone*.

The chromatographic procedure may be carried out using a glass column (1.8 m × 3.5 mm) packed with *silanised diatomaceous support* coated with 3 to 5% w/w of phenyl methyl silicone fluid (50% phenyl) (OV-17 is suitable) and maintained at 125°, with an inlet port temperature of 210°, a detector temperature of 230° and a flow rate of 30 ml per minute for the carrier gas. Allow the chromatography to proceed for three times the retention time (about 8 minutes) of chlorocresol.

The sum of the areas of any *secondary peaks* in the chromatogram is not greater than 1% of the total area of the peaks.

Non-volatile matter Evaporate 2 g to dryness on a water-bath and dry at 100° to 105°. The residue weighs not more than 2 mg (0.1%).

Assay Dissolve 70 mg in 30 ml of *glacial acetic acid*, add 25.0 ml of 0.0167M *potassium bromate VS*, 20 ml of a 15% w/v solution of *potassium bromide* and 10 ml of *hydrochloric acid*. Stopper the flask and allow to stand protected from light for 15 minutes. Add 1 g of *potassium iodide* and 100 ml of *water*. Titrate with 0.1M *sodium thiosulphate VS*, shaking vigorously and using 1 ml of *starch solution*, added towards the end of the titration, as indicator. Repeat the procedure without the substance being examined. The difference between the titrations represents the amount of potassium bromate required. Each ml of 0.0167M *potassium bromate VS* is equivalent to 0.003565 g of C_7H_7ClO.

Storage Chlorocresol should be kept in a well-closed container and protected from light.

Action and use Antiseptic; antimicrobial preservative.

Chloroform

CHCl$_3$ 119.4   *67-66-3*

Chloroform is trichloromethane to which 1.0 to 2.0 per cent v/v of ethanol has been added.

Characteristics A colourless, volatile liquid; odour, characteristic.

Solubility Slightly soluble in *water*; miscible with *absolute ethanol*, with *ether*, with fixed and volatile oils and with most organic solvents.

Identification A. Non-flammable. The vapour introduced into a flame imparts a green colour to the flame and gives rise to noxious vapours having a characteristic odour.
B. Warm 0.05 ml with 0.05 ml of *aniline* and 1 ml of 5M *sodium hydroxide*. The characteristic odour of phenyl isocyanide is produced.

Distillation range Not more than 5.0% v/v distils below 60° and the remainder distils at 60° to 62°, Appendix V C.

Weight per ml 1.474 to 1.479 g, Appendix V G.

Acidity or alkalinity Shake 10 ml with 20 ml of freshly boiled and cooled *water* for 3 minutes and allow to separate. To 5 ml of the aqueous layer add 0.1 ml of neutral *litmus solution*. The colour produced is the same as that produced on adding 0.1 ml of the neutral litmus solution to 5 ml of freshly boiled and cooled *water*.

Chloride To 5 ml of the aqueous layer obtained in the test for Acidity or alkalinity add 5 ml of *water* and 0.2 ml of *silver nitrate solution*. The solution is *clear*, Appendix IV A.

Free chlorine To 10 ml of the aqueous layer obtained in the test for Acidity or alkalinity add 1 ml of *cadmium iodide solution* and 0.1 ml of *starch mucilage*. No blue colour is produced.

Aldehyde Shake 5 ml with 5 ml of *water* and 0.2 ml of *alkaline potassium mercuri-iodide reagent* in a glass-stoppered flask and allow to stand in the dark for 15 minutes. Not more than a pale yellow colour is produced.

Decomposition products Carry out the following procedure in subdued light. Place 20 ml in a glass-stoppered flask previously rinsed with *sulphuric acid*, add 15 ml of *sulphuric acid* and 0.2 ml of *formaldehyde solution*, allow to stand for 30 minutes, shaking frequently, and allow to stand for a further 30 minutes. The acidic layer is not more than slightly coloured.

Foreign organic matter Shake 20 ml for 5 minutes with 10 ml of *sulphuric acid* in a glass-stoppered flask previously rinsed with *sulphuric acid* and allow to stand in the dark for 30 minutes. Both the acid and the chloroform remain colourless. Reserve the chloroform layer for the test for Foreign chlorine compounds. To 2 ml of the acid layer add 5 ml of *water*; the liquid remains colourless and clear and has no unpleasant odour. Add a further 10 ml of *water* and 0.2 ml of *silver nitrate solution*; no opalescence is produced.

Foreign chlorine compounds Shake 15 ml of the chloroform layer reserved in the test for Foreign organic matter with 30 ml of *water* in a glass-stoppered flask for 3 minutes and allow to separate. To the aqueous layer add 0.2 ml of *silver nitrate solution* and allow to stand in the dark for 5 minutes. No opalescence is produced.

Non-volatile matter 25 ml, when evaporated and dried at 105°, leaves not more than 1 mg of residue.

Storage Chloroform should be kept in a well-closed container with a glass stopper or other suitable closure and protected from light.

Preparations

Chloroform Spirit
Chloroform Water
Double-strength Chloroform Water

Action and use General anaesthetic; antimicrobial preservative.

Chloroquine Phosphate

$C_{18}H_{26}ClN_3,2H_3PO_4$ 515.9 *50-63-5*

Chloroquine Phosphate is 4-(7-chloro-4-quinolylamino)pentyldiethylamine diortho-phosphate. It contains not less than 98.0 per cent and not more than 101.0 per cent of $C_{18}H_{26}ClN_3,2H_3PO_4$, calculated with reference to the dried substance.

Characteristics A white or almost white powder; odourless or almost odourless.

Solubility Soluble in 4 parts of *water*; very slightly soluble in *ethanol (96%)*; practically insoluble in *chloroform* and in *ether*.

Identification A. Dissolve 0.1 g in 10 ml of *water*, add 2 ml of 2M *sodium hydroxide* and extract with two 20-ml quantities of *chloroform*, reserving the aqueous layer for test C. Wash the chloroform extracts with *water*, dry with *anhydrous sodium sulphate*, evaporate to dryness and dissolve the residue in 2 ml of *chloroform IR*. The *infra-red absorption spectrum* of the resulting solution, Appendix II A, is concordant with the *reference spectrum* of chloroquine.

B. The *light absorption*, Appendix II B, in the range 240 to 350 nm of a 0.003% w/v solution in 0.01M *hydrochloric acid* exhibits three maxima, at 257, 329 and 343 nm. The *absorbance* at 257 nm is about 0.87, at 329 nm, about 0.96 and at 343 nm, about 1.1.

C. Neutralise with 2M *nitric acid* the aqueous layer obtained in test A, add an equal volume of a 10% w/v solution of *ammonium molybdate* and warm. A yellow precipitate is produced.

D. Dissolve 25 mg in 20 ml of *water* and add 8 ml of *trinitrophenol solution*. The *melting point* of the precipitate, after washing successively with *water*, *ethanol (96%)* and *ether*, is about 207°, Appendix V A.

Acidity pH of a 10% w/v solution, 3.5 to 4.5, Appendix V L.

Lead Not more than 10 ppm when determined by the following method. Carefully heat 2.0 g for 10 minutes with 8 ml of *water* and 6 ml of *nitric acid* in a round-bottomed, long-necked flask. Cool, add 4 ml of *sulphuric acid* and heat until the mixture darkens. Continue heating, with the dropwise addition of *nitric acid*, until the liquid becomes colourless and white fumes of sulphur trioxide are produced. Add 3 ml of *water*, carefully evaporate until white fumes are again produced, cool and dilute to 18 ml with *water*. Add and dissolve 2 g of *citric acid*, make alkaline with 5M *ammonia* and add 1 ml of *potassium cyanide solution PbT*. Transfer to a separating funnel, add 10 ml of *dithizone solution*, shake vigorously and remove the lower layer. Repeat the extraction with two 5-ml quantities of *dithizone solution*. If, after the third extraction, the chloroform layer is bright red, continue the extraction with further 5-ml quantities of *dithizone solution* until the colour of the reagent no longer changes to bright red. Wash the combined chloroform solutions by shaking with 10 ml of *water* and then extract with two 10-ml quantities of 2M *hydrochloric acid*. Wash the combined acid solutions with 10 ml of *chloroform* and discard the chloroform. Transfer the solution to a *Nessler cylinder* and make alkaline with 5M *ammonia*. In a second *Nessler cylinder* mix 2 ml of 6M *acetic acid* with 20 ml of 2M *hydrochloric acid*, make alkaline with 5M *ammonia* and add 2 ml of *lead standard solution (10 ppm Pb)*.

Treat the contents of each cylinder as follows. Add 1 ml of *potassium cyanide solution PbT*; the solutions should not be more than faintly opalescent. If the colours of the solutions differ, equalise them by the addition of a few drops of a highly diluted solution of burnt sugar or other non-reactive substance. Dilute to 50 ml with *water*, add 0.1 ml of a solution prepared by dissolving 10 g of *sodium sulphide* in sufficient *water* to produce 100 ml and filtering and mix thoroughly.

Compare the colours of the two solutions by a suitable method, such as by light reflected from a white tile through the Nessler cylinders. The colour of the solution in the first cylinder is not more intense than that of the solution in the second cylinder.

Related substances Carry out the method for *thin-layer chromatography*, Appendix III A, using *silica gel GF254* as the coating substance and a mixture of 50 volumes of *chloroform*, 40 volumes of *cyclohexane* and 10 volumes of *diethylamine* as the mobile phase. Apply separately to the chromatoplate 2 μl of each of three solutions of the substance being examined in *water* containing (1) 5.0% w/v, (2) 0.050% w/v and (3) 0.025% w/v. After removal of the plate, allow it to dry in air and examine under *ultra-violet light (254 nm)*. Any *secondary spot* in the chromatogram obtained with solution (1) is not more intense than the spot in the chromatogram obtained with solution (2) and not more than one such spot is more intense than the spot in the chromatogram obtained with solution (3).

Loss on drying When dried to constant weight at 105°, loses not more than 1.5% of its weight. Use 1 g.

Assay Carry out Method I for *non-aqueous titration*, Appendix VIII A, using 0.5 g and determining the end-point potentiometrically. Each ml of 0.1M *perchloric acid VS* is equivalent to 0.02579 g of $C_{18}H_{26}ClN_3,2H_3PO_4$.

Preparations
Chloroquine Phosphate Injection
Chloroquine Phosphate Tablets

Action and use Antimalarial.

Chloroquine Sulphate

$C_{18}H_{26}ClN_3,H_2SO_4,H_2O$ 436.0   *132-73-0*

Chloroquine Sulphate is 4-(7-chloro-4-quinolylamino)pentyldiethylamine sulphate monohydrate. It contains not less than 98.0 per cent and not more than 101.0 per cent of $C_{18}H_{26}ClN_3,H_2SO_4$, calculated with reference to the anhydrous substance.

Characteristics A white or almost white, crystalline powder; odourless or almost odourless.

Solubility Soluble in 3 parts of *water*; practically insoluble in *ethanol (96%)*; sparingly soluble in *ether* and in *chloroform*.

Identification A. Dissolve 0.1 g in 10 ml of *water*, add 2 ml of 2M *sodium hydroxide* and extract with two 20-ml quantities of *chloroform*. Wash the chloroform extracts with *water*, dry with *anhydrous sodium sulphate*, evaporate to dryness and dissolve the residue in 2 ml of *chloroform IR*. The *infra-red absorption spectrum* of the resulting solution, Appendix II A, is concordant with the *reference spectrum* of chloroquine.

B. The *light absorption*, Appendix II B, in the range 240 to 350 nm of a 0.002% w/v solution in 0.01M *hydrochloric acid* exhibits three maxima, at 257, 329 and 343 nm. The *absorbance* at 257 nm is about 0.78, at 329 nm, about 0.88 and at 343 nm, about 0.92.

C. Dissolve 25 mg in 20 ml of *water* and add 8 ml of *trinitrophenol solution*. The *melting point* of the precipitate, after washing successively with *water*, *ethanol (96%)* and *ether*, is about 207°, Appendix V A.

D. Yields the *reactions* characteristic of sulphates, Appendix VI.

Acidity pH of a 10% w/v solution, 4.0 to 5.0, Appendix V L.

Lead Not more than 20 ppm when determined by the following method. Carefully heat 2.0 g for 10 minutes with 8 ml of *water* and 6 ml of *nitric acid* in a round-bottomed, long-necked flask. Cool, add 4 ml of *sulphuric acid* and heat until the mixture darkens. Continue heating, with the dropwise addition of *nitric acid*, until the liquid becomes colourless and white fumes of sulphur trioxide are produced. Add 3 ml of *water*, carefully evaporate until white fumes are again produced, cool and dilute to 18 ml with *water*. Add and dissolve 2 g of *citric acid*, make alkaline with 5M *ammonia* and add 1 ml of *potassium cyanide solution PbT*. Transfer to a separating funnel, add 10 ml of *dithizone solution*, shake vigorously and remove the lower layer. Repeat the extraction with two further 5-ml quantities of *dithizone solution*. If, after the third extraction, the chloroform layer is bright red, continue the extraction with further 5-ml quantities of *dithizone solution* until the colour of the reagent no longer changes to bright red. Wash the combined chloroform solutions by shaking with 10 ml of *water* and then extract with two 10-ml quantities of 2M *hydrochloric acid*. Wash the combined acid solutions with 10 ml of *chloroform* and discard the chloroform. Transfer the solution to a *Nessler cylinder* and make alkaline with 5M *ammonia*. In a second *Nessler cylinder* mix 2 ml of 6M *acetic acid* with 20 ml of 2M *hydrochloric acid*, make alkaline with 5M *ammonia* and add 4 ml of *lead standard solution (10 ppm Pb)*.

Treat the contents of each cylinder as follows. Add 1 ml of *potassium cyanide solution PbT*; the solutions should not be more than faintly opalescent. If the colours of the solutions differ, equalise them by the addition of a few drops of a highly diluted solution of burnt sugar or other non-reactive substance. Dilute to 50 ml with *water*, add 0.1 ml of a solution prepared by dissolving 10 g of *sodium sulphide* in sufficient *water* to produce 100 ml and filtering and mix thoroughly.

Compare the colours of the two solutions by a suitable method, such as by light reflected from a white tile through the Nessler cylinders. The colour of the solution in the first cylinder is not more intense than that of the solution in the second cylinder.

Chloride Dissolve 0.3 g in 30 ml of *water*. 15 ml of the resulting solution complies with the *limit test for chlorides*, Appendix VII (350 ppm).

Related substances Carry out the method for *thin-layer chromatography*, Appendix III A, using *silica gel GF254* as the coating substance and a mixture of 50 volumes of *chloroform*, 40 volumes of *cyclohexane* and 10 volumes of *diethylamine* as the mobile phase. Apply separately to the chromatoplate 2 μl of each of three solutions of the substance being examined in *water* containing (1) 5.0% w/v, (2) 0.050% w/v and (3) 0.025% w/v. After removal of the plate, allow it to dry in air and examine under *ultra-violet light (254 nm)*. Any *secondary spot* in the chromatogram obtained with solution (1) is not more intense than the spot in the chromatogram obtained with solution (2) and not more than one such spot is more intense than the spot in the chromatogram obtained with solution (3).

Sulphated ash Not more than 0.1%, Appendix IX A.

Water 3.0 to 5.0% w/w, Appendix IX C. Use 0.5 g.

Assay Dissolve 0.5 g in 10 ml of *water*, add 20 ml of 1M *sodium hydroxide* and extract with four 25-ml quantities of *chloroform*. Combine the chloroform extracts and evaporate to a volume of about 10 ml. Add 40 ml of *glacial acetic acid* and carry out Method I for *non-aqueous titration*, Appendix VIII A, using *oracet blue B solution* as indicator. Each ml of 0.1M *perchloric acid VS* is equivalent to 0.02090 g of $C_{18}H_{26}ClN_3,H_2SO_4$.

Preparations
Chloroquine Sulphate Injection
Chloroquine Sulphate Tablets
Action and use Antimalarial.

Chlorothiazide ☆

$C_7H_6ClN_3O_4S_2$ 295.7   *58-94-6*

Chlorothiazide is 6-chloro-2*H*-1,2,4-benzothia-diazine-7-sulphonamide 1,1-dioxide. It contains not less than 98.0 per cent and not more than 102.0 per cent of $C_7H_6ClN_3O_4S_2$, calculated with reference to the dried substance.

Characteristics A white or almost white, crystalline powder; odourless.

Solubility Very slightly soluble in *water*; slightly soluble in *ethanol (96%)*; sparingly soluble in *acetone*. It dissolves in dilute solutions of alkali hydroxides.

Identification *Test A may be omitted if tests B, C and D are carried out. Tests B and D may be omitted if tests A and C are carried out.*
A. The *infra-red absorption spectrum*, Appendix II A, is concordant with the spectrum of *chlorothiazide EPCRS*.
B. Dissolve 80 mg in 100 ml of 0.1M *sodium hydroxide*, add sufficient *water* to produce 1000 ml and dilute 10 ml to 100 ml with 0.01M *sodium hydroxide*. The *light absorption* of the resulting solution, Appendix II B, in the range 220 to 320 nm exhibits maxima at 225 nm and 292 nm and a shoulder at 310 nm. The A(1%, 1 cm) at 225 nm is 725 to 800 and the A(1%, 1 cm) at 292 nm is 425 to 455.
C. Carry out the method for *thin-layer chromatography*, Appendix III A, using *silica gel GF254* as the coating substance and *ethyl acetate* as the mobile phase but allowing the solvent front to ascend 10 cm above the line of application. Apply separately to the chromatoplate 2 µl of each of two solutions in *acetone* containing (1) 0.50% w/v of the substance being examined and (2) 0.50% w/v of *chlorothiazide EPCRS*. After removal of the plate, dry it in a current of air and examine under *ultra-violet light (254 nm)*. The principal spot in the chromatogram obtained with solution (1) is similar in position and size to that in the chromatogram obtained with solution (2).
D. To 0.1 g add a pellet of *sodium hydroxide* and heat strongly; a gas is evolved that turns *litmus paper* blue. Cool and dissolve the residue in 10 ml of 2M *hydrochloric acid*; a gas is evolved that turns *lead acetate paper* black.

Acidity or alkalinity Shake 1.0 g of the powdered substance being examined with 50 ml of *water* for 2 minutes and filter (solution A). To 10 ml of solution A add 0.2 ml of 0.01M *sodium hydroxide VS* and 0.15 ml of *methyl red solution*. The solution is yellow and not more than 0.4 ml of 0.01M *hydrochloric acid VS* is required to change the colour to red.

Heavy metals 1.0 g complies with *limit test C for heavy metals*, Appendix VII (20 ppm). Use 2 ml of *lead standard solution (10 ppm Pb)* to prepare the standard.

Chloride 15 ml of solution A complies with the *limit test for chlorides*, Appendix VII (170 ppm).

Related substances Carry out the method for *thin-layer chromatography*, Appendix III A, using *silica gel G* as the coating substance and a mixture of 85 volumes of *ethyl acetate* and 15 volumes of *propan-2-ol* as the mobile phase. Apply separately to the chromatoplate 5 µl of each of two solutions of the substance being examined in *acetone* containing (1) 0.50% w/v and (2) 0.0050% w/v. After removal of the plate, dry it in a current of air until the odour of solvent is no longer detectable (about 10 minutes) and spray with a 10% v/v solution of *sulphuric acid* in *ethanol (96%)*; use about 10 ml for a plate 200 mm × 200 mm in size and spray in small portions, allowing the solvent to evaporate each time to avoid excessive wetting. Heat at 100° to 105° for 30 minutes and immediately place above but not in 10 ml of a saturated solution of *sodium nitrite* in a glass tank. Add 0.5 ml of *sulphuric acid* to the sodium nitrite solution and allow to stand in the closed tank for 15 minutes. Remove the plate, heat it in a ventilated oven at 40° for 15 minutes, spray with three 5-ml quantities of a freshly prepared 0.5% w/v solution of N-*(1-naphthyl)ethylenediamine dihydrochloride* in *ethanol (96%)* and examine by transmitted light. Any *secondary spot* in the chromatogram obtained with solution (1) is not more intense than the spot in the chromatogram obtained with solution (2).

Loss on drying When dried to constant weight at 100° to 105°, loses not more than 1.0% of its weight. Use 1 g.

Sulphated ash Not more than 0.1%, Appendix IX A. Use 1 g.

Assay Dissolve 0.25 g in 50 ml of *dimethylformamide* and carry out Method II for *non-aqueous titration*, Appendix VIII A, using 0.1M *tetrabutylammonium hydroxide VS* as titrant and determining the end-point potentiometrically at the first inflection. Repeat the operation without the substance being examined. The difference between the titrations represents the amount of tetrabutylammonium hydroxide required. Each ml of 0.1M *tetrabutylammonium hydroxide VS* is equivalent to 0.02957 g of $C_7H_6ClN_3O_4S_2$.

Preparation
Chlorothiazide Tablets
Action and use Diuretic.

Chlorotrianisene

C$_{23}$H$_{21}$ClO$_3$ 380.9   569-57-3

Chlorotrianisene is chlorotris(4-methoxy-phenyl)ethylene. It contains not less than 98.0 per cent and not more than 102.0 per cent of C$_{23}$H$_{21}$ClO$_3$, calculated with reference to the dried substance.

Characteristics Small, white crystals or crystalline powder; odourless or almost odourless.

Solubility Slightly soluble in *water* and in *ethanol (96%)*; soluble in 7 parts of *acetone*, in 1.5 parts of *chloroform*, in 28 parts of *ether* and in 100 parts of fixed oils.

Identification A. Dissolve 20 mg in the minimum quantity of *absolute ethanol* and evaporate to dryness. The *infra-red absorption spectrum* of the residue, Appendix II A, is concordant with the *reference spectrum* of chlorotrianisene.

B. The *light absorption*, Appendix II B, in the range 230 to 350 nm of a 0.001% w/v solution in *chloroform* exhibits two maxima, at 247 nm and 310 nm. The *absorbance* at 247 nm is about 0.58 and at 310 nm is about 0.40.

C. Carry out the method for *thin-layer chromatography*, Appendix III A, using *silica gel G* as the coating substance and a mixture of 92 volumes of *1,2-dichloroethane*, 8 volumes of *methanol* and 0.5 volume of *water* as the mobile phase. Apply separately to the chromatoplate 5 μl of each of two solutions in *ethanol (96%)* containing (1) 0.04% w/v of the substance being examined and (2) 0.04% w/v of *chlorotrianisene BPCRS*. After removal of the plate, allow it to dry in air for a few minutes, heat at 110° for 10 minutes, spray while still warm with *ethanolic sulphuric acid (10%)* and heat at 110° for a further 10 minutes. The chromatogram obtained with solution (1) exhibits a pink spot corresponding in position and colour to the spot in the chromatogram obtained with solution (2).

D. *Melting point*, about 118°, Appendix V A.

Related substances Carry out the method for *high-performance liquid chromatography*, Appendix III D, using two solutions of the substance being examined in a mixture of 60 volumes of *hexane* and 40 volumes of *dichloromethane* containing (1) 0.00125% w/v and (2) 0.25% w/v.

The chromatographic procedure may be carried out using (a) a stainless steel column (20 cm × 4 mm) packed with *stationary phase A* (10 μm) (Partisil is suitable), (b) a mixture of 3 volumes of *hexane* and 2 volumes of *dichloromethane* as the mobile phase with a flow rate of 2 ml per minute and (c) a detection wavelength of 254 nm.

In the chromatogram obtained with solution (2) the sum of the areas of any *secondary peaks* is not greater than twice the area of the principal peak in the chromatogram obtained with solution (1).

Loss on drying When dried at 60° at a pressure not exceeding 0.7 kPa for 6 hours, loses not more than 1.0% of its weight. Use 1 g.

Sulphated ash Not more than 0.1%, Appendix IX A.

Assay Dissolve 0.5 g in 15 ml of *absolute ethanol* by heating gently under a reflux condenser, add 2 g of *sodium* in small pieces and continue heating for 1 hour, shaking frequently and dissolving any solid that may form by adding small quantities of *absolute ethanol*; ensure that free sodium is present throughout this period. Add sufficient *absolute ethanol* to dissolve the excess of sodium and continue heating for 15 minutes. Add 150 ml of *water*, cool, add 15 ml of *nitric acid* and 25 ml of 0.1M *silver nitrate VS*, shake vigorously, filter and wash the residue with *water*. Titrate the excess of silver nitrate in the combined filtrate and washings with 0.1M *ammonium thiocyanate VS* using *ammonium iron(III) sulphate solution* as indicator. Repeat the operation without the substance being examined. The difference between the titrations represents the amount of silver nitrate required. Each ml of 0.1M *silver nitrate VS* is equivalent to 0.03809 g of C$_{23}$H$_{21}$ClO$_3$.

Preparations
Chlorotrianisene Capsules
Chlorotrianisene Tablets
Action and use Oestrogen.

Chloroxylenol

C$_8$H$_9$ClO   156.6   88-04-0

Chloroxylenol is 4-chloro-3,5-xylenol.

Characteristics White or cream crystals or crystalline powder with a characteristic odour. It is volatile in steam.

Solubility Very slightly soluble in *water*; soluble in 1 part of *ethanol (96%)*; soluble in *ether*, in terpenes and in fixed oils. It dissolves in solutions of the alkali hydroxides.

Identification A. The *infra-red absorption spectrum*, Appendix II A, is concordant with the *reference spectrum* of chloroxylenol.

B. Dissolve 0.1 g in 5 ml of *chloroform* and add 0.5 ml of a filtered 1% w/v solution of *iron(III) chloride* in *chloroform* and 0.1 ml of *pyridine*. A blue colour is produced.

C. To 5 ml of a saturated solution in *water* add 0.5 ml of *iron(III) chloride test-solution*. No blue colour is produced.

D. Mix 50 mg with 0.5 g of *anhydrous sodium carbonate* and ignite strongly, cool, boil the residue with 5 ml of *water*, acidify with *nitric acid*, filter and add *silver nitrate solution*. A white precipitate is produced.

Melting point 114° to 116°, Appendix V A.

Related substances Carry out the method for *gas chromatography*, Appendix III B, using solutions in *chloroform* containing (1) 2.0% w/v of the substance being examined and (2) 2.0% w/v of the substance being examined and 0.040% w/v of *4-chloro-m-cresol* (internal standard).

The chromatographic procedure may be carried out using a glass column (1.5 m × 4 mm) packed with *acid-washed diatomaceous support* (80 to 100 mesh) coated with 3% w/w of polyethylene glycol (Carbowax 20M is suitable) and maintained at 160°.

In the chromatogram obtained with solution (2) the sum of the areas of any *secondary peaks* is not greater than the area of the peak due to the internal standard.

Preparation
Chloroxylenol Solution

Action and use Antiseptic; disinfectant.

Chlorpheniramine Maleate ☆

$C_{16}H_{19}ClN_2,C_4H_4O_4$ 390.9   *113-92-8*

Chlorpheniramine Maleate is 3-(4-chloro-phenyl)-3-(2-pyridyl)propyldimethylamine hydrogen maleate. It contains not less than 98.0 per cent and not more than of 101.0 per cent of $C_{16}H_{19}ClN_2, C_4H_4O_4$, calculated with reference to the dried substance.

Characteristics A white, crystalline powder; odourless.

Solubility Soluble in 4 parts of *water*, in 10 parts of *ethanol (96%)* and in 10 parts of *chloroform*; slightly soluble in *ether*.

Identification *Test A may be omitted if tests B, C, D and E are carried out. Tests B, C and D may be omitted if tests A and E are carried out.*
A. The *infra-red absorption spectrum*, Appendix II A, is concordant with the spectrum of *chlorphenamine maleate EPCRS*.
B. The *light absorption*, Appendix II B, in the range 230 to 350 nm of a 0.003% w/v solution in 0.1M *hydrochloric acid* exhibits a maximum at 265 nm. The A(1%, 1 cm) at 265 nm is 200 to 220.
C. To 0.2 g add 3 ml of *water* and 1 ml of 10M *sodium hydroxide* and extract with three 5-ml quantities of *ether*. To 0.1 ml of the aqueous layer add a solution of 10 mg of *resorcinol* in 3 ml of *sulphuric acid* and heat on a water-bath for 15 minutes; the solution is colourless. To the remainder of the aqueous layer add 2 ml of *bromine solution*, heat in a water-bath for 15 minutes, heat to boiling and cool. To 0.2 ml of the resulting solution add a solution of 10 mg of *resorcinol* in 3 ml of *sulphuric acid* and heat on a water-bath for 15 minutes; a blue colour is produced.
D. Dissolve 0.1 g in 10 ml of *water* and add dropwise with shaking 25 ml of a 1% w/v solution of *2,4,6-trinitrophenol*. Collect the precipitate on a sintered-glass filter, wash with 3 ml of *ethanol (96%)*, recrystallise from *ethanol (50%)* and dry at 100° to 105°. The *melting point* of the crystals is 196° to 200°, Appendix V A, Method I.
E. *Melting point*, 132° to 135°, Appendix V A, Method I.

Colour and clarity of solution A 10% w/v solution is *clear*, Appendix IV A, and not more intensely coloured than *reference solution BY₆*, Appendix IV B, Method II.

Heavy metals 1.0 g complies with *limit test C for heavy metals*, Appendix VII (20 ppm). Use 2 ml of *lead standard solution (10 ppm Pb)* to prepare the standard.

Related substances Carry out the method for *thin-layer chromatography*, Appendix III A, using *silica gel GF254* as the coating substance and a mixture of 50 volumes of *cyclohexane*, 40 volumes of *chloroform* and 10 volumes of *diethylamine* as the mobile phase but allowing the solvent front to ascend 12 cm above the line of application. Apply separately to the chromatoplate 10 μl of each of two solutions of the substance being examined in *chloroform* containing (1) 5% w/v and (2) 0.01% w/v. After removal of the plate, allow it to dry in air and examine under *ultra-violet light (254 nm)*. Any *secondary spot* in the chromatogram obtained with solution (1) is not more intense than the spot in the chromatogram obtained with solution (2). Disregard any spot remaining on the line of application.

Loss on drying When dried at 100° to 105° for 4 hours, loses not more than 0.5% of its weight. Use 1 g.

Sulphated ash Not more than 0.1%, Appendix IX A, Method II. Use 1 g.

Assay Dissolve 0.15 g in 25 ml of *anhydrous glacial acetic acid* and carry out Method I for *non-aqueous titration*, Appendix VIII A, determining the end-point potentiometrically. Each ml of 0.1M *perchloric acid VS* is equivalent to 0.01954 g of $C_{16}H_{19}ClN_2,C_4H_4O_4$.

Storage Chlorpheniramine Maleate should be kept in a well-closed container and protected from light.

Preparations
Chlorpheniramine Oral Solution
Chlorpheniramine Injection
Chlorpheniramine Tablets

Action and use Histamine H₁-receptor antagonist.

The title of the monograph in the European Pharmacopœia is Chlorphenamine Maleate.

Chlorpromazine

$C_{17}H_{19}ClN_2S$ 318.9   *50-53-3*

Chlorpromazine is [3-(2-chloro-phenothiazin-10-yl)propyl]dimethylamine. It contains not less than 99.0 per cent and not more than 101.0 per cent of $C_{17}H_{19}ClN_2S$, calculated with reference to the dried substance.

Characteristics A white or creamy-white powder or waxy solid; odourless or almost odourless.

Solubility Practically insoluble in *water*; soluble in 2 parts of *ethanol (96%)*, in less than 1 part of *chloroform* and in 1 part of *ether*.

Identification A. The *infra-red absorption spectrum*, Appendix II A, is concordant with the *reference spectrum* of chlorpromazine.

B. The *light absorption*, Appendix II B, in the range 230 to 350 nm of a 0.001% w/v solution in *ethanol (96%)* exhibits two maxima, at 258 nm and 312 nm. The *absorbance* at 258 nm is about 1.15.

C. Complies with the test for *identification of phenothiazines*, Appendix III A, using *chlorpromazine hydrochloride EPCRS* to prepare solution (2).

D. Dissolve 5 mg in 5 ml of *sulphuric acid*; a cherry red colour is produced which darkens slowly on standing. Warm a portion of the solution; the colour changes to red and finally to magenta. To the remainder of the solution add 0.2 ml of 0.0167M *potassium dichromate*; the colour changes to brownish-red.

Melting point 56° to 58°, Appendix V A.

Related substances Complies with the test for *related substances in phenothiazines*, Appendix III A, using *mobile phase A*.

Loss on drying When dried to constant weight over *phosphorus pentoxide* at a pressure not exceeding 0.7 kPa, loses not more than 0.5% of its weight. Use 1 g.

Sulphated ash Not more than 0.1%, Appendix IX A.

Assay Dissolve 0.8 g in 300 ml of *acetone* and carry out Method I for *non-aqueous titration*, Appendix VIII A, using 3 ml of a saturated solution of *methyl orange* in *acetone* as indicator. Each ml of 0.1M *perchloric acid VS* is equivalent to 0.03189 g of $C_{17}H_{19}ClN_2S$.

Storage Chlorpromazine should be kept in a well-closed container and protected from light.

Preparation
Chlorpromazine Suppositories

Action and use Antipsychotic.

D. Yields *reaction B* characteristic of chlorides, Appendix VI.

Acidity pH of a freshly prepared 10% w/v solution, 3.5 to 4.5, Appendix V L.

Heavy metals 1.0 g complies with *limit test C for heavy metals*, Appendix VII (10 ppm). Use 1 ml of *lead standard solution (10 ppm Pb)* to prepare the standard.

Related substances Complies with the test for *related substances in phenothiazines*, Appendix III A, using *mobile phase A* but allowing the solvent front to ascend 15 cm above the line of application.

Loss on drying When dried to constant weight at 100° to 105°, loses not more than 0.5% of its weight. Use 1 g.

Sulphated ash Not more than 0.1%, Appendix IX A, Method II. Use 1 g.

Assay Dissolve 0.25 g in a mixture of 5 ml of 0.01M *hydrochloric acid VS* and 50 ml of *ethanol (96%)* and titrate with 0.1M *sodium hydroxide VS* determining the end-point potentiometrically. Calculate the volume of 0.1M *sodium hydroxide VS* added between the two inflections. Each ml of 0.1M *sodium hydroxide VS* is equivalent to 0.03553 g of $C_{17}H_{19}ClN_2S,HCl$.

Storage Chlorpromazine Hydrochloride should be kept in an airtight container and protected from light.

Preparations
Chlorpromazine Oral Solution
Chlorpromazine Injection
Chlorpromazine Tablets

Action and use Antipsychotic; antiemetic.

Chlorpromazine Hydrochloride ☆

$C_{17}H_{19}ClN_2S,HCl$ 355.3   *69-09-0*

Chlorpromazine Hydrochloride is [3-(2-chloro-phenothiazin-10-yl)propyl]dimethylamine hydrochloride. It contains not less than 99.0 per cent and not more than 101.0 per cent of $C_{17}H_{19}ClN_2S,HCl$, calculated with reference to the dried substance.

Characteristics A white or almost white, crystalline powder. It decomposes on exposure to air and light becoming yellow, pink and finally violet. It melts at about 196°.

Solubility Soluble in 0.4 part of *water*, in 1.3 parts of *ethanol (96%)* and in 1 part of *chloroform*; practically insoluble in *ether*.

Identification *Test A may be omitted if tests B, C and D are carried out. Test B may be omitted if tests A, C and D are carried out.*

A. The *infra-red absorption spectrum*, Appendix II A, is concordant with the spectrum of *chlorpromazine hydrochloride EPCRS*. Examine the substances as 6% w/v solutions in *dichloromethane* using a 0.1 mm cell.

B. The *light absorption*, Appendix II B, in the range 230 to 340 nm of a 0.0005% w/v solution in 0.1M *hydrochloric acid* exhibits two maxima, at 254 nm and at 306 nm. The A(1%, 1 cm) at the maximum at 254 nm is 890 to 960.

C. Complies with the test for *identification of phenothiazines*, Appendix III A.

Chlorpropamide

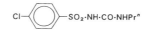

$C_{10}H_{13}ClN_2O_3S$ 276.7   *94-20-2*

Chlorpropamide is 1-(4-chlorobenzenesulph-onyl)-3-propylurea. It contains not less than 99.0 per cent and not more than 101.0 per cent of $C_{10}H_{13}ClN_2O_3S$, calculated with reference to the dried substance.

Characteristics A white, crystalline powder; odourless or almost odourless.

Solubility Practically insoluble in *water*; soluble in 12 parts of *ethanol (96%)*, in 9 parts of *chloroform* and in 5 parts of *acetone*; slightly soluble in *ether*. It dissolves in aqueous solutions of the alkali hydroxides.

Identification A. Dissolve 0.16 g in 50 ml of *methanol*, dilute 5 ml to 100 ml with 0.01M *hydrochloric acid* and dilute 10 ml of this solution to 100 ml with 0.01M *hydrochloric acid*. The *light absorption* of the resulting solution, Appendix II B, in the range 220 to 350 nm exhibits a maximum only at 232 nm. The *absorbance* at 232 nm is about 0.96.

B. Boil 0.1 g with 8 ml of a 50% w/w solution of *sulphuric acid* under a reflux condenser for 30 minutes, cool, filter and reserve the filtrate. The *melting point* of the precipitate, after recrystallisation from *water* and drying, is about 143°, Appendix V A.

C. Make the filtrate reserved in test B alkaline with 5M *sodium hydroxide* and heat. An ammoniacal odour is produced.

D. Heat 0.1 g with 1 g of *anhydrous sodium carbonate* at a dull red heat for 10 minutes. Cool, extract the residue with *water* and filter. Acidify the filtrate with 2M *nitric acid* and add *silver nitrate solution*. A white precipitate is produced.

Melting point 126° to 130°, Appendix V A.

Heavy metals Dissolve the residue obtained in the test for Sulphated ash in 10 ml of 2M *hydrochloric acid* with the aid of heat, cool and dilute to 20 ml with *water*. Make 5 ml alkaline with 5M *ammonia* and add 0.5 ml of a mixture of 1 volume of *sodium sulphide solution* and 19 volumes of *water*. No immediate darkening is produced.

Related substances Carry out the method for *thin-layer chromatography*, Appendix III A, using *silica gel G* as the coating substance and a mixture of 100 volumes of *chloroform*, 50 volumes of *methanol*, 30 volumes of *cyclohexane* and 11.5 volumes of 13.5M *ammonia* as the mobile phase. Apply separately to the chromatoplate 5 μl of each of four solutions in *acetone* containing (1) 6.0% w/v of the substance being examined, (2) 0.020% w/v of *4-chlorobenzenesulphonamide*, (3) 0.020% w/v of *1,3-dipropylurea BPCRS* and (4) 0.020% w/v of the substance being examined. After removal of the plate, dry it in a current of cold air, heat at 110° for 10 minutes, place the hot plate in a tank of chlorine gas prepared by the addition of *hydrochloric acid* to a 5% w/v solution of *potassium permanganate* contained in a beaker placed in the tank and allow to stand for 2 minutes. Dry it in a current of cold air until an area of the plate below the line of application gives at most a very faint blue colour with a 0.5% w/v solution of *potassium iodide* in *starch mucilage*; avoid prolonged exposure to cold air. Spray the plate with a 0.5% w/v solution of *potassium iodide* in *starch mucilage*. Any spots corresponding to 4-chlorobenzenesulphonamide and 1,3-dipropylurea in the chromatogram obtained with solution (1) are not more intense than the spots in the chromatograms obtained with solutions (2) and (3) respectively. Any other *secondary spot* in the chromatogram obtained with solution (1) is not more intense than the spot in the chromatogram obtained with solution (4).

Loss on drying When dried to constant weight at 105°, loses not more than 1.5% of its weight. Use 1 g.

Sulphated ash Not more than 0.1%, Appendix IX A. Use 2.0 g.

Assay Dissolve 0.5 g in 50 ml of *ethanol (96%)* previously neutralised to *phenolphthalein solution*, add 25 ml of *water* and titrate with 0.1M *sodium hydroxide VS* using *phenolphthalein solution* as indicator. Each ml of 0.1M *sodium hydroxide VS* is equivalent to 0.02767 g of $C_{10}H_{13}ClN_2O_3S$.

Preparation
Chlorpropamide Tablets

Action and use Hypoglycaemic.

Chlortetracycline Hydrochloride ☆

$C_{22}H_{23}ClN_2O_8,HCl$ 515.4   *64-72-2*

Chlortetracycline Hydrochloride is the hydrochloride of (4S,4aS,5aS,6S,12aS)-7-chloro-4-dimethylamino-1,4,4a,5,5a,6,11,12a-octahydro-3,6,10,12,12a-pentahydroxy-6-methyl-1,11-dioxonaphthacene-2-carboxamide, a substance produced by the growth of certain strains of *Streptomyces aureofaciens* or obtained by any other means. The potency is not less than 950 Units per mg, calculated with reference to the dried substance.

Characteristics Yellow crystals; odourless.

Solubility Slightly soluble in *water* and in *ethanol (96%)*.

Identification A. Complies with the test for *identification of tetracyclines*, Appendix III A, using the following solutions. Solution (1) contains 0.05% w/v each of the substance being examined, *demeclocycline hydrochloride EPCRS*, *doxycycline hyclate EPCRS*, *oxytetracycline hydrochloride EPCRS* and *tetracycline hydrochloride EPCRS*. Solution (2) contains 0.05% w/v each of *demeclocycline hydrochloride EPCRS*, *doxycycline hyclate EPCRS*, *oxytetracycline hydrochloride EPCRS* and *tetracycline hydrochloride EPCRS*.

B. A 0.1% w/v solution in 0.1M *sodium hydroxide* is yellow and exhibits a blue fluorescence when examined under ultra-violet light (365 nm).

C. To 2 mg add 5 ml of *sulphuric acid*; a deep blue colour is produced which changes to bluish-green. Add the solution to 2.5 ml of *water*; a brownish colour is produced.

D. Yields *reaction A* characteristic of chlorides, Appendix VI.

Acidity pH of a 1% w/v solution, 2.3 to 3.3, Appendix V L.

Light absorption Dissolve 10 mg in sufficient 0.01M *hydrochloric acid* to produce 100 ml and dilute 10 ml of the resulting solution to 100 ml with 0.01M *hydrochloric acid*. The A(1%, 1 cm) at 267 nm is 335 to 365 and the A(1%, 1 cm) at 367 nm is 195 to 220, Appendix II B.

Specific optical rotation In a 0.5% w/v solution, −235° to −250°, Appendix V F. Allow the solution to stand, protected from light, for 30 minutes before measurement.

Heavy metals 0.5 g complies with *limit test C for heavy metals*, Appendix VII (50 ppm). Use 2.5 ml of *lead standard solution (10 ppm Pb)* to prepare the standard.

Loss on drying When dried over *phosphorus pentoxide* at 60° at a pressure not exceeding 0.7 kPa for 3 hours, loses not more than 2.0% of its weight. Use 1 g.

Sulphated ash Not more than 0.5%, Appendix IX A, Method II. Use 1 g.

Assay Carry out the *biological assay of antibiotics*, Appendix XIV A. The precision of the assay is such that the fiducial limits of error are not less than 95% and not more than 105% of the estimated potency.

Storage Chlortetracycline Hydrochloride should be kept in a well-closed container and protected from light. If it is intended for use in the manufacture of a parenteral dosage form the container should be sterile, tamper-evident and sealed so as to exclude micro-organisms.

Labelling The label states (1) the date after which the material is not intended to be used; (2) the conditions under which it should be stored; (3) whether or not it is intended for use in the manufacture of a parenteral dosage form.

Preparations
Chlortetracycline Capsules
Chlortetracycline Eye Ointment

Action and use Antibacterial.

Chlortetracycline Hydrochloride intended for use in the manufacture of a parenteral dosage form complies with the following additional requirements.

Pyrogens Complies with the *test for pyrogens*, Appendix XIV K. Use per kg of the rabbit's weight 1 ml of *water for injections* containing 5 mg per ml of the substance being examined.

Sterility Complies with the *test for sterility*, Appendix XVI A.

Chlorthalidone

C₁₄H₁₁ClN₂O₄S   338.8   77-36-1

$C_{14}H_{11}ClN_2O_4S$ 338.8   77-36-1

Chlorthalidone is 2-chloro-5-(3-hydroxy-1-oxoisoindolin-3-yl)benzenesulphonamide. It contains not less than 98.0 per cent and not more than 102.0 per cent of $C_{14}H_{11}ClN_2O_4S$, calculated with reference to the dried substance.

Characteristics A white or creamy-white, crystalline powder; odourless or almost odourless.

Solubility Practically insoluble in *water*; slightly soluble in *ethanol (96%)*; soluble in 25 parts of *methanol*. It dissolves in solutions of alkali hydroxides.

Identification A. The *infra-red absorption spectrum*, Appendix II A, is concordant with the *reference spectrum* of chlorthalidone. If the spectra are not concordant, dissolve 0.1 g in 10 ml of warm *acetone* and cool. Add 20 ml of *water* and evaporate the acetone by heating on a water-bath for 20 minutes in a current of air. Cool to room temperature, allow to stand, filter, dry the crystals at 105° for 4 hours and prepare a new spectrum.
B. The *light absorption*, Appendix II B, in the range 230 to 350 nm of a 0.02% w/v solution in *ethanol (96%)* exhibits two maxima, at 275 nm and 284 nm. The *absorbance* at 275 nm is about 1.1 and at 284 nm is about 0.87.
C. Burn 20 mg by the method for *oxygen-flask combustion*, Appendix VIII C, using 5 ml of 1.25M *sodium hydroxide* as the absorbing liquid. When the process is complete, dilute the liquid to 25 ml with *water*. To 5 ml of the resulting solution add 0.1 ml of *hydrogen peroxide solution (100 vol)*

and 1 ml of 1M *hydrochloric acid*, mix and add 0.05 ml of *barium chloride solution*; the solution becomes turbid. Acidify a further 5 ml of the solution obtained as described above with 1M *sulphuric acid* and boil gently for 2 minutes; the solution yields *reaction A* characteristic of chlorides, Appendix VI.
D. Dissolve 50 mg in 3 ml of *sulphuric acid*. An intense yellow colour is produced.
E. *Melting point*, about 220°, with decomposition, Appendix V A.

Clarity and colour of solution Dissolve 1.0 g in sufficient 1.25M *sodium hydroxide* to produce 10 ml. The solution is *clear*, Appendix IV A, and not more intensely coloured than 10 ml of a solution prepared by mixing 1.50 ml of *iron(III) chloride solution CT*, 0.40 ml of *cobalt(II) chloride solution CT* and sufficient of a mixture of 1 volume of *hydrochloric acid* and 39 volumes of *water* to produce 100 ml.

Related substances Carry out the method for *thin-layer chromatography*, Appendix III A, using *silica gel GF254* as the coating substance and a mixture of 75 volumes of *butan-1-ol* and 15 volumes of 1M *ammonia* as the mobile phase. Apply separately to the chromatoplate 10 µl of each of two solutions in *acetone* containing (1) 1.0% w/v of the substance being examined and (2) 0.010% w/v of *2-(4-chloro-3-sulphamoylbenzoyl)benzoic acid BPCRS*. After removal of the plate, allow it to dry in air and examine under *ultra-violet light (254 nm)*. Any *secondary spot* in the chromatogram obtained with solution (1) is not more intense than the spot in the chromatogram obtained with solution (2).

Chloride Shake 0.30 g with 30 ml of *water* for 5 minutes and filter. 15 ml of the filtrate complies with the *limit test for chlorides*, Appendix VII (350 ppm).

Loss on drying When dried to constant weight at 105°, loses not more than 0.5% of its weight. Use 1 g.

Sulphated ash Not more than 0.1%, Appendix IX A.

Assay Dissolve 0.3 g in 50 ml of *anhydrous pyridine* and carry out Method II for *non-aqueous titration*, Appendix VIII A, using 0.1M *tetrabutylammonium hydroxide VS* as titrant and determining the end-point potentiometrically. Each ml of 0.1M *tetrabutylammonium hydroxide VS* is equivalent to 0.03388 g of $C_{14}H_{11}ClN_2O_4S$.

Preparation
Chlorthalidone Tablets

Action and use Diuretic.

In some countries the material described in this monograph may be known as Chlortalidone.

Cholecalciferol ☆

C$_{27}$H$_{44}$O   384.7   *67-97-0*

Cholecalciferol is (5*Z*,7*E*)-(3*S*)-9,10-secocholesta-5,7,10(19)-trien-3-ol.

Characteristics White or almost white crystals; odourless or almost odourless. It is sensitive to air, heat and light.

Solubility Practically insoluble in *water*; freely soluble in *ethanol (96%)*, in *acetone*, in *chloroform* and in *ether*; soluble in fixed oils. Solutions in volatile solvents are unstable and should be used immediately.

Identification A. The *infra-red absorption spectrum*, Appendix II A, is concordant with the spectrum of *cholecalciferol EPCRS*.

B. Dissolve 1 mg in 40 ml of *1,2-dichloroethane* and to 1 ml of the solution add 4 ml of *antimony trichloride reagent*. An orange colour is produced which gradually becomes pink.

C. *Melting point*, 82° to 87° when determined on the substance being examined without powdering and drying, Appendix V A, Method I.

Light absorption Dissolve 0.1 g, without warming, in *aldehyde-free ethanol (96%)* and dilute progressively with *aldehyde-free ethanol (96%)* to produce a solution containing 0.001% w/v of cholecalciferol. The *absorbance* of the solution at the maximum at 265 nm, measured within 30 minutes of preparation, is 0.46 to 0.50, Appendix II B. It does not differ by more than 3% from the *absorbance* of a reference solution prepared at the same time and in the same manner using 0.1 g of *cholecalciferol EPCRS*.

Specific optical rotation Dissolve 0.2 g rapidly and without heating in sufficient *aldehyde-free ethanol (96%)* to produce 25 ml. The *specific optical rotation*, determined in the resulting solution within 30 minutes of preparation, is +105° to +112°, Appendix V F.

7-Dehydrocholesterol Carry out the method for *thin-layer chromatography*, Appendix III A, using *silica gel G* as the coating substance and a 0.01% w/v solution of *butylated hydroxytoluene* in a mixture of equal volumes of *cyclohexane* and *peroxide-free ether* as the mobile phase. Apply separately to the chromatoplate 10 µl of each of solutions (1), (2) and (3) and 20 µl of solution (4), each solution being prepared immediately before use. Solution (1) contains 2.5% w/v of the substance being examined in *1,2-dichloroethane* containing 1% w/v of *squalane* and 0.01% w/v of *butylated hydroxytoluene* (solvent S). Solution (2) contains 0.0050% w/v of *7-dehydrocholesterol EPCRS* in solvent S. Solution (3) contains 2.5% w/v of *cholecalciferol EPCRS* in solvent S. For solution (4) mix equal volumes of solutions (2) and (3). Develop the chromatogram immediately, protected from light. After removal of the plate, allow it to dry in air, spray three times with *antimony trichloride reagent* and examine it for 3

to 4 minutes after spraying. The principal spot in the chromatogram obtained with solution (1) is initially yellowish-orange and then becomes brown (cholecalciferol); any violet spot immediately below the principal spot corresponding in Rf value to 7-dehydrocholesterol is not more intense than the spot due to 7-dehydrocholesterol in the chromatogram obtained with solution (2). The total number of spots in the chromatogram obtained with solution (1) is not more than the sum of the numbers of spots in the chromatograms obtained with solutions (2) and (3). The test is not valid unless the chromatogram obtained with solution (4) shows two clearly separated spots.

Storage Cholecalciferol should be kept in a hermetically sealed container, the air in which has been replaced by an inert gas, protected from light and stored at a temperature of 2° to 8°. The contents of an opened container should be used immediately.

In some countries the material described in this monograph may be known as Colecalciferol.

Preparations
Calciferol Oral Solution
Calciferol Injection
Calciferol Tablets

Cholecalciferol Concentrate (Oily Form) ☆

Cholecalciferol Concentrate (Oily Form) is a solution of Cholecalciferol in a suitable vegetable oil. It contains in 1 g not less than 500,000 Units and not less than 90.0 per cent and not more than 110.0 per cent of the number of Units stated on the label. It may contain suitable stabilising agents such as antioxidants.

Characteristics A clear, yellow liquid; odour, slight. Partial solidification may occur, depending on the temperature.

Solubility Practically insoluble in *water*; slightly soluble in *absolute ethanol*; miscible with solvents of fats.

Identification A. The *light absorption*, Appendix II B, in the range 250 to 300 nm of a solution in *cyclohexane UV* containing about 400 Units per ml exhibits a maximum only at 267 nm.

B. Carry out the method for *thin-layer chromatography*, Appendix III A, using *silica gel G* as the coating substance and a 0.01% w/v solution of *butylated hydroxytoluene* in a mixture of equal volumes of *cyclohexane* and *peroxide-free ether* as the mobile phase. Apply separately to the chromatoplate 20 µl of each of the following solutions prepared immediately before use. For solution (1) evaporate 100 ml of solution A obtained in the Assay to dryness at a pressure of 1.5 to 2.5 kPa by swirling the flask in a water-bath at 40°, cool under running water and restore atmospheric pressure with nitrogen. Dissolve the residue immediately in 0.4 ml of *1,2-dichloroethane* containing 1% w/v of *squalane* and 0.01% w/v of *butylated hydroxytoluene* (solvent S). For solution (2) dissolve 10 mg of *cholecalciferol EPCRS* in sufficient solvent S to produce 4 ml. For solution (3) dissolve 10 mg of *ergocalciferol*

EPCRS in sufficient solvent S to produce 4 ml. Develop the chromatogram immediately, protected from light. After removal of the plate, allow it to dry in air and spray with *sulphuric acid*. The chromatogram obtained with solution (1) immediately shows a bright yellow principal spot which rapidly becomes orange-brown, then gradually greenish-grey and remains so for 10 minutes. This spot corresponds in position, colour and size to the spot in the chromatogram obtained with solution (2). The chromatogram obtained with solution (3) immediately shows an orange principal spot with the same Rf value as the spot in the chromatogram obtained with solution (2); it gradually becomes reddish-brown and remains so for 10 minutes.

C. Dissolve a quantity containing 1000 Units in 1 ml of *1,2-dichloroethane* and add 4 ml of *antimony trichloride reagent*. An orange colour is rapidly produced which gradually becomes pink.

Irradiation by-products Carry out the test immediately after test B for Identification. Carry out the method for *thin-layer chromatography*, Appendix III A, using *silica gel G* as the coating substance and a 0.01% w/v solution of *butylated hydroxytoluene* in a mixture of equal volumes of *cyclohexane* and *peroxide-free ether* as the mobile phase. Apply separately to the chromatoplate 20 μl of each of solutions (1) and (2) prescribed in test B for Identification. Develop the chromatogram immediately, protected from light. After removal of the plate, allow it to dry in air and spray three times with *antimony trichloride reagent*. The principal spot in the chromatogram obtained with solution (1) is initially orange and then becomes brown (cholecalciferol); it corresponds in position, colour and size to the spot in the chromatogram obtained with solution (2). The chromatogram obtained with solution (1) also shows another spot of the same colour with an Rf value slightly higher than that of the principal spot, corresponding to precholecalciferol which in solution is in equilibrium with cholecalciferol. The chromatogram obtained with solution (1) does not show a greyish-blue spot on the line of application or streaking towards the principal spot.

Acid value Not more than 2.0, Appendix X B. Use 5 g dissolved in 25 ml of the prescribed mixture of solvents.

Peroxide value Not more than 20, Appendix X F.

Assay Carry out the assay as rapidly as possible avoiding exposure to light and air. Prepare two solutions, A and B, in the following manner.

To a quantity of the substance being examined containing 100,000 Units, weighed with an accuracy of 0.1%, add 20 ml of *absolute ethanol*, 1 ml of *sodium ascorbate solution* and 3 ml of a freshly prepared 50% w/w solution of *potassium hydroxide* and heat under a reflux condenser on a water-bath for 30 minutes. Cool rapidly under running water and transfer the liquid to a separating funnel using two 15-ml quantities of *water*, one 10-ml quantity of *ethanol (96%)* and two 50-ml quantities of n-*pentane*. Shake vigorously for 30 seconds, allow to stand until the two layers are clear and then transfer the lower, aqueous alcoholic layer to a second separating funnel and shake with a mixture of 10 ml of *ethanol (96%)* and 50 ml of n-*pentane*. After separation, transfer the aqueous alcoholic layer to a third separating funnel and the pentane layer to the first separating funnel, washing the second separating funnel with two 10-ml quantities of n-*pentane* and adding the washings to the first separating

funnel. Shake the aqueous alcoholic layer with 50 ml of n-*pentane* and add the pentane layer to the first funnel. Wash the pentane layers with two 50-ml quantities of a freshly prepared 3% w/v solution of *potassium hydroxide* in *ethanol (10%)*, shaking vigorously, and then wash with successive 50-ml quantities of *water* until the washings are neutral to *phenolphthalein*. Transfer the washed pentane extract to a graduated flask, rinsing the separating funnel with 10 ml of n-*pentane*, and dilute to 250 ml with the same solvent (solution A).

Evaporate 50 ml of solution A to dryness at a pressure of 1.5 to 2.5 kPa while swirling the flask in a water-bath at 40°, cool under running water and restore atmospheric pressure with nitrogen. Dissolve the residue immediately in 2 ml of a 5% w/v solution of *maleic anhydride* in *toluene*, allow to stand at room temperature in the dark for 30 minutes, add 50 ml of *2,2,4-trimethylpentane*, transfer the solution to a graduated flask using *2,2,4-trimethylpentane* and dilute to 100 ml with the same solvent (solution B).

Prepare a reference solution in the following manner. Dissolve 25 mg of *cholecalciferol EPCRS* in 2 ml of *toluene* and dilute to 100 ml with a 0.05% w/v solution of *butylated hydroxytoluene* in *2,2,4-trimethylpentane*. (This solution is stable for 1 month if kept in the dark at a temperature not exceeding 20°.) Dilute 2 ml of the solution to 100 ml with a 2% v/v solution of *toluene* in *2,2,4-trimethylpentane*.

Colorimetric determination Because of the sensitivity of *antimony trichloride reagent* to moisture, the spectrophotometer cells or colorimeter tubes used should be perfectly dry. If a spectrophotometer is employed, use matched 2-cm cells; if a colorimeter is used, it must be provided with an interference filter having a maximum transmission at about 500 nm and matched colorimeter tubes of internal diameter about 2 cm.

Introduce 2 ml of solution B into a tube and 2 ml of the reference solution into another identical tube. To each tube add quickly 5 ml of *antimony trichloride reagent* and mix. Using the reference solution, determine beforehand the time necessary for the development of maximum intensity of colour, which may vary from 45 seconds to 120 seconds. Measure, after the same interval, the *absorbance* of the two solutions at 500 nm, Appendix II B, using in the reference cell a mixture of 2 ml of a 2% v/v solution of *toluene* in *2,2,4-trimethylpentane* and 5 ml of *antimony trichloride reagent*. Repeat the determinations twice using fresh portions of solution B and the reference solution. Calculate the average absorbances obtained with solution B and with the reference solution.

Calculate the content of cholecalciferol in Units per g from the expression CVA_1/wA_2 where C is the number of Units per ml in the reference solution, w is the weight in g of the substance being examined, V is the volume of solution B corresponding to the whole of the solution being examined (500 ml) and A_1 and A_2 are the average absorbances of solution B and the reference solution respectively.

Storage Cholecalciferol Concentrate (Oily Form) should be kept in an airtight, well-filled container, protected from light and stored at a temperature of 8° to 15°. The contents of an opened container should be used as soon as possible; any unused part should be protected by an atmosphere of nitrogen.

Labelling The label states (1) the number of Units per g; (2) the method of restoring the solution if partial solidification occurs; (3) the nature and maximum concentration of any added stabilising agents.

Cholecalciferol Concentrate (Powder Form) ☆

Cholecalciferol Concentrate (Powder Form) is obtained by dispersing an oily solution of Cholecalciferol in an appropriate matrix which is usually a basis of gelatin and carbohydrates of suitable quality. It contains in 1 g not less than 100,000 Units and not less than 90.0 per cent and not more than 110.0 per cent of the number of Units stated on the label. It may contain suitable stabilising agents such as antioxidants.

Characteristics Almost white, small particles; odourless or almost odourless.

Solubility Depending on the formulation, may be practically insoluble in *water* or may swell or form a dispersion.

Identification A. The *light absorption*, Appendix II B, in the range 250 to 300 nm of solution A prepared as described under the Assay exhibits a maximum only at 265 nm. Use n-*pentane* in the reference cell.

B. Complies with test B for Identification described under Cholecalciferol Concentrate (Oily Form).

C. Evaporate a portion of solution A containing about 1000 Units to dryness under nitrogen, dissolve the residue in 1 ml of *1,2-dichloroethane* and add 4 ml of *antimony trichloride reagent*. An orange colour is rapidly produced which gradually becomes pink.

Irradiation by-products Complies with the test described under Cholecalciferol Concentrate (Oily Form).

Assay To a quantity of the substance being examined containing 100,000 Units, weighed with an accuracy of 0.1%, add 5 ml of *water* and carry out the Assay described under Cholecalciferol Concentrate (Oily Form), beginning at the words 'add 20 ml of *absolute ethanol*. . .'.

Storage Complies with the requirements stated under Cholecalciferol Concentrate (Oily Form).

Labelling The label on the container states (1) the number of Units per g; (2) the nature and maximum concentration of any added stabilising agents.

Choline Salicylate Solution

Choline Salicylate Solution is an aqueous solution of choline salicylate. It contains not less than 47.5 per cent w/v and not more than 52.5 per cent w/v of choline salicylate, $C_{12}H_{19}NO_4$. It may contain a suitable anti-microbial preservative.

Characteristics A clear, colourless liquid.

Identification A. Mix 0.5 ml with 10 ml of *methanol*, dry with *anhydrous sodium sulphate*, filter and evaporate the *methanol*. The *infra-red absorption spectrum* of the residue, Appendix II A, is concordant with the *reference spectrum* of choline salicylate.

B. To 2 ml add 3 ml of *5M sodium hydroxide* and heat to boiling. The odour of trimethylamine is produced.

C. Dilute 5 ml to 25 ml with *water*. The resulting solution yields the *reactions* characteristic of salicylates, Appendix VI.

Acidity Dilute 4 ml to 20 ml with *water* and add 0.1 ml of *phenol red solution*. The solution is yellow and not more than 0.4 ml of *0.1M sodium hydroxide VS* is required to change the colour of the solution to reddish-violet.

Clarity and colour of solution Dilute 1 volume of the solution to 5 volumes with *water*. The resulting solution is *clear*, Appendix IV A, and *colourless*, Appendix IV B, Method II.

Weight per ml 1.070 to 1.110 g, Appendix V G.

Chloride Mix 0.2 ml with 10 ml of *water* and add carefully, with mixing, 0.1 ml of a mixture of 10 volumes of *silver nitrate solution* and 1 volume of *nitric acid*. The resulting solution is not more opalescent than a standard prepared by treating 10 ml of a 0.00164% w/v solution of *sodium chloride* in the same manner beginning at the words 'add carefully . . .' (0.1%).

Assay To 1 g add 50 ml of *1,4-dioxan* and 5 ml of *acetic anhydride* and carry out Method I for *non-aqueous titration*, Appendix VIII A, using 0.25 ml of *methyl orange—xylene cyanol FF solution* as indicator. Each ml of *0.1M perchloric acid VS* is equivalent to 0.02413 g of $C_{12}H_{19}NO_4$. Use the *weight per ml* to calculate the percentage of $C_{12}H_{19}NO_4$, weight in volume.

Storage Choline Salicylate Solution should be kept in a well-closed container.

Preparations
Choline Salicylate Ear Drops
Choline Salicylate Dental Gel

Choline Theophyllinate

$C_{12}H_{21}N_5O_3$ 283.3   *4499-40-5*

Choline Theophyllinate is choline 1,2,3,6-tetrahydro-1,3-dimethyl-2,6-dioxo-7*H*-purin-7-ide. It contains not less than 41.9 per cent and not more than 43.6 per cent of choline, $C_5H_{15}NO_2$, and not less than 61.7 per cent and not more than 65.5 per cent of theophylline, $C_7H_9N_4O_2$, each calculated with reference to the dried substance.

Characteristics A white, crystalline powder; odourless or with a faint amine-like odour.

Solubility Very soluble in *water*; soluble in 10 parts of *ethanol (96%)*; very slightly soluble in *ether* and in *chloroform*.

Identification A. The *infra-red absorption spectrum*, Appendix II A, is concordant with the *reference spectrum* of choline theophyllinate.

B. The *light absorption*, Appendix II B, in the range 230 to 350 nm of a 0.002% w/v solution in 0.01M *sodium hydroxide* exhibits a maximum only at 275 nm. The *absorbance* at 275 nm is about 0.83.

C. Dissolve 0.5 g in 2 ml of *water*, add 3 ml of *5M sodium hydroxide* and heat to boiling. The odour of trimethylamine is produced.

D. Dissolve 10 mg in 1 ml of *hydrochloric acid*, add 0.1 g of *potassium chlorate* and evaporate to dryness in a porcelain dish. A reddish residue remains, which becomes purple on exposure to ammonia vapour.

Melting point 187° to 192°, Appendix V A.

Clarity and colour of solution 50 ml of a 10% w/v solution is *clear*, Appendix IV A, and not more intensely coloured than *reference solution GY₄*, Appendix IV B, Method I.

Related substances Carry out the method for *thin-layer chromatography*, Appendix III A, using *silica gel HF254* as the coating substance and a mixture of 95 volumes of *chloroform* and 5 volumes of *ethanol (96%)* as the mobile phase. Apply separately to the chromatoplate 5 µl of each of two solutions of the substance being examined in *ethanol (96%)* containing (1) 1.0% w/v and (2) 0.010% w/v. After removal of the plate, allow it to dry in air and examine under *ultra-violet light (254 nm)*. Any *secondary spot* in the chromatogram obtained with solution (1) is not more intense than the spot in the chromatogram obtained with solution (2).

Loss on drying When dried to constant weight at 105°, loses not more than 0.5% of its weight. Use 1 g.

Sulphated ash Not more than 0.1%, Appendix IX A.

Assay *For choline* Dissolve 0.6 g in 50 ml of *water* and titrate with 0.05M *sulphuric acid VS*, using *methyl red—methylene blue solution* as indicator, until a violet end-point is obtained. Each ml of 0.05M *sulphuric acid VS* is equivalent to 0.01212 g of choline, C₅H₁₅NO₂.

For theophylline To the solution obtained in the Assay for choline, add 25 ml of 0.1M *silver nitrate VS* and warm on a water-bath for 15 minutes. Cool in ice for 30 minutes, filter and wash the residue with three 10-ml quantities of *water*. Titrate the combined filtrate and washings with 0.1M *sodium hydroxide VS*. Each ml of 0.1M *sodium hydroxide VS* is equivalent to 0.01802 g of theophylline, C₇H₈N₄O₂.

Storage Choline Theophyllinate should be kept in a well-closed container, protected from light and stored at a temperature not exceeding 25°.

Preparation
Choline Theophyllinate Tablets

Action and use Xanthine bronchodilator.

Chorionic Gonadotrophin ☆

Chorionic Gonadotrophin is a dry, sterile preparation of placental glycoproteins that has luteinising activity. It is extracted from the urine of pregnant women. The purified material is sterilised by *Filtration* and dried under reduced pressure or freeze dried. It contains not less than 2500 Units per mg.

Characteristics A white or almost white, amorphous powder.

Solubility Soluble in *water*.

Identification Causes an increase in the weight of the seminal vesicles or of the prostate glands of immature male rats when administered as directed in the Assay.

Water Not more than 5% w/w when determined by the method for *gas chromatography*, Appendix III B, using

throughout dry glassware which may be siliconised and the following solutions. For solution (1) dilute 15 µl of *anhydrous methanol* (internal standard) with sufficient *anhydrous propan-2-ol* to produce 100 ml. For solution (2) dissolve 4 mg of the substance being examined in 0.5 ml of *anhydrous propan-2-ol*. For solution (3) dissolve 4 mg of the substance being examined in 0.5 ml of solution (1). For solution (4) add 10 µl of *water* to 50 ml of solution (1).

The chromatographic procedure may be carried out using a stainless-steel column (1 m × 2 mm) packed with porous polymer beads (60 to 80 mesh) (Chromosorb 102 is suitable), maintained at 120°, helium as the carrier gas and a thermal conductivity detector, maintained at 150°.

From the chromatograms obtained, and taking into account any water detectable in solution (1), calculate the percentage w/w of water taking 0.9972 g as the weight per ml at 20°.

Assay Carry out the *biological assay of chorionic gonadotrophin*, Appendix XIV C3. The estimated potency is not less than 80% and not more than 125% of the stated potency. The fiducial limits of error are not less than 64% and not more than 156% of the stated potency.

Storage Chorionic Gonadotrophin should be kept in an airtight container, protected from light and stored at a temperature not exceeding 20°. Under these conditions it may be expected to retain its potency for not less than 3 years.

If the contents are intended for use in the manufacture of a parenteral dosage form the container should be sterile, tamper-evident and sealed so as to exclude micro-organisms.

Labelling The label states (1) the number of Units in the container; (2) the number of Units per mg; (3) the date after which the material is not intended to be used; (4) the conditions under which it should be stored; (5) whether or not it is intended for use in the manufacture of a parenteral dosage form.

Preparation
Chorionic Gonadotrophin Injection

Action and use Gonadotrophic hormone.

Chorionic Gonadotrophin intended for use in the manufacture of a parenteral dosage form complies with the following additional requirements.

Abnormal toxicity Complies with the *test for abnormal toxicity*, Appendix XIV L. Use a quantity containing 1000 Units dissolved in 0.5 ml of *sodium chloride injection*.

Pyrogens Complies with the *test for pyrogens*, Appendix XIV K. Use per kg of the rabbit's weight, 1 ml of a solution in *sodium chloride injection* containing 300 Units per ml.

Sterility Complies with the *test for sterility*, Appendix XVI A.

Chymotrypsin ☆

Chymotrypsin is a proteolytic enzyme obtained by the activation of chymotrypsinogen extracted from ox (*Bos taurus* L.) pancreas. It contains not less than 5.0 microkatals per mg. In solution it has maximal enzymatic activity at about pH 8; the activity is reversibly inhibited at pH 3, at which pH it is most stable. It is prepared in conditions designed to minimise microbial contamination.

Characteristics A white, crystalline or amorphous powder. The amorphous form is hygroscopic.

Solubility Sparingly soluble in *water*.

Identification A. Prepare a substrate solution as follows. Add 0.2 ml of *ethanol (96%)* to 24.0 mg of *ethyl N-acetyl-L-tyrosinate*, swirl until the substance dissolves, add 2 ml of *0.067M mixed phosphate buffer pH 7.0* and 1 ml of *methyl red—methylene blue solution* and dilute to 10 ml with *water*. In a depression on a white spot plate mix 0.2 ml of this solution with 0.05 ml of a 0.1% w/v solution of the substance being examined in *carbon dioxide-free water*. A purple colour is produced.
B. To 5 ml of a 0.1% w/v solution in *carbon dioxide-free water* add 0.1 ml of a 2% w/v solution of *L-α-tosylaminophenethyl chloromethyl ketone* in *ethanol (96%)*. Adjust the pH to 7.0 and shake for 2 hours. In a depression on a white spot plate mix 0.05 ml of the resulting solution with 0.2 ml of the substrate solution prepared as described in test A. No colour is produced within 3 minutes of mixing.

Acidity pH of a 1% w/v solution, 3.0 to 5.0, Appendix V L.

Clarity of solution A 1% w/v solution in *carbon dioxide-free water* is not more than *slightly opalescent*, Appendix IV A, Method I.

Light absorption The *light absorption*, Appendix II B, of a 0.03% w/v solution in *0.001M hydrochloric acid* exhibits a maximum at 281 nm and a minimum at 250 nm. The A(1%, 1 cm) at 281 nm is 18.5 to 22.5 and at 250 nm is not more than 8.

Trypsin Prepare a substrate solution as follows. Add 5 ml of *tris—chloride buffer pH 8.1* to 98.5 mg of *methyl N-tosyl-L-arginate hydrochloride*, suitable for assaying trypsin, swirl until the substance dissolves, add 2.5 ml of *methyl red—methylene blue solution* and dilute to 25.0 ml with *water*. Transfer to a depression on a white-spot plate 0.05 ml of *tris—chloride buffer pH 8.1* and 0.10 ml of a 1.00% w/v solution of the substance being examined. Add 0.2 ml of the substrate solution and start a timer. No colour is produced within 3 to 5 minutes of the addition of the substrate solution. Carry out at the same time a control test using the substance being examined to which not more than 1% w/w of *trypsin EPBRP* has been added; a purple colour is produced.

Loss on drying When dried at 60° at a pressure not exceeding 0.7 kPa for 2 hours, loses not more than 5.0% of its weight. Use 0.1 g.

Histamine Not more than 1 μg (calculated as histamine base) per 5 microkatals of chymotrypsin activity, Appendix XIV N. Before carrying out the test, heat the solution of the substance being examined on a water-bath for 30 minutes.

Assay Carry out the *assay of chymotrypsin*, Appendix XIV E1.

Storage Chymotrypsin should be kept in an airtight container, protected from light and stored at a temperature of 2° to 8°.

Labelling The label states (1) the quantity of chymotrypsin and the total activity in microkatals in the container ; (2) when the contents are amorphous, that they are hygroscopic.

Action and use Proteolytic enzyme.

Cinchocaine Hydrochloride

$C_{20}H_{29}N_3O_2,HCl$ 379.9   *61-12-1*

Cinchocaine Hydrochloride is 2-butoxy-*N*-(2-diethylaminoethyl)quinoline-4-carboxamide hydrochloride. It contains not less than 99.0 per cent and not more than 101.0 per cent of $C_{20}H_{29}N_3O_2,HCl$, calculated with reference to the anhydrous substance.

Characteristics Fine, white crystals; odourless or almost odourless; hygroscopic.

Solubility Soluble in 0.5 part of *water*; freely soluble in *ethanol (96%)*; soluble in *chloroform*.

Identification A. The *infra-red absorption spectrum*, Appendix II A, is concordant with the *reference spectrum* of cinchocaine hydrochloride.
B. The *light absorption*, Appendix II B, in the range 230 to 350 nm of a 0.002% w/v solution in *1M hydrochloric acid* exhibits two maxima, at 247 nm and 319 nm. The *absorbance* at 247 nm is about 1.3 and at 319 nm is about 0.47.
C. Dissolve 0.1 g in 10 ml of *water*, add 1 ml of *5M sodium hydroxide* and shake with two 5-ml quantities of *petroleum spirit (boiling range, 40° to 60°)*. Wash the mixed extracts with *water* and remove the petroleum spirit in a current of air. The *melting point* of the residue is about 64°, Appendix V A.
D. To 5 ml of a 5% w/v solution add 10 ml of a saturated solution of *potassium perchlorate* and cool in ice for 10 minutes. The *melting point* of the precipitate, after recrystallisation from *water* and drying at 80° for 2 hours, is about 132°, Appendix V A.
E. Yields the *reactions* characteristic of chlorides, Appendix VI.

Acidity pH of a 2% w/v solution, 5.0 to 6.0, Appendix V L.

Related substances Carry out the method for *thin-layer chromatography*, Appendix III A, using a silica gel precoated chromatoplate (Merck silica gel 60 plates are suitable) and a mixture of 60 volumes of *butan-1-ol*, 30 volumes of *water* and 15 volumes of *glacial acetic acid* as the mobile phase. Apply separately to the plate 5 μl of each of two solutions of the substance being examined in *methanol* containing (1) 4.0% w/v and (2) 0.020% w/v. After removal of the plate, allow it to dry in a current of warm air, spray with *potassium dichromate reagent* and examine under *ultra-violet light (365 nm)*. Any *secondary spot* in the chromatogram obtained with solution (1) is not more intense than the spot in the chromatogram obtained with solution (2).

Water Not more than 2.5% w/w, Appendix IX C. Use 1 g.

Sulphated ash Not more than 0.1%, Appendix IX A.

Assay Carry out Method I for *non-aqueous titration*, Appendix VIII A, using 0.4 g and *crystal violet solution* as indicator. Each ml of 0.1M *perchloric acid VS* is equivalent to 0.01900 g of $C_{20}H_{29}N_3O_2,HCl$.

Storage Cinchocaine Hydrochloride should be kept in a well-closed container.

Action and use Local anaesthetic.

Cinchona Bark ☆

Cinchona; Red Cinchona Bark

Cinchona Bark consists of the dried bark of *Cinchona pubescens* Vahl (*Cinchona succirubra* Pavon) or of its varieties or its hybrids. It contains not less than 6.5 per cent of total alkaloids, of which 30 to 60 per cent are alkaloids of the quinine group.

Characteristics Odour, slight and characteristic.

Macroscopical The stem bark occurs in quills or curved pieces up to 30 cm or more long and 2 to 6 mm thick; outer surface dull, grey or brownish-grey, often bearing lichen, usually rough, being marked with transverse fissures, longitudinally furrowed or wrinkled and fissured; in some varieties the outer bark may be exfoliated; inner surface, deep reddish-brown, striated; fracture, short in the outer part, fibrous in the inner part. Root bark, irregularly channelled, curved or twisted pieces about 2 to 7 cm long; outer surface somewhat scaly, inner surface more or less striated; both surfaces deep reddish-brown, similar to the colour of the inner surface of the stem bark; fracture fibrous.

Microscopical In transverse section the cork shows several layers of relatively thin-walled cells with reddish-brown contents; cortex narrow, composed of tangentially elongated, pitted cells containing starch granules, 6 to 10 µm in diameter, or amorphous reddish-brown matter, with scattered idioblasts containing microprisms of calcium oxalate and large secretory cells, 100 to 350 µm in diameter, spaced at intervals near the inner part; phloem, sieve tubes narrow, with transverse sieve plates and phloem parenchyma which resembles that of the cortex and with large, characteristic spindle-shaped phloem fibres, up to 90 µm in diameter (usually 40 to 70 µm), with thick, conspicuously striated walls traversed by funnel-shaped pits occurring isolated or in irregular radial rows; medullary rays, two to three cells wide, with thin-walled, somewhat radially elongated cells; sclereids rare; secretory cells absent from the root bark.

Identification A. Carry out the method for *thin-layer chromatography*, Appendix III A, using *silica gel G* as the coating substance and a mixture of 90 volumes of *chloroform* and 10 volumes of *diethylamine* as the mobile phase. Apply separately to the chromatoplate, at 2-cm intervals, 1 µl and 2 µl of each of the following solutions. For solution (1) add 0.1 ml of 13.5M *ammonia* and 5 ml of *chloroform* to 0.1 g, in *No. 180 powder*, allow to stand for 30 minutes, occasionally shaking vigorously, and filter; evaporate the filtrate to dryness on a water-bath and dissolve the residue in 1 ml of *absolute ethanol*. For solution (2) dissolve 17.5 mg of *quinine*, 0.5 mg of *quinidine*, 10 mg of *cinchonine* and 10 mg of *cinchonidine* in 5 ml of *absolute ethanol*.

After removal of the plate, dry it at 100° to 105° for about 10 minutes, until the odour of diethylamine is no longer detectable, cool, spray with *anhydrous formic acid* and examine under *ultra-violet light (365 nm)*. The spots corresponding to quinine and quinidine show a distinct blue fluorescence. Spray with *potassium iodoplatinate reagent*. The chromatograms obtained with solution (2) show three violet spots, later becoming violet-grey, due to quinine (Rf value 0.2 to 0.3), quinidine (Rf value 0.3 to 0.4) and cinchonine (Rf value 0.4 to 0.5). Cinchonidine shows as an intense dark blue spot with an Rf value slightly less than that of quinidine. The chromatograms obtained with solution (1) show spots corresponding in position to, and having about the same intensity as, the spots due to quinine, quinidine, cinchonine and cinchonidine in the chromatograms obtained with the same volumes of solution (2).

B. Carefully heat 0.5 g, in powder, in a test-tube over an open flame; blood-red droplets condense on the side of the tube. Allow to cool and dissolve the drops in 10 ml of *ethanol (70%)*; the resulting solution shows a blue fluorescence when examined under ultra-violet light (365 nm).

C. Shake 0.1 g, in powder, for 1 minute with 5 ml of 1M *sulphuric acid* and filter. To 1 ml of the filtrate add 0.2 ml of *potassium mercuri-iodide solution*; a precipitate is produced. Dilute the remainder of the filtrate to 10 ml with *water*; the resulting solution, when examined under ultra-violet light (365 nm), shows a blue fluorescence which disappears on the addition of *hydrochloric acid*.

Foreign matter Not more than 2%, Appendix XI D, Test B.

Sulphated ash Not more than 4.0%, Appendix IX A, Method II. Use 1 g, in powder.

Assay Mix 1 g, in *No. 180 powder*, with 5 ml of a 10% w/v solution of *sodium hydroxide* in a 200-ml flask. Add 100 g of *benzene* and boil gently under a reflux condenser in a water-bath so that the water level is above that of the liquid in the flask and heat for 6 hours; cool and restore the original weight with benzene. Transfer 50 g of the benzene solution to a separating funnel and extract with at least six 15-ml quantities of 0.1M *hydrochloric acid*. Test 2 ml of the final extract for *complete extraction* of the alkaloids. Boil the combined acid extracts for 2 to 3 minutes to remove any remaining benzene, cool and dilute to 1000 ml with 0.1M *hydrochloric acid*. Prepare a 0.003% w/v solution of *quinine* in 0.1M *hydrochloric acid* and a 0.003% w/v solution of *cinchonine* in 0.1M *hydrochloric acid*. Measure the *absorbance* of the three solutions at the maxima at 316 nm and 348 nm, Appendix II B. Calculate the content, in mg, of alkaloids of the quinine group (x) and of alkaloids of the cinchonine group (y) in 0.5 g, from the expressions

$$x = \frac{[A_{316} \times A_{348}(c)] - [A_{316}(c) \times A_{348}]}{[A_{316}(q) \times A_{348}(c)] - [A_{316}(c) \times A_{348}(q)]}$$

and

$$y = \frac{[A_{316} \times A_{348}(q)] - [A_{316}(q) \times A_{348}]}{[A_{316}(c) \times A_{348}(q)] - [A_{316}(q) \times A_{348}(c)]}$$

where A_{316} and A_{348} are the absorbances of the solution being examined, $A_{316}(q)$ and $A_{348}(q)$ are the absorbances of the solution containing quinine calculated for a concentration of 0.0001% w/v and $A_{316}(c)$ and $A_{348}(c)$ are the absorbances of the solution containing cinchonine calculated for a concentration of 0.0001% w/v at the maxima at 316 nm and 348 nm respectively.

Storage Cinchona Bark should be kept in a well-closed container and protected from light.

Action and use Bitter.

Powdered Cinchona Bark

Powdered Cinchona Bark is Cinchona Bark in powder. It contains not less than 6.5 per cent of total alkaloids, of which 30 to 60 per cent are alkaloids of the quinine group.

Characteristics Reddish-brown. Diagnostic structures: thin-walled cork cells filled with reddish-brown matter; yellowish, spindle-shaped, striated phloem fibres, up to 90 μm in diameter (usually 40 to 70 μm) and up to 1300 μm in length (usually 600 to 700 μm), with conspicuous, funnel-shaped pits; a few starch granules, 6 to 10 μm in diameter; parenchymatous idioblasts containing microprisms of calcium oxalate.

Identification Complies with the tests decribed under Cinchona Bark.

Sulphated ash Not more than 4.0%, Appendix IX A, Method II. Use 1 g.

Assay Carry out the Assay described under Cinchona Bark.

Storage Powdered Cinchona Bark should be kept in a well-closed container and protected from light.

Action and use Bitter.

Cinnamic Acid

$C_9H_8O_2$ 148.2   *621-82-9*

Cinnamic Acid is (*E*)-3-phenylprop-2-enoic acid. It contains not less than 99.0 per cent and not more than 100.5 per cent of $C_9H_8O_2$, calculated with reference to the dried substance.

Characteristics Colourless crystals; odour, faint and balsamic.

Solubility Very slightly soluble in *water*; soluble in 6 parts of *ethanol (96%)*, in 15 parts of *chloroform* and in 15 parts of *ether*.

Identification A. The *infra-red absorption spectrum*, Appendix II A, is concordant with the *reference spectrum* of cinnamic acid.

B. The *light absorption*, Appendix II B, in the range 230 to 350 nm of a 0.0010% w/v solution in 0.1M *sodium hydroxide* exhibits a maximum only at 267 nm. The *absorbance* at 267 nm is about 1.4.

C. Warm 0.1 g with 0.1 g of *potassium permanganate* and 5 ml of 1M *sulphuric acid*. Benzaldehyde, recognisable by its odour, is produced.

Melting point 132° to 134°, Appendix V A.

Ethanol-insoluble matter A 10% w/v solution in *ethanol (96%)* is *clear*, Appendix IV A.

Related substances Carry out the method for *thin-layer chromatography*, Appendix III A, using *silica gel GF254* as the coating substance and a mixture of 90 volumes of *toluene* and 10 volumes of *glacial acetic acid* as the mobile phase. Apply separately to the chromatoplate 5 μl of each of two solutions of the substance being examined in *methanol* containing (1) 5.0% w/v and (2) 0.025% w/v. After removal of the plate, allow it to dry in air and examine under *ultra-violet light (254 nm)*. Any *secondary spot* in the chromatogram obtained with solution (1) is not more intense than the spot in the chromatogram obtained with solution (2).

Loss on drying When dried to constant weight at 60° at a pressure not exceeding 0.7 kPa, loses not more than 1.0% of its weight. Use 1 g.

Sulphated ash Not more than 0.1%, Appendix IX A.

Assay Dissolve 0.5 g in 15 ml of *ethanol (96%)* previously neutralised to *phenol red solution* and titrate with 0.1M *sodium hydroxide VS* using *phenol red solution* as indicator. Each ml of 0.1M *sodium hydroxide VS* is equivalent to 0.01482 g of $C_9H_8O_2$.

Action and use Antimicrobial preservative; pharmaceutical aid.

Cinnamon ☆

Cinnamon Bark; Ceylon Cinnamon

Cinnamon is the dried bark of the shoots of coppiced trees of *Cinnamomum zeylanicum* Nees freed from the outer cork and the underlying parenchyma.

Characteristics Odour, characteristic and aromatic; taste, characteristic, slightly sweet, warm and fragrant.

Macroscopical Bark about 0.2 to 0.8 mm thick occurring in closely packed compound quills made up of single or double quills. Outer surface smooth, yellowish-brown, showing faint scars, marking the positions of leaves and axillary buds, and with fine, whitish, wavy longitudinal striations; inner surface slightly darker, longitudinally striated. Fracture, short and fibrous.

Microscopical The outer surface shows a few discontinuous layers of cortical parenchyma within which is a wide, continuous layer of pericyclic sclerenchyma composed of groups of isodiametric or tangentially elongated sclereids, with thickened and pitted walls, and occasional groups of fibres. Phloem, fibres, singly or in small groups, thick-walled, 15 to 25 μm, occasionally up to 30 μm in diameter; sieve tissue; parenchyma with large secretory cells containing mucilage or volatile oil. Medullary rays uniseriate or biseriate, some cells containing small acicular crystals of calcium oxalate, the remainder, together with the phloem parenchyma, containing starch granules, simple or two- to four-compound and rarely more than 10 μm in diameter.

Identification Carry out the method for *thin-layer chromatography*, Appendix III A, using *silica gel GF254* as the coating substance and *dichloromethane* as the mobile phase, but allowing the solvent front to ascend 10 cm above the line of application. Apply separately to the chromatoplate, as bands 20 mm × 3 mm, 10 μl of each of the following solutions. For solution (1) shake 0.1 g, in *No. 500 powder*, for 15 minutes with 2 ml of *dichloromethane*, filter and evaporate almost to dryness on a water-bath; dissolve the residue in 0.4 ml of *toluene*. For solution (2) dissolve 50 μl of *cinnamaldehyde* and 10 μl of *eugenol* in 10 ml of *toluene*. After removal of the plate, allow it to dry in air, examine under *ultra-violet light (254 nm)*, marking the quenching bands, and under *ultra-violet light (365 nm)*, marking the fluorescent bands. When examined under ultra-violet light (254 nm) the chromatogram obtained with solution (1) shows a quenching band in the middle part of the chromatogram and, at a slightly higher Rf value, a weaker quenching band corresponding to the bands due to cinnamaldehyde and eugenol respectively in the chromatogram obtained with solution (2). When examined under ultra-violet light (365 nm) the chromatogram obtained with solution (1) shows a band of light blue fluorescence due to *o*-methoxycinnamaldehyde at an Rf value slightly lower than the band corresponding to cinnamaldehyde. Spray the plate with a solution of 2.5 g of *o-dianisidine* in 10 ml of *glacial acetic acid*; the bands due to cinnamaldehyde are yellowish-brown.

Volatile oil Not less than 1.2% v/w when determined by the method for the *determination of volatile oil in drugs*, Appendix XI E. Use a 500 ml flask, 200 ml of 0.1M *hydrochloric acid* as the distillation liquid and 0.50 ml of *xylene* in the graduated tube. Use 20 g, in *No. 710 powder*, and distil at a rate of 2.5 ml to 3.5 ml per minute for 3 hours.

Sulphated ash Not more than 6.0%, Appendix IX A, Method II. Use 2 g, in powder.

Storage Cinnamon should be kept in a well-closed container and protected from light.

Action and use Flavour.

Powdered Cinnamon

Powdered Cinnamon is Cinnamon in powder.

Characteristics Yellowish to reddish-brown. Diagnostic structures: groups of sclereids with pitted, channelled and moderately thickened walls; numerous colourless fibres with narrow lumen and thickened, lignified walls and few pits; occasional small acicular crystals of calcium oxalate; abundant starch granules. Cork fragments absent or very rare.

Identification Complies with the test for Identification described under Cinnamon.

Volatile oil Not less than 1.0% v/w when determined by the method for the *determination of volatile oil in drugs*, Appendix XI E. Use 40 g and distil for 5 hours.

Sulphated ash Not more than 6.0%, Appendix IX A, Method II. Use 2 g.

Storage Powdered Cinnamon should be kept in a well-closed container and protected from light.

Action and use Flavour.

Cinnamon Oil

Cinnamon Oil is obtained by distillation from Cinnamon.

Characteristics A clear, yellow liquid, gradually becoming reddish-brown with age; visibly free from water; odour, that of cinnamon.

Optical rotation 0° to −2°, Appendix V F.

Refractive index 1.573 to 1.600, Appendix V E.

Solubility in ethanol Dissolve 1 ml in 3 ml of *ethanol (70%)*. Any opalescence is not greater than that produced when 0.5 ml of 0.1M *silver nitrate VS* is added to a mixture of 0.5 ml of 0.1M *sodium chloride VS* and 50 ml of *water*.

Weight per ml 1.000 to 1.040 g, Appendix V G.

Content of aldehydes 60.0 to 80.0% w/w, calculated as cinnamaldehyde, C_9H_8O, Appendix X K. Each ml of 0.5M *potassium hydroxide in ethanol (60%) VS* is equivalent to 0.06661 g of C_9H_8O.

Eugenol Carry out the method for *gas chromatography*, Appendix III B, using three solutions in *butan-1-ol* containing (1) 0.25% w/v of *eugenol* and 0.75% w/v of *vanillin* (internal standard), (2) 5.0% w/v of the oil and (3) 5.0% w/v of the oil and 0.75% w/v of the internal standard.

The chromatographic procedure may be carried out using a column (2.0 m × 4 mm) packed with *acid-washed, silanised diatomaceous support* (80 to 100 mesh) coated with 20% w/w of dimethyl silicone fluid (OV-101 is suitable) and maintained at 150°.

In the chromatogram obtained with solution (3) the ratio of the area of any peak corresponding to eugenol to the area of the peak due to the internal standard is not greater than the corresponding ratio in the chromatogram obtained with solution (1).

Storage Cinnamon Oil should be kept in a well-filled, well-closed container, protected from light and stored at a temperature not exceeding 25°.

Preparation
Concentrated Cinnamon Water

Action and use Carminative; flavouring agent.

Anhydrous Citric Acid ☆
Citric Acid

$$CH_2 \cdot CO_2H$$
$$HOC \cdot CO_2H$$
$$CH_2 \cdot CO_2H$$

$C_6H_8O_7$ 192.1   77-92-9

Anhydrous Citric Acid* is 2-hydroxypropane-1,2,3-tricarboxylic acid. It contains not less than 99.5 per cent and not more than 101.0 per cent of $C_6H_8O_7$, calculated with reference to the anhydrous substance.

Characteristics Colourless crystals or a white, crystalline powder.

Solubility Soluble in 1 part of *water* and in 1.5 parts of *ethanol (96%)*; sparingly soluble in *ether*.

Identification A. Yields *reaction A* characteristic of citrates, Appendix VI.
B. A 10% w/v solution is strongly acidic.
C. Complies with the test for Water.

Clarity and colour of solution Dissolve 2.0 g in sufficient *water* to produce 10 ml. The solution is *clear*, Appendix IV A, and not more intensely coloured than *reference solution Y_7, BY_7 or GY_7*, Appendix IV B, Method II.

Barium Dissolve 5.0 g in several portions in 39 ml of 2M *sodium hydroxide* and dilute to 50 ml with *distilled water* (solution A). To 5 ml of solution A add 5 ml of 1M *sulphuric acid* and allow to stand for 1 hour. Any opalescence produced is not more intense than that of a mixture of 5 ml of solution A and 5 ml of *distilled water*.

Calcium 5 ml of solution A diluted to 10 ml with *distilled water* complies with the *limit test for calcium*, Appendix VII (200 ppm).

Heavy metals 12 ml of solution A complies with *limit test A for heavy metals*, Appendix VII (10 ppm). Use *lead standard solution (1 ppm Pb)* to prepare the standard.

Iron 2 ml of solution A diluted to 10 ml with *water* complies with the *limit test for iron*, Appendix VII (50 ppm).

Chloride To 10 ml of solution A add 1 ml of 2M *nitric acid* and dilute to 15 ml with *water*. The resulting solution complies with the *limit test for chlorides*, Appendix VII (50 ppm).

Oxalate Dissolve 0.8 g in 4 ml of *water*, add 3 ml of *hydrochloric acid* and boil for 1 minute with 1 g of *granulated zinc*. Allow to stand for 2 minutes, decant the liquid into a test-tube containing 0.25 ml of a 1% w/v solution of *phenylhydrazine hydrochloride* and heat to boiling. Cool rapidly, transfer to a graduated cylinder, add an equal volume of *hydrochloric acid* and 0.25 ml of a 5% w/v solution of *potassium hexacyanoferrate(III)*, shake and allow to stand for 30 minutes. Any pink colour produced is not more intense than that produced by treating 4 ml of a 0.01% w/v solution of *oxalic acid* at the same time and in the same manner (350 ppm, calculated as anhydrous oxalic acid).

Sulphate Dissolve 1.0 g in sufficient *distilled water* to produce 15 ml. The resulting solution complies with the *limit test for sulphates*, Appendix VII (150 ppm).

Readily carbonisable substances Dissolve 0.75 g, without heating, in 10 ml of *sulphuric acid (96% w/w)* and heat the solution in a water-bath at 89° to 91°. After 1 minute shake rapidly, replace in the water-bath, continue heating for a total of 60 minutes and immediately cool rapidly. The solution is not more intensely coloured than a mixture of 9 ml of *yellow primary solution* and 1 ml of *red primary solution*, Appendix IV B, Method I.

Sulphated ash Not more than 0.1%, Appendix IX A, Method II. Use 1 g.

Water Not more than 1.0% w/w, Appendix IX C. Use 2 g.

Assay Dissolve 0.55 g in 50 ml of *water* and titrate with 1M *sodium hydroxide VS* using 0.5 ml of *dilute phenolphthalein solution* as indicator. Each ml of 1M *sodium hydroxide VS* is equivalent to 0.06403 g of $C_6H_8O_7$.

Storage Anhydrous Citric Acid should be kept in an airtight container.

*In certain states party to the convention on the Elaboration of a European Pharmacopœia, Anhydrous Citric Acid intended for use in large-volume preparations for parenteral use may be required to comply with the *test for pyrogens*, Appendix XIV K. Use per kg of the rabbit's weight 20 mg of the substance being examined dissolved in a mixture of 0.3 ml of 1M *sodium hydroxide* and 9.7 ml of pyrogen-free *saline solution*.

Citric Acid Monohydrate ☆

$C_6H_8O_7,H_2O$ 210.1   *5949-29-1*

Citric Acid Monohydrate* contains not less than 99.5 per cent and not more than 101.0 per cent of $C_6H_8O_7$, calculated with reference to the anhydrous substance.

Characteristics Colourless crystals or a white, crystalline powder; efflorescent.

Solubility Soluble in less than 1 part of *water* and in 1.5 parts of *ethanol (96%)*; sparingly soluble in *ether*.

Identification A. Yields *reaction A* characteristic of citrates, Appendix VI.
B. A 10% w/v solution is strongly acidic.
C. Complies with the test for Water.

Clarity and colour of solution; Barium; Calcium; Heavy metals; Iron; Chloride; Oxalate; Sulphate; Readily carbonisable substances; Sulphated ash Complies with the requirements stated under Anhydrous Citric Acid.

Water 7.5 to 9.0%, Appendix IX C. Use 0.5 g.

Assay Dissolve 0.55 g in 50 ml of *water* and titrate with 1M *sodium hydroxide VS* using 0.5 ml of *dilute phenolphthalein solution* as indicator. Each ml of 1M *sodium hydroxide VS* is equivalent to 0.06403 g of $C_6H_8O_7$.

Storage Citric Acid Monohydrate should be kept in an airtight container.

*In certain states party to the convention on the Elaboration of a European Pharmacopœia, Citric Acid Monohydrate intended for use in large-volume preparations for parenteral use may be required to comply with the *test for pyrogens*, Appendix XIV K. Use per kg of the rabbit's weight 22 mg of the substance being examined dissolved in a mixture of 0.3 ml of 1M *sodium hydroxide* and 9.7 ml of pyrogen-free *saline solution*.

Clindamycin Hydrochloride

$C_{18}H_{33}ClN_2O_5S,HCl,H_2O$ 479.5   *21462-39-5*

Clindamycin Hydrochloride is methyl 6-amino-7-chloro-6,7,8-trideoxy-*N*-[(2S,4R)-1-methyl-4-propylprolyl]-1-thio-β-L-*threo*-D-*galacto*-octo-pyranoside hydrochloride monohydrate. It contains not less than 89.6 per cent and not more than 100.5 per cent of $C_{18}H_{33}ClN_2O_5S$, HCl, calculated with reference to the anhydrous substance.

Characteristics A white or almost white, crystalline powder.

Solubility Soluble in 2 parts of *water* and in 4 parts of *dimethylformamide*; slightly soluble in *ethanol (96%)*; very slightly soluble in *chloroform*.

Identification A. The *infra-red absorption spectrum*, Appendix II A, is concordant with the *reference spectrum* of clindamycin hydrochloride.
B. Yields *reaction B* characteristic of chlorides, Appendix VI.

Acidity pH of a 10% w/v solution, 3.0 to 5.5, Appendix V L.

Specific optical rotation In a 4% w/v solution, +135° to +150°, Appendix V F.

Related substances Carry out the method for *gas chromatography*, Appendix III B, using the following solution. Dissolve 50 mg of the substance being examined in 0.5 ml of *trifluoroacetic anhydride*, allow to stand at room temperature for 30 minutes, add 5 ml of *1,2-dichloroethane* and mix.

The chromatographic procedure may be carried out using a glass column (1.5 m × 4 mm) packed with *acid-washed, silanised diatomaceous support* (80 to 100 mesh) coated with 1% w/w of phenyl methyl silicone fluid (50% phenyl) (OV-17 is suitable) and maintained at 170°.

The sum of the areas of any *secondary peaks* is not greater than 5% and the area of any one such peak is not greater than 4.5% by *normalisation*.

Sulphated ash Not more than 0.5%, Appendix IX A.

Water 3.0 to 6.0% w/w, Appendix IX C. Use 1 g.

Assay Carry out the method for *gas chromatography*, Appendix III B, using the following solutions. For solution (1) add 1 ml of *trifluoroacetic anhydride* to 50 mg of *clindamycin hydrochloride BPCRS*, swirl to dissolve and allow to stand at room temperature for 30 minutes. Add 20 ml of a 0.15% w/v solution of *hexacosane* (internal standard) in *1,2-dichloroethane* and mix. For solution (2) add 1 ml of *trifluoroacetic anhydride* to 50 mg of the substance being examined, swirl to dissolve and allow to stand at room temperature for 30 minutes. Add 20 ml of *1,2-dichloroethane* and mix. Prepare solution (3) in the same manner as solution (1) but using 50 mg of the substance being examined in place of the clindamycin hydrochloride BPCRS.

The chromatographic procedure may be carried out using the conditions described in the test for Related substances.

Calculate the content of $C_{18}H_{33}ClN_2O_5S$,HCl using the declared content of $C_{18}H_{33}ClN_2O_5S$,HCl in *clindamycin hydrochloride BPCRS*.

Storage Clindamycin Hydrochloride should be kept in a well-closed container and stored at a temperature not exceeding 30°.

Labelling The label states (1) the date after which the material is not intended to be used; (2) the conditions under which it should be stored.

Preparation
Clindamycin Capsules

Action and use Antibacterial.

Clioquinol
Iodochlorhydroxyquin

C₉H₅ClINO   305.5   *130-26-7*

Clioquinol is 5-chloro-7-iodoquinolin-8-ol. It contains not less than 97.0 per cent and not more than 103.0 per cent of total phenols, calculated with reference to the dried substance.

Characteristics A yellowish-white to brownish-yellow, voluminous powder; odour, faint and characteristic.

Solubility Practically insoluble in *water* and in *ethanol (96%)*; freely soluble in *dimethylformamide* and in *pyridine*.

Identification A. The *infra-red absorption spectrum*, Appendix II A, is concordant with the *reference spectrum* of clioquinol.
B. Burn 20 mg by the method for *oxygen-flask combustion*, Appendix VIII C, using 5 ml of *2M sodium hydroxide* as the absorbing liquid and dilute to 25 ml with *water*. To 5 ml add 1 ml of *silver nitrate solution*; a yellow precipitate is produced. Add 5 ml of *5M ammonia*, shake, filter and acidify the filtrate with *nitric acid*; a white precipitate is produced.

Acidity or alkalinity Shake 0.5 g with 10 ml of *water* previously neutralised to *phenolphthalein solution*. The solution is colourless and not more than 0.05 ml of *0.1M sodium hydroxide VS* is required to change the colour of the solution to pink.

Free iodine Shake 1.0 g with a solution of 1 g of *potassium iodide* in 20 ml of *water* for 30 seconds, allow to stand for 5 minutes and filter. To 10 ml of the filtrate add 1 ml of *1M sulphuric acid* and 2 ml of *chloroform* and shake. Any colour in the chloroform layer is discharged on the addition of 0.1 ml of *0.005M sodium thiosulphate VS*.

Halide ions Shake 0.50 g with 25 ml of *water* for 1 minute and filter. To the filtrate add 0.5 ml of *2M nitric acid* and 0.5 ml of *0.1M silver nitrate* and allow to stand for 5 minutes. Any opalescence produced is not more intense than that produced by adding 0.5 ml of *0.1M silver nitrate* to 25 ml of *water* containing 0.5 ml of *2M nitric acid* and 0.2 ml of *0.01M hydrochloric acid VS* and allowing to stand for 5 minutes.

Related substances Carry out the method for *gas chromatography*, Appendix III B, protected from light, using the following solutions. For solution (1) add 0.5 ml of N,O-*bis(trimethylsilyl)acetamide* to 0.50 ml of a solution in *pyridine* containing 0.40% w/v each of *5-chloroquinolin-8-ol*, *5,7-dichloroquinolin-8-ol* and *5,7-di-iodoquinolin-8-ol* and 0.040% w/v of the substance being examined, mix, allow to stand for 15 minutes and add 5.0 ml of a 0.05% w/v solution of *dibutyl phthalate* (internal standard) in n-*hexane*. For solution (2) add 0.5 ml of N,O-*bis(trimethylsilyl)acetamide* to a mixture of 0.10 g of the substance being examined and 0.5 ml of *pyridine*, mix, allow to stand for 15 minutes and add 5.0 ml of n-*hexane*. For solution (3) treat a mixture of 0.10 g of the substance being examined and 0.5 ml of *pyridine* as described for solution (1).

The chromatographic procedure may be carried out using a glass column (1.5 m × 4 mm) packed with *silanised diatomaceous support* (100 to 120 mesh) coated with 3% w/w of methyl silicone gum (SE-30 is suitable) and maintained at 190°.

The peaks following the solvent peak in the chromatogram obtained with solution (1) are due to (a) 5-chloroquinolin-8-ol, (b) 5,7-dichloroquinolin-8-ol, (c) the internal standard, (d) clioquinol and (e) 5,7-di-iodo-quinolin-8-ol, in order of emergence.

Calculate the contents of 5-chloroquinolin-8-ol, 5,7-dichloroquinolin-8-ol and 5,7-di-iodoquinolin-8-ol in the chromatogram obtained with solution (3). The sum of the contents is not more than 4.0% w/w, the content of none of these impurities exceeds 3.0% w/w and the content of any other impurity does not exceed 0.2% w/w.

Loss on drying When dried over *phosphorus pentoxide* at a pressure not exceeding 0.7 kPa for 24 hours, loses not more than 0.5% of its weight. Use 1 g.

Sulphated ash Not more than 0.2%, Appendix IX A.

Assay Dissolve 0.6 g in 50 ml of *anhydrous pyridine* and carry out Method II for *non-aqueous titration*, Appendix VIII A, using 0.1M *tetrabutylammonium hydroxide VS* as titrant and determining the end-point potentiometrically. Each ml of 0.1M *tetrabutylammonium hydroxide VS* is equivalent to 0.03055 g of total phenols.

Storage Clioquinol should be protected from light.

Preparations
Clioquinol Cream
Hydrocortisone Acetate and Clioquinol Cream
Hydrocortisone and Clioquinol Ointment

Action and use Topical and intestinal antiseptic.

Clofazimine

C$_{27}$H$_{22}$Cl$_2$N$_4$ 473.4   *2030-63-9*

Clofazimine is 3-(4-chloroanilino)-10-(4-chloro-phenyl)-2,10-dihydrophenazin-2-ylidene-isopropylamine. It contains not less than 98.5 per cent and not more than 101.5 per cent of C$_{27}$H$_{22}$Cl$_2$N$_4$, calculated with reference to the dried substance.

Characteristics A reddish-brown, fine powder; odourless or almost odourless.

Solubility Practically insoluble in *water*; slightly soluble in *ethanol (96%)*; soluble in 15 parts of *chloroform*; very slightly soluble in *ether*.

Identification A. The *infra-red absorption spectrum*, Appendix II A, is concordant with the *reference spectrum* of clofazimine.

B. The *light absorption*, Appendix II B, in the range 230 to 600 nm of a 0.001% w/v solution in 0.01M *methanolic hydrochloric acid* exhibits two maxima, at 283 nm and 487 nm. The *absorbance* at 283 nm is about 1.30 and at 487 nm is about 0.64.

C. Dissolve 2 mg in 3 ml of *acetone* and add 0.1 ml of *hydrochloric acid*; an intense violet colour is produced. Add 0.5 ml of 5M *sodium hydroxide*; the colour changes to orange-red.

Related substances Carry out the method for *thin-layer chromatography*, Appendix III A, using a silica gel F254 precoated chromatoplate (Merck silica gel 60 F254 plates are suitable) exposed to ammonia vapour immediately before use by suspending the plate for 30 minutes in a tank containing a shallow layer of 0.2M *ammonia*. Use as the mobile phase, in another tank, a mixture of 85 volumes of *dichloromethane* and 4 volumes of *propan-1-ol*. Apply separately to the plate 5 μl of each of three solutions of the substance being examined in *chloroform* containing (1) 2.0% w/v, (2) 0.016% w/v and (3) 0.010% w/v. Allow the mobile phase to ascend 12 cm above the line of application, remove the plate from the tank, allow it to dry in air for 5 minutes and replace it in the tank. When the mobile phase has again ascended 12 cm above the line of application remove the plate from the tank, allow it to dry in air for 5 minutes and examine in daylight and then under *ultra-violet light (254 nm)*. Spray the plate with *sulphuric acid (50%)* and examine again in daylight. In the chromatogram obtained with solution (1), any *secondary spot* is not more intense than the spot in the chromatogram obtained with solution (2) and not more than two such spots are more intense than the spot in the chromatogram obtained with solution (3).

Loss on drying When dried to constant weight at 105°, loses not more than 0.5% of its weight. Use 1 g.

Sulphated ash Not more than 0.1%, Appendix IX A.

Assay Dissolve 0.4 g in 20 ml of *chloroform*, add 50 ml of *acetone* and carry out Method I for *non-aqueous titration*, Appendix VIII A, determining the end-point potentio-metrically. Each ml of 0.1M *perchloric acid VS* is equivalent to 0.04734 g of C$_{27}$H$_{22}$Cl$_2$N$_4$.

Preparation
Clofazimine Capsules

Action and use Antileprotic.

Clofibrate ☆

C$_{12}$H$_{15}$ClO$_3$ 242.7   *637-07-0*

Clofibrate is ethyl 2-(4-chlorophenoxy)-2-methylpropionate.

Characteristics A clear, almost colourless liquid; odour, characteristic and faintly acrid.

Solubility Very slightly soluble in *water*; miscible with *ethanol (96%)*, with *chloroform* and with *ether*.

Identification A. The *infra-red absorption spectrum*, Appendix II A, is concordant with the spectrum of *clofibrate EPCRS*.

B. The *light absorption*, Appendix II B, in the range 220 to 250 nm of a 0.001% w/v solution in *methanol* exhibits a maximum only at 226 nm. The A(1%, 1 cm) at 226 nm is about 460.

C. The *light absorption*, Appendix II B, in the range 250 to 350 nm of a 0.01% w/v solution in *methanol* exhibits two maxima, at 280 nm and 288 nm. The A(1%, 1 cm) at 280 nm is about 44 and at 288 nm is about 31.

Acidity To 1 g add 10 ml of *ethanol (96%)* and 0.1 ml of *phenol red solution*. Not more than 1.0 ml of 0.01M *sodium hydroxide VS* is required to change the colour of the solution.

Refractive index 1.500 to 1.505, Appendix V E.

Relative density 1.138 to 1.147, Appendix V G.

4-Chlorophenol Carry out the method for *gas chromatography*, Appendix III B, injecting 2 µl of each of the following solutions. Solution (1) contains 0.0025% w/v of *4-chlorophenol* in *chloroform*. For solution (2) extract 10.0 g of the substance being examined with 20 ml of 1M *sodium hydroxide*, wash the lower layer with 5 ml of *water*, add the washings to the aqueous layer and reserve the organic layer for the test for Volatile related substances. Extract the combined aqueous layer and washings with two 5-ml quantities of *chloroform*, discard the chloroform and acidify the aqueous layer by the dropwise addition of *hydrochloric acid*. Extract with three 3-ml quantities of *chloroform*, combine the organic extracts and dilute to 10 ml with *chloroform*.

The chromatographic procedure may be carried out using a glass column (1.5 m × 4 mm) maintained at 185° and packed with either *acid-washed, silanised diatomaceous support* (Gas Chrom Q is suitable) (40 to 60 mesh) coated with 30% w/w of dimethyl silicone fluid (E-301 and SE-30 are suitable) or *acid-washed, silanised diatomaceous support* (80 to 100 mesh) coated with 10% w/w of dimethyl silicone fluid.

The area of any peak corresponding to 4-chlorophenol in the chromatogram obtained with solution (2) is not greater than the area of the peak in the chromatogram obtained with solution (1).

Volatile related substances Carry out the method for *gas chromatography*, Appendix III B, injecting 2 µl of each of the following solutions. For solution (1) dry the organic layer reserved in the test for 4-Chlorophenol with *anhydrous sodium sulphate* and filter. Solution (2) contains 0.012% w/v of the substance being examined in *chloroform*. Solution (3) is a 0.012% w/v solution of *methyl 2-(4-chlorophenoxy)-2-methylpropionate EPCRS* in the substance being examined.

The chromatographic procedure may be carried out as described in the test for 4-Chlorophenol.

The sum of the areas of any *secondary peaks* in the chromatogram obtained with solution (1) is not greater than ten times the area of the peak due to clofibrate in the chromatogram obtained with solution (2).

In the chromatogram obtained with solution (3) measure from the baseline the height of the peak corresponding to methyl 2-(4-chlorophenoxy)-2-methyl-propionate (*x*) and the height of the lowest part of the curve separating this peak from the peak corresponding to clofibrate (*y*). The test is not valid unless *x* is equal to at least 30% of full-scale deflection and *x* − *y* is greater than 75% of *x*.

Preparation
Clofibrate Capsules

Action and use Antihyperlipidaemic.

Clomiphene Citrate

$C_{26}H_{28}ClNO, C_6H_8O_7$ 598.1   *50-41-9*

Clomiphene Citrate is a mixture of the *E*- and *Z*- isomers of 2-[4-(2-chloro-1,2-diphenylvinyl)-phenoxy]triethylamine dihydrogen citrate. It contains not less than 97.0 per cent and not more than 101.0 per cent of $C_{26}H_{28}ClNO$, $C_6H_8O_7$, calculated with reference to the anhydrous substance.

Characteristics A white to pale yellow powder; odourless or almost odourless.

Solubility Slightly soluble in *water* and in *chloroform*; sparingly soluble in *ethanol (96%)*; practically insoluble in *ether*.

Identification A. The *infra-red absorption spectrum*, Appendix II A, is concordant with the *reference spectrum* of clomiphene citrate.

B. The *light absorption*, Appendix II B, in the range 220 to 350 nm of a 0.0050% w/v solution in 0.1M *hydrochloric acid* exhibits two maxima, at 235 nm and 292 nm. The *absorbance* at 235 nm is about 1.58 and at 292 nm is about 0.88.

C. Dissolve 5 mg in 5 ml of a mixture of 1 volume of *acetic anhydride* and 5 volumes of *pyridine* and heat in a water-bath. A dark red colour is produced.

Z-**Isomer** 30.0 to 50.0% when determined in the following manner. Carry out the method for *high-performance liquid chromatography*, Appendix III D, protecting the solutions from light and using a solution prepared in the following manner. Dissolve 25 mg of the substance being examined in 25 ml of 0.1M *hydrochloric acid*, add 5 ml of 1M *sodium hydroxide* and extract with three 25-ml quantities of *ethanol-free chloroform*. Wash the combined extracts with 10 ml of *water*, dry over *anhydrous sodium sulphate* and add sufficient *ethanol-free chloroform* to produce 100 ml. To 20 ml of the solution add 0.1 ml of *triethylamine* and sufficient *hexane* to produce 100 ml.

The chromatographic procedure may be carried out using (a) a stainless steel column (30 cm × 4 mm) packed with *stationary phase A* (10 µm) (Porasil is suitable), (b) a mixture of *hexane* and *ethanol-free chloroform* each containing 0.10% v/v of *triethylamine* adjusted so that baseline separation is obtained between *E*- and *Z*-clomiphene (a mixture of 80 volumes of *hexane* and 20 volumes of *ethanol-free chloroform* is usually suitable) as the mobile phase with a flow rate of 2.0 ml per minute and (c) a detection wavelength of 302 nm. Passage of the mobile phase through the system should be maintained until stabilisation is achieved (about 250 ml).

In the chromatogram obtained with the solution being examined, a peak due to *E*-clomiphene precedes the peak due to *Z*-clomiphene. The test is not valid unless baseline separation is achieved between *E*- and *Z*-clomiphene and the *column efficiency* is greater than 10,000 theoretical plates per metre determined using the peak due to the *E*-isomer. Calculate the percentage of *Z*-isomer in the substance being examined from the expression

$$100A_Z(1.08A_E + A_Z)$$

where A_Z and A_E are the areas of the peaks due to the *Z*- and *E*-isomers, respectively.

Water Not more than 1.0% w/w, Appendix IX C. Use 2.5 g.

Assay Carry out Method I for *non-aqueous titration*, Appendix VIII A, using 1 g. Each ml of 0.1M *perchloric acid VS* is equivalent to 0.05981 g of $C_{26}H_{28}ClNO$, $C_6H_8O_7$.

Storage Clomiphene Citrate should be protected from light.

Preparation

Clomiphene Tablets

Action and use Induction of ovulation.

In some countries the material described in this monograph may be known as Clomifene Citrate.

Clomipramine Hydrochloride

$C_{19}H_{23}ClN_2,HCl$ 351.3   *17321-77-6*

Clomipramine Hydrochloride is 3-(3-chloro-10,11-dihydro-5*H*-dibenz[*b,f*]azepin-5-yl)-propyldimethylamine hydrochloride. It contains not less than 98.5 per cent and not more than 101.0 per cent of $C_{19}H_{23}ClN_2,HCl$, calculated with reference to the dried substance.

Characteristics A white or slightly yellow, crystalline powder; odourless or almost odourless.

Solubility Freely soluble in *water*, in *ethanol (96%)* and in *chloroform*; slightly soluble in *acetone*; practically insoluble in *ether*.

Identification A. The *infra-red absorption spectrum*, Appendix II A, is concordant with the *reference spectrum* of clomipramine hydrochloride.

B. The *light absorption*, Appendix II B, in the range 230 to 350 nm of a 0.003% w/v solution in 0.1M *hydrochloric acid* exhibits a maximum only at 252 nm and a shoulder at 270 nm. The *absorbance* at 252 nm is about 0.70.

C. Yields the *reactions* characteristic of chlorides, Appendix VI.

Acidity pH of a 10% w/v solution, 3.5 to 5.0, Appendix V L.

Clarity and colour of solution A 10.0% w/v solution is *clear*, Appendix IV A, and not more intensely coloured than *reference solution Y_5*, Appendix IV B, Method I.

Heavy metals 2.0 g complies with *limit test C for heavy metals*, Appendix VII (20 ppm). Use 4 ml of *lead standard solution (10 ppm Pb)* to prepare the standard.

Related substances Carry out the method for *thin-layer chromatography*, Appendix III A, using *silica gel G* as the coating substance and a mixture of 75 volumes of *ethyl acetate*, 25 volumes of *acetone* and 5 volumes of 13.5M *ammonia* as the mobile phase. Apply separately to the chromatoplate 5 µl of each of three solutions in *methanol* containing (1) 2.0% w/v of the substance being examined,

(2) 0.020% w/v solution of *imipramine hydrochloride EPCRS* and (3) 0.0040% w/v of the substance being examined. After removal of the plate, allow it to dry in air and spray with a 0.5% w/v solution of *potassium dichromate* in *sulphuric acid (20%)*. Any spot corresponding to imipramine in the chromatogram obtained with solution (1) is not more intense than the spot in the chromatogram obtained with solution (2) and any other *secondary spot* is not more intense than the spot in the chromatogram obtained with solution (3).

Loss on drying When dried to constant weight at 105°, loses not more than 0.5% of its weight. Use 1 g.

Sulphated ash Not more than 0.1%, Appendix IX A.

Assay Carry out Method I for *non-aqueous titration*, Appendix VIII A, using 0.26 g, adding 5 ml of *mercury (II) acetate solution* and *metanil yellow solution* as indicator. Each ml of 0.1M *perchloric acid VS* is equivalent to 0.03513 g of $C_{19}H_{23}ClN_2,HCl$.

Storage Clomipramine Hydrochloride should be kept in a well-closed container and protected from light.

Preparation

Clomipramine Capsules

Action and use Antidepressant.

Clonidine Hydrochloride ☆

$C_9H_9Cl_2N_3,HCl$ 266.6   *4205-91-8*

Clonidine Hydrochloride is 2-[(2,6-dichloro-phenyl)imino]imidazolidine hydrochloride. It contains not less than 98.5 per cent and not more than 101.0 per cent of $C_9H_9Cl_2N_3,HCl$, calculated with reference to the dried substance.

Characteristics A white or almost white, crystalline powder.

Solubility Soluble in 13 parts of *water*; soluble in *absolute ethanol*; slightly soluble in *chloroform*.

Identification *Test A may be omitted if tests B, C and D are carried out. Tests B and C may be omitted if tests A and D are carried out.*

A. The *infra-red absorption spectrum*, Appendix II A, is concordant with the spectrum of *clonidine hydrochloride EPCRS*.

B. The *light absorption*, Appendix II B, in the range 245 to 350 nm of a 0.03% w/v solution in 0.01M *hydrochloric acid* exhibits two maxima, at 272 nm and 279 nm, and an inflection at 265 nm. The A(1%, 1 cm) at 272 nm is about 18 and the A(1%, 1 cm) at 279 nm is about 16.

C. In the test for Related substances, the principal spot in the chromatogram obtained with solution (2) is similar in position, colour and size to that in the chromatogram obtained with solution (3).

D. Yields *reaction A* characteristic of chlorides, Appendix VI.

Acidity pH of a 5% w/v solution, 4.0 to 5.0, Appendix V L.

Colour and clarity of solution A 5.0% w/v solution in *carbon dioxide-free water* is *clear*, Appendix IV A, and not more intensely coloured than *reference solution Y₇*, Appendix IV B, Method II.

Related substances Carry out the method for *thin-layer chromatography*, Appendix III A, using *silica gel G* as the coating substance and as the mobile phase the filtered upper layer obtained by shaking together 50 volumes of *water*, 40 volumes of *butan-1-ol* and 10 volumes of *glacial acetic acid* and allowing the layers to separate. Apply separately to the chromatoplate 10 µl of each of four solutions in *methanol* containing (1) 1.0% w/v of the substance being examined, (2) 0.1% w/v of the substance being examined, (3) 0.1% w/v of *clonidine hydrochloride EPCRS* and (4) 0.0050% w/v of the substance being examined. After removal of the plate, allow it to dry in air and spray with *modified potassium iodobismuthate solution*. Allow to dry in air for 1 hour, spray again with the same reagent and immediately spray with a 5% w/v solution of *sodium nitrite*. Any *secondary spot* in the chromatogram obtained with solution (1) is not more intense than the spot in the chromatogram obtained with solution (4).

Loss on drying When dried to constant weight at 100° to 105°, loses not more than 0.5% of its weight. Use 1 g.

Sulphated ash Not more than 0.1%, Appendix IX A, Method II. Use 1 g.

Assay Dissolve 0.2 g in 70 ml of *ethanol (96%)* and titrate with 0.1M *ethanolic sodium hydroxide VS* determining the end-point potentiometrically. Each ml of 0.1M *ethanolic sodium hydroxide VS* is equivalent to 0.02666 g of $C_9H_9Cl_2N_3,HCl$.

Storage Clonidine Hydrochloride should be kept in a well-closed container.

Preparations
Clonidine Injection
Clonidine Tablets

Action and use Antihypertensive.

Clotrimazole

$C_{22}H_{17}ClN_2$ 344.8   *23593-75-1*

Clotrimazole is 1-(2-chlorotrityl)imidazole. It contains not less than 98.5 per cent and not more than 100.5 per cent of $C_{22}H_{17}ClN_2$, calculated with reference to the dried substance.

Characteristics A white to pale yellow, crystalline powder; odourless or almost odourless.

Solubility Practically insoluble in *water*; soluble in 10 parts of *ethanol (96%)*, in 10 parts of *chloroform* and in 100 parts of *ether*.

Identification A. The *infra-red absorption spectrum*, Appendix II A, is concordant with the *reference spectrum* of clotrimazole.

B. The *light absorption*, Appendix II B, in the range 230 to 350 nm of a 0.04% w/v solution in a mixture of 1 volume of 0.1M *hydrochloric acid* and 9 volumes of *methanol* exhibits two maxima, at 262 nm and 265 nm. The *absorbance* at 262 nm is about 0.90 and at 265 nm is about 0.92.

C. *Melting point*, about 143°, Appendix V A.

Clarity and colour of solution A 5.0% w/v solution in *chloroform* is *clear*, Appendix IV A, and not more intensely coloured than *reference solution BY₆*, Appendix IV B, Method I.

(2-Chlorotrityl)methanol Carry out the method for *thin-layer chromatography*, Appendix III A, using *silica gel G* as the coating substance and a mixture of 180 volumes of *toluene*, 20 volumes of *propan-1-ol* and 1 volume of 13.5M *ammonia* as the mobile phase. Apply separately to the chromatoplate 10 µl of each of two solutions in *chloroform* containing (1) 5.0% w/v of the substance being examined and (2) 0.010% w/v of *(2-chlorotrityl)methanol BPCRS*. After removal of the plate, allow it to dry in air, spray with *ethanolic sulphuric acid (10%)* and heat at 105° for 30 minutes. Any spot corresponding to (2-chlorotrityl)-methanol in the chromatogram obtained with solution (1) is not more intense than the spot in the chromatogram obtained with solution (2).

Imidazole Carry out the test for (2-Chlorotrityl)methanol but using as solution (2) a 0.010% w/v solution of *imidazole* in *chloroform*. After removal of the chromatoplate, allow it to dry in air, place in a tank of chlorine prepared by the addition of *hydrochloric acid* to a 5% w/v solution of *potassium permanganate* and allow to stand for 2 minutes. Remove any excess chlorine from the plate with a current of air and spray with *potassium iodide and starch solution*. Any spot corresponding to imidazole in the chromatogram obtained with solution (1) is not more intense than the spot in the chromatogram obtained with solution (2).

Loss on drying When dried to constant weight at 105°, loses not more than 0.5% of its weight. Use 1 g.

Sulphated ash Not more than 0.1%, Appendix IX A.

Assay Carry out Method I for *non-aqueous titration*, Appendix VIII A, using 0.3 g and determining the end-point potentiometrically. Each ml of 0.1M *perchloric acid VS* is equivalent to 0.03448 g of $C_{22}H_{17}ClN_2$.

Storage Clotrimazole should be stored in a well-closed container and protected from light.

Action and use Antifungal.

Preparations
Clotrimazole Cream
Clotrimazole Pessaries

Clove ☆

Clove consists of the flower buds of *Syzygium aromaticum* (L.) Merrill and L.M. Perry [(*Eugenia caryophyllus*) (C. Spreng.) Bull. and Harr.] dried until they turn reddish-brown.

Characteristics Odour, characteristic; taste, aromatic and pungent.

Macroscopical Flower buds reddish-brown, consisting of lower quadrangular stalked hypanthium, 10 to 12 mm × 2 to 3 mm, surmounted by four divergent sepal lobes surrounding a dome-shaped globular head, 4 to 6 mm in diameter, composed of four imbricated petals enclosing numerous incurved stamens and a short, erect style with a nectary disc at the base; bilocular ovary, containing numerous ovules, in upper part of hypanthium. The hypanthium exudes volatile oil when indented with the fingernail.

Microscopical Epidermis of hypanthium composed of small, polygonal cells with a thick cuticle and circular *anomocytic* stomata; underlying layers consisting of parenchyma with slightly thickened walls and numerous large, ovoid glands containing volatile oil; within this an area containing scattered fibro-vascular bundles which, below the ovary, is separated from the central area by a wide lacunose area of aerenchyma; the central area also contains fibro-vascular tissue. Calcium oxalate cluster crystals present in all parenchymatous tissue. Petals containing numerous oil glands; a single large gland occurring at the apex of each stamen.

Identification Carry out the method for *thin-layer chromatography*, Appendix III A, using *silica gel GF254* as the coating substance and *toluene* as the mobile phase. Use an unlined tank, develop the chromatogram immediately after introducing the mobile phase into the tank and allow the solvent front to ascend 10 cm above the line of application; allow the chromatoplate to stand for 5 minutes and again allow the solvent front to ascend 10 cm above the line of application under the same conditions. Apply separately to the plate, as bands 20 mm × 3 mm, 20 µl of solution (1) and 10 µl of solution (2). For solution (1) shake 0.1 g, in *No. 500 powder*, with 2 ml of *dichloromethane* for 15 minutes, filter, carefully evaporate the filtrate to dryness on a water-bath and dissolve the residue in 2 ml of *toluene*. For solution (2) dissolve 20 µl of *eugenol* in 2 ml of *toluene*. After removal of the plate following the second development, allow it to dry in air, examine under *ultra-violet light (254 nm)* and mark the quenching bands. In the chromatogram obtained with solution (1) there is a quenching band in the middle part corresponding to the quenching band due to eugenol in the chromatogram obtained with solution (2). A weak quenching band may also be present in the chromatogram obtained with solution (1) with an Rf value slightly lower than that of the band corresponding to eugenol (acetyleugenol). Spray the plate with about 10 ml of *anisaldehyde solution*, heat at 100° to 105° for 5 to 10 minutes and examine in daylight. In the chromatograms obtained with solutions (1) and (2) the bands corresponding to eugenol are strongly coloured brownish-violet; the band corresponding to acetyleugenol in the chromatogram obtained with solution (1) is faintly violet-blue. Other coloured bands may be visible in the chromatogram obtained with solution (1), in particular a faint red band in the lower part of the chromatogram and a reddish-violet band in the upper part (caryophyllene).

Foreign matter Not more than 4% of blown cloves, peduncles and fruits; not more than 2% of fermented cloves; not more than 0.5% of other foreign matter, Appendix XI D, Test B.

Volatile oil Not less than 15.0% v/w, Appendix XI E, using a 250-ml flask, 100 ml of *water* as the distillation liquid and 0.50 ml of *xylene* in the graduated tube. Grind 5 g of the material with 5 g of *diatomaceous earth* to form a fine, homogeneous powder and carry out the procedure immediately using 4 g of the mixture and distilling at a rate of 2.5 to 3.5 ml per minute for 2 hours.

Sulphated ash Not more than 8.0%, Appendix IX A, Method II. Use 1 g.

Storage Clove should be stored in a well-closed container and protected from light.

Action and use Carminative; flavouring agent.

Powdered Clove

Powdered Clove is Clove in powder.

Characteristics Dark brown; odour and taste, those of the unground material. Diagnostic structures: fragments of hypanthium showing epidermis and underlying parenchyma containing large oil glands; short fibres, occurring singly or in small groups, with thickened lignified walls and a few pits; abundant parenchyma containing calcium oxalate cluster crystals; numerous triangular pollen grains about 15 µm in diameter with three pores in the angles. Starch granules absent.

The powder turns blackish-blue when a 10.5% w/v solution of *iron(III) chloride hexahydrate* is added.

Identification Complies with the test for Identification described under Clove.

Volatile oil Not less than 12.0% v/w, Appendix XI E. Use 4 g and distil for 4 hours.

Sulphated ash Not more than 8.0%, Appendix IX A, Method II. Use 1 g.

Storage Powdered Clove should be stored in a well-closed container and protected from light.

Action and use Carminative; flavouring agent.

Clove Oil

Clove Oil is obtained by distillation from Clove.

Characteristics A clear, colourless or pale yellow liquid, visibly free from water; odour and taste, those of clove.

Optical rotation 0° to −1.5°, Appendix V F.

Refractive index 1.528 to 1.537, Appendix V E.

Solubility in ethanol Soluble in 2 volumes of *ethanol (70%)*, Appendix X M.

Weight per ml 1.041 to 1.054 g, Appendix V G.

Alkali-soluble matter Place 80 ml of a 5% w/v solution of *potassium hydroxide* in a 150-ml flask with a long neck which is graduated in tenths of a ml and is of such a diameter that not less than 15 cm in length has a capacity of 10 ml. Clean the flask with *sulphuric acid* and rinse well with *water* before use. Add 10 ml of the oil and shake thoroughly at 5-minute intervals for 30 minutes at ambient temperature. Raise the undissolved portion of the oil into the graduated part of the neck of the flask by the gradual addition of more of the potassium hydroxide solution; allow to stand for not less than 24 hours and read off the volume of the undissolved portion of the oil. The undissolved portion of the oil measures 1.0 to 1.5 ml.

Storage Clove Oil should be kept in a well-filled, well-closed container, protected from light and stored at a temperature not exceeding 25°. It darkens in colour with age or on exposure to air.

Action and use Local analgesic used in dentistry; flavour.

Cloxacillin Sodium

$C_{19}H_{17}ClN_3NaO_5S,H_2O$ 475.9   *7081-44-9*

Cloxacillin Sodium is sodium (6R)-6-[3-(2-chlorophenyl)-5-methylisoxazole-4-carboxamido]-penicillanate monohydrate. It contains not less than 95.0 per cent and not more than 100.5 per cent of $C_{19}H_{17}ClN_3NaO_5S$, calculated with reference to the anhydrous substance.

Characteristics A white, crystalline powder; hygroscopic.

Solubility Soluble in 2.5 parts of *water* and in 30 parts of *ethanol (96%)*; slightly soluble in *chloroform*.

Identification A. The *infra-red absorption spectrum*, Appendix II A, is concordant with the *reference spectrum* of cloxacillin sodium.
B. Yields the *reactions* characteristic of sodium salts, Appendix VI.

Acidity or alkalinity pH of a 10% w/v solution, 5.0 to 7.0, Appendix V L.

Specific optical rotation In a 1% w/v solution, +163° to +172°, Appendix V F.

Chlorine 7.0 to 8.0% when determined by the method for *oxygen-flask combustion*, Appendix VIII C, using 40 mg and using 20 ml of 0.01M *silver nitrate VS* and 0.01M *ammonium thiocyanate VS* in place of 10 ml of 0.05M *silver nitrate VS* and 0.05M *ammonium thiocyanate VS* respectively. Each ml of 0.01M *silver nitrate VS* is equivalent to 0.0003546 g of Cl.

Iodine-absorbing substances Not more than 5%, calculated with reference to the anhydrous substance, when determined by the following method. Dissolve 0.125 g in sufficient *mixed phosphate buffer pH 7.0* to produce 25 ml. To 10 ml add 10 ml of *mixed phosphate buffer pH 4.0* and 10 ml of 0.01M *iodine VS* and titrate immediately with 0.01M *sodium thiosulphate VS* using *starch mucilage*, added towards the end of the titration, as indicator. Repeat the operation without the substance being examined. The difference between the titrations represents the amount of iodine-absorbing substances present. Each ml of 0.01M *sodium thiosulphate VS* is equivalent to 0.000504 g of iodine-absorbing substances.

Water 3.0 to 4.5% w/w, Appendix IX C. Use 0.3 g.

Assay Dissolve 0.1 g in sufficient *water* to produce 500 ml and dilute 25 ml to 100 ml with *water*. Place two 2-ml quantities of the resulting solution in separate stoppered tubes. To one tube add 10 ml of *imidazole—mercury reagent*, mix, stopper the tube and immerse in a water-bath at 60° for exactly 25 minutes, swirling occasionally. Remove from the water-bath and cool rapidly to 20° (solution A). To the second tube add 10 ml of *water* and mix (solution B). Without delay measure the *absorbances* of solutions A and B at the maximum at 346 nm, Appendix II B, using in the reference cell a mixture of 2 ml of *water* and 10 ml of *imidazole—mercury reagent* for solution A and *water* for solution B. Calculate the content of $C_{19}H_{17}ClN_3NaO_5S$ from the difference between the absorbances of solutions A and B, from the difference obtained by repeating the operation using *cloxacillin sodium BPCRS* in place of the substance being examined and from the declared content of $C_{19}H_{17}ClN_3NaO_5S$ in *cloxacillin sodium BPCRS*.

Storage Cloxacillin Sodium should be kept in a well-closed container and stored at a temperature not exceeding 25°. If it is intended for use in the manufacture of a parenteral dosage form, the container should be sterile and sealed so as to exclude micro-organisms.

Labelling The label states (1) the date after which the material is not intended to be used; (2) the conditions under it which should be stored; (3) whether or not it is intended for use in the manufacture of a parenteral dosage form.

Preparations
Cloxacillin Capsules
Cloxacillin Oral Solution
Cloxacillin Injection

Action and use Antibacterial.

Cloxacillin Sodium intended for use in the manufacture of a parenteral dosage form complies with the following additional requirements.

Pyrogens Complies with the *test for pyrogens*, Appendix XIV K. Use per kg of the rabbit's weight 1 ml of *water for injections* containing 6 mg per ml.

Sterility When intended for use in the manufacture of a parenteral dosage form without further sterilisation complies with the *test for sterility*, Appendix XVI A.

Cocaine

$C_{17}H_{21}NO_4$ 303.4   *50-36-2*

Cocaine is (1R,2R,3s,5S)-2-methoxy-carbonyl-tropan-3-yl benzoate and may be obtained from the leaves of *Erythroxylum coca* Lam. and other species of *Erythroxylum* or by synthesis. It contains not less than 98.0 per cent and not more than 101.0 per cent of $C_{17}H_{21}NO_4$, calculated with reference to the dried substance.

Characteristics Colourless crystals or a white, crystalline powder. Slightly volatile.

Solubility Practically insoluble in *water*; soluble in 7 parts of *ethanol (96%)*, in 0.5 part of *chloroform*, in 4 parts of *ether* and in 30 parts of *arachis oil*; slightly soluble in *liquid paraffin*.

Identification A. The *light absorption*, Appendix II B, in the range 230 to 350 nm of a 0.002% w/v solution in 0.01M *hydrochloric acid* exhibits a well-defined maximum only at 233 nm. The *absorbance* at 233 nm is about 0.86.
B. Heat 0.1 g with 1 ml of *sulphuric acid* for 5 minutes at 100°, cool and cautiously mix with 2 ml of *water*. The aromatic odour of methyl benzoate is detectable and,

when the solution is cooled and allowed to stand for some hours, crystals of benzoic acid separate.

C. Dissolve 50 mg in 1.65 ml of 0.1M *hydrochloric acid*, add 8.5 ml of a 5.0% w/v solution of *alum* and 5 ml of *potassium permanganate solution* and stir briskly for several seconds. Characteristic rectangular, violet plates are produced.

D. A saturated solution is alkaline to *phenolphthalein solution*.

Melting point 96° to 98°, Appendix V A.

Specific optical rotation In a solution of 0.6 g in 2.5 ml of 1M *hydrochloric acid* and sufficient *water* to produce 25 ml, −79° to −81°, Appendix V F.

Cinnamylcocaine and reducing substances Dissolve 0.30 g in 1 ml of 1M *hydrochloric acid*, warming if necessary, and dilute to 15 ml with *water*. To 5 ml add 0.3 ml of 0.5M *sulphuric acid* and 0.5 ml of 0.004M *potassium permanganate* and reserve the remainder for the test for Truxillines. A clear violet solution is produced and the colour does not fade completely at a temperature not exceeding 20° within 30 minutes.

Truxillines Dilute 5 ml of the solution reserved in the test for Cinnamylcocaine and reducing substances to 100 ml with *water*, add while stirring 0.2 ml of 6M *ammonia* and allow to stand for 15 minutes, scratching the walls of the container occasionally with a glass rod. A crystalline precipitate is produced which on settling leaves a clear supernatant liquid.

Loss on drying When dried to constant weight at 80°, loses not more than 0.5% of its weight. Use 1 g.

Sulphated ash Not more than 0.1%, Appendix IX A.

Assay Carry out Method I for *non-aqueous titration*, Appendix VIII A, using 0.7 g dissolved in 50 ml of *1,4-dioxan* and *crystal violet solution* as indicator. Each ml of 0.1M *perchloric acid VS* is equivalent to 0.03034 g of $C_{17}H_{21}NO_4$.

Action and use Local anaesthetic.

Cocaine Hydrochloride ☆

$C_{17}H_{21}NO_4,HCl$ 339.8   *53-21-4*

Cocaine Hydrochloride is (1*R*,2*R*,3*s*,5*S*)-2-methoxycarbonyltropan-3-yl benzoate hydrochloride. It contains not less than 98.5 per cent and not more than 101.0 per cent of $C_{17}H_{21}NO_4,HCl$, calculated with reference to the dried substance.

Characteristics Colourless crystals or a white, crystalline powder; odourless; hygroscopic. It melts at about 197°, with decomposition.

Solubility Soluble in 0.5 part of *water*, in 4.5 parts of *ethanol (96%)* and in 18 parts of *chloroform*; practically insoluble in *ether* and in fixed oils.

Identification A. The *light absorption*, Appendix II B, in the range 220 to 350 nm of a 0.002% w/v solution in 0.01M *hydrochloric acid* exhibits two maxima, at 233 nm and 273 nm. The A(1%, 1 cm) at 233 nm is about 390 and at 273 nm is about 31.

B. To 5 ml of a 2% w/v solution add 1 ml of 2M *ammonia*; a white precipitate is produced. Induce crystallisation by scratching the walls of the container with a glass rod. The

melting point of the crystals, after washing with *water* and drying at a pressure not exceeding 0.7 kPa, is 96° to 99°, Appendix V A, Method I.

C. Yields the *reaction* characteristic of alkaloids, Appendix VI.

D. Yields the *reactions* characteristic of chlorides, Appendix VI.

Acidity To 10 ml of a 2% w/v solution add 0.05 ml of *methyl red solution*. Not more than 0.2 ml of 0.02M *sodium hydroxide VS* is required to change the colour of the solution.

Clarity and colour of solution A 2.0% w/v solution is *clear*, Appendix IV A, and *colourless*, Appendix IV B, Method II.

Specific optical rotation In a 2.5% w/v solution, −70° to −73°, Appendix V F.

Cinnamylcocaine and reducing substances To 5 ml of a 2.0% w/v solution add 0.3 ml of 0.5M *sulphuric acid* and 0.5 ml of 0.004M *potassium permanganate* and allow to stand, protected from light. After 30 minutes the colour of the permanganate is not completely discharged.

Readily carbonisable substances To 0.2 g add 2 ml of *sulphuric acid (96% w/w)* and allow to stand for 15 minutes. The solution is not more intensely coloured than *reference solution BY_5*, Appendix IV B, Method I.

Truxillines To 7.5 ml of a 2.0% w/v solution add 72.5 ml of *water* and 0.2 ml of 6M *ammonia*. Allow to stand for 15 minutes and then induce crystallisation by scratching the walls of the container with a glass rod. A crystalline precipitate is produced which on settling leaves a clear supernatant liquid.

Loss on drying When dried to constant weight at 100° to 105°, loses not more than 0.5% of its weight. Use 1 g.

Sulphated ash Not more than 0.1% when determined on the residue obtained in the test for Loss on drying, Appendix IX A, Method II.

Assay Dissolve 0.3 g in 10 ml of *anhydrous glacial acetic acid*, add 20 ml of *1,4-dioxan* and carry out Method I for *non-aqueous titration*, Appendix VIII A, using 7 ml of *mercury(II) acetate solution* and *crystal violet solution* as indicator. Each ml of 0.1M *perchloric acid VS* is equivalent to 0.03398 g of $C_{17}H_{21}NO_4,HCl$.

Storage Cocaine Hydrochloride should be kept in a well-closed container and protected from light and moisture.

Action and use Local anaesthetic.

Cochineal

Cochineal is the dried female insect, *Dactylopius coccus* Costa, containing eggs and larvae.

Characteristics Odour, characteristic.

Macroscopical Purplish-black or purplish-grey; about 3.5 to 5.5 mm long and 3 to 4.5 mm wide, plano-convex and somewhat oval in outline; the convex dorsal surface is transversely wrinkled and shows about 11 segments; the flat or slightly concave ventral surface carries upon the anterior part two seven-jointed straight antennae, three pairs of short legs, each terminating in a single claw, and a mouth from which projects the remains of a long filiform proboscis; these appendages are frequently more or less broken. Easily reduced to powder, which is dark red or puce.

Microscopical Scattered irregularly over the whole dermis are numerous solitary and grouped, short, tubular wax glands; within each insect are found numerous larvae, which are characterised by their proboscides appearing as two circular coils.

Colour value To 0.5 g in *moderately fine powder* add 60 ml of *phosphate buffer pH 8.0* and heat on a water-bath for 30 minutes. Cool, add sufficient *phosphate buffer pH 8.0* to produce 100 ml and filter. Dilute 5 ml of the filtrate to 100 ml with *phosphate buffer pH 8.0*. The *absorbance* of the resulting solution at the maximum at 530 nm is not less than 0.25, Appendix II B.

Ash Not more than 7.0%, Appendix XI J.

Foreign matter Not more than 2.0%, Appendix XI D.

Water-insoluble matter When the insects are placed in *water*, no insoluble powder separates.

Microbial contamination 1 g is free from *Escherichia coli*; 10 g is free from salmonellae, Appendix XVI B1.

Action and use Colouring agent.

Cocillana

Cocillana is the dried bark of *Guarea rusbyi* (Britton) Rusby and closely related species.

Characteristics Odour, slight and characteristic.

Macroscopical Large, flattish or curved pieces up to about 60 cm long and 15 cm wide and from 5 to 20 mm in thickness; outer surface showing shallow or deep longitudinal fissures according to age, colour greyish-brown or orange-brown where cork has been removed and often bearing whitish patches of lichen; inner surface longitudinally striated with straight or slightly wavy striae and easily detachable fibre strands; fracture short and granular in outer part, coarsely splintery, fibrous and soft in the much thicker inner part; transversely cut surface showing a narrow outer corky region and wider inner region with dark-coloured, narrow, wavy medullary rays.

Microscopical Cork cells in layers alternating with parenchyma containing yellowish sclereids, angular or irregular in shape and up to 150 μm long; fibres straight, thick walled and strongly sclerenchymatous in numerous tangentially elongated groups alternating with tangential bands of dark-coloured parenchyma and sieve tubes, each fibre group surrounded by a crystal sheath with prisms of calcium oxalate from 10 to 25 μm long; medullary rays one to three cells wide; cells of medullary rays and parenchyma with reddish-brown contents and single spheroidal or two- to four-compound starch granules, individual granules 5 to 20 μm in diameter.

Extractive soluble in ethanol (60%) Not less than 3.5%, Appendix XI B.

Action and use Expectorant.

Powdered Cocillana

Powdered Cocillana is Cocillana, in powder.

Characteristics Greyish-brown. Diagnostic structures: abundant thick-walled fibres occurring in groups accompanied by a calcium oxalate prism sheath; rectangular to irregularly-shaped sclereids containing yellowish pigment; reddish-brown fragments of parenchyma of the phloem and medullary rays; groups of dark brown cork cells; starch granules simple or compound with two to four components.

Extractive soluble in ethanol (60%) Not less than 3.5%, Appendix XI B.

Action and use Expectorant.

Coconut Oil

Coconut Oil is obtained by expression from the dried solid part of the endosperm of *Cocos nucifera* L.

Characteristics A white or pearl-white unctuous mass; odourless or with the odour of coconut. On exposure to air it readily becomes rancid, acquiring an unpleasant odour.

Solubility Soluble at 60° in 2 parts of *ethanol (96%)*, less soluble at lower temperatures; freely soluble in *ether* and in *chloroform*.

Acid value Not more than 0.2, Appendix X B. Use 20 g.

Iodine value 7.0 to 11.0 (*iodine monochloride method*), Appendix X E.

Melting point 23° to 26°, Appendix V A, Method IV.

Refractive index At 40°, 1.448 to 1.450, Appendix V E.

Saponification value 250 to 264, Appendix X G.

Unsaponifiable matter Not more than 0.8%, Appendix X H.

Peroxides Dissolve 5 g in 15 ml of *chloroform*, add 20 ml of *glacial acetic acid* and 0.5 ml of a saturated solution of *potassium iodide*, mix well, allow to stand in the dark for exactly 1 minute, add 30 ml of *water* and titrate with 0.01M *sodium thiosulphate VS* using *starch mucilage* as indicator. Not more than 0.5 ml of 0.01M *sodium thiosulphate VS* is required.

Storage Coconut Oil should be kept in a well-filled, well-closed container, protected from light and stored at a temperature not exceeding 25°.

Fractionated Coconut Oil

Fractionated Coconut Oil is prepared from the fixed oil obtained from the dried solid part of the endosperm of *Cocos nucifera* L. by hydrolysis, fractionation of the liberated fatty acids and re-esterification. It consists of a mixture of triglycerides containing only short- and medium-chain saturated fatty acids, mainly octanoic and decanoic acids.

Characteristics A clear, pale yellow liquid; odourless or almost odourless. It solidifies at about 0° and has a low viscosity even at temperatures near its solidification point.

Solubility Practically insoluble in *water*; miscible with *ethanol (96%)*, with *chloroform* and with *ether*.

Acid value Not more than 0.2, Appendix X B.

Iodine value Not more than 1.0 (*iodine monochloride method*), Appendix X E.

Refractive index 1.445 to 1.451, Appendix V E.

Saponification value 315 to 345, Appendix X G.

Weight per ml 0.940 to 0.950 g, Appendix V G.

Peroxides Dissolve 5 g in 15 ml of *chloroform*, add 20 ml of *glacial acetic acid* and 0.5 ml of a saturated solution of *potassium iodide*, mix well, allow to stand in the dark for exactly 1 minute, add 30 ml of *water* and titrate with 0.01M *sodium thiosulphate VS* using *starch mucilage* as indicator. Not more than 0.5 ml of 0.01M *sodium thiosulphate VS* is required.

Storage Fractionated Coconut Oil should be kept in a well-filled container, protected from light and stored at a temperature not exceeding 25°.

Codeine ☆

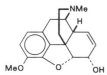

C₁₈H₂₁NO₃,H₂O   317.4   76-57-3

Codeine is (5*R*,6*S*)-7,8-didehydro-4,5-epoxy-3-methoxy-*N*-methylmorphinan-6-ol mono-hydrate. It contains not less than 99.0 per cent and not more than 101.0 per cent of C₁₈H₂₁NO₃, calculated with reference to the dried substance.

Characteristics Colourless crystals or a white, crystalline powder; odourless.

Solubility Slightly soluble in *water*; soluble in boiling *water* and in *ether*; freely soluble in *ethanol (96%)* and in *chloroform*.

Identification *Test A may be omitted if tests B, C, D and E are carried out. Tests B, C and D may be omitted if tests A and E are carried out.*

A. The *infra-red absorption spectrum*, Appendix II A, is concordant with the European Pharmacopœia reference spectrum of codeine. Prepare a dispersion in *potassium bromide IR*.

B. To 2 ml of a 0.5% w/v solution add 50 ml of *water* followed by 10 ml of 1M *sodium hydroxide* and dilute to 100 ml with *water*. The *light absorption* of the resulting solution, Appendix II B, in the range 250 to 350 nm exhibits a maximum only at 284 nm. The A(1%, 1 cm) at 284 nm is about 50.

C. Heat 10 mg on a water-bath with 1 ml of *sulphuric acid* and 0.05 ml of a 1.3% w/v solution of *iron(III) chloride hexahydrate*. A blue colour is produced which changes to red on the addition of 0.05 ml of *nitric acid*.

D. Yields the *reaction* characteristic of alkaloids, Appendix VI.

E. *Melting point*, 155° to 159°, Appendix V A, Method I.

Alkalinity pH of a 0.5% w/v solution, greater than 9, Appendix V L.

Clarity and colour of solution A 0.50% w/v solution in *carbon dioxide-free water* is *clear*, Appendix IV A, and *colourless*, Appendix IV B, Method II.

Specific optical rotation In a 2% w/v solution in *ethanol (96%)*, −142° to −146°, Appendix V F.

Foreign alkaloids Carry out the method for *thin-layer chromatography*, Appendix III A, using *silica gel G* as the coating substance and a mixture of 72 volumes of *absolute ethanol*, 30 volumes of *cyclohexane* and 6 volumes of 13.5M *ammonia* as the mobile phase. Apply separately to the chromatoplate 10 μl of each of three solutions of the substance being examined in *absolute ethanol* containing (1) 4% w/v, (2) 0.06% w/v and (3) 0.04% w/v. After removal of the plate, allow it to dry in air and spray with *acetic potassium iodobismuthate solution*. Any *secondary spot* in the chromatogram obtained with solution (1) is not more intense than the spot in the chromatogram obtained with solution (2) and not more than one such spot with an Rf value higher than that of the principal spot is more intense than the spot in the chromatogram obtained with solution (3).

Morphine Dissolve 0.10 g in sufficient 0.1M *hydrochloric acid* to produce 5 ml, add 2 ml of a 1% w/v solution of *sodium nitrite*, allow to stand for 15 minutes and add 3 ml of 6M *ammonia*. The resulting solution is not more intensely coloured than *reference solution B₄*, Appendix IV B, Method II (about 0.13% of morphine).

Loss on drying When dried to constant weight at 100° to 105°, loses 5.0 to 6.0% of its weight. Use 1 g.

Sulphated ash Not more than 0.1%, Appendix IX A, Method II. Use 1 g.

Assay Dissolve 0.25 g in 10 ml of *anhydrous glacial acetic acid*, add 20 ml of *1,4-dioxan* and carry out Method I for *non-aqueous titration*, Appendix VIII A, using *crystal violet solution* as indicator. Each ml of 0.1M *perchloric acid VS* is equivalent to 0.02994 g of C₁₈H₂₁NO₃.

Storage Codeine should be kept in a well-closed container and protected from light.

Action and use Antidiarrhoeal; cough suppressant; analgesic.

Codeine Hydrochloride

C₁₈H₂₁NO₃,HCl,2H₂O   371.9

Codeine Hydrochloride is 4,5-epoxy-3-methoxy-*N*-methylmorphin-7-en-6-ol hydrochloride dihydrate. It contains not less than 98.5 per cent and not more than 100.5 per cent of C₁₈H₂₁NO₃,HCl, calculated with reference to the dried substance.

Characteristics Small, colourless crystals or a white, crystalline powder.

Solubility Soluble in 20 parts of *water*; slightly soluble in *ethanol (96%)*; practically insoluble in *chloroform* and in *ether*.

Identification A. The *infra-red absorption spectrum*, Appendix II A, is concordant with the *reference spectrum* of codeine hydrochloride.

B. To 50 ml of a 0.04% w/v solution add 10 ml of 1M *sodium hydroxide* and dilute to 100 ml with *water*. The *light absorption* of the resulting solution, Appendix II B, in the range 230 to 350 nm exhibits a maximum only at 284 nm. The *absorbance* at 284 nm is about 0.88.

C. Yields *reaction A* characteristic of chlorides, Appendix VI.

Acidity or alkalinity To 10 ml of a 2% w/v solution add 0.05 ml of *methyl red solution*. Not more than 0.2 ml of either 0.02M *sodium hydroxide VS* or 0.02M *hydrochloric acid VS* is required to change the colour of the solution.

Clarity and colour of solution A 4.0% w/v solution is *clear*, Appendix IV A, and not more intensely coloured than *reference solution* Y_6, Appendix IV B, Method II.

Specific optical rotation In a 2% w/v solution, $-116°$ to $-120°$, Appendix V F.

Related substances Carry out the method for *thin-layer chromatography*, Appendix III A, using *silica gel G* as the coating substance and a mixture of 72 volumes of *absolute ethanol*, 30 volumes of *cyclohexane* and 6 volumes of 13.5M *ammonia* as the mobile phase. Apply separately to the chromatoplate 10 µl of each of three solutions of the substance being examined a mixture of 4 volumes of 0.01M *hydrochloric acid* and 1 volume of *absolute ethanol* containing (1) 5.0% w/v, (2) 0.075% w/v and (3) 0.05% w/v. After removal of the plate, allow it to dry in air and spray with *acetic potassium iodobismuthate solution*. Any *secondary spot* in the chromatogram obtained with solution (1) is not more intense than the spot in the chromatogram obtained with solution (2) and not more than one such spot with an Rf value higher than that of the principal spot is more intense than the spot in the chromatogram obtained with solution (3).

Sulphate 15 ml of a 1.0% w/v solution complies with the *limit test for sulphates*, Appendix VII (0.1%).

Morphine Dissolve 0.10 g in sufficient 0.1M *hydrochloric acid* to produce 5 ml, add 2 ml of a 1% w/v solution of *sodium nitrite*, allow to stand for 15 minutes and add 3 ml of 6M *ammonia*. The resulting solution is not more intensely coloured than *reference solution* B_4, Appendix IV B, Method II (about 0.1% of morphine).

Loss on drying When dried to constant weight at 100° to 105°, loses 8.0 to 10.5% of its weight. Use 1 g.

Sulphated ash Not more than 0.1%, Appendix IX A, Method II. Use 1 g.

Assay Dissolve 0.3 g in a mixture of 10 ml of *anhydrous glacial acetic acid* and 20 ml of *1,4-dioxan*. Carry out Method I for *non-aqueous titration*, Appendix VIII A, using 7 ml of *mercury(II) acetate solution* and determining the end-point potentiometrically. Each ml of 0.1M *perchloric acid VS* is equivalent to 0.03358 g of $C_{18}H_{21}NO_3,HCl$.

Storage Codeine Hydrochloride should be kept in a well-closed container and protected from light.

Action and use Analgesic.

Codeine Phosphate ☆

$C_{18}H_{21}NO_3,H_3PO_4,\frac{1}{2}H_2O$ 406.4   *41444-62-6*

Codeine Phosphate is (5*R*,6*S*)-7,8-didehydro-4,5-epoxy-3-methoxy-*N*-methylmorphinan-6-ol dihydrogen orthophosphate hemihydrate. It contains not less than 98.5 per cent and not more than 101.0 per cent of $C_{18}H_{21}NO_3,H_3PO_4$, calculated with reference to the dried substance.

Characteristics Small, colourless crystals or a white, crystalline powder; odourless.

Solubility Soluble in 4 parts of *water*; slightly soluble in *ethanol* (96%); practically insoluble in *chloroform* and in *ether*.

Identification *Test A may be omitted if tests B, C, D, E and F are carried out. Tests B, C, D and E may be omitted if tests A and F are carried out.*

A. To 5 ml of a 4% w/v solution add 1 ml of 2M *sodium hydroxide* and induce crystallisation, if necessary, by scratching the wall of the tube with a glass rod. The *infrared absorption spectrum*, Appendix II A, of the residue after washing with *water* and drying at 100° to 105° is concordant with the European Pharmacopœia reference spectrum of codeine. Prepare a dispersion in *potassium bromide IR*.

B. To 25 ml of a 0.04% w/v solution add 25 ml of *water* and 10 ml of 1M *sodium hydroxide* and dilute to 100 ml with *water*. The *light absorption* of the resulting solution, Appendix II B, in the range 250 to 350 nm exhibits a maximum only at 284 nm. The A(1%, 1 cm) at 284 nm is about 38.

C. Heat 10 mg on a water-bath with 1 ml of *sulphuric acid* and 0.05 ml of a 1.3% w/v solution of *iron(III) chloride hexahydrate*. A blue colour is produced which changes to red on the addition of 0.05 ml of *nitric acid*.

D. To 5 ml of a 4% w/v solution add 1 ml of 2M *sodium hydroxide* and initiate crystallisation if necessary, by scratching the wall of the tube with a glass rod. The *melting point* of the crystals, after washing and drying at 100° to 105°, is 155° to 159°, Appendix V A, Method I.

E. Yields the *reaction* characteristic of alkaloids, Appendix VI.

F. Yields *reaction A* characteristic of phosphates, Appendix VI.

Acidity pH of a 4% w/v solution in *carbon dioxide-free water* prepared from *distilled water*, 4.0 to 5.0, Appendix V L.

Clarity and colour of solution A 4.0% w/v solution in *carbon dioxide-free water* prepared from *distilled water* is *clear*, Appendix IV A, and not more intensely coloured than *reference solution* Y_6, Appendix IV B, Method II.

Specific optical rotation In a 2% w/v solution, $-98°$ to $-102°$, Appendix V F.

Sulphate 15 ml of a 1.0% w/v solution in *distilled water* complies with the *limit test for sulphates*, Appendix VII (0.1%).

Related substances Carry out the method for *thin-layer chromatography*, Appendix III A, using *silica gel G* as the coating substance and a mixture of 72 volumes of *absolute ethanol*, 30 volumes of *cyclohexane* and 6 volumes of 13.5M *ammonia* as the mobile phase. Apply separately to the chromatoplate 10 µl of each of the following solutions. For solution (1) dissolve 0.5 g of the substance being examined in sufficient of a mixture of 4 volumes of 0.01M *hydrochloric acid* and 1 volume of *absolute ethanol* to produce 10 ml. For solution (2) dilute 1.5 ml of solution (1) to 100 ml with the same solvent. For solution (3) dilute 1 ml of solution (1) to 100 ml with the same solvent. After removal of the plate, allow it to dry in air and spray with *acetic potassium iodobismuthate solution*. Any *secondary spot* in the chromatogram obtained with solution (1) is not more intense than the spot in the chromatogram obtained with solution (2) and not more than one such spot, with an Rf value higher than that of the principal spot, is more intense than the spot in the chromatogram obtained with solution (3).

Morphine Dissolve 0.10 g in sufficient 0.1M *hydrochloric acid* to produce 5 ml, add 2 ml of a 1% w/v solution of sodium nitrite, allow to stand for 15 minutes and add 3 ml of 6M ammonia. The resulting solution is not more intensely coloured than reference solution B_4, Appendix IV B, Method II (about 0.13% of morphine).

Loss on drying When dried to constant weight at 100° to 105°, loses 1.5 to 3.0% of its weight. Use 1 g.

Assay Dissolve 0.35 g in a mixture of 10 ml of anhydrous glacial acetic acid and 20 ml of 1,4-dioxan and carry out Method I for non-aqueous titration, Appendix VIII A, using crystal violet solution as indicator. Each ml of 0.1M perchloric acid VS is equivalent to 0.03974 g of $C_{18}H_{21}NO_3,H_3PO_4$.

Storage Codeine Phosphate should be kept in a well-closed container and protected from light.

Preparations
Codeine Linctus
Paediatric Codeine Linctus
Codeine Phosphate Tablets
Co-codaprin Tablets
Dispersible Co-codaprin Tablets

Action and use Antidiarrhoeal; cough suppressant; analgesic.

The title of the monograph in the European Pharmacopœia is Codeine Phosphate Hemihydrate.

Codeine Phosphate Sesquihydrate ☆

$C_{18}H_{21}NO_3,H_3PO_4,1\frac{1}{2}H_2O$ 424.4

Codeine Phosphate Sesquihydrate is (5R,6S)-7,8-didehydro-4,5-epoxy-3-methoxy-N-methyl-morphinan-6-ol dihydrogen orthophosphate sesquihydrate. It contains not less than 98.5 per cent and not more than 101.0 per cent of $C_{18}H_{21}NO_3,H_3PO_4$, calculated with reference to the dried substance.

Characteristics Small, colourless crystals or a white, crystalline powder; odourless.

Solubility Soluble in 4 parts of water; slightly soluble in ethanol (96%); practically insoluble in chloroform and in ether.

Identification Complies with the tests for Identification described under Codeine Phosphate.

Test A may be omitted if tests B, C, D, E and F are carried out. Tests B, C, D and E may be omitted if tests A and F are carried out.

Acidity; Clarity and colour of solution; Specific optical rotation; Sulphate; Related substances; Morphine Complies with the requirements stated under Codeine Phosphate.

Loss on drying When dried to constant weight at 100° to 105°, loses 5.0% to 7.5% of its weight. Use 0.5 g.

Assay Carry out the Assay described under Codeine Phosphate.

Storage Codeine Phosphate Sesquihydrate should be kept in a well-closed container and protected from light.

Preparations
Codeine Linctus
Paediatric Codeine Linctus
Codeine Phosphate Tablets

Action and use Antidiarrhoeal; cough suppressant; analgesic.

Co-dergocrine Mesylate

	R
dihydroergocristine mesylate	—CH$_2$Ph
dihydroergocryptine mesylate, α	—CH$_2$·CHMe$_2$
β	—CHMe·CH$_2$·CH$_3$
dihydroergocornine mesylate	—CHMe$_2$

8067-24-1

Co-dergocrine Mesylate consists of equal proportions of the methanesulphonates of dihydroergocornine ($C_{31}H_{41}N_5O_5,CH_4O_3S$; 659.8), dihydroergocristine ($C_{35}H_{41}N_5O_5$, CH_4O_3S; 707.8) and dihydroergocryptine ($C_{32}H_{43}N_5O_5,CH_4O_3S$; 673.8), the dihydroergocryptine being present as both the α and β forms in the ratio of not less than 1.5 to 1 and not more than 2.5 to 1. It contains not less than 97.0 per cent and not more than 103.0 per cent of co-dergocrine mesylate, calculated with reference to the dried substance, and not less than 30.0 per cent and not more than 36.5 per cent of each of the three components.

Characteristics A white to yellowish-white powder; odourless or almost odourless.

Solubility Soluble in 50 parts of water, in 30 parts of ethanol (96%), in 10 parts of acetone and in 100 parts of chloroform; practically insoluble in ether.

Identification A. In the Assay, the chromatogram obtained with solution (2) shows four major peaks having retention times corresponding to the peaks due to co-dergocrine mesylate in the chromatogram obtained with solution (1).
B. Dissolve 10 mg in 1 ml of methanol and add 5 ml of a 1% w/v solution of (+)-tartaric acid. To 1 ml of the resulting solution, add slowly 2 ml of dilute dimethylaminobenzaldehyde solution and mix. A deep blue colour is produced.
C. Mix 0.1 g with 0.5 g of powdered sodium hydroxide, heat to fusion and continue heating for a few seconds. Cool, add 0.5 ml of water and a slight excess of 2M hydrochloric acid and warm. Sulphur dioxide is evolved, which turns moistened starch—iodate paper blue.

Acidity pH of a 0.5% w/v solution, 4.2 to 5.2, Appendix V L.

Related substances Carry out in subdued light the method for thin-layer chromatography, Appendix III A, using a silica gel precoated chromatoplate (Merck silica gel 60 plates are suitable), scored at a distance of 15 cm from the line of application, and a freshly prepared mixture of 50 volumes of dichloromethane, 50 volumes of ethyl acetate, 3 volumes of methanol and 1 volume of 13.5M ammonia as the mobile phase. Use an unlined tank closed with an ungreased lid and develop the chromatogram immediately after introducing the mobile phase into the tank. Apply separately to the plate, in the order specified, 5 μl of each of the following solutions prepared immediately before use in a mixture of 9 volumes of *chloroform* and 1 volume of *methanol* containing (1) 0.0060% w/v of *dihydroergocristine mesylate BPCRS*, (2) 0.0040% w/v of *dihydroergocristine mesylate BPCRS*, (3) 0.0020% w/v of *dihydroergocristine mesylate BPCRS* and (4) 2.0% w/v of the substance being examined. Allow the solvent front to ascend for exactly 90 minutes, remove the plate and dry it in a current of cold air for not longer than 1 minute. Using a freshly prepared mobile phase, repeat the development for a further 90 minutes, remove the plate and dry it in a current of cold air for not longer than 1 minute. Spray with a 1% w/v solution of *dimethylaminobenzaldehyde* in a mixture of equal volumes of *hydrochloric acid* and *ethanol* (96%), dry in a current of cold air for not longer than 2 minutes and heat at 40° for 15 minutes. In the chromatogram obtained with solution (4), any *secondary spot* is not more intense than the spot in the chromatogram obtained with solution (1), not more than two such spots are more intense than the spot in the chromatogram obtained with solution (2) and not more than a total of four such spots are more intense than the spot in the chromatogram obtained with solution (3). Disregard any spot remaining on the line of application.

Loss on drying When dried to constant weight at 120° at a pressure of 14 Pa, loses not more than 6.0% of its weight. Use 1 g.

Assay Carry out the method for *high-performance liquid chromatography*, Appendix III D, using the following solutions. Solution (1) contains 0.060% w/v of *co-dergocrine mesylate BPCRS* in a mixture of 2 volumes of a 1% w/v solution of (+)-*tartaric acid* and 1 volume of *absolute ethanol*. Solution (2) contains 0.060% w/v of the substance being examined in the same solvent mixture.

The chromatographic procedure may be carried out using (a) a stainless steel column (10 cm × 4.6 mm) packed with *stationary phase C* (5 μm) (Spherisorb ODS1 is suitable), (b) a mixture of 150 volumes of *water*, 50 volumes of *acetonitrile* and 5 volumes of *triethylamine* as the mobile phase with a flow rate of 1.5 ml per minute and (c) a detection wavelength of 280 nm. The components are eluted in the following order: dihydroergocornine, dihydro-α-ergocryptine, dihydroergocristine and dihydro-β-ergocryptine.

The *resolution factor* between the peaks due to dihydro-α-ergocryptine and dihydroergocristine should be not less than 1.2; this value may be obtained by appropriate adjustment of the acetonitrile content of the mobile phase.

Calculate the content of co-dergocrine mesylate in the substance being examined using the following expression:

$$\frac{[A_1M_1 + A_2M_2 + A_3M_3 + A_4M_2]_S w_R p_R}{[A_1M_1 + A_2M_2 + A_3M_3 + A_4M_2]_R w_S [1 - 0.01L]}$$

where A_1, A_2, A_3, A_4 = the peak areas of the components in order of elution;

M_1, M_2, M_3 = the molecular weights of the methanesulphonates of dihydroergocornine, dihydroergocryptine (α and β forms) and dihydroergocristine;

w_R = the weight taken of *co-dergocrine mesylate BPCRS* ('R');

w_S = the weight taken of the substance being examined ('S');

L = the percentage loss on drying of the substance being examined;

p_R = the declared content of co-dergocrine mesylate in *co-dergocrine mesylate BPCRS*.

Calculate the percentage contents of the methane-sulphonates of dihydroergocornine, of dihydroergocryptine (α and β forms) and of dihydroergocristine with respect to the sum of these components in solution (2), using the products of the molecular weights and peak area figures, and determine the ratio of the peak area of dihydro-α-ergocryptine to that of dihydro-β-ergocryptine.

Storage Co-dergocrine Mesylate should be kept in a well-closed container, protected from light and stored at a temperature not exceeding 25°.

Preparation
Co-dergocrine Tablets

Action and use Vasodilator.

Cod-liver Oil

Cod-liver Oil is the oil obtained from the fresh liver of the cod, *Gadus callarias* L., and other species of *Gadus*, refined and clarified by filtration at about 0°. It contains in 1 g not less than 600 Units of vitamin A and not less than 85 Units of antirachitic activity (vitamin D). A quantity of Dodecyl Gallate, Octyl Gallate or Propyl Gallate or any mixture of these substances, not exceeding 0.01 per cent w/v, may be added as an antioxidant.

Characteristics A pale yellow liquid; odour and taste, slightly fishy, but not rancid.

Solubility Practically insoluble in *ethanol* (96%); miscible with *chloroform*, with *ether* and with *petroleum spirit* (*boiling range, 40° to 60°*).

Acid value Not greater than 1.2, Appendix X B.

Iodine value 150 to 180 (*iodine monochloride method*), Appendix X E.

Refractive index 1.477 to 1.482, Appendix V E.

Saponification value 180 to 190, Appendix X G.

Unsaponifiable matter Not more than 1.5%, Appendix X H.

Weight per ml 0.917 to 0.924 g, Appendix V G.

Stearin Remains bright when cooled to and kept at 0° for 3 hours.

Assay *For vitamin A* Determine the content of vitamin A by the *assay of vitamin A*, Appendix VIII K.

For antirachitic activity (vitamin D) Carry out the *biological assay of antirachitic vitamin (vitamin D)*, Appendix XIV G. For the purpose of the assay and calculations, assume the stated potency to be 100 Units per g. The estimated potency is not less than 85% of the stated potency. The fiducial limits of error are not less than 60% and not more than 170% of the stated potency.

Storage Cod-liver Oil should be kept in a well-filled, well-closed container and protected from light.

Action and use Source of vitamins A and D.

Colchicine

$C_{22}H_{25}NO_6$ 399.4 *64-86-8*

Colchicine is an alkaloid, (*S*)-*N*-(5,6,7,9-tetrahydro-1,2,3,10-tetramethoxy-9-oxo-benzo[α]heptalen-7-yl)acetamide, which occurs in the corm and seeds of *Colchicum autumnale* L. It contains not less than 97.0 per cent and not more than 103.0 per cent of $C_{22}H_{25}NO_6$, calculated with reference to the dried, solvent-free substance.

Characteristics Pale yellow crystals, amorphous scales or powder; odourless or almost odourless.

Solubility Freely soluble in *water*, but moderately concentrated solutions may deposit crystals of a sesquihydrate, which has a limited solubility in cold *water*; freely soluble in *ethanol (96%)* and in *chloroform*; slightly soluble at 15.5° in *ether*.

Identification A. The *infra-red absorption spectrum*, Appendix II A, is concordant with the *reference spectrum* of colchicine. If the spectra are not concordant, heat a sufficient quantity at 105° for 10 minutes and prepare a new spectrum. Disregard any peak at 1735 cm^{-1}.
B. The *light absorption*, Appendix II B, in the range 230 to 400 nm of a 0.001% w/v solution in *ethanol (96%)* exhibits two maxima, at 243 nm and 350 nm. The *absorbance* at 243 nm is about 0.73 and at 350 nm is about 0.42.
C. Dissolve 50 mg in 1.5 ml of *water*. A yellow colour is produced which is intensified on the addition of mineral acids.
D. Mix 1 mg with 0.2 ml of *sulphuric acid* in a white dish; a lemon colour is produced which on the addition of 0.05 ml of *nitric acid* changes to greenish-blue and then rapidly becomes reddish and finally yellow or almost colourless. On the addition of an excess of 5M *sodium hydroxide* the colour changes to red.
E. Dissolve 30 mg in 1 ml of *ethanol (96%)* and add 0.05 ml of *iron(III) chloride test-solution*. A red colour is produced immediately.

Specific optical rotation In a 1% w/v solution, −425° to −450°, Appendix V F.

Colchiceine To 5 ml of a 1.0% w/v solution add 0.1 ml of a 10.5% w/v solution of *iron(III) chloride hexahydrate*. Any colour produced is not more intense than that obtained by mixing 2 ml of *yellow primary solution* with 1 ml of *red primary solution* and 2 ml of *blue primary solution*, Appendix IV B.

Related substances Carry out the method for *thin-layer chromatography*, Appendix III A, using a suitable aluminium oxide containing a substance that fluoresces at about 254 nm as the coating substance and a mixture of 125 volumes of *chloroform*, 100 volumes of *acetone* and 2 volumes of 13.5M *ammonia* as the mobile phase. Apply separately to the chromatoplate 2 µl of each of two solutions of the substance being examined in *ethanol (96%)* containing (1) 5.0% w/v and (2) 0.25% w/v. After removal of the plate, allow it to dry in air and examine under *ultra-violet light (254 nm)*. Any *secondary spot* in the chromatogram obtained with solution (1) is not more intense than the spot in the chromatogram obtained with solution (2).

Loss on drying When dried over *phosphorus pentoxide* at a pressure not exceeding 0.7 kPa for 24 hours, loses not more than 2.0% of its weight. Use 1 g.

Solvent Carry out the method for *gas chromatography*, Appendix III B, using three solutions in *water* containing (1) 0.1% v/v of *ethanol-free chloroform*, 0.10% v/v of *ethyl acetate* and either 0.10% v/v (for the determination of ethyl acetate) or 0.020% v/v (for the determination of chloroform) of *absolute ethanol* (internal standard), (2) 1.0% w/v of the dried substance being examined and (3) 1.0% w/v of the dried substance being examined and the same concentration of the internal standard as in solution (1).

The chromatographic procedure may be carried out using a glass column (1.5 m × 4 mm) packed with *diatomaceous support* (100 to 120 mesh) coated with 10% w/w of *polyethylene glycol 1000* and maintained at 75°.

Calculate the percentage w/w of ethyl acetate or chloroform, taking 0.901 g or 1.477 g, respectively, as the weight per ml at 20°.

The sum of the content of chloroform or ethyl acetate and the percentage Loss on drying determined in the above test is not more than 10%.

Sulphated ash Not more than 0.1%, Appendix IX A.

Assay Dissolve 50 mg in a mixture of 10 ml of *acetic anhydride* and 20 ml of *toluene* and carry out Method I for *non-aqueous titration*, Appendix VIII A, but using 0.02M *perchloric acid VS* as titrant and determining the end-point potentiometrically. Each ml of 0.02M *perchloric acid VS* is equivalent to 0.007988 g of $C_{22}H_{25}NO_6$.

Storage Colchicine should be kept in a well-closed container and protected from light.

Preparation
Colchicine Tablets

Action and use Used in treatment of gout.

Colistin Sulphate ☆

1264-72-8

Colistin Sulphate is a mixture of the sulphates of polypeptides produced by certain strains of *Bacillus polymyxa* var. *colistinus* or obtained by any other means. The potency is not less than 19,000 Units per mg, calculated with reference to the dried substance.

Characteristics A white or almost white powder; almost odourless; hygroscopic.

Solubility Soluble in less than 2 parts of *water*; slightly soluble in *ethanol (96%)*; practically insoluble in *acetone*, in *chloroform* and in *ether*.

Identification A. Carry out the method for *thin-layer chromatography*, Appendix III A, protected from light, using *silica gel G* as the coating substance and a mixture of 75 parts of *phenol* and 25 parts of *water* as the mobile phase but allowing the solvent front to ascend 12 cm above the line of application. Apply separately to the chromatoplate 5 µl of each of the following solutions as bands 10 mm long. For solution (1) dissolve 5 mg of the substance being examined in a mixture of 0.5 ml of *hydrochloric acid* and 0.5 ml of *water*, heat in a sealed tube at 135° for 5 hours, evaporate to dryness on a water-bath, continue to heat until the odour of hydrogen chloride is no longer detectable and dissolve the residue in 0.5 ml of *water*. Solutions (2) to (5) are solutions in *water* containing 0.2% w/v of L-*leucine*, 0.2% w/v of L-*threonine*, 0.2% w/v of L-*phenylalanine* and 0.2% w/v of L-*serine*, respectively. Place the plate in the tank so that it is not in contact with the mobile phase and expose it to the vapour of the mobile phase for at least 12 hours. After removal of the plate, heat it at 100° to 105° and spray with a solution prepared by dissolving 1 g of *ninhydrin* in 50 ml of *ethanol* (96%) and adding 10 ml of *glacial acetic acid*. Heat the plate at 110° for 5 minutes.

The bands in the chromatogram obtained with solution (1) correspond to those in the chromatograms obtained with solutions (2) and (3) and do not correspond to those in the chromatograms obtained with solutions (4) and (5). The chromatogram obtained with solution (1) also shows a band with a very low Rf value (2,4-diaminobutanoic acid).
B. Dissolve 5 mg in 3 ml of *water* and add 3 ml of 2M *sodium hydroxide*. Shake and add 0.5 ml of a 1% w/v solution of *copper(II) sulphate*. A violet colour is produced.
C. Dissolve 50 mg in 1 ml of 1M *hydrochloric acid* and add 0.5 ml of 0.01M *iodine VS*. The colour is not discharged (distinction from colistin sulphomethate sodium).
D. Yields *reaction A* characteristic of sulphates, Appendix VI.

Acidity pH of a 1% w/v solution, 4.0 to 6.0, Appendix V L.

Specific optical rotation In a 5% w/v solution, −63° to −73°, Appendix V F.

Sulphate 16.0 to 18.0% of SO₄, calculated with reference to the dried substance, when determined by the following method. Dissolve 0.25 g in 100 ml of *water*, adjust the pH to 11 with 13.5M *ammonia* and add 10 ml of 0.1M *barium chloride VS*. Titrate with 0.1M *disodium edetate VS* using 0.5 mg of *metalphthalein* as indicator; add 50 ml of *ethanol* (96%) when the colour of the indicator begins to change and continue the titration until the violet-blue colour is discharged. Each ml of 0.1M *barium chloride VS* is equivalent to 0.009606 g of sulphate, SO₄.

Loss on drying When dried over *phosphorus pentoxide* at 60° at a pressure not exceeding 0.7 kPa for 3 hours, loses not more than 3.5% of its weight. Use 1 g.

Sulphated ash Not more than 1.0%, Appendix IX A, Method II. Use 1 g.

Assay Carry out the *biological assay of antibiotics*, Appendix XIV A. The precision of the assay is such that the fiducial limits of error are not less than 95% and not more than 105% of the estimated potency.

Storage Colistin Sulphate should be kept in an airtight container and protected from light.

Labelling The label states (1) the number of Units per mg; (2) the date after which the material is not intended to be used; (3) the conditions under which it should be stored.

Preparation
Colistin Tablets
Action and use Antibacterial.

Colistin Sulphomethate Sodium ☆

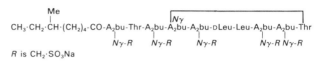

8068-28-8

Colistin Sulphomethate Sodium is prepared from colistin by the action of formaldehyde and sodium bisulphite, whereby amino groups of colistin are sulphomethylated. The potency is not less than 11,500 Units per mg, calculated with reference to the dried substance.

Characteristics A white or almost white powder; almost odourless; hygroscopic.

Solubility Soluble in less than 2 parts of *water*; slightly soluble in *ethanol* (96%); practically insoluble in *acetone*, in *chloroform* and in *ether*.

Identification A. Carry out the method for *thin-layer chromatography*, Appendix III A, protected from light, using *silica gel G* as the coating substance and a mixture of 75 parts of *phenol* and 25 parts of *water* as the mobile phase but allowing the solvent front to ascend 12 cm above the line of application. Apply separately to the chromatoplate 5 µl of each of the following solutions as bands 10 mm long. For solution (1) dissolve 5 mg of the substance being examined in a mixture of 0.5 ml of *hydrochloric acid* and 0.5 ml of *water*, heat in a sealed tube at 135° for 5 hours, evaporate to dryness on a water-bath, continue to heat until the odour of hydrogen chloride is no longer detectable and dissolve the residue in 0.5 ml of *water*. Solutions (2) to (5) are solutions in *water* containing 0.2% w/v of L-*leucine*, 0.2% w/v of L-*threonine*, 0.2% w/v of L-*phenylalanine* and 0.2% w/v of L-*serine*, respectively. Place the plate in the tank so that it is not in contact with the mobile phase and expose it to the vapour of the mobile phase for at least 12 hours. After removal of the plate, heat it at 100° to 105°, spray with a solution prepared by dissolving 1 g of *ninhydrin* in 50 ml of *ethanol* (96%) and adding 10 ml of *glacial acetic acid* and heat at 110° for 5 minutes.

The bands in the chromatogram obtained with solution (1) correspond to those in the chromatograms obtained with solutions (2) and (3) and do not correspond to those in the chromatograms obtained with solutions (4) and (5). The chromatogram obtained with solution (1) also shows a band with very low Rf value (2,4-diaminobutanoic acid).
B. Dissolve 5 mg in 3 ml of *water* and add 3 ml of 2M *sodium hydroxide*. Shake and add 0.5 ml of a 1% w/v solution of *copper(II) sulphate*. A violet colour is produced.
C. Dissolve 50 mg in 1 ml of 1M *hydrochloric acid* and add 0.5 ml of 0.01M *iodine VS*; the colour is discharged (distinction from colistin sulphate). The resulting solution yields *reaction A* characteristic of sulphates, Appendix VI.
D. Yields *reaction A* characteristic of sodium salts, Appendix VI.

Acidity or alkalinity pH of a 1% w/v solution, 6.2 to 7.7, Appendix V L.

Clarity of solution A 1.6% w/v solution is *clear*, Appendix IV A.

Specific optical rotation In a 5% w/v solution, −46° to −51°,Appendix V F.

Free colistin Dissolve 80 mg in 3 ml of *water*, add 0.1 ml of a 10% w/v solution of *silicotungstic acid* and allow to stand for 10 to 20 seconds. The resulting solution is not more opalescent than *reference suspension II*, Appendix IV A.

Total sulphite Dissolve 0.1 g in 50 ml of *water*, add 5 ml of 2.5M *sodium hydroxide* and 0.3 g of *potassium cyanide*, boil gently for 3 minutes and cool. Neutralise the solution with 0.5M *sulphuric acid* using 0.2 ml of *methyl orange solution* as indicator. Add 0.5 ml of 0.5M *sulphuric acid* and 0.2 g of *potassium iodide* and titrate with 0.05M *iodine VS* using *starch mucilage*, added towards the end of the titration, as indicator. The volume of 0.05M *iodine VS* required is 5.5 to 7.0 ml.

Loss on drying When dried over *phosphorus pentoxide* at 60° at a pressure not exceeding 0.7 kPa for 3 hours, loses not more than 1.5% of its weight. Use 1 g.

Sulphated ash 16 to 21%, Appendix IX A, Method II. Use 0.5 g.

Assay Carry out the *biological assay of antibiotics*, Appendix XIV A. The precision of the assay is such that the fiducial limits of error are not less than 95% and not more than 105% of the estimated potency.

Storage Colistin Sulphomethate Sodium should be kept in an airtight container and protected from light. If it is intended for use in the manufacture of a parenteral dosage form the container should be sterile, tamper-evident and sealed so as to exclude micro-organisms.

Labelling The label states (1) the number of Units per mg; (2) the date after which the material is not intended to be used; (3) the conditions under which it should be stored; (4) whether or not it is intended for use in the manufacture of a parenteral dosage form.

Preparation
Colistin Sulphomethate Injection

Action and use Antibacterial.

Colistin Sulphomethate Sodium intended for use in the manufacture of a parenteral dosage form complies with the following additional requirements.

Abnormal toxicity Complies with the *test for abnormal toxicity*, Appendix XIV L. Use 0.5 ml of *saline solution* containing 10 mg per ml.

Pyrogens Complies with the *test for pyrogens*, Appendix XIV K. Use per kg of the rabbit's weight 1 ml of *water for injections* containing 2.5 mg per ml.

Sterility Complies with the *test for sterility*, Appendix XVI A.

The title of the monograph in the European Pharmacopœia is Colistimethate Sodium.

Colophony
Resin

Colophony is the residue left after distilling the volatile oil from the oleo-resin obtained from various species of *Pinus*.

Characteristics Translucent, pale yellow or brownish-yellow, angular, brittle, readily fusible, glassy masses; odour, faintly terebinthinate.

Solubility Practically insoluble in *water*; soluble in *ethanol (96%)*, in *carbon disulphide* and in *ether*; partially soluble in *petroleum spirit (boiling range, 40° to 60°)*.

Identification Dissolve 0.1 g in 10 ml of *acetic anhydride* with the aid of gentle heat, cool and add 0.05 ml of *sulphuric acid*. A bright purplish-red colour, rapidly changing to violet, is produced.

Acid value 150 to 180, Appendix X B, using 1 g and 50 ml of *ethanol (96%)* as the solvent.

Sulphated ash Not more than 0.2%, Appendix IX A.

Coriander

Coriander consists of the dried ripe fruits of *Coriander sativum* L.

Characteristics Odour of the crushed fruit, aromatic; taste, spicy and characteristic.

Macroscopical Cremocarp glabrous, sub-globular, about 2 to 4 mm in diameter. Primary ridges ten, wavy and less prominent than the eight straight secondary ridges. Mericarps usually remaining united by their margins; generally brown, brownish-yellow or purplish-brown, apex with a small stylopod and the remains of sepals. Endosperm concave on the commissural side.

Microscopical Pericarp: many cells of the thin-walled epidermis, when present, can be seen to contain one or two small prisms of calcium oxalate. Mesocarp differentiated into outer, middle and inner zones. Outer zone, parenchymatous, containing degenerated vittae as tangentially flattened cavities. Two, or rarely more, normal vittae containing volatile oil also present on the commissural side of each mericarp. Middle zone sclerenchymatous, composed of sinuous rows of pitted fusiform cells often crossing one another at right angles and forming definite longitudinal strands in the secondary ridges. Inner mesocarp partially composed of thin-walled hexagonal sclereids; inner epidermis of mesocarp consisting of cells showing parquetry arrangement. Endosperm parenchymatous, with thickened cellulose walls; containing fixed oil and numerous aleurone grains about 4 to 8 μm in diameter with minute rosettes of calcium oxalate.

Acid-insoluble ash Not more than 1.5%, Appendix XI K.

Foreign matter Not more than 2.0%, Appendix XI D.

Volatile oil Not less than 0.3% v/w, Appendix XI E, Method I. Use 40 g, in *coarse powder*, and distil for 3 hours.

Storage Coriander should be stored in a dry place at a temperature not exceeding 25°.

Action and use Flavour.

Powdered Coriander

Powdered Coriander is Coriander in powder.

Characteristics Fawn to brown. Diagnostic structures: epidermal cells of the pericarp, if present, crossing layers of fusiform sclerenchymatous cells or thin-walled lignified cells of the mesocarp; inner epidermis; fragments of brown epithelium of vittae; endosperm containing fixed oil and aleurone grains containing calcium oxalate. Trichomes and starch absent.

Acid-insoluble ash Not more than 1.5%, Appendix XI K.

Volatile oil Not less than 0.2% v/w, Appendix XI E, Method I. Use 40 g and distil for 3 hours.

Storage Powdered Coriander should be kept in a well-closed container that prevents the loss of volatile oil and stored at a temperature not exceeding 25°.

Action and use Flavour.

Coriander Oil

Coriander Oil is obtained by distillation from Coriander.

Characteristics A clear, colourless or pale yellow liquid, visibly free from water; odour and taste, those of Coriander.

Optical rotation +8° to +12°, Appendix V F.

Refractive index 1.462 to 1.472, Appendix V E.

Solubility in ethanol Soluble, at 20°, in 3 volumes of *ethanol (70%)*, Appendix X M.

Weight per ml 0.863 to 0.870 g, Appendix V G.

Storage Coriander Oil should be kept in a well-filled, well-closed container, protected from light and stored at a temperature not exceeding 25°.

Action and use Flavour.

Cortisone Acetate ☆

$C_{23}H_{30}O_6$ 402.5   *50-04-4*

Cortisone Acetate is 17α,21-dihydroxypregn-4-ene-3,11,20-trione 21-acetate. It contains not less than 96.0 per cent and not more than 104.0 per cent of $C_{23}H_{30}O_6$, calculated with reference to the dried substance.

Characteristics A white or almost white, crystalline powder. It melts at about 240° with decomposition.

Solubility Practically insoluble in *water*; slightly soluble in *ethanol (96%)*, in *methanol* and in *ether*; freely soluble in *chloroform*; soluble in *1,4-dioxan*; sparingly soluble in *acetone*.

Identification *Tests A and B may be omitted if tests C, D and E are carried out. Tests C, D and E may be omitted if tests A and B are carried out.*

A. The *infra-red absorption spectrum*, Appendix II A, is concordant with the spectrum of *cortisone acetate EPCRS*. If the spectra are not concordant, prepare new spectra using 5% w/v solutions in *chloroform IR*.

B. Examine the chromatograms obtained in the test for Related substances under *ultra-violet light (254 nm)*. The principal spot in the chromatogram obtained with solution (2) is similar in position and size to the principal spot in the chromatogram obtained with solution (5). Spray the plate with *ethanolic sulphuric acid (20%)*, heat at 120° for 10 minutes or until the spots appear and allow to cool. Examine in daylight and under *ultra-violet light (365 nm)*. The principal spot in the chromatogram obtained with solution (2) is similar in colour in daylight, fluorescence in ultra-violet light (365 nm), position and size to the principal spot in the chromatogram obtained with solution (5).

C. Carry out the method for *thin-layer chromatography*, Appendix III A, using as the coating substance a suitable silica gel containing a fluorescent indicator with an optimal intensity at 254 nm (Merck silica gel 60 F254 is suitable) and a mixture of 77 volumes of *dichloromethane*, 15 volumes of *ether*, 8 volumes of *methanol* and 1.2 volumes of *water* as the mobile phase. Apply separately to the chromatoplate 5 μl of each of the following solutions. For solution (1) dissolve 25 mg of the substance being examined in *methanol* and dilute to 5 ml with the same solvent (solution A); dilute 2 ml of this solution to 10 ml with *chloroform*. For solution (2) transfer 2 ml of solution A to a stoppered 15-ml glass tube, add 10 ml of *saturated methanolic potassium hydrogen carbonate solution* and immediately pass a stream of nitrogen briskly through the solution for 5 minutes. Stopper the tube, heat in a water-bath at 45° protected from light for 150 minutes and allow to cool. For solution (3) dissolve 25 mg of *cortisone acetate EPCRS* in *methanol* with gentle heating and dilute to 5 ml with the same solvent (solution B); dilute 2 ml of this solution to 10 ml with *chloroform*. Prepare solution (4) in the same manner as solution (2) but using 2 ml of solution B in place of solution A.

After removal of the plate, allow it to dry in air and examine under *ultra-violet light (254 nm)*. The principal spot in the chromatogram obtained with solution (1) is similar in position and size to that in the chromatogram obtained with solution (3) and the principal spot in the chromatogram obtained with solution (2) is similar in position and size to that in the chromatogram obtained with solution (4). Spray with *ethanolic sulphuric acid (20%)*, heat at 120° for 10 minutes or until the spots appear and allow to cool. Examine the plate in daylight and under *ultra-violet light (365 nm)*. The principal spots in the chromatograms obtained with solutions (1) and (2) are similar in colour in daylight, fluorescence in ultra-violet light (365 nm), position and size to the principal spots obtained with solutions (3) and (4) respectively. The principal spots obtained with solutions (2) and (4) have Rf values distinctly lower than those of the principal spots in the chromatograms obtained with solutions (1) and (3).

D. Add 2 mg to 2 ml of *sulphuric acid* and shake to dissolve. A faint yellow colour is produced within 5 minutes. Add the solution to 10 ml of *water* and mix; the colour is discharged and a clear solution is produced.

E. 10 mg yields the *reaction* characteristic of acetyl groups, Appendix VI.

Light absorption Dissolve 10 mg in sufficient *ethanol (96%)* to produce 100 ml and dilute 10 ml to 100 ml with the same solvent. The A(1%, 1 cm) of the resulting solution at the maximum at 240 nm is 375 to 405, Appendix II B.

Specific optical rotation In a 1% w/v solution in *1,4-dioxan*, +211° to +220°, Appendix V F.

Related substances Carry out the method for *thin-layer chromatography*, Appendix III A, using *silica gel GF254* as the coating substance and a mixture of 77 volumes of *dichloromethane*, 15 volumes of *ether*, 8 volumes of *methanol* and 1.2 volumes of *water* as the mobile phase. Apply separately to the chromatoplate 5 µl of each of the following solutions in a mixture of 9 volumes of *chloroform* and 1 volume of *methanol*. Solutions (1), (2), (3) and (4) contain 1.0, 0.10, 0.020 and 0.010% w/v respectively of the substance being examined. Solution (5) contains 0.10% w/v of *cortisone acetate EPCRS*. Solution (6) contains 0.010% w/v each of the substance being examined and *hydrocortisone acetate EPCRS*. After removal of the plate, allow it to dry in air and examine under *ultra-violet light (254 nm)*. Any *secondary spot* in the chromatogram obtained with solution (1) is not more intense than the spot in the chromatogram obtained with solution (3) and not more than one such spot is more intense than the spot in the chromatogram obtained with solution (4). The test is not valid unless the chromatogram obtained with solution (6) shows two clearly separated principal spots.

Loss on drying When dried at 100° to 105° for 3 hours, loses not more than 0.5% of its weight. Use 0.5 g.

Assay Carry out the *tetrazolium assay of steroids*, Appendix VIII P, and calculate the content of $C_{23}H_{30}O_6$ from the *absorbance* obtained by repeating the operation using *cortisone acetate EPCRS* in place of the substance being examined.

Storage Cortisone Acetate should be kept in a well-closed container and protected from light.

Preparations
Cortisone Injection
Cortisone Tablets

Action and use Corticosteroid.

Cresol

Cresol is a mixture of cresols and other phenols obtained from coal tar.

Characteristics An almost colourless to pale brownish-yellow liquid; odour, resembling that of phenol but more tarry.

Solubility Almost completely soluble in 50 parts of *water*; freely soluble in *ethanol (96%)*, in *chloroform*, in *ether* and in fixed and volatile oils.

Identification Shake 0.5 ml with 300 ml of *water* and filter. The filtrate complies with the following tests.
A. Add *iron(III) chloride test-solution*. A transient blue colour is produced.
B. Add *bromine water*. A pale yellow flocculent precipitate is produced.

Acidity A 2.0% w/v solution is neutral to *bromocresol purple solution*.

Distillation range Not more than 2% v/v distils below 188° and not less than 80% v/v distils between 195° and 205°, Appendix V C.

Weight per ml 1.029 to 1.044 g, Appendix V G.

Hydrocarbons Place 50 ml in a 500-ml round-bottomed flask, add 150 ml of 5M *sodium hydroxide* and 30 ml of *water* and mix thoroughly. Connect the flask to a splash-bulb and air-condenser about 60 cm long, with the end of the air-condenser fitting closely into the neck of a 250-ml pear-shaped separating funnel and passing well into the separating funnel, which has a cylindrical graduated portion above the stopcock. Fill the graduated portion of the separating funnel with *water*. Distil rapidly until 75 ml of distillate has been collected, cooling the separating funnel in running water if necessary. Allow the separating funnel to stand in a vertical position until separation is complete and draw off the aqueous liquid into a titration flask for use in the test for Volatile bases.

Allow the separating funnel to stand for a few minutes, measure the volume of hydrocarbon oil in the graduated portion and warm, if necessary, to keep the oil in the liquid state. Subtract the volume of volatile bases in the hydrocarbon oil, as determined in the following test. Not more than 0.15% v/v of hydrocarbon oil is present.

Volatile bases To the aqueous liquid reserved in the test for Hydrocarbons add any aqueous liquid still remaining in the separating funnel and neutralise, if necessary, with 0.1M *hydrochloric acid* using *phenolphthalein solution* as indicator. Titrate with 1M *hydrochloric acid VS* using *methyl orange solution* as indicator. Wash the oil from the separating funnel into the titration flask with *water* and again titrate with 1M *hydrochloric acid VS*. From the volume of additional 1M *hydrochloric acid VS*, calculate the proportion of volatile bases in the hydrocarbon oil. From the total volume of 1M *hydrochloric acid VS* used in both titrations calculate the proportion of volatile bases in the substance being examined, each ml of 1M *hydrochloric acid VS* being taken as equivalent to 0.080 ml of volatile bases. Not more than 0.15% v/v of volatile bases is present.

Hydrocarbons and volatile bases The sum of the contents of hydrocarbon oil and volatile bases, as determined in the tests for Hydrocarbons and for Volatile bases, does not exceed 0.25% v/v.

Sulphur compounds Place 20 ml in a small conical flask and over the mouth of the flask fix a piece of filter paper moistened with a 10% w/v solution of *lead(II) acetate*. Heat the flask on a water-bath for 5 minutes. Not more than a light yellow colour is produced on the filter paper.

Non-volatile matter When evaporated on a water-bath and dried at 105°, leaves not more than 0.1% w/v of residue.

Storage Cresol should be kept in a well-closed container and protected from light. It darkens with age or on exposure to light.

Action and use Antiseptic; antimicrobial preservative.

Crotamiton

C₁₃H₁₇NO   203.3   483-63-6

Crotamiton is predominantly (*E*)-*N*-ethylcrotono-*o*-toluidide. It contains not less than 96.0 per cent and not more than 101.0 per cent of C₁₃H₁₇NO, calculated as the sum of the *E*- and *Z*-isomers.

Characteristics A colourless or pale yellow, oily liquid; odour, faint. At low temperatures it may solidify partly or completely.

Solubility Slightly soluble in *water*; miscible with *ethanol (96%)* and with *ether*.

Identification A. The *light absorption*, Appendix II B, in the range 220 to 350 nm of a 0.002% w/v solution in *cyclohexane UV* exhibits a maximum only at 242 nm. The *absorbance* at 242 nm is about 0.63.

B. Boil 2.5 ml under a reflux condenser for 2 hours with 20 ml of *sulphuric acid (50%)*, cool and add 20 ml of *water*. To 0.5 ml of the solution add 2 ml of *sodium carbonate solution* and a solution prepared by dissolving 0.05 g of *sulphanilic acid* in 2 ml of 2M *hydrochloric acid* and adding 0.2 ml of *sodium nitrite solution*. A reddish-orange colour is produced.

C. To the remainder of the solution obtained in test B add 20 ml of *water* and make alkaline to *phenolphthalein solution* with 5M *sodium hydroxide*. Extract with 50 ml of *ether*, wash the extract with three 20-ml quantities of *water*, shake with 1 g of *anhydrous sodium sulphate*, filter and evaporate the filtrate to dryness. Dissolve the residue in 0.5 ml of *ethanol (96%)* and add 3 ml of a saturated solution of *2,4,6-trinitrophenol* in *ethanol (96%)*, cooling in ice if necessary to induce crystallisation. The *melting point* of the precipitate, after drying for 1 hour at 105°, is about 158°, with decomposition, Appendix V A.

Refractive index 1.540 to 1.542, Appendix V E.

Weight per ml 1.004 to 1.009 g, Appendix V G.

Free amines Dissolve 5 g in 70 ml of *ether* and extract with two 10-ml quantities of 2M *hydrochloric acid*, washing each extract with two 50-ml quantities of *ether*. Evaporate the combined acid extracts to dryness on a water-bath and dry for 1 hour at 105°. The residue weighs not more than 2.5 mg.

Chloride Heat 5.0 g with 25 ml of *ethanol (96%)* and 5 ml of 5M *sodium hydroxide* under a reflux condenser for 1 hour. Cool, transfer to a separating funnel, add 25 ml of *ether* and 5 ml of *water*, shake and allow to separate. Transfer the lower layer to a *Nessler cylinder*, dilute to 20 ml with *water*, add 5 ml of *nitric acid*, dilute to 50 ml with *water* and add 1 ml of *silver nitrate solution*. Any opalescence produced is not greater than that produced by adding 1 ml of *silver nitrate solution* to a solution prepared by diluting 5 ml of 5M *sodium hydroxide* to 20 ml with *water* and adding 1.5 ml of 0.01M *hydrochloric acid VS*, 5 ml of *nitric acid* and sufficient *water* to produce 50 ml.

Related substances Carry out the method for *high-performance liquid chromatography*, Appendix III D, using three solutions in *hexane* containing (1) 0.00050% w/v of *crotamiton BPCRS*, (2) 0.050% w/v of *crotamiton BPCRS* and (3) 0.050% w/v of the substance being examined.

The chromatographic procedure may be carried out using (a) a stainless steel column (20 cm × 4.6 mm) packed with *stationary phase A* (70 μm) (Partisil is suitable), (b) a mixture of 200 volumes of *hexane* and 1.4 volumes of absolute *ethanol* as the mobile phase with a flow rate of 3 ml per minute and (c) a detection wavelength of 242 nm.

In the chromatogram obtained with solution (2) the principal peak, other than any peak due to solvent, is due to the *E*-isomer, the peak with a retention time of 0.6 relative to the principal peak is due to the *Z*-isomer and the peak with a retention time of 0.8 relative to the principal peak is due to *N*-ethyl-α-vinylaceto-*o*-toluidide. The content of *N*-ethyl-α-vinylaceto-*o*-toluidide in the substance being examined is not greater than 3.0% calculated using the declared content of *N*-ethyl-α-vinylaceto-*o*-toluidide in *crotamiton BPCRS*. In the chromatogram obtained with solution (3) the sum of the areas of any peaks, other than the solvent peak, the peaks due to the *E*- and *Z*-isomers and the peak due to *N*-ethyl-α-vinylaceto-*o*-toluidide, is not greater than the sum of the areas of the peaks due to the *E*- and *Z*-isomers in the chromatogram obtained with solution (1).

Z-Isomer Not more than 15% of the total content of *E*- and *Z*-isomers determined in the Assay.

Sulphated ash Not more than 0.1% w/w, Appendix IX A.

Assay Carry out the method for *high-performance liquid chromatography*, Appendix III D, using two solutions in *hexane* containing (1) 0.0025% w/v of *crotamiton BPCRS* and (2) 0.0025% w/v of the substance being examined.

The chromatographic procedure described under Related substances may be used.

In the chromatogram obtained with solution (1) the principal peak, other than any peak due to solvent, is due to the *E*-isomer and the peak with a retention time of 0.6 relative to the principal peak is due to the *Z*-isomer. Calculate the content of C₁₃H₁₇NO in the substance being examined as the sum of the *E*-and *Z*-isomers using the declared contents of *E*- and *Z*-crotamiton in *crotamiton BPCRS*.

Storage Crotamiton should be kept in small containers. When solidified, it should be completely liquefied before use by warming.

Preparations
Crotamiton Cream
Crotamiton Lotion

Action and use Antipruritic; used in treatment of scabies.

Cyanocobalamin ☆
Vitamin B$_{12}$

$C_{63}H_{88}CoN_{14}O_{14}P$ 1355   68-19-9

Cyanocobalamin is *Co*α-[α-(5,6-dimethylbenz-imidazolyl)]-*Co*β-cyanocobamide. It contains not less than 96.0 per cent and not more than 102.0 per cent of $C_{63}H_{88}CoN_{14}O_{14}P$, calculated with reference to the dried substance.

Characteristics Dark red crystals or crystalline powder; hygroscopic.

Solubility Sparingly soluble in *water* and in *ethanol (96%)*; practically insoluble in *acetone* and in *ether*.

Identification A. The *light absorption*, Appendix II B, in the range 260 to 610 nm of a 0.0025% w/v solution exhibits three maxima, at 278, 361 and 547 to 559 nm. The ratio of the *absorbance* at 361 nm to that at 547 to 559 nm is 3.15 to 3.45 and the ratio of the absorbance at 361 nm to that at 278 nm is 1.70 to 1.90.
B. Carry out the method for *thin-layer chromatography*, Appendix III A, protected from light, using *silica gel G* as the coating substance and a mixture of 60 volumes of *chloroform*, 40 volumes of *methanol* and 12 volumes of 6M *ammonia* as the mobile phase. Use an unlined tank and allow the mobile phase to ascend 12 cm above the line of application. Apply separately to the chromatoplate 10 μl of each of two solutions in *ethanol (50%)* containing (1) 0.2% w/v of the substance being examined and (2) 0.2% w/v of *cyanocobalamin EPCRS*. After removal of the plate, allow it to dry in air and examine in daylight. The principal spot in the chromatogram obtained with solution (1) corresponds in position, colour and size to that in the chromatogram obtained with solution (2).

Related substances Carry out the method for *high-performance liquid chromatography*, Appendix III D, injecting 20 μl of each of the following solutions. Solutions (1) to (3) are solutions of the substance being examined in the mobile phase containing (1) 0.0001% w/v, (2) 0.10% w/v and (3) 0.0030% w/v and should be used within 1 hour of preparation. For solution (4) dissolve 25 mg of the substance being examined in 10 ml of *water*, warming if necessary, allow to cool, add 5 ml of a 0.1% w/v solution of *chloramine* and 0.5 ml of 0.05M *hydrochloric acid*, dilute to 25 ml with *water*, shake and allow to stand for 5 minutes. Dilute 1 ml of this solution to 10 ml with the mobile phase and use immediately.

The chromatographic procedure may be carried out using (a) a stainless steel column (25 cm × 4 mm) packed with *stationary phase B* (5 μm), (b) a mixture of 147 volumes of a 1.0% w/v solution of *disodium hydrogen orthophosphate* and 53 volumes of *methanol* adjusted to pH 3.5 with *orthophosphoric acid* as the mobile phase with a flow rate of 0.8 ml per minute and (c) a detection wavelength of 361 nm. Use the mobile phase within 2 days of preparation. Allow the chromatography to proceed for three times the retention time of the peak due to cyanocobalamin.

In the chromatogram obtained with solution (2) the sum of the areas of any *secondary peaks* is not greater than the area of the principal peak in the chromatogram obtained with solution (3). Disregard any peak the area of which is less than that of the principal peak in the chromatogram obtained with solution (1). The test is not valid unless the chromatogram obtained with solution (4) exhibits two principal peaks, the *resolution factor* between those peaks is 2.5 or more and the chromatogram obtained with solution (3) exhibits one principal peak with a *signal-to-noise* ratio of 5 or more.

Loss on drying When dried at 100° to 105° at a pressure of 1.5 to 2.5 kPa for 2 hours, loses not more than 12.0% of its weight. Use 20 mg.

Assay Dissolve 25 mg in sufficient *water* to produce 1000 ml and measure the *absorbance* of the solution at the maximum at 361 nm, Appendix II B. Calculate the content of $C_{63}H_{88}CoN_{14}O_{14}P$ taking 207 as the value of A(1%, 1 cm) at the maximum at 361 nm.

Storage Cyanocobalamin should be kept in an airtight container and protected from light.

Preparation
Cyanocobalamin Injection

Action and use Used in treatment of vitamin B$_{12}$ deficiency.

Cyclizine

$C_{18}H_{22}N_2$ 266.4   82-92-8

Cyclizine is 1-benzhydryl-4-methylpiperazine. It contains not less than 98.5 per cent and not more than 101.0 per cent of $C_{18}H_{22}N_2$, calculated with reference to the dried substance.

Characteristics A white or creamy-white, crystalline powder.

Solubility Practically insoluble in *water*. It dissolves in most organic solvents and in dilute acids.

Identification A. The *infra-red absorption spectrum*, Appendix II A, is concordant with the *reference spectrum* of cyclizine.
B. The *light absorption*, Appendix II B, in the range 220 to 350 nm of a freshly prepared 0.002% w/v solution in 0.05M *sulphuric acid* exhibits a maximum at 227 nm with a series of ill-defined maxima between 258 and 272 nm. The *absorbance* at 227 nm is about 0.87.
C. *Melting point*, about 107°, Appendix V A.

Alkalinity Shake 1 g with 25 ml of *carbon dioxide-free water* for 5 minutes and filter. The pH of the filtrate is 7.6 to 8.6, Appendix V L.

Clarity of solution A 1.0% w/v solution in *ether* and a 1.0% w/v solution in 2M *hydrochloric acid* are *clear*, Appendix IV A.

Chloride Dissolve 0.20 g in 2 ml of *methanol* and dilute to 30 ml with 2M *nitric acid*. 15 ml of the resulting solution complies with the *limit test for chlorides*, Appendix VII (500 ppm).

N-Methylpiperazine Carry out the method for *thin-layer chromatography*, Appendix III A, using *silica gel G* as the coating substance and a mixture of 90 volumes of *chloroform*, 9 volumes of *methanol* and 1 volume of 13.5M *ammonia* as the mobile phase. Apply separately to the chromatoplate 20 μl of each of two freshly prepared solutions in *methanol* containing (1) 1.0% w/v of the substance being examined and (2) 0.0050% w/v of N-methylpiperazine. After removal of the plate, allow it to dry in air and expose to iodine vapour for 10 minutes. Any spot corresponding to N-methylpiperazine in the chromatogram obtained with solution (1) is not more intense than the spot in the chromatogram obtained with solution (2).

Loss on drying When dried to constant weight at 80°, loses not more than 1.0% of its weight. Use 1 g.

Sulphated ash Not more than 0.1%, Appendix IX A.

Assay Carry out Method I for *non-aqueous titration*, Appendix VIII A, using 0.1 g and determining the end-point potentiometrically. Each ml of 0.1M *perchloric acid VS* is equivalent to 0.01332 g of $C_{18}H_{22}N_2$.

Storage Cyclizine should be kept in a well-closed container.

Preparation
Cyclizine Injection

Action and use Antiemetic.

Cyclizine Hydrochloride

$C_{18}H_{22}N_2,HCl$ 302.9   *303-25-3*

Cyclizine Hydrochloride is 1-benzhydryl-4-methylpiperazine hydrochloride. It contains not less than 98.0 per cent and not more than 101.0 per cent of $C_{18}H_{22}N_2,HCl$, calculated with reference to the dried substance.

Characteristics A white, crystalline powder; odourless or almost odourless.

Solubility Slightly soluble in *water* and in *ethanol (96%)*; practically insoluble in *ether*.

Identification A. The *infra-red absorption spectrum*, Appendix II A, is concordant with the *reference spectrum* of cyclizine hydrochloride.
B. The *light absorption*, Appendix II B, in the range 220 to 350 nm of a freshly prepared 0.002% w/v solution in 0.05M *sulphuric acid* exhibits a maximum only at 225 nm. The *absorbance* at 225 nm is about 0.78.
C. Dissolve 0.5 g in 10 ml of *ethanol (60%)* using heat, cool in ice and add 1 ml of 5M *sodium hydroxide* and sufficient *water* to produce 20 ml. The *melting point* of the precipitate, after washing with *water* and drying at 60° at a

pressure not exceeding 0.7 kPa for 2 hours, is about 107°, Appendix V A.
D. Yields the *reactions* characteristic of chlorides, Appendix VI.

N-Methylpiperazine Carry out the method for *thin-layer chromatography*, Appendix III A, using *silica gel G* as the coating substance and a mixture of 90 volumes of *chloroform*, 8 volumes of *methanol* and 2 volumes of 13.5M *ammonia* as the mobile phase. Apply separately to the chromatoplate 20 μl of each of two freshly prepared solutions in *methanol* containing (1) 1.0% w/v of the substance being examined and (2) 0.0050% w/v of N-methylpiperazine. After removal of the plate, allow it to dry in air and expose to iodine vapour for 10 minutes. Any spot corresponding to N-methylpiperazine in the chromatogram obtained with solution (1) is not more intense than the spot in the chromatogram obtained with solution (2).

Loss on drying When dried to constant weight at 130°, loses not more than 1.0% of its weight. Use 1 g.

Sulphated ash Not more than 0.1%, Appendix IX A.

Assay Carry out Method I for *non-aqueous titration*, Appendix VIII A, using 0.4 g, adding 20 ml of *mercury (II) acetate solution* and determining the end-point potentiometrically. Each ml of 0.1M *perchloric acid VS* is equivalent to 0.01514 g of $C_{18}H_{22}N_2,HCl$.

Preparations
Cyclizine Tablets
Dipipanone and Cyclizine Tablets

Action and use Antiemetic.

Cyclobarbitone Calcium ☆

$C_{24}H_{30}CaN_4O_6$ 510.6   *5897-20-1*

Cyclobarbitone Calcium is calcium 5-(cyclohex-1-enyl)-5-ethylbarbiturate. It contains not less than 98.5 per cent and not more than 101.0 per cent of $C_{24}H_{30}CaN_4O_6$, calculated with reference to the dried substance.

Characteristics A white or slightly yellowish, crystalline powder.

Solubility Slightly soluble in *water*; very slightly soluble in *absolute ethanol (96%)*; practically insoluble in *chloroform* and in *ether*.

Identification *Test A may be omitted if tests B, C, D and E are carried out. Tests B and D may be omitted if tests A, C and E are carried out.*
A. Dissolve 0.1 g in sufficient *water* to produce 20 ml and acidify the solution with 2M *hydrochloric acid*. Shake with 20 ml of *ether*, separate the ether layer, wash with 10 ml of *water* and dry over *anhydrous sodium sulphate*. Filter, evaporate the filtrate to dryness and dry the residue at 100° to 105°. The *infra-red absorption spectrum* of the residue, Appendix II A, is concordant with the spectrum obtained

using the residue similarly prepared from 0.1 g of *cyclo-barbital calcium EPCRS*.

B. Complies with the test for *identification of barbiturates*, Appendix III A, but using solutions of the substance being examined in *water*. Heat to 60° to effect dissolution and disregard any slight residue.

C. Determine the *melting point*, Appendix V A, Method I, of the residue obtained from the substance being examined in test A. Mix equal parts of the residue with the residue obtained from *cyclobarbital calcium EPCRS* and determine the *melting point* of the mixture. The difference between the melting points, which are about 172°, is not greater than 2°.

D. To 10 mg add 1 ml of a 1% w/v solution of *vanillin* in *ethanol (96%)* and 2 ml of a cooled mixture of 2 volumes of *sulphuric acid* and 1 volume of *water*. Shake and allow to stand for 5 minutes. A greenish-yellow colour is produced which becomes dark red on heating on a water-bath for 10 minutes.

E. Yields *reaction A* characteristic of calcium salts, Appendix VI.

Free cyclobarbitone Shake 1 g with successive quantities of 50, 25 and 15 ml of *toluene*, filter and evaporate the solvent. The residue, after drying at 100° to 105°, weighs not more than 30 mg.

Oxidation products To 1.0 g add 2.5 ml of 2M *sodium hydroxide* and 2.5 ml of *water*. The mixture does not become coloured within 2 minutes.

Related substances Complies with the test for *related substances in barbiturates*, Appendix III A, but using solutions of the substance being examined in *water* containing (1) 0.50% w/v and (2) 0.0050% w/v. In preparing solution (1) heat to 60° to effect dissolution and disregard any slight residue.

Loss on drying When dried for 2 hours at 100° to 105°, loses not more than 1.0% of its weight. Use 1 g.

Assay To 0.25 g add 5 ml of *pyridine* and 10 ml of *silver nitrate—pyridine reagent* and heat on a water-bath at 80° for 5 minutes to obtain a clear solution. Cool and titrate with 0.1M *ethanolic sodium hydroxide VS*, using 0.5 ml of *thymolphthalein solution* as indicator, until a pure blue colour is obtained. Repeat the operation without the substance being examined. The difference between the titrations represents the amount of sodium hydroxide required. Each ml of 0.2M *ethanolic sodium hydroxide VS* is equivalent to 0.02553 g of $C_{24}H_{30}CaN_4O_6$.

Storage Cyclobarbitone Calcium should be kept in an airtight container.

Action and use Hypnotic.

The title of the monograph in the European Pharmacopœia is Cyclobarbital Calcium.

Cyclomethycaine Sulphate

$C_{22}H_{33}NO_3,H_2SO_4$ 457.6   *50978-10-4*

Cyclomethycaine Sulphate is 1-{3-[4-(cyclo-hexyloxy)benzoyloxy]propyl}-2-methyl-piperidine hydrogen sulphate. It contains not less than 98.0 per cent and not more than 101.0 per cent of $C_{22}H_{33}NO_3,H_2SO_4$, calculated with reference to the dried substance.

Characteristics A white, crystalline powder; odourless or almost odourless.

Solubility Soluble in 50 parts of *water* and in 50 parts of *ethanol (96%)*; slightly soluble in *chloroform* and in dilute mineral acids.

Identification A. The *infra-red absorption spectrum*, Appendix II A, is concordant with the *reference spectrum* of cyclomethycaine sulphate.

B. Disperse 0.5 g in 10 ml of *ethanol (96%)*, add 10 ml of 5M *sodium hydroxide* and heat under a reflux condenser for 1 hour. Cool and add 7 ml of *hydrochloric acid*. The *melting point* of the precipitate, after washing with *water*, drying and recrystallising from *ethanol (60%)*, is about 182°, Appendix V A.

C. Yields the *reactions* characteristic of sulphates, Appendix VI.

Melting point 162.5° to 165.5°, Appendix V A.

Related substances A. Carry out the method for *thin-layer chromatography*, Appendix III A, using *silica gel GF254* as the coating substance and a mixture of 96 volumes of *butan-1-ol* and 4 volumes of 13.5M *ammonia* as the mobile phase. Apply separately to the chromatoplate 10 µl of each of two freshly prepared solutions of the substance being examined in *ethanol (96%)* containing (1) 2.0% w/v and (2) 0.020% w/v. After removal of the plate, allow it to dry in air and examine under *ultra-violet light (254 nm)*. Any *secondary spot* in the chromatogram obtained with solution (1) is not more intense than the spot in the chromatogram obtained with solution (2).

B. Carry out the method for *gas chromatography*, Appendix III B, using the following solutions. For solution (1) suspend 20 mg of the substance being examined in 100 ml of *chloroform* containing 0.005% w/v of *tetraphenylethylene* (internal standard), add 0.2 ml of 13.5M *ammonia*, mix, add 2 g of *anhydrous sodium sulphate*, shake and filter. For solution (2) suspend 0.20 g of the substance being examined in 10 ml of *chloroform*, add 0.2 ml of 13.5M *ammonia*, mix, add 2 g of *anhydrous sodium sulphate*, shake and filter. Prepare solution (3) in the same manner as solution (2) but using 10 ml of *chloroform* containing 0.005% w/v of the internal standard.

The chromatographic procedure may be carried out using a glass column (1.5 m × 4 mm) packed with *acid-washed, silanised diatomaceous support* (80 to 100 mesh) coated with 3% w/w of phenyl methyl silicone fluid (50% phenyl) (OV-17 is suitable) and maintained at 250°.

Using the chromatogram obtained with solution (1) calculate the ratio of the area of the peak due to cyclomethycaine to the area of the peak due to the internal standard and using the chromatogram obtained with solution (3) calculate the ratio of the area of any *secondary peak* to the area of the peak due to the internal standard. The ratios calculated for solution (3) are not greater than the ratio calculated for solution (1).

Loss on drying When dried to constant weight at 105°, loses not more than 1.0% of its weight. Use 1 g.

Sulphated ash Not more than 0.1%, Appendix IX A.

Assay Dissolve 0.1 g in sufficient 0.01M *hydrochloric acid* to produce 500 ml, dilute 5 ml to 100 ml with 0.01M *hydrochloric acid* and measure the *absorbance* of the resulting solution at the maximum at 261 nm, Appendix II B. Calculate the content of $C_{22}H_{33}NO_3,H_2SO_4$ taking 400 as the value of A(1%, 1 cm) at the maximum at 261 nm.

Action and use Local anaesthetic.

Cyclopenthiazide

$C_{13}H_{18}ClN_3O_4S_2$ 379.9   *742-20-1*

Cyclopenthiazide is 6-chloro-3-cyclopentyl-methyl-3,4-dihydro-1,2,4-benzothiadiazine-7-sulphonamide 1,1-dioxide. It contains not less than 98.0 per cent and not more than 102.0 per cent of $C_{13}H_{18}ClN_3O_4S_2$, calculated with reference to the dried substance.

Characteristics A white powder; odourless or almost odourless.

Solubility Practically insoluble in *water*; soluble in 12 parts of *ethanol (96%)*; soluble in *acetone* and in *ether*; slightly soluble in *chloroform*.

Identification A. The *infra-red absorption spectrum*, Appendix II A, is concordant with the *reference spectrum* of cyclopenthiazide.
B. The *light absorption*, Appendix II B, in the range 230 to 350 nm of a 0.002% w/v solution in 0.01M *sodium hydroxide* exhibits two maxima, at 273 nm and 320 nm. The *absorbance* at 273 nm is about 0.88 and at 320 nm is about 0.12.
C. Carry out the method for *thin-layer chromatography*, Appendix III A, using *silica gel GF254* as the coating substance and *ethyl acetate* as the mobile phase. Apply separately to the chromatoplate 5 µl of each of two solutions in *acetone* containing (1) 0.1% w/v of the substance being examined and (2) 0.1% w/v of *cyclopenthiazide BPCRS*. After removal of the plate, dry it in a current of air, examine under *ultra-violet light (254 nm)* and then reveal the spots by *Method I*. By both methods of visualisation the principal spot in the chromatogram obtained with solution (1) corresponds in colour and intensity to that in the chromatogram obtained with solution (2).

Related substances Carry out the method for *thin-layer chromatography*, Appendix III A, using *silica gel G* as the coating substance and *ethyl acetate* as the mobile phase. Apply separately to the chromatoplate 5 µl of each of two

solutions of the substance being examined in *acetone* containing (1) 0.50% w/v and (2) 0.0050% w/v. After removal of the plate, dry it in a current of air and reveal the spots by *Method I*. Any *secondary spot* in the chromatogram obtained with solution (1) is not more intense than the spot in the chromatogram obtained with solution (2).

Loss on drying When dried to constant weight at 105°, loses not more than 0.5% of its weight. Use 1 g.

Sulphated ash Not more than 0.1%, Appendix IX A.

Assay Dissolve 0.5 g in 50 ml of *butylamine* and carry out Method II for *non-aqueous titration*, Appendix VIII A, using 0.1M *tetrabutylammonium hydroxide VS* as titrant and *magneson solution* as indicator; titrate to a pure blue end-point. Each ml of 0.1M *tetrabutylammonium hydroxide VS* is equivalent to 0.01899 g of $C_{13}H_{18}ClN_3O_4S_2$.

Preparation
Cyclopenthiazide Tablets

Action and use Diuretic.

Cyclopentolate Hydrochloride

$C_{17}H_{25}NO_3,HCl$ 327.9   *5870-29-1*

Cyclopentolate Hydrochloride is 2-dimethyl-aminoethyl 2-(1-hydroxycyclopentyl)-2-phenyl-acetate hydrochloride. It contains not less than 98.5 per cent and not more than 101.0 per cent of $C_{17}H_{25}NO_3,HCl$, calculated with reference to the dried substance.

Characteristics A white, crystalline powder; odourless or with an odour of phenylacetic acid.

Solubility Soluble in less than 1 part of *water* and in 5 parts of *ethanol (96%)*; insoluble in *ether*.

Identification A. The *infra-red absorption spectrum*, Appendix II A, is concordant with the *reference spectrum* of cyclopentolate hydrochloride. If the spectra are not concordant, dissolve a sufficient quantity in the minimum volume of *ethanol (96%)*, evaporate to dryness and prepare a new spectrum of the residue.
B. Dissolve 0.2 g in 2 ml of *water*, add 2 ml of 5M *sodium hydroxide*, boil for 1 minute and add 0.2 ml of *nitric acid*. A sweet odour resembling that of phenylacetic acid is produced.
C. Dissolve 0.5 g in 10 ml of *water*, add 2 g of *potassium carbonate*, extract with two 10-ml quantities of *ether*, dry the combined extracts with *anhydrous potassium carbonate* and filter. To the filtrate add carefully 0.2 ml of *dimethyl sulphate* and allow to stand for 2 hours. The *melting point* of the precipitate, after recrystallisation from *acetone* and drying at a pressure of 2 kPa for 2 hours, is about 141°, with decomposition, Appendix V A. Mix the residue with an equal quantity of the substance being examined; the *melting point* is lowered by not less than 15°.
D. Yields *reaction A* characteristic of chlorides, Appendix VI.

Acidity pH of a 1% w/v solution, 4.5 to 5.5, Appendix V L.

Melting point 135° to 137°, Appendix V A.

Related substances Carry out the method for *thin-layer chromatography*, Appendix III A, using *silica gel G* as the coating substance and a mixture of 50 volumes of *propan-2-ol*, 30 volumes of *butyl acetate*, 15 volumes of *water* and 5 volumes of 13.5M *ammonia* as the mobile phase. Apply separately to the chromatoplate 10 μl of each of two solutions of the substance being examined in *ethanol (96%)* containing (1) 2.0% w/v and (2) 0.010% w/v. After removal of the plate, allow it to dry in air, spray with *ethanolic sulphuric acid (10%)*, heat at 120° for 30 minutes and examine under *ultra-violet light (365 nm)*. Any *secondary spot* in the chromatogram obtained with solution (1) is not more intense than the spot in the chromatogram obtained with solution (2).

Loss on drying When dried at 60° at a pressure not exceeding 0.7 kPa for 2 hours, loses not more than 0.5% of its weight. Use 1 g.

Sulphated ash Not more than 0.1%, Appendix IX A.

Assay Carry out Method I for *non-aqueous titration*, Appendix VIII A, using 0.4 g, 10 ml of *mercury(II) acetate solution* and *crystal violet solution* as indicator. Each ml of 0.1M *perchloric acid VS* is equivalent to 0.03279 g of $C_{17}H_{25}NO_3,HCl$.

Preparation

Cyclopentolate Eye Drops

Action and use Mydriatic; cycloplegic.

Cyclophosphamide

O=P(O—)(NH)—N(CH₂·CH₂Cl)₂

$C_7H_{15}Cl_2N_2O_2P,H_2O$ 279.1   *6055-19-2*

Cyclophosphamide is 2-bis(2-chloroethyl)amino-perhydro-1,3,2-oxazaphosphorinane 2-oxide monohydrate. It contains not less than 98.0 per cent and not more than 100.5 per cent of $C_7H_{15}Cl_2N_2O_2P$, calculated with reference to the anhydrous substance.

Characteristics A fine, white, crystalline powder; odourless or almost odourless.

Solubility Soluble in 25 parts of *water* and in 1 part of *ethanol (96%)*; slightly soluble in *ether*.

Identification A. The *infra-red absorption spectrum*, Appendix II A, is concordant with the *reference spectrum* of cyclophosphamide.

B. Dissolve 0.1 g in 10 ml of *water* and add 5 ml of *silver nitrate solution*; no precipitate is produced. Boil; a white precipitate is produced which is insoluble in *nitric acid* but dissolves in 5M *ammonia* from which it is reprecipitated on the addition of *nitric acid*.

Acidity pH of a freshly prepared 2% w/v solution, 4.0 to 6.0, Appendix V L.

Melting point 49.5° to 53°, Appendix V A, determined on the substance without previous drying.

Chloride Dissolve 0.30 g in 30 ml of *water*. 15 ml of the resulting solution complies with the *limit test for chlorides*, Appendix VII (330 ppm). Carry out the test without delay and maintain at a temperature below 20°.

Water 6.0 to 7.0% w/w, Appendix IX C. Use 0.3 g.

Assay Heat 0.2 g in a long-necked flask with 2 ml of *sulphuric acid* and 2.5 ml of *nitric acid* until brown fumes cease to be evolved, cool, add 1 ml of *nitric acid* and heat again. Continue adding *nitric acid* and heating until brown fumes are no longer evolved and the solution is colourless when cold. Heat until dense white fumes are evolved, cool, transfer the solution to a flask with the aid of 150 ml of *water*, add 50 ml of *citric—molybdic acid solution* and heat slowly to boiling. Swirling the flask continuously, add 25 ml of *quinoline solution*, at first dropwise and then in a steady stream, heat on a water-bath for 5 minutes and cool. Filter, wash the precipitate with *water* until free from acid, transfer the precipitate to a flask with the aid of 100 ml of *water*, add 50 ml of 0.5M *sodium hydroxide VS* and shake until dissolved. Titrate the excess of alkali with 0.5M *hydrochloric acid VS* using *phenolphthalein—thymol blue solution* as indicator. Each ml of 0.5M *sodium hydroxide VS* is equivalent to 0.005021 g of $C_7H_{15}Cl_2N_2O_2P$.

Preparations

Cyclophosphamide Injection

Cyclophosphamide Tablets

Action and use Cytotoxic.

Cyclopropane

CH₂ / CH₂—CH₂

C_3H_6 42.08   *75-19-4*

Cyclopropane contains not less than 99.0 per cent v/v of C_3H_6. For convenience in use it is compressed in metal cylinders.

Characteristics A colourless gas at atmospheric temperature and pressure, boiling, at a pressure of 101.3 kPa, at about −34.5°; odour, characteristic. Flammable; mixtures with oxygen or air at certain concentrations are explosive.

Solubility 1 volume, measured at 0° and 101.3 kPa, dissolves in 2.85 volumes of *water*. Very soluble in *ethanol (96%)*, in *chloroform* and in *ether*.

Acidity or alkalinity Dilute 0.3 ml of *methyl red solution* with 400 ml of boiling *water* and boil the solution for 5 minutes. Cool to about 80° and pour 100 ml of the solution into each of three matched *Nessler cylinders* marked A, B and C respectively. To cylinder B add 0.2 ml of 0.01M *hydrochloric acid VS* and to cylinder C add 0.4 ml of 0.01M *hydrochloric acid VS*. Stopper each cylinder and cool to room temperature. Pass a volume of the gas equivalent to 2000 ml, measured at 0° and 101.3 kPa, through the solution in cylinder B, the time taken being about 30 minutes. The colour of the solution in cylinder B is not deeper red than that of the solution in cylinder C and not deeper yellow than that of the solution in cylinder A.

Acidity, carbon dioxide, ethanol and water Pass a volume of the gas equivalent to 1000 ml, measured at 0°

and 101.3 kPa, through a weighed tube containing *potassium hydroxide* in small pieces, the time taken being 40 to 60 minutes. The increase in weight of the tube does not exceed 5.6 mg (equivalent to 0.3% w/w of the cyclopropane used).

Unsaturated substances Pass the effluent gas in the test for Acidity, carbon dioxide and ethanol through a gas washing trap provided with a sintered-glass bubbler containing 20 ml of *iodine monochloride solution* and connected in series with two gas washing bottles containing, respectively, 5 ml of *iodine monochloride solution* and 10 ml of *potassium iodide solution*. Mix the contents of the trap and washing bottles and titrate the liberated iodine with 0.1M *sodium thiosulphate VS*. Add 10 ml of *potassium iodide solution* to 25 ml of *iodine monochloride solution* and titrate with 0.1M *sodium thiosulphate VS*. The difference between the titrations is not more than 1.8 ml, equivalent to 0.2% w/w of unsaturated substances calculated as propylene.

Carbon dioxide Pass a volume equivalent to 1000 ml, measured at 0° and 101.3 kPa, at a rate not exceeding 4000 ml per hour through 100 ml of a 3% w/v solution of *barium hydroxide* contained in a vessel such that the depth of the solution is between 12 and 14 cm, using a delivery tube with a bore of about 1 mm and extending to within 2 mm of the bottom of the vessel. Any turbidity produced is not greater than that produced by adding 1 ml of a 0.1% w/v solution of *sodium hydrogen carbonate* in *carbon dioxide-free water* to 100 ml of a 3% w/v solution of *barium hydroxide*.

Halogen-containing substances Pass a volume of gas equivalent to 1000 ml, measured at 0° and 101.3 kPa, with the necessary amount of air into a small mixing chamber and pass the resulting mixture through a heated quartz tube containing pieces of platinised quartz, or through a heated silica tube containing sintered silica plates or pieces of platinised quartz, the time taken being not less than 40 minutes. Absorb the products of combustion in 50 ml of a 3% w/v solution of *sodium peroxide*. Boil the solution for about 10 minutes, cool, neutralise with a solution of *nitric acid* (containing approximately 30% w/w of HNO_3) and add 5 ml of 2M *nitric acid* (test solution). To 50 ml of the same solution of *sodium peroxide* which has been boiled, cooled, neutralised and acidified in the same manner, add 7.5 ml of 0.001M *potassium bromide VS* (standard solution). Transfer the solutions to 100-ml matched *Nessler cylinders*, add 1.0 ml of 0.1M *silver nitrate* to each, dilute to 100 ml with *water*, mix well and allow to stand in the dark for 15 minutes. Compare the turbidities of the two solutions by viewing them both transversely and vertically against a black background. The turbidity of the test solution is not more intense than that of the standard solution.

Foreign odour Transfer 10 ml of the material liquefied under pressure to a cylinder cooled to a temperature not exceeding −40°, pour in successive small quantities onto a clean filter paper and allow it to evaporate spontaneously. No foreign odour is detectable at any stage of the evaporation.

Assay In a suitable nitrometer containing *mercury*, place a volume of the material liquefied under pressure equivalent to 80 to 100 ml of the gas, measured at 0° and 101.3 kPa, add 25 ml of *sulphuric acid* and allow to stand for 15 minutes. Not less than 99.0% of its volume is absorbed.

Labelling The metal cylinder is painted orange and carries a label stating 'Cyclopropane'. In addition, 'Cyclopropane' or the symbol 'C_3H_6' is stencilled in paint on the shoulder of the cylinder.

Action and use General anaesthetic.

Cycloserine

$C_3H_6N_2O_2$ 102.1   *68-41-7*

Cycloserine is (*R*)-4-aminoisoxazolidin-3-one, an antimicrobial substance produced by the growth of certain strains of *Streptomyces orchidaceus* or *S. garyphalus* or obtained by synthesis. It contains not less than 98.0 per cent and not more than 100.5 per cent of $C_3H_6N_2O_2$, calculated with reference to the dried substance.

Characteristics A white or pale yellow, crystalline powder; hygroscopic.

Solubility Soluble in 10 parts of *water* and in 50 parts of *ethanol (96%)*; slightly soluble in *chloroform* and in *ether*.

Identification A. The *light absorption*, Appendix II B, in the range 215 to 350 nm of a 0.0025% w/v solution in 0.1M *hydrochloric acid* exhibits a maximum only at 219 nm. The *absorbance* at 219 nm is about 0.86. Measure the absorbance within 15 minutes of preparing the solution.

B. To 1 ml of a 0.01% w/v solution in 0.1M *sodium hydroxide* add 3 ml of 1M *acetic acid* and 1 ml of a freshly prepared mixture of equal volumes of a 4% w/v solution of *sodium nitroprusside* and 5M *sodium hydroxide*. A blue colour is produced slowly.

Acidity pH of a 10% w/v solution, 5.7 to 6.3, Appendix V L.

Light absorption *Absorbance* of a 0.0025% w/v solution in 0.1M *hydrochloric acid* at the maximum at 219 nm, 0.84 to 0.88, Appendix II B. Measure the absorbance within 15 minutes of preparing the solution.

Specific optical rotation In a 5% w/v solution in 2M *sodium hydroxide*, +110° to +114°, Appendix V F.

Lead Not more than 10 ppm when determined by the following method. Heat 2.5 g with 8 ml of *nitric acid* in a long-necked digestion flask until the reaction has subsided, add 3 ml of *sulphuric acid* and continue heating until the solution is colourless, adding more *nitric acid* dropwise if necessary. Add 5 ml of *water*, evaporate to a small volume, cool and dilute to 25 ml with *water* (solution A). To 15 ml of solution A in a *Nessler cylinder* add 1 g of *citric acid* and make alkaline with 5M *ammonia* (solution B). To a further 5 ml of solution A in a second *Nessler cylinder* add 1 g of *citric acid*, make alkaline with 5M *ammonia* and add 1 ml of *lead standard solution (10 ppm Pb)* (solution C). Add 1 ml of *potassium cyanide solution PbT* to each of solutions B and C; the solutions should not be more than faintly opalescent. If the colours of the solutions differ, equalise them by the addition of a few drops of a highly diluted solution of burnt sugar or other non-reactive substance. Dilute the solutions to 50 ml with *water*. Add to each 0.1 ml of a filtered 10% w/v solution of *sodium sulphide* and mix thoroughly. Compare the colours of the two solutions by a suitable method, such as by light reflected from a white tile through the Nessler cylinders; the colour produced from solution B is not more intense than that produced from solution C.

Condensation products *Absorbance* of a 0.04% w/v solution in 0.1M *sodium hydroxide* at 285 nm, not more than 0.32, Appendix II B.

Loss on drying When dried at 60° at a pressure not exceeding 0.7 kPa for 3 hours, loses not more than 0.5% of its weight. Use 1 g.

Sulphated ash Not more than 0.5%, Appendix IX A.

Assay Dissolve 0.1 g in 5 ml of *water*, add 75 ml of *propan-2-ol* and titrate with 0.1M *sodium hydroxide VS* (carbonate-free) using *thymolphthalein solution* as indicator. Repeat the operation without the substance being examined. The difference between the titrations represents the amount of sodium hydroxide required. Each ml of 0.1M *sodium hydroxide VS* is equivalent to 0.01021 g of $C_3H_6N_2O_2$.

Storage Cycloserine should be kept in a well-closed container and stored at a temperature not exceeding 25°.

Preparations
Cycloserine Capsules
Cycloserine Tablets

Action and use Antibacterial.

Cyproheptadine Hydrochloride

$C_{21}H_{21}N,HCl,1\frac{1}{2}H_2O$ 350.9   *969-33-5*

Cyproheptadine Hydrochloride is 4-(dibenzo-[*a,d*]cyclohept-5-enylidene)-1-methylpiperidine hydrochloride sesquihydrate. It contains not less than 98.5 per cent and not more than 101.0 per cent of $C_{21}H_{21}N,HCl$, calculated with reference to the dried substance.

Characteristics A white or slightly yellow, crystalline powder; odourless or almost odourless.

Solubility Slightly soluble in *water*; soluble in 35 parts of *ethanol (96%)*, in 1.5 parts of *methanol* and in 16 parts of *chloroform* ; practically insoluble in *ether*.

Identification A. Dissolve 0.1 g in 10 ml of *water*, make alkaline with 1M *sodium hydroxide*, extract with 5 ml of *chloroform IR*, dry over *anhydrous sodium sulphate* and remove the solvent with the aid of a current of nitrogen. The *infra-red absorption spectrum* of the oily residue, Appendix II A, is concordant with the *reference spectrum* of cyproheptadine.

B. The *light absorption*, Appendix II B, in the range 230 to 350 nm of a 0.0032% w/v solution in *ethanol (96%)* exhibits a maximum only at 286 nm. The *absorbance* at 286 nm is about 1.05.

C. A saturated solution yields *reaction A* characteristic of chlorides, Appendix VI.

Dibenzocycloheptatriene Carry out the method for *thin-layer chromatography*, Appendix III A, using a silica gel F254 precoated chromatoplate (Merck silica gel 60 F254 plates are suitable) and a mixture of 90 volumes of *chloroform* and 10 volumes of *methanol* as the mobile phase. Apply separately to the plate 10 μl of each of two solutions in *chloroform* containing (1) 1.0% w/v of the substance being examined and (2) 0.0020% w/v of *dibenzocycloheptatriene BPCRS*. After removal of the plate, allow it to dry in air, spray with *ethanolic sulphuric acid (10%)*, heat at 110° for 30 minutes and examine under *ultra-violet light (365 nm)*. Any spot corresponding to dibenzocycloheptatriene in the chromatogram obtained with solution (1) is not more intense than the spot in the chromatogram obtained with solution (2).

Loss on drying When dried to constant weight at 100° at a pressure not exceeding 0.7 kPa, loses 7.0 to 9.0% of its weight. Use 1 g.

Sulphated ash Not more than 0.1%, Appendix IX A.

Assay Dissolve 0.5 g in 0.5 ml of *acetic anhydride* and 20 ml of *anhydrous glacial acetic acid*, add 10 ml of *mercury(II) acetate solution* and carry out Method I for *non-aqueous titration*, Appendix VIII A, using *crystal violet solution* as indicator. Each ml of 0.1M *perchloric acid VS* is equivalent to 0.03239 g of $C_{21}H_{21}N,HCl$.

Storage Cyproheptadine Hydrochloride should be kept in a well-closed container.

Preparation
Cyproheptadine Tablets

Action and use Histamine H_1-receptor antagonist.

Cytarabine

$C_9H_{13}N_3O_5$ 243.2   *147-94-4*

Cytarabine is 1-β-D-arabinofuranosylcytosine. It contains not less than 99.0 per cent and not more 100.5 per cent of $C_9H_{13}N_3O_5$, calculated with reference to the dried substance.

Characteristics A white or almost white, crystalline powder.

Solubility Soluble in 10 parts of *water*; very slightly soluble in *ethanol (96%)* and in *chloroform*.

Identification A. The *infra-red absorption spectrum*, Appendix II A, is concordant with the *reference spectrum* of cytarabine.

B. The *light absorption*, Appendix II B, in the range 230 to 350 nm of a 0.002% w/v solution in 0.1M *hydrochloric acid* exhibits a maximum only at 280 nm. The *absorbance* at 280 nm is about 1.11.

Specific optical rotation In a 1% w/v solution, +154° to +160°, Appendix V F.

Related substances Carry out the method for *thin-layer chromatography*, Appendix III A, using *silica gel GF254* as the coating substance and a mixture of 65 volumes of *butan-2-one*, 20 volumes of *acetone* and 15 volumes of *water* as the mobile phase. Apply separately to the chromatoplate 5 µl of each of three solutions in *water* containing (1) 4.0% w/v of the substance being examined, (2) 0.020% w/v of *uridine* and (3) 0.020% w/v of the substance being examined. After removal of the plate, allow it to dry in air and examine under *ultra-violet light (254 nm)*. Any spot in the chromatogram obtained with solution (1) with an Rf value of about 1.1 relative to the spot in the chromatogram obtained with solution (2) is not more intense than the spot in the chromatogram obtained with solution (2). Any other *secondary spot* in the chromatogram obtained with solution (1) is not more intense than the spot in the chromatogram obtained with solution (3).

Loss on drying When dried at 60° at a pressure not exceeding 0.7 kPa for 3 hours, loses not more than 1.0% of its weight. Use 1 g.

Sulphated ash Not more than 0.3%, Appendix IX A.

Assay Carry out Method I for *non-aqueous titration*, Appendix VIII A, using 0.5 g and *1-naphtholbenzein solution* as indicator. Each ml of 0.1M *perchloric acid VS* is equivalent to 0.02432 g of $C_9H_{13}N_3O_5$.

Storage Cytarabine should be kept in a well-closed container, protected from light and stored at a temperature not exceeding 15°.

Preparation
Cytarabine Injection

Action and use Cytotoxic.

Dacarbazine

$Me_2NN{=}N$ H
$H_2N{\cdot}CO$ N

$C_6H_{10}N_6O$ 182.2   *4342-03-4*

Dacarbazine is 5-(3,3-dimethyltriazeno)-imidazole-4-carboxamide. It contains not less than 98.5 per cent and not more than 101.0 per cent of $C_6H_{10}N_6O$, calculated with reference to the dried substance.

Characteristics A colourless or pale yellow, crystalline powder.

Solubility Slightly soluble in *water* and in *ethanol (96%)*.

Identification A. The *infra-red absorption spectrum*, Appendix II A, is concordant with the *reference spectrum* of dacarbazine.

B. The *light absorption*, Appendix II B, in the range 230 to 350 nm of a 0.0006% w/v solution in 0.1M *hydrochloric acid* exhibits a maximum at 323 nm and a pronounced shoulder at 275 nm. The *absorbance* at 323 nm is about 0.64.

Clarity and colour of solution A 2.0% w/v solution is *clear*, Appendix IV A, and not more intensely coloured than *reference solution BY₆*, Appendix IV B, Method II.

5-Aminoimidazole-4-carboxamide Carry out the method for *high-performance liquid chromatography*, Appendix III D, using two solutions in 0.1M *acetic acid* containing (1) 0.0024% w/v of *5-aminoimidazole-4-carboxamide hydrochloride* and (2) 0.40% w/v of the substance being examined.

The chromatographic procedure described under Related substances may be used but using 0.005M *dioctyl sodium sulphosuccinate* in a mixture of 110 volumes of *methanol*, 87 volumes of *water* and 3 volumes of *glacial acetic acid* as the mobile phase.

The area of any peak corresponding to 5-amino-imidazole-4-carboxamide hydrochloride in the chromatogram obtained with solution (2) is not greater than the area of the peak in the the chromatogram obtained with solution (1).

Related substances Carry out the method for *high-performance liquid chromatography*, Appendix III D, using two solutions in 0.1M *acetic acid* containing (1) 0.0040% w/v of *2-azahypoxanthine BPCRS* and (2) 0.40% w/v of the substance being examined.

The chromatographic procedure may be carried out using (a) a stainless steel column (20 cm × 4 mm) packed with *stationary phase C* (10 µm) (Nucleosil C18 is suitable), (b) 0.005M *dioctyl sodium sulphosuccinate* in a mixture of 98.5 volumes of *water* and 1.5 volumes of *glacial acetic acid* as the mobile phase with a flow rate of 1.5 ml per minute and (c) a detection wavelength of 254 nm.

In the chromatogram obtained with solution (2) the area of any *secondary peak* is not greater than the area of the principal peak in the chromatogram obtained with solution (1). Not more than one such peak has an area greater than half the area of the peak in the chromatogram obtained with solution (1) and the sum of the areas of all such peaks is not greater than three times the area of the peak in the chromatogram obtained with solution (1). After use the column should be thoroughly flushed with *methanol* to remove dacarbazine which does not elute with the mobile phase.

Loss on drying When dried to constant weight at 60° at a pressure not exceeding 0.7 kPa, loses not more than 0.5% of its weight. Use 1 g.

Sulphated ash Not more than 0.1%, Appendix IX A.

Assay Dissolve 0.4 g in 10 ml of *anhydrous glacial acetic acid* and carry out Method I for *non-aqueous titration*, Appendix VIII A, determining the end-point potentiometrically. Each ml of 0.1M *perchloric acid VS* is equivalent to 0.01822 g of $C_6H_{10}N_6O$.

Storage Dacarbazine should be kept in a well-closed container, protected from light and stored at a temperature of 2° to 8°.

Preparation
Dacarbazine Injection

Action and use Cytotoxic.

Danthron

$C_{14}H_8O_4$ 240.2   *117-10-2*

Danthron is mainly 1,8-dihydroxyanthra-quinone. It contains not less than 98.0 per cent and not more than 102.0 per cent of total phenols, calculated as $C_{14}H_8O_4$ and with reference to the dried substance.

Characteristics An orange, crystalline powder; odourless or almost odourless.

Solubility Practically insoluble in *water*; very slightly soluble in *ethanol (96%)*; soluble in *chloroform*; slightly soluble in *ether*. It dissolves in solutions of alkali hydroxides.

Identification A. The *infra-red absorption spectrum*, Appendix II A, is concordant with the *reference spectrum* of danthron.

B. The *light absorption*, Appendix II B, in the range 230 to 350 nm of a 0.001% w/v solution in *chloroform* exhibits maxima at 255 nm and 285 nm and a less well-defined maximum at 275 nm. The *absorbance* at 255 nm is about 0.82 and at 285 nm is about 0.48.

C. Dissolve 5 mg in 5 ml of 1M *sodium hydroxide*. A clear red solution is produced immediately.

Mercury To 0.50 g in a long-necked flask add 2.5 ml of *nitric acid* and allow to stand until the initial vigorous reaction has subsided. Add 2.5 ml of *sulphuric acid* and heat until dense white fumes are evolved. Cool, add 2.5 ml of *nitric acid* and heat until fumes are again evolved. Repeat the procedure with a further 2.5 ml of *nitric acid*, cool, add 50 ml of *water*, boil the solution until the volume has been reduced to about 25 ml and cool. Transfer to a separating funnel using *water*, dilute to about 50 ml with *water* and add 50 ml of 0.5M *sulphuric acid*. Add 100 ml of *water*, 2 g of *hydroxylamine hydrochloride*, 1 ml of 0.05M *disodium edetate*, 1 ml of *glacial acetic acid* and 5 ml of *chloroform*, shake, allow to separate and discard the chloroform layer. Titrate the aqueous layer with a 0.0008% w/v solution of *dithizone* in *chloroform*, shaking vigorously after each addition, allowing the layers to separate and discarding the chloroform layer, until the chloroform layer remains green. Repeat the operation using a solution prepared by diluting 1 ml of *mercury standard solution (5 ppm Hg)* to 100 ml with 0.5M *sulphuric acid* and beginning at the words 'Add 100 ml of *water* . . .'. The volume of the dithizone solution required by the substance being examined does not exceed that required by the mercury standard solution.

Related substances Carry out the method for *high-performance liquid chromatography*, Appendix III D, using the following solutions. For solution (1) dilute 20 ml of a 0.00125% w/v solution of *1-hydroxyanthraquinone* in *tetrahydrofuran* to 100 ml with the mobile phase. For solution (2) dissolve 50 mg of the substance being examined in 20 ml of *tetrahydrofuran* and dilute to 100 ml with the mobile phase. For solution (3) dilute 1 volume of solution (2) to 200 volumes with the mobile phase. For solution (4) dissolve 50 mg of *danthron BPCRS* in 20 ml of a 0.00125% w/v solution of *1-hydroxyanthraquinone* in *tetrahydrofuran* and dilute to 100 ml with the mobile phase.

The chromatographic procedure may be carried out using (a) a stainless steel column (20 cm × 4.6 mm) packed with *stationary phase C* (5 μm) (Nucleosil C18 is suitable), (b) a mixture of 60 volumes of *water*, 40 volumes of *tetrahydrofuran* and 2.5 volumes of *glacial acetic acid* as the mobile phase with a flow rate of 1 ml per minute and (c) a detection wavelength of 254 nm. For solution (2) allow the chromatography to proceed for 1.5 times the retention time of the principal peak.

In the chromatogram obtained with solution (2) the area of any *secondary peak* is not greater than the area of the principal peak in the chromatogram obtained with solution (3) and the sum of the areas of any *secondary peaks* is not greater than twice the area of the principal peak in the chromatogram obtained with solution (3).

The test is not valid unless, in the chromatogram obtained with solution (4), a peak due to 1-hydroxy-anthraquinone appears immediately before the principal peak and the height of the trough separating the two peaks is not greater than one-third of the height of the peak due to 1-hydroxyanthraquinone.

Loss on drying When dried to constant weight at 105°, loses not more than 0.5% of its weight. Use 1 g.

Assay Dissolve 0.2 g in 50 ml of *anhydrous pyridine* and carry out Method II for *non-aqueous titration*, Appendix VIII A, using 0.1M *tetrabutylammonium hydroxide VS* as titrant and determining the end-point potentiometrically. Each ml of 0.1M *tetrabutylammonium hydroxide VS* is equivalent to 0.02402 g of total phenols, calculated as $C_{14}H_8O_4$.

Action and use Laxative.

In some countries the material described in this monograph may be known as Dantron.

Dapsone ☆

$C_{12}H_{12}N_2O_2S$ 248.3   *80-08-0*

Dapsone is bis(4-aminophenyl) sulphone. It contains not less than 99.0 per cent and not more than 101.0 per cent of $C_{12}H_{12}N_2O_2S$, calculated with reference to the dried substance.

Characteristics A white or slightly yellowish-white, crystalline powder; odourless.

Solubility Very slightly soluble in *water*; soluble in 30 parts of *ethanol (96%)*; freely soluble in *acetone*. It dissolves in dilute mineral acids.

Identification A. The *light absorption*, Appendix II B, in the range 230 to 350 nm of a 0.0005% w/v solution in *methanol* exhibits two maxima, at 260 nm and 295 nm. The A(1%, 1 cm) at 260 nm is about 720 and at 295 nm is about 1200.

B. Carry out the method described under Related substances applying separately to the chromatoplate 1 μl of each of two solutions in *methanol* containing (1) 0.1% w/v of the substance being examined and (2) 0.1% w/v of *dapsone EPCRS*. The principal spot in the chromatogram obtained with solution (1) corresponds to that in the chromatogram obtained with solution (2).

C. 2 ml of a 0.005% w/v solution in 0.1M *hydrochloric acid* yields the *reaction* characteristic of primary aromatic amines, Appendix VI.

D. *Melting point*, 175° to 181°, Appendix V A, Method I.

Related substances Carry out the method for *thin-layer chromatography*, Appendix III A, using *silica gel G* as the coating substance and a mixture of 80 volumes of *toluene* and 40 volumes of *acetone* as the mobile phase. Apply separately to the chromatoplate 10 μl of each of three solutions of the substance being examined in *methanol* containing (1) 1.0% w/v, (2) 0.010% w/v and (3) 0.0020% w/v. After removal of the plate, allow it to dry in air and spray with a 0.5% w/v solution of *sodium nitrite* in 0.1M *hydrochloric acid* and, while still damp, with a 0.1% w/v solution of N-(1-naphthyl)ethylenediamine dihydrochloride. Any *secondary spot* in the chromatogram obtained with solution (1) is not more intense than the spot in the chromatogram obtained with solution (2) and not more than two such spots are more intense than the spot in the chromatogram obtained with solution (3).

Loss on drying When dried to constant weight at 100° to 105°, loses not more than 1.5% of its weight. Use 1 g.

Sulphated ash Not more than 0.1%, Appendix IX A, Method II. Use 1 g.

Assay Dissolve 0.2 g in 50 ml of 2M *hydrochloric acid*, add 3 g of *potassium bromide*, cool if necessary in ice and carry out the method for *amperometric titration*, Appendix VIII B. Each ml of 0.1M *sodium nitrite VS* is equivalent to 0.01242 g of $C_{12}H_{12}N_2O_2S$.

Preparation
Dapsone Tablets

Action and use Antileprotic.

Debrisoquine Sulphate

$(C_{10}H_{13}N_3)_2,H_2SO_4$ 448.5   *581-88-4*

Debrisoquine Sulphate is 1,2,3,4-tetrahydro-isoquinoline-2-carboxamidine sulphate. It contains not less than 99.0 per cent and not more than 101.0 per cent of $(C_{10}H_{13}N_3)_2,H_2SO_4$, calculated with reference to the dried substance.

Characteristics A white, crystalline powder; odourless or almost odourless.

Solubility Soluble in 40 parts of *water*; very slightly soluble in *ethanol* (96%); almost insoluble in *chloroform* and in *ether*.

Identification A. The *light absorption*, Appendix II B, in the range 230 to 350 nm of a 0.05% w/v solution in 0.05M *sulphuric acid* exhibits two maxima, at 262 nm and 270 nm. The *absorbance* at 262 nm is about 0.69 and at 270 nm is about 0.51.

B. Carry out the method described under Related substances, applying separately to the chromatoplate 10 μl of each of the following solutions in *water*. Solution (1) contains 0.25% w/v of the substance being examined. Solution (2) contains 0.25% w/v of *debrisoquine sulphate BPCRS*. Solution (3) is a mixture of equal volumes of solutions (1) and (2). The principal spot in the chromatogram obtained with solution (1) corresponds to that in the chromatogram obtained with solution (2). The principal spot in the chromatogram obtained with solution (3) appears as a single compact spot.

C. Yields the *reactions* characteristic of sulphates, Appendix VI.

D. *Melting point*, about 274°, with decomposition, Appendix V A.

Acidity pH of a 3% w/v solution, 5.3 to 6.8, Appendix V L.

Related substances Carry out the method for *thin-layer chromatography*, Appendix III A, using *silica gel G* as the coating substance and a mixture of 60 volumes of *butan-1-ol*, 25 volumes of *water* and 15 volumes of *glacial acetic acid* as the mobile phase. Apply separately to the chromatoplate 10 μl of each of two solutions in *water* containing (1) 2.0% w/v of the substance being examined and (2) 0.010% w/v of *debrisoquine sulphate BPCRS*. After removal of the plate, allow it to dry in air and spray with a solution prepared by adding 1 ml of *sulphuric acid* to 40 ml of a freshly prepared mixture of equal volumes of a 0.135% w/v solution of *chloroplatinic(IV) acid* and a 1.1% w/v solution of *potassium iodide*. Any *secondary spot* in the chromatogram obtained with solution (1) is not more intense than the spot in the chromatogram obtained with solution (2).

Loss on drying When dried to constant weight at 105°, loses not more than 0.5% of its weight. Use 1 g.

Sulphated ash Not more than 0.1%, Appendix IX A.

Assay Carry out Method I for *non-aqueous titration*, Appendix VIII A, using 1 g and determining the end-point potentiometrically. Each ml of 0.1M *perchloric acid VS* is equivalent to 0.04485 g of $(C_{10}H_{13}N_3)_2,H_2SO_4$.

Storage Debrisoquine Sulphate should be kept in a well-closed container and protected from light.

Preparation
Debrisoquine Tablets

Action and use Adrenergic neurone blocking agent.

Demeclocycline Hydrochloride ☆
Demethylchlortetracycline Hydrochloride

$C_{21}H_{21}ClN_2O_8,HCl$ 501.3   *64-73-3*

Demeclocycline Hydrochloride is the hydrochloride of (4*S*,4a*S*,5a*S*,6*S*,12a*S*)-7-chloro-4-dimethylamino-1,4,4a,5,5a,6,11,12a-octahydro-3,6,10,12,12a-pentahydroxy-1,11-dioxonaphthacene-2-carboxamide, a substance produced by the growth of certain strains of *Streptomyces aureofaciens* or obtained by any other means. The potency is not less than 950 Units per mg, calculated with reference to the dried substance.

Characteristics A yellow, crystalline powder; odourless.

Solubility Soluble in 30 parts of *water*; slightly soluble in *ethanol (96%)*; very slightly soluble in *acetone* and in *chloroform*; practically insoluble in *ether*. It dissolves in aqueous solutions of alkali hydroxides and carbonates.

Identification A. Complies with the test for *identification of tetracyclines*, Appendix III A. Solution (1) contains 0.05% w/v each of the substance being examined, *chlortetracycline hydrochloride EPCRS*, *doxycycline hyclate EPCRS*, *oxytetracycline hydrochloride EPCRS* and *tetracycline hydrochloride EPCRS*. Solution (2) contains 0.05% w/v each of *chlortetracycline hydrochloride EPCRS*, *doxycycline hyclate EPCRS*, *oxytetracycline hydrochloride EPCRS* and *tetracycline hydrochloride EPCRS*.
B. To 2 mg add 5 ml of *sulphuric acid*; a violet colour is produced. Add the solution to 2.5 ml of *water*; the colour changes to yellow.
C. Yields *reaction A* characteristic of chlorides, Appendix VI.

Acidity pH of a 1% w/v solution, 2.0 to 3.0, Appendix V L.

Light absorption Dissolve 10 mg in sufficient *0.001M hydrochloric acid* to produce 100 ml. To 10 ml of the resulting solution add 75 ml of *water*, 12 ml of *2M sodium hydroxide* and sufficient *water* to produce 100 ml. The A(1%, 1 cm) at 385 nm is 340 to 370, Appendix II B.

Specific optical rotation In a 1% w/v solution in *0.1M hydrochloric acid*, −248° to −263°, Appendix V F.

Heavy metals 0.5 g complies with *limit test C for heavy metals*, Appendix VII (50 ppm). Use 2.5 ml of *lead standard solution (10 ppm Pb)* to prepare the standard.

Loss on drying When dried over *phosphorus pentoxide* at 60° at a pressure not exceeding 0.7 kPa for 3 hours, loses not more than 2.0% of its weight. Use 1 g.

Sulphated ash Not more than 0.5%, Appendix IX A, Method II. Use 1 g.

Assay Carry out the *biological assay of antibiotics*, Appendix XIV A. The precision of the assay is such that the fiducial limits of error are not less than 95% and not more than 105% of the estimated potency.

Storage Demeclocycline Hydrochloride should be kept in a well-closed container and protected from light.

Labelling The label states (1) the date after which the material is not intended to be used; (2) the conditions under which it should be stored.

Preparation
Demeclocycline Capsules

Action and use Antibacterial.

Deoxycortone Acetate ☆

C₂₃H₃₂O₄   372.5   56-47-3

$C_{23}H_{32}O_4$ 372.5 56-47-3

Deoxycortone Acetate is 3,20-dioxopregn-4-en-21-yl acetate. It contains not less than 96.0 per cent and not more than 104.0 per cent of $C_{23}H_{32}O_4$, calculated with reference to the dried substance.

Characteristics Colourless crystals or a white, crystalline powder.

Solubility Practically insoluble in *water*; soluble in 50 parts of *ethanol (96%)* and in 30 parts of *acetone*; freely soluble in *chloroform*; slightly soluble in *propane-1,2-diol* and in fixed oils.

Identification *Test A may be omitted if tests B, C, D and E are carried out. Tests C, D and E may be omitted if tests A and B are carried out.*
A. The *infra-red absorption spectrum*, Appendix II A, is concordant with the spectrum of *desoxycortone acetate EPCRS*. If the spectra are not concordant, prepare new spectra using 5% w/v solutions in *chloroform IR*.
B. Examine the chromatograms obtained in the test for Related substances under *ultra-violet light (254 nm)*. The principal spot in the chromatogram obtained with solution (2) is similar in position and size to the principal spot in the chromatogram obtained with solution (5). Spray the plate with *ethanolic sulphuric acid (20%)* and heat at 120° for 10 minutes or until the spots are visible. Allow to cool and examine in daylight and under *ultra-violet light (365 nm)*. The principal spot in the chromatogram obtained with solution (2) is similar in colour in daylight, fluorescence under ultra-violet light (365 nm), position and size to that in the chromatogram obtained with solution (5).
C. Add 2 mg to 2 ml of *sulphuric acid* and shake to dissolve; a yellow colour is produced within 5 minutes. Add the solution to 2 ml of *water* and shake; the resulting solution is dichroic showing an intense blue colour by transparency and a red fluorescence which is particularly intense under ultra-violet light (365 nm).
D. Yields the *reaction* characteristic of acetyl groups, Appendix VI. Use 10 mg.
E. *Melting point*, 157° to 161°, Appendix V A, Method I.

Light absorption Dissolve 5 mg in sufficient *ethanol (96%)* to produce 100 ml and dilute 1 ml to 50 ml with the same solvent. The A(1%, 1 cm) in the resulting solution at the maximum at 240 nm is 430 to 460, Appendix II B.

Specific optical rotation In a 1% w/v solution in *1,4-dioxan*, +171° to +179°, Appendix V F.

Related substances Carry out the method for *thin-layer chromatography*, Appendix III A, using as the coating substance a suitable silica gel containing a fluorescent indicator with an optimal intensity at 254 nm (Merck silica gel 60 F254 is suitable) and a mixture of 77 volumes of *dichloromethane*, 15 volumes of *ether*, 8 volumes of *methanol* and 1.2 volumes of *water* as the mobile phase. Apply separately to the chromatoplate 5 μl of each of the following solutions in a mixture of 9 volumes of *chloroform* and 1 volume of *methanol*. Solutions (1), (2), (3) and (4) contain 1.0%, 0.10%, 0.020% and 0.010% w/v respectively of the substance being examined. Solution (5) contains 0.10% w/v of *desoxycortone acetate EPCRS*. Solution (6) contains 0.010% w/v each of *cortisone acetate EPCRS* and *hydrocortisone acetate EPCRS*. After removal of the plate, allow it to dry in air and examine under *ultra-violet light (254 nm)*. Any *secondary spot* in the chromatogram obtained with solution (1) is not more intense than the spot in the chromatogram obtained with solution (3) and not more than one such spot is more intense than the spot in the chromatogram obtained with solution (4). The test is not valid unless the chromatogram obtained with solution (6) shows two clearly separated principal spots.

Loss on drying When dried at 100° to 105° for 3 hours, loses not more than 0.5% of its weight. Use 0.5 g.

Assay Carry out the *tetrazolium assay of steroids*, Appendix VIII P, and calculate the content of $C_{23}H_{32}O_4$ from the *absorbance* obtained by repeating the operation using *desoxycortone acetate EPCRS* in place of the substance being examined.

Storage Deoxycortone Acetate should be kept in a well-closed container and protected from light.

Action and use Corticosteroid.

The title of the monograph in the European Pharmacopœia is Desoxycortone Acetate.

Dequalinium Chloride

$C_{30}H_{40}Cl_2N_4$　　527.6　　*522-51-0*

Dequalinium Chloride is 4,4′-diamino-2,2′-dimethyl-*N,N′*-decamethylenedi(quinolinium chloride). It contains not less than 95.0 per cent and not more than 101.0 per cent of $C_{30}H_{40}Cl_2N_4$, calculated with reference to the dried substance.

Characteristics A creamy-white powder; odourless or almost odourless.

Solubility Slightly soluble in *water*; soluble in 30 parts of boiling *water*; slightly soluble in *propane-1,2-diol*.

Identification A. The *light absorption*, Appendix II B, in the range 230 to 350 nm of a 0.0016% w/v solution exhibits three maxima, at 240, 326 and 335 nm. The *absorbance* at 240 nm is about 1.3, at 326 nm, about 0.75 and at 335 nm, about 0.65.

B. Yields *reaction A* characteristic of chlorides, Appendix VI.

C. *Melting point*, about 315°, with decomposition, Appendix V A.

Acidity or alkalinity Shake 0.1 g with 100 ml of *carbon dioxide-free water* for 10 minutes and add *bromocresol purple solution* as indicator. Not more than 0.2 ml of either 0.1M *hydrochloric acid VS* or 0.1M *sodium hydroxide VS* is required to change the colour of the solution.

Non-quaternised amines Not more than 1.0%, calculated as 4-aminoquinaldine, $C_{10}H_{10}N_2$, when determined by the following method. Shake 1 g with 45 ml of *water* for 5 minutes, add 5 ml of 2M *nitric acid*, shake for 10 minutes and filter through absorbent cotton. Transfer 20 ml of the filtrate to a separating funnel, add 20 ml of 1M *sodium hydroxide*, extract with two 50-ml quantities of *ether*, washing each extract in turn with the same 5 ml of *water*, and then extract each ether solution successively with quantities of 20, 20 and 5 ml of 1M *hydrochloric acid*. Combine the acid extracts, dilute to 50 ml with 1M *hydrochloric acid* and measure the *absorbance* of the resulting solution at 319 nm and 326.5 nm, Appendix II B. The absorbance at 319 nm is not less than that at 326.5 nm. Calculate the percentage of $C_{10}H_{10}N_2$ from the expression $0.387a - 0.306b$, where a is the A(1%, 1 cm) at 319 nm and b is the A(1%, 1 cm) at 326.5 nm.

Loss on drying When dried at 105° at a pressure not exceeding 0.7 kPa for 3 hours, loses not more than 5.0% of its weight. Use 1 g.

Sulphated ash Not more than 0.1%, Appendix IX A.

Assay Dissolve 0.7 g in 80 ml of *anhydrous glacial acetic acid* by warming gently under a reflux condenser, add 20 ml of *mercury(II) acetate solution* while hot, cool and titrate with 0.1M *perchloric acid VS*, using 0.2 ml of *crystal violet solution* as indicator, until the colour changes from violet-blue to pure blue. Repeat the operation without the substance being examined. The difference between the titrations represents the amount of perchloric acid required. Each ml of 0.1M *perchloric acid VS* is equivalent to 0.02638 g of $C_{30}H_{40}Cl_2N_4$.

Action and use Antiseptic.

Desferrioxamine Mesylate

$C_{25}H_{48}N_6O_8,CH_4SO_3$　　656.8　　*138-14-7*

Desferrioxamine Mesylate is 30-amino-3,14,25-trihydroxy-3,9,14,20,25-penta-azatriacontane-2,10,13,21,24-pentaone methanesulphonate. It contains not less than 98.0 per cent and not more than 102.0 per cent of $C_{25}H_{48}N_6O_8$, CH_4SO_3, calculated with reference to the anhydrous substance.

Characteristics A white to cream powder; odourless or almost odourless.

Solubility Soluble in 5 parts of *water* and in 20 parts of *ethanol (96%)*; insoluble in *absolute ethanol*, in *chloroform* and in *ether*.

Identification A. The *infra-red absorption spectrum*, Appendix II A, is concordant with the *reference spectrum* of desferrioxamine mesylate.

B. In a 1% w/v solution in a buffer solution prepared by mixing 15 volumes of *formic acid* and 10 volumes of *glacial acetic acid* and diluting to 200 volumes with *water*, its mobility on paper in a suitable electrophoretic field corresponds with that of a 1% w/v solution of *desferrioxamine mesylate BPCRS* in the same buffer solution. The spots may be revealed by spraying with a solution prepared by dissolving 16 g of *iron(III) chloride* in 20 ml of 0.05M *sulphuric acid* and adding sufficient *water* to produce 1000 ml.

C. The titrated solution obtained in the Assay is reddish-brown. The colour is extracted by *benzyl alcohol* but not by *ether*.

Acidity pH of a 10% w/v solution, 3.5 to 5.5, Appendix V L.

Clarity and colour of solution A 10.0% w/v solution is not more than *slightly opalescent*, Appendix IV A. The *absorbance* of the solution at 425 nm is not more than 0.10, Appendix II B.

Chloride Dissolve 0.3 g in 30 ml of *water*. 15 ml of the resulting solution complies with the *limit test for chlorides*, Appendix VII (330 ppm).

Sulphate 0.25 g complies with the *limit test for sulphates*, Appendix VII (600 ppm).

Sulphated ash Not more than 0.1%, Appendix IX A.

Water Not more than 2.0% w/w, Appendix IX C. Use 1 g.

Assay Dissolve 0.3 g in 15 ml of *water* and add 2 ml of 0.05M *sulphuric acid*. Titrate slowly with 0.1M *ammonium iron(III) sulphate VS* determining the end-point potentiometrically using a platinum electrode and a calomel reference electrode. Each ml of 0.1M *ammonium iron(III) sulphate VS* is equivalent to 0.06568 g of $C_{25}H_{48}N_6O_8,CH_4SO_3$.

Storage Desferrioxamine Mesylate should be kept in a well-closed container, protected from light and stored at a temperature not exceeding 4°.

Preparation
Desferrioxamine Injection

Action and use Iron chelating agent.

In some countries the material described in this monograph may be known as Desferoxamine Mesilate.

Desipramine Hydrochloride ☆

$C_{18}H_{22}N_2,HCl$ 302.8   58-28-6

Desipramine Hydrochloride is 3-(10,11-dihydro-5*H*-dibenz[*b,f*]azepin-5-yl)propyl-(methyl)amine hydrochloride. It contains not less than 99.0 per cent and not more than 101.0 per cent of $C_{18}H_{22}N_2,HCl$, calculated with reference to the dried substance.

Characteristics A white or almost white, crystalline powder. It melts at about 214°.

Solubility Soluble in 20 parts of *water*, in 20 parts of *ethanol (96%)* and in 4 parts of *chloroform*; practically insoluble in *ether*.

Identification *Test A may be omitted if tests B, C, D and E are carried out. Tests B, C and D may be omitted if tests A and E are carried out.*

A. The *infra-red absorption spectrum*, Appendix II A, is concordant with the spectrum of *desipramine hydrochloride EPCRS*.

B. The *light absorption*, Appendix II B, in the range 230 to 350 nm of a 0.002% w/v solution in 0.01M *hydrochloric acid* exhibits a maximum at 251 nm and a shoulder at 270 nm. The A(1%, 1 cm) at 251 nm is 255 to 285.

C. In the test for Related substances, the principal spot in the chromatogram obtained with solution (2) is similar in position, colour and size to that in the chromatogram obtained with solution (3).

D. Dissolve 50 mg in 3 ml of *water* and add 0.05 ml of a 2.5% w/v solution of *quinhydrone* in *methanol*. An intense pink colour is produced within about 15 minutes (distinction from imipramine hydrochloride).

E. Dissolve 1.25 g in *carbon dioxide-free water*, warming to not more than 30° if necessary, and dilute to 25 ml with the same solvent (solution A). To 0.5 ml add 1.5 ml of *water*. The solution yields *reaction A* characteristic of chlorides, Appendix VI.

Acidity pH of solution A, 4.0 to 5.5, Appendix V L.

Colour of solution Solution A, examined immediately after preparation, is not more intensely coloured than *reference solution BY₆*, Appendix IV B, Method I.

Heavy metals 2.0 g complies with *limit test C for heavy metals*, Appendix VII (20 ppm). Use 4 ml of *lead standard solution (10 ppm Pb)* to prepare the standard.

Related substances Carry out the method for *thin-layer chromatography*, Appendix III A, protected from light, using *silica gel G* as the coating substance and a mixture of 50 volumes of *glacial acetic acid*, 50 volumes of *toluene* and 5 volumes of *water* as the mobile phase but allowing the solvent front to ascend 7 cm above the line of application. Apply separately to the chromatoplate 5 μl of each of four solutions prepared immediately before use in a mixture of equal volumes of *chloroform* and *absolute ethanol* containing (1) 1.0% w/v of the substance being examined, (2) 0.1% w/v of the substance being examined, (3) 0.1% w/v of *desipramine hydrochloride EPCRS* and (4) 0.0020% w/v of *desipramine hydrochloride EPCRS*. After removal of the plate, dry it for 10 minutes in a current of air, spray with a 0.5% w/v solution of *potassium dichromate* in a mixture of 1 volume of *sulphuric acid* and 4 volumes of *water* and examine immediately. Any *secondary spot* in the chromatogram obtained with solution (1) is not more intense than the spot in the chromatogram obtained with solution (4).

Loss on drying When dried to constant weight at 100° to 105°, loses not more than 0.5% of its weight. Use 1 g.

Sulphated ash Not more than 0.1%, Appendix IX A, Method II. Use 1 g.

Assay Dissolve 0.25 g in a mixture of 5 ml of 0.01M *hydrochloric acid VS* and 50 ml of *ethanol (96%)* and titrate with 0.01M *sodium hydroxide VS* determining the end-point potentiometrically. Record the volume added between the two inflections. Each ml of 0.01M *sodium hydroxide VS* is equivalent to 0.03028 g of $C_{18}H_{22}N_2,HCl$.

Storage Desipramine Hydrochloride should be kept in a well-closed container and protected from light.

Preparation
Desipramine Tablets

Action and use Antidepressant.

Deslanoside ☆

$C_{47}H_{74}O_{19}$ 943.1   *17598-65-1*

Deslanoside is 3-[(*O*-β-D-glucopyranosyl-(1→4)-*O*-2,6-dideoxy-β-D-*ribo*-hexopyranosyl-(1→4)-*O*-2,6-dideoxy-β-D-*ribo*-hexopyranosyl-(1→4)-*O*-2,6-dideoxy-β-D-*ribo*-hexopyranosyl)-oxy]-12,14-dihydroxy-3β,5β,12β-card-20(22)-enolide. It contains not less than 95.0 per cent and not more than 105.0 per cent of $C_{47}H_{74}O_{19}$, calculated with reference to the dried substance.

Characteristics A white, crystalline or finely crystalline powder; hygroscopic. It loses water in an atmosphere of low relative humidity.

Solubility Practically insoluble in *water*, in *chloroform* and in *ether*; very slightly soluble in *ethanol (96%)*.

Identification *Test A may be omitted if tests B, C and D are carried out. Tests B, C and D may be omitted if test A is carried out.*

A. The *infra-red absorption spectrum*, Appendix II A, is concordant with the spectrum of *deslanoside EPCRS*. Examine the substances as dispersions prepared by dissolving 1 mg in 0.3 ml of *methanol* and triturating with 0.4 g of dry, finely powdered *potassium bromide IR* until the mixture is uniform and completely dry. When comparing the spectra special attention should be given to the absence of a distinct maximum at 1260 cm^{-1} and to the intensity of the maximum at 1740 cm^{-1}.

B. In the test for Related substances, the principal band in the chromatogram obtained with solution (2) is similar in position, colour and size to that in the chromatogram obtained with solution (3).

C. Suspend 0.5 mg in 0.2 ml of *ethanol (60%)* and add 0.1 ml of a 2.0% w/v solution of *3,5-dinitrobenzoic acid* in *ethanol (96%)* and 0.1 ml of 2M *sodium hydroxide*. A violet colour is produced.

D. Dissolve 5 mg in 5 ml of *glacial acetic acid*, add 0.05 ml of a 10.5% w/v solution of *iron(III) chloride hexahydrate*. Cautiously add 2 ml of *sulphuric acid* without mixing and allow to stand. A brown but not reddish ring is produced at the interface and a greenish-yellow, changing to bluish-green, colour diffuses from it into the upper layer.

Clarity and colour of solution A 2.0% w/v solution in a mixture of equal volumes of *chloroform* and *methanol* is

clear, Appendix IV A, and *colourless*, Appendix IV B, Method II.

Specific optical rotation In a 2% w/v solution in *anhydrous pyridine*, +6.5° to +8.5°, Appendix V F.

Related substances Carry out the method for *thin-layer chromatography*, Appendix III A, using *silica gel G* as the coating substance and a mixture of 130 volumes of *dichloromethane*, 36 volumes of *methanol* and 3 volumes of *water* as the mobile phase. Apply separately to the chromatoplate as 10-mm bands 5 μl of each of five solutions in a mixture of equal volumes of *chloroform* and *methanol* containing (1) 2.0% w/v of the substance being examined, (2) 0.2% w/v of the substance being examined, (3) 0.2% w/v of *deslanoside EPCRS*, (4) 0.050% w/v of *deslanoside EPCRS* and (5) 0.020% w/v of *deslanoside EPCRS*. After removal of the plate, allow it to dry in a current of warm air, spray with *ethanolic sulphuric acid (5%)*, heat at 140° for 15 minutes and examine in daylight. Any *secondary band* in the chromatogram obtained with solution (1) is not more intense than the band in the chromatogram obtained with solution (4) and not more than two such bands are more intense than the band in the chromatogram obtained with solution (5).

Loss on drying When dried to constant weight over *phosphorus pentoxide* at 100° to 105° at a pressure of 1.5 to 2.5 kPa, loses not more than 5.0% of its weight. Use 0.5 g.

Sulphated ash Not more than 0.1%, Appendix IX A, Method II. Use the residue obtained in the test for Loss on drying.

Assay Carry out the following procedure in subdued light. Dissolve 50 mg in sufficient *ethanol (96%)* to produce 50 ml and dilute 5 ml to 100 ml with the same solvent. To 5 ml of the resulting solution add 3 ml of *alkaline trinitrophenol solution* and allow to stand in a water-bath at 19° to 21° for 40 minutes. Measure the *absorbance* of the solution at the maximum at 484 nm, Appendix II B, using in the reference cell a mixture of 5 ml of *ethanol (96%)* and 3 ml of *alkaline trinitrophenol solution* prepared at the same time. Calculate the content of $C_{47}H_{74}O_{19}$ from the *absorbance* obtained by carrying out the procedure at the same time using *deslanoside EPCRS* in place of the substance being examined.

Storage Deslanoside should be kept in an airtight, glass container, protected from light and stored at a temperature not exceeding 10°.

Action and use Cardiac glycoside.

Desmopressin

S·CH₂·CH₂·CO·Tyr-Phe-Gln-Asn-Cys-Pro-DArg-Gly-NH₂

$C_{46}H_{64}N_{14}O_{12}S_2$ 1069.1   *16679-58-6*

Desmopressin is a synthetic analogue of the cyclic nonapeptide arginine vasopressin; it has a selective and prolonged antidiuretic action. It contains not less than 900 Units per mg, calculated with reference to the anhydrous, acetic acid-free substance. It is available in the acetate trihydrate form.

Characteristics A white, fluffy powder.

Solubility Soluble in *water*, in *ethanol (96%)*, in *glacial acetic acid* and in *methanol*; slightly soluble in *chloroform* and in *ethyl acetate*.

Identification A. Causes an antidiuretic response when administered as directed in the Assay.
B. In the test for Related peptides, the principal spot in the chromatogram obtained with solution (1) corresponds to that in the chromatogram obtained with solution (4).

Light absorption *Absorbance* of a 0.02% w/v solution in 0.1M *sodium hydroxide* at the maximum at 293 nm, 0.34 to 0.43, Appendix II B.

Specific optical rotation In a 0.5% w/v solution containing 1% v/v of *glacial acetic acid*, −60° to −70°, Appendix V F.

Acetic acid Not more than 6% w/w when determined by the method for *gas chromatography*, Appendix III B, using solutions in *water* containing (1) 0.1% w/v of *glacial acetic acid* and 0.1% v/v of *1,4-dioxan* (internal standard), (2) 2.0% w/v of the substance being examined and (3) 2.0% w/v of the substance being examined and 0.1% v/v of the internal standard.

The chromatographic procedure may be carried out using a glass column (2 m × 3 mm) packed with porous polymer beads (100 to 110 mesh) (Porapak Q is suitable) and maintained at 150°.

Amino acids Carry out the method for *amino acid analysis*, Appendix III G, using 1 mg. Use 0.03% of DL-*norleucine* (internal standard) and heat for 24 hours. Express the content of each amino acid, except cystine, in moles and calculate the relative proportions of the amino acids, taking that for arginine to be 1. The values for aspartic acid, glutamic acid, proline, glycine, tyrosine and phenylalanine are between 0.9 and 1.1. Not more than traces of other amino acids, apart from cystine and ornithine, are present in the hydrolysate.

Peptide Not less than 90% of the peptide $C_{46}H_{64}N_{14}O_{12}S_2$, calculated with reference to the anhydrous, acetic acid-free substance, when determined by the following method. Carry out the method for *high-performance liquid chromatography*, Appendix III D, using two solutions in *water* containing (1) 0.1% w/v of the substance being examined and (2) 0.1% w/v of *desmopressin BPCRS*.

The chromatographic procedure may be carried out using (a) a stainless steel column (10 cm × 5 mm) packed with *stationary phase C* (5 μm) (Nucleosil C18 is suitable), (b) as the mobile phase with a flow rate of 2 ml per minute a mixture of *0.067M phosphate buffer pH 7* and *acetonitrile*, the mixture being adjusted so that the retention time of desmopressin is about 5 minutes (a mixture of 80 volumes of *0.067M phosphate buffer pH 7* and 20 volumes of *acetonitrile* is usually suitable) and (c) a detection wavelength of 220 nm.

Calculate the content of the peptide, $C_{46}H_{64}N_{14}O_{12}S_2$, using the declared content of $C_{46}H_{64}N_{14}O_{12}S_2$ in *desmopressin BPCRS*.

Related peptides Carry out the method for *thin-layer chromatography*, Appendix III A, using *silica gel HF254* as the coating substance and a mixture of 60 volumes of *chloroform*, 40 volumes of *methanol*, 12 volumes of *water* and 8 volumes of *glacial acetic acid* as the mobile phase. Apply separately to the chromatoplate 5 μl of each of four solutions in *water* containing (1) 1.0% w/v of the substance being examined, (2) 0.030% w/v of the substance being examined, (3) 0.010% w/v of the

substance being examined and (4) 1.0% w/v of *desmopressin BPCRS*. After removal of the plate, allow it to dry in air for 1 hour, heat at 110° for 10 minutes, place the hot plate in a closed tank of chlorine gas prepared by the addition of *hydrochloric acid* to a 5% w/v solution of *potassium permanganate* in a container placed at the bottom of the tank and allow to stand for 2 minutes. Dry in a current of cold air until a sprayed area of the plate below the line of application gives at most a very faint blue colour with 0.05 ml of a 0.5% w/v solution of *potassium iodide* in *strong starch mucilage*; avoid prolonged exposure to cold air. Spray the plate with a 0.5% w/v solution of *potassium iodide* in *strong starch mucilage*. Any *secondary spot* in the chromatogram obtained with solution (1) is not more intense than the principal spot in the chromatogram obtained with solution (2) and not more than two such spots are more intense than the principal spot in the chromatogram obtained with solution (3).

Water Not more than 6% w/w when determined by the following method. Use dry glassware throughout; siliconised glassware may be used. Carry out the method for *gas chromatography*, Appendix III B, using the following solutions. For solution (1) dilute 50 μl of *anhydrous methanol* (internal standard) with sufficient *anhydrous propan-2-ol* to produce 100 ml. For solution (2) dissolve 4 mg of the substance being examined in 1 ml of *anhydrous propan-2-ol*. For solution (3) dissolve 4 mg of the substance being examined in 1 ml of solution (1). For solution (4) add 10 μl of *water* to 50 ml of solution (1).

The chromatographic procedure may be carried out using (a) a stainless steel column (1 m × 2 mm) packed with porous polymer beads (Chromosorb 102 is suitable) (60 to 80 mesh), maintained at 120°, (b) helium as the carrier gas and (c) a thermal conductivity detector maintained at 150°.

From the chromatograms obtained and taking into account any water detectable in solution (1), calculate the percentage w/w of water taking 0.9972 g as its weight per ml at 20°.

Assay Carry out the *biological assay of desmopressin*, Appendix XIV C17. The estimated potency is not less than 80% and not more than 125% of the stated potency. The fiducial limits of error are not less than 64% and not more than 156% of the stated potency.

Storage Desmopressin should be kept in a well-closed container, protected from light and stored at a temperature not exceeding 25°. Under these conditions it may be expected to retain its potency for not less than 3 years.

Labelling The label states (1) the number of Units per mg; (2) the weight of the peptide in the container; (3) the date after which the material is not intended to be used; (4) the conditions under which it should be stored.

Preparations
Desmopressin Intranasal Solution
Desmopressin Injection

Action and use Antidiuretic and factor VIII-increasing peptide.

Dexamethasone ☆

C$_{22}$H$_{29}$FO$_5$ 392.5   *50-02-2*

Dexamethasone is 9α-fluoro-11β,17α,21-trihydroxy-16α-methylpregna-1,4-diene-3,20-dione. It contains not less than 96.0 per cent and not more than 104.0 per cent of C$_{22}$H$_{29}$FO$_5$, calculated with reference to the dried substance.

Characteristics A white or almost white powder. It melts at about 255°, with decomposition.

Solubility Practically insoluble in *water*; sparingly soluble in *ethanol (96%)*; slightly soluble in *chloroform*.

Identification *Test A may be omitted if tests B, C, D and E are carried out. Tests B, D and E may be omitted if tests A and C are carried out.*

A. The *infra-red absorption spectrum*, Appendix II A, is concordant with the spectrum of *dexamethasone EPCRS*. If the spectra are not concordant dissolve the substances in the minimum volume of *acetone*, evaporate to dryness on a water-bath and prepare new spectra of the residues as dispersions in either *potassium bromide IR* or *liquid paraffin*.

B. To 2 ml of a 0.010% w/v solution in *absolute ethanol* in a stoppered tube add 10 ml of *phenylhydrazine sulphate solution*, mix, place in a water-bath at 60° for 20 minutes and cool immediately. The *absorbance* of the resulting solution at the maximum at 419 nm is not less than 0.4, Appendix II B.

C. Complies with the test for *identification of steroids*, Appendix III A, Method B, using *betamethasone EPCRS* to prepare solution (4).

D. Heat 0.5 ml of *chromic—sulphuric acid mixture* in a small test-tube in a naked flame until white fumes appear in the upper part of the tube; the solution wets the sides of the tube readily and there is no greasiness. Add 2 mg of the substance being examined and again heat in a naked flame until white fumes appear; the solution does not wet the sides of the tube.

E. To 2 ml of *sulphuric acid* add 2 mg and shake to dissolve; a faint reddish-brown colour is produced within 5 minutes. Add 10 ml of *water* and mix; the colour is discharged.

Light absorption The A(1%, 1 cm) of a 0.001% w/v solution in *ethanol (96%)* at the maximum at 240 nm is 380 to 410, Appendix II B.

Specific optical rotation In a 1% w/v solution in *1,4-dioxan*, +75° to +80°, Appendix V F.

Related substances Carry out the method for *thin-layer chromatography*, Appendix III A, using *silica gel GF254* as the coating substance and a mixture of 77 volumes of *dichloromethane*, 15 volumes of *ether*, 8 volumes of *methanol* and 1.2 volumes of *water* as the mobile phase. Apply separately to the chromatoplate 5 µl of each of the following solutions in a mixture of 9 volumes of *chloroform* and 1 volume of *methanol*. Solutions (1), (2) and (3)

contain 1.0% w/v, 0.020% w/v and 0.010% w/v respectively of the substance being examined. Solution (4) contains 0.10% w/v each of *hydrocortisone EPCRS* and *prednisolone EPCRS*. After removal of the plate, allow it to dry in air and examine under *ultra-violet light (254 nm)*. Any *secondary spot* in the chromatogram obtained with solution (1) is not more intense than the spot in the chromatogram obtained with solution (2) and not more than one such spot is more intense than the spot in the chromatogram obtained with solution (3). The test is not valid unless the chromatogram obtained with solution (4) shows two clearly separated principal spots.

Loss on drying When dried at 100° to 105° at a pressure not exceeding 0.7 kPa for 3 hours, loses not more than 0.5% of its weight. Use 0.5 g.

Assay Carry out the *tetrazolium assay of steroids*, Appendix VIII P, and calculate the content of C$_{22}$H$_{29}$FO$_5$ from the *absorbance* obtained by repeating the operation using *dexamethasone EPCRS* in place of the substance being examined.

Storage Dexamethasone should be kept in a well-closed container and protected from light.

Preparation
Dexamethasone Tablets

Action and use Corticosteroid.

Dexamethasone Sodium Phosphate

C$_{22}$H$_{28}$FNa$_2$O$_8$P   516.4   *2392-39-4*

Dexamethasone Sodium Phosphate is disodium 9α-fluoro-11β,17α-dihydroxy-16α-methyl-3,20-dioxopregna-1,4-dien-21-yl orthophosphate. It contains not less than 96.0 per cent and not more than 103.0 per cent of C$_{22}$H$_{28}$FNa$_2$O$_8$P, calculated with reference to the anhydrous, ethanol-free substance.

Characteristics A white or almost white powder; hygroscopic.

Solubility Soluble in 2 parts of *water*; sparingly soluble in *absolute ethanol*; practically insoluble in *chloroform*.

Identification *Test A may be omitted if tests B, C, D, E and F are carried out. Tests B, C, D and E may be omitted if tests A and F are carried out.*

A. Dissolve 50 mg in 1 ml of *deuterium oxide* containing 0.1% w/v of *sodium 3-trimethylsilylpropanesulphonate*. The *nuclear magnetic resonance spectrum*, Appendix II C, is concordant with that of a similar solution of *dexamethasone sodium phosphate BPCRS*.

B. Carry out the method for *thin-layer chromatography*, Appendix III A, using *silica gel G* as the coating substance and a freshly prepared mixture of 60 volumes of *butan-1-ol*, 20 volumes of *acetic anhydride* and 20 volumes of *water* as the mobile phase. Apply separately to the chromatoplate 2 µl of each of two solutions in *methanol* containing (1) 0.25% w/v of the substance being examined and (2) 0.25% w/v of *dexamethasone sodium phosphate BPCRS*. Solution (3) contains equal volumes of solutions (1) and (2). Solution (4) contains equal volumes of solution (1) and a 0.25% w/v solution of *prednisolone sodium phosphate BPCRS* in *methanol*. After removal of the plate, allow it to dry in air until the solvents have evaporated, spray with *ethanolic sulphuric acid (20%)*, heat at 120° for 10 minutes, allow to cool and examine under *ultra-violet light (365 nm)*. The principal spot in the chromatogram obtained with solution (1) corresponds to that in the chromatogram obtained with solution (2). The principal spot in the chromatogram obtained with solution (3) appears as a single compact spot and the chromatogram obtained with solution (4) shows two principal spots with almost identical Rf values.

C. To 2 ml of a 0.013% w/v solution in *ethanol (96%)* add 10 ml of *phenylhydrazine sulphate solution*, mix, place in a water-bath at 60° for 20 minutes and cool immediately. The *absorbance* of the resulting solution at the maximum at 423 nm is not less than 0.25, Appendix II B.

D. Dissolve 2 mg in 2 ml of *sulphuric acid* and allow to stand for 2 minutes. A pale straw colour is produced (distinction from prednisolone sodium phosphate).

E. Heat 0.5 ml of *chromic—sulphuric acid mixture* in a small test-tube in a naked flame until white fumes appear in the upper part of the tube. The solution wets the sides of the tube readily and there is no greasiness. Add 2 to 3 mg of the substance being examined and again heat in a naked flame until white fumes appear; the solution does not wet the sides of the tube and does not pour easily from the tube.

F. Gently heat 40 mg with 2 ml of *sulphuric acid* until white fumes are evolved, add *nitric acid* dropwise until oxidation is complete and cool. Add 2 ml of *water*, heat until white fumes are again evolved, cool, add 10 ml of *water* and neutralise to *litmus paper* with 5M *ammonia*. The solution yields *reaction A* characteristic of sodium salts and *reaction B* characteristic of phosphates, Appendix VI.

Alkalinity pH of a 1% w/v solution, 7.5 to 9.5, Appendix V L.

Specific optical rotation In a 1% w/v solution, +74° to +79°, Appendix V F.

Inorganic phosphate Dissolve 25 mg in 10 ml of *water*, add 4 ml of 1M *sulphuric acid*, 1 ml of a 10% w/v solution of *ammonium molybdate* and 2 ml of *methylaminophenol—sulphite reagent* and allow to stand for 15 minutes. Add sufficient *water* to produce 25 ml and allow to stand for a further 15 minutes. The *absorbance* of a 4-cm layer of the resulting solution at 730 nm, Appendix II B, is not more than the *absorbance* of a 4-cm layer of a solution prepared by treating 10 ml of a 0.0036% w/v solution of *potassium dihydrogen orthophosphate* in the same manner, beginning at the words 'add 4 ml . . .'.

Free dexamethasone and other derivatives Carry out the method for *thin-layer chromatography*, Appendix III A, using *silica gel GF254* as the coating substance and *methanol* as the mobile phase. Apply separately to the chromatoplate 2 µl of each of three solutions in *methanol* containing (1) 1.0% w/v of the substance being examined, (2) 1.0% w/v of *dexamethasone sodium phosphate BPCRS* and (3) 0.020% w/v of *dexamethasone EPCRS*. After removal of the plate, allow it to dry in air for 5 minutes, spray with a 30% w/v solution of *zinc chloride* in *methanol*,

heat at about 125° for 1 hour and examine under *ultra-violet light (254 nm)*. Any *secondary spot* in the chromatogram obtained with solution (1) is not more intense than the spot in the chromatogram obtained with solution (3).

Ethanol Not more than 8% w/w when determined by the method for *gas chromatography*, Appendix III B, using solutions in *water* containing (1) 1.0% v/v of *propan-1-ol* (internal standard) and 1.0% v/v of *absolute ethanol*, (2) 10.0% w/v of the substance being examined and (3) 10.0% w/v of the substance being examined and 1.0% v/v of the internal standard. If necessary adjust the content of *absolute ethanol* in solution (1) to produce a peak of similar height to the corresponding peak in the chromatogram obtained with solution (2).

The chromatographic procedure may be carried out using a glass column (1.5 m × 4 mm) packed with porous polymer beads (80 to 100 mesh) (Porapak Q is suitable) and maintained at 135°.

Calculate the percentage w/w of ethanol taking 0.790 g as its weight per ml at 20°.

Total ethanol and water Determine the content of water, Appendix IX C, using 0.3 g. The sum of the percentage of ethanol found by the method described above and the percentage of water is not more than 16.0%.

Assay Dissolve 0.2 g in sufficient *water* to produce 200 ml. Dilute 5 ml to 250 ml with *water* and measure the *absorbance* of the resulting solution at the maximum at 241 nm, Appendix II B. Calculate the content of $C_{22}H_{28}FNa_2O_8P$ taking 297 as the value of A(1%, 1 cm) at the maximum at 241 nm.

Storage Dexamethasone Sodium Phosphate should be kept in a well-closed container and protected from light.

Action and use Corticosteroid.

Dexamphetamine Sulphate
Dextro Amphetamine Sulphate

$(C_{19}H_{13}N)_2,H_2SO_4$ 368.5   *51-63-8*

Dexamphetamine Sulphate is (S)-α-methyl-phenethylamine sulphate. It contains not less than 99.0 per cent and not more than 100.5 per cent of $(C_9H_{13}N)_2,H_2SO_4$, calculated with reference to the dried substance.

Characteristics A white or almost white, crystalline powder; odourless or almost odourless.

Solubility Soluble in 9 parts of *water*; slightly soluble in *ethanol (96%)*; practically insoluble in *ether*.

Identification A. Dissolve 1 g in 50 ml of *water*, add 10 ml of 5M *sodium hydroxide* and 0.5 ml of *benzoyl chloride* and shake. Repeat the addition of *benzoyl chloride* in 0.5-ml quantities until no further precipitate is produced. The *melting point* of the precipitate, after recrystallisation twice from *ethanol (50%)*, is about 157°, Appendix V A.

B. Dissolve 2 mg in 4 ml of *water*, add 1 ml of 1M *hydrochloric acid*, 2 ml of *diazotised nitroaniline solution*,

4 ml of 1M *sodium hydroxide* and 2 ml of *butan-1-ol*, shake and allow to separate. A red colour is produced in the butanol layer (distinction from methylamphetamine).
C. Yields the *reactions* characteristic of sulphates, Appendix VI.

Acidity or alkalinity Dissolve 0.5 g in 10 ml of *water* and titrate with 0.01M *hydrochloric acid VS* or 0.01M *sodium hydroxide VS* using *methyl red solution* as indicator. Not more than 0.1 ml of 0.01M *hydrochloric acid VS* or 0.01M *sodium hydroxide VS* is required to change the colour of the solution.

Specific optical rotation In an 8.0% w/v solution, +19.5° to +22°, Appendix V F.

Loss on drying When dried to constant weight at 105°, loses not more than 1.0% of its weight. Use 1 g.

Sulphated ash Not more than 0.1%, Appendix IX A.

Assay Dissolve 0.4 g in 120 ml of *water*, add 2 ml of 5M *sodium hydroxide* and distil into 50 ml of 0.1M *hydrochloric acid VS*, continuing the distillation until only 5 ml of liquid is left in the distillation flask. Titrate the excess of acid with 0.1M *sodium hydroxide VS* using *methyl red solution* as indicator. Each ml of 0.1M *hydrochloric acid VS* is equivalent to 0.01842 g of $(C_9H_{13}N)_2,H_2SO_4$.

Preparation
Dexamphetamine Tablets

Action and use Central nervous system stimulant.

Dextrin

Dextrin is maize starch or potato starch partially hydrolysed by heat with or without the aid of suitable acids and buffers.

Characteristics A white or pale yellow powder; odour, slight and characteristic.

Microscopical Granules similar in appearance to the starch from which the dextrin has been prepared except that in dextrin prepared from maize starch many of the granules show concentric striations and in dextrin prepared from potato starch concentric striations are not clearly visible; the hilum is frequently bicleft and a small proportion of the granules are distorted.

Solubility Very soluble in boiling *water* forming a mucilaginous solution; slowly soluble in cold *water*; practically insoluble in *ethanol (96%)* and in *ether*.

Identification A. Boil 1 g in 50 ml of *water*, cool and to a quantity of the cloudy suspension add 0.05 ml of 0.005M *iodine VS* and mix. A purple colour is produced.
B. To a mixture of 5 ml of the suspension produced in test A and 2 ml of 2M *sodium hydroxide* add dropwise with shaking 0.5 ml of *copper sulphate solution* and boil. A red precipitate is produced.

Acidity Add 10 g to 100 ml of *ethanol (70%)* previously neutralised to *phenolphthalein solution*, shake for 1 hour, filter and titrate 50 ml of the filtrate with 0.1M *sodium hydroxide VS*. Not more than 1.0 ml is required to change the colour of the solution.

Heavy metals 1.0 g complies with *limit test C for heavy metals*, Appendix VII (40 ppm). Use 4 ml of *lead standard solution (10 ppm Pb)* to prepare the standard.

Chloride Dissolve 2.5 g in 50 ml of boiling *water*, cool, dilute to 100 ml with *water* and filter. 1 ml of the filtrate

diluted to 15 ml complies with the *limit test for chlorides*, Appendix VII (0.2%).

Protein Not more than 0.5% when determined by the following method. Carry out Method I for the *determination of nitrogen*, Appendix VIII H, using 5 g and 30 ml of *nitrogen-free sulphuric acid*. Calculate the content of protein by multiplying the percentage of nitrogen in the substance being examined by 6.25.

Reducing substances To a quantity of the substance being examined containing the equivalent of 2.0 g of the dried substance add 100 ml of *water*, shake for 30 minutes, dilute to 200 ml with *water* and filter. To 10 ml of *potassium cupri-tartrate solution* add 20 ml of the filtrate, mix and heat on a hot plate to bring the solution to the boil in 3 minutes. Boil for a further 2 minutes and cool quickly. Add 5 ml of a 30% w/v solution of *potassium iodide* and 10 ml of 1M *sulphuric acid*, mix and titrate immediately with 0.1M *sodium thiosulphate VS* using *starch mucilage*, added towards the end of the titration, as indicator. Repeat the procedure using 20 ml of a 0.1% w/v solution of *D-glucose* in place of the filtrate and beginning at the words 'To 10 ml of . . .'. Carry out a blank titration. The difference between the blank titre and the titre obtained with the sample filtrate is not more than the difference between the blank titre and the titre obtained with the glucose solution (10%, calculated as glucose, $C_6H_{12}O_6$).

Loss on drying When dried to constant weight at 110°, loses not more than 11.0% of its weight. Use 1 g.

Ash Not more than 0.5%, Appendix XI J.

Action and use Pharmaceutical aid.

Dextromethorphan Hydrobromide ☆

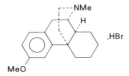

$C_{18}H_{25}NO,HBr,H_2O$ 370.3   *6700-34-1*

Dextromethorphan Hydrobromide is (+)-3-methoxy-9a-methylmorphinan hydrobromide monohydrate. It contains not less than 99.0 per cent and not more than 101.0 per cent of $C_{18}H_{25}NO,HBr$, calculated with reference to the dried substance.

Characteristics A white or almost white, crystalline powder; odourless. It melts at about 125°, with decomposition.

Solubility Soluble in 60 parts of *water* and in 10 parts of *ethanol (96%)*; freely soluble in *chloroform* with the separation of water; practically insoluble in *ether*.

Identification A. The *light absorption*, Appendix II B, in the range 230 to 350 nm of a 0.01% w/v solution exhibits a maximum only at 278 nm. The A(1%, 1 cm) at 278 nm is about 54.
B. The *light absorption*, Appendix II B, in the range 230 to 350 nm of a 0.01% w/v solution in 0.1M *sodium hydroxide* exhibits a maximum at 280 nm. The A(1%, 1 cm) at 280 nm is about 59.

C. Dissolve 50 mg in 2 ml of 1M *sulphuric acid* and add dropwise, with shaking, 1 ml of a mixture of 1 volume of *mercury—nitric acid solution* and 9 volumes of *water*; a white, crystalline precipitate consisting of platelets is produced and the solution does not immediately turn red. Heat on a water bath for about 10 minutes; a yellow to red colour is produced.

D. Yields the *reactions* characteristic of bromides, Appendix VI.

Acidity Dissolve 0.4 g in *carbon dioxide-free water* using gentle heat, dilute to 20 ml with the same solvent and cool to 20°. The pH of the resulting solution, measured immediately, is 5.2 to 6.5, Appendix V L.

Specific optical rotation In a 2% w/v solution in 0.1M *hydrochloric acid*, +28.0° to +30.0°, Appendix V F.

Dimethylaniline Dissolve 0.5 g in 20 ml of *water* using heat, cool and add 2 ml of 2M *acetic acid*, 1 ml of a 1% w/v solution of *sodium nitrite* and sufficient *water* to produce 25 ml. The colour of the resulting solution is not more intense than that obtained by treating a solution of 5 μg of N,N-*dimethylaniline* in 20 ml of *water* in the same manner (10 ppm).

Related substances Carry out the method for *thin-layer chromatography*, Appendix III A, using *silica gel G* as the coating substance and a mixture of 55 volumes of *toluene*, 20 volumes of *ethyl acetate*, 13 volumes of *methanol*, 10 volumes of *dichloromethane* and 2 volumes of 13.5M *ammonia* as the mobile phase. Apply separately to the chromatoplate 5 μl of each of two solutions of the substance being examined in *methanol* containing (1) 5.0% w/v and (2) 0.025% w/v. After removal of the plate, allow it to dry in air, spray with *potassium iodobismuthate solution* until spots appear and then immediately spray with a mixture of 10 volumes of *hydrogen peroxide solution (100 vol)* and 20 volumes of *water*. Any *secondary spot* in the chromatogram obtained with solution (1) is not more intense than the spot in the chromatogram obtained with solution (2).

Loss on drying When dried over *phosphorus pentoxide* at 80° at a pressure of 1.5 to 2.5 kPa for 4 hours, loses 4.0 to 5.5% of its weight. Use 0.5 g.

Sulphated ash Not more than 0.1%, Appendix IX A, Method II. Use 1 g.

Assay Dissolve 0.5 g in 40 ml of *anhydrous glacial acetic acid*, add 10 ml of *mercury(II) acetate solution* and carry out Method I for *non-aqueous titration*, Appendix VIII A, using *crystal violet solution* as indicator. Each ml of 0.1M *perchloric acid VS* is equivalent to 0.03523 g of $C_{18}H_{25}NO,HBr$.

Storage Dextromethorphan Hydrobromide should be kept in a well-closed container.

Action and use Cough suppressant.

Dextromoramide Tartrate ☆

$C_{25}H_{32}N_2O_2,C_4H_6O_6$ 542.6   *2922-44-3*

Dextromoramide Tartrate is (+)-3-methyl-4-morpholino-2,2-diphenyl-1-pyrrolidinobutan-1-one hydrogen tartrate. It contains not less than 98.0 per cent and not more than 101.0 per cent of $C_{25}H_{32}N_2O_2,C_4H_6O_6$, calculated with reference to the dried substance.

Characteristics A white, crystalline or amorphous powder; odourless. It melts at about 190°, with slight decomposition.

Solubility Soluble in 25 parts of *water* and in 85 parts of *ethanol (96%)*; slightly soluble in *chloroform*; very slightly soluble in *ether*.

Identification A. The *light absorption*, Appendix II B, in the range 230 to 350 nm of a 0.075% w/v solution in 1M *hydrochloric acid* exhibits three maxima, at 254, 259 and 264 nm. The A(1%, 1 cm) at 254 nm is about 6.9, at 259 nm, about 7.7 and at 264 nm, about 6.5.

B. To 2 ml of a 0.5% w/v solution add 3 ml of *ammoniacal silver nitrate solution* and heat on a water-bath. A grey or black precipitate is produced.

C. Yields *reaction B* characteristic of tartrates, Appendix VI.

Acidity pH of a 1% w/v solution, 3.0 to 4.0, Appendix V L.

Specific optical rotation In a 5% w/v solution in 0.1M *hydrochloric acid*, +21.0° to +23.0°, Appendix V F.

Related substances Carry out the method for *thin-layer chromatography*, Appendix III A, using *silica gel G* as the coating substance and *methanol* as the mobile phase. Apply separately to the chromatoplate 10 μl of each of two solutions of the substance being examined in *methanol* containing (1) 2.0% w/v and (2) 0.020% w/v. After removal of the plate, allow it to dry in air and spray with *dilute potassium iodobismuthate solution*. Any *secondary spot* in the chromatogram obtained with solution (1) is not more intense than the spot in the chromatogram obtained with solution (2).

Loss on drying When dried to constant weight at 100° to 105°, loses not more than 0.5% of its weight. Use 1 g.

Sulphated ash Not more than 0.1%, Appendix IX A, Method II. Use 1 g.

Assay Dissolve 0.25 g in 30 ml of *anhydrous glacial acetic acid* and carry out Method I for *non-aqueous titration*, Appendix VIII A, using 0.05M *perchloric acid VS* as titrant and 0.15 ml of *1-naphtholbenzein solution* as indicator. Each ml of 0.05M *perchloric acid VS* is equivalent to 0.02713 g of $C_{25}H_{32}N_2O_2,C_4H_6O_6$.

Preparations
Dextromoramide Injection
Dextromoramide Tablets

Action and use Narcotic analgesic.

Dextropropoxyphene Hydrochloride

$$Me_2NCH_2-\overset{\overset{\displaystyle Me}{|}}{\underset{\underset{\displaystyle H}{|}}{C}}-\overset{\overset{\displaystyle OCOEt}{|}}{C}-CH_2-\bigcirc \quad ,HCl$$

$C_{22}H_{29}NO_2,HCl$ 375.9   *1639-60-7*

Dextropropoxyphene Hydrochloride is (1*S*,2*R*)-1-benzyl-3-dimethylamino-2-methyl-1-phenyl-propyl propionate hydrochloride. It contains not less than 98.5 per cent and not more than 101.0 per cent of $C_{22}H_{29}NO_2,HCl$, calculated with reference to the dried substance.

Characteristics A white or slightly yellow powder; odourless or almost odourless.

Solubility Soluble in 0.3 part of *water*, in 1.5 parts of *ethanol (96%)* and in 0.6 part of *chloroform*; practically insoluble in *ether*.

Identification A. The *infra-red absorption spectrum*, Appendix II A, is concordant with the *reference spectrum* of dextropropoxyphene hydrochloride.
B. Dissolve 25 mg in 5 ml of *water*, evaporate 0.05 ml of the solution in a porcelain dish and streak the spot with *sulphuric acid* containing 5% v/v of *formaldehyde solution*. A purple colour is produced.
C. Yields the *reactions* characteristic of chlorides, Appendix VI.
D. *Melting point*, about 165°, Appendix V A.

Specific optical rotation In a 10% w/v solution, +36° to +40°, Appendix V F.

Related substances Dissolve 10 mg of *triphenylamine* (internal standard) in sufficient *chloroform* to produce 50 ml (solution A). Carry out the method for *gas chromatography*, Appendix III B, using the following solutions. For solution (1) add 5 ml of solution A, 10 ml of *water*, 2 ml of 1.25M *sodium hydroxide* and 15 ml of *chloroform* to 5 ml of a solution in *chloroform* containing 0.022% w/v of *(1S,2R)-1-benzyl-3-dimethylamino-2-methyl-1-phenylpropyl acetate BPCRS* and 0.020% w/v of *4-dimethylamino-3-methyl-1,2-diphenylbutan-2-ol hydrochloride BPCRS* and shake. Extract the aqueous layer with two 20-ml quantities of *chloroform*. Shake the combined chloroform extracts with 5 g of *anhydrous sodium sulphate*, filter and evaporate to dryness at a temperature not exceeding 40° using a rotary evaporator. Dissolve the residue in 10 ml of *chloroform*. For solution (2) dissolve 0.2 g of the substance being examined in 5 ml of *chloroform*, add 10 ml of *water*, 2 ml of 1.25M *sodium hydroxide* and 15 ml of *chloroform* and shake. Extract the aqueous layer with two 20-ml quantities of *chloroform*. Shake the combined chloroform extracts with 5 g of *anhydrous sodium sulphate*, filter and evaporate to dryness at a temperature not exceeding 40° using a rotary evaporator. Dissolve the residue in 10 ml of *chloroform*. Prepare solution (3) in the same manner as solution (2) but add 5 ml of solution A to the initial solution of the substance being examined.

The chromatographic procedure may be carried out using a glass column (60 cm × 3 mm) packed with *acid-washed, silanised diatomaceous support* (100 to 120 mesh) coated with 3% w/w of dimethyl silicone fluid (OV-101 is suitable) and maintained at 160° with an inlet port temperature of 150° and using 60 ml per minute as the flow rate of the carrier gas.

The peaks, other than the solvent peak, in the chromatogram obtained with solution (1) are due, in order of emergence, to (a) the internal standard, (b) (1*S*,2*R*)-1-benzyl-3-dimethylamino-2-methyl-1-phenylpropyl acetate and (c) 4-dimethylamino-3-methyl-1,2-diphenylbutan-2-ol hydrochloride. In the chromatogram obtained with solution (3) the ratio of the area of any peak corresponding to (c) to that of the peak due to (a) and the ratio of the area of any peak corresponding to (b) to that of the peak due to (a) are not greater than the corresponding ratios in the chromatogram obtained with solution (1).

Loss on drying When dried to constant weight at 105°, loses not more than 1.0% of its weight. Use 1 g.

Sulphated ash Not more than 0.1%, Appendix IX A.

Assay Carry out Method I for *non-aqueous titration*, Appendix VIII A, using 0.5 g, adding 10 ml of *mercury(II) acetate solution* and using *1-naphtholbenzein solution* as indicator. Each ml of 0.1M *perchloric acid VS* is equivalent to 0.03759 g of $C_{22}H_{29}NO_2,HCl$.

Storage Dextropropoxyphene Hydrochloride should be kept in a well-closed container.

Action and use Analgesic.

Dextropropoxyphene Napsylate

$$Me_2NCH_2-\overset{\overset{\displaystyle Me}{|}}{\underset{\underset{\displaystyle H}{|}}{C}}-\overset{\overset{\displaystyle OCOEt}{|}}{C}-CH_2-\bigcirc \qquad \bigcirc\!\!\bigcirc-SO_3H$$

$C_{22}H_{29}NO_2,C_{10}H_8O_3S,H_2O$ 565.8   *26570-10-5*

Dextropropoxyphene Napsylate is (1*S*,2*R*)-1-benzyl-3-dimethylamino-2-methyl-1-phenyl-propyl propionate naphthalene-2-sulphonate monohydrate. It contains not less than 98.0 per cent and not more than 101.0 per cent of $C_{22}H_{29}NO_2,C_{10}H_8O_3S$, calculated with reference to the anhydrous substance.

Characteristics A white powder; odourless or almost odourless.

Solubility Practically insoluble in *water*; soluble in 13 parts of *ethanol (96%)* and in 3 parts of *chloroform*.

Identification A. The *infra-red absorption spectrum*, Appendix II A, is concordant with the *reference spectrum* of dextropropoxyphene napsylate. If the spectra are not concordant, dissolve a sufficient quantity in the minimum volume of *chloroform IR*, evaporate to dryness, dry the residue at 105° for 1 hour and prepare a new spectrum.
B. Dissolve 25 mg in 5 ml of *chloroform*, evaporate 0.05 ml of the solution in a porcelain dish and streak the spot with *sulphuric acid* containing 5% v/v of *formaldehyde solution*. A purple colour is produced.
C. Burn 20 mg by the method for *oxygen-flask combustion*, Appendix VIII C, using 5 ml of 1.25M *sodium hydroxide* as the absorbing liquid. When the process is complete, dilute the liquid to 25 ml with *water*. To 5 ml of the solution so obtained add 1 ml of *hydrogen peroxide solution (100 vol)*

and 1 ml of 1M *hydrochloric acid*, mix and add 0.05 ml of *barium chloride solution*. The solution becomes turbid.

D. *Melting point*, about 160°, Appendix V A.

Specific optical rotation In a 5% w/v solution in *ethanol (96%)*, +26° to +31°, Appendix V F.

Related substances Complies with the test described under Dextropropoxyphene Hydrochloride using in the preparation of solutions (2) and (3) 0.3 g of the substance being examined.

Sulphated ash Not more than 0.1%, Appendix IX A.

Water 3.0 to 5.0% w/w, Appendix IX C. Use 0.5 g.

Assay To 0.75 g add 50 ml of *water*, swirl to disperse, add 5 ml of 5M *sodium hydroxide* and extract with five 25-ml quantities of *chloroform*, washing each extract with the same 20 ml of *water*. Dry the combined extracts with *anhydrous sodium sulphate*, evaporate to about 3 ml on a water-bath in a current of air and allow to evaporate to dryness at room temperature. Carry out Method I for *non-aqueous titration* on the residue, Appendix VIII A, using *1-naphtholbenzein solution* as indicator. Each ml of 0.1M *perchloric acid VS* is equivalent to 0.05477 g of $C_{22}H_{29}NO_2,C_{10}H_8O_3S$.

Preparation
Dextropropoxyphene Capsules

Action and use Analgesic.

Diamorphine Hydrochloride

$C_{21}H_{23}NO_5,HCl,H_2O$ 423.9   *1502-95-0*

Diamorphine Hydrochloride is 4,5-epoxy-17-methylmorphinan-3,6-diyl diacetate hydrochloride monohydrate. It contains not less than 98.0 per cent and not more than 101.0 per cent of $C_{21}H_{23}NO_5,HCl$, calculated with reference to the dried substance.

Characteristics An almost white, crystalline powder; odourless when freshly prepared but an odour characteristic of acetic acid is produced on storage.

Solubility Soluble in 1.6 parts of *water*, in 12 parts of *ethanol (96%)* and in 1.6 parts of *chloroform*; practically insoluble in *ether*.

Identification *Test A may be omitted if tests B, C, D, E, F and G are carried out. Tests B, C, D, E and F may be omitted if tests A and G are carried out.*

A. Dissolve a sufficient quantity in the minimum volume of *dichloromethane* and evaporate to dryness. The *infra-red absorption spectrum* of the residue, Appendix II A, is concordant with the *reference spectrum* of diamorphine hydrochloride.

B. The *light absorption*, Appendix II B, in the range 230 to 350 nm of a 0.02% w/v solution exhibits a maximum only at 279 nm. The *absorbance* at 279 nm is about 0.80.

C. The *light absorption*, Appendix II B, in the range 230 to 350 nm of a 0.015% w/v solution in 0.1M *sodium hydroxide* exhibits a maximum only at 299 nm. The *absorbance* at 299 nm is about 0.9.

D. Moisten 10 mg with 0.2 ml of *nitric acid*. A yellow colour is produced which changes to greenish-blue on warming and reverts to yellow on cooling.

E. Dissolve 0.1 g in 2 ml of *ethanol (96%)*, add 1 ml of *sulphuric acid* and warm. The odour of ethyl acetate is produced.

F. Dissolve 0.1 g in 1 ml of *sulphuric acid*; a colourless solution is produced. Warm on a water-bath, cool and add 6 ml of *water* and 0.5 ml of a mixture of 19 volumes of *potassium hexacyanoferrate(III) solution* and 1 volume of *iron(III) chloride test-solution*; a deep blue colour is produced.

G. Yields *reaction A* characteristic of chlorides, Appendix VI.

Acidity Dissolve 0.2 g in 10 ml of *carbon dioxide-free water* and titrate with 0.02M *sodium hydroxide VS* using *methyl red solution* as indicator. Not more than 0.2 ml of 0.02M *sodium hydroxide VS* is required.

Melting point 229° to 233°, Appendix V A.

Phenolic substances Dissolve 10.0 mg in 10 ml of 0.1M *hydrochloric acid*, immediately add 5 ml of a freshly prepared 0.5% w/v solution of *sodium nitrite*, allow to stand for 15 minutes and add 2.5 ml of 5M *ammonia* and sufficient *water* to produce 25 ml. Measure the *absorbance* of the resulting solution at the maximum at 435 nm, Appendix II B. The absorbance is not more than that obtained by treating 10 ml of a 0.0020% w/v solution of *anhydrous morphine* in 0.1M *hydrochloric acid* in the same manner, beginning at the words 'add 5 ml . . .'.

Loss on drying When dried to constant weight at 105°, loses not more than 4.5% of its weight. Use 1 g.

Sulphated ash Not more than 0.1%, Appendix IX A.

Assay Carry out Method I for *non-aqueous titration*, Appendix VIII A, using 0.5 g, adding 10 ml of *mercury(II) acetate solution* and using *crystal violet solution* as indicator. Each ml of 0.1M *perchloric acid VS* is equivalent to 0.04059 g of $C_{21}H_{23}NO_5,HCl$.

Storage Diamorphine Hydrochloride should be kept in a well-closed container and protected from light.

Preparation
Diamorphine Injection

Action and use Narcotic analgesic.

Diazepam ☆

$C_{16}H_{13}ClN_2O$ 284.7   *439-14-5*

Diazepam is 7-chloro-1,3-dihydro-1-methyl-5-phenyl-1,4-benzodiazepin-2-one. It contains not less than 99.0 per cent and not more than 101.0 per cent of $C_{16}H_{13}ClN_2O$, calculated with reference to the dried substance.

Characteristics A white or almost white, crystalline powder; odourless or almost odourless.

Solubility Very slightly soluble in *water*; soluble in *ethanol (96%)*; freely soluble in *chloroform*.

Identification A. Carry out the following procedure in subdued light and measure the *absorbances* immediately. The *light absorption*, Appendix II B, in the range 230 to 330 nm of a 0.0005% w/v solution in 0.05M *methanolic sulphuric acid* exhibits two maxima, at 242 nm and 285 nm; the A(1%, 1 cm) at 242 nm is about 1020. The *light absorption* in the range 325 to 400 nm of a 0.0025% w/v solution in 0.05M *methanolic sulphuric acid* exhibits a maximum only at 366 nm; the A(1%, 1 cm) at 366 nm is 140 to 155.

B. A solution of 10 mg in 3 ml of *sulphuric acid* exhibits a greenish-yellow fluorescence when examined under ultra-violet light (365 nm).

C. Burn 20 mg by the method for *oxygen-flask combustion*, Appendix VIII C, using 5 ml of 2M *sodium hydroxide* as the absorbing liquid. Acidify with 1M *sulphuric acid* and boil gently for 2 minutes. The solution yields *reaction A* characteristic of chlorides, Appendix VI.

D. *Melting point*, 131° to 135°, Appendix V A, Method I.

Heavy metals 2.0 g complies with *limit test C for heavy metals*, Appendix VII (20 ppm). Use 4 ml of *lead standard solution (10 ppm Pb)* to prepare the standard.

Related substances and decomposition products Carry out in subdued light the method for *thin-layer chromatography*, Appendix III A, using *silica gel GF254* as the coating substance and a mixture of 50 volumes of *ethyl acetate* and 50 volumes of *hexane* as the mobile phase but allowing the solvent front to ascend 12 cm above the line of application. Apply separately to the chromatoplate 5 μl of each of two freshly prepared solutions of the substance being examined in *acetone* containing (1) 10% w/v and (2) 0.01% w/v. After removal of the plate, allow it to dry in air and examine under *ultra-violet light (254 nm)*. Any *secondary spot* in the chromatogram obtained with solution (1) is not more intense than the spot in the chromatogram obtained with solution (2).

Loss on drying When dried over *phosphorus pentoxide* at 60° at a pressure of 1.5 to 2.5 kPa for 4 hours, loses not more than 0.5% of its weight. Use 1 g.

Sulphated ash Not more than 0.1%, Appendix IX A, Method II. Use 1 g.

Assay Dissolve 0.5 g in 50 ml of *acetic anhydride* and carry out Method I for *non-aqueous titration*, Appendix VIII A, using 0.3 ml of *nile blue A solution* as indicator and titrating until a yellowish-green colour is obtained. Each ml of 0.1M *perchloric acid VS* is equivalent to 0.02847 g of $C_{16}H_{13}ClN_2O$.

Storage Diazepam should be kept in a well-closed container and protected from light.

Preparations
Diazepam Capsules
Diazepam Oral Solution
Diazepam Injection
Diazepam Tablets

Action and use Anxiolytic.

Diazoxide

$C_8H_7ClN_2O_2S$ 230.7   *364-98-7*

Diazoxide is 7-chloro-3-methyl-2*H*-1,2,4-benzo-thiadiazine 1,1-dioxide. It contains not less than 98.0 per cent and not more than 101.0 per cent of $C_8H_7ClN_2O_2S$, calculated with reference to the dried substance.

Characteristics A white or almost white, crystalline powder; odourless or almost odourless.

Solubility Practically insoluble in *water*, in *ether* and in *chloroform*; slightly soluble in *ethanol (96%)*; very soluble in solutions of alkali hydroxides.

Identification A. The *infra-red absorption spectrum*, Appendix II A, is concordant with the *reference spectrum* of diazoxide.

B. The *light absorption*, Appendix II B, in the range 230 to 350 nm of a 0.001% w/v solution in 0.1M *sodium hydroxide* exhibits a maximum only at 280 nm. The *absorbance* at 280 nm is about 0.59.

C. Carry out the method for *thin-layer chromatography*, Appendix III A, using *silica gel GF254* as the coating substance and a mixture of 50 volumes of *toluene*, 30 volumes of *ether* and 20 volumes of *acetone* as the mobile phase. Apply separately to the chromatoplate 20 μl of each of two solutions in *methanol* containing (1) 0.02% w/v of the substance being examined and (2) 0.02% w/v of *diazoxide BPCRS*. After removal of the plate, allow it to dry in air until the odour of the solvent is no longer detectable and examine under *ultra-violet light (254 nm)*. The principal spot in the chromatogram obtained with solution (1) corresponds in colour and intensity to that in the chromatogram obtained with solution (2).

Related substances Carry out the method for *thin-layer chromatography*, Appendix III A, using *silica gel GF254* as the coating substance and a mixture of 85 volumes of *ethyl acetate*, 20 volumes of *methanol* and 15 volumes of 13.5M *ammonia* as the mobile phase. Apply separately to the chromatoplate 10 μl of each of two solutions in 0.1M *sodium hydroxide* containing (1) 1.5% w/v of the substance being examined and (2) 0.0075% w/v of *diazoxide BPCRS*. After removal of the plate, allow it to dry in air until the odour of ammonia is no longer detectable and examine under *ultra-violet light (254 nm)*. Any *secondary spot* in the chromatogram obtained with solution (1) is not more intense than the spot in the chromatogram obtained with solution (2).

Loss on drying When dried to constant weight at 105°, loses not more than 0.5% of its weight. Use 1 g.

Sulphated ash Not more than 0.1%, Appendix IX A.

Assay Dissolve 0.5 g in 100 ml of a mixture of 2 volumes of *dimethylformamide* and 1 volume of *water* and titrate with 0.1M *sodium hydroxide VS* determining the end-point potentiometrically. Each ml of 0.1M *sodium hydroxide VS* is equivalent to 0.02307 g of $C_8H_7ClN_2O_2S$.

Preparations
Diazoxide Injection
Diazoxide Tablets

Action and use Vasodilator.

Dibromopropamidine Isethionate

$C_{17}H_{18}Br_2N_4O_2,2C_2H_6O_4S$ 722.4   *614-87-9*

Dibromopropamidine Isethionate is 3,3'-dibromo-4,4'-trimethylenedioxydibenzamidine bis(2-hydroxyethanesulphonate). It contains not less than 97.0 per cent and not more than 101.0 per cent of $C_{17}H_{18}Br_2N_4O_2,2C_2H_6O_4S$, calculated with reference to the dried substance.

Characteristics A white or almost white, crystalline powder; odourless or almost odourless.

Solubility Soluble in 2 parts of *water*, in 60 parts of *ethanol (96%)* and in 20 parts of *glycerol*; practically insoluble in *chloroform*, in *ether*, in *liquid paraffin* and in fixed oils.

Identification A. The *infra-red absorption spectrum*, Appendix II A, is concordant with the *reference spectrum* of dibromopropamidine isethionate.

B. The *light absorption*, Appendix II B, in the range 230 to 350 nm of a 0.003% w/v solution in 0.01M *hydrochloric acid* exhibits a maximum only at 261 nm. The *absorbance* at 261 nm is about 1.0.

C. To 10 ml of a 0.05% w/v solution add 1 ml of a 0.1% w/v solution of *glyoxal sodium bisulphite* and 1 ml of a solution prepared by dissolving 4 g of *boric acid* in a mixture of 27 ml of 1M *sodium hydroxide* and sufficient *water* to produce 100 ml. Heat on a water-bath for 10 minutes. A magenta colour is produced.

D. Mix 0.1 g with 0.5 g of *anhydrous sodium carbonate*, ignite and extract the residue with 20 ml of *water*. Filter and neutralise the filtrate to *litmus paper* with *nitric acid*. The solution yields *reaction A* characteristic of bromides, Appendix VI.

Acidity or alkalinity pH of a 5% w/v solution, 5.0 to 7.0, Appendix V L.

Light absorption *Absorbance* of a 0.0015% w/v solution in 0.01M *hydrochloric acid* at the maximum at 261 nm, 0.50 to 0.52, Appendix II B.

Ammonium isethionate To 1 g in a test-tube about 4 cm in diameter add 10 ml of *water* and 20 ml of 1M *sodium hydroxide*. Immediately insert a stopper carrying a splash head and an aspirator tube about 5 mm in diameter. Connect the splash head to two test-tubes in series, each containing 20 ml of 0.01M *sulphuric acid VS*. Heat the tube containing the substance being examined in a water-bath at 45° to 50° and, maintaining this temperature, draw a current of air, previously passed through 1M *sulphuric acid*, through the liquids in the series of tubes for 3 hours at such a rate that the bubbles are just too rapid to count. Titrate the combined solutions from the two absorption tubes with 0.02M *sodium hydroxide VS* using *methyl red—methylene blue solution* as indicator. Not less than 36.5 ml is required.

Related substances Carry out the method for *thin-layer chromatography*, Appendix III A, using a silica gel F254 precoated chromatoplate (Merck silica gel 60 F254 plates are suitable) activated at 105° for 1 hour and a mixture of 90 volumes of *propan-1-ol*, 5 volumes of *formic acid* and 5 volumes of *water* as the mobile phase. Apply separately to the plate 10 µl of each of two solutions of the substance being examined in *methanol (90%)* containing (1) 1.0% w/v and (2) 0.0050% w/v. After removal of the plate, allow it to dry in air and examine under *ultra-violet light (254 nm)*. Any *secondary spot* in the chromatogram obtained with solution (1) is not more intense than the spot in the chromatogram obtained with solution (2).

Loss on drying When dried to constant weight at 105°, loses not more than 2.0% of its weight. Use 1 g.

Sulphated ash Not more than 0.1%, Appendix IX A.

Assay Heat 0.4 g with 70 ml of *amyl alcohol* and 4 g of *sodium* under a reflux condenser until the sodium has dissolved. Continue heating for a further 30 minutes, cool, add 50 ml of *water* and shake. Add 15 ml of *nitric acid* and 25 ml of 0.1M *silver nitrate VS*, keeping the mixture cold. Shake vigorously and titrate the excess of silver nitrate with 0.1M *ammonium thiocyanate VS* using *ammonium iron(III) sulphate solution* as indicator. Each ml of 0.1M *silver nitrate VS* is equivalent to 0.03612 g of $C_{17}H_{18}Br_2N_4O_2,2C_2H_6O_4S$.

Storage Dibromopropamidine Isethionate should be kept in a well-closed container.

Action and use Antiseptic.

In some countries the material described in this monograph may be known as Dibrompropamidine Isetionate.

Dichloralphenazone

$C_{15}H_{18}Cl_6N_2O_5$ 519.0   *480-30-8*

Dichloralphenazone is a complex of chloral hydrate and phenazone. It contains not less than 97.0 per cent and not more than 100.5 per cent of $C_{15}H_{18}Cl_6N_2O_5$, when determined by both methods described under Assay; the difference between the results is not more than 1.5 per cent.

Characteristics A white, microcrystalline powder; odour, slight, characteristic of chloral hydrate.

Solubility Soluble in 10 parts of *water*, in 1 part of *ethanol (96%)* and in 2 parts of *chloroform*. It dissolves in dilute acids and is decomposed by dilute alkalis.

Identification A. The *infra-red absorption spectrum*, Appendix II A, is concordant with the *reference spectrum* of dichloralphenazone.

B. Decomposes when treated with caustic alkalis, liberating chloroform.

C. Dissolve 0.1 g in 10 ml of *water* containing 0.1 g of *sodium nitrite* and add 1 ml of 1M *sulphuric acid*. A green colour is produced.

Melting point 64° to 67°, Appendix V A.

Heavy metals Ignite 4.0 g gently until thoroughly charred, cool, add 2 ml of *nitric acid* and 0.25 ml of *sulphuric acid*, heat cautiously until fumes are evolved and ignite until the residue is free of carbon. Cool, add 2 ml of *hydrochloric acid*, evaporate to dryness on a water-bath, dissolve the residue in a mixture of 5 ml of 6M *acetic acid* and 10 ml of hot *water*, neutralise with 5M *ammonia* and add sufficient *water* to produce 20 ml. 12 ml of the resulting solution complies with *limit test A for heavy metals*, Appendix VII (10 ppm). Use *lead standard solution (2 ppm Pb)* to prepare the standard.

Sulphated ash Not more than 0.1%, Appendix IX A.

Assay To 1.5 g add 10 ml of *water* and 20 ml of 0.5M *sodium hydroxide VS*. Allow to stand for 2 minutes and titrate with 0.25M *sulphuric acid VS* using *phenolphthalein solution* as indicator. Titrate the neutralised solution with 0.1M *silver nitrate VS* using a 1% w/v solution of *potassium chromate* as indicator. To the volume of 0.25M *sulphuric acid VS* used in the first titration add four-fifteenths of the volume of 0.1M *silver nitrate VS* used in the second titration and subtract the figure obtained from the volume of 0.5M *sodium hydroxide VS* added. Each ml of 0.5M *sodium hydroxide VS* represented by the difference is equivalent to 0.1298 g of $C_{15}H_{18}Cl_6N_2O_5$.

Dissolve 0.4 g in 20 ml of a 10% w/v solution of *sodium acetate*, add 25 ml of 0.05M *iodine VS* and allow to stand for 20 minutes, shaking occasionally. Add 10 ml of *chloroform*, shake until the precipitate is dissolved and titrate the excess of iodine with 0.1M *sodium thiosulphate VS* using *starch mucilage*, added towards the end of the titration, as indicator. Repeat the operation without the substance being examined. The difference between the titrations represents the amount of iodine required. Each ml of 0.05M *iodine VS* is equivalent to 0.02595 g of $C_{15}H_{18}Cl_6N_2O_5$.

Storage Dichloralphenazone should be kept in a well-closed container.

Preparations
Dichloralphenazone Oral Solution
Dichloralphenazone Tablets

Action and use Sedative; hypnotic.

Dichlorodifluoromethane
Propellant 12

CCl_2F_2 120.9   *75-71-8*

Dichlorodifluoromethane is a gas at ordinary temperatures. For convenience in use it is compressed in metal cylinders.

Characteristics A colourless, non-flammable gas; odour, faintly ethereal. The compressed liquid form has a weight per ml of about 1.50 g at −35° and about 1.35 g at 15°.

Solubility In the liquid state, immiscible with *water*; miscible with *absolute ethanol*.

Identification It boils at about −29.8°.

Acidity Not more than 2 ppm, calculated as HCl, when determined by the following method. Transfer 200 ml of *water* previously neutralised to *bromocresol purple solution* to a gas-washing bottle fitted with a sintered-glass distribution tube, pass 200 g of the gas being examined through the water and titrate with 0.02M *sodium hydroxide VS* using *bromocresol purple solution* as indicator. Each ml of 0.02M *sodium hydroxide VS* is equivalent to 0.000729 g of HCl.

Distillation range 0.2°, Appendix V C, Method II, using a water-bath at 20° and correcting the temperatures by ±0.233° per kPa.

Chloride Mix 5 ml of the liquid with 5 ml of *methanol* and add 0.2 ml of a saturated solution of *silver nitrate* in *methanol*. The solution is *clear*, Appendix IV A.

High-boiling matter Not more than 0.01% v/v when determined by the following method. Allow the boiling tube containing the remaining 15 ml of liquid from the determination of Distillation range to stand in ice for 30 minutes and measure the volume.

Water Not more than 0.001% w/w, Appendix IX C, Method I C.

Storage Dichlorodifluoromethane should be kept compressed in a metal cylinder and stored at a temperature of 8° to 15°.

Action and use Aerosol propellant.

Dichlorophen

$C_{13}H_{10}Cl_2O_2$ 269.1   *97-23-4*

Dichlorophen is 4,4′-dichloro-2,2′-methylene-diphenol. It contains not less than 97.0 per cent and not more than 101.0 per cent of $C_{13}H_{10}Cl_2O_2$, calculated with reference to the dried substance.

Characteristics A white or not more than slightly cream powder; odour, not more than slightly phenolic.

Solubility Practically insoluble in *water*; soluble in 1 part of *ethanol (96%)* and in less than 1 part of *ether*.

Identification A. The *light absorption*, Appendix II B, in the range 220 to 350 nm of a 0.002% w/v solution in 0.1M *sodium hydroxide* exhibits two maxima, at 245 nm and 304 nm. The *absorbance* at 245 nm is about 1.3 and at 304 nm is about 0.54.
B. Dissolve 0.2 g in a mixture of 5 ml of *water* and 5 ml of 5M *sodium hydroxide*, cool in ice and add a solution prepared by mixing 1 ml of *sodium nitrite solution* with a cold solution containing 0.15 ml of *aniline* in a mixture of 4 ml of *water* and 1 ml of *hydrochloric acid*. A reddish-brown precipitate is produced.
C. Fuse 0.5 g with 2 g of *anhydrous sodium carbonate*, cool, extract the residue with *water* and filter. The filtrate yields *reaction A* characteristic of chlorides, Appendix VI.
D. *Melting point*, about 175°, Appendix V A.

Chloride Dissolve 1.0 g in 2 ml of *ethanol (96%)*, dilute to 100 ml with *water*, allow to stand for 5 minutes and filter through a slow filter paper (Whatman No. 42 is suitable). 15 ml of the filtrate complies with the *limit test for chlorides*, Appendix VII (350 ppm).

Sulphate Shake 0.8 g with 16 ml of *water* for 2 minutes, filter and dilute 5 ml of the filtrate to 15 ml with *water*. The solution complies with the *limit test for sulphates*, Appendix VII (600 ppm).

Related substances Prepare a solution in *methanol* containing 0.0060% w/v of *4-hydroxybenzoic acid* and 0.21% w/v of *triphenylamine* (internal standards) (solution A). Carry out the method for *high-performance* *liquid chromatography*, Appendix III D, using the following solutions. For solution (1) add 10 ml of solution A, 1 ml of *glacial acetic acid* and 25 ml of *water* to 10 ml of a 0.010% w/v solution of *4-chlorophenol* in *methanol*, mix and add sufficient *methanol* to produce 100 ml. Solution (2) contains 1.0% w/v of the substance being examined in the mobile phase. For solution (3) dissolve 1.0 g of the substance being examined in 10 ml of solution A, add 1 ml of *glacial acetic acid* and 25 ml of *water*, mix and add sufficient *methanol* to produce 100 ml.

The chromatographic procedure may be carried out using (a) a stainless steel column (20 cm × 5 mm) packed with *stationary phase C* (10 μm) (Spherisorb ODS 1 is suitable), (b) a mixture of 75 volumes of *methanol*, 25 volumes of *water* and 1 volume of *glacial acetic acid* as the mobile phase with a flow rate of 1.5 ml per minute and (c) a detection wavelength of 280 nm.

In the chromatogram obtained with solution (1) the peaks, in order of their emergence, are due to 4-hydroxy-benzoic acid, 4-chlorophenol and triphenylamine. In the chromatogram obtained with solution (3) any peak due to 4-chloro-2,6-bis(5-chloro-2-hydroxybenzyl)phenol emerges just before the peak due to triphenylamine. In the chromatogram obtained with solution (3) the areas of any peaks corresponding to 4-chlorophenol and 4-chloro-2,6-bis(5-chloro-2-hydroxybenzyl)phenol are not greater than the areas of the peaks due to 4-hydroxybenzoic acid and triphenylamine respectively. The sum of the areas of any other *secondary peaks* with a retention time of up to twice that of triphenylamine is not greater than 25% of the area of the peak due to triphenylamine.

Loss on drying When dried to constant weight at 105°, loses not more than 1.0% of its weight. Use 1 g.

Sulphated ash Not more than 0.1%, Appendix IX A.

Assay Dissolve 0.5 g in 20 ml of *propan-2-ol* and carry out Method II for *non-aqueous titration*, Appendix VIII A, using 0.1M *tetrabutylammonium hydroxide VS* as titrant and determining the end-point potentiometrically. Each ml of 0.1M *tetrabutylammonium hydroxide VS* is equivalent to 0.02691 g of $C_{13}H_{10}Cl_2O_2$.

Preparation
Dichlorophen Tablets

Action and use Anthelmintic.

Dichlorotetrafluoroethane
Propellant 114

CClF₂·CClF₂

$C_2Cl_2F_4$ 170.9   *76-14-2*

Dichlorotetrafluoroethane is 1,2-dichloro-1,1,2,2-tetrafluoroethane. It is a gas at ordinary temperatures. For convenience in use it is compressed in metal cylinders.

Characteristics A colourless, non-flammable gas; odour, faintly ethereal. The compressed liquid form has a weight per ml of about 1.63 g at −35° and about 1.49 g at 15°.

Solubility In the liquid state, immiscible with *water*; miscible with *absolute ethanol*.

Identification It boils at about 3.5°.

Acidity Not more than 2 ppm, calculated as HCl, when determined by the following method. Transfer 200 ml of *water* previously neutralised to *bromocresol purple solution* to a gas-washing bottle fitted with a sintered-glass distribution tube, pass 200 g of the gas being examined through the water and titrate with 0.02M *sodium hydroxide VS* using *bromocresol purple solution* as indicator. Each ml of 0.02M *sodium hydroxide VS* is equivalent to 0.000729 g of HCl.

Distillation range 0.3°, Appendix V C, Method II, using a water-bath at 34° and correcting the temperatures by ±0.251° per kPa.

Chloride Mix 5 ml of the liquid with 5 ml of *methanol* and add 0.2 ml of a saturated solution of *silver nitrate* in *methanol*. The solution is *clear*, Appendix IV A.

High-boiling matter Not more than 0.01% v/v when determined by the following method. Allow the boiling tube containing the remaining 15 ml of liquid from the determination of Distillation range to stand in a water-bath at 34° for 30 minutes and measure the volume.

Water Not more than 0.001% w/w, Appendix IX C, Method I C.

Storage Dichlorotetrafluoroethane should be kept compressed in a metal cylinder and stored at a temperature of 8° to 15°.

Action and use Aerosol propellant.

Dichlorphenamide

$C_6H_6Cl_2N_2O_4S_2$ 305.2   *120-97-8*

Dichlorphenamide is 4,5-dichlorobenzene-1,3-disulphonamide. It contains not less than 98.0 per cent and not more than 101.0 per cent of $C_6H_6Cl_2N_2O_4S_2$, calculated with reference to the dried substance.

Characteristics A white or almost white, crystalline powder; odour, slight.

Solubility Practically insoluble in *water* and in *chloroform*; soluble in 30 parts of *ethanol (96%)*. It dissolves in solutions of the alkali hydroxides.

Identification A. The *infra-red absorption spectrum*, Appendix II A, is concordant with the *reference spectrum* of dichlorphenamide. If the spectra are not concordant, dissolve a sufficient quantity in the minimum volume of *methanol*, evaporate to dryness and prepare a new spectrum.
B. The *light absorption*, Appendix II B, in the range 275 to 350 nm of a 0.02% w/v solution in 0.1M *sodium hydroxide* exhibits two maxima, at 285 nm and at 294 nm. The *absorbance* at 285 nm is about 0.85 and at 294 nm is about 0.72.
C. Burn 20 mg by the method for *oxygen-flask combustion*, Appendix VIII C, using 5 ml of 2M *sodium hydroxide* as the absorbing liquid. When the process is complete, dilute the liquid to 25 ml with *water*. To 5 ml of the resulting solution add 0.1 ml of *hydrogen peroxide solution (100 vol)*

and 1 ml of 1M *hydrochloric acid*, mix and add 0.05 ml of *barium chloride solution*. The solution becomes turbid.

D. Acidify a further 5 ml of the solution obtained in test B with 1M *sulphuric acid* and boil gently for 2 minutes. The solution yields *reaction A* characteristic of chlorides, Appendix VI.

E. *Melting point*, about 240°, Appendix V A.

Chloride Shake 0.23 g with 60 ml of *water* for 5 minutes and filter. 15 ml of the filtrate complies with the *limit test for chlorides*, Appendix VII (0.09%).

Related substances Carry out the method for *thin-layer chromatography*, Appendix III A, using *silica gel GF254* as the coating substance and a mixture of 80 volumes of *chloroform*, 25 volumes of *methanol* and 5 volumes of 13.5M *ammonia* as the mobile phase. Apply separately to the chromatoplate, as single applications, 10 µl of each of two solutions of the substance being examined in *methanol* containing (1) 2.0% w/v and (2) 0.040% w/v. After removal of the plate, allow it to dry in air and examine under *ultra-violet light (254 nm)*. Any *secondary spot* in the chromatogram obtained with solution (1) is not more intense than the spot in the chromatogram obtained with solution (2).

Loss on drying When dried to constant weight at 100° at a pressure not exceeding 0.7 kPa, loses not more than 1.0% of its weight. Use 1 g.

Sulphated ash Not more than 0.1%, Appendix IX A.

Assay Dissolve 0.5 g in 50 ml of *anhydrous pyridine* and titrate with 0.1M *sodium methoxide VS*, using 0.25 ml of *thymolphthalein solution* as indicator, until a blue colour is produced. Repeat the operation without the substance being examined. The difference between the titrations represents the amount of sodium methoxide required. Each ml of 0.1M *sodium methoxide VS* is equivalent to 0.01526 g of $C_6H_6Cl_2N_2O_4S_2$.

Preparation
Dichlorphenamide Tablets

Action and use Used in treatment of glaucoma.

In some countries the material described in this monograph may be known as Diclofenamide.

Dicyclomine Hydrochloride

CO·OCH₂·CH₂·NEt₂ ,HCl

$C_{19}H_{35}NO_2,HCl$ 346.0   67-92-5

Dicyclomine Hydrochloride is 2-diethylamino-ethyl bicyclohexyl-1-carboxylate hydrochloride. It contains not less than 99.0 per cent and not more than 101.0 per cent of $C_{19}H_{35}NO_2,HCl$, calculated with reference to the dried substance.

Characteristics A white or almost white, crystalline powder; odourless or almost odourless.

Solubility Soluble in 20 parts of *water*, in 5 parts of *ethanol (96%)* and in 2 parts of *chloroform*; insoluble in *ether*.

Identification A. Dissolve a suitable quantity in *acetone* and evaporate to dryness. The *infra-red absorption spectrum* of the residue, Appendix II A, is concordant with the *reference spectrum* of dicyclomine hydrochloride.

B. To 3 ml of a 0.1% w/v solution of *sodium dodecyl sulphate* add 5 ml of *chloroform* and 0.05 ml of a 0.25% w/v solution of *methylene blue*, mix gently and allow to separate; the chloroform layer is blue. Add 20 mg of the substance being examined dissolved in 2 ml of *water*, mix gently and allow to separate; the aqueous layer is blue and the chloroform layer is colourless.

C. Dissolve 10 mg in 5 ml of *water* and add 0.2 ml of 2M *nitric acid* and 0.5 ml of *silver nitrate solution*. A white precipitate is produced.

Melting point 172° to 174°, Appendix V A.

Related substances Carry out the method for *thin-layer chromatography*, Appendix III A, using *silica gel G* as the coating substance and a mixture of 50 volumes of *propan-1-ol*, 30 volumes of *ethyl acetate*, 15 volumes of *water* and 5 volumes of 13.5M *ammonia* as the mobile phase. Apply separately to the chromatoplate 10 µl of each of two solutions of the substance being examined in *methanol* containing (1) 5.0% w/v and (2) 0.010% w/v. After removal of the plate, allow it to dry in air and spray with *dilute potassium iodobismuthate solution*. Any *secondary spot* in the chromatogram obtained with solution (1) is not more intense than the spot in the chromatogram obtained with solution (2).

Loss on drying When dried to constant weight at 105°, loses not more than 1.0% of its weight. Use 1 g.

Sulphated ash Not more than 0.1%, Appendix IX A.

Assay Carry out Method I for *non-aqueous titration*, Appendix VIII A, using 0.6 g and *crystal violet solution* as indicator. Each ml of 0.1M *perchloric acid VS* is equivalent to 0.03460 g of $C_{19}H_{35}NO_2,HCl$.

Preparations
Dicyclomine Oral Solution
Dicyclomine Tablets

Action and use Antispasmodic.

In some countries the material described in this monograph may be known as Dicycloverine Hydrochloride.

Dienoestrol ☆

Me   OH

HO   Me

$C_{18}H_{18}O_2$ 266.3   84-17-3

Dienoestrol is (Z,Z)-4,4'-[bis(ethylidene)-ethylene]diphenol. It contains not less than 98.5 per cent and not more than 101.5 per cent of $C_{18}H_{18}O_2$, calculated with reference to the dried substance.

Characteristics A white or almost white, crystalline powder.

Solubility Practically insoluble in *water*; soluble in 8 parts of *ethanol (96%)*, in 5 parts of *acetone* and in 15 parts of *ether*. It dissolves in solutions of the alkali hydroxides.

Identification *Test A may be omitted if tests B, C and D are carried out. Test B and C may be omitted if tests A and D are carried out.*

A. The *infra-red absorption spectrum*, Appendix II A, is concordant with the spectrum of *dienestrol EPCRS*.

B. In the test for Related substances, the principal spot in the chromatogram obtained with solution (2) is similar in position, colour and size to that in the chromatogram obtained with solution (3).

C. Dissolve 1 mg in 5 ml of *glacial acetic acid*, add 1 ml of a 1% v/v solution of *bromine* in *glacial acetic acid* and heat in a water-bath for 2 minutes. To 0.5 ml of the solution in a dry test-tube add 0.5 ml of *absolute ethanol*, mix and add 10 ml of *water*; a reddish-violet colour is produced. Add 5 ml of *chloroform*, shake vigorously and allow to separate; the chloroform layer is deep orange-red and the aqueous layer is almost colourless.

D. Dissolve 0.5 mg in 0.2 ml of *glacial acetic acid*, add 1 ml of *orthophosphoric acid* and heat in a water-bath for 3 minutes. A reddish-violet colour is produced.

Melting point 227° to 234°, Appendix V A, Method I. The temperature interval between the formation of a definite meniscus in the melt and the disappearance of the last particle does not exceed 3°.

Related substances Carry out the method for *thin-layer* chromatography, Appendix III A, using *silica gel G* as the coating substance and 90 volumes of *toluene* and 10 volumes of *diethylamine* as the mobile phase. Apply separately to the chromatoplate 1 µl of each of the following solutions in *ethanol (96%)*. Solutions (1) and (2) contain 10% w/v and 0.50% w/v respectively of the substance being examined. Solutions (3) and (4) contain 0.50% w/v and 0.050% w/v respectively of *dienestrol EPCRS*. Solution (5) contains 0.25% w/v each of *dienestrol EPCRS* and *diethylstilbestrol EPCRS*. After removal of the plate, allow it to dry in air, spray with *ethanolic sulphuric acid (20%)* and heat at 110° for 10 minutes. Any *secondary spot* in the chromatogram obtained with solution (1) is not more intense than the spot in the chromatogram obtained with solution (4). The test is not valid unless the chromatogram obtained with solution (5) shows two clearly separated spots having approximately the same intensity.

Loss on drying When dried to constant weight at 100° to 105°, loses not more than 0.5% of its weight. Use 1 g.

Sulphated ash Not more than 0.1%, Appendix IX A, Method II. Use 1 g.

Assay Dissolve 25 mg in sufficient *absolute alcohol* to produce 100 ml. To 5 ml of the solution add 10 ml of *absolute ethanol*, dilute with 0.1M *sodium hydroxide* to 250 ml and measure the *absorbance* of the resulting solution at the maximum at 245 nm, Appendix II B. Calculate the content of $C_{18}H_{18}O_2$ from the *absorbance* obtained by repeating the procedure using *dienestrol EPCRS*.

Storage Dienoestrol should be kept in a well-closed container and protected from light.

Action and use Oestrogen.

The title of the monograph in the European Pharmacopœia is Dienestrol.

Diethyl Phthalate

$C_{12}H_{14}O_4$ 222.2   *84-66-2*

Diethyl Phthalate contains not less than 99.0 per cent and not more than 100.5 per cent w/w of $C_{12}H_{14}O_4$.

Characteristics A clear, colourless or faintly coloured liquid; odourless or almost odourless.

Solubility Practically insoluble in *water*; miscible with *ethanol (96%)*, with *ether* and with aromatic hydrocarbons.

Identification A. The *infra-red absorption spectrum*, Appendix II A, is concordant with the *reference spectrum* of diethyl phthalate.

B. Gently boil 1 g with 5 ml of a 10% w/v solution of *potassium hydroxide* in *methanol* for 10 minutes, add 5 ml of *water* and evaporate to half its volume. Add 1 ml of *hydrochloric acid*, filter, melt the dried precipitate in a small tube, add 0.5 g of *resorcinol* and 0.05 ml of *chloroform* and heat at about 180° for 3 minutes. Cool, add 1 ml of 5M *sodium hydroxide* and pour into *water*. An intense yellowish-green fluorescence is produced.

Acidity Mix 20 ml with 50 ml of *ethanol (96%)* previously neutralised to *phenolphthalein solution*. Not more than 0.1 ml of 0.1M *sodium hydroxide VS* is required to neutralise the solution using *phenolphthalein solution* as indicator.

Refractive index 1.500 to 1.505, Appendix V E.

Weight per ml 1.115 to 1.119 g, Appendix V G.

Related substances Prepare a 0.030% w/v solution of *biphenyl* (internal standard) in *chloroform* (solution A). Carry out the method for *gas chromatography*, Appendix III B, using solutions of the substance being examined containing (1) 0.050% w/v in solution A, (2) 5.0% w/v in *chloroform* and (3) 5.0% w/v in solution A.

The chromatographic procedure may be carried out using a glass column (1.5 m × 4 mm) packed with *acid-washed, silanised diatomaceous support* (80 to 100 mesh) coated with 3% w/w of phenyl methyl silicone fluid (50% phenyl) (OV-17 is suitable) and maintained at 165°.

In the chromatogram obtained with solution (3) the ratio of the sum of the areas of any *secondary peaks* to the area of the peak due to the internal standard is not greater than the ratio of the area of the peak due to diethyl phthalate to the area of the peak due to the internal standard in the chromatogram obtained with solution (1).

Sulphated ash Not more than 0.02%, Appendix IX A.

Water Not more than 0.2% w/w, Appendix IX C. Use 12.5 g.

Assay Carry out the method for the *determination of esters*, Appendix VIII L, using 1.5 g and 50 ml of 0.5M *ethanolic potassium hydroxide VS*. Each ml of 0.5M *ethanolic potassium hydroxide VS* is equivalent to 0.05556 g of $C_{12}H_{14}O_4$.

Action and use Pharmaceutical aid.

Diethylamine Salicylate

$C_{11}H_{17}NO_3$ 211.3   *4419-92-5*

Diethylamine Salicylate contains not less than 99.0 per cent and not more than 101.0 per cent of $C_{11}H_{17}NO_3$.

Characteristics White or almost white crystals; odourless or almost odourless.

Solubility Soluble in less than 1 part of *water*, in 2 parts of *ethanol (96%)* and in 1.5 parts of *chloroform*.

Identification A. The *infra-red absorption spectrum*, Appendix II A, is concordant with the *reference spectrum* of diethylamine salicylate.
B. To 0.2 g add 5 ml of 1M *sodium hydroxide* and boil. Diethylamine, detectable by its odour, is produced.
C. Cool the solution obtained in test B and acidify with 2M *hydrochloric acid*; a white precipitate is produced. Reserve a sufficient quantity of the precipitate for test D. Add 10 ml of *water* and 0.05 ml of *iron(III) chloride test-solution*; a deep violet colour is produced.
D. *Melting point* of the precipitate obtained in test C, after recrystallisation from *water* and drying at 105°, about 160°, Appendix V A.

Acidity Dissolve 2 g in 25 ml of *water* and titrate with 0.1M *sodium hydroxide VS* using *phenol red solution* as indicator. Not more than 0.2 ml of 0.1M *sodium hydroxide VS* is required to change the colour of the solution.

Clarity and colour of solution A 50% w/v solution is *clear*, Appendix IV A, and not more intensely coloured than *reference solution BY$_5$*, Appendix IV B, Method II.

Melting point 100° to 102°, Appendix V A.

Heavy metals 12 ml of a 10.0% w/v solution complies with *limit test A for heavy metals*, Appendix VII (10 ppm). Use *lead standard solution (1 ppm Pb)* to prepare the standard.

Sulphate 0.6 g complies with the *limit test for sulphates*, Appendix VII (250 ppm).

Loss on drying When dried at 60° for 3 hours, loses not more than 0.1% of its weight. Use 1 g.

Assay Carry out Method I for *non-aqueous titration*, Appendix VIII A, using 0.4 g and *1-naphtholbenzein solution* as indicator. Each ml of 0.1M *perchloric acid VS* is equivalent to 0.02113 g of $C_{11}H_{17}NO_3$.

Storage Diethylamine Salicylate should be kept in a well-closed container and protected from light. It should not be allowed to come into contact with iron or iron salts.

Preparation
Diethylamine Salicylate Cream

Action and use Counter-irritant.

Diethylcarbamazine Citrate ☆

$C_{10}H_{21}N_3O,C_6H_8O_7$ 391.4   *1642-54-2*

Diethylcarbamazine Citrate is *N,N*-diethyl-4-methylpiperazine-1-carboxamide dihydrogen citrate. It contains not less than 98.0 per cent and not more than 101.0 per cent of $C_{10}H_{21}N_3O,C_6H_8O_7$, calculated with reference to the dried substance.

Characteristics A white, crystalline powder; odourless; slightly hygroscopic. It melts at about 138° with decomposition.

Solubility Very soluble in *water*; soluble in 35 parts of *ethanol (96%)*; practically insoluble in *acetone*, in *chloroform* and in *ether*.

Identification *Test A may be omitted if tests B and C are carried out. Test B may be omitted if tests A and C are carried out.*
A. The *infra-red absorption spectrum*, Appendix II A, is concordant with the spectrum of *diethylcarbamazine citrate EPCRS*.
B. In the test for *N,N'*-Dimethylpiperazine and *N*-methylpiperazine, the principal spot in the chromatogram obtained with solution (1) corresponds in position, colour and size to that in the chromatogram obtained with solution (2).
C. A 2% w/v solution yields *reaction A* characteristic of citrates, Appendix VI.

Clarity and colour of solution A 10.0% w/v solution is not more opalescent than *reference suspension II*, Appendix IV A, and not more intensely coloured than *reference solution BY$_6$*, Appendix IV B, Method II.

Heavy metals A 10.0% w/v solution complies with *limit test A for heavy metals*, Appendix VII (20 ppm). Use 10 ml of *lead standard solution (2 ppm Pb)* to prepare the standard.

***N,N'*-Dimethylpiperazine and *N*-methylpiperazine** Carry out the method for *thin-layer chromatography*, Appendix III A, using *silica gel G* as the coating substance and a mixture of 65 volumes of *methanol*, 30 volumes of *butan-2-one* and 5 volumes of 13.5M *ammonia* as the mobile phase but allowing the solvent front to ascend 12 cm above the line of application. Apply separately to the chromatoplate 10 μl of each of four solutions in *methanol* containing (1) 5.0% w/v of the substance being examined, (2) 5% w/v of *diethylcarbamazine citrate EPCRS*, (3) 0.010% w/v of *N,N'-dimethylpiperazine* and (4) 0.010% w/v of *N-methylpiperazine*. After removal of the plate, allow it to dry at 100° to 105° and expose it to iodine vapour for 30 minutes. Any spots corresponding to *N,N'*-dimethylpiperazine and *N*-methylpiperazine in the chromatogram obtained with solution (1) are not more intense than the spots in the chromatograms obtained with solutions (3) and (4) respectively.

Loss on drying When dried over *phosphorus pentoxide* at 60° at a pressure of 1.5 to 2.5 kPa for 4 hours, loses not more than 0.5% of its weight. Use 1 g.

Sulphated ash Not more than 0.1%, Appendix IX A, Method II. Use 1 g.

Assay Dissolve 0.35 g in 25 ml of *anhydrous glacial acetic acid* and add 25 ml of *acetic anhydride*. Carry out Method I for *non-aqueous titration*, Appendix VIII A, using 0.2 ml of *crystal violet solution* as indicator until a greenish-blue colour is produced. Each ml of 0.1M *perchloric acid VS* is equivalent to 0.03914 g of $C_{10}H_{21}N_3O,C_6H_8O_7$.

Storage Diethylcarbamazine Citrate should be kept in an airtight container.

Preparation
Diethylcarbamazine Tablets

Action and use Anthelmintic.

Diethylpropion Hydrochloride

CH₃·CH·CO—⟨ ⟩ ,HCl
  |
  NEt₂

$C_{13}H_{19}NO,HCl$ 241.8   *134-80-5*

Diethylpropion Hydrochloride is α-diethyl-aminopropiophenone hydrochloride. It may contain 1 per cent of Tartaric Acid as a stabilising agent. It contains not less than 98.0 per cent and not more than 101.0 per cent of $C_{13}H_{19}NO,HCl$, calculated with reference to the dried substance.

Characteristics A white or almost white, crystalline powder; odourless or almost odourless.

Solubility Freely soluble in *water*, in *ethanol (96%)* and in *chloroform*; practically insoluble in *ether*.

Identification A. The *infra-red absorption spectrum*, Appendix II A, is concordant with the *reference spectrum* of diethylpropion hydrochloride.
B. The *light absorption*, Appendix II B, in the range 230 to 350 nm of a 0.002% w/v solution in 0.1M *hydrochloric acid* exhibits a maximum only at 253 nm. The *absorbance* at 253 nm is about 1.14.
C. Yields the *reactions* characteristic of chlorides, Appendix VI.

Free bromine Place 0.05 ml of a 10% w/v solution on *starch—iodide paper*. No colour is produced.

Hydrobromic acid and bromide Dissolve 1.0 g in 10 ml of *water*, add 1 ml of 2M *sodium hydroxide*, mix well and extract with 25 ml of *chloroform*. Discard the chloroform layer, acidify the aqueous solution with 2M *hydrochloric acid*, add 0.5 ml of *chloroform* and 0.5 ml of a 10% w/v solution of *chloramine T* and shake. No yellow or brownish-red colour is produced in the chloroform layer.

Related substances Carry out the method for *thin-layer chromatography*, Appendix III A, using *silica gel GF254* as the coating substance and a mixture of 50 volumes of *propan-2-ol*, 30 volumes of *butyl acetate*, 15 volumes of *water* and 5 volumes of 13.5M *ammonia* as the mobile phase. Apply separately to the chromatoplate 20 μl of each of two freshly prepared solutions of the substance being examined in *chloroform* containing (1) 2.0% w/v and (2) 0.010% w/v. After removal of the plate, allow it to dry in air and examine under *ultra-violet light (254 nm)*. Any *secondary spot* in the chromatogram obtained with solution (1) is not more intense than the spot in the chromatogram obtained with solution (2).

Secondary amines Adjust the pH of a 1% w/v solution to 9.0 to 10.5 by the addition of a 20% w/v solution of *sodium carbonate*. To 0.5 ml of the resulting solution add 0.1 ml of a freshly prepared mixture of 4 volumes of *acetaldehyde*, 3 volumes of *ethanol (96%)* and 1 volume of *water* and 0.05 ml of a 1.0% w/v solution of *sodium nitroprusside*. No blue colour is produced within 5 minutes.

Loss on drying When dried to constant weight over *phosphorus pentoxide* at 60° at a pressure not exceeding 0.7 kPa, loses not more than 0.5% of its weight. Use 1 g.

Assay Carry out Method I for *non-aqueous titration*, Appendix VIII A, using 0.4 g, adding 15 ml of *mercury(II) acetate solution* and using *1-naphtholbenzein solution* as indicator. Each ml of 0.1M *perchloric acid VS* is equivalent to 0.02418 g of $C_{13}H_{19}NO,HCl$.

Storage Diethylpropion Hydrochloride should be kept in a well-closed container, protected from light and stored at a temperature not exceeding 25°.

Action and use Appetite suppressant.

In some countries the material described in this monograph may be known as Amfepramone Hydrochloride.

Diflunisal

F—⟨ ⟩—⟨ ⟩—OH
   | CO₂H
   F

$C_{13}H_8F_2O_3$ 250.2   *22494-42-4*

Diflunisal is 5-(2,4-difluorophenyl)salicylic acid. It contains not less than 98.5 per cent and not more than 101.0 per cent of $C_{13}H_8F_2O_3$, calculated with reference to the dried substance.

Characteristics A white or almost white, crystalline powder.

Solubility Practically insoluble in *water*; soluble in *ethanol (96%)* and in *ether*.

Identification A. The *infra-red absorption spectrum*, Appendix II A, is concordant with the *reference spectrum* of diflunisal (form A).
B. The *light absorption*, Appendix II B, in the range 230 to 350 nm of a 0.002% w/v solution in 0.1M *methanolic hydrochloric acid* exhibits two maxima, at 251 nm and 315 nm. The *absorbance* at 251 nm is about 1.12 and at 315 nm is about 0.26.
C. Dissolve 2 mg in 10 ml of *ethanol (96%)* and add 0.1 ml of *iron(III) chloride solution*. A deep purple colour is produced.

Heavy metals 2.0 g complies with *limit test C for heavy metals*, Appendix VII (10 ppm). Use 2 ml of *lead standard solution (10 ppm Pb)* to prepare the standard.

Related substances A. Carry out the method for *thin-layer chromatography*, Appendix III A, using a silica gel F254 precoated chromatoplate (Merck silica gel 60 F254 plates are suitable) and a mixture of 70 volumes of *carbon tetrachloride*, 20 volumes of *acetone* and 10 volumes of *glacial acetic acid* as the mobile phase. Apply separately to the plate 5 µl of each of two solutions in *methanol* containing (1) 2.0% w/v of the substance being examined and (2) 0.0030% w/v of *4-hydroxybiphenyl*. After removal of the plate, allow it to dry in a current of warm air and examine under *ultra-violet light (254 nm)*. Any *secondary spot* in the chromatogram obtained with solution (1) is not more intense than the spot in the chromatogram obtained with solution (2).

B. Carry out the method for *high-performance liquid chromatography*, Appendix III D, using the following solutions in a mixture of 4 volumes of *acetonitrile* and 1 volume of *water*. Solution (1) contains 0.00055% w/v of *fluoranthene* (internal standard). Solution (2) contains 0.50% w/v of the substance being examined and 0.00055% w/v of the internal standard.

The chromatographic procedure may be carried out using (a) a stainless steel column (30 cm × 4 mm) packed with *stationary phase C* (10 µm) (µBondapak C18 is suitable), (b) a mixture of 70 volumes of *acetonitrile*, 55 volumes of *water*, 25 volumes of *methanol* and 2 volumes of *glacial acetic acid* as the mobile phase with a flow rate of 2 ml per minute and (c) a detection wavelength of 254 nm.

In the chromatogram obtained with solution (2) the sum of the areas of any peaks with retention times greater than that of the internal standard is not greater than the area of the peak due to the internal standard.

Loss on drying When dried at 60° at a pressure not exceeding 0.7 kPa for 2 hours, loses not more than 0.3% of its weight. Use 1 g.

Sulphated ash Not more than 0.1%, Appendix IX A.

Assay Dissolve 0.45 g in 80 ml of *methanol*, add 10 ml of *water* and titrate with 0.1M *sodium hydroxide VS* using *phenol red solution* as indicator. Each ml of 0.1M *sodium hydroxide VS* is equivalent to 0.02502 g of $C_{13}H_8F_2O_3$.

Storage Diflunisal should be kept in a well-closed container and protected from light.

Preparation
Diflunisal Tablets

Action and use Anti-inflammatory; analgesic.

Digitalis Leaf ☆
Digitalis

Digitalis Leaf is the dried leaf of *Digitalis purpurea* L. It contains not less than 0.3 per cent of cardenolic glycosides, calculated as digitoxin, $C_{41}H_{64}O_{13}$, with reference to the dried material.

Characteristics Odour, slight and characteristic.

Macroscopical Leaf, simple, brittle and often broken, about 10 to 40 cm long and 4 to 15 cm wide. Upper surface green, rugose and pubescent; lower surface greyish-green, reticulated with raised veinlets and densely pubescent. Lamina, ovate-lanceolate to broadly ovate, with irregularly crenate, dentate or serrate margin, decurrent base and subacute apex; winged petiole 2.5 to 10 cm long. Venation pinnate, lateral veins prominent especially on the lower surface, leaving the midrib at about 45° and anastomosing near the margin; a veinlet terminates in each tooth of the margin and the lower veins run down the winged petiole.

Microscopical Epidermal cells, about 30 to 75 µm long, anticlinal walls straight or slightly sinuous on the upper surface, markedly sinuous on the lower surface; cuticle smooth. Stomata *anomocytic*; occasional on the upper surface, frequent on the lower surface. Trichomes, of two types: covering trichomes, uniseriate, bluntly pointed, three to five cells long, walls occasionally smooth, usually finely warty or faintly striated, adjacent cells often collapsed at right angles; glandular trichomes, with a unicellular or more rarely a multicellular uniseriate stalk and a unicellular or bicellular head; mesophyll dorsiventral with a single layer (rarely double) of short palisade cells and a spongy mesophyll; midrib prominent on the lower surface, containing an arc of radiate xylem, a narrow phloem and a narrow band of collenchyma, all enclosed within a single layer of endodermal cells containing starch granules. Calcium oxalate and sclerenchyma absent.

Identification A. Carry out the method for *thin-layer chromatography*, Appendix III A, using *silica gel G* as the coating substance and a mixture of 75 volumes of *ethyl acetate*, 10 volumes of *methanol* and 7.5 volumes of *water* as the mobile phase, but allowing the solvent front to ascend 10 cm above the line of application. Apply separately, as bands 2 cm × 3 mm, 20 µl of each of the following solutions. For solution (1) evaporate 10 ml of solution A to dryness and dissolve the residue in 1 ml of a mixture of equal volumes of *chloroform* and *methanol*. For solution (2) dissolve 5 mg of *purpureaglycoside A EPCRS*, 2 mg of *purpureaglycoside B EPCRS*, 5 mg of *digitoxin* and 2 mg of *gitoxin* in a mixture of equal volumes of *chloroform* and *methanol* and dilute to 10 ml with the same solvent. After removal of the plate, allow it to dry in air, spray with a mixture of 8 volumes of a 25% w/v solution of *trichloroacetic acid* in *ethanol (96%)* and 2 volumes of a 1% w/v solution of *chloramine T*, heat at 100° to 105° for 10 minutes and examine under *ultra-violet light (365 nm)*. The chromatogram obtained with solution (2) shows bands at an Rf value of about 0.2 with a light blue fluorescence (purpureaglycoside B), at an Rf value of about 0.25 with a brownish-yellow fluorescence (purpureaglycoside A), at an Rf value of about 0.5 with a light blue fluorescence (gitoxin) and at an Rf value of about 0.6 with a brownish-yellow fluorescence (digitoxin). The bands in the chromatogram obtained with solution (1) correspond in position, size and colour to those in the chromatogram obtained with solution (2); other fluorescent bands may also be present.

B. To 1 g, in *No. 180 powder*, add 20 ml of *ethanol (50%)* and 10 ml of *lead acetate solution*, boil for 2 minutes, allow to cool, centrifuge and extract the clear supernatant liquid with two 15-ml quantities of *chloroform*, separating the layers, if necessary, by centrifugation. Dry the combined chloroform extracts over *anhydrous sodium sulphate* and filter (solution A). Reserve 15 ml of solution A for use in tests B and C and evaporate 5 ml of the remainder to dryness on a water-bath. To the residue add 2 ml of a 2% w/v solution of *3,5-dinitrobenzoic acid* in *ethanol (96%)* and 1 ml of 1M *sodium hydroxide*. A reddish-violet colour is produced within 5 minutes.

C. Evaporate 5 ml of solution A to dryness on a water-bath, add 3 ml of *xanthydrol solution* and heat for 3 minutes on a water-bath. A red colour is produced.

Acid-insoluble ash Not more than 5.0%, Appendix XI K, Method II. Use 1 g, in powder.

Foreign matter Leaves having few or no trichomes and epidermal cells showing, in surface view, beaded anticlinal walls are absent (*Digitalis lanata*).

Loss on drying When dried to constant weight at 100° to 105°, loses not more than 6.0% of its weight. Use 1 g.

Assay Shake 0.25 g, in *No. 180 powder*, for 1 hour with 50 ml of *water*. Add 5 ml of a 15% w/v solution of *lead acetate* and shake. After a few minutes add 7.5 ml of a 4% w/v solution of *disodium hydrogen orthophosphate* and filter. To 50 ml of the filtrate add 5 ml of 4M *hydrochloric acid*, heat under a reflux condenser on a water-bath for 1 hour and transfer to a separating funnel, rinsing the flask with two 5-ml quantities of *water*. Extract with three 25-ml quantities of *chloroform*, dry the combined chloroform extracts over *anhydrous sodium sulphate* and dilute to 100 ml with *chloroform*. Evaporate 40 ml of the chloroform solution and add to the residue 7 ml of *ethanol (50%)*, 2 ml of a 2% w/v solution of *3,5-dinitrobenzoic acid* in *ethanol (96%)* and 1 ml of 1M *sodium hydroxide*. Measure the *absorbance* of the resulting solution, Appendix II B, at 540 nm at intervals during the first 12 minutes until the maximum is reached, using in the reference cell a mixture of 7 ml of *ethanol (50%)*, 2 ml of a 2% w/v solution of *3,5-dinitrobenzoic acid* in *ethanol (96%)* and 1 ml of 1M *sodium hydroxide*. Calculate the content of digitoxin from the absorbance obtained by carrying out the operation at the same time using a solution prepared in the following manner. Dissolve 50 mg of *digitoxin EPCRS* in sufficient *ethanol (96%)* to produce 50 ml and dilute 5 ml to 50 ml with *ethanol (96%)*; to 5 ml of the resulting solution add 25 ml of *water* and 3 ml of 4M *hydrochloric acid* and complete the procedure described above, beginning at the words 'heat under a reflux condenser . . .'.

Storage Digitalis Leaf should be kept in a well-closed container and protected from light and moisture.

Preparation
Prepared Digitalis

Action and use Cardiac glycoside.

Powdered Digitalis Leaf

Powdered Digitalis Leaf is Digitalis Leaf in powder. It contains not less than 0.3 per cent of cardenolic glycosides, calculated as digitoxin, $C_{41}H_{64}O_{13}$, with reference to the dried material.

Characteristics Green to greyish-green. Diagnostic structures: numerous trichomes, whole or broken; fragments of leaf showing cicatrices and epidermal cells with straight or sinuous anticlinal walls and smooth cuticle; stomata *anomocytic*; whole or partial cross sections with short palisade cells or undifferentiated mesophyll and narrow, spirally-thickened vessels; wider vessels from the midrib and main veins, accompanied by elongated parenchyma. Calcium oxalate and sclerenchyma absent.

Identification Complies with the tests for Identification described under Digitalis Leaf.

Acid-insoluble ash Not more than 5.0%, Appendix XI K.

Microbial contamination 1.0 g is free from *Escherichia coli*, Appendix XVI B1.

Assay Carry out the Assay described under Digitalis Leaf.

Storage Powdered Digitalis Leaf should be kept in a well-closed container and protected from light and moisture.

Action and use Cardiac glycoside.

Prepared Digitalis

Prepared Digitalis is Digitalis Leaf reduced to a powder not more coarse than a *moderately coarse powder*, no portion being discarded, and assayed by the method described under Assay.

For therapeutic administration, Prepared Digitalis is adjusted to contain not less than 0.36 per cent and not more than 0.44 per cent of cardenolic glycosides, calculated as digitoxin, by thorough mixture, if necessary, with Prepared Digitalis of lower glycoside content or with powdered grass.

Characteristics Green; odour, slight.

Microscopical Exhibits the diagnostic structures described under Powdered Digitalis Leaf.

If powdered grass is present the histological details vary with the species but for those most likely to occur the following characteristics are diagnostic. Trichomes represented by scarce to abundant, long or short, unicellular hairs with thin or thick walls and by prickles with bulbous bases and short barbs. Epidermis typically consisting of parallel, longitudinal files of cells, the cells in many or all of the files being of two distinct sizes referred to as 'long' and 'short' respectively. Short cells commonly solitary or in pairs, many of them containing solitary silica bodies, the shapes of which are diagnostic for the species of grass concerned. Short cells in which no silica bodies are present usually have suberised walls. Stomata with characteristic dumb-bell shaped guard cells, restricted to certain files of cells in the intercostal zones. Crystals absent. Pollen grains spherical, each with a single pore.

Identification Complies with the tests for Identification described under Digitalis Leaf.

Loss on drying When dried to constant weight at 105°, loses not more than 6.0% of its weight. Use 1 g.

Microbial contamination 1 g is free from *Escherichia coli* and 10 g is free from salmonellae, Appendix XVI B1.

Assay Shake 0.25 g, in *fine powder*, for 1 hour with 50 ml of *water*. Add 5 ml of a 15% w/v solution of *lead acetate* and shake. After a few minutes add 7.5 ml of a 4% w/v solution of *disodium hydrogen orthophosphate* and filter. To 50 ml of the filtrate add 5 ml of 4M *hydrochloric acid*, heat under a reflux condenser on a water-bath for 1 hour and transfer to a separating funnel, rinsing the flask with two 5-ml quantities of *water*. Extract with three 25-ml quantities of *chloroform*, dry the combined chloroform extracts over *anhydrous sodium sulphate* and dilute to 100 ml with *chloroform*. Evaporate 40 ml of the chloroform solution and add to the residue 7 ml of *ethanol (50%)*, 2 ml of a 2% w/v solution of *3,5-dinitrobenzoic acid* in *ethanol (96%)* and 1 ml of 1M *sodium hydroxide*. Measure the *absorbance* of the resulting solution, Appendix II B, at 540 nm at intervals during the first 12 minutes until the maximum is reached, using in the reference cell a mixture of 7 ml of *ethanol (50%)*, 2 ml of a 2% w/v solution of *3,5-dinitrobenzoic acid* in *ethanol (96%)* and 1 ml of 1M *sodium hydroxide*. Calculate the content of cardenolic glycosides, as digitoxin, from the *absorbance* obtained by carrying out the operation at the same time using a solution prepared in the following manner. Dissolve 50 mg of *digitoxin EPCRS* in sufficient *ethanol (96%)* to produce 50 ml and dilute 10 ml to 50 ml with *ethanol (96%)*. To 5 ml of the resulting solution add 25 ml of *water* and 3 ml of 4M *hydrochloric acid* and complete the procedure described above, beginning at the words 'heat under a reflux condenser . . .'.

Storage Prepared Digitalis should be kept in a container that prevents access of moisture.

Preparation
Digitalis Tablets

Action and use Cardiac glycoside.

Digitoxin ☆

$C_{41}H_{64}O_{13}$ 765   71-63-6

Digitoxin is 3β-[(*O*-2,6-dideoxy-β-D-*ribo*-hexopyranosyl-(1→4)-*O*-2,6-dideoxy-β-D-*ribo*-hexopyranosyl-(1→4)-2,6-dideoxy-β-D-*ribo*-hexopyranosyl)oxy]-14β-hydroxy-5β-card-20(22)-enolide. It contains not less than 95.0 per cent and not more than 103.0 per cent of $C_{41}H_{64}O_{13}$, calculated with reference to the dried substance.

Characteristics A white or almost white powder.

Solubility Practically insoluble in *water*; slightly soluble in *ethanol (96%)*, in *methanol* and in *ether*; soluble in 40 parts of *chloroform*; freely soluble in a mixture of equal volumes of *chloroform* and *methanol*.

Identification *Test A may be omitted if tests B, C and D are carried out. Tests B, C and D may be omitted if test A is carried out.*

A. The *infra-red absorption spectrum*, Appendix II A, is concordant with the spectrum of *digitoxin EPCRS*.

B. In the test for Related substances, the principal spot in the chromatogram obtained with solution (1) is similar in position, colour and size to that in the chromatogram obtained with solution (2).

C. Suspend 0.5 mg in 0.2 ml of *ethanol (60%)* and add 0.1 ml of a 2% w/v solution of *3,5-dinitrobenzoic acid* in *ethanol (96%)* and 0.1 ml of 2M *sodium hydroxide*. A violet colour is produced.

D. Dissolve 0.5 mg in 1 ml of *glacial acetic acid* with the aid of gentle heat, cool and add 0.05 ml of a 10.5% w/v solution of *iron(III) chloride hexahydrate*. Cautiously add 1 ml of *sulphuric acid* without mixing. A brown ring is produced at the interface and a green colour, which changes to blue, passes to the upper layer.

Clarity and colour of solution A 0.50% w/v solution in a mixture of equal volumes of *chloroform* and *methanol* is *clear*, Appendix IV A, and *colourless*, Appendix IV B, Method I.

Specific optical rotation In a 2.5% w/v solution in *chloroform*, +16.0° to +18.5°, Appendix V F.

Related substances Carry out the method for *thin-layer chromatography*, Appendix III A, using *silica gel G* as the coating substance and a mixture of 90 volumes of *chloroform*, 40 volumes of *cyclohexane* and 15 volumes of *methanol* as the mobile phase and developing the chromatograms immediately after application of the solutions. Apply separately to the chromatoplate 5 μl of each of six solutions in a mixture of equal volumes of *chloroform* and *methanol* containing (1) 1.0% w/v of the substance being examined, (2) 1.0% w/v of *digitoxin EPCRS*, (3) 0.010% w/v of *digitoxin EPCRS*, (4) 0.020% w/v of *gitoxin EPCRS*, (5) 0.0050% w/v of *digitoxin EPCRS* and (6) 0.50% w/v of *digitoxin EPCRS* and 0.010% w/v of *gitoxin EPCRS*. After removal of the plate, dry it in a current of cold air for 5 minutes. Repeat the development and again dry the plate in a current of cold air for 5 minutes. Spray with *ethanolic sulphuric acid (10%)* and heat at 130° for 15 minutes. Examine the chromatograms in daylight. Any spot in the chromatogram obtained with solution (1) corresponding to gitoxin is not more intense than the spot in the chromatogram obtained with solution (4). Any other *secondary spot* in the chromatogram obtained with solution (1) is not more intense than the spot in the chromatogram obtained with solution (3). The test is not valid unless the chromatogram obtained with solution (6) shows clearly separated spots corresponding to digitoxin, gitoxin and other glycosides and the spot in the chromatogram obtained with solution (5) is clearly visible.

Loss on drying When dried for 2 hours at 100° to 105°, loses not more than 1.5% of its weight. Use 0.5 g.

Sulphated ash Not more than 0.1%, Appendix IX A, Method II. Use the residue obtained in the test for Loss on drying.

Assay Dissolve 40 mg in sufficient *ethanol (96%)* to produce 50 ml and dilute 5 ml to 100 ml with the same solvent. To 5 ml of this solution add 3 ml of *alkaline trinitrophenol solution*, allow to stand in subdued light for 30 minutes and measure the *absorbance* of the resulting solution at the maximum at 495 nm, Appendix II B, using in the reference cell a mixture of 5 ml of *ethanol (96%)* and 3 ml of *alkaline trinitrophenol solution*. Calculate the content of $C_{41}H_{64}O_{13}$ from the *absorbance* obtained by repeating the operation using *digitoxin EPCRS* in place of the substance being examined.

Storage Digitoxin should be kept in a well-closed container, protected from light and stored at a temperature not exceeding 15°.

Preparation
Digitoxin Tablets

Action and use Cardiac glycoside.

Digoxin ☆

$C_{41}H_{64}O_{14}$ 781   20830-75-5

Digoxin is 3β-[(O-2,6-dideoxy-β-D-ribo-hexopyranosyl-(1→4)-O-2,6-dideoxy-β-D-ribo-hexopyranosyl-(1→4)-2,6-dideoxy-β-D-ribo-hexopyranosyl)oxy]-12β,14β-dihydroxy-5β-card-20(22)-enolide. It contains not less than 95.0 per cent and not more than the 103.0 per cent of $C_{41}H_{64}O_{14}$, calculated with reference to the dried substance.

Characteristics Colourless crystals or a white or almost white powder.

Solubility Practically insoluble in *water*; slightly soluble in *ethanol (96%)* and in *chloroform*; freely soluble in a mixture of equal volumes of *chloroform* and *methanol*.

Identification *Test A may be omitted if tests B, C and D are carried out. Tests B, C and D may be omitted if test A is carried out.*
A. The *infra-red absorption spectrum*, Appendix II A, is concordant with the spectrum of *digoxin EPCRS*.
B. In the test for Related substances, the principal spot in the chromatogram obtained with solution (1) is similar in position, colour and size to that in the chromatogram obtained with solution (2).
C. Suspend 0.5 mg in 0.2 ml of *ethanol (60%)* and add 0.1 ml of a 2% w/v solution of *3,5-dinitrobenzoic acid* in *ethanol (96%)* and 0.1 ml of 2M *sodium hydroxide*. A violet colour is produced.
D. Dissolve 0.5 mg in 1 ml of *glacial acetic acid* with the aid of gentle heat, cool and add 0.05 ml of a 10.5% w/v solution of *iron(III) chloride hexahydrate*. Cautiously add 1 ml of *sulphuric acid* without mixing. A brown ring is produced at the interface and a green colour, which changes to blue, passes to the upper layer.

Clarity and colour of solution A 0.50% w/v solution in a mixture of equal volumes of *chloroform* and *methanol* is *clear*, Appendix IV A, and *colourless*, Appendix IV B, Method I.

Specific optical rotation In a 2% w/v solution in *anhydrous pyridine*, +10.0° to +13.0°, Appendix V F.

Related substances Carry out the method for *thin-layer chromatography*, Appendix III A, using *kieselguhr G* as the coating substance, but allowing the solvent front to ascend 12 cm above the line of application. Impregnate the dry chromatoplate by placing it in a closed tank containing the necessary quantity of a mixture of 90 volumes of *acetone* and 10 volumes of *formamide* so that the plate dips about 5 mm into the liquid and allow the impregnating solvent to ascend at least 15 cm. Remove the plate from the tank, allow to stand for 30 minutes and then use immediately. Use as the mobile phase a mixture of 50 volumes of *butan-2-one*, 50 volumes of *xylene* and 4 volumes of *formamide*. Apply separately to the plate 2 µl of each of six solutions in a mixture of equal volumes of *chloroform* and *methanol* containing (1) 1.0% w/v of the substance being examined, (2) 1.0% w/v of *digoxin EPCRS*, (3) 0.020% of *digoxin EPCRS*, (4) 0.010% w/v of *digoxin EPCRS*, (5) 0.010% w/v of *digitoxin EPCRS* and (6) 0.010% w/v of *gitoxin EPCRS*.

After removal of the plate, dry it in a current of cold air until only the lower edge is still visibly moist. Repeat the development and dry the plate at 115° for 20 minutes. Allow to cool, spray with a mixture of 15 volumes of a 25% w/v solution of *trichloroacetic acid* in *ethanol (96%)* and 1 volume of a freshly prepared 3% w/v solution of *chloramine T* and heat at 115° for 5 minutes. Examine under *ultra-violet light (365 nm)*. Any spot corresponding to digitoxin in the chromatogram obtained with solution (1) is not more intense than the spot in the chromatogram obtained with solution (5). Any spot corresponding to gitoxin in the chromatogram obtained with solution (1) is not more intense than the spot in the chromatogram obtained with solution (6). Any other *secondary spot* in the chromatogram obtained with solution (1) is not more intense than the spot in the chromatogram obtained with solution (3) and not more than one such spot is more intense than the spot in the chromatogram obtained with solution (4).

Loss on drying When dried to constant weight over *phosphorus pentoxide* at a pressure not exceeding 2.7 kPa, loses not more than 1.0% of its weight. Use 0.5 g.

Sulphated ash Not more than 0.1%, Appendix IX A, Method II. Use the residue obtained in the test for Loss on drying.

Assay Dissolve 40 mg, heating if necessary, in sufficient *ethanol (96%)* to produce 50 ml and dilute 5 ml to 100 ml with the same solvent. To 5 ml of this solution add 3 ml of *alkaline trinitrophenol solution*, allow to stand in subdued light for 30 minutes and measure the *absorbance* of the resulting solution at the maximum at 495 nm, Appendix II B, using in the reference cell a mixture of 5 ml of *ethanol (96%)* and 3 ml of *alkaline trinitrophenol solution*. Calculate the content of $C_{41}H_{64}O_{14}$ from the *absorbance* obtained by repeating the operation using *digoxin EPCRS* in place of the substance being examined.

Storage Digoxin should be kept in a well-closed container and protected from light.

Preparations
Paediatric Digoxin Oral Solution
Digoxin Injection
Paediatric Digoxin Injection
Digoxin Tablets

Action and use Cardiac glycoside.

Dihydrocodeine Tartrate

$C_{18}H_{23}NO_3,C_4H_6O_6$ 451.5   5965-13-9

Dihydrocodeine Tartrate is 4,5-epoxy-3-methoxy-17-methylmorphinan-6-ol hydrogen tartrate. It contains not less than 98.0 per cent and not more than 101.0 per cent of $C_{18}H_{23}NO_3,C_4H_6O_6$, calculated with reference to the dried substance.

Characteristics Colourless crystals or a white, crystalline powder; odourless or almost odourless.

Solubility Soluble in 4.5 parts of *water*; sparingly soluble in *ethanol (96%)*; practically insoluble in *ether*.

Identification A. The *light absorption*, Appendix II B, in the range 230 to 350 nm of a 0.02% w/v solution exhibits a maximum only at 284 nm. The *absorbance* at 284 nm is about 0.72.
B. Add 10 mg, in powder, to 1 ml of *sulphuric acid* containing 0.05 ml of *formaldehyde solution*. A purple colour is produced (distinction from pholcodine).
C. Add 5M *ammonia* to a 2% w/v solution. No precipitate is produced.
D. Dissolve 10 mg in 0.05 ml of *nitric acid*. A yellow but no red colour is produced (distinction from morphine).
E. Dissolve 0.1 g in 1 ml of *sulphuric acid*, add 0.05 ml of *iron(III) chloride test-solution* and warm gently. A brownish-yellow colour is produced which does not become red on the addition of 0.05 ml of 2M *nitric acid* (distinction from codeine and morphine).
F. Yields *reaction B* characteristic of tartrates, Appendix VI.

Acidity pH of a 10% w/v solution, 3.2 to 4.2, Appendix V L.

Colour of solution A 10% w/v solution is not more intensely coloured than *reference solution BY_5*, Appendix IV B, Method II.

Specific optical rotation In a 5% w/v solution, −71.5° to −73.5°, Appendix V F.

Codeine To 0.1 g add 5 ml of *sulphuric acid (80%)* and 0.05 ml of *iron(III) chloride test-solution* and heat on a water-bath for 2 minutes. Any blue or green colour produced is not more intense than that produced when a mixture of 0.5 mg of *codeine phosphate* and 30 mg of *(+)-tartaric acid* is treated in the same manner, beginning at the words 'add 5 ml . . .'.

Morphine To 5 ml of a 2.0% w/v solution in 0.1M *hydrochloric acid*, add 2 ml of a 1% w/v solution of *sodium nitrite*, allow to stand for 15 minutes and add 3 ml of 5M *ammonia*. The *absorbance* of a 2-cm layer of the solution at 510 nm is not more than that obtained when 5 ml of a 0.0020% w/v solution of *anhydrous morphine* in 0.1M *hydrochloric acid* is treated in the same manner, Appendix II B.

Other foreign alkaloids Carry out the method for *thin-layer chromatography*, Appendix III A, using *silica gel GF254* as the coating substance and a mixture of 90 volumes of *dichloromethane*, 10 volumes of *methanol* and 1 volume of 13.5M *ammonia* as the mobile phase. Apply separately to the chromatoplate 10 μl of each of three solutions of the substance being examined in *water* containing (1) 2.0% w/v, (2) 0.020% w/v and (3) 0.010% w/v. After removal of the plate, allow it to dry in air and spray with *dilute potassium iodobismuthate solution*. Any *secondary spot* in the chromatogram obtained with solution (1) is not more intense than the spot in the chromatogram obtained with solution (2) and not more than one such spot is more intense than the spot in the chromatogram obtained with solution (3).

Loss on drying When dried to constant weight at 105°, loses not more than 0.5% of its weight. Use 1 g.

Sulphated ash Not more than 0.1%, Appendix IX A.

Assay Carry out Method I for *non-aqueous titration*, Appendix VIII A, using 0.5 g and *crystal violet solution* as indicator. Each ml of 0.1M *perchloric acid VS* is equivalent to 0.04515 g of $C_{18}H_{23}NO_3,C_4H_6O_6$.

Storage Dihydrocodeine Tartrate should be protected from light.

Preparations
Dihydrocodeine Injection
Dihydrocodeine Tablets

Action and use Analgesic.

Dihydroergotamine Mesylate

$C_{33}H_{37}N_5O_5,CH_4O_3S$ 679.8   6190-39-2

Dihydroergotamine Mesylate is (5′S)-5′-benzyl-9,10-dihydro-12′-hydroxy-2′-methylergotaman-3′,6′,18-trione methanesulphonate. It contains not less than 97.0 per cent and not more than 103.0 per cent of $C_{33}H_{37}N_5O_5,CH_4O_3S$, calculated with reference to the dried substance.

Characteristics Colourless crystals or a white or almost white, crystalline powder; odourless or almost odourless.

Solubility Slightly soluble in *water* and in *ethanol (96%)*; sparingly soluble in *methanol* and in *chloroform*.

Identification A. The *infra-red absorption spectrum*, Appendix II A, is concordant with the *reference spectrum* of dihydroergotamine mesylate.
B. The *light absorption*, Appendix II B, in the range 230 to 350 nm of a 0.01% w/v solution in *methanol* exhibits two maxima, at 281 nm and 291 nm, and a shoulder at 275 nm. The *absorbance* at 281 nm is about 1.0.
C. In the test for Related substances, the principal spot in the chromatogram obtained with solution (1) corresponds to that in the chromatogram obtained with solution (2).
D. Fuse 0.1 g with 0.5 g of powdered *sodium hydroxide* and moisten with *hydrochloric acid*. Sulphur dioxide is evolved which turns moistened *starch—iodate paper* blue.

Acidity pH of a 0.1% w/v solution, 4.4 to 5.4, Appendix V L.

Clarity and colour of solution Dissolve 0.1 g in 50 ml of a 0.014% w/v solution of *methanesulphonic acid*. The resulting solution is *clear*, Appendix IV A, and not more intensely coloured than *reference solution BY₇ or Y₇*, Appendix IV B, Method II.

Related substances Carry out the method for *thin-layer chromatography*, Appendix III A, protected from light, using *silica gel G* as the coating substance and a mixture of 50 volumes of *dichloromethane*, 50 volumes of *ethyl acetate*, 6 volumes of *methanol* and 1 volume of 13.5M *ammonia* as the mobile phase. Apply separately to the chromatoplate 5 µl of each of the following solutions freshly prepared in a mixture of 9 volumes of *chloroform* and 1 volume of *methanol*. Solution (1) contains 2.0% w/v of the substance being examined. Solutions (2), (3) and (4) contain 2.0% w/v, 0.010% w/v and 0.0040% w/v respectively of *dihydroergotamine mesylate BPCRS*. After removal of the plate, dry it in a current of cold air for not more than 1 minute, then repeat the development using freshly prepared mobile phase. After removal of the plate, dry it in a current of cold air and spray with a recently prepared 1% w/v solution of *4-dimethylaminobenzaldehyde* in a mixture of equal volumes of *hydrochloric acid* and *ethanol (96%)*. Warm the plate at 40° for 20 minutes and cool. Any *secondary spot* in the chromatogram obtained with solution (1) is not more intense than the spot in the chromatogram obtained with solution (3) and not more than two such spots are more intense than the spot in the chromatogram obtained with solution (4).

Loss on drying When dried to constant weight at 105° at a pressure not exceeding 14 Pa, loses not more than 4.0% of its weight. Use 0.5 g.

Assay Dissolve 10 mg in 2 ml of *methanol* and add sufficient of a 1% w/v solution of *(+)-tartaric acid* to produce 200 ml. To 3 ml add 6 ml of *dilute dimethylamino-benzaldehyde solution*, allow to stand in subdued light for 20 minutes and measure the *absorbance* of the resulting solution at 585 nm, Appendix II B, using in the reference cell a mixture of 3 ml of a 1% w/v solution of *(+)-tartaric acid* and 6 ml of *dilute dimethylaminobenzaldehyde solution*. Calculate the content of $C_{33}H_{37}N_5O_5,CH_4O_3S$ from the *absorbance* obtained by repeating the operation using 10 mg of *dihydroergotamine mesylate BPCRS* in place of the substance being examined and using the declared content of $C_{33}H_{37}N_5O_5,CH_4O_3S$ in *dihydroergotamine mesylate BPCRS*.

Storage Dihydroergotamine Mesylate should be kept in a well-closed container and protected from light.

Preparations
Dihydroergotamine Oral Solution
Dihydroergotamine Injection
Dihydroergotamine Tablets

Action and use Used in treatment of migraine.

Dihydroergotamine Tartrate

$(C_{33}H_{37}N_5O_5)_2,C_4H_6O_6$ 1317   *5989-77-5*

Dihydroergotamine Tartrate is (5′*S*,8*R*)-5′-benzyl-9,10-dihydro-12′-hydroxy-2′-methyl-3′,6′,18-trioxoergotaman tartrate. It contains not less than 98.0 per cent and not more than 101.0 per cent of $(C_{33}H_{37}N_5O_5)_2,C_4H_6O_6$, calculated with reference to the dried substance.

Characteristics Colourless crystals or a white or almost white, crystalline powder; odourless or almost odourless.

Solubility Very slightly soluble in *water*; sparingly soluble in *ethanol (96%)*; soluble in *pyridine*.

Identification A. The *light absorption*, Appendix II B, in the range 250 to 350 nm of a 0.01% w/v solution in *methanol* exhibits a principal maximum at 280 nm and negligible absorption at wavelengths greater than 320 nm. The *absorbance* at 280 nm is about 1.0.

B. Dissolve 1 mg in 1 ml of 5M *acetic acid* and add 1 ml of *dimethylaminobenzaldehyde reagent*. A dark blue colour is produced.

C. Yields the *reactions* characteristic of tartrates, Appendix VI.

D. *Melting point*, about 203°, with decomposition, Appendix V A, Method I.

Acidity pH of a 0.25% w/v suspension, 4.0 to 5.5, Appendix V L.

Clarity and colour of solution A freshly prepared 0.5% w/v solution in *ethanol (85%)*, prepared by warming carefully at 40°, is *clear*, Appendix IV A, and not more intensely coloured than *reference solution Y₆*, Appendix IV B, Method I.

Specific optical rotation In a 1% w/v solution in *pyridine*, −52° to −57°, Appendix V F.

Related substances Carry out the method for *thin-layer chromatography*, Appendix III A, using *silica gel G* as the coating substance and a mixture of 89 volumes of *chloroform*, 10 volumes of *absolute ethanol* and 1 volume of 13.5M *ammonia* as the mobile phase but allowing the solvent front to ascend 10 cm above the line of application. Apply separately to the chromatoplate 10 µl of each of three solutions of the substance being examined in a mixture of 95 volumes of *methanol*, 95 volumes of *chloroform* and 10 volumes of *pyridine* containing (1) 0.50% w/v, (2) 0.010% w/v and (3) 0.00250% w/v. After removal of the plate, allow it to dry in air and examine under *ultra-violet light (365 nm)*. No bluish fluorescence is visible in the chromatogram obtained with solution (1). Spray with *dimethylaminobenzaldehyde reagent*. Any *secondary spot* in the chromatogram obtained with solution (1) is not more intense than the spot in the chromatogram obtained with solution (2) and not more than one such spot is more intense than the spot in the chromatogram obtained with solution (3).

Loss on drying When dried to constant weight at 100° to 105°, loses not more than 5.0% of its weight. Use 0.1 g.

Assay Carry out Method I for *non-aqueous titration*, Appendix VIII A, using 0.3 g and *1-naphtholbenzein solution* as indicator. Each ml of 0.05M *perchloric acid VS* is equivalent to 0.03294 g of $(C_{33}H_{37}N_5O_5)_2,C_4H_6O_6$.

Storage Dihydroergotamine Tartrate should be kept in a well-closed container and protected from light.

Action and use Used in treatment of migraine.

Dihydrotachysterol

$C_{28}H_{46}O$ 398.7   67-96-9

Dihydrotachysterol is (5Z,7E)-(3S,10S)-9,10-secoergosta-5,7,22-trien-3-ol.

Characteristics Colourless crystals or a white, crystalline powder; odourless or almost odourless.

Solubility Practically insoluble in water; soluble in 20 parts of ethanol (96%), in 50 parts of arachis oil, in 0.7 part of chloroform and in 3 parts of ether.

Identification A. The light absorption, Appendix II B, in the range 230 to 350 nm of a 0.001% w/v solution in methanol exhibits three maxima, at 242, 251 and 261 nm. The absorbance at 242 nm is about 0.87, at 251 nm, about 1.0 and at 261 nm, about 0.65.
B. To 5 mg add 2 ml of antimony trichloride solution and warm in a water-bath. A red colour is produced.

Melting point 126° to 129°, Appendix V A. It may also occur in a form melting at about 113°.

Specific optical rotation In a freshly prepared 2% w/v solution in absolute ethanol, +100° to +103°, Appendix V F.

Tachysterol Absorbance of a 0.01% w/v solution in methanol at 280 nm, not more than 0.08, Appendix II B.

Loss on drying When dried over phosphorus pentoxide at a pressure not exceeding 0.7 kPa for 24 hours, loses not more than 0.2% of its weight. Use 1 g.

Sulphated ash Not more than 0.1%, Appendix IX A.

Storage Dihydrotachysterol should be kept in an atmosphere of nitrogen, protected from light and stored at a temperature not exceeding 15°.

Action and use Used in treatment of hypocalcaemia.

Dill Oil

Dill Oil is obtained by distillation from the dried ripe fruits of Anethum graveolens L.

Characteristics A clear, colourless or pale yellow liquid, visibly free from water; odour, characteristic of the crushed fruit.

Optical rotation +70° to +80°, Appendix V F.
Refractive index 1.481 to 1.492, Appendix V E.
Solubility in ethanol Soluble, at 20°, in 1 volume or more of ethanol (90%) and in 10 volumes or more of ethanol (80%), Appendix X M.
Weight per ml 0.895 to 0.910 g, Appendix V G.
Content of carvone 43.0 to 63.0% w/w, Appendix X L.
Storage Dill Oil should be kept in a well-filled, well-closed container, protected from light and stored at a temperature not exceeding 25°. It darkens in colour on storage.
Action and use Carminative.

Diloxanide Furoate

$C_{14}H_{11}Cl_2NO_4$ 328.2   3736-81-0

Diloxanide Furoate is 4-(N-methyl-2,2-dichloroacetamido)phenyl 2-furoate. It contains not less than 98.0 per cent and not more than 102.0 per cent of $C_{14}H_{11}Cl_2NO_4$, calculated with reference to the dried substance.

Characteristics A white or almost white, crystalline powder; odourless or almost odourless.

Solubility Very slightly soluble in water; slightly soluble in ethanol (96%) and in ether; soluble in 2.5 parts of chloroform.

Identification A. The infra-red absorption spectrum, Appendix II A, is concordant with the reference spectrum of diloxanide furoate.
B. The light absorption, Appendix II B, in the range 240 to 350 nm of a 0.0014% w/v solution in ethanol (96%) exhibits a maximum only at 258 nm. The absorbance at 258 nm is about 0.98.
C. Burn 20 mg by the method for oxygen-flask combustion, Appendix VIII C, using 10 ml of 1M sodium hydroxide as the absorbing liquid. When the process is complete, acidify the liquid with nitric acid and add silver nitrate solution. A white precipitate is produced.

Melting point 114° to 116°, Appendix V A.

Free acidity Shake 3 g with 50 ml of water, filter and wash the residue with three 20-ml quantities of water. Titrate the combined filtrate and washings with 0.1M sodium hydroxide VS using phenolphthalein solution as indicator. Not more than 1.3 ml is required.

Related substances Carry out the method for thin-layer chromatography, Appendix III A, using silica gel HF254 as the coating substance and a mixture of 96 volumes of dichloromethane and 4 volumes of methanol as the mobile phase. Apply separately to the chromatoplate 5 μl of each of two solutions of the substance being examined in chloroform containing (1) 10.0% w/v and (2) 0.025% w/v. After removal of the plate, allow it to dry in air and examine under ultra-violet light (254 nm). Any secondary spot in the chromatogram obtained with solution (1) is not more intense than the spot in the chromatogram obtained with solution (2).

Loss on drying When dried to constant weight at 105°, loses not more than 0.5% of its weight. Use 1 g.

Sulphated ash Not more than 0.1%, Appendix IX A.

Assay Dissolve 0.3 g in 50 ml of *anhydrous pyridine* and carry out Method II for *non-aqueous titration*, Appendix VIII A, using 0.1M *tetrabutylammonium hydroxide VS* as titrant and determining the end-point potentiometrically. Each ml of 0.1M *tetrabutylammonium hydroxide VS* is equivalent to 0.03282 g of $C_{14}H_{11}Cl_2NO_4$.

Storage Diloxanide Furoate should be protected from light.

Preparation
Diloxanide Tablets

Action and use Antiprotozoal.

Dimenhydrinate

$C_{17}H_{21}NO,C_7H_7ClN_4O_2$ 470.0   *523-87-5*

Dimenhydrinate is the diphenhydramine salt of 8-chlorotheophylline. It contains not less than 97.5 per cent and not more than 102.0 per cent of $C_{17}H_{21}NO,C_7H_7ClN_4O_2$, calculated with reference to the dried substance, when determined by both methods described under Assay.

Characteristics A white, crystalline powder; odourless or almost odourless.

Solubility Soluble in 95 parts of *water*, in 2 parts of *ethanol (96%)* and in 2 parts of *chloroform*; sparingly soluble in *ether*.

Identification A. The *infra-red absorption spectrum*, Appendix II A, is concordant with the *reference spectrum* of dimenhydrinate.
B. Dissolve 0.25 g in 15 ml of *ethanol (50%)*, add 15 ml of *water* and 2 ml of 1M *sulphuric acid* and cool in ice for 30 minutes. Dissolve 10 mg of the precipitate in 1 ml of *hydrochloric acid*, add 0.1 g of *potassium chlorate* and evaporate to dryness in a porcelain dish. A reddish residue remains, which becomes purple when exposed to the vapour of 5M *ammonia*.
C. Fuse 50 mg of the precipitate obtained in test B with 0.5 g of *anhydrous sodium carbonate*, boil with 5 ml of *water*, acidify to *litmus paper* with *nitric acid* and filter. The filtrate yields *reaction A* characteristic of chlorides, Appendix VI.

Melting point 102° to 107°, Appendix V A.

Related substances Carry out the method for *thin-layer chromatography*, Appendix III A, using *silica gel H* as the coating substance and a mixture of 80 volumes of *chloroform* and 20 volumes of *methanol* as the mobile phase. Apply separately to the chromatoplate 5 µl of each of two solutions of the substance being examined in *chloroform* containing (1) 4.0% w/v and (2) 0.020% w/v. After removal of the plate, allow it to dry in air and spray with *dilute potassium iodobismuthate solution*. Any *secondary*

spot in the chromatogram obtained with solution (1) is not more intense than the spot in the chromatogram obtained with solution (2).

Loss on drying When dried over *phosphorus pentoxide* at a pressure not exceeding 0.7 kPa for 24 hours, loses not more than 0.5% of its weight. Use 1 g.

Sulphated ash Not more than 0.2%, Appendix IX A.

Assay Dissolve 0.5 g in 100 ml of *water*, add 10 g of *sodium chloride* and 5 ml of 5M *sodium hydroxide* and extract with successive 20-ml quantities of *ether* until complete extraction is effected. Wash the combined extracts with two 5-ml quantities of *water*, extract the combined washings with two 10-ml quantities of *ether*, add the ether to the combined ether extracts and evaporate to about 10 ml. Add 15 ml of 0.1M *hydrochloric acid VS*, warm gently to complete the removal of the ether, cool and titrate the excess of acid with 0.1M *sodium hydroxide VS* using *methyl red solution* as indicator. Each ml of 0.1M *hydrochloric acid VS* is equivalent to 0.04700 g of $C_{17}H_{21}NO,C_7H_7ClN_4O_2$.

To 0.8 g add 50 ml of *water*, 3 ml of 5M *ammonia* and 6 ml of a 10% w/v solution of *ammonium nitrate* and warm on a water-bath for 5 minutes. Add 25 ml of 0.1M *silver nitrate VS*, warm on a water-bath for 15 minutes, shaking frequently, cool, add sufficient *water* to produce 200 ml and allow to stand for 16 hours. Filter, wash the residue with *water*, neutralise the combined filtrate and washings to *litmus paper* with *nitric acid*, add a further 3 ml of *nitric acid* and titrate the excess of silver nitrate with 0.1M *ammonium thiocyanate VS* using *ammonium iron(III) sulphate solution* as indicator. Each ml of 0.1M *silver nitrate VS* is equivalent to 0.04700 g of $C_{17}H_{21}NO,C_7H_7ClN_4O_2$.

Storage Dimenhydrinate should be kept in a well-closed container.

Preparations
Dimenhydrinate Injection
Dimenhydrinate Tablets

Action and use Antiemetic.

Dimercaprol ☆
B.A.L.

CH₂OH
|
CHSH
|
CH₂SH

$C_3H_8OS_2$ 124.2   *59-52-9*

Dimercaprol is 2,3-dimercaptopropan-1-ol. It contains not less than 98.5 per cent w/w and not more than 101.5 per cent w/w of $C_3H_8OS_2$.

Characteristics A clear, colourless or slightly yellow liquid; odour, alliaceous.

Solubility Soluble in 20 parts of *water* and in 18 parts of *arachis oil*; miscible with *ethanol (96%)* and with *benzyl benzoate*.

Identification A. Dissolve 0.05 ml in 2 ml of *water* and add 1 ml of *iodine solution*. The colour of the iodine is immediately discharged.
B. Dissolve 0.1 ml in 5 ml of *water* and add 2 ml of 0.5M *copper(II) sulphate*. A bluish-black precipitate is produced which quickly becomes dark grey.

C. In a stoppered glass tube suspend 0.6 g of *sodium bismuthate*, previously heated to 200° for 2 hours, in a mixture of 6 ml of *water* and 2.8 ml of a 10% w/w solution of *orthophosphoric acid*. Add 0.2 ml of the substance being examined, mix and allow to stand for 10 minutes shaking frequently. To 1 ml of the supernatant liquid add 5 ml of a 0.4% w/v solution of *chromotropic acid sodium salt* in *sulphuric acid*, mix and heat for 15 minutes in a water-bath. A violet-red colour is produced.

Acidity or alkalinity Dissolve 0.2 g in sufficient *carbon dioxide-free water* to produce 10 ml. Add 0.25 ml of *bromocresol green solution* and 0.3 ml of 0.01M *hydrochloric acid VS*. The solution is yellow and not more than 0.5 ml of 0.01M *sodium hydroxide VS* is required to change the colour of the solution to blue.

Clarity and colour The substance being examined is *clear*, Appendix IV A, and not more intensely coloured than *reference solution B$_6$* or *BY$_6$*, Appendix IV B, Method II.

Refractive index 1.568 to 1.574, Appendix V E.

Halides Boil 2 g under a reflux condenser for 2 hours with 25 ml of *ethanolic potassium hydroxide solution*. Remove the ethanol by evaporation in a current of warm air, add 20 ml of *water* and cool. Add a mixture of 10 ml of *hydrogen peroxide solution (100 vol)* and 40 ml of *water*, boil gently for 10 minutes, cool and filter rapidly. Add 10 ml of 2M *nitric acid* and 5 ml of 0.1M *silver nitrate VS* and titrate with 0.1M *ammonium thiocyanate VS* using 1 ml of a 10% w/v solution of *ammonium iron(III) sulphate* as indicator. Repeat the operation without the substance being examined. The difference between the titrations does not exceed 1.0 ml.

Assay Dissolve 0.1 g in 40 ml of *methanol* and add 20 ml of 0.1M *hydrochloric acid* and 50 ml of 0.05M *iodine VS*. Allow to stand for 10 minutes and titrate with 0.1M *sodium thiosulphate VS*. Repeat the operation without the substance being examined. The difference between the titrations represents the amount of iodine required. Each ml of 0.05M *iodine VS* is equivalent to 0.00621 g of $C_3H_8OS_2$.

Storage Dimercaprol should be kept in a well-filled, airtight container, protected from light and stored at a temperature of 2° to 8°.

Preparation
Dimercaprol Injection

Action and use Used in treatment of arsenic, gold and mercury poisoning.

Dimethicones ☆

$$Me\!-\!\!\begin{bmatrix} Me \\ | \\ Si\!-\!O \\ | \\ Me \end{bmatrix}_n\!\!-\!SiMe$$

Dimethicones are poly(dimethylsiloxanes) obtained by hydrolysis and polycondensation of dichlorodimethylsilane, $(CH_3)_2SiCl_2$, and chlorotrimethylsilane, $(CH_3)_3SiCl$. The various grades are distinguished by a number indicating the declared viscosity* which in terms of kinematic viscosity falls between 20 and 1000 mm^2 s^{-1}.

Characteristics Clear, colourless liquids; odourless.

Solubility Practically insoluble in *water* and in *methanol*; very slightly soluble in *absolute ethanol*; miscible with *butan-2-one*, with *carbon tetrachloride*, with *chloroform*, with *ether*, with *ethyl acetate* and with *toluene*.

Identification A. The *infra-red absorption spectrum*, Appendix II A, is concordant with the spectrum of *dimeticone EPCRS*. Disregard the region of the spectrum from 850 to 750 cm^{-1} since slight differences may be observed depending on the degree of polymerisation.
B. Gently heat 0.5 g in a test-tube until white fumes are evolved. Invert the test-tube over a second tube containing 1 ml of a 0.1% w/v solution of *chromotropic acid sodium salt* in *sulphuric acid* so that the fumes reach the solution. Shake the second tube for about 10 seconds and heat on a water-bath for 5 minutes. A violet solution is produced.
C. Prepare the *sulphated ash*, Appendix IX A, Method II, using 50 mg and a platinum crucible. The residue is white and yields the *reaction* characteristic of silicates, Appendix VI.
D. Comply with the test for Kinematic viscosity.

Acidity Shake 2 g with 25 ml of a mixture of equal volumes of *absolute ethanol* and *ether* and 0.2 ml of *aqueous bromothymol blue solution*. Not more than 0.15 ml of 0.01M *sodium hydroxide VS* is required to change the colour of the resulting solution to blue.

Kinematic viscosity At 25°, for Dimethicones having a declared kinematic viscosity of 50 mm^2 s^{-1} or less, 90 to 110% of the declared value; for Dimethicones having a declared kinematic viscosity of more than 50 mm^2 s^{-1}, 95 to 105% of the declared value, Appendix V H, Method II.

Heavy metals Dissolve 1.0 g in sufficient *chloroform* to produce 20 ml, add 1 ml of a freshly prepared 0.002% w/v solution of *dithizone* in *chloroform*, 0.5 ml of *water* and 0.5 ml of a mixture of 1 volume of 2M *ammonia* and 9 volumes of a 0.2% w/v solution of *hydroxylamine hydrochloride* and shake immediately for 1 minute. Any red colour produced is not more intense than that obtained by treating at the same time and in the same manner a mixture of 0.5 ml of *lead standard solution (10 ppm Pb)* and 20 ml of *chloroform* (5 ppm).

Mineral oils Place 2 ml in a glass tube and examine under ultra-violet light (365 nm). Any fluorescence produced is not greater than that of a solution containing 0.1 ppm of *quinine sulphate* in 0.005M *sulphuric acid* examined under the same conditions.

Phenylated compounds The *absorbance* of a solution of 5 g in 10 ml of *cyclohexane UV* in the range 250 to 270 nm is not more than 0.2, Appendix II B.

Labelling The label states the nominal kinematic viscosity in mm^2 s^{-1} in the form of a numerical suffix to the name of the product.

Dimethicones with a nominal viscosity of more than 50 mm^2 s^{-1} comply with the following additional test.

Volatile matter When heated at 150° for 2 hours in a dish 60 mm in diameter and 10 mm deep, lose not more than 0.3% of their weight. Use 1 g.

The title of the monograph in the European Pharmacopœia is Dimeticone.

*Dimethicones with a nominal viscosity of 50 mm^2 s^{-1} or less are intended for external use only.

Dimethyl Phthalate

C₁₀H₁₀O₄   194.2   *131-11-3*

$C_{10}H_{10}O_4$ 194.2   *131-11-3*

Dimethyl Phthalate contains not less than 99.0 per cent and not more than 100.5 per cent w/w of $C_{10}H_{10}O_4$.

Characteristics A colourless or faintly coloured liquid; odourless or almost odourless.

Solubility Slightly soluble in *water*; miscible with *ethanol (96%)*, with *ether* and with most organic solvents.

Identification A. The *infra-red absorption spectrum*, Appendix II A, is concordant with the *reference spectrum* of dimethyl phthalate.

B. Gently boil 1 g with 5 ml of 2M *methanolic potassium hydroxide* for 10 minutes, add 5 ml of *water*, evaporate the mixture to half its volume and cool. Add 1 ml of *hydrochloric acid*, filter, melt the dried precipitate in a small tube, add 0.5 g of *resorcinol* and 0.05 ml of *chloroform* and heat to about 180° for 3 minutes. Cool, add 1 ml of 5M *sodium hydroxide* and pour into *water*. An intense yellowish-green fluorescence is produced.

Acidity Mix 20 ml with 50 ml of *ethanol (96%)* previously neutralised to *phenolphthalein solution*. Not more than 0.1 ml of 0.1M *sodium hydroxide VS* is required to neutralise the solution using *phenolphthalein solution* as indicator.

Refractive index 1.515 to 1.517, Appendix V E.

Weight per ml 1.186 to 1.192 g, Appendix V G.

Related substances Prepare a 0.075% w/v solution of *phenyl benzoate* (internal standard) in *chloroform* (solution A). Carry out the method for *gas chromatography*, Appendix III B, using solutions of the substance being examined containing (1) 0.10% w/v in solution A, (2) 5.0% w/v in *chloroform* and (3) 5.0% w/v in solution A.

The chromatographic procedure may be carried out using a glass column (1.5 m × 4 mm) packed with *acid-washed, silanised diatomaceous support* (80 to 100 mesh) coated with 3% w/w of phenyl methyl silicone fluid (50% phenyl) (OV-17 is suitable) and maintained at 145°.

In the chromatogram obtained with solution (3) the ratio of the sum of the areas of any *secondary peaks* to the area of the peak due to the internal standard is not greater than the ratio of the area of the peak due to dimethyl phthalate to the area of the peak due to the internal standard in the chromatogram obtained with solution (1).

Sulphated ash Not more than 0.02%, Appendix IX A.

Water Not more than 0.1% w/w, Appendix IX C. Use 20 g.

Assay Carry out the method for the *determination of esters*, Appendix VIII L, using 1.5 g and 50 ml of 0.5M *ethanolic potassium hydroxide VS*. Each ml of 0.5M *ethanolic potassium hydroxide VS* is equivalent to 0.04855 g of $C_{10}H_{10}O_4$.

Action and use Insect repellent.

Dimethyl Sulphoxide

CH₃·SO·CH₃

C_2H_6OS 78.1   *67-68-5*

Characteristics A colourless liquid; odourless or almost odourless; hygroscopic.

Solubility Completely miscible with *water*, with *ethanol (96%)*, with *ether* and with most organic solvents; immiscible with paraffin hydrocarbons.

Identification Cautiously add 1.5 ml dropwise to 2.5 ml of *hydriodic acid* cooled in ice and filter rapidly. The residue, after drying at a pressure of 2 kPa, is an unstable, deep violet, crystalline solid with an unpleasant odour and which is soluble in *chloroform* producing a red solution.

Light absorption The *absorbance*, Appendix II B, after purging with dry nitrogen for 15 minutes and using *water* in the reference cell, is not more than 0.3 at 275 nm and not more than 0.2 at 285 nm and 295 nm. The absorption spectrum is smooth and shows no maxima in the range 270 to 350 nm.

Freezing point Not lower than 18.3°, Appendix V B.

Refractive index 1.478 to 1.479, Appendix V E.

Weight per ml 1.099 to 1.101 g, Appendix V G.

Dimethyl sulphone Carry out the method for *gas chromatography*, Appendix III B, using solutions in *acetone* containing (1) 0.050% w/v of *dimethyl sulphone* and 0.025% w/v of *dibenzyl* (internal standard), (2) 50% w/v of the substance being examined and (3) 50% w/v of the substance being examined and 0.025% w/v of the internal standard.

The chromatographic procedure may be carried out using a glass column (1.5 m × 4 mm) packed with *acid-washed diatomaceous support* (100 to 120 mesh) coated with 10% w/w of *polyethylene glycol adipate* and maintained at 165°.

In the chromatogram obtained with solution (3) the ratio of the area of the peak corresponding to dimethyl sulphone to that of the peak due to the internal standard is not greater than the corresponding ratio in the chromatogram obtained with solution (1).

Water Not more than 0.2% w/w, Appendix IX C. Use 10 g.

Storage Dimethyl Sulphoxide should be kept free from contact with plastics and protected from light and moisture.

Action and use Pharmaceutical aid.

Diphenhydramine Hydrochloride ☆

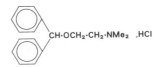

$C_{17}H_{21}NO,HCl$ 291.8   *147-24-0*

Diphenhydramine Hydrochloride is 2-benzhydryloxyethyldimethylamine hydrochloride. It contains not less than 99.0 per cent and not more than 101.0 per cent of $C_{17}H_{21}NO,HCl$, calculated with reference to the dried substance.

Characteristics A white or almost white, crystalline powder; odourless or almost odourless.

Solubility Soluble in 1 part of *water*, in 2 parts of *ethanol (96%)* and in 2 parts of *chloroform*; practically insoluble in *ether*.

Identification *Test A may be omitted if tests B, C, D and E are carried out. Tests B and C may be omitted if tests A, D and E are carried out.*

A. The *infra-red absorption spectrum*, Appendix II A, is concordant with the spectrum of *diphenhydramine hydrochloride EPCRS*.

B. The *light absorption*, Appendix II B, in the range 230 to 350 nm of a 0.05% w/v solution in *ethanol (96%)* exhibits three maxima, at 253, 258 and 264 nm. The A(1%, 1 cm) at 253 nm is about 12, at 258 nm, about 15 and at 264 nm, about 12.

C. To 0.05 ml of a 5% w/v solution add 2 ml of *sulphuric acid*; an intense yellow colour is produced which changes to cherry red on the addition of 0.5 ml of *nitric acid*. Add 15 ml of *water*, cool, add 5 ml of *chloroform* and shake; an intense violet colour is produced in the chloroform layer.

D. Yields the *reactions* characteristic of chlorides, Appendix VI.

E. *Melting point*, 168° to 172°, Appendix V A, Method I.

Acidity pH of a 5% w/v solution, 4.0 to 6.0, Appendix V L.

Clarity and colour of solution A 5.0% w/v solution in *carbon dioxide-free water*, and a fivefold dilution thereof, are both *clear*, Appendix IV A. The 5.0% solution is not more intensely coloured than *reference solution BY6*, Appendix IV B, Method II.

Related substances Carry out the method for *thin-layer chromatography*, Appendix III A, using *silica gel H* as the coating substance and a mixture of 80 volumes of *chloroform*, 20 volumes of *methanol* and 1 volume of *diethylamine* as the mobile phase, but allowing the solvent front to ascend 10 cm above the line of application. Apply separately to the chromatoplate 5 μl of each of two freshly prepared solutions of the substance being examined in *methanol* containing (1) 2.0% w/v and (2) 0.020% w/v. After removal of the plate, allow it to dry in air for 5 minutes, spray with *sulphuric acid* and heat at 120° for about 10 minutes until the spots appear. Any *secondary spot* in the chromatogram obtained with solution (1) is not more intense than the spot in the chromatogram obtained with solution (2).

Loss on drying When dried to constant weight at 100° to 105°, loses not more than 0.5% of its weight. Use 1 g.

Sulphated ash Not more than 0.1%, Appendix IX A, Method II. Use 1 g.

Assay Dissolve 0.25 g in 20 ml of *anhydrous glacial acetic acid*, add 10 ml of *mercury(II) acetate solution* and carry out Method I for *non-aqueous titration*, Appendix VIII A, using *crystal violet solution* as indicator. Each ml of 0.1M *perchloric acid VS* is equivalent to 0.02918 g of $C_{17}H_{21}NO,HCl$.

Storage Diphenhydramine Hydrochloride should be kept in a well-closed container and protected from light.

Preparations
Diphenhydramine Capsules
Diphenhydramine Oral Solution

Action and use Histamine H_1-receptor antagonist.

Diphenoxylate Hydrochloride

$C_{30}H_{32}N_2O_2,HCl$ 489.1   *3810-80-8*

Diphenoxylate Hydrochloride is ethyl 1-(3-cyano-3,3-diphenylpropyl)-4-phenylpiperidine-4-carboxylate hydrochloride. It contains not less than 98.0 per cent and not more than 101.0 per cent of $C_{30}H_{32}N_2O_2,HCl$, calculated with reference to the dried substance.

Characteristics A white or almost white powder; odourless or almost odourless.

Solubility Sparingly soluble in *water*; soluble in 50 parts of *ethanol (96%)*, in 40 parts of *acetone* and in 2.5 parts of *chloroform*; practically insoluble in *ether*.

Identification A. The *infra-red absorption spectrum*, Appendix II A, is concordant with the *reference spectrum* of diphenoxylate hydrochloride.

B. The *light absorption*, Appendix II B, in the range 230 to 350 nm of a 0.1% w/v solution in a mixture of 1 volume of 1M *hydrochloric acid* and 99 volumes of *methanol* exhibits three maxima, at 252, 258 and 264 nm. The *absorbance* at 252 nm is about 1.1, at 258 nm, about 1.3 and at 264 nm, about 1.0.

C. To 5 ml of a 0.1% w/v solution add 0.1 ml of *potassium mercuri-iodide solution*. A cream precipitate is produced.

D. Yields *reaction A* characteristic of chlorides, Appendix VI.

Melting point 221° to 226°, Appendix V A.

Related substances Carry out the method for *thin-layer chromatography*, Appendix III A, using *silica gel G* as the coating substance and a mixture of 92 volumes of *chloroform*, 5 volumes of *glacial acetic acid* and 3 volumes of *methanol* as the mobile phase. Apply separately to the chromatoplate 10 μl of each of two solutions of the substance being examined in *chloroform* containing (1) 5.0% w/v and (2) 0.050% w/v. After removal of the plate, allow it to dry in air and expose it to iodine vapour. Any *secondary spot* in the chromatogram obtained with solution (1) is not more intense than the spot in the chromatogram obtained with solution (2).

Loss on drying When dried to constant weight at 105°, loses not more than 0.5% of its weight. Use 1 g.

Sulphated ash Not more than 0.1%, Appendix IX A.

Assay Carry out Method I for *non-aqueous titration*, Appendix VIII A, using 0.6 g, adding 10 ml of *mercury(II) acetate solution* and using *crystal violet solution* as indicator. Each ml of 0.1M *perchloric acid VS* is equivalent to 0.04891 g of $C_{30}H_{32}N_2O_2,HCl$.

Action and use Antidiarrhoeal.

Diphenylpyraline Hydrochloride

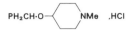

PH₂CH·O—⟨ ⟩NMe ,HCl

C₁₉H₂₃NO,HCl   317.9   *132-18-3*

Diphenylpyraline Hydrochloride is 4-benz-hydryloxy-1-methylpiperidine hydrochloride. It contains not less than 98.0 per cent and not more than 101.0 per cent of C₁₉H₂₃NO,HCl, calculated with reference to the dried substance.

Characteristics A white or almost white powder; odourless or almost odourless.

Solubility Soluble in 1 part of *water*, in 3 parts of *ethanol (96%)* and in 2 parts of *chloroform*; practically insoluble in *ether*.

Identification A. The *infra-red absorption spectrum*, Appendix II A, is concordant with the *reference spectrum* of diphenylpyraline hydrochloride.
B. Dissolve 10 mg in 10 ml of *sulphuric acid*; an orange solution is produced. To 5 ml of the solution add 0.2 ml of *potassium dichromate solution*, warm and allow to stand; the colour of the solution changes slowly from red to brown. Pour the remainder of the solution into about 10 ml of *water*; a colourless, opalescent solution is produced.
C. To 10 ml of a hot 1% w/v solution add dropwise *trinitrophenol solution* until precipitation is complete. The *melting point* of the precipitate, after recrystallisation from *ethanol (96%)*, is about 168°, Appendix V A.
D. Yields the *reactions* characteristic of chlorides, Appendix VI.
E. *Melting point*, about 206°, Appendix V A.

Related substances Carry out the method for *gas chromatography*, Appendix III B, using the following solutions. For solution (1) dissolve 45 mg of *dibenzyl* (internal standard) in sufficient *chloroform* to produce 100 ml. For solution (2) dissolve 0.20 g of the substance being examined in 20 ml of *water*, make the solution alkaline with 5M *ammonia* and extract with three 25-ml quantities of *chloroform*. Shake the combined extracts with 10 g of *anhydrous sodium sulphate*, filter, evaporate the filtrate to dryness at about 30° and dissolve the residue in 2 ml of *chloroform*. Prepare solution (3) in the same manner as solution (2) but dissolve the residue in 2 ml of solution (1).

The chromatographic procedure may be carried out using a glass column (1.5 m × 4 mm) packed with *acid-washed, silanised diatomaceous support* (80 to 100 mesh) coated with 3% w/w of *phenyl methyl silicone fluid (50% phenyl)* (OV-17 is suitable) and maintained at 165°. After allowing chromatography to proceed for three times the retention time of dibenzyl, increase the oven temperature to 240° to elute the diphenylpyraline from the column.

In the chromatogram obtained with solution (3) the sum of the areas of any *secondary peaks* is not greater than the area of the peak due to the internal standard.

Loss on drying When dried to constant weight at 105°, loses not more than 1.0% of its weight. Use 1 g.

Sulphated ash Not more than 0.1%, Appendix IX A.

Assay Carry out Method I for *non-aqueous titration*, Appendix VIII A, using 0.2 g, adding 5 ml of *mercury(II) acetate solution* and using *oracet blue B solution* as indicator. Each ml of 0.1M *perchloric acid VS* is equivalent to 0.03179 g of C₁₉H₂₃NO,HCl.

Action and use Histamine H₁-receptor antagonist.

Dipipanone Hydrochloride

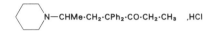

⟨ ⟩N—CHMe·CH₂·CPh₂·CO·CH₂·CH₃ ,HCl

C₂₄H₃₁NO,HCl,H₂O   404.0   *856-87-1*

Dipipanone Hydrochloride is 4,4-diphenyl-6-piperidinoheptan-3-one hydrochloride mono-hydrate. It contains not less than 99.0 per cent and not more than 101.0 per cent of C₂₄H₃₁NO, HCl, calculated with reference to the anhydrous substance.

Characteristics A white, crystalline powder; odourless or almost odourless.

Solubility Soluble in 40 parts of *water*, in 1.5 parts of *ethanol (96%)* and in 6 parts of *acetone*; practically insoluble in *ether*.

Identification A. Dissolve 20 mg in 5 ml of *water* and make alkaline to *litmus paper* with 2M *sodium hydroxide*. Extract with two 10-ml quantities of *chloroform*, evaporate the chloroform extracts and dry at 50° at a pressure not exceeding 0.7 kPa for 2 hours. The *infra-red absorption spectrum* of a thin film of the oily residue, Appendix II A, is concordant with the *reference spectrum* of dipipanone.
B. Dissolve 0.2 g in 10 ml of *water* and add 1 ml of *potassium mercuri-iodide solution*. A white precipitate is produced.
C. Dissolve 0.1 g in 10 ml of *water*, add 10 ml of a 1% w/v solution of *2,4,6-trinitrophenol* and 0.05 ml of *hydrochloric acid* and shake vigorously. The *melting point* of the precipitate, after recrystallisation from *ethanol (70%)* and drying at 105°, is about 141°, Appendix V A.
D. Yields the *reactions* characteristic of chlorides, Appendix VI.

Acidity pH of a 2.5% w/v solution, 4.0 to 6.0, Appendix V L.

Melting point 124° to 127°, determined on the undried substance, Appendix V A.

Related substances Carry out the method for *thin-layer chromatography*, Appendix III A, using a silica gel precoated chromatoplate (Merck silica gel 60 plates are suitable) and *methanol* as the mobile phase. Apply separately to the plate 5 µl of each of two solutions freshly prepared in *methanol* containing (1) 2.0% w/v of the substance being examined and (2) 0.020% w/v of *3-methyl-2,2-diphenyl-4-piperidinobutyronitrile BPCRS*. After removal of the plate, allow it to dry in air and expose to iodine vapour for 10 minutes. Any *secondary spot* in the chromatogram obtained with solution (1) is not more intense than the spot in the chromatogram obtained with solution (2).

Sulphated ash Not more than 0.1%, Appendix IX A.

Water 4.0 to 5.0% w/w, Appendix IX C. Use 0.5 g.

Assay Carry out Method I for *non-aqueous titration*, Appendix VIII A, using 0.8 g and determining the end-point potentiometrically. Each ml of 0.1M *perchloric acid VS* is equivalent to 0.03860 g of $C_{24}H_{31}NO,HCl$.

Preparation
Dipipanone and Cyclizine Tablets

Action and use Narcotic analgesic.

Diprophylline ☆

$C_{10}H_{14}N_4O_4$ 254.2   *479-18-5*

Diprophylline is 7-(2,3-dihydroxypropyl)-theophylline. It contains not less than 98.5 per cent and not more than 101.0 per cent of $C_{10}H_{14}N_4O_4$, calculated with reference to the dried substance.

Characteristics A white, crystalline powder.

Solubility Freely soluble in *water*; slightly soluble in *ethanol (96%)* and in *chloroform*; practically insoluble in *ether*.

Identification *Test A may be omitted if tests B, C and D are carried out. Tests C and D may be omitted if tests A and B are carried out.*
A. The *infra-red absorption spectrum*, Appendix II A, is concordant with the spectrum of *diprophylline EPCRS*. Examine as dispersions of 0.5 to 1 mg in 0.3 g of *potassium bromide IR*.
B. Dissolve 1 g in 5 ml of *acetic anhydride* and boil under a reflux condenser for 15 minutes. Allow to cool, add 100 ml of a mixture of 4 volumes of *petroleum spirit (boiling range, 50° to 70°)* and 1 volume of *ether* and cool in ice for not less than 20 minutes, with occasional shaking. Filter, wash the precipitate with the same solvent mixture and recrystallise from *ethanol (96%)*. The *melting point* of the crystals, after drying over *phosphorus pentoxide* at a pressure of 1.5 to 2.5 kPa, is 142° to 148°, Appendix V A, Method I.
C. Yields the *reaction* characteristic of xanthines, Appendix VI.
D. *Melting point*, 160° to 165°, Appendix V A, Method I.

Acidity or alkalinity To 10 ml of a 5.0% w/v solution in *carbon dioxide-free water* (solution A) add 0.25 ml of *bromothymol blue solution*. The solution is yellow or green and not more than 0.4 ml of 0.01M *sodium hydroxide VS* is required to change the colour of the solution to blue.

Clarity and colour of solution Solution A is *clear*, Appendix IV A, and *colourless*, Appendix IV B, Method II.

Heavy metals 12 ml of solution A complies with *limit test A for heavy metals*, Appendix VII (20 ppm). Use *lead standard solution (1 ppm Pb)* to prepare the standard.

Chloride Dilute 2.5 ml of solution A to 15 ml with *water*. The resulting solution complies with the *limit test for chlorides*, Appendix VII (400 ppm).

Related substances Carry out the method for *thin-layer chromatography*, Appendix III A, using *silica gel HF254* as the coating substance and a mixture of 90 volumes of *chloroform*, 10 volumes of *absolute ethanol* and 1 volume of 13.5M *ammonia* as the mobile phase. Apply separately to the chromatoplate 10 μl of each of the following freshly prepared solutions. For solution (1) dissolve 0.3 g of the substance being examined in sufficient *methanol (60%)* to produce 10 ml. For solution (2) dilute 1 volume of solution (1) to 100 volumes with *methanol*. For solution (3) dilute 1 volume of solution (1) to 500 volumes with *methanol*. For solution (4) dissolve 10 mg of *theophylline* in *methanol*, add 0.3 ml of solution (1) and dilute to 10 ml with *methanol*. After removal of the plate, allow it to dry in air and examine under *ultra-violet light (254 nm)*. Any *secondary spot* in the chromatogram obtained with solution (1) is not more intense than the spot in the chromatogram obtained with solution (2) and not more than one such spot is more intense than the spot in the chromatogram obtained with solution (3). The test is not valid unless the chromatogram obtained with solution (4) shows two clearly separated principal spots.

Loss on drying When dried to constant weight at 100° to 105°, loses not more than 0.5% of its weight. Use 1 g.

Sulphated ash Not more than 0.1%, Appendix IX A, Method II. Use 1 g.

Assay Dissolve 0.2 g in 3 ml of *anhydrous formic acid*, add 50 ml of *acetic anhydride* and carry out Method I for *non-aqueous titration*, Appendix VIII A, determining the end-point potentiometrically. Each ml of 0.1M *perchloric acid VS* is equivalent to 0.02542 g of $C_{10}H_{14}N_4O_4$.

Storage Diprophylline should be kept in a well-closed container and protected from light.

Action and use Xanthine bronchodilator.

Dipyridamole

$C_{24}H_{40}N_8O_4$ 504.6   *58-32-2*

Dipyridamole is 2,2′,2″,2‴-[(4,8-dipiperidino-pyrimido[5,4-*d*]pyrimidine-2,6-diyl)dinitrilo]-tetraethanol. It contains not less than 98.0 per cent and not more than 101.0 per cent of $C_{24}H_{40}N_8O_4$, calculated with reference to the dried substance.

Characteristics A bright yellow, crystalline powder; odourless or almost odourless.

Solubility Practically insoluble in *water*; freely soluble in *chloroform*; soluble in *ethanol (96%)*.

Identification A. The *infra-red absorption spectrum*, Appendix II A, is concordant with the *reference spectrum* of dipyridamole.

B. The *light absorption*, Appendix II B, in the range 220 to 450 nm of a 0.002% w/v solution in 0.01M *methanolic hydrochloric acid* exhibits three maxima, at 230, 285 and 405 nm. The *absorbance* at 230 nm is about 1.0, at 285 nm, about 1.3 and at 405 nm, about 0.28.

C. To 10 mg add 2 ml of *sulphuric acid* and 0.1 ml of *nitric acid*. An intense violet colour is produced.

Melting point 164° to 167°, Appendix V A.

Related substances Carry out the method for *thin-layer chromatography*, Appendix III A, using a silica gel precoated chromatoplate (Merck silica gel 60 plates are suitable) and *acetone* as the mobile phase. Apply separately to the plate 10 µl of each of two freshly prepared solutions of the substance being examined in a mixture of equal volumes of *chloroform* and *methanol* containing (1) 2.0% w/v and (2) 0.010% w/v. After removal of the plate, allow it to dry in air and spray thoroughly with a solution prepared by dissolving a mixture of 1 g of *iodine* and 3 g of *potassium iodide* in 10 ml of *ethanol (96%)* and adding 20 ml of 1M *sulphuric acid* and sufficient *water* to produce 100 ml. Any *secondary spot* in the chromatogram obtained with solution (1) is not more intense than the spot in the chromatogram obtained with solution (2).

Loss on drying When dried to constant weight at 120°, loses not more than 1.0% of its weight. Use 1 g.

Sulphated ash Not more than 0.1%, Appendix IX A.

Assay Dissolve 0.4 g in 70 ml of *anhydrous methanol* and titrate with 0.1M *perchloric acid VS* determining the end-point potentiometrically. Each ml of 0.1M *perchloric acid VS* is equivalent to 0.05046 g of $C_{24}H_{40}N_8O_4$.

Storage Dipyridamole should be protected from light.

Preparation
Dipyridamole Tablets

Action and use Antiplatelet aggregating agent.

Disodium Edetate ☆

NaO$_2$CCH$_2$\ /CH$_2$·CO$_2$Na
　　　NCH$_2$·CH$_2$N
HO$_2$CCH$_2$/ \CH$_2$·CO$_2$H

$C_{10}H_{14}N_2Na_2O_8,2H_2O$ 372.2   *139-33-3*

Disodium Edetate is disodium ethylenediamine-tetra-acetate dihydrate. It contains not less than 98.5 per cent and not more than 101.0 per cent of $C_{10}H_{14}N_2Na_2O_8,2H_2O$.

Characteristics A white, crystalline powder; odourless.

Solubility Soluble in 11 parts of *water*; slightly soluble in *ethanol (96%)*; practically insoluble in *chloroform* and in *ether*.

Identification A. The *infra-red absorption spectrum*, Appendix II A, is concordant with the spectrum of *disodium edetate EPCRS*.

B. Dissolve 2 g in 25 ml of *water*, add 2 ml of a 10% w/v solution of *lead(II) nitrate*, shake and add 3 ml of *potassium iodide solution*; no yellow precipitate is produced. Make alkaline to *litmus paper* with 2M *ammonia* and add 3 ml of a 4% w/v solution of *ammonium oxalate*; no precipitate is produced.

C. Dissolve 0.5 g in 10 ml of *water*, add 0.5 ml of a 10% w/v solution of *calcium chloride*, make alkaline to *litmus paper* with 2M *ammonia* and add 3 ml of a 4% w/v solution of *ammonium oxalate*. No precipitate is produced.

D. Yields *reactions A* and *B* characteristic of sodium salts, Appendix VI.

Acidity pH of a 5% w/v solution, 4.0 to 5.5, Appendix V L.

Clarity and colour of solution A 5.0% w/v solution in *carbon dioxide-free water* is *clear*, Appendix IV A, and *colourless*, Appendix IV B, Method II.

Iron Dissolve 0.25 g in 20 ml of *water*. 10 ml of the resulting solution complies with the *limit test for iron*, Appendix VII (80 ppm). Add 0.25 g of *calcium chloride* to both solutions before the mercaptoacetic acid.

Heavy metals 1.0 g complies with *limit test D for heavy metals*, Appendix VII (20 ppm). Use 2 ml of *lead standard solution (10 ppm Pb)* to prepare the standard.

Assay Dissolve 0.5 g in sufficient *water* to produce 300 ml and add 2 g of *hexamine* and 2 ml of 2M *hydrochloric acid*. Titrate with 0.1M *lead nitrate VS* using 50 mg of *xylenol orange mixture* as indicator. Each ml of 0.1M *lead(II) nitrate VS* is equivalent to 0.03722 g of $C_{10}H_{14}N_2Na_2O_8,2H_2O$.

Preparation
Trisodium Edetate Intravenous Infusion

Disopyramide

Ph
ᶦPr$_2$NCH$_2$·CH$_2$—C—CO·NH$_2$
　　　　　　　　|
　　　　　　　(N)

$C_{21}H_{29}N_3O$ 339.5   *3737-09-5*

Disopyramide is 4-di-isopropylamino-2-phenyl-2-(2-pyridyl)butyramide. It contains not less than 98.5 per cent and not more than 101.5 per cent of $C_{21}H_{29}N_3O$, calculated with reference to the dried substance.

Characteristics A white powder; odourless or almost odourless.

Solubility Slightly soluble in *water*; soluble in 10 parts of *ethanol (96%)*, in 5 parts of *chloroform* and in 5 parts of *ether*.

Identification A. The *infra-red absorption spectrum*, Appendix II A, is concordant with the *reference spectrum* of disopyramide.

B. The *light absorption*, Appendix II B, in the range 230 to 350 nm of a 0.004% w/v solution in 0.05M *methanolic sulphuric acid* exhibits a maximum only at 269 nm. The *absorbance* at 269 nm is about 0.8.

Related substances Carry out the method for *thin-layer chromatography*, Appendix III A, using *silica gel G* as the coating substance and a mixture of 80 volumes of *butan-1-ol*, 15 volumes of *water* and 5 volumes of 13.5M *ammonia* as the mobile phase; use the upper layer if the mixture separates. Apply separately to the chromatoplate 10 µl of each of two solutions of the substance being examined in *methanol* containing (1) 2.0% w/v and (2) 0.0050% w/v. After removal of the plate, allow it to dry in air and spray with *dilute potassium iodobismuthate solution*. Any *secondary spot* in the chromatogram obtained with solution (1) is not more intense than the spot in the chromatogram obtained with solution (2).

Loss on drying When dried at 80° at a pressure not exceeding 0.7 kPa for 2 hours, loses not more than 0.5% of its weight. Use 1 g.

Sulphated ash Not more than 0.2%, Appendix IX A.

Assay Carry out Method I for *non-aqueous titration*, Appendix VIII A, using 0.35 g and *1-naphtholbenzein solution* as indicator. Each ml of 0.1M *perchloric acid VS* is equivalent to 0.01697 g of $C_{21}H_{29}N_3O$.

Preparation
Disopyramide Capsules

Action and use Anti-arrhythmic.

Disopyramide Phosphate

$C_{21}H_{29}N_3O,H_3PO_4$ 437.5   *22059-60-5*

Disopyramide Phosphate is 4-di-isopropyl-amino-2-phenyl-2-(2-pyridyl)butyramide dihydrogen orthophosphate. It contains not less than 98.0 per cent and not more than 102.0 per cent of $C_{21}H_{29}N_3O,H_3PO_4$, calculated with reference to the dried substance.

Characteristics A white powder; odourless or almost odourless.

Solubility Soluble in 20 parts of *water* and in 50 parts of *ethanol (96%)*; practically insoluble in *chloroform*.

Identification A. Suspend 0.25 g in 50 ml of *chloroform*, add 2 ml of 13.5M *ammonia*, shake and filter through *anhydrous sodium sulphate*. Evaporate the filtrate to dryness using a rotary evaporator and dissolve the residue in 2 ml of *chloroform*. The *infra-red absorption spectrum* of the resulting solution, Appendix II A, is concordant with the *reference spectrum* of disopyramide.
B. The *light absorption*, Appendix II B, in the range 230 to 350 nm of a 0.005% w/v solution in 0.05M *methanolic sulphuric acid* exhibits a maximum only at 269 nm and a shoulder at 263 nm. The *absorbance* at 269 nm is about 0.8.
C. A 5% w/v solution yields the *reactions* characteristic of phosphates, Appendix VI.

Acidity pH of a 5% w/v solution, 4.0 to 5.0, Appendix V L.

Related substances Carry out the method for *thin-layer chromatography*, Appendix III A, using *silica gel G* as the coating substance and a mixture of 80 volumes of *butan-1-ol*, 15 volumes of *water* and 5 volumes of 13.5M *ammonia* as the mobile phase; use the upper layer if the mixture separates. Apply separately to the chromatoplate 10 µl of each of two solutions of the substance being examined in *methanol* containing (1) 2.6% w/v and (2) 0.0013% w/v. After removal of the plate, allow it to dry in air and spray with *dilute potassium iodobismuthate solution*. Any *secondary spot* in the chromatogram obtained with solution (1) is not more intense than the spot in the chromatogram obtained with solution (2).

Loss on drying When dried to constant weight at 105°, loses not more than 0.5% of its weight. Use 1 g.

Assay Carry out Method I for *non-aqueous titration*, Appendix VIII A, using 0.45 g and *1-naphtholbenzein solution* as indicator. Each ml of 0.1M *perchloric acid VS* is equivalent to 0.02188 g of $C_{21}H_{29}N_3O,H_3PO_4$.

Preparation
Disopyramide Phosphate Capsules

Action and use Anti-arrhythmic.

Disulfiram

$Et_2N \cdot CS \cdot S \cdot S \cdot CS \cdot NEt_2$

$C_{10}H_{20}N_2S_4$ 296.5   *97-77-8*

Disulfiram is tetraethylthiuram disulphide. It contains not less than 98.0 per cent and not more than 101.0 per cent of $C_{10}H_{20}N_2S_4$, calculated with reference to the dried substance.

Characteristics A white or almost white powder; odourless or almost odourless.

Solubility Practically insoluble in *water*; soluble in 65 parts of *ethanol (96%)*, in 2 parts of *chloroform* and in 20 parts of *ether*.

Identification A. The *infra-red absorption spectrum*, Appendix II A, is concordant with the *reference spectrum* of disulfiram.
B. In the test for Related substances, the principal spot in the chromatogram obtained with solution (2) corresponds to that in the chromatogram obtained with solution (3).
C. Dissolve 50 mg in 5 ml of *ethanol (96%)* and add 1 ml of *potassium cyanide solution*. A yellow colour is produced which becomes green and then darkens to bluish-green.

Melting point 70° to 73°, Appendix V A.

Acidity or alkalinity Shake 1 g with 30 ml of *carbon dioxide-free water* and filter. Not more than 0.1 ml of 0.1M *sodium hydroxide VS* or 0.1M *hydrochloric acid VS* is required to bring the pH to 7.0.

Diethyldithiocarbamate Dissolve 0.1 g in 10 ml of *chloroform*, add 10 ml of 0.1M *sodium hydroxide*, shake, discard the chloroform layer and wash the aqueous layer with three 10-ml quantities of *chloroform*. To the aqueous layer add 0.25 ml of a 0.4% w/v solution of *copper(II) sulphate* and 2 ml of *carbon tetrachloride*, shake and allow to separate. The lower layer is not more intensely coloured than *reference solution BY_4*, Appendix IV B, Method I.

Related substances Carry out the method for *thin-layer chromatography*, Appendix III A, using *silica gel GF254* as the coating substance and a mixture of 70 volumes of *hexane* and 30 volumes of *butyl acetate* as the mobile phase. Apply separately to the chromatoplate 10 µl of each of four solutions in *ethyl acetate* containing (1) 2.5% w/v of the substance being examined, (2) 0.025% w/v of the substance being examined, (3) 0.025% w/v of *disulfiram BPCRS* and (4) 0.050% w/v of *monosulfiram BPCRS*. After removal of the plate, allow it to dry in air and examine under *ultra-violet light (254 nm)*. In the chromatogram obtained with solution (1) any spot corresponding to monosulfiram is not more intense than the spot in the chromatogram obtained with solution (4) and any other *secondary spot* is not more intense than the spot in the chromatogram obtained with solution (2).

Loss on drying When dried to constant weight at 50° at a pressure not exceeding 0.7 kPa, loses not more than 0.5% of its weight. Use 1 g.

Sulphated ash Not more than 0.1%, Appendix IX A.

Assay Carry out Method I for the *determination of nitrogen*, Appendix VIII H, using 0.35 g and 8 ml of *nitrogen-free sulphuric acid*. Each ml of 0.05M *sulphuric acid VS* is equivalent to 0.01482 g of $C_{10}H_{20}N_2S_4$.

Storage Disulfiram should be kept in a well-closed container and protected from light.

Preparation
Disulfiram Tablets

Action and use Used in treatment of alcoholism.

Dithranol

$C_{14}H_{10}O_3$ 226.2   *1143-38-0*

Dithranol is 1,8-dihydroxyanthrone. It contains not less than 97.5 per cent and not more than 101.0 per cent of $C_{14}H_{10}O_3$, calculated with reference to the dried substance.

Characteristics A yellow to orange-yellow, microcrystalline powder; odourless or almost odourless.

Solubility Practically insoluble in *water*; slightly soluble in *ethanol (96%)* and in *ether*; soluble in *chloroform*; slightly soluble in fixed oils.

Identification A. The *infra-red absorption spectrum*, Appendix II A, is concordant with the *reference spectrum* of dithranol.

B. The *light absorption*, Appendix II B, in the range 240 to 450 nm of a 0.002% w/v solution in *chloroform* exhibits three maxima, at 255, 287 and 354 nm. The *absorbance* at 255 nm is about 1.1, at 287 nm, about 1.0 and at 354 nm, about 0.90.

C. *Melting point*, about 178°, Appendix V A.

Dihydroxyanthraquinone and dithranol dimer Not more than 3.0%, calculated as the sum of the amounts of dihydroxyanthraquinone and dithranol dimer, when determined by the following methods.

DIHYDROXYANTHRAQUINONE Carry out the method for *high-performance liquid chromatography*, Appendix III D, using solutions in *hexane* containing (1) 0.0010% w/v of *1,8-dihydroxyanthraquinone* and (2) 0.050% w/v of the substance being examined.

The chromatographic procedure may be carried out using (a) a stainless steel column (20 cm × 4.6 mm) packed with *stationary phase A* (10 µm) (Partisil is suitable), (b) a mixture of 100 volumes of *hexane*, 0.3 volume of *glacial acetic acid* and 0.075 volume of *absolute ethanol* as the mobile phase with a flow rate of 2 ml per minute and (c) a detection wavelength of 434 nm.

Calculate the amount of dihydroxyanthraquinone in the substance being examined.

DITHRANOL DIMER Carry out the method for *high-performance liquid chromatography*, Appendix III D, using solutions in *toluene* containing (1) 0.0010% w/v of *dithranol dimer BPCRS* and (2) 0.050% w/v of the substance being examined.

The chromatographic conditions described under the test for dihydroxyanthraquinone may be used but using a mixture of 100 volumes of *hexane*, 0.3 volume of *glacial acetic acid* and 0.2 volume of *absolute ethanol* as the mobile phase and a detection wavelength of 360 nm.

Calculate the amount of dithranol dimer in the substance being examined.

Loss on drying When dried to constant weight at 105°, loses not more than 0.5% of its weight. Use 1 g.

Sulphated ash Not more than 0.1%, Appendix IX A.

Assay Dissolve 0.2 g in 50 ml of *anhydrous pyridine* and carry out Method II for *non-aqueous titration*, Appendix VIII A, in an atmosphere of nitrogen using 0.1M *tetrabutylammonium hydroxide VS* as titrant and determining the end-point potentiometrically. Each ml of 0.1M *tetrabutylammonium hydroxide VS* is equivalent to 0.02262 g of $C_{14}H_{10}O_3$.

Storage Dithranol should be kept in a well-closed container and protected from light.

Preparations
Dithranol Ointment
Dithranol Paste

Action and use Used in treatment of psoriasis.

Docusate Sodium

Dioctyl Sodium Sulphosuccinate

$C_{20}H_{37}NaO_7S$ 444.6   *577-11-7*

Docusate Sodium is sodium 1,4-bis(2-ethyl-hexyl)sulphosuccinate. It contains not less than 98.5 per cent and not more than 100.5 per cent of $C_{20}H_{37}NaO_7S$, calculated with reference to the dried substance.

Characteristics White or almost white, waxy masses or flakes; odour, characteristic; hygroscopic.

Solubility Soluble in 70 parts of *water*, higher concentrations forming a thick gel; soluble in 3 parts of *ethanol (96%)*, in 1 part of *chloroform* and in 1 part of *ether*.

Identification A. The *infra-red absorption spectrum*, Appendix II A, is concordant with the *reference spectrum* of docusate sodium.

B. To 5 ml of a 0.1% w/v solution add 1 ml of 1M *sulphuric acid*, 10 ml of *chloroform* and 0.2 ml of *dimethyl yellow solution* and shake; a red colour is produced in the chloroform layer. Add 50 mg of *cetrimide* and shake; the chloroform layer is yellow.

Alkalinity Dissolve 1 g in 100 ml of *methanol (50%)* previously neutralised to *methyl red solution*. Not more than 0.5 ml of 0.1M *hydrochloric acid VS* is required to change the colour of the solution.

Heavy metals 12 ml of a 20% w/v solution in *ethanol (80%)* complies with *limit test A for heavy metals*, Appendix VII (10 ppm). Use *lead standard solution (2 ppm Pb)* to prepare the standard.

Chloride Dissolve 5.0 g in 50 ml of *ethanol (50%)* and titrate with 0.1M *silver nitrate VS* using *potassium dichromate solution* as indicator. Not more than 0.5 ml of 0.1M *silver nitrate VS* is required to change the colour of the solution.

Related non-ionic substances Dissolve 10 mg of *methyl docosanoate* (internal standard) in sufficient n-*hexane* to produce 50 ml (solution A). Carry out the method for *gas chromatography*, Appendix III B, using two solutions prepared in the following manner. For solution (1) dissolve 0.1 g of the substance being examined in 3 ml of n-*hexane* and 2 ml of solution A and pass it at a rate of about 1.5 ml per minute through a column 1 cm in diameter, packed with 5 g of *basic aluminium oxide* (Brockmann grade I is suitable) and prewashed with 25 ml of n-*hexane*. Elute with 5 ml of n-*hexane* and discard the eluate. Elute with 20 ml of a mixture of equal volumes of n-*hexane* and *ether*, evaporate the eluate to dryness and dissolve the residue in 2 ml of n-*hexane*. Prepare solution (2) in the same manner as solution (1) but dissolving the substance being examined in 5 ml of n-*hexane* and using a second column.

The chromatographic procedure may be carried out using a glass column (1.5 m × 4 mm) packed with *acid-washed, silanised diatomaceous support* (80-100 mesh) coated with 3% w/w of phenyl methyl silicone fluid (50% phenyl) (OV-17 is suitable) and maintained at 230°.

In the chromatogram obtained with solution (1) the area of any *secondary peak* with a retention time less than 2.5 times that of the internal standard peak is not greater than the area of the peak due to the internal standard.

Sodium sulphate Dissolve 0.25 g in 40 ml of a mixture of 8 volumes of *propan-2-ol* and 2 volumes of *water* and adjust to pH 2.5 to 4.0 by the addition of 1M *perchloric acid*. Titrate with 0.02M *barium perchlorate VS*, using 0.1 ml of a 0.2% w/v solution of *naphtharson* and 0.1 ml of a 0.0125% w/v solution of *methylene blue* as indicator, until the colour changes from yellowish-green to yellowish-pink. Not more than 1.8 ml is required (2.0%).

Loss on drying When dried to constant weight at 105°, loses not more than 3.0% of its weight. Use 1 g.

Assay To 3 g add 50 ml of hot *water* and stir until a paste is produced. Add, with stirring, two further 50-ml quantities of hot *water* and continue stirring until solution is complete. Cool and dilute to 1000 ml with *water*. To 25 ml of 0.01M *tetrabutylammonium iodide VS* add a solution containing 5 g of *anhydrous sodium sulphate* and 0.5 g of *sodium carbonate* in 50 ml of *water*, 25 ml of *chloroform* and 0.4 ml of *bromophenol blue solution*. Shake well until the chloroform layer is blue. Titrate with the solution of the substance being examined until about 1 ml from the end-point. Shake the stoppered flask vigorously for 2 minutes and continue the titration in 0.05-ml increments, shaking vigorously and allowing the flask to stand for about 10 seconds after each addition. Continue the titration until the chloroform layer is colourless. Each ml of 0.01M *tetrabutylammonium iodide VS* is equivalent to 0.004446 g of $C_{20}H_{37}NaO_7S$.

Storage Docusate Sodium should be kept in a well-closed container.

Preparation
Docusate Tablets

Action and use Faecal softener.

Dodecyl Gallate

$C_{19}H_{30}O_5$ 338.4   *1166-52-5*

Dodecyl Gallate is dodecyl 3,4,5-trihydroxy-benzoate.

Characteristics A white or creamy-white powder; odourless or almost odourless.

Solubility Practically insoluble in *water*; soluble in 3.5 parts of *ethanol (96%)*, in 2 parts of *acetone*, in 1.5 parts of *methanol*, in 60 parts of *propane-1,2-diol*, in 60 parts of *chloroform*, in 4 parts of *ether* and in 30 parts of *arachis oil*.

Identification A. The *light absorption*, Appendix II B, in the range 230 to 350 nm of a 0.002% w/v solution in *methanol* exhibits a maximum only at 275 nm. The *absorbance* at 275 nm is about 0.60.
B. Carry out the method for *gas chromatography*, Appendix III B, using a solution prepared in the following manner. Boil 0.5 g with 50 ml of 5M *sodium hydroxide* under a reflux condenser for 10 minutes, cool and extract with 50 ml of *ether*.

The chromatographic procedure may be carried out using a glass column (1.5 m × 4 mm) packed with *acid-washed, silanised diatomaceous support* (80 to 100 mesh) coated with 10% w/w of free fatty acid phase (Supelco FFAP is suitable) and maintained at 180°.

The principal peak in the chromatogram has the same retention time as that of *dodecan-1-ol*, examined under the same conditions.
C. Dissolve 5 mg in a mixture of 25 ml of *acetone* and 25 ml of *water* and add 0.05 ml of *iron(III) chloride solution*. A purplish-blue colour is produced which rapidly becomes bluish-black.

Acidity Dissolve 0.4 g in 50 ml of *acetone*, add 50 ml of *carbon dioxide-free water* and titrate with 0.1M *sodium hydroxide VS*, using *bromocresol green solution* as indicator, to the blue colour indicative of pH 5.0. Repeat the operation without the substance being examined. The difference between the titrations does not exceed 0.1 ml.

Melting point 96° to 97.5°, Appendix V A.

Chloride Shake 0.50 g with 100 ml of *water* at 60° for 10 minutes, cool and filter. 15 ml of the filtrate complies with the *limit test for chlorides*, Appendix VII (0.07%).

Sulphate Shake 0.25 g with 30 ml of *water* at 60° for 10 minutes, cool and filter. 15 ml of the filtrate complies with the *limit test for sulphates*, Appendix VII (0.12%).

Loss on drying When dried to constant weight at 70°, loses not more than 0.5% of its weight. Use 1 g.

Sulphated ash Not more than 0.1%, Appendix IX A.

Storage Dodecyl Gallate should be kept in a well-closed container and protected from light. Contact with metals should be avoided.

Action and use Antioxidant.

Domiphen Bromide

C₂₂H₄₀BrNO   414.5   *538-71-6*

Domiphen Bromide consists chiefly of dodecyl-dimethyl-2-phenoxyethylammonium bromide. It contains not less than 97.0 per cent and not more than 100.5 per cent of $C_{22}H_{40}BrNO$, calculated with reference to the dried substance.

Characteristics Colourless or faintly yellow, crystalline flakes.

Solubility Soluble in less than 2 parts of *water*, in less than 2 parts of *ethanol (96%)* and in 30 parts of *acetone*.

Identification A. The *light absorption*, Appendix II B, in the range 230 to 350 nm of a 0.04% w/v solution exhibits two maxima, at 268 nm and 274 nm. The *absorbance* at 268 nm is about 1.2 and at 274 nm, about 1.0.
B. Dissolve 10 mg in 10 ml of *water* and add 0.1 ml of a 0.5% w/v solution of *eosin* and 100 ml of *water*. An intense pink colour is produced.
C. Yields the *reactions* characteristic of bromides, Appendix VI.
D. *Melting point*, 106° to 116°, Appendix V A.

Acidity or alkalinity Dissolve 0.10 g in 10 ml of *carbon dioxide-free water* and add 0.5 ml of *bromothymol blue solution*. Add 0.5 ml of *bromothymol blue solution* to each of 10 ml of *phosphate buffer pH 6.4* (solution A) and 10 ml of *phosphate buffer pH 7.6* (solution B). The solution is not more yellow than solution A and not more blue than solution B.

Clarity and colour of solution Dissolve 1.0 g in 10 ml of *carbon dioxide-free water*. The solution is not more than *slightly opalescent*, Appendix IV A, and not more intensely coloured than *reference solution Y₇*, Appendix IV B, Method I.

Non-quaternary amines Carry out the Assay described below using a further 25 ml of the original solution and 10 ml of 0.1M *hydrochloric acid* in place of the 0.1M *sodium hydroxide*. The difference between the volume of 0.05M *potassium iodate VS* required in this titration and that required in the Assay is not more than 0.5 ml for each g of substance taken.

Loss on drying When dried to constant weight at 70° at a pressure not exceeding 0.7 kPa, loses not more than 1.0% of its weight. Use 1 g.

Sulphated ash Not more than 0.1%, Appendix IX A.

Assay Dissolve 2 g in sufficient *water* to produce 100 ml. Transfer 25 ml to a separating funnel and add 25 ml of *chloroform*, 10 ml of 0.1M *sodium hydroxide* and 10.0 ml of a freshly prepared 5% w/v solution of *potassium iodide*. Shake well, allow to separate and discard the chloroform layer. Wash the aqueous layer with three 10-ml quantities of *chloroform* and discard the chloroform solutions. Add 40 ml of *hydrochloric acid*, allow to cool and titrate with 0.05M *potassium iodate VS* until the deep brown colour is discharged. Add 2 ml of *chloroform* and continue the titration, shaking vigorously, until the chloroform layer no longer changes colour. Carry out a blank titration on a mixture of 10.0 ml of the freshly prepared potassium iodide solution, 20 ml of *water* and 40 ml of *hydrochloric acid*. The difference between the titrations represents the amount of potassium iodate required. Each ml of 0.05M *potassium iodate VS* is equivalent to 0.04145 g of $C_{22}H_{40}BrNO$.

Action and use Antiseptic detergent.

Dopamine Hydrochloride

C₈H₁₁NO₂,HCl   189.6   *62-31-7*

Dopamine Hydrochloride is 4-(2-aminoethyl)-pyrocatechol hydrochloride. It contains not less than 97.0 per cent and not more than 101.0 per cent of $C_8H_{11}NO_2$,HCl, calculated with reference to the dried substance.

Characteristics A white or almost white, crystalline powder; odourless or almost odourless.

Solubility Freely soluble in *water*; sparingly soluble in *ethanol (96%)*; practically insoluble in *chloroform* and in *ether*.

Identification A. The *infra-red absorption spectrum*, Appendix II A, is concordant with the *reference spectrum* of dopamine hydrochloride.
B. The *light absorption*, Appendix II B, in the range 220 to 350 nm of a 0.004% w/v solution in a 0.1% w/v solution of *sodium metabisulphite* exhibits a maximum only at 280 nm. The *absorbance* at 280 nm is about 0.55.
C. Dissolve 10 mg in 2 ml of *water* and add 0.05 ml of *iron(III) chloride test-solution*. An intense green colour is produced.

Acidity pH of a 4% w/v solution in a 1.0% w/v solution of *sodium metabisulphite*, 2.5 to 5.5, Appendix V L.

Clarity and colour of solution A 4.0% w/v solution is *clear*, Appendix IV A, and not more intensely coloured than *reference solution Y₇*, Appendix IV B, Method I.

Heavy metals Dissolve 2.0 g in 20 ml of *water*. 12 ml of the resulting solution complies with *limit test A for heavy metals*, Appendix VII (20 ppm). Use 10 ml of *lead standard solution (2 ppm Pb)* to prepare the standard.

Related substances Carry out the method for *thin-layer chromatography*, Appendix III A, using *silica gel G* as the coating substance and a mixture of 52 volumes of *chloroform*, 36 volumes of *methanol*, 7 volumes of *water* and 2 volumes of *formic acid* as the mobile phase. Apply separately to the chromatoplate 10 μl of each of two solutions in *methanol* containing (1) 2.0% w/v of the substance being examined and (2) 0.0033% w/v of *3,4-dimethoxyphenethylamine*. After removal of the plate, allow it to dry in a current of warm air and spray with a freshly prepared mixture of equal volumes of a 10% w/v solution of *iron(III) chloride hexahydrate* and a 5% w/v solution of *potassium hexacyanoferrate(III)*. Any *secondary spot* in the chromatogram obtained with solution (1) is not more intense than the spot in the chromatogram obtained with solution (2).

Readily carbonisable substances Dissolve 0.1 g in 5 ml of *sulphuric acid*. The solution is not more intensely coloured than *reference solution BY₃*, Appendix IV B, Method I.

Loss on drying When dried to constant weight at 105°, loses not more than 0.5% of its weight. Use 1 g.

Sulphated ash Not more than 0.1%, Appendix IX A.

Assay Carry out Method I for *non-aqueous titration*, Appendix VIII A, using 0.4 g and *crystal violet solution* as indicator. Each ml of 0.1M *perchloric acid VS* is equivalent to 0.01896 g of $C_8H_{11}NO_2,HCl$.

Storage Dopamine Hydrochloride should be kept in a well-closed container and protected from light.

Preparation
Dopamine Intravenous Infusion

Action and use Sympathomimetic.

Dothiepin Hydrochloride

$C_{19}H_{21}NS,HCl$ 331.9   1897-15-4

Dothiepin Hydrochloride is 3-(6*H*-dibenzo[*b*,*e*]-thiepin-11-ylidene)propyldimethylamine hydrochloride; it consists predominantly of the *E*-isomer. It contains not less than 98.0 per cent and not more than 101.0 per cent of $C_{19}H_{21}NS,HCl$, calculated with reference to the dried substance.

Characteristics A white to faintly yellow, crystalline powder; odourless or almost odourless.

Solubility Soluble in 2 parts of *water*, in 8 parts of *ethanol* (96%) and in 2 parts of *chloroform*; practically insoluble in *ether*.

Identification A. The *infra-red absorption spectrum*, Appendix II A, is concordant with the *reference spectrum* of dothiepin hydrochloride.
B. Dissolve 1 mg in 5 ml of *sulphuric acid*. A dark red colour is produced.
C. Burn 20 mg by the method for *oxygen-flask combustion*, Appendix VIII C, using a mixture of 15 ml of *water* and 1 ml of *hydrogen peroxide solution (20 vol)* as the absorbing liquid. The solution yields *reaction A* characteristic of sulphates, Appendix VI.
D. Yields *reaction A* characteristic of chlorides, Appendix VI.
E. *Melting point*, about 224°, with decomposition, Appendix V A.

Heavy metals Dissolve the residue obtained in the test for Sulphated ash in 0.5 ml of *hydrochloric acid*, evaporate to dryness, dissolve the residue in 2 ml of *water*, neutralise to *phenolphthalein solution* with *dilute sodium hydroxide solution* and dilute to 15 ml with *water*. 12 ml of the resulting solution complies with *limit test A for heavy metals*, Appendix VII (20 ppm). Use *lead standard solution (2 ppm Pb)* to prepare the standard.

Related compounds Carry out the method for *thin-layer chromatography*, Appendix III A, using *silica gel HF254* as the coating substance and a mixture of 90 volumes of *1,2-dichloroethane*, 10 volumes of *propan-2-ol* and 1 volume of 13.5M *ammonia* as the mobile phase. Apply separately to the chromatoplate 5 μl of each of three solutions in *chloroform* containing (1) 10.0% w/v of the substance being examined, (2) 4.0% w/v of the substance being examined and (3) 0.020% each of *11-(3-dimethylaminopropylidene)-6H-dibenzo[b,e]thiepin 5-oxide BPCRS* and *6H-dibenzo-[b,e]thiepin-11-one BPCRS*. After removal of the plate, allow it to dry in air and examine under *ultra-violet light (254 nm)*. In the chromatogram obtained with solution (3) the spot with the lower Rf value is more intense than any corresponding spot in the chromatogram obtained with solution (2). In the chromatogram obtained with solution (1) any *secondary spot* other than any spot corresponding to the spot with the lower Rf value in the chromatogram obtained with solution (3) is not more intense than the proximate spot in the chromatogram obtained with solution (3).

Z-isomer Carry out the method for *gas chromatography*, Appendix III B, using two solutions in *methanol* containing (1) 0.50% w/v of *dothiepin hydrochloride BPCRS* and (2) 0.50% w/v of the substance being examined.

The chromatographic procedure may be carried out using a glass column (1.8 m × 3 mm) packed with *acid-washed, silanised diatomaceous support* (100 to 120 mesh) coated with 3% w/w of cyanopropylmethyl phenyl methyl silicone fluid (OV-225 is suitable) and maintained at 200°.

In the chromatogram obtained with solution (1) a peak due to *Z*-dothiepin is present with a retention time of approximately 0.83 relative to the retention time of the principal peak which is due to *E*-dothiepin. In the chromatogram obtained with solution (2) the area of any peak corresponding to *Z*-dothiepin is not greater than 7.5% of the sum of the areas of the peaks due to *Z*-dothiepin and *E*-dothiepin.

Loss on drying When dried to constant weight at 105°, loses not more than 0.5% of its weight. Use 1 g.

Sulphated ash Not more than 0.1%, Appendix IX A. Use 1.5 g.

Assay Dissolve 0.6 g in 100 ml of *acetone*, add 15 ml of *mercury(II) acetate solution* and carry out Method I for *non-aqueous titration*, Appendix VIII A, using 3 ml of a saturated solution of *methyl orange in acetone* as indicator. Each ml of 0.1M *perchloric acid VS* is equivalent to 0.03319 g of $C_{19}H_{21}NS,HCl$.

Storage Dothiepin Hydrochloride should be kept in a well-closed container and protected from light.

Preparation
Dothiepin Capsules

Action and use Antidepressant.

In some countries the material described in this monograph may be known as Dosulepin Hydrochloride.

Doxapram Hydrochloride

$C_{24}H_{30}N_2O_2,HCl,H_2O$ 432.9   *7081-53-0*

Doxapram Hydrochloride is l-ethyl-4-(2-morpholinoethyl)-3,3-diphenyl-2-pyrrolidone hydrochloride monohydrate. It contains not less than 98.0 per cent and not more than 100.5 per cent of $C_{24}H_{30}N_2O_2,HCl$, calculated with reference to the dried substance.

Characteristics A white or almost white, crystalline powder; odourless or almost odourless.

Solubility Soluble in *water* and in *chloroform*; sparingly soluble in *ethanol (96%)*; practically insoluble in *ether*.

Identification A. The *infra-red absorption spectrum*, Appendix II A, is concordant with the *reference spectrum* of doxapram hydrochloride.
B. The *light absorption*, Appendix II B, in the range 230 to 350 nm of a 0.08% w/v solution exhibits three maxima, at 253, 258 and 265 nm. The *absorbance* at 253 nm is about 0.68, at 258 nm, about 0.80 and at 265 nm, about 0.65.
C. Yields the *reactions* characteristic of chlorides, Appendix VI.

Acidity pH of a 1% w/v solution, 3.5 to 5.0, Appendix V L.

Clarity and colour of solution A 2.0% w/v solution is *clear*, Appendix IV A, and *colourless*, Appendix IV B, Method I.

Related substances Carry out the method for *thin-layer chromatography*, Appendix III A, using a silica gel F254 precoated chromatoplate (Merck silica gel 60 F254 plates are suitable) and a mixture of 80 volumes of *propan-2-ol* and 20 volumes of 1M *ammonia* as the mobile phase. Apply separately to the plate 10 µl of each of four solutions in *methanol* containing (1) 6.0% w/v of the substance being examined, (2) 0.012% w/v of the substance being examined, (3) 0.030% w/v of *4-(2-chloroethyl)-1-ethyl-3,3-diphenyl-2-pyrrolidone BPCRS* and (4) 0.012% w/v of *1-ethyl-4-[2-(2-hydroxyethyl)aminoethyl]-3,3-diphenyl-2-pyrrolidone BPCRS*. After removal of the plate, allow it to dry in air, spray with *dilute potassium iodobismuthate solution* and examine immediately. In the chromatogram obtained with solution (1) any spot corresponding to 4-(2-chloroethyl)-1-ethyl-3,3-diphenyl-2-pyrrolidone is not more intense than the spot in the chromatogram obtained with solution (3) and any spot corresponding to 1-ethyl-4-[2-(2-hydroxyethyl)aminoethyl]-3,3-diphenyl-2-pyrrolidone is not more intense than the spot in the chromatogram obtained with solution (4). Any other *secondary spot* in the chromatogram obtained with solution (1) is not more intense than the spot in the chromatogram obtained with solution (2).

Loss on drying When dried to constant weight at 105°, loses 3.0 to 4.5% of its weight. Use 1 g.

Sulphated ash Not more than 0.1%, Appendix IX A.

Assay Carry out Method I for *non-aqueous titration*, Appendix VIII A, using 0.4 g, adding 7 ml of *mercury(II) acetate solution* and using *crystal violet solution* as indicator.

Each ml of 0.1M *perchloric acid VS* is equivalent to 0.04148 g of $C_{24}H_{30}N_2O_2,HCl$.

Storage Doxapram Hydrochloride should be kept in a well-closed container.

Preparation
Doxapram Injection

Action and use Respiratory stimulant.

Doxepin Hydrochloride

$C_{19}H_{21}NO,HCl$ 315.8   *1229-29-4*

Doxepin Hydrochloride is 3-(6*H*-dibenz[*b*,*e*]-oxepin-11-ylidene)propyldimethylamine hydrochloride; it consists of a mixture of *Z*- and *E*-isomers. It contains not less than 98.0 per cent and not more than 101.0 per cent of $C_{19}H_{21}NO,HCl$, calculated with reference to the dried substance.

Characteristics A white, crystalline powder; odour, slight and amine-like.

Solubility Soluble in 1.5 parts of *water*, in 1 part of *ethanol (96%)* and in 2 parts of *chloroform*.

Identification A. The *infra-red absorption spectrum*, Appendix II A, is concordant with the *reference spectrum* of doxepin hydrochloride.
B. The *light absorption*, Appendix II B, in the range 230 to 350 nm of a 0.008% w/v solution in 0.01M *methanolic hydrochloric acid* exhibits a maximum only at 297 nm. The *absorbance* at 297 nm is about 1.05.
C. Dissolve 5 mg in 2 ml of *nitric acid*. A red colour is produced.
D. Yields *reaction A* characteristic of chlorides, Appendix VI.

Melting point 185° to 191°, Appendix V A.

Heavy metals Dissolve the residue obtained in the test for Sulphated ash in 0.5 ml of *hydrochloric acid*, evaporate to dryness, dissolve the residue in 2 ml of *water*, neutralise to *phenolphthalein solution* with 2M *sodium hydroxide* and dilute to 15 ml with *water*. 12 ml of the resulting solution complies with *limit test A for heavy metals*, Appendix VII (20 ppm). Use *lead standard solution (2 ppm Pb)* to prepare the standard.

Z-Isomer 13.0 to 18.5% when determined by the following method. Carry out the method for *gas chromatography*, Appendix III B, using two solutions in *methanol* containing (1) 0.5% w/v of *doxepin hydrochloride BPCRS* and (2) 0.5% w/v of the substance being examined.

The chromatographic procedure may be carried out using a glass column (1.5 m × 4 mm) packed with *acid-washed, silanised diatomaceous support* (100 to 120 mesh) coated with 3% w/w of cyanopropylmethyl phenyl methyl silicone fluid (OV-225 is suitable) and maintained at 200°.

In the chromatogram obtained with solution (1) a peak due to *Z*-doxepin immediately precedes and is adequately separated from the principal peak which is due to *E*-doxepin. Measure the areas or heights of the peaks due to *Z*- and *E*-isomers in the chromatograms obtained with solutions (1) and (2) and calculate the content of *Z*-isomer in the substance being examined using the declared content of *Z*-isomer in *doxepin hydrochloride BPCRS*.

Loss on drying When dried to constant weight at 105°, loses not more than 1.0% of its weight. Use 1 g.

Sulphated ash Not more than 0.2%, Appendix IX A. Use 1.5 g.

Assay Dissolve 0.6 g in 100 ml of *acetone*, add 15 ml of *mercury(II) acetate solution* and carry out Method I for *non-aqueous titration*, Appendix VIII A, using 3 ml of a saturated solution of *methyl orange* in *acetone* as indicator. Each ml of 0.1M *perchloric acid VS* is equivalent to 0.03158 g of $C_{19}H_{21}NO,HCl$.

Storage Doxepin Hydrochloride should be protected from light.

Preparation
Doxepin Capsules

Action and use Antidepressant.

Doxycycline Hydrochloride ☆

$C_{22}H_{24}N_2O_8,HCl,\frac{1}{2}C_2H_5OH,\frac{1}{2}H_2O$ 512.9   *24390-14-5*

Doxycycline Hydrochloride is the hydrochloride hemihydrate hemiethanolate of (4*S*,4a*R*,5*S*,5a*R*,6*R*,12a*S*)-4-dimethylamino-1,4,4a,5,5a,6,11,12a-octahydro-3,5,10,12,12a-pentahydroxy-6-methyl-1,11-dioxonaphthacene-2-carboxamide, an antimicrobial substance obtained from oxytetracycline or methacycline or by any other means. The potency is not less than 880 Units per mg, calculated with reference to the anhydrous, ethanol-free substance.

Characteristics A yellow, crystalline powder; hygroscopic.

Solubility Soluble in 3 parts of *water* and in 4 parts of *methanol*; sparingly soluble in *ethanol (96%)*; practically insoluble in *chloroform* and in *ether*. It dissolves in aqueous solutions of alkali hydroxides and carbonates.

Identification A. Complies with the test for *identification of tetracyclines*, Appendix III A, using the following solutions. Solution (1) contains 0.05% w/v each of the substance being examined, *chlortetracycline hydrochloride EPCRS*, *demeclocycline hydrochloride EPCRS*, *oxytetracycline hydrochloride EPCRS* and *tetracycline hydrochloride EPCRS*. Solution (2) contains 0.05% w/v each of *chlortetracycline hydrochloride EPCRS*, *demeclocycline hydrochloride EPCRS*, *oxytetracycline hydrochloride EPCRS* and *tetracycline hydrochloride EPCRS*.
B. To 2 mg add 5 ml of *sulphuric acid*. A yellow colour is produced.

C. Yields *reaction A* characteristic of chlorides, Appendix VI.

Acidity pH of a 1% w/v solution, 2.0 to 3.0, Appendix V L.

Light absorption Prepare a 0.001% w/v solution in a mixture of 1 volume of 1M *hydrochloric acid* and 99 volumes of *methanol* and measure the *absorbance* at 349 nm within 1 hour of preparation, Appendix II B. The A(1%, 1 cm) at 349 nm is 300 to 335.

Specific optical rotation In a 1% w/v solution in a mixture of 1 volume of 1M *hydrochloric acid* and 99 volumes of *methanol*, −105° to −120°, Appendix V F. Measure the angle of rotation within 5 minutes of preparing the solution.

Fluorine Burn 0.30 g, in three equal portions, by the method for *oxygen-flask combustion*, Appendix VIII C, using a 1000-ml flask and a separate 20-ml portion of *water* as the absorbing liquid for each combustion, shaking the flask vigorously for about 15 minutes and transferring to the same 100-ml *Nessler cylinder*. Add 5 ml of *acid zirconyl alizarin solution* to the combined liquids, adjust the volume to 100 ml with *water* and allow to stand for 1 hour. The colour of the resulting solution is greater than that obtained by repeating the operation with no substance enclosed in the successive portions of filter paper burnt in the method for oxygen-flask combustion, but adding 3.0 ml of *fluoride standard solution (10 ppm F)* to the combined absorption liquids before adding the acid zirconyl alizarin solution.

Heavy metals 0.5 g complies with *limit test C for heavy metals*, Appendix VII (50 ppm). Use 2.5 ml of *lead standard solution (10 ppm Pb)* to prepare the standard.

Sulphur Burn 50.0 mg by the method for *oxygen-flask combustion*, Appendix VIII C, using a 1-litre flask and a mixture of 0.25 ml of *hydrogen peroxide solution (100 vol)* and 10 ml of *water* as the absorbing liquid. When the process is complete, shake the flask vigorously for about 15 minutes, transfer to a beaker, rinse the stopper, platinum wire, platinum gauze and sides of the flask with *water*, transfer the washings to the beaker and dilute to 15 ml with *water*. The solution complies with the *limit test for sulphates*, Appendix VII (0.1% of S).

Light-absorbing impurities Dissolve 0.1 g in sufficient of a mixture of 1 volume of 1M *hydrochloric acid* and 99 volumes of *methanol* to produce 10 ml. The *absorbance* at 490 nm, measured within 1 hour of preparing the solution, is not more than 0.07, Appendix II B.

Related substances Carry out in subdued light the method for *thin-layer chromatography* using the mobile phase and the chromatoplate prepared as described under the test for *identification of tetracyclines*, Appendix III A, but using 0.1M *disodium edetate* previously adjusted to pH 7.0 with 2M *sodium hydroxide* in place of the citro-phosphate buffer. Apply separately to the plate 1 μl of each of five solutions in *methanol* containing (1) 1.0% w/v of the substance being examined, (2) 0.010% w/v of *oxytetracycline hydrochloride EPCRS*, (3) 0.020% w/v of *6-epidoxycyline hydrochloride EPCRS*, (4) 0.020% w/v of *metacycline hydrochloride EPCRS* and (5) 0.010% w/v of *oxytetracycline hydrochloride EPCRS*, 0.020% w/v of *6-epidoxycyline hydrochloride EPCRS*, 0.020% w/v of *metacycline hydrochloride EPCRS* and 0.050% w/v of *doxycyline hyclate EPCRS*. Spray the plate evenly and very finely with a 5% w/v solution of *2,4,6-collidine*, freshly prepared at 5°, until traces of moisture appear (about 8 ml for a plate 200 mm × 200 mm in size) and if necessary allow to dry at room temperature before allowing the chromatography to proceed.

After removal of the plate, allow it to dry in air, expose it to ammonia vapour and examine immediately under *ultra-violet light (365 nm)*; the lamp and the conditions of visualisation used in the test should be sufficient to reveal the spots due to the reference substances.

In the chromatogram obtained with solution (1) any spots corresponding to oxytetracycline hydrochloride, 6-epidoxycycline hydrochloride and metacycline hydrochloride are not more intense than the spots in the chromatograms obtained with solutions (2), (3) and (4), respectively. The test is not valid unless the chromatogram obtained with solution (5) shows four clearly separated principal spots.

Ethanol 4.3 to 6.0% w/w of C_2H_6O when determined by the following method. Prepare a 0.05% v/v solution of *propan-1-ol* (internal standard) in *water* (solution A). Carry out the method for *gas chromatography*, Appendix III B, using the following solutions. For solution (1) dissolve 0.1 g of the substance being examined in sufficient of solution A to produce 10 ml. For solution (2) dissolve 0.1 g of the substance being examined in sufficient *water* to produce 10 ml. For solution (3) dilute 0.5 ml of *absolute ethanol* to 100 ml with solution A and dilute 1 ml of the resulting solution to 10 ml with solution A.

The chromatographic procedure may be carried out using a column (1.5 m × 4 mm) packed with porous polymer beads (80 to 100 mesh) (Porapak Q is suitable) and maintained at 135°.

Calculate the content of C_2H_6O taking as 0.790 g its weight per ml at 20°.

Sulphated ash Not more than 0.4%, Appendix IX A. Use 1 g.

Water 1.4 to 2.8% w/w, Appendix IX C. Use 1.2 g.

Assay Carry out the *biological assay of antibiotics*, Appendix XIV A. The precision of the assay is such that the fiducial limits of error are not less than 95% and not more than 105% of the estimated potency.

Storage Doxycycline Hydrochloride should be kept in an airtight container and protected from light. If it is intended for use in the manufacture of a parenteral dosage form, the container should be sterile, tamper-evident and sealed so as to exclude micro-organisms.

Labelling The label states (1) the date after which the material is not intended to be used; (2) the conditions under which it should be stored; (3) whether or not it is intended for use in the manufacture of a parenteral dosage form.

Preparation
Doxycycline Capsules

Action and use Antibacterial.

Doxycycline Hydrochloride intended for use in the manufacture of a parenteral dosage form complies with the following additional requirements.

Pyrogens Complies with the *test for pyrogens*, Appendix XIV K. Use per kg of the rabbit's weight 1 ml of *water for injections* containing 7.5 mg per ml of the substance being examined.

Sterility Complies with the *test for sterility*, Appendix XVI A.

The title of the monograph in the European Pharmacopœia is Doxycycline Hyclate.

Drostanolone Propionate

$C_{23}H_{36}O_3$ 360.5   *521-12-0*

Drostanolone Propionate is 2α-methyl-3-oxo-5α-androstan-17β-yl propionate. It contains not less than 97.0 per cent and not more than 103.0 per cent of $C_{23}H_{36}O_3$, calculated with reference to the dried substance.

Characteristics A white or almost white, crystalline powder.

Solubility Practically insoluble in *water*; soluble in *ethanol (96%)*; soluble in 2 parts of *chloroform* and in 20 parts of *ether*.

Identification A. The *infra-red absorption spectrum*, Appendix II A, is concordant with the *reference spectrum* of drostanolone propionate. If the spectra are not concordant dissolve a sufficient quantity in the minimum volume of *chloroform IR*, evaporate the chloroform, dry the residue at 40° at a pressure not exceeding 0.7 kPa for 1 hour and prepare a new spectrum of the residue.

B. Carry out the method for *thin-layer chromatography*, Appendix III A, using *silica gel G* as the coating substance and a mixture of 180 volumes of *cyclohexane*, 15 volumes of *ethyl acetate* and 5 volumes of *methanol* as the mobile phase. Apply separately to the chromatoplate 2 µl of each of the following three solutions in *chloroform*. Solutions (1) and (2) contain 0.25% w/v of the substance being examined and of *drostanolone propionate BPCRS* respectively. Solution (3) is a mixture of equal volumes of solutions (1) and (2). After removal of the plate, allow the solvent to evaporate, heat at 120° for 15 minutes and spray the hot plate with *ethanolic sulphuric acid (20%)*. Heat at 120° for a further 10 minutes, allow to cool and examine under *ultra-violet light (365 nm)*. The principal spot in the chromatogram obtained with solution (1) corresponds to that in the chromatogram obtained with solution (2). The test is not valid unless the principal spot in the chromatogram obtained with solution (3) appears as a single, compact spot.

C. *Melting point*, about 130°, Appendix V A.

Specific optical rotation In a 2% w/v solution in *chloroform*, +22° to +28°, Appendix V F.

Related substances Carry out the method for *thin-layer chromatography*, Appendix III A, using a silica gel F254 precoated chromatoplate (Merck silica gel 60 F254 plates are suitable) and a mixture of 90 volumes of *heptane* and 10 volumes of *ethyl acetate* as the mobile phase. Apply separately to the plate 10 µl of each of three solutions of the substance being examined in *chloroform* containing (1) 1.0% w/v, (2) 0.010% w/v and (3) 0.0050% w/v. After removal of the plate, allow it to dry in air, develop again over a path-length of 15 cm, remove the plate and allow it to dry in air. Heat at 120° for 15 minutes and spray the hot plate with *ethanolic sulphuric acid (20%)*. Heat at 120° for a further 10 minutes, allow to cool and examine under *ultra-violet light (365 nm)*. Any *secondary spot* in the chromatogram obtained with solution (1) is not more intense than the spot in the chromatogram obtained with solution (2) and not more than one such spot is more intense than the spot in the chromatogram obtained with solution (3).

Loss on drying When dried to constant weight at 40° at a pressure not exceeding 0.7 kPa, loses not more than 1.0% of its weight. Use 1 g.

Sulphated ash Not more than 0.1%, Appendix IX A.

Assay Carry out the method for *gas chromatography*, Appendix III B, using solutions in *chloroform* containing (1) 0.3% w/v of *cholesterol* (internal standard) and 0.2% w/v of *drostanolone propionate BPCRS*, (2) 0.2% w/v of the substance being examined and (3) 0.2% w/v of the substance being examined and 0.3% w/v of the internal standard.

The chromatographic procedure may be carried out using a glass column (1.5 m × 4 mm) packed with *acid- and alkali-washed, silanised, diatomaceous support* (100 to 120 mesh) coated with 3% w/v of dimethyl silicone fluid (OV-101 is suitable) and maintained at 240°.

Calculate the content of $C_{23}H_{36}O_3$ using the declared content of $C_{23}H_{36}O_3$ in *drostanolone propionate BPCRS*.

Storage Drostanolone Propionate should be kept in a well-closed container and protected from light.

Preparation
Drostanolone Injection

Action and use Androgen.

Dydrogesterone

$C_{21}H_{28}O_2$ 312.5   *152-62-5*

Dydrogesterone is 9β,10α-pregna-4,6-diene-3,20-dione. It contains not less than 97.0 per cent and not more than 103.0 per cent of $C_{21}H_{28}O_2$, calculated with reference to the dried substance.

Characteristics A white or almost white, crystalline powder; odourless or almost odourless.

Solubility Practically insoluble in *water*; soluble in 52 parts of *ethanol (96%)*, in 17 parts of *acetone*, in 2 parts of *chloroform* and in 40 parts of *methanol*; slightly soluble in *ether* and in fixed oils.

Identification A. The *infra-red absorption spectrum*, Appendix II A, is concordant with the *reference spectrum* of dydrogesterone.
B. Complies with the test for *identification of steroids*, Appendix III A, using *impregnating solvent II* and *mobile phase E*.

Light absorption The *light absorption*, Appendix II B, in the range 230 to 350 nm of the solution obtained in the Assay exhibits a maximum only at 286 nm. The ratio of the *absorbance* at 240 nm to that at the maximum at 286 nm is not more than 0.12.

Melting point 167° to 171°, Appendix V A.

Specific optical rotation In a 1% w/v solution in *1,4-dioxan*, −446° to −464°, Appendix V F.

Related substances Carry out the method for *gas chromatography*, Appendix III B, using three solutions in *chloroform* containing (1) 0.040% w/v of the substance being examined and 0.020% w/v of *1,2,3,4-tetraphenyl-cyclopenta-1,3-diene* (internal standard), (2) 2.0% w/v of the substance being examined and (3) 2.0% w/v of substance being examined and 0.020% w/v of the internal standard.

The chromatographic procedure may be carried out using a glass column (1.5 m × 2.5 mm) packed with *acid-washed, silanised diatomaceous support* (100 to 120 mesh) coated with 3% w/w of cyanopropyl methyl silicone fluid (SP-2300 is suitable) and maintained at 240°.

In the chromatogram obtained with solution (3) the ratio of the sum of the areas of any *secondary peaks* to the area of the peak due to the internal standard is not greater than the ratio of the area of the peak due to the substance being examined to the area of the peak due to the internal standard in the chromatogram obtained with solution (1).

Loss on drying When dried at 105° for 3 hours, loses not more than 0.5% of its weight. Use 1 g.

Sulphated ash Not more than 0.1%, Appendix IX A.

Assay Dissolve 40 mg in sufficient *methanol* to produce 200 ml, dilute 5 ml to 100 ml with *methanol* and measure the *absorbance* of the resulting solution at the maximum at 286 nm, Appendix II B. Calculate the content of $C_{21}H_{28}O_2$ taking 845 as the value of A(1%, 1 cm) at the maximum at 286 nm.

Storage Dydrogesterone should be kept in a well-closed container and protected from light.

Preparation
Dydrogesterone Tablets

Action and use Progestogen.

Econazole Nitrate

$C_{18}H_{15}Cl_3N_2O,HNO_3$ 444.7   *68797-31-9*

Econazole Nitrate is 1-[2,4-dichloro-β-(*p*-chloro-benzyloxy)phenethyl]imidazole nitrate. It contains not less than 98.5 per cent and not more than 101.0 per cent of $C_{18}H_{15}Cl_3N_2O$, HNO_3, calculated with reference to the dried substance.

Characteristics A white or almost white, crystalline powder; odourless or almost odourless.

Solubility Very slightly soluble in *water* and in *ether*; slightly soluble in *ethanol (96%)*; soluble in 60 parts of *chloroform* and in 25 parts of *methanol*.

Identification A. The *infra-red absorption spectrum*, Appendix II A, is concordant with the *reference spectrum* of econazole nitrate.

B. The *light absorption*, Appendix II B, in the range 230 to 350 nm of a 0.08% w/v solution in a mixture of 1 volume of 0.1M *hydrochloric acid* and 9 volumes of *methanol* exhibits maxima at 265, 271 and 280 nm. The *absorbance* at 265 nm is about 0.84, at 271 nm, about 0.86 and at 280 nm, about 0.52.
C. Shake 10 mg with 5 ml of *water* and cool the resulting suspension in ice. Keeping the suspension cool, add 0.4 ml of a 10% w/v solution of *potassium chloride* and 0.1 ml of *diphenylamine solution* and dropwise, with shaking, 5 ml of *sulphuric acid*. An intense blue colour is produced.
D. *Melting point*, about 164°, with decomposition, Appendix V A.

Related substances Carry out the method for *thin-layer chromatography*, Appendix III A, using *silica gel G* as the coating substance and a mixture of 70 volumes of *chloroform*, 20 volumes of *methanol* and 10 volumes of an 85% w/v solution of *formic acid* as the mobile phase. Apply separately to the chromatoplate 20 µl of each of two solutions of the substance being examined in *methanol* containing (1) 2.0% w/v and (2) 0.0075% w/v. After removal of the plate, allow it to dry in air and expose to iodine vapour for 1 hour. Any *secondary spot* in the chromatogram obtained with solution (1) is not more intense than the spot in the chromatogram obtained with solution (2).

Loss on drying When dried to constant weight at 105°, loses not more than 0.5% of its weight. Use 1 g.

Sulphated ash Not more than 0.1%, Appendix IX A.

Assay Carry out Method I for *non-aqueous titration*, Appendix VIII A, using 0.4 g and determining the end-point potentiometrically. Each ml of 0.1M *perchloric acid VS* is equivalent to 0.04447 g of $C_{18}H_{15}Cl_3N_2O,HNO_3$.

Storage Econazole Nitrate should be kept in a well-closed container and protected from light.

Preparations
Econazole Cream
Econazole Pessaries

Action and use Antifungal.

Ecothiopate Iodide

Me₃ÑCH₂·CH₂·SP(OEt)₂   I⁻

$C_9H_{23}INO_3PS$ 383.2   *513-10-0*

Ecothiopate Iodide is (2-diethoxyphosphinyl-thioethyl)trimethylammonium iodide. It contains not less than 92.5 per cent and not more than 100.5 per cent of $C_9H_{23}INO_3PS$.

Characteristics A white, crystalline powder; odour, alliaceous; hygroscopic.

Solubility Soluble in 1 part of *water*, in 25 parts of *ethanol* (96%) and in 3 parts of *methanol*; practically insoluble in other organic solvents.

Identification A. Carry out the method for *thin-layer chromatography*, Appendix III A, using a sandwich chamber. Use *silica gel G* as the coating substance and a mixture of 40 volumes of *absolute ethanol*, 40 volumes of *water* and 20 volumes of 13.5M *ammonia* as the mobile phase. Apply separately to the chromatoplate 1 µl of each of two solutions in *water* containing (1) 0.25% w/v of the substance being examined and (2) 0.25% w/v of *ecothiopate iodide BPCRS*. After removal of the plate, allow it to dry in air and expose to iodine vapour overnight. The principal spot in the chromatogram obtained with solution (1) corresponds to that in the chromatogram obtained with solution (2).
B. Dissolve 0.1 g in 2 ml of *water* and add 1 ml of *nitric acid*; a brown precipitate of iodine is produced. To 0.05 ml of the mixture add 1 ml of *carbon tetrachloride* and shake; a pink colour is produced in the carbon tetrachloride layer.
C. Heat the remainder of the mixture obtained in test B until colourless, cool and dilute with *water* to 10 ml. The resulting solution yields the *reactions* characteristic of phosphates and of sulphates, Appendix VI.
D. *Melting point*, about 119°, with decomposition, Appendix V A.

Loss on drying When dried at 50° at a pressure not exceeding 0.7 kPa for 3 hours, loses not more than 1.0% of its weight. Use 1 g.

Assay Dissolve 0.12 g in sufficient *water* to produce 100 ml. To 25 ml add 2 ml of 1.25M *sodium hydroxide* and allow to stand for 30 minutes. Add 2 ml of *glacial acetic acid* and titrate with 0.02M *iodine VS* using *starch mucilage* as indicator. To a further 25 ml add 2 ml of *glacial acetic acid* and titrate with 0.02M *iodine VS* using *starch mucilage* as indicator. The difference between the titrations represents the amount of iodine required. Each ml of 0.02M *iodine VS* is equivalent to 0.01533 g of $C_9H_{23}INO_3PS$.

Storage Ecothiopate Iodide should be kept in a well-closed container, protected from light and stored at a temperature of 2° to 8°.

Action and use Used in treatment of glaucoma.

Edrophonium Chloride

$C_{10}H_{16}ClNO$ 201.7   *116-38-1*

Edrophonium Chloride is ethyl(3-hydroxyphenyl)dimethylammonium chloride. It contains not less than 98.5 per cent and not more than 101.0 per cent of $C_{10}H_{16}ClNO$, calculated with reference to the dried substance.

Characteristics A white, crystalline powder; odourless or almost odourless.

Solubility Soluble in 0.5 part of *water* and in 5 parts of *ethanol* (96%); practically insoluble in *chloroform* and in *ether*.

Identification A. The *infra-red absorption spectrum*, Appendix II A, is concordant with the *reference spectrum* of edrophonium chloride.
B. The *light absorption*, Appendix II B, in the range 220 to 350 nm of a 0.01% w/v solution in 0.1M *hydrochloric acid*

VS exhibits a maximum only at 273 nm. The *absorbance* at 273 nm is about 1.1.

C. Dissolve 50 mg in 2 ml of *water* and add 0.05 ml of *iron(III) chloride test-solution*. A reddish-violet colour is produced.

D. Yields the *reactions* characteristic of chlorides, Appendix VI.

E. *Melting point*, about 168°, with decomposition, Appendix V A.

Dimethylaminophenol Dissolve 0.1 g in 10 ml of *water*, add 5 ml of *phosphate buffer pH 8.0* and extract with two 20-ml quantities of *chloroform*. Wash the extracts successively with two 10-ml quantities of *water*, extract with 10 ml of 0.1M *sodium hydroxide* and discard the chloroform. The *absorbance* of the resulting solution at 293 nm is not greater than 0.25, Appendix II B.

Loss on drying When dried over *phosphorus pentoxide* at a pressure not exceeding 0.7 kPa for 24 hours, loses not more than 0.5% of its weight. Use 1 g.

Sulphated ash Not more than 0.1%, Appendix IX A.

Assay Carry out Method I for *non-aqueous titration*, Appendix VIII A, using 0.6 g, adding 20 ml of *mercury(II) acetate solution* and using a 0.1% w/v solution of *quinaldine red* in *absolute ethanol* as indicator. Each ml of 0.1M *perchloric acid VS* is equivalent to 0.02017 g of $C_{10}H_{16}ClNO$.

Storage Edrophonium Chloride should be kept in a well-closed container and protected from light.

Preparation
Edrophonium Injection

Action and use Anticholinesterase.

Emetine Hydrochloride ☆

$C_{29}H_{40}N_2O_4,2HCl,7H_2O$ 679.7   *316-42-7 (anhydrous)*

Emetine Hydrochloride is 6′,7′,10,11-tetra-methoxyemetan dihydrochloride heptahydrate. It contains not less than 98.0 per cent and not more than 102.0 per cent of $C_{29}H_{40}N_2O_4,2HCl$, calculated with reference to the dried substance.

Characteristics A white or slightly yellow, crystalline powder; odourless.

Solubility Freely soluble in *water*, in *ethanol (96%)* and in *chloroform*.

Identification *Test A may be omitted if tests B, C, D and E are carried out. Tests B, C and D may be omitted if tests A and E are carried out.*

A. The *infra-red absorption spectrum*, Appendix II A, is concordant with the spectrum of *emetine hydrochloride EPCRS*.

B. In the test for Other alkaloids, the principal spot in the chromatogram obtained with solution (1) corresponds to that in the chromatogram obtained with solution (5).

C. Dissolve 10 mg in 2 ml of *hydrogen peroxide solution (10 vol)*, add 1 ml of *hydrochloric acid* and heat. An orange colour is produced.

D. Sprinkle 5 mg on the surface of 1 ml of a 5% w/v solution of *ammonium molybdate* in *sulphuric acid*. A bright green colour is produced.

E. Yields *reaction A* characteristic of chlorides, Appendix VI.

Acidity pH of a 2% w/v solution, 4.0 to 6.0, Appendix V L.

Clarity and colour of solution A 5.0% w/v solution is *clear*, Appendix IV A, and not more intensely coloured than *reference solution Y_5 or BY_5*, Appendix IV B, Method II.

Specific optical rotation In a solution prepared by dissolving a quantity of the substance being examined equivalent to 1.25 g of the dried substance in sufficient *water* to produce 25 ml, +16° to +19°, Appendix V F.

Other alkaloids Carry out the method for *thin-layer chromatography*, Appendix III A, using *silica gel G* as the coating substance and a mixture of 200 volumes of *chloroform*, 40 volumes of *2-methoxyethanol*, 10 volumes of *methanol*, 4 volumes of *water* and 1 volume of *diethylamine* as the mobile phase. Apply separately to the chromatoplate 10 µl of each of five solutions prepared immediately before use in a 1% v/v solution of 2M *ammonia* in *methanol* containing (1) 0.050% w/v of the substance being examined, (2) 0.0010% w/v of *isoemetine hydrobromide EPCRS*, (3) 0.0010% w/v of *cephaeline hydrochloride EPCRS*, (4) 0.00050% w/v of *emetine hydrochloride EPCRS* and (5) 0.05% w/v of *emetine hydrochloride EPCRS*. Also apply 30 µl of solution (6) prepared immediately before use by mixing 1 ml of solution (5), 1 ml of solution (2) and 1 ml of solution (3). After removal of the plate, allow it to dry in air until the odour of solvent is no longer detectable, spray with a 0.5% w/v solution of *iodine* in *chloroform*, heat at 60° for 15 minutes and examine under *ultra-violet light (365 nm)*. Any spots corresponding to isoemetine and cephaeline in the chromatogram obtained with solution (1) are not more intense than the spots in the chromatograms obtained with solutions (2) and (3) respectively. Any other *secondary spot* in the chromatogram obtained with solution (1) is not more intense than the spot in the chromatogram obtained with solution (4). The test is not valid unless the chromatogram obtained with solution (6) shows three clearly separated principal spots.

Loss on drying When dried at 100° to 105° for 3 hours, loses 15.0 to 19.0% of its weight. Use 1 g.

Sulphated ash Not more than 0.1%, Appendix IX A, Method II. Use 1 g.

Assay Dissolve 0.2 g in 20 ml of *anhydrous glacial acetic acid* and carry out Method I for *non-aqueous titration*, Appendix VIII A, using 7 ml of *mercury(II) acetate solution* and *crystal violet solution* as indicator. Each ml of 0.1M *perchloric acid VS* is equivalent to 0.02768 g of $C_{29}H_{40}N_2O_4,2HCl$.

Storage Emetine Hydrochloride should be kept in a well-closed container and protected from light.

Preparation
Emetine Injection

Action and use Antiprotozoal.

The title of the monograph in the European Pharmacopœia is Emetine Hydrochloride Heptahydrate.

Emetine Hydrochloride Pentahydrate ☆

$C_{29}H_{40}N_2O_4,2HCl,5H_2O$ 643.6   _316-42-7 (anhydrous)_

Emetine Hydrochloride Pentahydrate is 6′,7′,10,11-tetramethoxyemetan dihydro-chloride pentahydrate. It contains not less than 98.0 per cent and not more than 102.0 per cent of $C_{29}H_{40}N_2O_4,2HCl$, calculated with reference to the dried substance.

Characteristics A white or slightly yellow, crystalline powder; odourless.

Solubility Freely soluble in _water_, in _ethanol (96%)_ and in _chloroform_.

Identification; Acidity; Clarity and colour of solution; Specific optical rotation; Other alkaloids; Sulphated ash Complies with the requirements stated under Emetine Hydrochloride.

Loss on drying When dried at 100° to 105° for 3 hours, loses 11.0 to 15.0% of its weight. Use 1 g.

Assay Carry out the Assay described under Emetine Hydrochloride. Each ml of 0.1M _perchloric acid VS_ is equivalent to 0.02768 g of $C_{29}H_{40}N_2O_4,2HCl$.

Storage Emetine Hydrochloride Pentahydrate should be kept in a well-closed container and protected from light.

Preparation
Emetine Injection

Action and use Antiprotozoal.

Ephedrine ☆

$C_{10}H_{15}NO,\frac{1}{2}H_2O$ 174.2   _50906-05-3_

Ephedrine is (1R,2S)-2-methylamino-1-phenyl-propan-1-ol hemihydrate. It contains not less than 99.0 per cent and not more than 101.0 per cent of $C_{10}H_{15}NO$, calculated with reference to the anhydrous substance.

Characteristics Colourless crystals or a white, crystalline powder. The undried substance melts at about 42°.

Solubility Soluble in _water_; very soluble in _ethanol (96%)_; freely soluble in _ether_.

Identification _Test A may be omitted if tests B, C, D and E are carried out. Tests B, C and E may be omitted if tests A and D are carried out._
A. The _infra-red absorption spectrum_, Appendix II A, is concordant with the spectrum of the base isolated from _ephedrine hydrochloride EPCRS_. Examine the substances as discs prepared in the following manner. Separately dissolve 40 mg of the substance being examined and 50 mg of _ephedrine hydrochloride EPCRS_ in 1 ml of _water_, add 1 ml of 2M _sodium hydroxide_ and 4 ml of _chloroform_, shake and dry the organic layer with 0.2 g of _anhydrous sodium sulphate_. Prepare the discs using about 0.3 g of _potassium bromide IR_, apply dropwise to the discs 0.1 ml of the chloroform layers, allowing the solvent to evaporate between applications, and dry the discs at 50° for 2 minutes.
B. Complies with the test for Specific optical rotation.
C. In the test for Related substances, the principal spot in the chromatogram obtained with solution (2) is similar in position, colour and size to the principal spot in the chromatogram obtained with solution (3).
D. Dissolve 10 mg in 1 ml of _water_, add 0.2 ml of 10M _sodium hydroxide_ and 0.2 ml of 0.5M _copper(II) sulphate_; a violet colour is produced. Add 2 ml of _ether_ and shake; the ether layer is purple and the aqueous layer blue.
E. Complies with the test for Water.

Clarity and colour of solution A 2.5% w/v solution is _clear_, Appendix IV A, and _colourless_, Appendix IV B, Method II.

Specific optical rotation Dissolve 2.25 g in 15 ml of 2M _hydrochloric acid_ and dilute to 50 ml with _water_. The _specific optical rotation_ in the resulting solution is −41° to −43°, Appendix V F.

Chloride Dissolve 0.18 g in 10 ml of _water_, add 5 ml of 2M _nitric acid_ and 0.5 ml of 0.25M _silver nitrate_ and allow to stand for 2 minutes in subdued light. Any opalescence produced is not more intense than that obtained by repeating the operation at the same time and in the same manner using 10 ml of _chloride standard solution (5 ppm Cl)_ in place of the solution of the substance being examined (280 ppm).

Related substances Carry out the method for _thin-layer chromatography_, Appendix III A, using _silica gel G_ as the coating substance and a mixture of 80 volumes of _propan-2-ol_, 15 volumes of 13.5M _ammonia_ and 5 volumes of _chloroform_ as the mobile phase. Apply separately to the chromatoplate 10 μl of each of four solutions in _methanol_ containing (1) 2.0% w/v of the substance being examined, (2) 0.2% w/v of the substance being examined, (3) 0.25% w/v of _ephedrine hydrochloride EPCRS_ and (4) 0.010% w/v of the substance being examined. After removal of the plate, allow it to dry in air, spray with _ninhydrin solution_ and heat at 110° for 5 minutes. Any _secondary spot_ in the chromatogram obtained with solution (1) is not more intense than the spot in the chromatogram obtained with solution (4). Disregard any spot of lighter colour than the background.

Sulphated ash Not more than 0.1%, Appendix IX A, Method II. Use 1 g.

Water 4.5 to 5.5% w/w, Appendix IX C. Use 0.3 g.

Assay Dissolve 0.2 g in 5 ml of _ethanol (96%)_, add 20 ml of 0.1M _hydrochloric acid VS_ and titrate with 0.1M _sodium hydroxide VS_, using _methyl red solution_ as indicator, until a yellow colour is obtained. Each ml of 0.1M _hydrochloric acid VS_ is equivalent to 0.01652 g of $C_{10}H_{15}NO$.

Storage Ephedrine should be kept in a well-closed container and protected from light.

Action and use Beta-adrenoceptor agonist.

The title of the monograph in the European Pharmacopœia is Ephedrine Hemihydrate.

Anhydrous Ephedrine ☆

$C_{10}H_{15}NO$ 165.2   *299-42-3*

Anhydrous Ephedrine is (1*R*,2*S*)-2-methyl-amino-1-phenylpropan-1-ol. It contains not less than 99.0 per cent and not more than 101.0 per cent of $C_{10}H_{15}NO$, calculated with reference to the anhydrous substance.

Characteristics Colourless crystals or a white, crystalline powder. It melts at about 36°.

Solubility Soluble in *water* and in *chloroform*; very soluble in *ethanol (96%)*; freely soluble in *ether*.

Identification; Clarity and colour of solution; Specific optical rotation; Chloride; Related substances; Sulphated ash Complies with the requirements stated under Ephedrine.

Water Not more than 0.5% w/w, Appendix IX C. Use 2 g.

Assay Dissolve 0.2 g in 5 ml of *ethanol (96%)* and add 20 ml of 0.1M *hydrochloric acid VS*. Titrate with 0.1M *sodium hydroxide VS*, using *methyl red solution* as indicator, until a yellow colour is obtained. Each ml of 0.1M *hydrochloric acid VS* is equivalent to 0.01652 g of $C_{10}H_{15}NO$.

Storage Anhydrous Ephedrine should be kept in a well-closed container and protected from light.

Action and use Beta-adrenoceptor agonist.

Ephedrine Hydrochloride ☆

$C_{10}H_{15}NO,HCl$ 201.7   *50-98-6*

Ephedrine Hydrochloride is (1*R*,2*S*)-2-methyl-amino-1-phenylpropan-1-ol hydrochloride. It contains not less than 99.0 per cent and not more than 101.0 per cent of $C_{10}H_{15}NO,HCl$, calculated with reference to the dried substance.

Characteristics Colourless crystals or a white, crystalline powder. It melts at about 219°.

Solubility Soluble in 4 parts of *water* and in 17 parts of *ethanol (96%)*; very slightly soluble in *chloroform*; practically insoluble in *ether*.

Identification *Test A may be omitted if tests B, C, D and E are carried out. Tests B, C and D may be omitted if tests A and E are carried out.*

A. The *infra-red absorption spectrum*, Appendix II A, is concordant with the spectrum of *ephedrine hydrochloride EPCRS*.

B. Complies with the test for Specific optical rotation.

C. In the test for Related substances, the principal spot in the chromatogram obtained with solution (2) is similar in position, colour and size to the spot in chromatogram obtained with solution (3).

D. To 0.1 ml of a 10% w/v solution add 1 ml of *water*, 0.2 ml of 0.5M *copper(II) sulphate* and 1 ml of 10M *sodium hydroxide*; a violet colour is produced. Add 2 ml of *ether* and shake; the ether layer is purple and the aqueous layer blue.

E. A 5% w/v solution yields *reaction A* characteristic of chlorides, Appendix VI.

Acidity or alkalinity To 10 ml of a 10.0% w/v solution in *distilled water* add 0.1 ml of *methyl red solution* and 0.2 ml of 0.01M *sodium hydroxide VS*; the solution is yellow. Add 0.4 ml of 0.01M *hydrochloric acid VS*; the solution is red.

Clarity and colour of solution A 10.0% w/v solution in *distilled water* is *clear*, Appendix IV A, and *colourless*, Appendix IV B, Method II.

Specific optical rotation In a 5% w/v solution in *distilled water*, −33.5° to −35.5°, Appendix V F.

Sulphate A 10.0% w/v solution in *distilled water* complies with the *limit test for sulphates*, Appendix VII (100 ppm).

Related substances Carry out the method for *thin-layer chromatography*, Appendix III A, using *silica gel G* as the coating substance and a mixture of 80 volumes of *propan-2-ol*, 15 volumes of 13.5M *ammonia* and 5 volumes of *chloroform* as the mobile phase. Apply separately to the chromatoplate 10 µl of each of four solutions in *methanol* containing (1) 2.0% w/v of the substance being examined, (2) 0.2% w/v of the substance being examined, (3) 0.2% w/v of *ephedrine hydrochloride EPCRS* and (4) 0.010% w/v of the substance being examined. After removal of the plate, allow it to dry in air, spray with *ninhydrin solution* and heat at 110° for 5 minutes. Any *secondary spot* in the chromatogram obtained with solution (1) is not more intense than the spot in the chromatogram obtained with solution (4). Disregard any spot of lighter colour than the background.

Loss on drying When dried to constant weight at 100° to 105°, loses not more than 0.5% of its weight. Use 1 g.

Sulphated ash Not more than 0.1%, Appendix IX A, Method II. Use 1 g.

Assay Dissolve 0.17 g in 10 ml of warm *mercury(II) acetate solution*, add 50 ml of *acetone* and carry out Method I for *non-aqueous titration*, Appendix VIII A, using 1 ml of a saturated solution of *methyl orange* in *acetone* as indicator, until a red colour is obtained. Each ml of 0.1M *perchloric acid VS* is equivalent to 0.02017 g of $C_{10}H_{15}NO,HCl$.

Storage Ephedrine Hydrochloride should be protected from light.

Preparations
Ephedrine Elixir
Ephedrine Hydrochloride Tablets

Action and use Beta-adrenoceptor agonist.

Ergocalciferol ☆
Calciferol; Vitamin D_2

$C_{28}H_{44}O$ 396.7   *50-14-6*

Ergocalciferol is (5*Z*,7*E*,22*E*)-(3*S*)-9,10-seco-ergosta-5,7,10(19),22-tetraen-3-ol.

Characteristics Colourless or slightly yellow crystals or a white or slightly yellow, crystalline powder; odourless or almost odourless. It is sensitive to air, heat and light.

Solubility Practically insoluble in *water*; soluble in 2 parts of *ethanol (96%)*, in 10 parts of *acetone*, in 0.7 part of *chloroform* and in 2 parts of *ether*; slightly soluble in fixed oils.

Identification A. The *infra-red absorption spectrum*, Appendix II A, is concordant with the spectrum of *ergocalciferol EPCRS*.

B. Dissolve 1 mg in 40 ml of *1,2-dichloroethane* and to 1 ml of the solution add 4 ml of *antimony trichloride reagent*. An orange colour is produced which gradually becomes pink.

C. *Melting point*, 112° to 117° when determined without powdering and drying, Appendix V A, Method I.

Light absorption Dissolve 50 mg rapidly and without heating in sufficient *aldehyde-free ethanol (96%)* to produce 100 ml and dilute 5 ml of the solution to 250 ml with *aldehyde-free ethanol (96%)*. The *absorbance* of the resulting solution at the maximum at 265 nm measured within 30 minutes of dissolution is 0.45 to 0.50, Appendix II B. It does not differ by more than 3% from the *absorbance* of a solution prepared at the same time and in the same manner using 50 mg of *ergocalciferol EPCRS*.

Specific optical rotation Dissolve 0.2 g rapidly and without heating in sufficient *aldehyde-free ethanol* to produce 25 ml. The *specific optical rotation*, determined in the resulting solution within 30 minutes of preparation, is $+103°$ to $+107°$, Appendix V F.

Ergosterol Carry out the method for *thin-layer chromatography*, Appendix III A, using *silica gel G* as the coating substance and as the mobile phase a 0.01% w/v solution of *butylated hydroxytoluene* in a mixture of equal volumes of *cyclohexane* and *peroxide-free ether*. Carry out the development in the dark immediately after application of the solutions. Apply separately to the chromatoplate 10 µl each of solutions (1), (2) and (3) and 20 µl of solution (4), each solution being prepared immediately before use. For solution (1) dissolve 0.25 g of the substance being examined in sufficient *1,2-dichloroethane* containing 1% w/v of *squalane* and 0.01% w/v of *butylated hydroxytoluene* (solvent A) to produce 5 ml. For solution (2) dissolve 0.10 g of *ergocalciferol EPCRS* in sufficient solvent A to produce 2 ml. For solution (3) dissolve 5 mg of *ergosterol EPCRS* in sufficient solvent A to produce 50 ml. For solution (4) mix equal volumes of solution (2) and solution (3). After removal of the plate, allow it to dry in air and spray three times with *antimony trichloride reagent*. Examine the chromatograms for 3 to 4 minutes after spraying. The principal spot in the chromatogram obtained with solution (1) is initially orange-yellow and then becomes brown; it corresponds in position, colour and size to the principal spot in the chromatogram obtained with solution (2). In the chromatogram obtained with solution (1) any violet spot with an Rf value slightly lower than that of the principal spot (corresponding to ergosterol and appearing slowly) is not more intense than the spot in the chromatogram obtained with solution (3). The total number of spots in the chromatogram obtained with solution (1) is not more than the sum of the numbers of spots in the chromatograms obtained with solution (2) and solution (3). The test is not valid unless the chromatogram obtained with solution (4) shows two clearly separated principal spots.

Reducing substances To 10 ml of a 1.0% w/v solution in *aldehyde-free ethanol (96%)* add 0.5 ml of a 0.5% w/v solution of *tetrazolium blue* in *aldehyde-free ethanol (96%)*,

followed by 0.5 ml of *dilute tetramethylammonium hydroxide solution*. Allow to stand for exactly 5 minutes and then add 1 ml of *glacial acetic acid*. Measure the *absorbance* of the resulting solution at 525 nm, Appendix II B, using in the reference cell a solution prepared by treating 10 ml of *aldehyde-free ethanol (96%)* in the same manner. The absorbance is not more than that obtained by repeating the operation using a solution of *hydroquinone* in *aldehyde-free ethanol (96%)* containing 0.2 µg per ml.

Storage Ergocalciferol should be kept in a hermetically sealed container in which the air has been replaced by an inert gas, protected from light and stored at a temperature of 2° to 8°. The contents of an opened container should be used immediately.

Preparations
Calciferol Oral Solution
Calciferol Injection
Calciferol Tablets

Ergometrine Maleate ☆
Ergonovine Maleate

$C_{19}H_{23}N_3O_2,C_4H_4O_4$ 441.5   *129-51-1*

Ergometrine Maleate is 9,10-didehydro-*N*-[(*S*)-2-hydroxy-1-methylethyl]-6-methylergoline-8β-carboxamide hydrogen maleate. It contains not less than 98.0 per cent and not more than 101.0 per cent of $C_{19}H_{23}N_3O_2,C_4H_4O_4$, calculated with reference to the dried substance.

Characteristics A white or slightly coloured, crystalline powder.

Solubility Soluble in 40 parts of *water* and in 100 parts of *ethanol (96%)*; practically insoluble in *chloroform* and in *ether*.

Identification *Test A may be omitted if tests B, C, D and E are carried out. Tests B, D and E may be omitted it tests A and C are carried out.*

A. The *infra-red absorption spectrum*, Appendix II A, is concordant with the spectrum of *ergometrine maleate EPCRS*.

B. Dissolve 30 mg in sufficient 0.01M *hydrochloric acid* to produce 100 ml and dilute 10 ml of the solution to 100 ml with 0.01M *hydrochloric acid*. The *light absorption* of the resulting solution, Appendix II B, in the range 250 to 360 nm exhibits a maximum at 311 nm and a minimum at 265 to 272 nm. The A(1%, 1 cm) at 311 nm is 175 to 195.

C. In the test for Related substances, the principal spot in the chromatogram obtained with solution (2) is similar in position, colour and size to the principal spot in the chromatogram obtained with solution (3).

D. Dissolve 0.100 g without heating and protected from light in sufficient *carbon dioxide-free water* to produce 10 ml (solution A). To 0.1 ml of solution A add 1 ml of *glacial acetic acid*, 0.05 ml of a 10.5% w/v solution of *iron(III) chloride hexahydrate* and 1 ml of *orthophosphoric acid* and heat on a water-bath at 80°. After about 10 minutes a blue or violet colour is produced, which becomes more intense on standing.

E. Dissolve 0.1 g in a mixture of 0.5 ml of 1M *sulphuric acid* and 2.5 ml of *water*, add 1 ml of 10M *sodium hydroxide* and extract with three 5-ml quantities of *ether*. Heat 0.1 ml of the aqueous layer on a water-bath for 15 minutes with a solution of 10 mg of *resorcinol* in 3 ml of *sulphuric acid*; no colour is produced. To the remainder of the aqueous layer add 1 ml of *bromine water*, heat on a water-bath for 10 minutes, then bring to the boil and allow to cool. Heat 0.2 ml of the resulting solution with a solution of 10 mg of *resorcinol* in 3 ml of *sulphuric acid*; a pinkish-violet colour is produced.

Acidity pH of solution A, 3.6 to 4.4, Appendix V L.

Clarity and colour of solution Solution A is *clear*, Appendix IV A, and not more intensely coloured than *reference solution Y5 or BY5*, Appendix IV B, Method II.

Specific optical rotation In solution A, +50° to +56°, Appendix V F.

Related substances Carry out the operations as rapidly as possible, protected from light. Carry out the method for *thin-layer chromatography*, Appendix III A, using *silica gel G* as the coating substance and a mixture of 75 volumes of *chloroform*, 25 volumes of *methanol* and 3 volumes of *water* as the mobile phase, but allowing the solvent front to ascend 14 cm above the line of application. Apply separately to the chromatoplate 5 µl of each of five solutions, prepared immediately before use, in a mixture of 1 volume of 13.5M *ammonia* and 9 volumes of *ethanol (80%)* and containing (1) 1.00% w/v of the substance being examined, (2) 0.1% w/v of the substance being examined, (3) 0.1% w/v of *ergometrine maleate EPCRS*, (4) 0.010% w/v of *ergometrine maleate EPCRS* and (5) 0.0050% w/v of *ergometrine maleate EPCRS*. After removal of the plate, allow it to dry in a current of cold air and spray with a solution prepared by dissolving 1.0 g of *4-dimethylaminobenzaldehyde* in 50 ml of *hydrochloric acid* and adding 50 ml of *ethanol (96%)*. Dry in a current of warm air for 2 minutes. Any *secondary spot* in the chromatogram obtained with solution (1) is not more intense than the principal spot in the chromatogram obtained with solution (4) and not more than one such spot is more intense than the principal spot in the chromatogram obtained with solution (5).

Loss on drying When dried over *phosphorus pentoxide* at 80° at a pressure of 1.5 to 2.5 kPa for 2 hours, loses not more than 2.0% of its weight. Use 0.2 g.

Assay Dissolve 0.15 g in 40 ml of *anhydrous glacial acetic acid* and carry out Method I for *non-aqueous titration*, Appendix VIII A, using 0.05M *perchloric acid VS* and determining the end-point potentiometrically. Each ml of 0.05M *perchloric acid VS* is equivalent to 0.02207 g of $C_{19}H_{23}N_3O_2,C_4H_4O_4$.

Storage Ergometrine Maleate should be kept in an airtight, glass container, protected from light and stored at a temperature of 2° to 8°.

Preparations
Ergometrine Injection
Ergometrine Tablets
Ergometrine and Oxytocin Injection

Action and use Uterine stimulant.

Ergotamine Tartrate ☆

$(C_{33}H_{35}N_5O_5)_2,C_4H_6O_6$ 1313   *379-79-3*

Ergotamine Tartrate is (5′S)-12′-hydroxy-2′-methyl-3′,6′,18-trioxo-5-benzylergotaman (+)-tartrate. It contains not less than 98.0 per cent and not more than 101.0 per cent of $(C_{33}H_{35}N_5O_5)_2,C_4H_6O_6$, calculated with reference to the dried substance. It may contain two molecular equivalents of methanol of crystallisation.

Characteristics Colourless crystals or a white or almost white, crystalline powder; slightly hygroscopic.

Solubility Dissolves in *water*; the solution may become turbid but this may be prevented by the addition of tartaric acid. Slightly soluble in *ethanol (96%)* and in *chloroform*; practically insoluble in *ether*.

Identification *Test A may be omitted if tests B, C, D and E are carried out. Tests B, D and E may be omitted if tests A and C are carried out.*

A. The *infra-red absorption spectrum*, Appendix II A, is concordant with the spectrum of *ergotamine tartrate EPCRS*. Examine the substances as discs but triturate with 0.2 ml of *methanol* before triturating with *potassium bromide IR*.

B. Dissolve 50 mg in sufficient 0.01M *hydrochloric acid* to produce 100 ml and dilute 10 ml of the solution to 100 ml with 0.01M *hydrochloric acid*. The *light absorption* of the resulting solution, Appendix II B, in the range 250 to 360 nm exhibits a maximum at 311 to 321 nm and a minimum at 265 to 275 nm. The A(1%, 1 cm) at the maximum is 118 to 128.

C. In the test for Related substances, the principal spot in the chromatogram obtained with solution (5) is similar in position and intensity to the spot in the chromatogram obtained with solution (1) when examined for not more than 1 minute under *ultra-violet light (365 nm)*. It is also similar in position, colour and size to the spot in the chromatogram obtained with solution (1) when examined in daylight after spraying with a solution prepared by dissolving 1.0 g of *4-dimethylaminobenzaldehyde* in 50 ml of *hydrochloric acid* and adding 50 ml of *ethanol (96%)*.

D. Dissolve 10 mg in 1 ml of 0.01M *sodium hydroxide*, shake with 5 ml of *chloroform*, discard the chloroform layer and neutralise the aqueous layer with 2M *hydrochloric acid*. The resulting solution yields *reaction B* characteristic of tartrates, Appendix VI. A dark blue colour is produced which changes to red or brownish-red when the solution is poured into 1 ml of *water*.

E. Finely triturate 30 mg with 15 mg of *(+)-tartaric acid* and dissolve the mixture in 6 ml of *water* with shaking (solution A). Heat 0.1 ml in a water-bath at 80° with 1 ml of *glacial acetic acid*, 0.05 ml of a 10.5% w/v solution of *iron(III) chloride hexahydrate* and 1 ml of *orthophosphoric acid*. After about 10 minutes a blue or violet colour is produced, which becomes more intense on standing.

Acidity Shake 10 mg of the finely powdered substance with 4 ml of *water*. The pH of the suspension is 4.0 to 5.5, Appendix V L.

Clarity and colour of solution Solution A is *clear*, Appendix IV A, and not more intensely coloured than *reference solution* Y_6, Appendix IV B, Method II.

Specific optical rotation Carry out the following procedure as rapidly as possible, protected from light. Dissolve 0.4 g in 40 ml of a 1% w/v solution of (+)-*tartaric acid*, cautiously add 0.5 g of *sodium hydrogen carbonate* in several portions and mix. Wash 100 ml of *chloroform* by shaking with five 50-ml quantities of *water* and extract the solution of the substance being examined with four 10-ml quantities of the washed chloroform. Filter the combined chloroform extracts, dilute to 50 ml with the same solvent and measure the *optical rotation*, Appendix V F.

To 25 ml of the chloroform solution add 50 ml of *anhydrous glacial acetic acid* and carry out Method I for *non-aqueous titration*, Appendix VIII A, using 0.05M *perchloric acid VS* and determining the end-point potentiometrically. Each ml of 0.05M *perchloric acid VS* is equivalent to 0.02908 g of ergotamine base, $C_{33}H_{35}N_5O_5$. The *specific optical rotation* of the base is $-154°$ to $-165°$.

Related substances Carry out as rapidly as possible and protected from light the method for *thin-layer chromatography*, Appendix III A, using *silica gel G* as the coating substance and a mixture of 70 volumes of *ether*, 15 volumes of *dimethylformamide*, 10 volumes of *chloroform* and 5 volumes of *absolute ethanol* as the mobile phase, but allowing the solvent front to ascend 17 cm above the line of application. Apply separately to the chromatoplate 5 μl of each of five solutions, prepared immediately before use in the order stated, in a mixture of 9 volumes of *chloroform* and 1 volume of *methanol* containing (1) 0.1% w/v of *ergotamine tartrate EPCRS*, (2) 0.015% w/v of *ergotamine tartrate EPCRS*, (3) 0.0050% w/v of *ergotamine tartrate EPCRS*, (4) 1.0% w/v of the substance being examined and (5) 0.1% w/v of the substance being examined. Immediately after applying the solutions to the plate, expose it to an atmosphere saturated with ammonia vapour for exactly 20 seconds, dry the plate at the line of application in a current of cold air for exactly 20 seconds and start the chromatography immediately. After removal of the plate, allow it to dry in a current of cold air for 2 minutes and examine under *ultra-violet light (365 nm)* for not more than 1 minute. Spray with a solution prepared by dissolving 1.0 g of *4-dimethylaminobenzaldehyde* in 50 ml of *ethanol (96%)* and adding 50 ml of *hydrochloric acid* and allow it to dry in a current of warm air for 2 minutes. Any *secondary spot* in the chromatogram obtained with solution (4) is not more intense than the spot in the chromatogram obtained with solution (2) and not more than one such spot is more intense than the principal spot in the chromatogram obtained with solution (3).

Loss on drying When dried over *phosphorus pentoxide* at 95° at a pressure of 1.5 to 2.5 kPa for 6 hours, loses not more than 6.0% of its weight. Use 0.1 g.

Assay Dissolve 0.2 g in 40 ml of *anhydrous glacial acetic acid* and carry out Method I for *non-aqueous titration*, Appendix VIII A, using 0.05M *perchloric acid VS* and determining the end-point potentiometrically. Each ml of 0.05M *perchloric acid VS* is equivalent to 0.03284 g of $(C_{33}H_{35}N_5O_5)_2,C_4H_6O_6$.

Storage Ergotamine Tartrate should be kept in an airtight, glass container, protected from light and stored at a temperature of 2° to 8°.

Preparations
Ergotamine Injection
Ergotamine Tablets

Action and use Used in treatment of migraine.

Erythromycin ☆

Erythromycin	R	R_1
A	OH	Me
B	H	Me
C	OH	H

$C_{37}H_{67}NO_{13}$ 734   *114-07-8*

Erythromycin is a mixture of macrolide antibiotics consisting largely of erythromycin A, (2R,3S,4S,5R,6R,8R,10R,11R,12S,13R)-5-(3-amino-3,4,6-trideoxy-N,N-dimethyl-β-D-*xylo*-hexopyranosyloxy)-3-(2,6-dideoxy-3-C,3-O-dimethyl-α-L-*ribo*-hexopyranosyloxy)-13-ethyl-6,11,12-trihydroxy-2,4,6,8,10,12-hexamethyl-9-oxotridecan-13-olide. It is produced by the growth of a strain of *Streptomyces erythreus*. The potency is not less than 920 Units per mg, calculated with reference to the anhydrous substance.

Characteristics White or slightly yellow crystals or powder; odourless; slightly hygroscopic.

Solubility Slightly soluble in *water* but less soluble in hot *water*; soluble in 5 parts of *ethanol (96%)*; soluble in *chloroform* and in *methanol*. It dissolves in 2M *hydrochloric acid*.

Identification *Test A may be omitted if tests B, C and D are carried out. Tests B and D may be omitted if tests A and C are carried out.*
A. The *infra-red absorption spectrum*, Appendix II A, is concordant with the spectrum of *erythromycin EPCRS*. Examine the substances as 5% w/v solutions in *chloroform*.
B. Carry out the method for *thin-layer chromatography*, Appendix III A, using *silica gel G* as the coating substance and, as the mobile phase, the upper layer obtained by shaking together 45 volumes of *ethyl acetate*, 40 volumes of a 15% w/v solution of *ammonium acetate* previously adjusted to pH 9.6 with 9M *ammonia* and 20 volumes of *propan-2-ol* and allowing to separate. Apply separately to the chromatoplate 10 μl of each of three solutions in *methanol* containing (1) 0.10% w/v of the substance being examined, (2) 0.10% w/v of *erythromycin EPCRS* and (3) 0.20% w/v of *spiramycin EPCRS*. After removal of the plate, allow it to dry in air, spray with *ethanolic anisaldehyde solution*, heat at 110° for 5 minutes and allow

to cool. The principal spot in the chromatogram obtained with solution (1) is similar in position, colour and size to that in the chromatogram obtained with solution (2) and is different in position and colour from the spots in the chromatogram obtained with solution (3).

C. Dissolve 3 mg in 2 ml of *acetone* and add 2 ml of *hydrochloric acid*; an orange colour is produced which changes to red and then to deep violet-red. Add 2 ml of *chloroform* and shake; the chloroform layer becomes violet-red.

D. To 5 mg add 5 ml of a 0.02% w/v solution of *xanthydrol* in a mixture of 1 volume of *hydrochloric acid* and 99 volumes of 5M *acetic acid* and heat on a water-bath. A red colour is produced.

Alkalinity pH of a solution containing 0.1 g in 150 ml of *carbon dioxide-free water*, 8.0 to 10.5, Appendix V L.

Specific optical rotation In a 2% w/v solution in *absolute ethanol*, −71° to −78°, Appendix V F. Measure the angle of rotation at least 30 minutes after preparing the solution.

Related substances Carry out the method for *thin-layer chromatography*, Appendix III A, using *silanised silica gel H* as the coating substance and a mixture of 75 volumes of *methanol* and 45 volumes of a 5% w/v solution of *ammonium acetate* as the mobile phase. Apply separately to the chromatoplate 10 µl of each of three solutions in *methanol* containing (1) 0.20% w/v of the substance being examined, (2) 0.20% w/v of *erythromycin EPCRS* and (3) 0.010% w/v of *erythromycin EPCRS*. After removal of the plate, allow it to dry in air, spray with *anisaldehyde solution*, heat at 110° for 5 minutes and allow to cool. In the chromatogram obtained with solution (1) any *secondary spot* with an Rf value lower than that of the principal spot is not more intense than the corresponding spot in the chromatogram obtained with solution (2) and any *secondary spot* with an Rf value higher than that of the principal spot is not more intense than the principal spot in the chromatogram obtained with solution (3).

Sulphated ash Not more than 0.2%, Appendix IX A, Method II. Use 1 g.

Water Not more than 6.5%, Appendix IX C, Method I B. Use 0.2 g.

Assay Carry out the *biological assay of antibiotics*, Appendix XIV A. The precision of the assay is such that the fiducial limits of error are not less than 95% and not more than 105% of the estimated potency.

Storage Erythromycin should be kept in a well-closed container, protected from light and stored at a temperature not exceeding 30°.

Preparation
Erythromycin Tablets

Action and use Antibacterial.

Erythromycin Estolate

$C_{40}H_{71}NO_{14},C_{12}H_{26}O_4S$ 1056.4   *3521-62-8*

Erythromycin Estolate is the 2'-propionate dodecyl sulphate of erythromycin, an antimicrobial substance produced by the growth of certain strains of *Streptomyces erythreus* Waksman. The potency is not less than 610 Units per mg, calculated with reference to the anhydrous substance.

Characteristics A white, crystalline powder.

Solubility Practically insoluble in *water*; soluble in 2 parts of *ethanol* (96%); freely soluble in *chloroform*; practically insoluble in 2M *hydrochloric acid*.

Identification A. The *infra-red absorption spectrum*, Appendix II A, is concordant with the *reference spectrum* of erythromycin estolate.

B. Dissolve 15 mg in 2 ml of *acetone* and add 2 ml of *hydrochloric acid*; an orange-red colour is produced which changes to red and then to deep purple. Add 2 ml of *chloroform* and shake; the chloroform layer becomes purple.

Acidity or alkalinity Stir 0.4 g with 10 ml of *carbon dioxide-free water* for 5 minutes. The pH of the clear supernatant liquid is 4.5 to 7.0, Appendix V L.

Acetone To 1 ml of a 0.1% w/v solution in *methanol* add 0.1 ml of *salicylaldehyde* and mix. Add 1.5 ml of a saturated solution of *potassium hydroxide*, allow to stand for 20 minutes and add 6 ml of *methanol*. The *absorbance* of the resulting solution at 490 nm, Appendix II B, is not more than the *absorbance* of the solution obtained when 1 ml of a 0.0020% w/v solution of *acetone* in *methanol* is treated in the same manner.

Thiocyanate Dissolve 0.10 g in a few ml of *ethanol* (96%) and add 5 ml of a solution prepared by dissolving 3.35 g of *iron(III) chloride hexahydrate* in *water* and adding 52.5 ml of *nitric acid* and sufficient *water* to produce 200 ml. Dilute to 100 ml with *ethanol* (96%). The *absorbance* of the resulting solution at 470 nm, Appendix II B, is not more than the *absorbance* of the solution obtained when 2 ml of a 0.0417% w/v solution of *potassium thiocyanate* is treated in the same manner.

Sulphated ash Not more than 0.5%, Appendix IX A.

Water Not more than 4.0% w/w, Appendix IX C. Use 0.6 g.

Content of $C_{12}H_{26}O_4S$ 22.0 to 25.5%, calculated with reference to the anhydrous substance, when determined by the following method. Dissolve 0.5 g in 25 ml of *dimethylformamide* and carry out Method II for *non-aqueous titration*, Appendix VIII A, using 0.1M *sodium methoxide VS* and a 0.3% w/v solution of *thymol blue* in *methanol* as indicator. Each ml of 0.1M *sodium methoxide VS* is equivalent to 0.02664 g of $C_{12}H_{26}O_4S$.

Assay Dissolve 0.4 g in 400 ml of *methanol* and add 200 ml of sterile *phosphate buffer pH 7.0* and sufficient *water for injections* to produce 1000 ml. Maintain the solution at 60° for 3 hours, cool and carry out the *biological assay of antibiotics* for erythromycin, Appendix XIV A. The precision of the assay is such that the fiducial limits of error are not less than 95% and not more than 105% of the estimated potency.

Preparation
Erythromycin Estolate Capsules

Action and use Antibacterial.

Erythromycin Ethyl Succinate ☆

$C_{43}H_{75}NO_{16}$ 862   *41342-53-4*

Erythromycin Ethyl Succinate is (2*R*,3*S*,4*S*, 5*R*,6*R*,8*R*,10*R*,11*R*,12*S*,13*R*)-5-[3-amino-3,4,6-trideoxy-2-*O*-(3-ethoxycarbonylpropionyl)-*N*,*N*-dimethyl-β-D-*xylo*-hexopyranosyloxy]-3-(2,6-dideoxy-3-*C*,3-*O*-dimethyl-α-L-*ribo*-hexopyranosyloxy)-13-ethyl-6,11,12-trihydroxy-2,4,6,8,10,12-hexamethyl-9-oxotridecan-13-olide. The potency is not less than 780 Units per mg, calculated with reference to the anhydrous substance.

Characteristics A white, crystalline powder; hygroscopic.

Solubility Practically insoluble in *water*; freely soluble in *absolute ethanol*, in *acetone*, in *chloroform* and in *methanol*.

Identification *Test A may be omitted if tests B, C and D are carried out. Tests B, C and D may be omitted if test A is carried out.*
A. The *infra-red absorption spectrum*, Appendix II A, is concordant with the spectrum of *erythromycin ethylsuccinate EPCRS*.
B. In the test for Related substances, the principal spot in the chromatogram obtained with solution (2) is similar in position and colour to the principal spot in the chromatogram obtained with solution (3). The test is not valid unless the chromatogram obtained with solution (4) shows two clearly separated principal spots.
C. Dissolve 3 mg in 2 ml of *acetone* and add 2 ml of *hydrochloric acid*; an orange colour is produced which changes to red and then to deep violet-red. Add 2 ml of *chloroform* and shake; the chloroform layer becomes violet.
D. To 5 mg add 5 ml of a 0.02% w/v solution of *xanthydrol* in a mixture of 1 volume of *hydrochloric acid* and 99 volumes of 5M *acetic acid* and heat on a water-bath. A red colour is produced.

Acidity or alkalinity pH of a 1% w/v suspension, 6.0 to 8.5, Appendix V L.

Clarity and colour of solution A 10% w/v solution in *absolute ethanol* is clear, Appendix IV A, and not more intensely coloured than *reference solution B₆*, Appendix IV B, Method II.

Specific optical rotation In a 1% w/v solution in *acetone*, −70° to −82°, Appendix V F. Measure the angle of rotation at least 30 minutes after preparing the solution.

Related substances Carry out the method for *thin-layer chromatography*, Appendix III A, using *silica gel G* as the coating substance and a mixture of 85 volumes of *chloroform*, 15 volumes of *ethanol (96%)* and 1 volume of a 15% w/v solution of *ammonium acetate* previously adjusted to pH 7.0 as the mobile phase. Apply separately to the chromatoplate 10 µl of each of five solutions in *acetone* containing (1) 0.40% w/v of the substance being examined, (2) 0.1% w/v of the substance being examined, (3) 0.1% w/v of *erythromycin ethylsuccinate EPCRS*, (4) 0.1% w/v of *erythromycin ethylsuccinate EPCRS* and 0.1% w/v of *erythromycin estolate EPCRS* and (5) 0.020% w/v of *erythromycin EPCRS*. After removal of the plate, allow it to dry in air, spray with *anisaldehyde solution*, heat at 110° for 5 minutes and allow to cool. Any *secondary spot* in the chromatogram obtained with solution (1) is not more intense than the spot in the chromatogram obtained with solution (5).

Sulphated ash Not more than 0.3%, Appendix IX A, Method II. Use 1 g.

Water Not more than 3.0%, Appendix IX C. Use 0.3 g.

Assay Dissolve 0.1 g in 40 ml of *methanol* and add sufficient *phosphate buffer pH 8.0* to produce 100 ml. Allow to stand at room temperature for 2 hours and carry out the *biological assay of antibiotics* for erythromycin, Appendix XIV A. The precision of the assay is such that the fiducial limits of error are not less than 95% and not more than 105% of the estimated potency.

Storage Erythromycin Ethyl Succinate should be kept in an airtight container, protected from light and stored at a temperature not exceeding 30°.

Action and use Antibacterial.

The title of the monograph in the European Pharmacopœia is Erythromycin Ethylsuccinate.

Erythromycin Stearate ☆

$C_{37}H_{67}NO_{13},C_{18}H_{36}O_2$ 1018   *643-22-1*

Erythromycin Stearate is a mixture of the stearate of (2*R*,3*S*,4*S*,5*R*,6*R*,8*R*,10*R*,11*R*,12*S*, 13*R*)-5-(3-amino-3,4,6-trideoxy-*N*,*N*-dimethyl-β-D-*xylo*-hexopyranosyloxy)-3-(2,6-dideoxy-3-*C*,3-*O*-dimethyl-α-L-*ribo*-hexopyranosyloxy)-13-ethyl-6,11,12-trihydroxy-2,4,6,8,10,12-hexamethyl-9-oxotridecan-13-olide, a substance produced by the growth of certain strains of *Streptomyces erythreus* or by other means, and stearic acid. The potency is not less than 600 Units per mg, calculated with reference to the anhydrous substance.

Characteristics A white, crystalline powder.

Solubility Practically insoluble in *water*; soluble in *absolute ethanol*, in *methanol*, in *acetone* and in *chloroform*. Solutions in *absolute ethanol*, in *methanol*, in *acetone* and in *chloroform* may be opalescent.

Identification A. Carry out the method for *thin-layer chromatography*, Appendix III A, using *silica gel G* as the coating substance and as the mobile phase the upper layer of a mixture of 45 volumes of *ethyl acetate*, 40 volumes of a 15% w/v solution of *ammonium acetate*, previously adjusted to pH 9.6 with 9M *ammonia*, and 20 volumes of *propan-2-ol*. Apply separately to the chromatoplate 5 µl of each of three solutions in *methanol* containing (1) 0.28% w/v of the substance being examined, (2) 0.20% w/v of *erythromycin EPCRS* and (3) 0.10% w/v of *stearic acid*. After removal of the plate, allow it to dry in air, spray with a solution containing 0.02% w/v of 2,7-*dichlorofluorescein* and 0.01% of *rhodamine B* in *ethanol (96%)*, allow the plate to stand for a few seconds in the vapour above a water-bath and examine under *ultra-violet light (365 nm)*. The chromatogram obtained with solution (1) exhibits two spots, one of which corresponds in position to the principal spot in the chromatogram obtained with solution (2) and the other to the principal spot in the chromatogram obtained with solution (3). Spray the plate with *ethanolic anisaldehyde solution*, heat at 110° for 5 minutes and examine in daylight. The coloured spot in the chromatogram obtained with solution (1) corresponds in position, colour and size to the principal spot in the chromatogram obtained with solution (2).

B. Dissolve 3 mg in 2 ml of *acetone* and add 2 ml of *hydrochloric acid*; an orange colour is produced, which changes to red and then to deep violet-red. Add 2 ml of *chloroform* and shake; the chloroform layer becomes violet.

C. To 5 mg add 5 ml of a 0.02% w/v solution of *xanthydrol* in a mixture of 1 volume of *hydrochloric acid* and 99 volumes of 5.4M *acetic acid* and heat on a water-bath. A red colour is produced.

Acidity or alkalinity pH of a 1% w/v suspension, 7.0 to 10.5, Appendix V L.

Related substances Carry out the method for *thin-layer chromatography*, Appendix III A, using *silanised silica gel H* as the coating substance and a mixture of 100 volumes of *methanol* and 60 volumes of a 15% w/v solution of *ammonium acetate* as the mobile phase. Apply separately to the chromatoplate 10 µl of each of three solutions in *methanol* containing (1) 0.28% w/v of the substance being examined, (2) 0.20% w/v of *erythromycin EPCRS* and (3) 0.010% w/v of *erythromycin EPCRS*. After removal of the plate, allow it to dry in air, spray with *anisaldehyde solution*, heat at 110° for 5 minutes and allow to cool. In the chromatogram obtained with solution (1) any spot with an Rf value lower than that of the principal spot is not more intense than the corresponding spot in the chromatogram obtained with solution (2) and any spot with an Rf value higher than that of the principal spot is not more intense than the principal spot in the chromatogram obtained with solution (3).

Sulphated ash Not more than 0.5%, Appendix IX A, Method II. Use 1 g.

Water Not more than 4.0% w/w, Appendix IX C. Use 0.3 g.

Erythromycin stearate Not less than 84.0% of $C_{37}H_{67}NO_{13},C_{18}H_{36}O_2$, calculated with reference to the anhydrous substance, when determined by the following method. Dissolve 0.5 g in 30 ml of *chloroform*. If the solution is opalescent, filter and shake the residue with three 25-ml quantities of *chloroform*. Filter if necessary and wash the filter with *chloroform*. Evaporate the combined filtrate and washings on a water-bath to about 30 ml, add 50 ml of *anhydrous glacial acetic acid* and titrate with 0.1M *perchloric acid VS* determining the end-point potentiometrically. Each ml of 0.1M *perchloric acid VS* is equivalent to 0.1018 g of $C_{37}H_{67}NO_{13},C_{18}H_{36}O_2$.

Free stearic acid Not more than 14.0% of $C_{18}H_{36}O_2$, calculated with reference to the anhydrous substance, when determined by the following method. Dissolve 0.4 g in 50 ml of *methanol* and titrate with 0.1M *sodium hydroxide VS* determining the end-point potentio-metrically. Calculate the volume of 0.1M *sodium hydroxide VS* required for each g of the substance and subtract the volume of 0.1M *perchloric acid VS* required for each g of the substance in the test for Erythromycin stearate. Each ml of the difference is equivalent to 0.02845 g of $C_{18}H_{36}O_2$.

Erythromycin stearate and free stearic acid 98.0 to 103.0%, calculated by adding together the percentages of erythromycin stearate and free stearic acid determined as described above.

Assay Dissolve 50 mg in sufficient *methanol* to produce 100 ml and carry out the *biological assay of antibiotics* for erythromycin, Appendix XIV A. The precision of the assay is such that the fiducial limits of error are not less than 95% and not more than 105% of the estimated potency.

Storage Erythromycin Stearate should be kept in a well-closed container, protected from light and stored at a temperature below 30°.

Preparation

Erythromycin Stearate Tablets

Action and use Antibacterial.

Estramustine Sodium Phosphate

$C_{23}H_{30}Cl_2NNa_2O_6P$ 564.4   *52205-73-9*

Estramustine Sodium Phosphate is disodium 3-[bis(2-chloroethyl)carbamoyloxy]estra-1,3,5(10)-trien-17β-yl orthophosphate. It contains not less than 97.0 per cent and not more than 103.0 per cent of $C_{23}H_{30}Cl_2NNa_2O_6P$, calculated with reference to the anhydrous substance.

Characteristics A white or almost white powder.

Solubility Freely soluble in *water* and in *methanol*; very slightly soluble in *absolute ethanol* and in *chloroform*.

Identification A. The *infra-red absorption spectrum*, Appendix II A, is concordant with the *reference spectrum* of estramustine sodium phosphate. In preparing the potassium bromide disc precautions should be taken to exclude moisture and avoid excessive grinding; if necessary heat the prepared disc at 90° for 2 minutes.

B. The *light absorption*, Appendix II B, in the range 230 to 350 nm of a 0.05% w/v solution exhibits maxima at 267 nm and at 275 nm. The *absorbance* at 267 nm is about 0.76 and at 275 nm is about 0.71.

C. A 1% w/v solution yields the *reactions* characteristic of sodium salts, Appendix VI.

Alkalinity pH of a 0.5% w/v solution, 8.5 to 10.0, Appendix V L.

Clarity and colour of solution A 5.0% w/v solution is not more opalescent than *reference suspension II*, Appendix IV A, and is *colourless*, Appendix IV B, Method I.

Specific optical rotation In a 2% w/v solution, +11° to +13°, Appendix V F.

Ionisable chlorine Dissolve 0.10 g in 10 ml of *water*, add carefully, with mixing, 0.1 ml of a mixture of 10 volumes of *silver nitrate solution* and 1 volume of *nitric acid* and examine immediately. Any opalescence produced is not more intense than that obtained by treating 10 ml of a 0.000134% w/v solution of *sodium chloride* in the same manner (0.1%).

Estradiol 17β-phosphate Dissolve 50 mg in 5 ml of 0.2M *sodium hydroxide*, add sufficient *ethanol (96%)* to produce 10 ml, mix and immediately measure the *absorbance* at the maxima at 300 nm and 350 nm, Apppendix II B. The difference between the two absorbances is not more than 0.34 (1.0%).

Inorganic phosphate Dissolve 25 mg in 10 ml of *water*, add 4 ml of 1M *sulphuric acid*, 1 ml of a 10% w/v solution of *ammonium molybdate* and 2 ml of *methylaminophenolsulphite reagent* and allow to stand for 15 minutes. Add sufficient *water* to produce 25 ml, allow to stand for 15 minutes and filter. The *absorbance* of the filtrate at 730 nm, Appendix II B, is not more than the *absorbance* at 730 nm of a solution obtained by repeating the operation using 10 ml of a 0.00180% w/v solution of *potassium dihydrogen orthophosphate* and beginning at the words 'add 4 ml of 1M *sulphuric acid* . . .'.

Volatile matter Carry out the method for *gas chromatography*, Appendix III B, using solutions in *water* containing (1) 0.0040% v/v of *pyridine*, 0.020% v/v of *absolute ethanol* and 0.020% v/v of *butan-1-ol* (internal standard), (2) 4.0% w/v of the substance being examined and (3) 4.0% w/v of the substance being examined and 0.020% v/v of the internal standard.

The chromatographic procedure may be carried out using a glass column (1.5 m × 4 mm) packed with *acid-washed, silanised diatomaceous support* (80 to 100 mesh) coated with 20% w/w of polyethylene glycol (Carbowax 20M is suitable) and maintained at 120°.

In the chromatogram obtained with solution (1) the area of the peak due to pyridine is greater than the area of any corresponding peak in the chromatogram obtained with solution (3). In the chromatogram obtained with solution (1) the area of the peak due to ethanol is greater than the sum of the areas of any peaks having a retention time less than that of the peak due to the internal standard in the chromatogram obtained with solution (3).

Related substances Carry out the method for *thin-layer chromatography*, Appendix III A, using *silica gel G* as the coating substance and a mixture of equal volumes of *butan-2-one, propan-2-ol* and 0.5M *triethylamine hydrogen carbonate solution* as the mobile phase. Apply separately to the chromatoplate 10 μl of each of four freshly prepared solutions in a mixture of 49 volumes of *methanol* and 1 volume of *triethylamine* containing (1) 4.0% w/v of the substance being examined, (2) 0.020% w/v of the substance being examined, (3) 0.080 % w/v of *17β,17'β-bis{3-[bis(2-chloroethyl)carbamoyloxy]estra-1,3,5(10)-trienyl} pyrophosphate BPCRS* and (4) 0.040% of *estramustine BPCRS*. After removal of the plate allow it to dry in air, spray with *methanolic sulphuric acid (20%)* and heat at 110° for 10 minutes. The principal spots in the chromatograms obtained with solutions (3) and (4) are more intense than any corresponding spots in the chromatogram obtained with solution (1) in which any other *secondary spot* is not more intense than the spot in the chromatogram obtained with solution (2).

Water Not more than 5.0% w/w, Appendix IX C. Use 0.2 g.

Assay To 0.5 g add 40 ml of 1M *sodium hydroxide* and boil under a reflux condenser for 60 minutes. Cool and transfer the mixture to a 250-ml graduated flask with the aid of *water*. Add 100 ml of 0.1M *silver nitrate VS* and 10 ml of *nitric acid*, dilute to 250 ml with *water* and mix. Filter and titrate the excess of silver nitrate in 50 ml of the filtrate with 0.1M *ammonium thiocyanate VS* using 3 ml of *ammonium iron(III) sulphate solution* as indicator. Each ml of 0.1M *silver nitrate VS* is equivalent to 0.02822 g of $C_{23}H_{30}Cl_2NNa_2O_6P$.

Storage Estramustine Sodium Phosphate should be kept in a well-closed container and protected from light.

Preparation
Estramustine Phosphate Capsules

Action and use Cytotoxic substance.

Etamiphylline Camsylate

$C_{13}H_{21}N_5O_2,C_{10}H_{16}O_4S$ 511.6   *19326-29-5*

Etamiphylline Camsylate is 7-(2-diethylaminoethyl)theophylline camphorsulphonate. It contains not less than 98.0 per cent and not more than 102.0 per cent of $C_{13}H_{21}N_5O_2$, $C_{10}H_{16}O_4S$, calculated with reference to the dried substance, when determined by both methods described under the Assay.

Characteristics A white or almost white powder; odour, faint and camphoraceous.

Solubility Very soluble in *water*; soluble in *ethanol (96%)* and in *chloroform*; very slightly soluble in *ether*.

Identification A. The *infra-red absorption spectrum*, Appendix II A, is concordant with the *reference spectrum* of etamiphylline camsylate.
B. The *light absorption*, Appendix II B, in the range 230 to 350 nm of a 0.004% w/v solution exhibits a maximum only at 274 nm. The *absorbance* at 274 nm is about 0.70.
C. Fuse 0.1 g with a pellet of *sodium hydroxide*, dissolve in *water* and neutralise with *hydrochloric acid*. The resulting solution yields *reaction A* characteristic of sulphates, Appendix VI.

Melting point 198° to 202°, Appendix V A.

Acidity pH of a 10% w/v solution, 3.9 to 5.4, Appendix V L.

Free etamiphylline Not more than 2.0% w/w when determined by Method I for *non-aqueous titration*, Appendix VIII A, using 2 g dissolved in 75 ml of *acetic anhydride* and determining the end-point potentiometrically. Each ml of 0.1M *perchloric acid VS* is equivalent to 0.02793 g of free etamiphylline.

Related substances Carry out the method for *thin-layer chromatography*, Appendix III A, using *silica gel HF254* as the coating substance and a mixture of 80 volumes of *chloroform*, 20 volumes of *ethanol (96%)* and 1 volume of 13.5M *ammonia* as the mobile phase. Apply separately to the chromatoplate 10 μl of each of two solutions of the substance being examined in *water* containing (1) 4.0% w/v and (2) 0.0080% w/v. After removal of the plate, allow it to dry in air and examine under *ultra-violet light (254 nm)*. Any *secondary spot* in the chromatogram obtained with solution (1) is not more intense than the spot in the chromatogram obtained with solution (2).

Loss on drying When dried to constant weight at 105°, loses not more than 0.5% of its weight. Use 1 g.

Sulphated ash Not more than 0.2%, Appendix IX A.

Assay *For camphorsulphonic acid* Dissolve 1 g in 25 ml of *methanol*, previously neutralised with 1M *sodium hydroxide*

VS, and titrate with 0.1M *sodium hydroxide VS* using *thymol blue solution* as indicator. Each ml of 0.1M *sodium hydroxide VS* is equivalent to 0.05116 g of $C_{13}H_{21}N_5O_2,C_{10}H_{16}O_4S$.

For etamiphylline Dissolve 0.15 g in 20 ml of 2M *hydrochloric acid*, add 12 ml of a 5% w/v solution of *silicotungstic acid* and allow to stand for 5 hours. Filter, wash the residue with 2M *hydrochloric acid* until the filtrate yields no precipitate with a 1% w/v solution of *quinine hydrochloride* and dry at 110°. Each g of residue is equivalent to 0.2830 g of $C_{13}H_{21}N_5O_2,C_{10}H_{16}O_4S$.

Storage Etamiphylline Camsylate should be kept in a well-closed container.

Preparations
Etamiphylline Injection
Etamiphylline Suppositories

Action and use Xanthine bronchodilator.

In some countries the material described in this monograph may be known as Etamiphylline Camsilate.

Ethacrynic Acid ☆

$C_{13}H_{12}Cl_2O_4$ 303.1   *58-54-8*

Ethacrynic Acid is [(*E*)-2,3-dichloro-4-(2-ethyl-acryloyl)phenoxy]acetic acid. It contains not less than 98.0 per cent and not more than 102.0 per cent of $C_{13}H_{12}Cl_2O_4$, calculated with reference to the dried substance.

Characteristics A white or almost white, crystalline powder.

Solubility Very slightly soluble in *water*; soluble in 1.6 parts of *ethanol (96%)*, in 6 parts of *chloroform* and in 3.5 parts of *ether*. It dissolves in ammonia and in dilute aqueous solutions of alkali hydroxides and carbonates.

Identification *Test A may be omitted if tests B, C, D and E are carried out. Tests B, C and D may be omitted if tests A and E are carried out.*
A. The *infra-red absorption spectrum*, Appendix II A, is concordant with the spectrum of *etacrynic acid EPCRS*.
B. Dissolve 50 mg in a mixture of 99 ml of *methanol* and 1 ml of 1M *hydrochloric acid* and dilute 10 ml to 100 ml with the same mixture of solvents. The *light absorption* of the resulting solution, Appendix II B, in the range 230 to 350 nm exhibits a maximum only at 270 nm and a shoulder at 285 nm. The (A1%, 1 cm) at 270 nm is 110 to 120.
C. Dissolve 70 mg of *hydroxylamine hydrochloride* in 0.1 ml of *water*, add 7 ml of *ethanolic potassium hydroxide solution* and dilute to 10 ml with *aldehyde-free ethanol (96%)*. Allow to stand and add 1 ml of the supernatant liquid to a solution of 30 mg of the substance being examined in 2 ml of *aldehyde-free ethanol (96%)*. Heat the mixture on a water-bath for 3 minutes, cool, add 3 ml of *water* and 0.15 ml of *hydrochloric acid* and examine under ultra-violet light (254 nm). The mixture shows an intense blue fluorescence.

D. Dissolve 25 mg in 2 ml of 1M *sodium hydroxide* and heat on a water-bath for 5 minutes. Cool and add 0.25 ml of a 50% v/v solution of *sulphuric acid*. Add 0.5 ml of a 10% w/v solution of *chromotropic acid sodium salt* and, carefully, 2 ml of *sulphuric acid*. An intense violet colour is produced.
E. *Melting point*, 121° to 124°, Appendix V A, Method I.

Heavy metals 1.0 g complies with *limit test C for heavy metals*, Appendix VII (20 ppm). Use 2 ml of *lead standard solution (10 ppm Pb)* to prepare the standard.

Related substances Carry out the method for *thin-layer chromatography*, Appendix III A, using *silica gel GF254* as the coating substance and a mixture of 60 volumes of *chloroform*, 50 volumes of *ethyl acetate* and 20 volumes of *glacial acetic acid* as the mobile phase. Apply separately to the chromatoplate 10 µl of each of three solutions of the substance being examined in *ethanol (96%)* containing (1) 2.0% w/v, (2) 0.030% w/v and (3) 0.010% w/v. After removal of the plate, allow it to dry in air and examine under *ultra-violet light (254 nm)*. Any *secondary spot* in the chromatogram obtained with solution (1) is not more intense than the spot in the chromatogram obtained with solution (2) and not more than one such spot is more intense than the spot in the chromatogram obtained with solution (3).

Loss on drying When dried to constant weight over *phosphorus pentoxide* at 60° at a pressure of 0.1 to 0.5 kPa, loses not more than 0.5% of its weight. Use 2 g.

Sulphated ash Not more than 0.1%, Appendix IX A, Method II. Use 1 g.

Assay Dissolve 0.25 g in 100 ml of *methanol* and add 5 ml of *water*. Titrate with 0.1M *sodium hydroxide VS* determining the end-point potentiometrically. Each ml of 0.1M *sodium hydroxide VS* is equivalent to 0.03031 g of $C_{13}H_{12}Cl_2O_4$.

Storage Ethacrynic Acid should be kept in a well-closed container.

Preparations
Ethacrynic Acid Tablets
Sodium Ethacrynate Injection

Action and use Diuretic.

The title of the monograph in the European Pharmacopœia is Etacrynic Acid.

Ethambutol Hydrochloride

$C_{10}H_{24}N_2O_2,2HCl$ 277.3   *1070-11-7*

Ethambutol Hydrochloride is (*R,R*)-*N,N'*-ethylenebis(2-aminobutan-1-ol) dihydrochloride. It contains not less than 98.0 per cent and not more than 100.5 per cent of $C_{10}H_{24}N_2O_2,2HCl$, calculated with reference to the dried substance.

Characteristics A white, crystalline powder; odourless or almost odourless.

Solubility Soluble in 1 part of *water* and in 4 parts of *ethanol (96%)*; slightly soluble in *chloroform*; practically insoluble in *ether*.

Identification A. The *infra-red absorption spectrum*, Appendix II A, is concordant with the *reference spectrum* of ethambutol hydrochloride.

B. Dissolve 0.1 g in 10 ml of *water* and add 2 ml of a 1% w/v solution of *copper(II) sulphate* followed by 1 ml of 1M *sodium hydroxide*. A blue colour is produced.

C. Yields the *reactions* characteristic of chlorides, Appendix VI.

Specific optical rotation In a 10% w/v solution, +5.8° to +6.6°, Appendix V F, determined at a temperature of 25°.

Melting point 199° to 204°, Appendix V A.

Heavy metals A 5.0% w/v solution complies with *limit test A for heavy metals*, Appendix VII (20 ppm). Use *lead standard solution (1 ppm Pb)* to prepare the standard.

(+)-2-Aminobutan-1-ol Carry out the method for *thin-layer chromatography*, Appendix III A, using *silica gel G* as the coating substance and a mixture of 55 volumes of *ethyl acetate*, 35 volumes of *glacial acetic acid*, 5 volumes of *hydrochloric acid* and 5 volumes of *water* as the mobile phase. Apply separately to the chromatoplate 2 μl of each of two solutions in *methanol* containing (1) 5.0% w/v of the substance being examined and (2) 0.050% w/v of *(+)-2-aminobutan-1-ol*. After removal of the plate, allow it to dry in air, heat at 105° for 5 minutes, cool, spray with *cadmium and ninhydrin solution* and heat at 90° for 5 minutes. Any spot corresponding to (+)-2-aminobutan-1-ol in the chromatogram obtained with solution (1) is not more intense than the spot in the chromatogram obtained with solution (2).

Loss on drying When dried to constant weight at 105°, loses not more than 0.5% of its weight. Use 1 g.

Sulphated ash Not more than 0.1%, Appendix IX A.

Assay Dissolve 0.2 g in 10 ml of 2M *sodium hydroxide* and extract with five 25-ml quantities of *chloroform*. Evaporate the combined extracts to about 25 ml, filter, add 100 ml of *anhydrous glacial acetic acid* and carry out Method I for *non-aqueous titration*, Appendix VIII A, using *1-naphthol-benzein solution* as indicator. Each ml of 0.1M *perchloric acid VS* is equivalent to 0.01386 g of $C_{10}H_{24}N_2O_2,2HCl$.

Preparation
Ethambutol Tablets

Action and use Antituberculous.

Ethamivan

$C_{12}H_{17}NO_3$ 223.3   *304-84-7*

Ethamivan is *N,N*-diethylvanillamide. It contains not less than 99.0 per cent and not more than 101.0 per cent of $C_{12}H_{17}NO_3$, calculated with reference to the dried substance.

Characteristics A white, crystalline powder; odourless or almost odourless.

Solubility Soluble in 100 parts of *water*, in 2 parts of *ethanol (96%)*, in 3 parts of *acetone*, in 1.5 parts of *chloroform* and in 50 parts of *ether*.

Identification A. The *infra-red absorption spectrum*, Appendix II A, is concordant with the *reference spectrum* of ethamivan.

B. The *light absorption*, Appendix II B, in the range 230 to 350 nm of a 0.006% w/v solution in 0.01M *hydrochloric acid* exhibits a maximum only at 280 nm. The *absorbance* at 280 nm is about 0.92.

C. Dissolve 5 mg in 1 ml of *ethanol (96%)*, add 3 ml of *water* and 1 ml of *iron(III) chloride test-solution*. A blue colour is produced.

D. Boil 0.5 g with 1 ml of 25% v/v *sulphuric acid*, cool, make alkaline with 5M *sodium hydroxide* and heat. The odour of diethylamine is produced.

Acidity or alkalinity pH of a 1% w/v solution, 5.5 to 7.0, Appendix V L.

Melting point 96° to 99°, Appendix V A.

Related substances Carry out the method for *thin-layer chromatography*, Appendix III A, using *silica gel G* as the coating substance and a mixture of 80 volumes of *chloroform* and 20 volumes of *methanol* as the mobile phase. Apply separately to the chromatoplate 10 μl of each of two solutions in *ethanol (96%)* containing (1) 2.0% w/v of the substance being examined and (2) 0.0050% w/v of *vanillic acid*. After removal of the plate, dry it in a current of air, spray with *diazotised sulphanilic acid*, allow to dry and spray with *sodium carbonate solution*. Any *secondary spot* in the chromatogram obtained with solution (1) is not more intense than the spot in the chromatogram obtained with solution (2).

Loss on drying When dried to constant weight over *phosphorus pentoxide* at a pressure not exceeding 0.7 kPa, loses not more than 1.0% of its weight. Use 1 g.

Sulphated ash Not more than 0.1%, Appendix IX A.

Assay Dissolve 0.4 g in 50 ml of *dimethylformamide* and carry out Method II for *non-aqueous titration*, Appendix VIII A, using *magneson solution* as indicator and 0.1M *tetrabutylammonium hydroxide VS*. Each ml of 0.1M *tetrabutylammonium hydroxide VS* is equivalent to 0.02233 g of $C_{12}H_{17}NO_3$.

Preparation
Ethamivan Oral Solution

Action and use Respiratory stimulant.

In some countries the material described in this monograph may be known as Etamivan.

Ethanol

Absolute Alcohol; Dehydrated Alcohol

$CH_3 \cdot CH_2OH$

C_2H_6O 46.07   *64-17-5*

Ethanol contains not less than 99.4 per cent v/v or 99.0 per cent w/w and not more than 100.0 per cent v/v or 100.0 per cent w/w of C_2H_6O.

Characteristics A colourless, clear, mobile and volatile liquid, boiling at 78°; odour, characteristic and spirituous; readily flammable, burning with a blue, smokeless flame; hygroscopic.

Solubility Miscible with *water*, with *chloroform* and with *ether*.

Identification; Acidity or alkalinity; Clarity of solution; Aldehydes; Benzene; Volatile impurities; Non-volatile matter Complies with the requirements stated under Ethanol (96 per cent).

Density 788.16 to 791.2 kg m⁻³, Appendix V G.

Reducing substances Carry out the test described under Ethanol (96 per cent). Not less than 20 minutes elapses between the addition of the permanganate and the colour match.

Storage Ethanol should be protected from moisture and stored at a temperature of 8° to 15°.

Ethanol (96 per cent)
Alcohol (96 per cent)

Ethanol (96 per cent) is a mixture of ethanol and water. It contains not less than 96.0 per cent v/v or 93.8 per cent w/w and not more than 96.6 per cent v/v or 94.7 per cent w/w of C_2H_6O.

Characteristics A colourless, clear, mobile and volatile liquid, boiling at about 78°; odour, characteristic and spirituous; readily flammable, burning with a blue, smokeless flame.

Solubility Miscible with *water*, with *chloroform*, with *ether* and with *glycerol*.

Identification A. Mix 0.25 ml in a small beaker with 1 ml of *potassium permanganate solution* and 0.25 ml of 1M *sulphuric acid* and immediately cover the beaker with a filter paper moistened with a solution recently prepared by dissolving 0.1 g of *sodium nitroprusside* and 0.5 g of *piperazine hydrate* in 5 ml of *water*. An intense blue colour is produced on the filter paper which fades after a few minutes.

B. To 5 ml of a 0.5% v/v solution add 1 ml of 1M *sodium hydroxide* and then, slowly, 2 ml of *iodine solution*. The odour of iodoform is detectable and a yellow precipitate is produced.

Acidity or alkalinity To 20 ml add 0.25 ml of *phenolphthalein solution*. The solution remains colourless and not more than 0.2 ml of 0.1M *sodium hydroxide VS* is required to change the colour of the solution to pink.

Clarity of solution Dilute 5.0 ml to 100 ml with *water*. The solution is *clear*, Appendix IV A, Method I.

Density 803.8 to 806.3 kg m⁻³, Appendix V G.

Aldehydes To 5.0 ml add 5 ml of *water* and 1 ml of *decolorised magenta solution* and allow to stand for 30 minutes. Any colour produced is not more intense than that produced by treating in the same manner 5 ml of a 0.001% w/v solution of redistilled *acetaldehyde* in *aldehyde-free ethanol (96%)* (10 ppm).

Benzene Record the *light absorption*, Appendix II B, of a 4-cm layer over the range 245 to 265 nm. If benzene is present, maxima occur at 249, 254 and 261 nm. Draw a perpendicular through the maximum at 254 nm and draw a line between the minima at 253 nm and 259 nm. The difference between the *absorbance* at the maximum at 254 nm and that at the intercept of the perpendicular with the line joining the minima is not greater than 0.035 (5 ppm).

Reducing substances Carry out the following test in subdued light. Rinse two glass-stoppered measuring cylinders with 15 ml of *hydrochloric acid*, six times with tap water, twice with *water* and finally with the substance being examined. Into one of the cylinders place 50 ml of a colour-standard solution containing 0.5% w/v of *cobalt(II) chloride* and 0.56% w/v of *uranyl nitrate*. Add 50 ml of the substance being examined to the second cylinder and allow to stand for 15 minutes in a water-bath at 14.8° to 15.2°, the water level being approximately 2.5 cm below the neck of the cylinder. Add 2.0 ml of a 0.02% w/v solution of *potassium permanganate* prepared with *water* previously boiled for 30 minutes with sufficient diluted potassium permanganate solution to maintain a faint pink colour. Note the time, stopper the cylinder, shake and return it to the water-bath. Observe the change of colour of the solution and periodically compare with the colour-standard solution by viewing both tubes vertically downwards against a white background. Note the time at which the colour of the solution being examined is concordant with that of the colour-standard solution. Not less than 30 minutes elapse between the addition of the permanganate solution and the colour match.

Volatile impurities Carry out the method for *gas chromatography*, Appendix III B, using the following solutions. Solution (1) contains 0.020% v/v of *butan-2-one* (internal standard). Solution (2) is the substance being examined. Solution (3) is the substance being examined containing 0.020% v/v of the internal standard.

The chromatographic procedure may be carried out using a glass column (1.5 m × 4 mm) packed with porous polymer beads (100 to 120 mesh) (Porapak N or Q and Chromosorb 102 are suitable) and maintained at 130°.

Allow the chromatography to proceed for twice the retention time of the internal standard. In the chromatogram obtained with solution (3) the area of any *secondary peak* is not greater than the area of the peak due to the internal standard and the sum of the areas of the *secondary peaks* is not greater than twice the area of the peak due to the internal standard.

Non-volatile matter 100 ml, evaporated and dried at 105°, leaves not more than 5 mg of residue.

Dilute Ethanols

The official Dilute Ethanols contain 90, 80, 70, 60, 50, 45, 25 and 20 per cent v/v respectively of ethanol. They may be prepared as described below, the final adjustment of volume being made at the same temperature, 20°, as that at which the Ethanol (96 per cent) is measured.

Note On mixing ethanol and water, contraction of volume and rise of temperature occur.

The Dilute Ethanols comply with the tests for Acidity or alkalinity, Clarity of solution, Aldehydes and Non-volatile matter stated under Ethanol (96 per cent).

ETHANOL (90 PER CENT)
Alcohol (90 per cent); Rectified Spirit

Dilute 934 ml of Ethanol (96 per cent) to 1000 ml with Purified Water.

Content of ethanol 89.6 to 90.5% v/v.

Density 826.4 to 829.4 kg m⁻³, Appendix V G.

ETHANOL (80 PER CENT)
Alcohol (80 per cent)

Dilute 831 ml of Ethanol (96 per cent) to 1000 ml with Purified Water.

Content of ethanol 79.5 to 80.3% v/v.

Density 857.4 to 859.6 kg m^{-3}, Appendix V G.

ETHANOL (70 PER CENT)
Alcohol (70 per cent)

Dilute 727 ml of Ethanol (96 per cent) to 1000 ml with Purified Water.

Content of ethanol 69.5 to 70.4% v/v.

Density 883.5 to 885.8 kg m^{-3}, Appendix V G.

ETHANOL (60 PER CENT)
Alcohol (60 per cent)

Dilute 623 ml of Ethanol (96 per cent) to 1000 ml with Purified Water.

Content of ethanol 59.7 to 60.2% v/v.

Density 907.6 to 908.7 kg m^{-3}, Appendix V G.

ETHANOL (50 PER CENT)
Alcohol (50 per cent)

Dilute 519 ml of Ethanol (96 per cent) to 1000 ml with Purified Water.

Content of ethanol 49.6 to 50.2% v/v.

Density 928.6 to 929.8 kg ml^{-3}, Appendix V G.

ETHANOL (45 PER CENT)
Alcohol (45 per cent)

Dilute 468 ml of Ethanol (96 per cent) to 1000 ml with Purified Water.

Content of ethanol 44.7 to 45.3% v/v.

Density 938.0 to 939.0 kg m^{-3}, Appendix V G.

ETHANOL (25 PER CENT)
Alcohol (25 per cent)

Dilute 259 ml of Ethanol (96 per cent) to 1000 ml with Purified Water.

Content of ethanol 24.6 to 25.4% v/v.

Density 966.6 to 967.5 kg m^{-3}, Appendix V G.

ETHANOL (20 PER CENT)
Alcohol (20 per cent)

Dilute 207 ml of Ethanol (96 per cent) to 1000 ml with Purified Water.

Content of ethanol 19.5 to 20.5% v/v.

Density 972.0 to 973.1 kg m^{-3}, Appendix V G.

Ethanolamine
Monoethanolamine

$H_2NCH_2 \cdot CH_2OH$

C_2H_7NO 61.08   *141-43-5*

Ethanolamine is 2-aminoethanol. It contains not less than 98.0 per cent and not more than 100.5 per cent of C_2H_7NO.

Characteristics A clear, colourless or pale yellow liquid; odour, slight.

Solubility Miscible with *water* and with *ethanol (96%)*; slightly soluble in *ether*.

Identification A. To 0.1 ml add 0.3 g of *2,4,6-trinitrophenol* and 1 ml of *water* and evaporate to dryness on a water-bath. The *melting point* of the residue, after recrystallisation from *ethanol (96%)* and drying at 105°, is about 160°, Appendix V A.
B. When freshly distilled the second half of the distillate freezes at about 10°.
C. It is alkaline to *litmus solution*.

Refractive index 1.453 to 1.459, Appendix V E.

Weight per ml 1.014 to 1.023 g, Appendix V G.

Related substances Carry out the method for *gas chromatography*, Appendix III B, using the substance being examined.

The chromatographic procedure may be carried out using a glass column (1.5 m × 4 mm) packed with porous polymer beads (Tenax-GC, 60 to 80 mesh, is suitable), with a temperature rise of 8° per minute from 120° to 190° and maintaining this latter temperature for 15 minutes.

The sum of the areas of the *secondary peaks* is not greater than 2.0% of the area of the principal peak.

Assay Dissolve 2.5 g in 50 ml of 1M *hydrochloric acid VS* and titrate the excess of acid with 1M *sodium hydroxide VS* using *methyl red solution* as indicator. Each ml of 1M *hydrochloric acid VS* is equivalent to 0.06108 g of C_2H_7NO.

Preparation
Ethanolamine Oleate Injection

Action and use Sclerosant.

Anaesthetic Ether ☆
Ether

$(CH_3 \cdot CH_2)_2O$

$C_4H_{10}O$ 74.1   *60-29-7*

Anaesthetic Ether is diethyl ether to which an appropriate quantity of a suitable non-volatile antioxidant may have been added.

Characteristics A clear, colourless, volatile, very mobile liquid; highly flammable.

Solubility Soluble in 15 parts of *water*; miscible with *ethanol (96%)*, with *chloroform* and with fixed and volatile oils.

Identification Complies with the tests for Distillation range and Relative density.

Acidity To 20 ml of *ethanol (96%)* add 0.25 ml of *bromothymol blue solution* and 0.02M *sodium hydroxide VS* dropwise until the blue colour persists for 30 seconds. Add 25 ml of the substance being examined, shake and add 0.02M *sodium hydroxide VS* dropwise until the blue colour reappears and persists for 30 seconds. Not more than 0.4 ml of 0.02M *sodium hydroxide VS* is required.

Distillation range *Do not distil if the substance being examined does not comply with the test for Peroxides.* It distils completely between 34.0° and 35.0°, Appendix V C, using an appropriate heating device and taking precautions to avoid superheating the distillation flask above the level of the liquid.

Relative density 0.714 to 0.716, Appendix V G.

Acetone and aldehydes Shake 10 ml for 10 seconds with 1 ml of *alkaline potassium mercuri-iodide reagent* and allow to stand for 5 minutes protected from light. Only a slight opalescence is produced in the lower layer.

If the substance does not comply with the test, distil 40 ml, after ensuring that it complies with the test for Peroxides, until only 5 ml remains. Collect the distillate in a receiver cooled in ice and repeat the test using 10 ml of the distillate.

Foreign odour Moisten a circle of filter paper 8 cm in diameter with 5 ml of the substance being examined and allow to evaporate. No foreign odour is detectable immediately after the evaporation.

Peroxides Transfer 8 ml of *potassium iodide and starch solution* to a stoppered tube of about 12-ml capacity and about 1.5 cm in diameter. Fill completely with the substance being examined, shake vigorously and allow to stand protected from light for 30 minutes. No colour is produced.

Non-volatile matter *Do not carry out this test unless the substance being examined complies with the test for Peroxides.* Evaporate 50 ml to dryness on a water-bath and dry at 100° to 105°. Not more than 1 mg of residue remains (0.002% w/v).

Water Not more than 0.2% w/v, Appendix IX C. Use 20 ml.

Storage Anaesthetic Ether should be kept in an airtight container, protected from light and stored at a temperature of 8° to 15°. Anaesthetic Ether remaining in a partially filled container may deteriorate rapidly.

Labelling The label states the nature and the quantity of any added antioxidant.

Action and use General anaesthetic.

Solvent Ether

$C_4H_{10}O$ 74.12   *60-29-7*

Solvent Ether is diethyl ether.

Characteristics A clear, colourless, volatile, very mobile liquid; odour, characteristic. Highly flammable; mixtures of its vapour with oxygen, air, or nitrous oxide in certain concentrations are explosive.

Solubility Soluble in 15 parts of *water*; miscible with *ethanol (96%)*, with *chloroform* and with fixed and volatile oils.

Acidity To 20 ml of *ethanol (96%)* add 0.25 ml of *bromothymol blue solution* and 0.02M *sodium hydroxide VS* dropwise until the blue colour persists for 30 seconds. Add 25 ml of the substance being examined, shake and

add 0.02M *sodium hydroxide VS* dropwise until the blue colour reappears and persists for 30 seconds. Not more than 0.4 ml of 0.02M *sodium hydroxide VS* is required.

Distillation range *Do not distil if the substance being examined does not comply with the test for Peroxides.* It distils completely between 34° and 36°, Appendix V C, using an appropriate heating device and taking precautions to avoid superheating the distillation flask above the level of the liquid.

Weight per ml 0.714 to 0.718 g, Appendix V G.

Peroxides Transfer 8 ml of *potassium iodide solution* to a stoppered tube of about 12-ml capacity and about 1.5 cm in diameter. Fill completely with the substance being examined, shake vigorously and allow to stand protected from light for 30 minutes. Any yellow colour produced is not more intense than that of 0.5 ml of 0.0005M *iodine* diluted with 8 ml of *potassium iodide solution*.

Methanol Shake vigorously 2 volumes with 1 volume of *ethanol (20%)* and 1 volume of *water* and allow the mixture to separate. To 5 ml of the lower layer add 2 ml of *potassium permanganate—orthophosphoric acid reagent*, allow to stand for 10 minutes and add 2.0 ml of *oxalic acid—sulphuric acid reagent*. To the colourless solution add 5 ml of *decolorised magenta solution*, allow to stand at 15° to 30° and examine after 30 minutes. No colour is produced.

Non-volatile matter *Do not carry out this test unless the substance being examined complies with the test for Peroxides.* Evaporate 70 ml to dryness on a water-bath and dry at 100° to 105°. Not more than 1 mg of residue remains.

Storage Solvent Ether should be kept in a well-closed container, protected from light and stored at a temperature not exceeding 15°.

Ethinyloestradiol ☆

$C_{20}H_{24}O_2$ 296.4   *57-63-6*

Ethinyloestradiol is 19-nor-17α-pregna-1,3,5(10)-trien-20-yne-3,17β-diol. It contains not less than 97.0 per cent and not more than 102.0 per cent of $C_{20}H_{24}O_2$, calculated with reference to the dried substance.

Characteristics A white or slightly yellowish-white, crystalline powder.

Solubility Practically insoluble in *water*; soluble in 6 parts of *ethanol (96%)*; freely soluble in *ether*; sparingly soluble in *chloroform*. It dissolves in dilute solutions of alkali hydroxides.

Identification *Test A may be omitted if tests B, C and D are carried out. Tests C and D may be omitted if tests A and B are carried out.*

A. The *infra-red absorption spectrum*, Appendix II A, is concordant with the spectrum of *ethinylestradiol EPCRS*. If the spectra are not concordant, prepare new spectra using 3% w/v solutions in *chloroform IR*.

B. In the test for Related substances the principal spot in the chromatogram obtained with solution (2) corresponds to that in the chromatogram obtained with solution (4) when examined in daylight and under *ultra-violet light (365 nm)*.

C. Dissolve 1 mg in 1 ml of *sulphuric acid*; an orange-red colour develops which exhibits a greenish fluorescence when examined under ultra-violet light (365 nm). Add the solution to 10 ml of *water*; the colour changes to violet and a violet precipitate is produced.

D. *Melting point*, 181° to 185°, Appendix V A, Method I.

Clarity and colour of solution A 5.0% w/v solution in *absolute ethanol* is *clear*, Appendix IV A, and not more intensely coloured than *reference solution BY₆*, Appendix IV B, Method I.

Light absorption Dissolve 0.1 g in sufficient *ethanol (96%)* to produce 100 ml and dilute 10 ml to 100 ml with *ethanol (96%)*. The A(1%, 1 cm) of the resulting solution at the maximum at 281 nm is 69 to 73, Appendix II B.

Specific optical rotation In a 5% w/v solution in *pyridine*, −27° to −30°, Appendix V F.

Related substances Carry out the method for *thin-layer chromatography*, Appendix III A, using *silica gel G* as the coating substance and a mixture of 90 volumes of *toluene* and 10 volumes of *ethanol (96%)* as the mobile phase. Apply separately to the chromatoplate 5 µl of each of five solutions in a mixture of 9 volumes of *chloroform* and 1 volume of *methanol* containing (1) 2.0% w/v of the substance being examined, (2) 0.10% w/v of the substance being examined, (3) 0.020% w/v of the substance being examined, (4) 0.10% w/v of *ethinylestradiol EPCRS* and (5) 0.020% w/v of *estrone EPCRS*. After removal of the plate, allow it to dry in air until the odour of the solvent is no longer detectable, heat at 110° for 10 minutes and spray the hot plate with *ethanolic sulphuric acid (20%)*. Heat again at 110° for 10 minutes and examine under *ultra-violet light (365 nm)*. In the chromatogram obtained with solution (1) any spot corresponding to estrone is not more intense than the spot in the chromatogram obtained with solution (5) and any other *secondary spot* is not more intense than the spot in the chromatogram obtained with solution (3).

Loss on drying When dried at 100° to 105° for 3 hours, loses not more than 1.0% of its weight. Use 0.5 g.

Assay Dissolve 0.2 g in 40 ml of *tetrahydrofuran*, add 5 ml of a 10% w/v solution of *silver nitrate* and titrate with 0.1M *sodium hydroxide VS* determining the end-point potentiometrically. Repeat the operation without the substance being examined. The difference between the titrations represents the amount of sodium hydroxide required. Each ml of 0.1M *sodium hydroxide VS* is equivalent to 0.02964 g of $C_{20}H_{24}O_2$.

Storage Ethinyloestradiol should be kept in a well-closed container and protected from light.

Preparation

Ethinyloestradiol Tablets

Action and use Oestrogen.

The title of the monograph in the European Pharmacopœia is Ethinylestradiol.

Ethionamide ☆

$C_8H_{10}N_2S$ 166.2   *536-33-4*

Ethionamide is 2-ethylpyridine-4-carbothio-amide. It contains not less than 98.5 per cent and not more than 101.0 per cent of $C_8H_{10}N_2S$, calculated with reference to the dried substance.

Characteristics Small yellow crystals or a yellow, crystalline powder; odour, slight.

Solubility Practically insoluble in *water*; soluble in 30 parts of *ethanol (96%)*; soluble in *methanol*; slightly soluble in *chloroform* and in *ether*.

Identification *Test A may be omitted if tests B, C and D are carried out. Tests B and C may be omitted if tests A and D are carried out.*

A. The *infra-red absorption spectrum*, Appendix II A, is concordant with the spectrum of *ethionamide EPCRS*.

B. The *light absorption*, Appendix II B, in the range 230 to 350 nm of a 0.001% w/v solution in *methanol* exhibits a maximum only at 290 nm. The A(1%, 1 cm) at 290 nm is 380 to 440.

C. Dissolve 10 mg in 5 ml of *methanol* and add 5 ml of 0.1M *silver nitrate*. A dark brown precipitate is produced.

D. *Melting point*, 158° to 164°, Appendix V A, Method I.

Acidity Dissolve 2 g in 20 ml of *methanol*, heat to about 50° and add 20 ml of *water*. Cool slightly, shake until crystallisation occurs and allow to cool to room temperature. Add 60 ml of *water* and titrate with 0.1M *sodium hydroxide VS* using 0.2 ml of *cresol red solution* as indicator. Not more than 0.2 ml is required to change the colour of the solution to red.

Clarity of solution Dissolve 0.5 g in 10 ml of *methanol*, heat to about 50° and allow to cool to room temperature. The solution is not more opalescent than *reference suspension II*, Appendix IV A.

Heavy metals 1.0 g complies with *limit test D for heavy metals*, Appendix VII (20 ppm). Use 2 ml of *lead standard solution (10 ppm Pb)* to prepare the standard.

Related substances Carry out the method for *thin-layer chromatography*, Appendix III A, using *silica gel GF254* as the coating substance and a mixture of 90 volumes of *chloroform* and 10 volumes of *methanol* as the mobile phase. Apply separately to the chromatoplate 10 µl of each of three solutions of the substance being examined in *acetone* containing (1) 2.0% w/v, (2) 0.010% w/v and (3) 0.0040% w/v. After removal of the plate, allow it to dry in air and examine under *ultra-violet light (254 nm)*. Any *secondary spot* in the chromatogram obtained with solution (1) is not more intense than the spot in the chromatogram obtained with solution (2) and not more than one such spot is more intense than the spot in the chromatogram obtained with solution (3).

Loss on drying When dried at 100° to 105° for 3 hours, loses not more than 0.5% of its weight. Use 1 g.

Sulphated ash Not more than 0.1%, Appendix IX A, Method II. Use 1 g.

Assay Dissolve 0.15 g in 50 ml of *anhydrous glacial acetic acid* and carry out Method I for *non-aqueous titration*, Appendix VIII A, determining the end-point potentiometrically. Each ml of 0.1M *perchloric acid VS* is equivalent to 0.01662 g of $C_8H_{10}N_2S$.

Action and use Antituberculous.

Ethisterone ☆

$C_{21}H_{28}O_2$ 312.5   *434-03-7*

Ethisterone is 17β-hydroxy-17α-pregn-4-en-20-yn-3-one. It contains not less than 98.0 per cent and not more than 102.0 per cent of $C_{21}H_{28}O_2$, calculated with reference to the dried substance.

Characteristics A white or almost white, crystalline powder; odourless or almost odourless. It melts at about 274°, with slight decomposition.

Solubility Practically insoluble in *water*; slightly soluble in *ethanol (96%)* and in *chloroform*; sparingly soluble in *pyridine*.

Identification *Test A may be omitted if tests B, C, D and E are carried out. Tests C and D may be omitted if tests A, B and E are carried out.*

A. The *infra-red absorption spectrum*, Appendix II A, is concordant with the spectrum of *ethisterone EPCRS*. If the spectra are not concordant, dissolve the substances in *chloroform IR*, evaporate to dryness on a water-bath and prepare new spectra of the residues.

B. Carry out the test for *identification of steroids*, Appendix III A, using *impregnating solvent I* and *mobile phase G* and applying separately to the chromatoplate 2 μl of each of two solutions in a mixture of 3 volumes of *chloroform* and 1 volume of *absolute ethanol* containing (1) 0.1% w/v of the substance being examined and (2) 0.1% w/v of *ethisterone EPCRS*. The principal spot in the chromatogram obtained with solution (1) is similar in position, colour, fluorescence and size to that in the chromatogram obtained with solution (2).

C. Dissolve 2 mg in 2 ml of *ethanol (96%)*, add 1 ml of *ammoniacal silver nitrate solution* and heat on a water-bath. The solution becomes turbid and a white precipitate is produced which becomes grey on heating with the deposition of a silver mirror on the walls of the tube.

D. Dissolve 2 mg in a cooled mixture of 2 ml of *absolute ethanol* and 2 ml of *sulphuric acid* and heat to 70°. The resulting solution appears bluish-violet when examined under transmitted light and red in reflected light and exhibits a bright red fluorescence when examined under ultra-violet light (365 nm).

E. Dissolve 2 mg in 2 ml of *ethanol (96%)* and add 1 ml of a 1% w/v solution of *butylated hydroxytoluene* in *ethanol (96%)* and 2 ml of 1M *sodium hydroxide*. Heat at 80° for 30 minutes and cool. An intense blue colour develops.

Light absorption Dissolve 10 mg in sufficient *absolute ethanol* to produce 100 ml and dilute 10 ml to 100 ml with the same solvent. The A(1%, 1 cm) of the resulting solution at the maximum at 240 nm is 500 to 540, Appendix II B.

Specific optical rotation In a 1% w/v solution in *pyridine*, +29° to +33°, Appendix V F.

Related substances Carry out the method for *thin-layer chromatography*, Appendix III A, using *silica gel H* as the coating substance and a mixture of 95 volumes of *chloroform* and 5 volumes of *methanol* as the mobile phase. Apply separately to the chromatoplate 10 μl, as two 5-μl applications, of each of two solutions of the substance being examined in a mixture of 3 volumes of *chloroform* and 1 volume of *absolute ethanol* containing (1) 1.0% w/v and (2) 0.0050% w/v. After removal of the plate, allow it to dry in air, spray with *ethanolic sulphuric acid (20%)* and heat at 120° for 15 minutes. Examine in daylight and under *ultra-violet light (365 nm)*. Any *secondary spot* in the chromatogram obtained with solution (1) is not more intense than the spot in the chromatogram obtained with solution (2).

Loss on drying When dried to constant weight at 100° to 105°, loses more than 0.5% of its weight. Use 1 g.

Assay Dissolve 0.2 g in 40 ml of *tetrahydrofuran*, add 10 ml of a 10% w/v solution of *silver nitrate* and titrate with 0.1M *sodium hydroxide VS*, using *bromocresol green solution* as indicator, until a violet colour is produced. Repeat the operation without the substance being examined. The difference between the titrations represents the amount of sodium hydroxide required. Each ml of 0.1M *sodium hydroxide VS* is equivalent to 0.03125 g of $C_{21}H_{28}O_2$.

Storage Ethisterone should be kept in a well-closed container and protected from light.

Action and use Progestogen.

Ethosuximide

$C_7H_{11}NO_2$ 141.2   *77-67-8*

Ethosuximide is 2-ethyl-2-methylsuccinimide. It contains not less than 98.5 per cent and not more than 101.0 per cent of $C_7H_{11}NO_2$, calculated with reference to the anhydrous substance.

Characteristics A white or almost white powder or waxy solid; odourless or almost odourless.

Solubility Soluble in 4.5 parts of *water* and in less than 1 part of *ethanol (96%)*, of *chloroform* and of *ether*.

Identification A. The *infra-red absorption spectrum*, Appendix II A, is concordant with the *reference spectrum* of ethosuximide. Melt a sufficient quantity, prepare a thin film between two previously warmed potassium bromide plates and record the spectrum immediately.

B. The *light absorption*, Appendix II B, in the range 230 to 350 nm of a 0.10% w/v solution in *ethanol (96%)* exhibits a maximum only at 248 nm. The *absorbance* at 248 nm is about 0.85.

C. Heat 0.1 g with 0.2 g of *resorcinol* and 0.1 ml of *sulphuric acid* at 140° for 5 minutes, add 5 ml of *water*, make alkaline with 5M *sodium hydroxide* and add 0.2 ml to a large volume of *water*. A bright green fluorescence is produced.

D. *Melting point*, about 46°, Appendix V A.

Cyanide To 1.0 g add 1 ml of 1M *sodium hydroxide*, warm on a water-bath for 2 minutes, cool and add 1 ml of 1M *hydrochloric acid*, 25 ml of *water* and 1 ml of *bromine water*. Allow to stand for 2 minutes, add 2 ml of *arsenic trioxide solution* and remove the bromine vapour with a current of air. Add 10 ml of *barbituric acid and pyridine solution*, warm in a water-bath at 40° for 45 minutes, cool and add sufficient *water* to produce 50 ml. The *absorbance* of the resulting solution at the maximum at 586 nm is not more than 0.88, Appendix II B.

2-Ethyl-2-methylsuccinic acid and anhydride Carry out the method for *gas chromatography*, Appendix III B, using solutions in *chloroform* containing (1) 0.010% w/v of *2-ethyl-2-methylsuccinic acid BPCRS* and (2) 5.0% w/v of the substance being examined.

The chromatographic procedure may be carried out using a glass column (1.5 m × 4 mm) packed with *acid-washed, silanised diatomaceous support* (80 to 100 mesh) coated with 3% w/w of cyanopropylmethyl phenyl methyl silicone fluid (OV-225 is suitable) and maintained at 165° with an inlet port temperature of 240°.

The area of the peak in the chromatogram obtained with solution (1) is greater than the area of any corresponding peak in the chromatogram obtained with solution (2).

Sulphated ash Not more than 0.1%, Appendix IX A.

Water Not more than 0.5% w/w, Appendix IX C. Use 1 g.

Assay Dissolve 0.2 g in 30 ml of *dimethylformamide* and carry out Method II for *non-aqueous titration*, Appendix VIII A, using *magneson solution* as indicator and 0.1M *tetrabutylammonium hydroxide VS*. Each ml of 0.1M *tetrabutylammonium hydroxide VS* is equivalent to 0.01412 g of $C_7H_{11}NO_2$.

Preparations
Ethosuximide Capsules
Ethosuximide Oral Solution

Action and use Anticonvulsant.

Ethyl Chloride

$CH_3 \cdot CH_2Cl$

C_2H_5Cl 64.52   *75-00-3*

Ethyl Chloride may be prepared by the action of hydrogen chloride on Ethanol or on Industrial Methylated Spirit; in the latter case it contains a small variable proportion of methyl chloride.

Characteristics Gaseous at ambient temperatures and pressures, but usually compressed to a colourless, mobile, flammable and very volatile liquid; odour, ethereal.

Solubility Slightly soluble in *water*; miscible with *ethanol* (96%) and with *ether*.

Identification A. Burns with a luminous flame with the production of hydrogen chloride.

B. Shake vigorously 2 ml with 5M *sodium hydroxide* and warm on a water-bath. Reserve a portion of the solution for test C. To the resulting solution add 2 ml of *iodine solution* and warm. Crystals of iodoform are produced.

C. The solution reserved in test B yields the *reactions* characteristic of chlorides, Appendix VI.

Acidity or alkalinity Shake 10 ml with 10 ml of ice-cold *water* and allow the ethyl chloride to evaporate spontaneously. The residual liquid is neutral to *litmus solution*.

Ethanol Warm 5 ml of the residual liquid obtained in the test for Acidity or alkalinity with *iodine solution* and *sodium carbonate*. No yellow crystals of iodoform are produced.

Ionisable chloride 5 ml of the residual liquid obtained in the test for Acidity or alkalinity yields no turbidity with *silver nitrate solution*.

Distillation range Fit a dry 100-ml measuring cylinder with a stopper carrying a short exit tube not less than 6 mm in internal diameter and an accurately standardised short-bulb thermometer covering the range −20° to +30° and graduated in increments of 0.1°. Cover the bulb of the thermometer with a piece of very fine muslin, free from grease and sizing materials, so that one end hangs down about 10 mm below the bulb. Cool the cylinder in ice, transfer to it 100 ml of the sample, previously cooled in ice, insert the stopper and adjust the thermometer so that the end of the muslin dips into the liquid and the bulb is above the surface. Replace the ice with water at 24° to 26° and observe the temperature when 5 ml of sample has evaporated and again when 5 ml remains. Continually lower the thermometer to maintain its position relative to the liquid surface throughout the test. Correct the observed temperature by adding 0.26° for every kPa that the barometric pressure is below 101.3 kPa or by subtracting 0.26° for every kPa above. The corrected temperature range is 12.0° to 12.5°.

Apparent specific gravity (0°/15°) Cool a sufficient quantity to about −5° by surrounding the container with a mixture of methanol and solid carbon dioxide. Transfer the cooled substance being examined to a hydrometer cylinder standing in melting ice and insert a hydrometer and thermometer. The reading on the hydrometer when the temperature has risen to 0° is 0.921 to 0.926.

Other organic compounds On evaporation, no foreign odour is detectable at any stage.

Non-volatile matter When evaporated and dried at 105°, leaves not more than 0.01% w/w of residue.

Storage Ethyl Chloride should be protected from light and stored at a temperature not exceeding 15°.

Action and use Anaesthetic.

Ethyl Cinnamate

C₁₁H₁₂O₂   176.2   *103-36-6*

Ethyl Cinnamate is predominantly ethyl (*E*)-3-phenylprop-2-enoate. It contains not less than 99.0 per cent and not more than 100.5 per cent of $C_{11}H_{12}O_2$, calculated with reference to the anhydrous substance.

Characteristics A clear, colourless or almost colourless liquid; odour, fruity, balsamic.

Solubility Practically insoluble in *water*; miscible with most organic solvents.

Identification A. The *infra-red absorption spectrum*, Appendix II A, is concordant with the *reference spectrum* of ethyl cinnamate.
B. The *light absorption*, Appendix II B, in the range 230 to 350 nm of a 0.001% w/v solution in *ethanol (96%)* exhibits a maximum only at 276 nm. The *absorbance* at 276 nm is about 1.23.
C. To 1 g add 25 ml of 1M *sodium hydroxide*, boil under a reflux condenser for 1 hour, cool and acidify with *hydrochloric acid*. The *melting point* of the resulting precipitate, after filtration, washing with *water* and drying at 60° at a pressure not exceeding 0.7 kPa, is about 133°, Appendix V A.

Acidity Mix 30 g with 150 ml of *ethanol (96%)* previously neutralised to *phenolphthalein solution*. Not more than 1.0 ml of 0.1M *sodium hydroxide VS* is required for neutralisation using *phenolphthalein solution* as indicator.

Refractive index 1.558 to 1.560, Appendix V E.

Weight per ml 1.048 to 1.051 g, Appendix V G.

Related substances Carry out the method for *gas chromatography*, Appendix III B, using the following solutions. Solution (1) contains 1.0% w/v of the substance being examined in *chloroform*. Solution (2) is the substance being examined.

The chromatographic procedure may be carried out using a glass column (1.5 m × 4 mm) packed with *acid-washed, silanised diatomaceous support* coated with 3% w/w of cyanopropylmethyl phenyl methyl silicone fluid (OV-225 is suitable) and maintained at 150°.

In the chromatogram obtained with solution (2) the sum of the areas of any *secondary peaks* is not greater than 1% by *normalisation*.

Sulphated ash Not more than 0.1%, Appendix IX A.

Water Not more than 0.1% w/w, Appendix IX C. Use 5 g.

Assay Carry out the method for the *determination of esters*, Appendix VIII L, using 2.5 g and 50 ml of 0.5M *ethanolic potassium hydroxide VS*. Each ml of 0.5M *ethanolic potassium hydroxide VS* is equivalent to 0.08811 g of $C_{11}H_{12}O_2$.

Ethyl Gallate

C₉H₁₀O₅   198.2   *831-61-8*

Ethyl Gallate is ethyl 3,4,5-trihydroxybenzoate.

Characteristics A white to creamy-white, crystalline powder, odourless or almost odourless.

Solubility Slightly soluble in *water*; soluble in 3 parts of *ethanol (96%)* and in 3 parts of *ether*; practically insoluble in *arachis oil*.

Identification A. The *light absorption*, Appendix II B, in the range 230 to 350 nm of a 0.002% w/v solution in *methanol* exhibits a maximum only at 275 nm. The *absorbance* at 275 nm is about 1.08.
B. Carry out the method for *gas chromatography*, Appendix III B, using a solution prepared in the following manner. Boil 0.5 g with 50 ml of 5M *sodium hydroxide* under a reflux condenser for 10 minutes and distil 5 ml.

The chromatographic procedure may be carried out using a glass column (1.5 m × 4 mm) packed with *acid-washed, silanised diatomaceous support* (80 to 100 mesh) coated with 10% w/w of free fatty acid phase (Supelco 'FFAP' is suitable) and maintained at 80°.

The principal peak in the chromatogram has the same retention time as that of *absolute ethanol*, examined under the same conditions.
C. Dissolve 5 mg in a mixture of 25 ml of *acetone* and 25 ml of *water* and add 0.05 ml of *iron(III) chloride solution*. A purplish-black colour is produced which rapidly becomes bluish-black.

Melting point 151° to 154°, Appendix V A.

Acidity Dissolve 0.4 g in 100 ml of warm *carbon dioxide-free water*, cool and titrate with 0.1M *sodium hydroxide VS* using *bromocresol green solution* as indicator. Not more than 0.1 ml of 0.1M *sodium hydroxide VS* is required.

Chloride Shake 0.50 g with 50 ml of *water* for 5 minutes and filter. 15 ml of the resulting solution complies with the *limit test for chlorides*, Appendix VII (330 ppm).

Loss on drying When dried to constant weight at 105°, loses not more than 1.0% of its weight. Use 1 g.

Sulphated ash Not more than 0.1%, Appendix IX A.

Storage Ethyl Gallate should be kept in a well-closed container and protected from light. Contact with metals should be avoided.

Action and use Antioxidant.

Ethyl Hydroxybenzoate
Ethylparaben

C₉H₁₀O₃   166.2   *120-47-8*

Ethyl Hydroxybenzoate is ethyl 4-hydroxybenzoate. It contains not less than 99.0 per cent and not more than 101.0 per cent of $C_9H_{10}O_3$.

Characteristics A white, crystalline powder; odourless or almost odourless.

Solubility Very slightly soluble in *water*; soluble in 2 parts of *ethanol (96%)* and in 3.5 parts of *ether*; slightly soluble in *glycerol*. It dissolves in solutions of the alkali hydroxides.

Identification A. The *infra-red absorption spectrum*, Appendix II A, is concordant with the *reference spectrum* of ethyl hydroxybenzoate.

B. The *light absorption*, Appendix II B, in the range 230 to 350 nm of a 0.001% w/v solution in *ethanol (96%)* exhibits a maximum only at 259 nm. The *absorbance* at 259 nm is about 0.96.

C. Dissolve 0.1 g in 2 ml of *ethanol (96%)*, boil and add 0.5 ml of *mercury—nitric acid solution*. A precipitate is produced slowly and the supernatant liquid becomes red.

C. *Melting point*, about 117°, Appendix V A.

Acidity Dissolve 0.2 g in 10 ml of *ethanol (50%)* previously neutralised to *methyl red solution* and titrate with 0.1M *sodium hydroxide VS* using *methyl red solution* as indicator. Not more than 0.1 ml of 0.1M *sodium hydroxide VS* is required to change the colour of the solution.

Related substances Carry out the method for *thin-layer chromatography*, Appendix III A, using a silica gel F254 precoated chromatoplate the surface of which has been modified by chemically-bonded octadecylsilyl groups (Whatman KC18F plates are suitable) and a mixture of 70 volumes of *methanol*, 30 volumes of *water* and 1 volume of *glacial acetic acid* as the mobile phase. Apply separately to the plate 2 µl of each of two solutions of the substance being examined in *acetone* containing (1) 1.0% w/v and (2) 0.010% w/v. After removal of the plate, allow it to dry in air and examine under *ultra-violet light (254 nm)*. Any *secondary spot* in the chromatogram obtained with solution (1) is not more intense than the spot in the chromatogram obtained with solution (2).

Sulphated ash Not more than 0.1%, Appendix IX A.

Assay Gently boil 0.1 g under a reflux condenser with 15 ml of 2M *sodium hydroxide* for 30 minutes. Allow to cool, add 25 ml of 0.0333M *potassium bromate VS*, 5 ml of a 12.5% w/v solution of *potassium bromide* and 10 ml of *hydrochloric acid* and immediately stopper the flask. Shake for 15 minutes and allow to stand for 15 minutes. Add 25 ml of *potassium iodide solution* and shake vigorously. Titrate the liberated iodine with 0.1M *sodium thiosulphate VS* using *starch mucilage*, added towards the end of the titration, as indicator. The volume of 0.0333M *potassium bromate VS* used is equivalent to half of the volume of 0.1M *sodium thiosulphate VS* required for the titration. Each ml of 0.0333M *potassium bromate VS* is equivalent to 0.005539 g of $C_9H_{10}O_3$.

Action and use Antimicrobial preservative.

Ethyl Oleate

HC·(CH₂)₇CO₂Et
‖
HC·(CH₂)₇·CH₃

$C_{20}H_{38}O_2$ 310.5   *111-62-6*

Ethyl Oleate contains the equivalent of not less than 100.0 per cent w/w and not more than 105.0 per cent w/w of the ethyl esters of oleic and related acids, calculated as $C_{20}H_{38}O_2$.

Characteristics A pale yellow oil; odour, slight but not rancid.

Solubility Practically insoluble in *water*; miscible with *ethanol (96%)*, with *chloroform*, with *ether* and with fixed oils.

Acid value Not more than 0.5, Appendix X B.

Iodine value 75 to 84 (*iodine monochloride method*), Appendix X E.

Weight per ml 0.869 to 0.874 g, Appendix V G.

Peroxides Dissolve 5 g in 15 ml of *chloroform*, add 20 ml of *glacial acetic acid* and 0.5 ml of a saturated solution of *potassium iodide*, mix well, allow to stand in the dark for exactly 1 minute, add 30 ml of *water* and titrate with 0.01M *sodium thiosulphate VS* using *starch mucilage* as indicator. Not more than 2.5 ml of 0.01M *sodium thiosulphate VS* is required.

Assay Carry out the method for the *determination of esters*, Appendix VIII L. Each ml of 0.5M *ethanolic potassium hydroxide VS* is equivalent to 0.1553 g of $C_{20}H_{38}O_2$.

Storage Ethyl Oleate should be kept in a small, well-filled and well-closed container or under an atmosphere of nitrogen. It should be protected from light.

Ethylenediamine

CH₂·NH₂
|
CH₂·NH₂

$C_2H_8N_2$ 60.1   *107-15-3*

Ethylenediamine is ethane-1,2-diamine. It contains not less than 97.5 per cent w/w and not more than 101.5 per cent w/w of $C_2H_8N_2$.

Characteristics A clear, colourless or slightly yellow liquid; odour, ammoniacal.

Solubility Miscible with *water* and with *ethanol (96%)*.

Identification A. The *infra-red absorption spectrum*, Appendix II A, is concordant with the *reference spectrum* of ethylenediamine.

B. Mix 1 ml with 5 ml of *water*. To 0.2 ml of the mixture add 2 ml of a 1% w/v solution of *copper(II) sulphate* and shake. A purplish-blue colour is produced.

C. Strongly alkaline.

Ammonia and other bases Dissolve 1.2 g in 20 ml of *ethanol (96%)* and add, dropwise with stirring, 4.5 ml of *hydrochloric acid*. Evaporate to dryness on a water-bath, breaking up any resulting cake with a glass rod, and dry at 105° for 1 hour. Each g of residue is equivalent to 0.4518 g of $C_2H_8N_2$. Calculate the percentage of $C_2H_8N_2$. The result is within 0.5 of the percentage determined in the Assay.

Heavy metals Evaporate 5.0 g to dryness on a water-bath, add 1 ml of *hydrochloric acid* and 0.5 ml of *nitric acid* and again evaporate to dryness. Dissolve the residue in 20 ml of warm *water* and dilute to 50 ml with *water*. 12 ml of the resulting solution complies with *limit test A for heavy metals*, Appendix VII (10 ppm). Use *lead standard solution (1 ppm Pb)* to prepare the standard.

Iron To the residue obtained in the test for Non-volatile matter add 1 ml of *hydrochloric acid* and 0.5 ml of *nitric acid*, evaporate to dryness on a water-bath, dissolve the residue in 20 ml of warm *water* and dilute to 100 ml with *water*. 10 ml of the resulting solution complies with the *limit test for iron*, Appendix VII (20 ppm).

Non-volatile matter Evaporate 4 ml to dryness on a water-bath and dry at 105° for 1 hour. The residue weighs not more than 0.11 g.

Assay Dissolve 1.2 g in 60 ml of *water* and titrate with 1M *hydrochloric acid VS*, using *bromophenol blue solution* as indicator, until a yellow colour is produced. Each ml of 1M *hydrochloric acid VS* is equivalent to 0.03005 g of $C_2H_8N_2$.

Storage Ethylenediamine should be kept in a well-closed container and protected from light.

Ethylenediamine Hydrate

$C_2H_8N_2,H_2O$ 78.11

Ethylenediamine Hydrate contains not less than 97.5 per cent w/w and not more than 101.5 per cent w/w of $C_2H_8N_2,H_2O$.

Characteristics A clear, colourless or slightly yellow liquid; odour, ammoniacal.

Solubility Miscible with *water* and with *ethanol (96%)*.

Identification A. Mix 1 ml with 5 ml of *water*. To 0.15 ml of the mixture add 2 ml of a 1% w/v solution of *copper(II) sulphate* and shake. A purplish-blue colour is produced.
B. Strongly alkaline.

Ammonia and other bases Transfer 1.5 g to a small dish with the aid of *ethanol (96%)*, add, with stirring, 20 ml of 2M *hydrochloric acid*, rinse the stirring rod with 5 ml of *ethanol (96%)*, evaporate the solution to dryness on a water-bath and dry at 105° for 1 hour. Each g of residue is equivalent to 0.5872 g of $C_2H_8N_2,H_2O$. Calculate the percentage of $C_2H_8N_2,H_2O$; the result is within 0.5 of the percentage determined in the Assay.

Heavy metals Evaporate 5.0 g to dryness on a water-bath, add 1 ml of *hydrochloric acid* and 0.5 ml of *nitric acid* and again evaporate to dryness. Dissolve the residue in 20 ml of warm *water* and dilute to 50 ml with *water*. 12 ml of the resulting solution complies with *limit test A for heavy metals*, Appendix VII (10 ppm). Use *lead standard solution (1 ppm Pb)* to prepare the standard.

Iron To the residue obtained in the test for Non-volatile matter add 1 ml of *hydrochloric acid* and 0.5 ml of *nitric acid* and evaporate to dryness on a water-bath; dissolve the residue in 20 ml of warm *water* and dilute to 100 ml with *water*. 10 ml of the resulting solution complies with the *limit test for iron*, Appendix VII (20 ppm).

Non-volatile matter Evaporate 5 ml to dryness on a water-bath and dry at 105° for 1 hour. The residue weighs not more than 1 mg.

Assay Dissolve 1.5 g in 75 ml of *water* and titrate with 1M *hydrochloric acid VS*, using *bromophenol blue solution* as indicator, until a yellow colour is produced. Each ml of 1M *hydrochloric acid VS* is equivalent to 0.03906 g of $C_2H_8N_2,H_2O$.

Storage Ethylenediamine Hydrate should be kept in a well-closed container and protected from light.

Ethylmorphine Hydrochloride ☆

$C_{19}H_{23}NO_3,HCl,2H_2O$ 385.9   *125-30-4*

Ethylmorphine Hydrochloride is 7,8-didehydro-4,5-epoxy-3-ethyl-17-methylmorphinan-6-ol hydrochloride dihydrate. It contains not less than 99.0 per cent and not more than 100.5 per cent of $C_{19}H_{23}NO_3,HCl$, calculated with reference to the anhydrous substance.

Characteristics A white or almost white, crystalline powder.

Solubility Soluble in *water* and in *ethanol (96%)*; slightly soluble in *chloroform*; practically insoluble in *ether*.

Identification *Test A may be omitted if tests B, C and D are carried out. Tests B and C may be omitted if tests A and D are carried out.*
A. The *infra-red absorption spectrum*, Appendix II A, is concordant with the European Pharmacopœia reference spectrum of ethylmorphine hydrochloride.
B. To 10 mg add 1 ml of *sulphuric acid* and 0.05 ml of a 1.3% w/v solution of *iron(III) chloride hexahydrate* and heat on a water-bath. A blue colour is produced which changes to red on the addition of 0.05 ml of *nitric acid*.
C. Dissolve 0.5 g in 6 ml of *water* and add 15 ml of 0.1M *sodium hydroxide*. A white crystalline precipitate is produced on scratching the walls of the tube with a glass rod. Collect the precipitate, wash it with *water*, dissolve in 20 ml of *water* at 80°, filter and cool in ice. The *melting point* of the crystals, after drying over *phosphorus pentoxide* at a pressure of 1.5 to 2.5 kPa for 12 hours, is 85° to 89°, Appendix V A, Method I.
D. A 2% w/v solution yields *reaction A* characteristic of chlorides, Appendix VI.

Acidity pH of a 2% w/v solution, 4.3 to 5.7, Appendix V L.

Clarity and colour of solution A 2.0% w/v solution in *carbon dioxide-free water* is *clear*, Appendix IV A, and not more intensely coloured than *reference solution BY₆*, Appendix IV B, Method II.

Specific optical rotation In a 2% w/v solution in *carbon dioxide-free water*, −102° to −105°, Appendix V F.

Related substances Carry out the method for *thin-layer chromatography*, Appendix III A, using *silica gel G* as the coating substance and a mixture of 70 volumes of *toluene*, 65 volumes of *acetone*, 35 volumes of *ethanol (96%)* and 5 volumes of 13.5M *ammonia* as the mobile phase. Apply separately to the chromatoplate 10 µl of each of two solutions of the substance being examined in a mixture of equal volumes of *ethanol (96%)* and *water* containing (1) 2.5% w/v and (2) 0.0125% w/v. After removal of the plate, allow it to dry in a current of air and spray with *dilute potassium iodobismuthate solution*. Any *secondary spot* in the chromatogram obtained with solution (1) is not more intense than the spot in the chromatogram obtained with solution (2).

Sulphated ash Not more than 0.1%, Appendix IX A, Method II. Use 1 g.

Water 8.0 to 10.0% w/w, Appendix IX C. Use 0.25 g.

Assay Dissolve 0.3 g in 30 ml of *anhydrous glacial acetic acid*, add 20 ml of *acetic anhydride* and 5 ml of *mercury(II) acetate solution* and carry out Method I for *non-aqueous titration*, Appendix VIII A, determining the end-point potentiometrically. Each ml of 0.1M *perchloric acid VS* is equivalent to 0.03499 g of $C_{19}H_{23}NO_3,HCl$.

Storage Ethylmorphine Hydrochloride should be kept in a well-closed container and protected from light.

Action and use Narcotic analgesic.

Ethyloestrenol

$C_{20}H_{32}O$ 288.5   *965-90-2*

Ethyloestrenol is 17α-ethylestr-4-en-17β-ol containing a variable amount of methanol of crystallisation. It contains not less than 95.0 per cent and not more than 103.0 per cent of $C_{20}H_{32}O$, calculated with reference to the anhydrous and methanol-free substance.

Characteristics A white or almost white, crystalline powder; odourless or almost odourless.

Solubility Practically insoluble in *water*; soluble in 9 parts of *ethanol (96%)*, in 2 parts of *chloroform* and in 6 parts of *ether*.

Identification A. The *infra-red absorption spectrum*, Appendix II A, is concordant with the *reference spectrum* of ethyloestrenol. If the spectra are not concordant dissolve 50 mg of the substance being examined in 5 ml of hot *methanol*, allow to cool in ice for 15 minutes and evaporate to dryness using a rotary evaporator and a temperature not exceeding 40°. Dry the residue at room temperature at a pressure not exceeding 0.7 kPa and prepare a new spectrum.

B. Carry out the method for *thin-layer chromatography*, Appendix III A, using *silica gel G* as the coating substance and a mixture of 80 volumes of *heptane* and 20 volumes of *acetone* as the mobile phase but allowing the solvent front to ascend 10 cm above the line of application. Apply separately to the chromatoplate 2 μl of each of the following three solutions in a mixture of 9 volumes of *chloroform* and 1 volume of *methanol*. Solution (1) contains 0.25% w/v of the substance being examined. Solution (2) contains 0.25% w/v of *ethyloestrenol BPCRS*. Solution (3) is a mixture of equal volumes of solutions (1) and (2). After removal of the plate, heat it at 105° for 10 minutes, spray with *ethanolic sulphuric acid (20%)*, heat at 105° for a further 10 minutes, allow to cool and examine in daylight and under *ultra-violet light (365 nm)*. The principal spot in the chromatogram obtained with solution (1) corresponds in colour, size and fluorescence to that in the chromatogram obtained with solution (2). The principal spot in the chromatogram obtained with solution (3) appears as a single, compact spot.

Specific optical rotation In a 1% w/v solution in *1,4-dioxan*, +29° to +33°, Appendix V F.

17α-Ethylestran-17β-ol Carry out the method for *thin-layer chromatography*, Appendix III A, using *silica gel G* containing 20% w/w of *silver nitrate* as the coating substance and a mixture of 75 volumes of *toluene* and 25 volumes of *nonan-5-one* as the mobile phase. Apply separately to the chromatoplate 5 μl of each of two solutions in a mixture of 9 volumes of *chloroform* and 1 volume of *methanol* containing (1) 4.0% w/v of the substance being examined and (2) 0.080% w/v of *17α-ethylestran-17β-ol BPCRS*. After removal of the plate, heat it at 105° for 10 minutes, spray with *ethanolic sulphuric acid (20%)*, heat at 105° for a further 10 minutes and allow to cool. Any spot corresponding to 17α-ethylestran-17β-ol in the chromatogram obtained with solution (1) is not more intense than the spot in the chromatogram obtained with solution (2).

Methanol Not more than 4% w/w when determined by the following method. Carry out the method for *gas chromatography*, Appendix III B, using solutions in *acetone* containing (1) 0.40% v/v of *methanol* and 0.40% v/v of *absolute ethanol* (internal standard), (2) 10.0% w/v of the substance being examined and (3) 10.0% w/v of the substance being examined and 0.40% v/v of the internal standard.

The chromatographic procedure may be carried out using a glass column (2.0 m × 4 mm) packed with porous polymer beads (100 to 120 mesh) (Porapak Q is suitable) and maintained at 170°.

Calculate the percentage w/w of methanol taking 0.792 g as its weight per ml at 20°.

Related substances Carry out the method for *thin-layer chromatography*, Appendix III A, using *silica gel G* as the coating substance and a mixture of 80 volumes of *heptane* and 20 volumes of *acetone* as the mobile phase. Apply separately to the chromatoplate 10 μl of each of three solutions of the substance being examined in a mixture of 9 volumes of *chloroform* and 1 volume of *methanol* containing (1) 1.0% w/v, (2) 0.010% w/v and (3) 0.0050% w/v. After removal of the plate, heat it at 105° for 10 minutes, spray with *ethanolic sulphuric acid (20%)*, heat at 105° for a further 10 minutes, allow to cool and examine under *ultra-violet light (365 nm)*. Any *secondary spot* in the chromatogram obtained with solution (1) is not more intense than the spot in the chromatogram obtained with solution (2) and not more than one such spot is more intense than the spot in the chromatogram obtained with solution (3).

Sulphated ash Not more than 0.1%, Appendix IX A.

Water Not more than 0.5% w/w, Appendix IX C. Use 5.0 g.

Assay Carry out the method for *gas chromatography*, Appendix III B, using three solutions in *chloroform* containing (1) 0.2% w/v of *ethyloestrenol BPCRS* and 0.1% w/v of *arachidic alcohol* (internal standard), (2) 0.2% w/v of the substance being examined and (3) 0.2% w/v of the substance being examined and 0.1% w/v of the internal standard.

The chromatographic procedure may be carried out using (a) a glass column (1.0 m × 4 mm) packed with *acid-washed, silanised diatomaceous support* (80 to 100 mesh) coated with 3% w/w of phenyl methyl silicone fluid (50% phenyl) (OV-17 is suitable) and maintained at 200°.

Calculate the content of $C_{20}H_{32}O$ using the declared content of $C_{20}H_{32}O$ in *ethyloestrenol BPCRS*.

Storage Ethyloestrenol should be kept in a well-closed container, protected from light and stored at a temperature not exceeding 15°.

Preparation
Ethyloestrenol Tablets

Action and use Anabolic steroid.

In some countries the material described in this monograph may be known as Ethylestrenol.

Ethynodiol Diacetate

$C_{24}H_{32}O_4$ 384.5   297-76-7

Ethynodiol Diacetate is 19-nor-17α-pregn-4-en-20-yne-3β,17β-diol diacetate. It contains not less than 97.0 per cent and not more than 102.0 per cent of $C_{24}H_{32}O_4$, calculated with reference to the dried substance.

Characteristics A white or almost white, crystalline powder; odourless or almost odourless.

Solubility Very slightly soluble in *water*; soluble in 15 parts of *ethanol* (96%), in 1 part of *chloroform* and in 3.5 parts of *ether*.

Identification A. The *infra-red absorption spectrum*, Appendix II A, is concordant with the *reference spectrum* of ethynodiol diacetate.
B. The *light absorption*, Appendix II B, in the range 220 to 350 nm of the solution obtained in the test for Light absorption exhibits a maximum only at 236 nm and shoulders at 229 and 243 nm.
C. Yields the *reaction* characteristic of acetyl groups, Appendix VI.

Light absorption Dissolve 50 mg in sufficient *methanol* to produce 50 ml. To 10 ml add 40 ml of *methanol* and a mixture of 3 ml of *hydrochloric acid* and 2 ml of *water*, mix and boil on a water-bath for exactly 10 minutes. Cool, dilute to 100 ml with *methanol* and dilute 10 ml of the solution to 100 ml with *methanol*. The *absorbance* of the resulting solution at the maximum at 236 nm, Appendix II B, is 0.47 to 0.50, using in the reference cell a solution prepared by diluting 1 ml of the initial 0.1% w/v solution to 100 ml with *methanol*.

Melting point 126° to 131°, Appendix V A.

Specific optical rotation In a 1% w/v solution in *chloroform*, −70° to −76°, Appendix V F.

Conjugated compounds *Absorbance* of a 0.050% w/v solution in *methanol* at 236 nm, not more than 0.47, Appendix II B.

Loss on drying When dried to constant weight at 105°, loses not more than 0.5% of its weight. Use 1 g.

Sulphated ash Not more than 0.1%, Appendix IX A.

Assay Dissolve 0.2 g in 40 ml of *tetrahydrofuran*, add 10 ml of a 10% w/v solution of *silver nitrate* and titrate with 0.1M *sodium hydroxide VS*, determining the end-point potentiometrically. Each ml of 0.1M *sodium hydroxide VS* is equivalent to 0.03845 g of $C_{24}H_{32}O_4$.

Storage Ethynodiol Diacetate should be kept in a well-closed container and protected from light.

Action and use Progestogen.

In some countries the material described in this monograph may be known as Etynodiol Diacetate.

Etofylline ☆

$C_9H_{12}N_4O_3$ 224.2   519-37-9

Etofylline is 3,7-dihydro-7-(2-hydroxyethyl)-1,3-dimethyl-1*H*-purine-2,6-dione. It contains not less than 98.5 per cent and not more than 101.0 per cent of $C_9H_{12}N_4O_3$, calculated with reference to the dried substance.

Characteristics A white, crystalline powder.

Solubility Soluble in *water*; slightly soluble in *ethanol* (96%); sparingly soluble in *chloroform*; practically insoluble in *ether*.

Identification *Test A may be omitted if tests B, C and D are carried out. Tests C and D may be omitted if tests A and B are carried out.*
A. The *infra-red absorption spectrum*, Appendix II A, is concordant with the spectrum of *etophylline EPCRS*. Examine as dispersions of 0.5 to 1 mg in 0.3 g of *potassium bromide IR*.
B. Dissolve 1 g in 5 ml of *acetic anhydride* and boil under a reflux condenser for 15 minutes. Allow to cool, add 100 ml of a mixture of 4 volumes of *petroleum spirit* (*boiling range, 50° to 70°*) and 1 volume of *ether* and cool in ice for not less than 20 minutes, with occasional shaking. Filter, wash the precipitate with the same solvent mixture and recrystallise from *ethanol* (96%). The *melting point* of the crystals, after drying over *phosphorus pentoxide* at a pressure of 1.5 to 2.5 kPa, is 101° to 105°, Appendix V A, Method I.
C. Yields the *reaction* characteristic of xanthines, Appendix VI.
D. *Melting point*, 161° to 166°, Appendix V A, Method I.

Acidity or alkalinity To 10 ml of a 5.0% w/v solution in *carbon dioxide-free water* (solution A) add 0.25 ml of *bromothymol blue solution*. The solution is yellow or green and not more than 0.4 ml of 0.01M *sodium hydroxide VS* is required to change the colour of the solution to blue.

Clarity and colour of solution Solution A is *clear*, Appendix IV A, and *colourless*, Appendix IV B, Method II.

Heavy metals 12 ml of solution A complies with *limit test A for heavy metals*, Appendix VII (20 ppm). Use *lead standard solution (1 ppm Pb)* to prepare the standard.

Chloride Dilute 2.5 ml of solution A to 15 ml with *water*. The solution complies with the *limit test for chlorides*, Appendix VII (400 ppm).

Related substances Carry out the method for *thin-layer chromatography*, Appendix III A, using *silica gel HF254* as the coating substance and a mixture of 90 volumes of *chloroform*, 10 volumes of *absolute ethanol* and 1 volume of 13.5M *ammonia* as the mobile phase. Apply separately to the chromatoplate 10 μl of each of the following freshly prepared solutions. For solution (1) dissolve 0.3 g of the substance being examined in sufficient of a mixture of 3 volumes of *methanol* and 2 volumes of *water* to produce 10 ml. For solution (2) dilute 1 volume of solution (1) to 100 volumes with *methanol*. For solution (3) dilute 1 volume of solution (1) to 500 volumes with *methanol*. For solution (4) dissolve 10 mg of *theophylline* in *methanol*, add 0.3 ml of solution (1) and dilute to 10 ml with *methanol*. After removal of the plate, allow it to dry in air and examine under *ultra-violet light (254 nm)*. Any *secondary spot* in the chromatogram obtained with solution (1) is not more intense than the spot in the chromatogram obtained with solution (2) and not more than one such spot is more intense than the spot in the chromatogram obtained with solution (3). The test is not valid unless the chromatogram obtained with solution (4) shows two clearly separated principal spots.

Loss on drying When dried to constant weight at 100° to 105°, loses not more than 0.5% of its weight. Use 1 g.

Sulphated ash Not more than 0.1%, Appendix IX A, Method II. Use 1 g.

Assay Dissolve 0.2 g in 3 ml of *anhydrous formic acid*, add 50 ml of *acetic anhydride* and carry out Method I for *non-aqueous titration*, Appendix VIII A, determining the end-point potentiometrically. Each ml of 0.1M *perchloric acid VS* is equivalent to 0.02242 g of $C_9H_{12}N_4O_3$.

Storage Etofylline should be kept in a well-closed container and protected from light.

Action and use Xanthine bronchodilator.

Eucalyptus Oil ☆

Eucalyptus Oil is obtained by steam distillation and rectification from the fresh leaves or the fresh terminal branches of various species of eucalyptus that are rich in cineole. The species used are *Eucalyptus globulus* Labill., *E. fruticetorum* F. von Muell. (*E. polybractea* R. T. Baker) and *E. smithii* (R. T. Baker).

Eucalyptus Oil contains not less than 70.0 per cent w/w of cineole, $C_{10}H_{18}O$.

Characteristics A colourless or pale yellow liquid; odour, aromatic and camphoraceous; taste, pungent and camphoraceous, followed by a sensation of cold.

Identification Carry out the method for *thin-layer chromatography*, Appendix III A, using *silica gel G* as the coating substance and a mixture of 90 volumes of *toluene* and 10 volumes of *ethyl acetate* as the mobile phase. Apply separately to the chromatoplate 2 μl of each of two solutions in *toluene* containing (1) 1% w/v of the oil and (2) 1% w/v solution of o-*cineole*. After removal of the plate, allow it to dry in air, spray with *anisaldehyde solution*, using about 10 ml for a 200 mm × 200 mm plate, heat at 100° to 105° for 10 minutes and examine in daylight and under *ultra-violet light (365 nm)*. In the chromatogram

obtained with solution (2) a dark brown spot due to cineole is visible in daylight in the middle part; when examined under ultra-violet light (365 nm), the spot shows a brown fluorescence. The principal spot in the chromatogram obtained with solution (1) corresponds to that of cineole; no carmine-brown spot appears in daylight in the upper third of the chromatogram and when examined under ultra-violet light (365 nm) no spot showing a greenish-brown fluorescence appears in the upper third (citronellal). Other spots may be visible in the upper and lower thirds of the chromatogram.

Optical rotation 0° to +10°, Appendix V F.

Refractive index 1.458 to 1.470, Appendix V E.

Relative density 0.906 to 0.925, Appendix V G.

Solubility in ethanol Soluble in 5 volumes of *ethanol (70%)*, Appendix X M.

Aldehydes Place 10 ml in a glass-stoppered tube, 150 mm × 25 mm, add 5 ml of *toluene* and 4 ml of *hydroxylamine solution in ethanol (60%)*, shake vigorously and titrate immediately with 0.5M *potassium hydroxide in ethanol (60%) VS* until the red colour changes to yellow. Continue the shaking and neutralising until the pure yellow colour of the indicator is permanent in the lower layer after shaking vigorously for 2 minutes and allowing separation to take place; the reaction is complete in about 15 minutes. Repeat the operation using a further 10 ml of the oil and, as the standard for the end-point, the titrated liquid of the first determination with the addition of 0.5 ml of 0.5M *potassium hydroxide in ethanol (60%) VS*. Not more than 2 ml of 0.5M *potassium hydroxide in ethanol (60%) VS* is required in the second determination.

Phellandrene Mix 1 ml with 2 ml of *glacial acetic acid* and 5 ml of *petroleum spirit (boiling range, 40° to 60°)*, add 2 ml of a saturated solution of *sodium nitrite* and shake gently. No crystalline precipitate is produced in the upper layer within 1 hour.

Assay Carry out the method for the *determination of cineole*, Appendix X J.

Storage Eucalyptus Oil should be kept in a well-filled, airtight container and stored at a temperature not exceeding 25°.

Hard Fat ☆

Hard Fat is a mixture of mono-, di- and triglycerides of the saturated fatty acids $C_{10}H_{20}O_2$ to $C_{18}H_{36}O_2$.

Characteristics A white, brittle mass; almost odourless and free from rancid odour; greasy to the touch. On warming, it melts to give a colourless or slightly yellowish liquid. When the molten material is shaken with an equal quantity of hot *water*, a white emulsion is produced.

Solubility Practically insoluble in *water*; freely soluble in *ether*; slightly soluble in *absolute ethanol*.

Melting point 33° to 36°, Appendix V A, Method IV. Introduce the melted substance into the capillary tubes and allow to stand below 10° for 24 hours before carrying out the determination.

Acid value Not more than 0.5, Appendix X B. Dissolve 5 g in 50 ml of the prescribed mixture of solvents.

Hydroxyl value Not more than 50, Appendix X D, Method II.

Iodine value Not more than 3 (*iodine bromide method*), Appendix X E.

Peroxide value Not more than 6, Appendix X F.

Saponification value 225 to 245, Appendix X G, Method II.

Unsaponifiable matter Not more than 0.5%, Appendix X H, Method II.

Alkaline impurities Dissolve 2 g in a mixture of 1.5 ml of *ethanol* (96%) and 3 ml of *ether* and add 0.05 ml of *bromophenol blue solution*. Not more than 0.15 ml of 0.01M *hydrochloric acid VS* is required to change the colour of the solution to yellow.

Decomposition products Shake 1.00 g with 1 ml of *hydrochloric acid* for 1 minute, add 1 ml of *resorcinol solution*, shake for 5 seconds and allow to stand for 5 minutes. The aqueous layer is not more intensely coloured than 1 ml of a mixture of 0.4 ml of 0.002M *potassium permanganate VS* and 9.6 ml of *water*.

Ash Not more than 0.05%, Appendix XI J. Use 2 g.

Storage Hard Fat should be protected from light.

Action and use Pharmaceutical aid.

The standards of this monograph encompass several different suppository bases. The selection of a basis for a particular suppository formulation should be appropriate to the product concerned and it may be necessary to apply more restricted standards for a particular application.

Fenfluramine Hydrochloride

CH₂·CHMe·NHEt ,HCl

F₃C

$C_{12}H_{16}F_3N,HCl$ 267.7   *404-82-0*

Fenfluramine Hydrochloride is ethyl(α-methyl-3-trifluoromethylphenethyl)amine hydrochloride. It contains not less than 98.5 per cent and not more than 101.0 per cent of $C_{12}H_{16}F_3N,HCl$, calculated with reference to the dried substance.

Characteristics A white, crystalline powder; odourless or almost odourless.

Solubility Soluble in 20 parts of *water*, in 10 parts of *ethanol* (96%) and in 10 parts of *chloroform*; practically insoluble in *ether*.

Identification A. The *infra-red absorption spectrum*, Appendix II A, is concordant with the *reference spectrum* of fenfluramine hydrochloride.

B. Carry out the method for *thin-layer chromatography*, Appendix III A, using *silica gel G* as the coating substance and a mixture of 200 volumes of *methanol* and 3 volumes of 13.5M *ammonia* as the mobile phase. Apply separately to the chromatoplate 10 µl of each of two solutions in *chloroform* containing (1) 1% w/v of the substance being examined and (2) 1% w/v of *fenfluramine hydrochloride BPCRS*. After removal of the plate, allow it to dry in air and spray with *dilute potassium iodobismuthate solution*. The principal spot in the chromatogram obtained with solution (1) corresponds to that in the chromatogram obtained with solution (2).

C. Yields the *reactions* characteristic of chlorides, Appendix VI.

Melting point 168° to 172°, Appendix V A.

Ethyl(α-methyl-4-trifluoromethylphenethyl)amine Carry out the method for *gas chromatography*, Appendix III B, using the following solutions. For solution (1) dissolve 8 mg of *fenfluramine hydrochloride BPCRS* in 100 ml of *water*, add 10 ml of a 20% w/v solution of *potassium hydroxide*, extract with four 25-ml quantities of *chloroform*, filter and evaporate the combined filtrates to dryness, removing the final solvent in a current of *nitrogen*. Dissolve the residue in 10 ml of a 0.01% v/v solution of N,N-*diethylaniline* (internal standard) in *chloroform*. For solution (2) treat 0.40 g of the substance being examined in the same manner but dissolve the residue from the chloroform extraction in 10 ml of *chloroform*. For solution (3) treat 0.40 g of the substance being examined in the same manner as solution (1).

The chromatographic procedure may be carried out using (a) a glass column (2.75 m × 4 mm) packed with *acid-washed diatomaceous support* (80 to 100 mesh) coated with 10% w/w of polyethylene glycol compound (Carbowax 20M is suitable) and 2% w/w of *potassium hydroxide* and maintained at 135° with a detector temperature of 200°.

In the chromatogram obtained with solution (2) a peak due to ethyl(α-methyl-4-trifluoromethylphenethyl)amine may appear immediately after the principal peak. In the chromatogram obtained with solution (3) the ratio of the area of any peak corresponding to ethyl(α-methyl-4-trifluoromethylphenethyl)amine to that of the peak due to the internal standard is not greater than the ratio of the area of the peak due to fenfluramine to that of the peak due to the internal standard in the chromatogram obtained with solution (1).

The *column efficiency*, determined using the peak due to the internal standard in the chromatogram obtained with solution (1), should be not less than 1500 theoretical plates per metre.

Loss on drying When dried to constant weight at 105°, loses not more than 1.0% of its weight. Use 1 g.

Sulphated ash Not more than 0.1%, Appendix IX A.

Assay Carry out Method I for *non-aqueous titration*, Appendix VIII A, using 0.3 g, adding 10 ml of *mercury(II) acetate solution* and determining the end-point potentiometrically. Each ml of 0.1M *perchloric acid VS* is equivalent to 0.02677 g of $C_{12}H_{16}F_3N,HCl$.

Preparation

Fenfluramine Tablets

Action and use Appetite suppressant.

Fenoprofen Calcium

$(C_{15}H_{13}O_3)_2Ca,2H_2O$ 558.6   53746-45-5

Fenoprofen Calcium is calcium 2-(3-phenoxy-phenyl)propionate dihydrate. It contains not less than 97.5 per cent and not more than 101.0 per cent of $(C_{15}H_{13}O_3)_2Ca$, calculated with reference to the anhydrous substance.

Characteristics A white or almost white, crystalline powder; odourless or almost odourless.

Solubility Slightly soluble in *water* and in *chloroform*; soluble in 15 parts of *ethanol (96%)*.

Identification A. The *infra-red absorption spectrum*, Appendix II A, is concordant with the *reference spectrum* of fenoprofen calcium.

B. Dissolve 0.1 g in 5 ml of *glacial acetic acid* and add sufficient *methanol* to produce 100 ml. Dilute 5 ml of this solution to 50 ml with *methanol*. The *light absorption* of the resulting solution, Appendix II B, in the range 230 to 350 nm exhibits two maxima, at 272 nm and 278 nm, and a shoulder at 266 nm. The *absorbance* at 272 nm is about 0.70 and at 278 nm is about 0.65.

C. The residue on ignition yields the *reactions* characteristic of calcium salts, Appendix VI.

Related substances Carry out the method for *thin-layer chromatography*, Appendix III A, using a silica gel F254 precoated chromatoplate (Merck silica gel 60 F254 plates are suitable) and a mixture of 90 volumes of *toluene* and 10 volumes of *glacial acetic acid* as the mobile phase. Apply separately to the plate 20 µl of each of two solutions of the substance being examined in a 10% v/v solution of *glacial acetic acid* in *methanol* containing (1) 5.0% w/v and (2) 0.025% w/v. After removal of the plate, allow it to dry in air and examine under *ultra-violet light (254 nm)*. Any *secondary spot* in the chromatogram obtained with solution (1) is not more intense than the spot in the chromatogram obtained with solution (2).

Water 5.0 to 8.0% w/w, Appendix IX C. Use 0.2 g.

Assay Carry out Method I for *non-aqueous titration*, Appendix VIII A, using 0.5 g and determining the end-point potentiometrically. Each ml of 0.1M *perchloric acid VS* is equivalent to 0.02613 g of $(C_{15}H_{13}O_3)_2Ca$.

Storage Fenoprofen Calcium should be kept in a well-closed container.

Preparation
Fenoprofen Tablets

Action and use Anti-inflammatory; analgesic.

Fenoterol Hydrobromide

$C_{17}H_{21}NO_4,HBr$ 384.3   1944-12-3

Fenoterol Hydrobromide is a mixture of (R)-1-(3,5-dihydroxyphenyl)-2-[(R)-4-hydroxy-α-methylphenethylamino]ethanol hydrobromide and its enantiomer. It contains not less than 98.0 per cent and not more than 102.0 per cent of $C_{17}H_{21}NO_4,HBr$, calculated with reference to the dried substance.

Characteristics A white, crystalline powder.

Solubility Soluble in *water* and in *ethanol (96%)*; practically insoluble in *chloroform* and in *ether*.

Identification A. The *infra-red absorption spectrum*, Appendix II A, is concordant with the *reference spectrum* of fenoterol hydrobromide.

B. The *light absorption*, Appendix II B, in the range 230 to 350 nm of a 0.01% w/v solution in 0.01M *hydrochloric acid* exhibits a maximum only at 275 nm and a shoulder at 280 nm. The *absorbance* at 275 nm is about 0.83.

C. Yields the *reactions* characteristic of bromides, Appendix VI.

Acidity pH of a 4% w/v solution, 4.2 to 5.2, Appendix V L.

Clarity and colour of solution A 4.0% w/v solution is *clear*, Appendix IV A, and not more intensely coloured than *reference solution* Y_7, Appendix IV B, Method I.

Heavy metals 4.0 g complies with *limit test C for heavy metals*, Appendix VII. Use 4 ml of *lead standard solution (10 ppm Pb)* to prepare the standard.

Iron Dissolve the residue from the test for Sulphated ash in sufficient 0.5M *hydrochloric acid* to produce 10 ml. The resulting solution complies with the *limit test for iron*, Appendix VII (5 ppm).

Phenone The *absorbance* of a 4% w/v solution at 330 nm is not more than 0.42, Appendix II B.

(SR)- and (RS)-Enantiomers Not more than 4% when determined by the following method. Carry out the method for *high-performance liquid chromatography*, Appendix III D, using solutions in *water* containing (1) 0.25% w/v of *fenoterol hydrobromide BPCRS* and (2) 0.25% w/v of the substance being examined.

The chromatographic procedure may be carried out using (a) a stainless steel column (20 cm × 4.6 mm) packed with *stationary phase C* (10 µm) (Lichrosorb RP-18 is suitable), (b) as the mobile phase a methanolic phosphate buffer adjusted to a suitable pH (a mixture of 105 volumes of 0.067M *disodium hydrogen orthophosphate*, 46 volumes of *methanol* and 1 volume of 0.067M *potassium dihydrogen orthophosphate*, adjusted to pH 8.5 with *orthophosphoric acid*, is usually suitable) and (c) a detection wavelength of 280 nm.

In the chromatogram obtained with solution (1) a peak due to the (SR)- and (RS)-enantiomers appears immediately after the principal peak. Adjust the sensitivity of the instrument so that in the chromatogram obtained with solution (1) the height of the peak due to the (SR)- and (RS)-enantiomers is not less than 10% of full-scale deflection on the chart paper. In both chromatograms measure the height of the peak due to the (SR)-and (RS)-enantiomers by dropping a perpendicular from the apex of the peak to a line drawn tangentially from the trough between the two peaks to the baseline. Calculate the content of (SR)-and (RS)-enantiomers in the substance being examined using the declared content of (SR)- and (RS)-enantiomers in *fenoterol hydrobromide BPCRS*.

The test is not valid unless the height of the trough separating the (SR)- and (RS)-enantiomers from the principal peak is less than 4% of full-scale deflection and the retention time of the principal peak is less than 20 minutes.

Loss on drying When dried to constant weight at 105°, loses not more than 0.5% of its weight. Use 1 g.

Sulphated ash Not more than 0.1%, Appendix IX A. Use 2.0 g.

Assay Dissolve 0.6 g in *water* and add 5 ml of 2M *nitric acid*, 25 ml of 0.1M *silver nitrate VS* and 2 ml of *ammonium iron(III) sulphate solution*. Shake and titrate with 0.1M *ammonium thiocyanate VS* until the colour becomes reddish-yellow. Repeat the operation without the substance being examined. The difference between the titrations represents the amount of silver nitrate required. Each ml of 0.1M *silver nitrate VS* is equivalent to 0.03843 g of $C_{17}H_{21}NO_4$,HBr.

Storage Fenoterol Hydrobromide should be kept in a well-closed container and protected from light.

Action and use Beta-adrenoceptor agonist.

Fentanyl Citrate

PhCH₂·CH₂—N ⟨ring⟩ NCO·Et   Ph

CH₂·CO₂H
,HOCCO₂H
CH₂·CO₂H

$C_{22}H_{28}N_2O,C_6H_8O_7$ 528.6   *990-73-8*

Fentanyl Citrate is *N*-(1-phenethyl-4-piperidyl)-propionanilide dihydrogen citrate. It contains not less than 98.0 per cent and not more than 101.0 per cent of $C_{22}H_{28}N_2O,C_6H_8O_7$, calculated with reference to the dried substance.

Characteristics A white, crystalline powder or white granules.

Solubility Soluble in 40 parts of *water*; slightly soluble in *ethanol (96%)*, in *chloroform* and in *ether*; soluble in *methanol*.

Identification A. The *infra-red absorption spectrum*, Appendix II A, is concordant with the *reference spectrum* of fentanyl citrate.
B. The *light absorption*, Appendix II B, in the range 230 to 350 nm of a 0.1% w/v solution exhibits three maxima, at 251, 257 and 262 nm. The *absorbance* at 251 nm is about 0.72, at 257 nm, about 0.82 and at 262 nm, about 0.64.
C. Boil a 0.1% w/v neutral solution with an excess of *mercury(II) sulphate solution* and filter if necessary. To the resulting solution add 0.15 ml of *potassium permanganate solution* and boil. The solution becomes colourless and a white precipitate is produced.

Melting point 148° to 150°, Appendix V A.

Loss on drying When dried to constant weight at 60° at a pressure not exceeding 0.7 kPa, loses not more than 0.5% of its weight. Use 1 g.

Sulphated ash Not more than 0.1%, Appendix IX A.

Assay Dissolve 75 mg in 25 ml of *anhydrous glacial acetic acid* and carry out Method I for *non-aqueous titration*, Appendix VIII A, using 0.02M *perchloric acid VS* as titrant and *crystal violet solution* as indicator. Each ml of 0.02M *perchloric acid VS* is equivalent to 0.01057 g of $C_{22}H_{28}N_2O$, $C_6H_8O_7$.

Action and use Narcotic analgesic.

Ferrous Fumarate

⎡ HCCO₂— ⎤
⎢   ‖   ⎥ Fe
⎣ —O₂CCH ⎦

$C_4H_2FeO_4$ 169.9   *141-01-5*

Ferrous Fumarate is iron(II) fumarate. It contains not less than 93.0 per cent of $C_4H_2FeO_4$, calculated with reference to the dried substance.

Characteristics A fine, reddish-orange to reddish-brown powder; odour, slight.

Solubility Slightly soluble in *water*; very slightly soluble in *ethanol (96%)*.

Identification A. Heat 1 g with 25 ml of a mixture of equal volumes of *hydrochloric acid* and *water* on a water-bath for 15 minutes, cool and filter. Reserve the residue for test B. The filtrate yields *reaction A* characteristic of iron salts, Appendix VI.
B. Wash the residue reserved in test A with a mixture of 1 volume of 2M *hydrochloric acid* and 9 volumes of *water* and dry at 105°. Suspend 0.1 g of the residue in 2 ml of *sodium carbonate solution* and add *potassium permanganate solution* dropwise. The permanganate is decolorised and a brownish solution is produced.
C. Mix 0.5 g with 1 g of *resorcinol*. To 0.5 g of the mixture in a crucible add 0.15 ml of *sulphuric acid* and heat gently; a deep red, semi-solid mass is produced. Add the mass to a large volume of *water*; an orange-yellow solution is produced which exhibits no fluorescence.

Arsenic Mix 0.2 g with 1.5 g of *anhydrous sodium carbonate*, add 10 ml of *bromine water* and mix thoroughly. Evaporate to dryness on a water-bath, ignite gently and dissolve the cooled residue in 20 ml of *brominated hydrochloric acid* and 10 ml of *water*. Transfer to a small flask, add sufficient *tin(II) chloride solution AsT* to remove the yellow colour, connect to a condenser and distil 22 ml. The distillate complies with the *limit test for arsenic*, Appendix VII (5 ppm).

Ferric iron Not more than 2.0% when determined by the following method. Dissolve 3 g in a mixture of 100 ml of *water* and 10 ml of *hydrochloric acid* by heating rapidly to the boiling point. Boil for 15 seconds, cool rapidly, add 3 g of *potassium iodide*, stopper, allow to stand in the dark for 15 minutes and titrate the liberated iodine with 0.1M *sodium thiosulphate VS* using *starch mucilage* as indicator. Repeat the operation without the substance being examined. The difference between the titrations represents the amount of iodine liberated by the ferric iron. Each ml of 0.1M *sodium thiosulphate VS* is equivalent to 0.005585 g of ferric iron.

Heavy metals Ignite 1.0 g gently until free from carbon, dissolve in 5 ml of *hydrochloric acid* by heating on a water-bath and evaporate to dryness. Dissolve the residue in a mixture of 15 ml of *hydrochloric acid*, 4 ml of *nitric acid* and 6 ml of *water*, boil gently for 1 minute, cool and extract with three 20-ml quantities of *ether*. If the aqueous layer is more than slightly yellow carry out a fourth extraction with a further 20 ml of *ether*. Discard the ether extracts, heat the aqueous solution gently to remove dissolved ether, add 1 g of *citric acid*, make alkaline with 5M *ammonia* and add 1 ml of *potassium cyanide solution PbT* and sufficient *water* to produce 50 ml. 12 ml of the resulting solution complies with *limit test A for heavy metals*, Appendix VII (100 ppm). Use *lead standard solution (2 ppm Pb)* to prepare the standard.

Sulphate Boil 0.15 g with 8 ml of 2M *hydrochloric acid* and 20 ml of *water*, cool in ice, filter and dilute to 30 ml with *water*. The filtrate complies with the *limit test for sulphates*, Appendix VII (0.2%).

Loss on drying When dried to constant weight at 105°, loses not more than 1.0% of its weight. Use 1 g.

Assay Dissolve 0.3 g in 7.5 ml of 1M *sulphuric acid* with gentle heating. Cool, add 25 ml of *water* and titrate immediately with 0.1M *ammonium cerium(IV) sulphate VS* using *ferroin sulphate solution* as indicator. Each ml of 0.1M *ammonium cerium(IV) sulphate VS* is equivalent to 0.01699 g of $C_4H_2FeO_4$.

Preparation

Ferrous Fumarate Tablets

Action and use Used in prevention and treatment of anaemias.

Ferrous Fumarate contains in 200 mg about 65 mg of iron.

Ferrous Gluconate ☆

$C_{12}H_{22}FeO_{14},xH_2O$ 446.1 (*anhydrous*)
299-29-6 (anhydrous)

Ferrous Gluconate★ is iron(II) di(D-gluconate). It contains not less than 11.8 per cent and not more than 12.5 per cent of iron(II), calculated with reference to the dried substance.

Characteristics A greenish-yellow to grey powder or granules. It may have a faint odour of burnt sugar.

Solubility Slowly soluble in 10 parts of *water*, producing a greenish-brown solution; more readily soluble in hot *water*; practically insoluble in *ethanol (96%)*.

Identification A. Carry out the method for *thin-layer chromatography*, Appendix III A, using *silica gel G* as the coating substance and a mixture of 50 volumes of *ethanol (96%)*, 30 volumes of *water*, 10 volumes of 13.5M *ammonia* and 10 volumes of *ethyl acetate* as the mobile phase but allowing the solvent front to ascend 10 cm above the line of application. Apply separately to the chromatoplate 5 μl of each of the following solutions which may be heated, if necessary, to effect solution in a water-bath at 60°. For solution (1) dissolve 20 mg of the substance being examined in 2 ml of *water*. For solution (2) dissolve 20 mg of *ferrous gluconate EPCRS* in 2 ml of *water*. After removal of the plate, dry it at 100° to 105° for 20 minutes, allow to cool and spray it with a 5% w/v solution of *potassium dichromate* in a 40% w/w solution of *sulphuric acid*. After 5 minutes the principal spot in the chromatogram obtained with solution (1) corresponds in position, colour and size to that in the chromatogram obtained with solution (2).

B. Dissolve 5.0 g in *carbon dioxide-free water* prepared from *distilled water*, at 60°, cool and dilute to 50 ml with the same solvent (solution A). 1 ml of solution A yields *reaction A* characteristic of iron salts, Appendix VI.

Acidity pH of solution A, measured 3 to 4 hours after preparation, 4.0 to 5.5, Appendix V L.

Clarity of solution Dilute 2 ml of solution A to 10 ml with *water*. When examined against the light, the resulting solution is *clear*, Appendix IV A.

Arsenic 0.5 g complies with the *limit test for arsenic*, Appendix VII (2 ppm).

Barium Dilute 10 ml of solution A to 50 ml with *distilled water* and add 5 ml of 1M *sulphuric acid*. The solution, after not less than 5 minutes, is not more opalescent than a mixture of 10 ml of solution A and 45 ml of *distilled water*. Examine the solutions against the light.

Ferric iron Dissolve 5 g in a mixture of 100 ml of *carbon dioxide-free water* and 10 ml of *hydrochloric acid*. Add 3 g of *potassium iodide*, stopper the flask, allow to stand in the dark for 5 minutes and titrate with 0.1M *sodium thiosulphate VS* using 0.5 ml of *starch solution*, added towards the end of the titration, as indicator. Repeat the operation without the substance being examined. The difference between the titrations represents the amount of iodine liberated by the ferric iron. Not more than 9.0 ml of 0.1M *sodium thiosulphate VS* is required.

Heavy metals Thoroughly mix 2.5 g with 0.5 g of *magnesium oxide* in a silica crucible and ignite at dull redness until a homogeneous mass is obtained. Heat at 800° for 1 hour, cool, dissolve the residue in 20 ml of hot *hydrochloric acid*, cool and transfer to a separating funnel. Extract with three 20-ml quantities of a solution prepared by shaking 100 ml of freshly distilled *4-methylpentan-2-one* with 1 ml of *hydrochloric acid*, shaking for 3 minutes for each extraction. Discard the extracts, evaporate the aqueous layer to half its volume, allow to cool and dilute to 25 ml with *water*. To 7.5 ml add 6M *ammonia* until the solution is neutral to *litmus paper* and dilute to 15 ml with *water*. 12 ml of the resulting solution complies with *limit test A for heavy metals*, Appendix VII (20 ppm). Use *lead standard solution (1 ppm Pb)* to prepare the standard.

Chloride 0.8 ml of solution A diluted to 15 ml with *water* complies with the *limit test for chlorides*, Appendix VII (600 ppm).

Oxalate Dissolve 5.0 g in a mixture of 10 ml of 1M *sulphuric acid* and 40 ml of *water*. Shake the solution with 50 ml of *ether* for 5 minutes, separate the aqueous layer and shake with a further 20 ml of *ether* for 5 minutes. Combine the ether layers, evaporate the ether and dissolve the residue in 15 ml of *water*. Filter, evaporate the filtrate to 5 ml and add 1 ml of 2M *acetic acid* and 1.5 ml of a 7.35% w/v solution of *calcium chloride*. No precipitate is produced within 30 minutes.

Sulphate To 3 ml of solution A add 3 ml of 6M *acetic acid* and dilute to 15 ml with *distilled water*. The resulting solution complies with the *limit test for sulphates*, Appendix VII (500 ppm). Examine the solutions against the light.

Sucrose and reducing sugars Dissolve 0.5 g in 10 ml of warm *water*, add 1 ml of 6M *ammonia*, pass *hydrogen sulphide* through the solution and allow to stand for 30 minutes. Filter the resulting precipitate and wash with two 5-ml quantities of *water*, acidify the combined filtrate and washings to *litmus paper* with 2M *hydrochloric acid* and add a further 2 ml. Boil until the vapour no longer darkens *lead acetate paper* and continue boiling, if necessary, until the volume is reduced to about 10 ml. Cool, add 15 ml of a 10.6% w/v solution of *anhydrous sodium carbonate*, allow to stand for 5 minutes, filter and dilute the filtrate to 100 ml with *water*. To 5 ml of the resulting solution add 2 ml of *potassium cupri-tartrate solution*, boil for 1 minute and allow to stand for 1 minute. No red precipitate is produced.

Loss on drying When dried at 100° to 105° for 5 hours, loses 7.0 to 10.5% of its weight. Use 0.5 g.

Assay Dissolve 0.5 g of *sodium hydrogen carbonate* in a mixture of 70 ml of *water* and 30 ml of 1M *sulphuric acid*. When effervescence ceases, add 1 g of the substance being examined, shake gently to dissolve and titrate with 0.1M *ammonium cerium(IV) nitrate VS*, using 0.1 ml of *ferroin sulphate solution* as indicator, until the red colour disappears. Each ml of 0.1M *ammonium cerium(IV) nitrate VS* is equivalent to 0.005585 g of iron(II).

Storage Ferrous Gluconate should be kept in a well-closed container and protected from light.

Preparation
Ferrous Gluconate Tablets

Action and use Used in prevention and treatment of iron deficiency.

Ferrous Gluconate contains in 600 mg about 70 mg of iron.

*In certain states party to the Convention on the Elaboration of a European Pharmacopœia, Ferrous Gluconate may be required to comply with a limit for total viable aerobic count of 10^2 micro-organisms per gram, determined by plate count, Appendix XVI B2.

Ferrous Succinate

10030-90-7

Ferrous Succinate contains not less than 34.0 per cent and not more than 36.0 per cent of iron(II), calculated with reference to the dried substance.

Characteristics A brownish-yellow to brown, amorphous powder; odour, slight.

Solubility Practically insoluble in *water* and in *ethanol* (96%). It dissolves in dilute mineral acids.

Identification A. Mix 0.5 g with 1 g of *resorcinol*. To 0.5 g of the mixture in a crucible add 0.15 ml of *sulphuric acid* and heat gently; a deep red, semi-solid mass is produced. Add the mass to a large volume of *water*; an orange-yellow solution exhibiting an intense green fluorescence is produced. Add an excess of 5M *sodium hydroxide*; the fluorescence intensifies and the solution becomes red.

B. Dissolve 2 g in the minimum quantity of 2M *hydrochloric acid* by heating, cool and filter. The *melting point* of the precipitate, after washing with small amounts of 2M *hydrochloric acid* and *water* and drying at 105°, is about 186°, Appendix V A.

C. Yields *reaction A* characteristic of iron salts, Appendix VI.

Arsenic To 0.5 g add 15 ml of *water* and 15 ml of *stannated hydrochloric acid* and distil 22 ml. The distillate complies with the *limit test for arsenic*, Appendix VII (2 ppm).

Ferric iron Not more than 2.0 per cent when determined by the following method. Dissolve 3 g in a mixture of 100 ml of *carbon dioxide-free water* and 10 ml of *hydrochloric acid*, add 3 g of *potassium iodide*, close the vessel, allow to stand in the dark for 5 minutes and titrate the liberated iodine with 0.1M *sodium thiosulphate VS* using *starch mucilage* as indicator. Repeat the operation without the substance being examined. The difference between the titrations represents the amount of iodine liberated by the ferric iron. Each ml of 0.1M *sodium thiosulphate VS* is equivalent to 0.005585 g of ferric iron.

Heavy metals Gently warm 2.5 g with 10 ml of *nitric acid* until reaction begins and allow to stand until the evolution of nitrous fumes subsides. Boil gently to complete oxidation, adding a further 5 ml of *nitric acid*, if necessary, and continue boiling until the volume is reduced to about 5 ml. Add 20 ml of *hydrochloric acid*, boil gently for 1 minute, cool and extract with three 20-ml quantities of *ether*. If the aqueous layer is still more than slightly yellow carry out a fourth extraction with a further 20 ml of *ether*. Discard the ether extracts, transfer the aqueous solution to a narrow-necked flask, rinse the separating funnel with 5 ml of *water* and add the rinsings to the flask. Heat to remove dissolved ether and part of the hydrochloric acid and dilute to 50 ml with *water*. 12 ml of the resulting solution complies with *limit test A for heavy metals*, Appendix VII (40 ppm). Use *lead standard solution (2 ppm Pb)* to prepare the standard.

Sulphate Boil 0.25 g with 5 ml of 2M *hydrochloric acid* and 15 ml of *water*, cool in ice, filter and dilute the filtrate to 30 ml with *water*. 15 ml of the resulting solution complies with the *limit test for sulphates*, Appendix VII (0.12%).

Loss on drying When dried to constant weight at 105°, loses not more than 1.0% of its weight. Use 1 g.

Assay Dissolve 0.5 g in a mixture of 30 ml of *water* and 20 ml of 1M *sulphuric acid* and titrate immediately with 0.1M *ammonium cerium(IV) sulphate VS* using *ferroin sulphate solution* as indicator. Each ml of 0.1M *ammonium cerium(IV) sulphate VS* is equivalent to 0.005585 g of iron(II).

Storage Ferrous Succinate should be kept in a well-closed container and protected from light.

Preparations
Ferrous Succinate Capsules
Ferrous Succinate Tablets

Action and use Used in prevention and treatment of anaemias.

Ferrous Succinate contains in 200 mg about 70 mg of iron.

Ferrous Sulphate ☆

FeSO₄,7H₂O   278.0   7720-78-7

Ferrous Sulphate contains not less than 98.0 per cent and not more than 105.0 per cent of FeSO₄,7H₂O.

Characteristics Bluish-green crystals or a light green, crystalline powder; odourless. Efflorescent in air. It oxidises in moist air, becoming brown.

Solubility Freely soluble in *water*; very soluble in boiling *water*; practically insoluble in *ethanol (96%)*.

Identification Yields *reaction A* characteristic of iron salts and the *reactions* characteristic of sulphates, Appendix VI.

Acidity pH of a 5% w/v solution, 3.0 to 4.0, Appendix V L.

Clarity of solution Dissolve 2.5 g in *carbon dioxide-free water*, add 0.5 ml of *1M sulphuric acid* and dilute to 50 ml with *water*. The solution is not more opalescent than *reference suspension II*, Appendix IV A.

Ferric iron Dissolve 5 g in a mixture of 10 ml of *hydrochloric acid* and 100 ml of *carbon dioxide-free water* and add 3 g of *potassium iodide*. Close the flask and allow to stand in the dark for 5 minutes. Titrate the liberated iodine with *0.1M sodium thiosulphate VS* using 0.5 ml of *starch solution*, added towards the end of the titration, as indicator. Repeat the operation without the substance being examined. The difference between the titrations represents the amount of iodine liberated by the ferric iron. Not more than 4.5 ml of *0.1M sodium thiosulphate VS* is required (0.5%).

Heavy metals Dissolve 1.0 g in 10 ml of *7M hydrochloric acid*, add 2 ml of *hydrogen peroxide solution (100 vol)* and evaporate to 5 ml. Allow to cool, dilute to 20 ml with *7M hydrochloric acid* and extract with three successive 20-ml quantities of a solution prepared by shaking 100 ml of freshly distilled *4-methylpentan-2-one* with 1 ml of *7M hydrochloric acid*. Evaporate the aqueous layer to half its volume, allow to cool and dilute to 25 ml with *water* (solution A). Neutralise 7.5 ml of solution A to *litmus paper* using *6M ammonia* and dilute to 15 ml with *water*. 12 ml of the resulting solution complies with *limit test A for heavy metals*, Appendix VII (50 ppm). Use *lead standard solution (1 ppm Pb)* to prepare the standard.

Manganese Dissolve 1.0 g in 40 ml of *water*, add 10 ml of *nitric acid* and boil until red fumes are evolved. Add 0.5 g of *ammonium persulphate* and boil for 10 minutes. Discharge any pink colour by the dropwise addition of a 5% w/v solution of *sodium sulphite* and boil to remove any odour of sulphur dioxide. Add 10 ml of *water*, 5 ml of *orthophosphoric acid* and 0.5 g of *sodium metaperiodate*, boil for 1 minute and allow to cool. The resulting solution is not more intensely coloured than a solution prepared at the same time and in the same manner using 1.0 ml of

0.02M *potassium permanganate VS* in place of the substance being examined (0.1%).

Zinc To 5 ml of solution A prepared in the test for Heavy metals add 1 ml of *potassium hexacyanoferrate(II) solution*, dilute to 13 ml with *water* and allow to stand for 5 minutes. Any turbidity produced is not more intense than that of a solution prepared by mixing 10 ml of *zinc standard solution (10 ppm Zn)*, 2 ml of *7M hydrochloric acid* and 1 ml of *potassium hexacyanoferrate(II) solution* (500 ppm).

Chloride Dilute 3.3 ml of the solution prepared for the test for Clarity of solution to 10 ml with *water* and add 5 ml of *2M nitric acid*. The resulting solution complies with the *limit test for chlorides*, Appendix VII (300 ppm). Use 0.15 ml of *dilute silver nitrate solution* in the test.

Assay Dissolve 2.5 g of *sodium hydrogen carbonate* in a mixture of 150 ml of *water* and 10 ml of *sulphuric acid*. When effervescence ceases, add 0.5 g of the substance being examined, shake gently to dissolve and titrate with *0.1M ammonium cerium(IV) nitrate VS*, using 0.1 ml of *ferroin sulphate solution* as indicator, until the red colour disappears. Each ml of *0.1M ammonium cerium(IV) nitrate VS* is equivalent to 0.02780 g of FeSO₄,7H₂O.

Storage Ferrous Sulphate should be kept in a well-closed container.

Preparation
Paediatric Ferrous Sulphate Oral Solution

Action and use Used in prevention and treatment of anaemias.

Ferrous Sulphate contains in 300 mg about 60 mg of iron.

Dried Ferrous Sulphate

13463-43-9

Dried Ferrous Sulphate is Ferrous Sulphate from which part of the water of crystallisation has been removed by drying at a temperature of 40°. It contains not less than 80.0 per cent and not more than 90.0 per cent of FeSO₄.

Characteristics A greyish-white powder.

Solubility It dissolves slowly, but almost completely, in freshly boiled and cooled *water*.

Identification Yields *reaction A* characteristic of iron salts and the *reactions* characteristic of sulphates, Appendix VI.

Arsenic Dissolve 1.0 g in 10 ml of *water* and 15 ml of *stannated hydrochloric acid* and distil 20 ml. To the distillate add 0.15 ml of *bromine water*, remove the excess bromine with 0.15 ml of *tin(II) chloride solution AsT* and dilute to 75 ml with *water*. 25 ml of the resulting solution complies with the *limit test for arsenic*, Appendix VII (3 ppm).

Copper Dissolve 5.0 g in 40 ml of *hydrochloric acid* by warming, add 10 ml of *nitric acid* and 15 ml of *water*, boil gently for 5 minutes and cool. Shake with four 30-ml quantities of *ether* and discard the ether. Heat the acid solution on a water-bath to remove dissolved ether, cool and add sufficient *water* to produce 100 ml (solution A). To 10 ml of solution A add 1 g of *citric acid*, make alkaline with *5M ammonia* and add 25 ml of *water* and 5 ml of *sodium diethyldithiocarbamate solution*. Extract with successive quantities of 5, 3 and 2 ml of *carbon tetrachloride* and adjust the combined extracts to 10 ml with *carbon tetrachloride*. The colour of the solution is not more intense than that produced by treating in the same manner a solution prepared by mixing 2.5 ml of *copper standard solution (10 ppm Cu)* and 7.5 ml of *water* (50 ppm).

Lead Not more than 50 ppm when determined by the following method. For solution (1) use 40 ml of solution A and for solution (2) use a mixture of 10 ml of *hydrochloric acid*, 0.5 ml of *nitric acid* and 10 ml of *lead standard solution (10 ppm Pb)*. Make solutions (1) and (2) alkaline with 5M *ammonia* and to each add 1 ml of *potassium cyanide solution PbT*; the solutions should be not more than faintly opalescent. If the colours of the solutions differ, equalise by the addition of about 0.2 ml of a highly diluted solution of burnt sugar or other non-reactive substance. Dilute each solution to 50 ml with *water*, add 0.1 ml of a 10 per cent w/v solution of *sodium sulphide* to each and mix thoroughly. The colour produced in solution (1) is not more intense than that produced in solution (2) when viewed against a white background.

Manganese Dissolve 1.0 g in 40 ml of *water*, add 10 ml of *nitric acid* and boil until red fumes cease to be evolved. Add 0.5 g of *ammonium persulphate* and boil for 10 minutes. If any pink colour is produced, decolorise the solution by the dropwise addition of a 5% w/v solution of *sodium sulphite* and boil until the odour of sulphur dioxide is no longer detectable. Add 10 ml of *water*, 5 ml of *orthophosphoric acid* and 0.5 g of *sodium metaperiodate*, boil for 1 minute and cool. The colour of the solution is not more intense than that of a solution containing the same quantities of the same reagents and 1.0 ml of 0.02M *potassium permanganate VS*.

Zinc To 10 ml of solution A add 1 g of *citric acid* and 0.1 g of *resorcinol*, neutralise with 5M *ammonia*, using *thymol blue solution* as indicator, and shake for 1 minute with two successive 20-ml quantities of *dithizone solution*. To the combined extracts add 10 ml of 0.1M *hydrochloric acid*, shake for 1 minute, separate the acid layer and wash with 2 ml of *chloroform*. To the acid layer add 3 ml of 1M *hydrochloric acid* and 20 ml of a 10% w/v solution of *ammonium chloride* and adjust the volume to 50 ml with *water*. Add 1 ml of *potassium hexacyanoferrate(II) solution* and allow to stand for 15 minutes. Any turbidity produced is not greater than that produced in 15 minutes by the addition of 1 ml of *potassium hexacyanoferrate(II) solution* to a freshly prepared mixture of 4 ml of *zinc standard solution (25 ppm Zn)*, 4 ml of 1M *hydrochloric acid*, 20 ml of a 10% w/v solution of *ammonium chloride* and sufficient *water* to produce 50 ml.

Basic sulphate 2.0 g dissolves slowly in a mixture of 7.5 ml of freshly boiled and cooled *water* and 0.5 ml of 0.5M *sulphuric acid*, producing a solution that is not more than faintly turbid.

Assay Dissolve 0.5 g in a mixture of 30 ml of *water* and 20 ml of 1M *sulphuric acid* and titrate with 0.1M *ammonium cerium(IV) sulphate VS* using *ferroin sulphate solution* as indicator. Each ml of 0.1M *ammonium cerium(IV) sulphate VS* is equivalent to 0.01519 g of $FeSO_4$.

Storage Dried Ferrous Sulphate should be kept in a well-closed container.

Preparation
Ferrous Sulphate Tablets

Action and use Used in prevention and treatment of anaemias.

Fig

Fig is the sun-dried succulent fruit of *Ficus carica* L.

Characteristics Odour, pleasantly fruity; taste, sweet.

Macroscopical Fruit compound, soft, fleshy, brown or yellowish-brown, sometimes covered with a saccharine efflorescence; at the summit a small opening surrounded by scales and at the base a short, stalk-like prolongation; fruit up to about 5 cm in length and breadth, consisting of a hollow receptacle bearing on the inner surface numerous drupelets, each containing a stone about 1.5 to 2.0 mm long; seed containing endosperm and a curved embryo.

Microscopical Receptacle: epidermal cells polyhedral, stomata raised, trichomes unicellular, thick walled, of varying length up to about 300 μm; hypodermis composed of rounded polyhedral cells, some containing small rosette crystals of calcium oxalate; aerenchyma made up of large, irregular cells, forming the greater part of the receptacle, containing large rosette crystals of calcium oxalate and interspersed with numerous latex tubes, about 30 to 50 μm wide, and slender vascular bundles. Pericarp: epicarp consisting of radially elongated cells with mucilaginous outer walls; mesocarp of delicate, often disorganised cells; endocarp of radially elongated sclereids with pitted walls. Endosperm and embryo: small cells containing aleurone grains and fixed oil; starch absent.

Water-soluble extractive Not less than 60.0% when determined by the following method. To 25 g, minced, add 500 ml of *water*, boil under a reflux condenser for 1 hour, cool and filter. To 20 ml of the filtrate add 20 g of washed and ignited sand, evaporate to dryness in a tared, flat-bottomed shallow dish and dry the residue to constant weight at 100°. Calculate the water-soluble extractive by subtracting the weight of sand from the weight of the residue obtained.

Storage Fig should be stored in a dry place.

Preparation
Compound Fig Elixir

Action and use Demulcent.

Fluclorolone Acetonide

$C_{24}H_{29}Cl_2FO_5$ 487.4   *3693-39-9*

Fluclorolone Acetonide is 9α,11β-dichloro-6α-fluoro-21-hydroxy-16α,17α-isopropylidene-dioxypregna-1,4-diene-3,20-dione. It contains not less than 97.0 per cent and not more than the equivalent of 102.0 per cent of $C_{24}H_{29}Cl_2FO_5$, calculated with reference to the dried substance.

Characteristics A white or creamy white, crystalline powder; odourless or almost odourless.

Solubility Practically insoluble in *water*; soluble in *ethanol (96%)* and in *chloroform*; slightly soluble in *ether*.

Identification A. The *infra-red absorption spectrum*, Appendix II A, is concordant with the *reference spectrum* of fluclorolone acetonide.

B. The *light absorption*, Appendix II B, in the range 220 to 350 nm of a 0.003% w/v solution in *methanol* exhibits a maximum only at 236 nm. The *absorbance* at 236 nm is about 0.96.

Specific optical rotation In a 1% w/v solution in *chloroform*, +148° to +158°, Appendix V F.

Foreign steroids and other impurities Carry out the method for *thin-layer chromatography*, Appendix III A, using *silica gel G* as the coating substance and a mixture of 97 volumes of *toluene* and 3 volumes of *absolute ethanol* as the mobile phase. Apply separately to the chromatoplate 10 μl of each of three solutions of the substance being examined in a mixture of equal volumes of *methanol* and *chloroform* containing (1) 2.0% w/v, (2) 0.020% w/v and (3) 0.010% w/v. After removal of the plate, allow it to dry in air, return the plate to the tank and again allow the solvent front to ascend 15 cm above the line of application. Remove the plate, allow it to dry in air and spray with *alkaline tetrazolium blue solution*. Any *secondary spot* in the chromatogram obtained with solution (1) is not more intense than the spot in the chromatogram obtained with solution (2) and not more than one such spot is more intense than the spot in the chromatogram obtained with solution (3).

Loss on drying When dried at 105° at a pressure not exceeding 0.7 kPa for 3 hours, loses not more than 1.0% of its weight. Use 1 g.

Assay Carry out the method for *high-performance liquid chromatography*, Appendix III D, using solutions in the mobile phase containing (1) 0.0025% w/v of *fluclorolone acetonide BPCRS* and 0.00030% w/v of *propyl 4-hydroxybenzoate* (internal standard), (2) 0.0025% w/v of the substance being examined and (3) 0.0025% w/v of the substance being examined and 0.00030% w/v of the internal standard.

The chromatographic procedure may be carried out using (a) a stainless steel column (30 cm × 3.9 mm) packed with *stationary phase C* (10 μm) (μBondapak C18 is suitable), (b) a mixture of *methanol* and *water* as the mobile phase with a flow rate of 2 ml per minute (a mixture of 62 volumes of *methanol* and 38 volumes of *water* is usually suitable) and (c) a detection wavelength of 254 nm.

Calculate the content of $C_{24}H_{29}Cl_2FO_5$ using the declared content of $C_{24}H_{29}Cl_2FO_5$ in *fluclorolone acetonide BPCRS*.

Storage Fluclorolone Acetonide should be protected from light.

Preparation
Fluclorolone Ointment

Action and use Corticosteroid.

Flucloxacillin Magnesium

$(C_{19}H_{16}ClFN_3O_5S)_2Mg,8H_2O$ 1074.2   58486-36-5

Flucloxacillin Magnesium is magnesium (6*R*)-6-[3-(2-chloro-6-fluorophenyl)-5-methylisoxazole-4-carboxamido]penicillanate octahydrate. It contains not less than 95.0 per cent and not more than 100.5 per cent of $(C_{19}H_{16}ClFN_3O_5S)_2Mg$, calculated with reference to the anhydrous substance.

Characteristics A white or almost white powder.

Solubility Slightly soluble in *water* and in *chloroform*; soluble in 1 part of *methanol*.

Identification A. The *infra-red absorption spectrum*, Appendix II A, is concordant with the *reference spectrum* of flucloxacillin magnesium.

B. Carry out the method for *thin-layer chromatography*, Appendix III A, using a silanised silica gel F254 precoated chromatoplate (Merck silanised silica gel 60 F254 plates are suitable) and a mixture of 70 volumes of a 15.4% w/v solution of *ammonium acetate* previously adjusted to pH 5.0 with *glacial acetic acid* and 30 volumes of *acetone* as the mobile phase. Apply separately to the plate 1 μl of each of three solutions in *water* containing (1) 0.5% w/v of the substance being examined, (2) 0.5% w/v of *flucloxacillin sodium BPCRS* and (3) 0.5% w/v each of *cloxacillin sodium BPCRS*, *dicloxacillin sodium BPCRS* and *flucloxacillin sodium BPCRS*. After removal of the plate, allow it to dry in air and expose to iodine vapour until spots appear. The principal spot in the chromatogram obtained with solution (1) corresponds in colour, position and size to the principal spot in the chromatogram obtained with solution (2). The test is not valid unless the chromatogram obtained with solution (3) shows three clearly separated principal spots.

C. Yields *reaction B* characteristic of magnesium salts, Appendix VI.

Acidity pH of a 0.5% w/v solution, 4.5 to 6.5, Appendix V L.

Specific optical rotation In a 0.5% w/v solution, +163° to +173°, Appendix V F.

Iodine-absorbing substances Not more than 5.0%, calculated with reference to the anhydrous substance, when determined by the following method. Dissolve 0.125 g in sufficient *mixed phosphate buffer pH 7.0* to produce 25 ml. To 10 ml add 10 ml of *mixed phosphate buffer pH 4.0* and 10 ml of 0.01M *iodine VS* and titrate immediately with 0.01M *sodium thiosulphate VS* using *starch mucilage*, added towards the end of the titration, as indicator. Repeat the operation without the substance being examined. The difference between the titrations represents the amount of iodine-absorbing substances present. Each ml of 0.01M *sodium thiosulphate VS* is equivalent to 0.000524 g of iodine-absorbing substances.

Water 12.0 to 15.0% w/w, Appendix IX C. Use 0.3 g.

Assay Dissolve 0.1 g in sufficient *water* to produce 500 ml and dilute 25 ml to 100 ml with *water*. Place two 2-ml aliquots of the resulting solution in separate stoppered tubes. To one tube add 10 ml of *imidazole—mercury reagent*, mix, stopper the tube and immerse in a water-bath at 60° for exactly 25 minutes, swirling occasionally. Remove from the water-bath and cool rapidly to 20° (solution A). To the second tube add 10 ml of *water* and mix (solution B). Without delay measure the *absorbances* of solutions A and B at the maximum at 346 nm, Appendix II B, using in the reference cell a mixture of 2 ml of *water* and 10 ml of *imidazole—mercury reagent* for solution A and *water* for solution B. Calculate the content of $(C_{19}H_{16}ClFN_3O_5S)_2Mg$ from the difference between the absorbances of solutions A and B, from the difference obtained by repeating the procedure using *flucloxacillin sodium BPCRS* in place of the substance being examined and from the declared content of $C_{19}H_{17}ClFN_3O_5S$ in *flucloxacillin sodium BPCRS*. Each mg of $C_{19}H_{17}ClFN_3O_5S$ is equivalent to 1.025 mg of $(C_{19}H_{16}ClFN_3O_5S)_2Mg$.

Storage Flucloxacillin Magnesium should be kept in a well-closed container, protected from moisture and stored at a temperature not exceeding 25°.

Labelling The label states (1) the date after which the material is not intended to be used; (2) the conditions under which it should be stored.

Preparation
Flucloxacillin Oral Suspension

Action and use Antibacterial.

Flucloxacillin Sodium

$C_{19}H_{16}ClFN_3NaO_5S,H_2O$ 493.9   *1847-24-1*

Flucloxacillin Sodium is sodium (6*R*)-6-[3-(2-chloro-6-fluorophenyl)-5-methylisoxazole-4-carboxamido]penicillanate monohydrate. It contains not less than 95.0 per cent and not more than 100.5 per cent of $C_{19}H_{16}ClFN_3NaO_5S$, calculated with reference to the anhydrous substance.

Characteristics A white or almost white powder; hygroscopic.

Solubility Soluble in 1 part of *water*, in 2 parts of *methanol*, in 8 parts of *ethanol (96%)* and in 8 parts of *acetone*.

Identification A. The *infra-red absorption spectrum*, Appendix II A, is concordant with the *reference spectrum* of flucloxacillin sodium.
B. Yields *reactions B* and *C* characteristic of sodium salts, Appendix VI.

Acidity or alkalinity pH of a 10% w/v solution, 5.0 to 7.0, Appendix V L.

Specific optical rotation In a 1% w/v solution, +158° to +168°, Appendix V F.

Dichloromethane Not more than 0.2% w/w when determined by the method for *gas chromatography*, Appendix III B, using solutions in *water* containing (1)

0.020% v/v of *dichloromethane* and 0.020% v/v of *1,2-dichloroethane* (internal standard), (2) 10% w/v of the substance being examined and (3) 10% w/v of the substance being examined and 0.020% v/v of the internal standard.

The chromatographic procedure may be carried out using a glass column (1.5 m × 4 mm) packed with *acid-washed, silanised diatomaceous support* (100 to 120 mesh) coated with 10% w/w of polyethylene glycol 1000 and maintained at 60°.

Calculate the percentage w/w of dichloromethane taking 1.325 g as its weight per ml at 20°.

Iodine-absorbing substances Not more than 5.0%, calculated with reference to the anhydrous substance, when determined by the following method. Dissolve 0.125 g in sufficient *mixed phosphate buffer pH 7.0* to produce 25 ml. To 10 ml add 10 ml of *mixed phosphate buffer pH 4.0* and 10 ml of 0.01M *iodine VS* and titrate immediately with 0.01M *sodium thiosulphate VS* using *starch mucilage*, added towards the end of the titration, as indicator. Repeat the operation without the substance being examined. The difference between the titrations represents the amount of iodine-absorbing substances present. Each ml of 0.01M *sodium thiosulphate VS* is equivalent to 0.000524 g of iodine-absorbing substances.

Water 3.0 to 4.3% w/w, Appendix IX C. Use 0.3 g.

Assay Dissolve 0.1 g in sufficient *water* to produce 500 ml and dilute 25 ml to 100 ml with *water*. Place two 2-ml aliquots of the resulting solution in separate stoppered tubes. To one tube add 10 ml of *imidazole—mercury reagent*, mix, stopper the tube and immerse in a water-bath at 60° for exactly 25 minutes, swirling occasionally. Remove from the water-bath and cool rapidly to 20° (solution A). To the second tube add 10 ml of *water* and mix (solution B). Without delay measure the *absorbances* of solutions A and B at the maximum at 346 nm, Appendix II B, using in the reference cell a mixture of 2 ml of *water* and 10 ml of *imidazole—mercury reagent* for solution A and *water* for solution B. Calculate the content of $C_{19}H_{16}ClFN_3NaO_5S$ from the difference between the absorbances of solutions A and B, from the difference obtained by repeating the procedure using *flucloxacillin sodium BPCRS* in place of the substance being examined and from the declared content of $C_{19}H_{16}ClFN_3NaO_5S$ in *flucloxacillin sodium BPCRS*.

Storage Flucloxacillin Sodium should be kept in a well-closed container, protected from moisture and stored at a temperature not exceeding 25°. If it is intended for use in the manufacture of a parenteral dosage form the container should be sterile and sealed so as to exclude micro-organisms.

Labelling The label states (1) the date after which the material is not intended to be used; (2) the conditions under which it should be stored; (3) whether or not it is intended for use in the manufacture of a parenteral dosage form.

Preparations
Flucloxacillin Capsules
Flucloxacillin Oral Solution
Flucloxacillin Injection

Action and use Antibacterial.

Flucloxacillin Sodium intended for use in the manufacture of a parenteral dosage form complies with the following additional requirements.

Pyrogens Complies with the *test for pyrogens*, Appendix XIV K. Use per kg of the rabbit's weight 1 ml of *water for injections* containing 6 mg per ml of the substance being examined.

Sterility When intended for use in the manufacture of a parenteral dosage form without further sterilisation, complies with the *test for sterility*, Appendix XVI A.

Flucytosine

$C_4H_4FN_3O$ 129.1   *2022-85-7*

Flucytosine is 4-amino-5-fluoropyrimidin-2(1*H*)-one. It contains not less than 98.5 per cent and not more than 101.0 per cent of $C_4H_4FN_3O$, calculated with reference to the dried substance.

Characteristics A white or almost white, crystalline powder; odourless or almost odourless.

Solubility Sparingly soluble in *water*; slightly soluble in *ethanol (96%)*; practically insoluble in *chloroform* and in *ether*.

Identification A. The *infra-red absorption spectrum*, Appendix II A, is concordant with the *reference spectrum* of flucytosine.
B. The *light absorption*, Appendix II B, in the range 230 to 350 nm of a 0.001% w/v solution in 0.1M *hydrochloric acid* exhibits a maximum only at 286 nm. The *absorbance* at 286 nm is about 0.71.
C. To 5 ml of a 1% w/v solution add 0.15 ml of *bromine water*. The colour is discharged or almost discharged.

Free fluoride 0.10 g complies with the *limit test for fluorides*, Appendix VII (500 ppm).

Heavy metals To the residue obtained in the test for Sulphated ash add 1 ml of 2M *hydrochloric acid* and evaporate to dryness on a water-bath. Dissolve the residue in 15 ml of *water* and dilute to 20 ml with *water*. 12 ml of the resulting solution complies with *limit test A for heavy metals*, Appendix VII (20 ppm). Use *lead standard solution (1 ppm Pb)* to prepare the standard.

Fluorouracil Carry out the method for *thin-layer chromatography*, Appendix III A, using a silica gel F254 precoated chromatoplate (Merck silica gel 60 F254 plates are suitable) and a mixture of 86 volumes of *ethyl acetate*, 7 volumes of *formic acid* and 7 volumes of *water* as the mobile phase but allowing the solvent front to ascend 10 cm above the line of application. Apply separately to the plate 50 μl of each of the following solutions. For solution (1) shake 0.10 g of the substance being examined with 10 ml of a mixture of equal volumes of *methanol* and 13.5M *ammonia*. Solution (2) contains 1.0% w/v of *5-fluorouracil* in the same solvent mixture. After removal of the plate, dry it in a current of warm air and examine under *ultra-violet light (254 nm)*. Any spot corresponding to 5-fluorouracil in the chromatogram obtained with solution (1) is not more intense than the spot in the chromatogram obtained with solution (2).

Loss on drying When dried at 105° for 4 hours, loses not more than 1.5% of its weight. Use 1 g.

Sulphated ash Not more than 0.1%, Appendix IX A. Use 1.0 g.

Assay Dissolve 0.3 g in a mixture of 50 ml of *acetic anhydride* and 100 ml of *anhydrous glacial acetic acid*, warming if necessary, and carry out Method I for *non-aqueous titration*, Appendix VIII A, determining the end-point potentiometrically. Each ml of 0.1M *perchloric acid VS* is equivalent to 0.01291 g of $C_4H_4FN_3O$.

Storage Flucytosine should be kept in a well-closed container and protected from light.

Preparation
Flucytosine Tablets

Action and use Antifungal.

Fludrocortisone Acetate

$C_{23}H_{31}FO_6$ 422.5   *514-36-3*

Fludrocortisone Acetate is 9α-fluoro-11β,17α,21-trihydroxypregn-4-ene-3,20-dione 21-acetate (9α-fluorohydrocortisone 21-acetate). It contains not less than 96.0 per cent and not more than 104.0 per cent of $C_{23}H_{31}FO_6$, calculated with reference to the dried substance.

Characteristics A white or almost white crystalline powder; odourless or almost odourless; hygroscopic.

Solubility Practically insoluble in *water*; soluble in 50 parts of *ethanol (96%)* and in 50 parts of *chloroform*; slightly soluble in *ether*.

Identification A. The *infra-red absorption spectrum*, Appendix II A, is concordant with the *reference spectrum* of fludrocortisone acetate. If the spectra are not concordant dissolve a sufficient quantity in the minimum volume of *chloroform IR*, evaporate to dryness in a current of nitrogen and prepare a new spectrum of the residue.
B. Complies with the test for *identification of steroids*, Appendix III A, using *impregnating solvent I* and *mobile phase B*.
C. Heat 0.5 ml of *chromic—sulphuric acid mixture* in a naked flame until white fumes appear in the upper part of the tube; the solution wets the sides of the tube readily and there is no greasiness. Add 2 or 3 mg of the substance being examined and again heat in a naked flame until white fumes appear; the solution does not wet the sides of the tube and does not pour easily from the tube.
D. Yields the *reaction* characteristic of acetyl groups, Appendix VI.

Light absorption *Absorbance* of a 0.001% w/v solution in *absolute ethanol* at the maximum at 240 nm, 0.39 to 0.42, Appendix II B.

Specific optical rotation In a 1% w/v solution in *1,4-dioxan*, +148° to +156°, Appendix V F.

Related foreign steroids Complies with the test for *related foreign steroids*, *Method B*, Appendix III A.

Loss on drying When dried to constant weight at 105°, loses not more than 1.0% of its weight. Use 1 g.

Sulphated ash Not more than 0.1%, Appendix IX A.

Assay Carry out the *tetrazolium assay of steroids*, Appendix VIII P, using a quantity dissolved in sufficient *aldehyde-free absolute ethanol* to produce a solution containing between 440 and 460 μg in 10 ml and calculate the content of $C_{23}H_{31}FO_6$ from the *absorbance* obtained by repeating the operation using *fludrocortisone acetate BPCRS* in place of the substance being examined.

Storage Fludrocortisone Acetate should be kept in a well-closed container.

Preparation
Fludrocortisone Tablets

Action and use Corticosteroid.

Fluocinolone Acetonide ☆

$C_{24}H_{30}F_2O_6$ 452.5   67-73-2

Fluocinolone Acetonide is 6α,9a-difluoro-11β,21-dihydroxy-16α,17α-isopropylidene-dioxypregna-1,4-diene-3,20-dione. It contains not less than 96.0 per cent and not more than 104.0 per cent of $C_{24}H_{30}F_2O_6$, calculated with reference to the dried substance.

Characteristics A white or almost white, crystalline powder; odourless.

Solubility Practically insoluble in *water*; soluble in 10 parts of *acetone*, in 26 parts of *absolute ethanol* and in 15 parts of *chloroform*; practically insoluble in light petroleum.

Identification *Test A may be omitted if tests B, C and D are carried out. Tests C and D may be omitted if tests A and B are carried out.*

A. The *infra-red absorption spectrum*, Appendix II A, is concordant with the spectrum of *fluocinolone acetonide EPCRS*.

B. Complies with the test for *identification of steroids*, Appendix III A, using *impregnating solvent I* and *mobile phase H*. Apply 5 μl of each of the three solutions.

C. Complies with the test for *identification of steroids*, Appendix III A, using the conditions specified in test B but using solutions prepared in the following manner. For solution (1) dissolve 10 mg in 1.5 ml of *glacial acetic acid* in a separating funnel, add 0.5 ml of a 2% w/v solution of *chromium trioxide* and allow to stand for 30 minutes. Add 5 ml of *water* and 2 ml of *dichloromethane* and shake vigorously for 2 minutes. Allow to separate and use the lower layer. Prepare solution (2) in the same manner but using 10 mg of *fluocinolone acetonide EPCRS*.

D. Heat 0.5 ml of *chromic—sulphuric acid mixture* in a small test-tube in a naked flame until white fumes appear in the upper part of the tube; the solution wets the sides of the tube readily and there is no greasiness. Add 2 to 3 mg of the substance being examined and again heat in a naked flame until white fumes appear; the solution does not wet the sides of the tube and does not pour easily from the tube.

Light absorption Dissolve 15 mg in *absolute ethanol* and dilute to 100 ml with the same solvent. Dilute 10 ml of the solution to 100 ml with *absolute ethanol*. The A(1%, 1 cm) of the resulting solution at the maximum at 239 nm is 345 to 375, Appendix II B.

Specific optical rotation In a 1% w/v solution in *1,4-dioxan*, +92° to +96°, Appendix V F.

Related substances Carry out the method for *thin-layer chromatography*, Appendix III A, using *silica gel GF254* as the coating substance and a mixture of 77 volumes of *dichloromethane*, 15 volumes of *ether*, 8 volumes of *methanol* and 1.2 volumes of *water* as the mobile phase. Apply separately to the chromatoplate 5 μl of each of three solutions of the substance being examined in *chloroform* containing (1) 1.0% w/v, (2) 0.020% w/v and (3) 0.010% w/v. After removal of the plate, allow it to dry in air and examine under *ultra-violet light (254 nm)*. Any *secondary spot* in the chromatogram obtained with solution (1) is not more intense than the spot in the chromatogram obtained with solution (2) and not more than one such spot is more intense than the spot in the chromatogram obtained with solution (3).

Loss on drying When dried at 100° to 105° for 3 hours, loses not more than 1.0% of its weight. Use 1 g.

Assay Carry out the *tetrazolium assay of steroids*, Appendix VIII P, and calculate the content of $C_{24}H_{30}F_2O_6$ from the *absorbance* obtained by repeating the operation using *fluocinolone acetonide EPCRS* in place of the substance being examined.

Storage Fluocinolone Acetonide should be kept in a well-closed container and protected from light.

Preparations
Fluocinolone Cream
Fluocinolone Ointment

Action and use Corticosteroid.

Fluocortolone Hexanoate
Fluocortolone Caproate

$C_{28}H_{39}FO_5$ 474.6   303-40-2

Fluocortolone Hexanoate is 6α-fluoro-11β,21-dihydroxy-16α-methylpregna-1,4-diene-3,20-dione 21-hexanoate. It contains not less than 97.0 per cent and not more than 103.0 per cent of $C_{28}H_{39}FO_5$, calculated with reference to the dried substance.

Characteristics A white to creamy-white, crystalline powder; odourless or almost odourless.

Solubility Practically insoluble in *water* and in *ether*; very slightly soluble in *ethanol (96%)* and in *methanol*; slightly soluble in *acetone* and in *1,4-dioxan*; sparingly soluble in *chloroform*.

Identification A. The *infra-red absorption spectrum*, Appendix II A, is concordant with the *reference spectrum* of fluocortolone hexanoate.

B. Complies with the test for *identification of steroids*, Appendix III A, using *impregnating solvent II* and *mobile phase D*.

C. To 1 mg add 2 ml of a mixture of 3 volumes of *sulphuric acid* and 2 volumes of *glacial acetic acid* and heat for 1 minute on a water-bath; a red colour is produced. Add 5 ml of *water*; the colour changes to violet-red.

D. Heat 0.5 ml of *chromic—sulphuric acid mixture* in a small test-tube in a naked flame until white fumes appear in the upper part of the tube; the solution wets the sides of the tube readily and there is no greasiness. Add 2 to 3 mg of the substance being examined and again heat in a naked flame until white fumes appear; the solution does not wet the sides of the tube and does not pour easily from the tube.

E. Heat 50 mg with 2 ml of 0.5M *ethanolic potassium hydroxide* in a water-bath for 5 minutes. Add 3 ml of *water*, evaporate the ethanol, add 2 ml of *sulphuric acid (50%)* and heat on a water-bath. The odour of hexanoic acid is produced.

F. *Melting point*, about 244°, Appendix V A.

Light absorption Ratio of the *absorbance* of the solution prepared as directed in the Assay at the maximum at 242 nm to that at 263 nm, 2.15 to 2.35, Appendix II B.

Specific optical rotation In a 1% w/v solution in *1,4-dioxan*, prepared with the aid of heat, +97° to +103°, Appendix V F.

Related foreign steroids Complies with the test for *related foreign steroids, Method B*, Appendix III A, using as solution (1) a 0.50% w/v solution of the substance being examined in *acetone* and applying 3 µl of this solution to the chromatoplate.

Loss on drying When dried to constant weight at 105°, loses not more than 0.5% of its weight. Use 1 g.

Sulphated ash Not more than 0.1%, Appendix IX A.

Assay Dissolve 15 mg in sufficient *methanol* to produce 100 ml, dilute 20 ml to 100 ml with *methanol* and measure the *absorbance* of the resulting solution at the maximum at 242 nm, Appendix II B. Calculate the content of $C_{28}H_{39}FO_5$ taking 340 as the value of A(1%, 1 cm) at the maximum at 242 nm.

Storage Fluocortolone Hexanoate should be protected from light.

Preparations
Fluocortolone Cream
Fluocortolone Ointment

Action and use Corticosteroid.

Fluocortolone Pivalate

Fluocortolone Trimethylacetate

$C_{27}H_{37}FO_5$ 460.6   *29205-06-9*

Fluocortolone Pivalate is 6α-fluoro-11β,21-dihydroxy-16α-methylpregna-1,4-diene-3,20-dione 21-pivalate. It contains not less than 97.0 per cent and not more than 103.0 per cent of $C_{27}H_{37}FO_5$, calculated with reference to the dried substance.

Characteristics A white to creamy-white, crystalline powder; odourless or almost odourless.

Solubility Practically insoluble in *water*; sparingly soluble in *ethanol (96%)* and in *methanol*; freely soluble in *chloroform* and in *1,4-dioxan*; slightly soluble in *ether*.

Identification A. The *infra-red absorption spectrum*, Appendix II A, is concordant with the *reference spectrum* of fluocortolone pivalate.

B. Complies with the test for *identification of steroids*, Appendix III A, using *impregnating solvent II* and *mobile phase D*.

C. To 1 mg add 2 ml of a mixture of 3 volumes of *sulphuric acid* and 2 volumes of *glacial acetic acid* and heat for 1 minute on a water-bath; a red colour is produced. Add 5 ml of *water*; the colour changes to violet-red.

D. Heat 0.5 ml of *chromic—sulphuric acid mixture* in a small test-tube in a naked flame until white fumes appear in the upper part of the tube. The solution wets the sides of the tube readily and there is no greasiness. Add 2 to 3 mg of the substance being examined and again heat in the naked flame until white fumes appear; the solution does not wet the sides of the tube and does not pour easily from the tube.

E. Heat 50 mg with 2 ml of 0.5M *ethanolic potassium hydroxide* in a water-bath for 5 minutes. Add 2 ml of *water*, evaporate the alcohol, add 2 ml of *sulphuric acid (50%)*, extract with 5 ml of *ether* and evaporate the ether. The odour of pivalic acid is produced.

F. *Melting point*, about 187°, Appendix V A.

Light absorption Ratio of the *absorbance* of the solution prepared as directed in the Assay at the maximum at 242 nm to that at 263 nm, 2.15 to 2.35, Appendix II B.

Specific optical rotation In a 1% w/v solution in *1,4-dioxan*, +100° to +105°, Appendix V F.

Related foreign steroids Complies with the test for *related foreign steroids, Method B*, Appendix III A.

Loss on drying When dried to constant weight at 105°, loses not more than 0.5% of its weight. Use 1 g.

Sulphated ash Not more than 0.1%, Appendix IX A.

Assay Dissolve 15 mg in sufficient *absolute ethanol* to produce 100 ml, dilute 20 ml to 100 ml with *absolute ethanol* and measure the *absorbance* of the resulting solution at the maximum at 242 nm, Appendix II B. Calculate the content of $C_{27}H_{37}FO_5$ taking 350 as the value of A(1%, 1 cm) at the maximum at 242 nm.

Storage Fluocortolone Pivalate should be protected from light.

Preparations
Fluocortolone Cream
Fluocortolone Ointment

Action and use Corticosteroid.

Fluorescein Sodium
Soluble Fluorescein

$C_{20}H_{10}Na_2O_5$ 376.3   *518-47-8*

Fluorescein Sodium is disodium 3'6'-dihydroxy-spiro[isobenzofuran-1-(3*H*),9'(9*H*)-xanthen]-3-one. It contains not less than 98.5 per cent and not more than 100.5 per cent of $C_{20}H_{10}Na_2O_5$, calculated with reference to the dried substance.

Characteristics An orange-red powder; odourless or almost odourless; hygroscopic.

Solubility Soluble in 1.5 parts of *water* and in 10 parts of *ethanol (96%)*.

Identification A. The *infra-red absorption spectrum*, Appendix II A, is concordant with the *reference spectrum* of fluorescein sodium.
B. A solution is strongly fluorescent, even in extreme dilution. The fluorescence disappears when the solution is made acidic and reappears when it is made alkaline.
C. One drop of a 0.05% w/v solution, absorbed by a piece of filter paper, colours the paper yellow. On exposing the moist paper to bromine vapour for 1 minute and then to ammonia vapour the yellow colour becomes deep pink.
D. The residue after incineration yields the *reactions* characteristic of sodium salts, Appendix VI.

Acidity or alkalinity pH of a 2% w/v solution, 7.0 to 9.0, Appendix V L.

Chloroform-soluble matter Dissolve 0.2 g in 10 ml of 0.1M *sodium hydroxide* and extract with 10 ml of *chloroform*. Allow to separate, dry the chloroform layer over *anhydrous sodium sulphate* and filter. The *absorbance* of the resulting solution at 480 nm is not more than 0.10, Appendix II B, using *chloroform* in the reference cell.

Zinc Dissolve 0.10 g in 10 ml of *water*, add 2 ml of *hydrochloric acid*, filter and add 0.1 ml of *potassium hexacyanoferrate(II) solution*. No turbidity or precipitate is produced immediately.

Chloride Dissolve 0.10 g in 100 ml of *water*, add 1 ml of *nitric acid* and filter. 15 ml of the filtrate complies with the *limit test for chlorides*, Appendix VII (0.33%).

Sulphate Dissolve 0.10 g in 120 ml of *water* containing 2.5 ml of 2M *hydrochloric acid* and filter. The filtrate complies with the *limit test for sulphates*, Appendix VII (1.2%).

Dimethylformamide Prepare a 0.020% v/v solution of *dimethylacetamide* (internal standard) (solution A) and carry out the method for *gas chromatography*, Appendix III B, using the following solutions. Solution (1) is a mixture of 10 ml of a 0.020% v/v solution of *dimethylformamide* and 10 ml of solution A. For solution (2) dissolve 1.0 g of the substance being examined in 10 ml of *water*, add, with stirring, 10 ml of 0.6M *hydrochloric acid*, allow to stand for 15 minutes and centrifuge; dissolve 0.1 g of *trisodium orthophosphate* in 5 ml of the supernatant liquid. Prepare solution (3) in the same manner as solution (2) but use 10 ml of solution A in place of the water.

The chromatographic procedure may be carried out using a glass column (1.5 m × 4 mm) packed with *acid-washed, silanised diatomaceous support* (80 to 100 mesh) coated with 10% w/w of polyethylene glycol 1000 and maintained at 120°.

In the chromatogram obtained with solution (3) the ratio of the area of any peak corresponding to dimethylformamide to the area of the peak due to the internal standard is not greater than the corresponding ratio in the chromatogram obtained with solution (1).

Resorcinol Carry out the method for *thin-layer chromatography*, Appendix III A, using a silica gel F254 precoated chromatoplate (Merck silica gel 60 F254 plates are suitable) and a mixture of 60 volumes of *hexane* and 40 volumes of *ethyl acetate* as the mobile phase. Apply separately to the plate 5 µl of each of the following solutions. For solution (1) dissolve 1.0 g of the substance being examined in 10 ml of *water*, add slowly, with constant stirring, 10 ml of 0.6M *hydrochloric acid*, allow to stand for 15 minutes, centrifuge and use the supernatant liquid. Solution (2) contains 0.025% w/v of *resorcinol* in *water*. After removal of the plate, allow it to dry in air and expose to iodine vapour for 30 minutes. Any spot corresponding to resorcinol in the chromatogram obtained with solution (1) is not more intense than the spot in the chromatogram obtained with solution (2).

Related substances Carry out the method for *thin-layer chromatography*, Appendix III A, using a silica gel F254 precoated chromatoplate (Merck silica gel 60 F254 plates are suitable) and a mixture of 80 volumes of *chloroform* and 20 volumes of *methanol* as the mobile phase. Apply separately to the plate 5 µl of each of two solutions of the substance being examined in 0.1M *methanolic hydrochloric acid* containing (1) 1.0% w/v and (2) 0.0020% w/v. After removal of the plate, allow it to dry in air and examine under *ultra-violet light (365 nm)*. Expose the plate to iodine vapour for 30 minutes and re-examine. Any *secondary spot* in the chromatogram obtained with solution (1) is not more intense than the spot in the chromatogram obtained with solution (2).

Loss on drying When dried to constant weight at 105°, loses not more than 10.0% of its weight. Use 1 g.

Assay Dissolve 0.5 g in 20 ml of *water*, add 5 ml of 2M *hydrochloric acid* and extract with four 20-ml quantities of a mixture of equal volumes of *2-methylpropan-1-ol* and *chloroform*. Wash the combined extracts with 10 ml of *water*, extract the washings with 5 ml of the mixture and add to the combined extracts. Evaporate the combined extracts to dryness on a water-bath in a current of air, dissolve the residue in 10 ml of *ethanol (96%)*, evaporate to dryness on a water-bath and dry to constant weight at 105°. Each g of residue is equivalent to 1.132 g of $C_{20}H_{10}Na_2O_5$.

Storage Fluorescein Sodium should be kept in a well-closed container and protected from light.

Preparations
Fluorescein Eye Drops
Fluorescein Injection

Action and use Dye used for detection of abrasions of the cornea.

Fluorouracil

$C_4H_3FN_2O_2$ 130.1   *51-21-8*

Fluorouracil is 5-fluoropyrimidine-2,4(1*H*,3*H*)-dione. It contains not less than 98.5 per cent and not more than 101.0 per cent of $C_4H_3FN_2O_2$, calculated with reference to the dried substance.

Characteristics A white or almost white, crystalline powder.

Solubility Sparingly soluble in *water*; slightly soluble in *ethanol (96%)*; practically insoluble in *chloroform* and in *ether*.

Identification A. The *infra-red absorption spectrum*, Appendix II A, is concordant with the *reference spectrum* of fluorouracil.
B. The *light absorption*, Appendix II B, in the range 230 to 350 nm of a 0.002% w/v solution in 0.1M *hydrochloric acid* exhibits a maximum at 266 nm. The *absorbance* at 266 nm is about 1.1.
C. To 5 ml of a 1% w/v solution add 1 ml of *bromine water*. The colour is discharged.

Acidity pH of a 1% w/v solution, 4.3 to 5.3, Appendix V L.

Related substances Carry out the method for *thin-layer chromatography*, Appendix III A, using a silica gel F254 precoated chromatoplate (Merck silica gel 60 F254 plates are suitable) and a mixture of 70 volumes of *ethyl acetate*, 15 volumes of *methanol* and 15 volumes of *water* as the mobile phase. Apply separately to the plate 10 μl of each of three solutions in a mixture of equal volumes of *methanol* and *water* containing (1) 2.0% w/v of the substance being examined, (2) 0.0050% w/v of the substance being examined and (3) 0.0050% w/v of *5-hydroxyuracil*. After removal of the plate, allow it to dry in a current of air and examine under *ultra-violet light (254 nm)*. Any *secondary spot* in the chromatogram obtained with solution (1) is not more intense than the spot in the chromatogram obtained with solution (2). Spray with a freshly prepared 0.5% w/v solution of *fast blue B salt* and then with 0.1M *sodium hydroxide*. Any spot corresponding to 5-hydroxyuracil in the chromatogram obtained with solution (1) is not more intense than the spot in the chromatogram obtained with solution (3).

Loss on drying When dried to constant weight over *phosphorus pentoxide* at 80° at a pressure not exceeding 0.7 kPa for 4 hours, loses not more than 0.5% of its weight. Use 1 g.

Sulphated ash Not more than 0.1%, Appendix IX A.

Assay Dissolve 0.25 g in 50 ml of *dimethylformamide* with the aid of gentle heat and carry out Method II for *non-aqueous titration*, Appendix VIII A, using 0.1M *tetrabutyl-ammonium hydroxide VS* as titrant and determining the end-point potentiometrically. Each ml of 0.1M *tetrabutylammonium hydroxide VS* is equivalent to 0.01301 g of $C_4H_3FN_2O_2$.

Storage Fluorouracil should be kept in a well-closed container and protected from light.

Preparations
Fluorouracil Cream
Fluorouracil Injection

Action and use Cytotoxic.

Fluoxymesterone

$C_{20}H_{29}FO_3$ 336.5   *76-43-7*

Fluoxymesterone is 9α-fluoro-11β,17β-dihydroxy-17α-methylandrost-4-en-3-one. It contains not less than 97.0 per cent and not more than 103.0 per cent of $C_{20}H_{29}FO_3$, calculated with reference to the dried substance.

Characteristics A white or creamy white, crystalline powder; odourless or almost odourless.

Solubility Practically insoluble in *water*; sparingly soluble in *ethanol (96%)*; slightly soluble in *chloroform*.

Identification A. The *infra-red absorption spectrum*, Appendix II A, is concordant with the *reference spectrum* of fluoxymesterone.
B. Complies with the test for *identification of steroids*, Appendix III A, using *impregnating solvent II* and *mobile phase C*.
C. Heat 0.5 ml of *chromic—sulphuric acid mixture* in a small test-tube in heat in a naked flame until white fumes appear in the upper part of the tube; the solution wets the sides of the tube readily and there is no greasiness. Add 2 or 3 mg of the substance being examined and again heat in heat in a naked flame until white fumes appear; the solution does not wet the sides of the tube and does not pour easily from the tube.
D. *Melting point*, about 278°, Appendix V A.

Specific optical rotation In a 1% w/v solution in *ethanol (96%)*, +102° to +112°, Appendix V F.

Related substances Carry out the method for *thin-layer chromatography*, Appendix III A, using *silica gel G* as the coating substance and a mixture of 45 volumes of *cyclohexane*, 45 volumes of *ethyl acetate* and 10 volumes of *methanol* as the mobile phase. Apply separately to the chromatoplate 10 μl of each of two solutions of the substance being examined in *methanol* containing (1) 1.0% w/v and (2) 0.010% w/v. After removal of the plate, allow it to dry in air for 10 minutes, spray with a 0.5% w/v solution of *vanillin in ethanolic sulphuric acid*

(80%) and heat at 105° for 5 minutes. Any *secondary spot* in the chromatogram obtained with solution (1) is not more intense than the spot in the chromatogram obtained with solution (2).

Loss on drying When dried over *phosphorus pentoxide* at a pressure not exceeding 0.7 kPa for 24 hours, loses not more than 1.0% of its weight. Use 1 g.

Sulphated ash Not more than 0.1%, Appendix IX A.

Assay Dissolve 10 mg in sufficient *absolute ethanol* to produce 100 ml, dilute 10 ml to 50 ml with *absolute ethanol* and measure the *absorbance* of the resulting solution at the maximum at 240 nm, Appendix II B. Calculate the content of $C_{20}H_{29}FO_3$ taking 495 as the value of A(1%, 1 cm) at the maximum at 240 nm.

Storage Fluoxymesterone should be kept in a well-closed container and protected from light.

Preparation
Fluoxymesterone Tablets

Action and use Anabolic steroid.

Fluphenazine Decanoate

$C_{32}H_{44}F_3N_3O_2S$　591.8　*5002-47-1*

Fluphenazine Decanoate is 2-{4-[3-(2-trifluoro-methylphenothiazin-10-yl)propyl]piperazin-1-yl}ethyl decanoate. It contains not less than 98.5 per cent and not more than 101.5 per cent of $C_{32}H_{44}F_3N_3O_2S$, calculated with reference to the dried substance.

Characteristics A pale yellow, viscous liquid or a yellow, crystalline, oily solid; odour, faint and ester-like.

Solubility Practically insoluble in *water*; miscible with *absolute ethanol*, with *chloroform* and with *ether*. It dissolves in fixed oils.

Identification A. The *infra-red absorption spectrum*, Appendix II A, is concordant with the *reference spectrum* of fluphenazine decanoate.
B. The *light absorption*, Appendix II B, in the range 230 to 350 nm of a 0.001% w/v solution in *absolute ethanol* exhibits a maximum at 261 nm and a less well-defined maximum at 310 nm. The *absorbance* at 261 nm is about 0.60.
C. Carry out the method for *thin-layer chromatography*, Appendix III A, using *silica gel GF254* as the coating substance. Impregnate the dry chromatoplate by placing it in a tank containing a 5% v/v solution of n-*tetradecane* in n-*hexane*, allowing the impregnating solvent to ascend to the top and allowing to dry. Use *methanol (90%)* as the mobile phase. Apply separately to the chromatoplate 1 μl of each of two solutions in *ethanol (96%)* containing (1) 2.0% w/v of the substance being examined and (2) 2.0% w/v of *fluphenazine decanoate BPCRS*. After removal of the plate, allow it to dry in air and examine under *ultra-violet light (254 nm)*. The principal spot in the

chromatogram obtained with solution (1) corresponds to that in the chromatogram obtained with solution (2).
D. Burn 20 mg by the method for *oxygen-flask combustion*, Appendix VIII C, using 5 ml of 2M *sodium hydroxide* as the absorbing liquid. When the process is complete, dilute the liquid to 25 ml with *water*. To 0.2 ml of the resulting solution add 0.5 ml of *aminomethylalizarindiacetic acid solution*, sufficient 0.02M *hydrochloric acid* to give a full yellow colour and 0.02M *sodium hydroxide* dropwise until the solution just begins to turn pink. Add 0.2 ml of a solution containing 12% w/v of *sodium acetate* and 6% v/v of *glacial acetic acid*, dilute with *water* to 4 ml and add 0.5 ml of *cerium(III) nitrate solution*. A deep lilac-blue colour is produced.
E. Dissolve 5 mg in 2 ml of *sulphuric acid* and allow to stand for 5 minutes. A reddish-brown colour is produced.

Related substances Carry out the method for *thin-layer chromatography*, Appendix III A, using a silica gel F254 precoated chromatoplate (Merck silica gel 60 F254 plates are suitable) and a mixture of 80 volumes of *acetone*, 30 volumes of *cyclohexane* and 5 volumes of 13.5M *ammonia* as the mobile phase. Apply separately to the plate 20 μl of each of two solutions in *methanol* containing (1) 2.5% w/v of the substance being examined and (2) 0.025% w/v of *fluphenazine hydrochloride BPCRS*. After removal of the plate, allow it to dry in air and examine under *ultra-violet light (254 nm)*. Spray the plate with *sulphuric acid (50%)* and examine in daylight. By both methods of visualisation, any *secondary spot* in the chromatogram obtained with solution (1) is not more intense than the spot in the chromatogram obtained with solution (2).

Loss on drying When dried at 60° at a pressure not exceeding 0.7 kPa for 3 hours, loses not more than 1.0% of its weight. Use 1 g.

Sulphated ash Not more than 0.2%, Appendix IX A.

Assay Carry out Method I for *non-aqueous titration*, Appendix VIII A, using 0.6 g and *crystal violet solution* as indicator. Each ml of 0.1M *perchloric acid VS* is equivalent to 0.02959 g of $C_{32}H_{44}F_3N_3O_2S$.

Storage Fluphenazine Decanoate should be protected from light.

Preparation
Fluphenazine Decanoate Injection

Action and use Antipsychotic.

Fluphenazine Enanthate

$C_{29}H_{38}F_3N_3O_2S$　549.7　*2746-81-8*

Fluphenazine Enanthate is 2-{4-[3-(2-trifluoro-methylphenothiazin-10-yl)propyl]piperazin-1-yl}ethyl heptanoate. It contains not less than 98.5 per cent and not more than 101.5 per cent of $C_{29}H_{38}F_3N_3O_2S$, calculated with reference to the dried substance.

Characteristics A pale yellow, viscous liquid or a yellow, crystalline, oily solid; odour, faint and ester-like.

Solubility Practically insoluble in *water*; miscible with *absolute ethanol*, with *chloroform* and with *ether*. It dissolves in fixed oils.

Identification A. The *infra-red absorption spectrum*, Appendix II A, is concordant with the *reference spectrum* of fluphenazine enanthate.

B. The *light absorption*, Appendix II B, in the range 230 to 350 nm of a 0.001% w/v solution in *absolute ethanol* exhibits a maximum at 261 nm and a less well-defined maximum at 310 nm. The *absorbance* at 261 nm is about 0.64.

C. Complies with test C for Identification described under Fluphenazine Decanoate using as solution (2) a 2.0% w/v solution of *fluphenazine enanthate BPCRS* in *ethanol (96%)*.

D. Burn 20 mg by the method for *oxygen-flask combustion*, Appendix VIII C, using 5 ml of 2M *sodium hydroxide* as the absorbing liquid. When the process is complete, dilute the liquid to 25 ml with *water*. To 0.2 ml of the resulting solution add 0.5 ml of *aminomethylalizarindiacetic acid solution*, sufficient 0.02M *hydrochloric acid* to give a full yellow colour and 0.02M *sodium hydroxide* dropwise until the solution just begins to turn pink. Add 0.2 ml of a solution containing 12% w/v of *sodium acetate* and 6% v/v of *glacial acetic acid*, dilute to 4 ml with *water* and add 0.5 ml of *cerium(III) nitrate solution*. A deep lilac-blue colour is produced.

E. Dissolve 5 mg in 2 ml of *sulphuric acid* and allow to stand for 5 minutes. A reddish-brown colour is produced.

Related substances Complies with the test described under Fluphenazine Decanoate.

Loss on drying When dried at 60° at a pressure not exceeding 0.7 kPa for 3 hours, loses not more than 1.0% of its weight. Use 1 g.

Sulphated ash Not more than 0.2%, Appendix IX A.

Assay Carry out Method I for *non-aqueous titration*, Appendix VIII A, using 0.6 g and *crystal violet solution* as indicator. Each ml of 0.1M *perchloric acid VS* is equivalent to 0.02749 g of $C_{29}H_{38}F_3N_3O_2S$.

Storage Fluphenazine Enanthate should be protected from light.

Preparation
Fluphenazine Enanthate Injection

Action and use Antipsychotic.

Fluphenazine Hydrochloride

(CH₂)₃—N   N—CH₂·CH₂OH

CF₃   ,2HCl

$C_{22}H_{26}F_3N_3OS,2HCl$ 510.4   *146-56-5*

Fluphenazine Hydrochloride is 2-{4-[3-(2-trifluoromethylphenothiazin-10-yl)propyl]-piperazin-1-yl}ethanol dihydrochloride.

It contains not less than 98.5 per cent and not more than 101.0 per cent of $C_{22}H_{26}F_3N_3OS$, 2HCl, calculated with reference to the dried substance.

Characteristics A white or almost white, crystalline powder; odourless or almost odourless.

Solubility Soluble in 10 parts of *water*; sparingly soluble in *ethanol (96%)* and in *ether*.

Identification A. Dissolve 0.1 g in 10 ml of *water*, make alkaline with 1M *sodium hydroxide*, extract with 5 ml of

chloroform, filter through *anhydrous sodium sulphate* and evaporate the solvent in a current of nitrogen. The *infrared absorption spectrum* of the oily residue, Appendix II A, is concordant with the *reference spectrum* of fluphenazine.

B. The *light absorption*, Appendix II B, in the range 230 to 350 nm of a 0.002% w/v solution in a mixture of 1 volume of 1M *hydrochloric acid* and 99 volumes of *ethanol (80%)* exhibits a maximum at 258 nm and a less well-defined maximum at 310 nm. The *absorbance* at 258 nm is about 1.2.

C. Carry out in subdued light the method for *thin-layer chromatography*, Appendix III A, using *kieselguhr G* as the coating substance. Impregnate the dry chromatoplate by placing it in a tank containing a shallow layer of a mixture of 180 volumes of *acetone*, 15 volumes of *formamide* and 5 volumes of *2-phenoxyethanol*, allowing the impregnating solvent to ascend to the top, removing the plate from the tank and using it immediately. Use a mixture of 100 volumes of *petroleum spirit (boiling range, 40° to 60°)* saturated with *2-phenoxyethanol* and 2 volumes of *diethylamine* as the mobile phase. Apply separately to the plate 2 μl of each of two solutions in *methanol* containing (1) 0.2% w/v of the substance being examined and (2) 0.2% w/v of *fluphenazine hydrochloride BPCRS*. After removal of the plate, allow it to dry in air, examine under *ultra-violet light (365 nm)* and observe the fluorescence produced after about 2 minutes. Heat the plate at 120° for 20 minutes, cool, spray with *ethanolic sulphuric acid (20%)* and observe the colour produced. The principal spot in the chromatogram obtained with solution (1) corresponds in position, fluorescence and colour to that in the chromatogram obtained with solution (2).

D. Dissolve 5 mg in 2 ml of *sulphuric acid* and allow to stand for 5 minutes. An orange colour is produced.

E. Heat 0.5 ml of *chromic—sulphuric acid mixture* in a small test-tube in a water-bath for 5 minutes; the solution wets the sides of the tube readily and there is no greasiness. Add 2 or 3 mg of the substance being examined and again heat in a water-bath for 5 minutes; the solution does not wet the sides of the tube and does not pour easily from the tube.

F. Yields *reaction A* characteristic of chlorides, Appendix VI.

Acidity pH of a 5% w/v solution, 1.9 to 2.3, Appendix V L.

Related substances Carry out in subdued light the method for *thin-layer chromatography*, Appendix III A, using *silica gel GF254* as the coating substance and a mixture of 80 volumes of *acetone*, 30 volumes of *cyclohexane* and 5 volumes of 13.5M *ammonia* as the mobile phase. Apply separately to the chromatoplate 10 μl of each of three solutions of the substance being examined in 0.1M *methanolic sodium hydroxide* containing (1) 1.0% w/v, (2) 0.010% w/v and (3) 0.0050% w/v. After removal of the plate, allow it to dry in air and examine under *ultra-violet light (254 nm)*. Any *secondary spot* in the chromatogram obtained with solution (1) is not more intense than the spot in the chromatogram obtained with solution (2) and not more than one such spot is more intense than the spot in the chromatogram obtained with solution (3). Disregard any spot on the line of application.

Loss on drying When dried to constant weight at 105°, loses not more than 1.0% of its weight. Use 1 g.

Sulphated ash Not more than 0.1%, Appendix IX A.

Assay Carry out Method I for *non-aqueous titration*, Appendix VIII A, using 0.6 g and *crystal violet solution* as indicator. Each ml of 0.1M *perchloric acid VS* is equivalent to 0.02552 g of $C_{22}H_{26}F_3N_3OS,2HCl$.

Storage Fluphenazine Hydrochloride should be kept in a well-closed container and protected from light.

Preparation
Fluphenazine Tablets

Action and use Antipsychotic.

Flurazepam Monohydrochloride

$C_{21}H_{23}ClFN_3O,HCl$ 424.3   *36105-20-1*

Flurazepam Monohydrochloride is 7-chloro-1-[2-(diethylamino)ethyl]-5-(*o*-fluorophenyl)-1,3-dihydro-2*H*-1,4-benzodiazepin-2-one monohydrochloride. It contains not less than 99.0 per cent and not more than 101.0 per cent of $C_{21}H_{23}ClFN_3O,HCl$ and not less than 8.2 per cent and not more than 8.5 per cent of ionic Cl, both calculated with reference to the dried substance.

Characteristics A white or almost white, crystalline powder; odourless or almost odourless.

Solubility Very soluble in *water*; freely soluble in *ethanol (96%)*; practically insoluble in *ether*.

Identification A. The *infra-red absorption spectrum*, Appendix II A, is concordant with the *reference spectrum* of flurazepam monohydrochloride.
B. The *light absorption*, Appendix II B, in the range 220 to 350 nm of a 0.002% w/v solution in 0.5M *methanolic sulphuric acid*, prepared using *anhydrous methanol*, exhibits two maxima, at 240 nm and 284 nm. The *absorbance* at 240 nm is about 1.3 and at 284 nm is about 0.6.
C. Yields *reaction A* characteristic of chlorides, Appendix VI.

Acidity pH of a 5% w/v solution, 5.0 to 6.0, Appendix V L.

Fluorides 0.10 g complies with *limit test B for fluorides*, Appendix VII (500 ppm).

Related substances and decomposition products Carry out the method for *thin-layer chromatography*, Appendix III A, using a silica gel F254 precoated chromatoplate (Merck silica gel 60 F254 plates are suitable) and a mixture of 195 volumes of *ether* and 5 volumes of *diethylamine* as the mobile phase. Apply separately to the plate 10 μl of each of two solutions of the substance being examined in a mixture of 98 volumes of *methanol* and 2 volumes of 13.5M *ammonia* containing (1) 5.0% w/v and (2) 0.010% w/v. After removal of the plate, allow it to dry in a current of air and examine under *ultra-violet light*

(254 nm). Any *secondary spot* in the chromatogram obtained with solution (1) is not more intense than the spot in the chromatogram obtained with solution (2).

Loss on drying When dried at 105° for 4 hours, loses not more than 0.5% of its weight. Use 1 g.

Sulphated ash Not more than 0.1%, Appendix IX A.

Assay *For flurazepam monohydrochloride* Dissolve 0.45 g in 90 ml of *anhydrous glacial acetic acid* and carry out Method I for *non-aqueous titration*, Appendix VIII A, determining the end-point potentiometrically. Each ml of 0.1M *perchloric acid VS* is equivalent to 0.02122 g of $C_{21}H_{23}ClFN_3O,HCl$.
  For chloride Dissolve 0.4 g in 80 ml of *water*, add 2 ml of *glacial acetic acid* and titrate with 0.1M *silver nitrate VS* determining the end-point potentiometrically. Each ml of 0.1M *silver nitrate VS* is equivalent to 0.003545 g of ionic Cl.

Storage Flurazepam Monohydrochloride should be kept in a well-closed container and stored at a temperature of 8° to 15°.

Preparation
Flurazepam Capsules

Action and use Anxiolytic.

Flurbiprofen

$C_{15}H_{13}FO_2$ 244.3   *5104-49-4*

Flurbiprofen is 2-(2-fluorobiphenyl-4-yl)propionic acid. It contains not less than 99.0 per cent and not more than 100.5 per cent of $C_{15}H_{13}FO_2$, calculated with reference to the dried substance.

Characteristics A white or almost white, crystalline powder.

Solubility Practically insoluble in *water*; soluble in 3 parts of *ethanol (96%)*, in 4 parts of *chloroform* and in 4.5 parts of *ether*. It dissolves in aqueous solutions of alkali hydroxides and carbonates.

Identification A. The *infra-red absorption spectrum*, Appendix II A, is concordant with the *reference spectrum* of flurbiprofen.
B. The *light absorption*, Appendix II B, in the range 230 to 350 nm of a 0.001% w/v solution in 0.1M *sodium hydroxide* exhibits a maximum only at 247 nm. The *absorbance* at the maximum at 247 nm is about 0.8.
C. Heat 0.5 ml of *chromic—sulphuric acid mixture* in a small test-tube in a water-bath for 5 minutes; the solution wets the sides of the tube readily and there is no greasiness. Add 2 or 3 mg of the substance being examined and heat in a water-bath for 5 minutes; the solution does not wet the sides of the tube and does not pour easily from the tube.

Melting point 114° to 117°, Appendix V A.

Heavy metals 12 ml of a 20% w/v solution in *methanol* complies with *limit test A for heavy metals*, Appendix VII (10 ppm). Use 10 ml of the solution obtained by diluting

10 ml of *lead standard solution (20 ppm Pb)* to 100 ml with *methanol* to prepare the standard.

Related substances Carry out the method for *high-performance liquid chromatography*, Appendix III D, using three solutions in a mixture of 45 volumes of *acetonitrile* and 55 volumes of *water* containing (1) 0.0010% w/v of *2-(biphenyl-4-yl)propionic acid BPCRS*, (2) 0.20% w/v of the substance being examined and (3) 0.20% w/v of the substance being examined and 0.0010% w/v of *2-(biphenyl-4-yl)propionic acid BPCRS*.

The chromatographic procedure may be carried out using (a) a stainless steel column (15 cm × 3.9 mm) packed with *stationary phase C* (5 μm) (Resolve 5μ is suitable), (b) a mixture of 60 volumes of *water*, 35 volumes of *acetonitrile* and 5 volumes of *glacial acetic acid* as the mobile phase with a flow rate of 1 ml per minute and (c) a detection wavelength of 254 nm. Adjust the sensitivity of the instrument so that with solution (1) the height of the peak due to 2-(biphenyl-4-yl)propionic acid is about 40% of full-scale deflection on the chart paper.

In the chromatogram obtained with solution (2) the area of any *secondary peak* is not greater than the area of the peak in the chromatogram obtained with solution (1) and the sum of the areas of the *secondary peaks* is not greater than twice the area of the peak in the chromatogram obtained with solution (1).

The test is not valid unless a peak due to 2-(biphenyl-4-yl)propionic acid appears immediately before the principal peak in the chromatogram obtained with solution (3) and the height of the trough separating the two peaks is less than 4% of full-scale deflection on the chart paper.

Loss on drying When dried to constant weight at 60° at a pressure not exceeding 0.7 kPa, loses not more than 0.5% of its weight. Use 1 g.

Sulphated ash Not more than 0.1%, Appendix IX A.

Assay Dissolve 0.5 g in 100 ml of *ethanol (96%)* previously neutralised to *phenolphthalein solution* and titrate with 0.1M *sodium hydroxide VS* using *phenolphthalein solution* as indicator. Each ml of 0.1M *sodium hydroxide VS* is equivalent to 0.02443 g of $C_{15}H_{13}FO_2$.

Preparation
Flurbiprofen Tablets

Action and use Anti-inflammatory; analgesic.

Folic Acid ☆

$C_{19}H_{19}N_7O_6$ 441.4   *59-30-3*

Folic Acid is 4-(2-amino-4-hydroxypteridin-6-yl)methylaminobenzoyl-L-glutamic acid. It contains not less than 96.0 per cent and not more than 102.0 per cent of $C_{19}H_{19}N_7O_6$, calculated with reference to the dried substance.

Characteristics A yellow to orange, crystalline powder; odourless or almost odourless.

Solubility Practically insoluble in *water* and in most organic solvents. It dissolves in dilute acids and in alkaline solutions.

Identification A. The *light absorption*, Appendix II B, in the range 230 to 380 nm of a 0.001% w/v solution in 0.1M *sodium hydroxide* exhibits three maxima, at 256, 283 and 365 nm. The A(1%, 1 cm) at 256 nm is about 590, at 283 nm, about 575 and at 365 nm, about 206. The ratio of the *absorbance* at 256 nm to that at 365 nm is 2.8 to 3.0.

B. Carry out the method for *thin-layer chromatography*, Appendix III A, using *silica gel G* as the coating substance and a mixture of 60 volumes of *ethanol (96%)*, 20 volumes of 13.5M *ammonia* and 20 volumes of *propan-1-ol* as the mobile phase. Apply separately to the chromatoplate 2 μl of each of two solutions in a mixture of 9 volumes of *methanol* and 2 volumes of 13.5M *ammonia* containing (1) 0.05% w/v of the substance being examined and (2) 0.05% w/v of *folic acid EPCRS*. After removal of the plate, allow it to dry in air and examine under *ultra-violet light (365 nm)*. The principal spot in the chromatogram obtained with solution (1) is similar in position, fluorescence and size to that in the chromatogram obtained with solution (2).

C. *Specific optical rotation*, in a 1.0% w/v solution in 0.1M *sodium hydroxide*, about +20°, Appendix V F.

Free amines The *absorbance* of the unreduced solution as determined in the Assay is not more than one-sixth of the *absorbance* of the reduced solution.

Loss on drying When dried at 100° to 105° at a pressure not exceeding 0.7 kPa for 3 hours, loses 5.0 to 8.5% of its weight. Use 1 g.

Sulphated ash Not more than 0.2%, Appendix IX A, Method II. Use 1 g.

Assay Dissolve 50 mg in 50 ml of 0.1M *sodium hydroxide* and add sufficient 0.1M *sodium hydroxide* to produce 100 ml (solution A). Add 20 ml of 2M *hydrochloric acid* to 3 ml of solution A and dilute to 100 ml with *water*. To 50 ml of the resulting solution add 0.5 g of *zinc powder*, allow to stand protected from light for 20 minutes, shaking frequently, and filter. Discard the first 10 ml of the filtrate and then dilute 10 ml to 25 ml with *water*, add 5 ml of 2M *hydrochloric acid* and 5 ml of a 0.1% w/v solution of *sodium nitrite*, mix and allow to stand for 2 minutes. Add 5 ml of a 0.5% w/v solution of *ammonium sulphamate*, mix and allow to stand for 2 minutes. Add 5 ml of a 0.1% w/v solution of *N-(1-naphthyl)ethylene-diamine dihydrochloride*, mix and allow to stand for 10 minutes. Add sufficient *water* to produce 50 ml and measure the *absorbance* of the resulting solution at the maximum at 550 nm, Appendix II B, using in the reference cell a solution prepared in the same manner but using 25 ml of *water* and beginning at the words 'add 5 ml of 2M *hydrochloric acid* . . .'. To a further 30 ml of solution A add 20 ml of 2M *hydrochloric acid* and sufficient *water* to produce 100 ml. Mix 10 ml of this solution with 15 ml of *water* and carry out the above procedure, beginning at the words 'add 5 ml of 2M *hydrochloric acid* . . .'. Subtract one-tenth of the *absorbance* of the unreduced solution from that of the reduced solution and from the result calculate the amount of $C_{19}H_{19}N_7O_6$ using the result obtained by repeating the operation using *folic acid EPCRS* in place of the substance being examined and the declared content of $C_{19}H_{19}N_7O_6$ in *folic acid EPCRS*.

Storage Folic Acid should be kept in a well-closed container and protected from light.

Preparation
Folic Acid Tablets

Action and use Used in treatment and prevention of megaloblastic anaemias.

Formaldehyde Solution

Formalin

Note The name Formalin as a synonym for Formaldehyde Solution may be used freely in many countries, including Great Britain and Northern Ireland, but in other countries exclusive proprietary rights in this name are claimed.

CH₂O   30.03   *50-00-0*

Formaldehyde Solution is an aqueous solution of formaldehyde containing methanol as a stabilising agent. It contains not less than 34.0 per cent w/w and not more than 38.0 per cent w/w of CH_2O.

Characteristics A colourless liquid; odour, characteristic, pungent and irritating. A slight white deposit may form during storage.

Solubility Miscible with *water* and with *ethanol (96%)*.

Identification A. Dilute 1 ml with sufficient *water* to produce 1000 ml. To 10 ml of this solution add 2 ml of a freshly prepared 1% w/v solution of *phenylhydrazine hydrochloride*, 1 ml of *potassium hexacyanoferrate(III) solution* and 5 ml of *hydrochloric acid*. A brilliant red colour is produced.
B. Evaporate on a water-bath. A white, amorphous residue is produced.

Acidity Dilute 10 ml with 10 ml of *carbon dioxide-free water* and titrate with 0.1M *sodium hydroxide VS* using *bromothymol blue solution* as indicator. Not more than 5 ml of 0.1M *sodium hydroxide VS* is required.

Methanol Add 3 g to a mixture of 10 ml of 5M *sodium hydroxide*, 25 ml of *hydrogen peroxide solution (20 vol)* and 200 ml of *water* and distil 150 ml, collecting the distillate in 50 ml of *chromic acid solution* through a delivery tube which dips below the surface. Heat the distillate at 60° for 1 hour, cool and dilute to 1000 ml with *water*. To 25 ml add 2 g of *potassium iodide* and titrate with 0.1M *sodium thiosulphate VS* using *starch mucilage* as indicator. Dilute a further 50 ml of *chromic acid solution* to 1000 ml with *water*. To 25 ml add 2 g of *potassium iodide* and titrate with 0.1M *sodium thiosulphate VS* using *starch mucilage* as indicator. The difference between the titrations is not less than 12.7 ml.

Assay Add 3 g to a mixture of 25 ml of *hydrogen peroxide solution (20 vol)* and 50 ml of 1M *sodium hydroxide VS*, warm on a water-bath until effervescence ceases and titrate the excess of alkali with 1M *hydrochloric acid VS* using *phenolphthalein solution* as indicator. Repeat the operation without the solution being examined. The difference between the titrations represents the amount of sodium hydroxide required to neutralise the formic acid produced by the oxidation of the formaldehyde. Each ml

of 1M *sodium hydroxide VS* is equivalent to 0.03003 g of CH₂O.

Storage Formaldehyde Solution should be kept in a well-closed container and stored at a temperature not exceeding 25°.

Action and use Used in treatment of warts.

Fosfestrol Sodium

$C_{18}H_{18}Na_4O_8P_2, xH_2O$ 516.2 *(anhydrous)*   23519-26-8

Fosfestrol Sodium is a hydrate of tetrasodium (*E*)-4,4'-(1,2-diethylvinylene)bis(phenyl orthophosphate). It contains not less than 98.0 per cent and not more than 101.0 per cent of $C_{18}H_{18}Na_4O_8P_2$, calculated with reference to the anhydrous substance.

Characteristics A white or almost white powder.

Solubility Freely soluble in *water*; practically insoluble in *ether* and in *absolute ethanol*.

Identification A. The *infra-red absorption spectrum*, Appendix II A, is concordant with the *reference spectrum* of fosfestrol sodium.
B. The *light absorption*, Appendix II B, in the range 230 to 350 nm of a 0.0050% w/v solution in 0.1M *sodium hydroxide* exhibits a maximum only at 242 nm.
C. Gently heat 40 mg with 2 ml of *sulphuric acid* until white fumes are evolved, add *nitric acid* dropwise until oxidation is complete and allow to cool. Add 2 ml of *water*, heat until white fumes are again evolved, allow to cool and add 10 ml of *water*. The resulting solution yields the *reactions* characteristic of phosphates, Appendix VI.
D. Yields the *reactions* characteristic of sodium salts, Appendix VI.

Acidity or alkalinity pH of a 5% w/v solution, 7.0 to 9.0, Appendix V L.
    To 20 ml of a 2.5% w/v solution, add 3.0 ml of 0.01M *sodium hydroxide VS*. The pH of the resulting solution is not less than 8.8.

Light absorption Measure the *absorbance* of the solution obtained in test B for Identification at the maximum at 242 nm, Appendix II B. The A(1%, 1 cm) at 242 nm is 280 to 320.

Chloride Dissolve 1.0 g in 10 ml of *water*, add 10 ml of 2M *nitric acid*, filter, wash the precipitate with 25 ml of *water* and dilute the combined filtrate and washings to 100 ml with *water*. 15 ml of the resulting solution complies with the *limit test for chlorides*, Appendix VII (350 ppm).

Inorganic phosphate Dissolve 0.5 g in 20 ml of *water*, add 5 ml of 2M *hydrochloric acid* and extract with four 30-ml quantities of *ether*. Discard the ether extracts and heat the aqueous solution on a water-bath until any remaining ether has evaporated. Allow to cool, add sufficient *water* to produce 100 ml (solution A) and then add 4 ml of *sulphomolybdic acid solution*, shake, add 0.1 ml of a mixture of 1 volume of freshly prepared *tin(II) chloride solution* and 9 volumes of 2M *hydrochloric acid*, shake again and examine 20 ml. Any colour produced is not more intense than that of 20 ml of a solution obtained by repeating the operation using a mixture of 5 ml of a 0.01% w/v solution of *potassium dihydrogen orthophosphate* and 95 ml of *water* in place of solution A.

Free stilboestrol Dissolve 1 g in 25 ml of *water* and extract with successive quantities of 15 ml and 5 ml of *chloroform*. Filter the combined chloroform extracts through *anhydrous sodium sulphate*, wash the filter with 5 ml of *chloroform* and evaporate the combined filtrates to dryness on a water-bath. Dissolve the residue in 10 ml of *absolute ethanol* and add 10 ml of a solution prepared by dissolving 1 g of *dipotassium hydrogen orthophosphate* in 55 ml of *water*. Transfer a portion of the mixture to a 1-cm closed silica cell, place the cell 10 cm from a 15-watt, short wave ultra-violet lamp, and irradiate for 30 minutes. The *absorbance* of the irradiated solution measured at the maximum at 418 nm, Appendix II B, is not greater than that obtained by repeating the operation using 10 ml of a 0.0015% w/v solution of *diethylstilboestrol EPCRS* in *absolute ethanol*, beginning at the words 'add 10 ml of a solution . . .'.

Water 13.0 to 16.5% w/w, Appendix IX C. Use 0.2 g.

Assay Heat 0.2 g in a long-necked flask with 2 ml of *sulphuric acid* and 2.5 ml of *nitric acid* until brown fumes cease to be evolved, allow to cool, add 1 ml of *nitric acid* and heat again. Continue adding *nitric acid* and heating until brown fumes are no longer evolved and the solution is colourless when cold. Heat until dense, white fumes are evolved, cool, transfer the solution to a flask with the aid of 150 ml of *water*, add 50 ml of *citric—molybdic acid solution* and heat slowly to boiling point. Swirling the flask continuously, add 25 ml of *quinoline solution*, at first dropwise and then in a steady stream, heat on a water-bath for 5 minutes and cool. Filter, wash the precipitate with *water* until free from acid, transfer the precipitate to a flask with the aid of 100 ml of *water*, add 50 ml of 0.5M *sodium hydroxide VS* and shake until dissolved. Titrate the excess of alkali with 0.5M *hydrochloric acid VS* using *phenolphthalein—thymol blue solution* as indicator. Each ml of 0.5M *sodium hydroxide VS* is equivalent to 0.004964 g of $C_{18}H_{18}Na_4O_8P_2$.

Storage Fosfestrol Sodium should be kept in a well-closed container and protected from light.

Action and use Oestrogen.

Framycetin Sulphate ☆

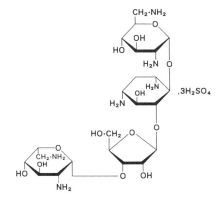

$C_{23}H_{46}N_6O_{13},3H_2SO_4$　　908.9　　*4146-30-9*

Framycetin Sulphate is the sulphate of 2-deoxy-4-*O*-(2,6-diamino-2,6-dideoxy-α-D-glucopyranosyl)-5-*O*-[3-*O*-(2,6-diamino-2,6-dideoxy-β-L-idopyranosyl)-β-D-ribofuranosyl]-streptamine (neomycin B), a substance produced by the growth of selected strains of *Streptomyces fradiae* or *Streptomyces decaris* or by any other means. The potency is not less than 630 Units of neomycin B per mg, calculated with reference to the dried substance.

Characteristics A white or yellowish-white powder; odourless or almost odourless; hygroscopic.

Solubility Soluble in 1 part of *water*; very slightly soluble in *ethanol* (96%); practically insoluble in *acetone*, in *chloroform* and in *ether*.

Identification A. Carry out the method for *thin-layer chromatography*, Appendix III A, using a chromatoplate prepared immediately before use as described in the test for Neamine and a 10% w/v solution of *potassium dihydrogen orthophosphate* as the mobile phase. Apply separately to the plate 10 µl of each of three solutions in *water* containing (1) 0.1% w/v of the substance being examined, (2) 0.1% w/v of *framycetin sulphate EPCRS* and (3) 0.1% w/v each of *framycetin sulphate EPCRS*, *kanamycin monosulphate EPCRS* and *streptomycin sulphate EPCRS*. Allow the solvent front to ascend 15 cm above the line of application but if a precoated plate is used allow the solvent front to reach the top of the plate. After removal of the plate, dry it in a current of warm air, spray with a mixture of equal volumes of a 46% w/v solution of *sulphuric acid* and of a 0.2% w/v solution of *naphthalene-1,3-diol* in *ethanol* (96%) and heat at 150° for 5 to 10 minutes. The principal spot in the chromatogram obtained with solution (1) is similar in position, colour and size to that in the chromatogram obtained with solution (2). The test is not valid unless the chromatogram obtained with solution (3) shows three clearly separated principal spots.
B. Dissolve 10 mg in 5 ml of *water*, add 0.1 ml of *pyridine* and 2 ml of a 0.1% w/v solution of *ninhydrin* and heat in a water-bath at 65° to 70° for 10 minutes. An intense violet colour is produced.
C. Yields *reaction A* characteristic of sulphates, Appendix VI.

Acidity or alkalinity pH of a 1% w/v solution, 6.0 to 7.0, Appendix V L.

Specific optical rotation In a 10% w/v solution, +52.5° to +55.5°, Appendix V F.

Sulphate 27.0 to 31.0% of SO_4, calculated with reference to the dried substance, when determined by the following method. Dissolve 0.25 g in 100 ml of *water*, adjust the pH to 11 with 13.5M *ammonia* and add 10 ml of 0.1M *barium chloride VS*. Titrate with 0.1M *disodium edetate VS* using 0.5 mg of *metalphthalein* as indicator; add 50 ml of *ethanol (96%)* when the colour of the solution begins to change and continue the titration until the violet blue colour disappears. Each ml of 0.1M *barium chloride VS* is equivalent to 0.009606 g of sulphate, SO_4.

Neamine Carry out the method for *thin-layer chromatography*, Appendix III A, using a 10% w/v solution of *potassium dihydrogen orthophosphate* as the mobile phase and a chromatoplate prepared in the following manner. Mix 0.3 g of *carbomer* (Carbopol 934 is suitable) with 240 ml of *water*, allow to stand for 1 hour with moderate shaking, adjust to pH 7 by the gradual addition, with constant shaking, of 2M *sodium hydroxide* and add 30 g of *silica gel H*. Spread a uniform layer of the suspension 0.75 mm thick, heat at 110° for 1 hour, allow to cool and use the plate immediately. Apply separately to the plate 10 µl of each of two solutions in *water* containing (1) 0.50% w/v of the substance being examined and (2) 0.005% w/v of *neamine EPCRS*. Allow the solvent front to ascend 15 cm above the line of application but if a precoated plate is used allow the solvent front to reach the top of the plate. After removal of the plate, dry it in a current of warm air, spray with *ninhydrin and stannous chloride reagent* and heat at 110° for 15 minutes. Any spot corresponding to neamine in the chromatogram obtained with solution (1) is not more intense than the spot in the chromatogram obtained with solution (2).

Neomycin C Use a chromatographic column (40 cm × 6 mm), maintained at a constant uniform temperature (±1°) between 10° and 20° and provided with a suitable means of passing the mobile phase down the column at a constant rate. Introduce into the column to within 1 cm of the top successive portions of a suspension of an anion-exchange resin (Bio-Rad AG1-X2 is suitable) in *water* and wash the column with *water* for 90 minutes. Apply to the surface of the resin 0.1 ml of a 1% w/v solution of the substance being examined in *water* and use *water* adjusted to pH 7.5 with 0.01M *sodium hydroxide* as the mobile phase with a flow rate of 1 ml per minute. Collect the eluate in 1-ml fractions. Add 2 ml of *ninhydrin reagent* to each fraction, heat in a water-bath for 15 minutes, allow to cool and measure the *absorbance* at 570 nm, Appendix II B, using in the reference cell 1 ml of *water* treated in the same manner. If the absorbance is more than 0.6, dilute the contents of the tube by the addition of 6 ml of a mixture of equal volumes of *ethanol (96%)* and *water* and repeat the measurement. Plot a graph from the results obtained, correcting the absorbances for dilution if necessary, and determine the areas of the peaks corresponding to neomycin B and neomycin C.

Neamine is eluted first from the column, showing as a single peak or as a partly-resolved double peak, followed by neomycin C and then neomycin B. The area of the peak corresponding to neomycin C is less than 3.0% of the sum of the areas of the peaks corresponding to neomycin B and neomycin C. The test is not valid unless the *resolution factor* between the peaks corresponding to neomycin B and neomycin C is greater than 1.4.

Alcohols Not more than 2% w/w calculated as methanol, CH_4O, when determined by the following method. Dissolve 0.2 g in 5 ml of *water* and add 0.05 ml of 0.05M *sulphuric acid*. Distil the solution and collect about 2.5 ml of distillate. Transfer the distillate to a flask with two 1-ml quantities of *water* and add 25 ml of 0.0167M *potassium dichromate VS* in a mixture of 3 volumes of *water* and 2 volumes of *sulphuric acid*. Heat on a water-bath for 30 minutes, cool and add sufficient *water* to produce 500 ml. Add 10 ml of *potassium iodide solution*, allow to stand for 5 minutes and titrate with 0.1M *sodium thiosulphate VS*, using *starch mucilage* as indicator, until the solution becomes pale green. Repeat the operation without the substance being examined. The difference between the titrations represents the amount of potassium dichromate equivalent to the alcohols present. Each ml of 0.0167M *potassium dichromate VS* is equivalent to 0.000534 g of CH_4O.

Loss on drying When dried over *phosphorus pentoxide* at 60° at a pressure not exceeding 0.7 kPa for 3 hours, loses not more than 8.0% of its weight. Use 1 g.

Sulphated ash Not more than 1.0%, Appendix IX A, Method II. Use 1 g.

Assay Carry out the *biological assay of antibiotics*, Appendix XIV A, using the Standard Preparation of neomycin B. The precision of the assay is such that the fiducial limits of error are not less than 95% and not more than 105% of the estimated potency.

Storage Framycetin Sulphate should be kept in a well-closed container, protected from light and stored at a temperature not exceeding 30°. If it is intended for introduction into body cavities, the container should be sterile, tamper-evident and sealed so as to exclude micro-organisms.

Labelling The label states (1) the number of Units per mg; (2) the conditions under which the material should be stored; (3) whether or not it is intended for introduction into body cavities.

Preparation
Framycetin Gauze Dressing

Action and use Antibacterial.

Framycetin Sulphate intended for introduction into body cavities complies with the following additional requirements.

Abnormal toxicity Complies with the *test for abnormal toxicity*, Appendix XIV L. Use a quantity containing 100 Units dissolved in 0.5 ml of *water for injections* or *saline solution*.

Depressor substances Complies with the *test for depressor substances*, Appendix XIV M. Use per kg of the cat's weight 1 ml of *saline solution* containing 5 mg per ml of the substance being examined.

Pyrogens Complies with the *test for pyrogens*, Appendix XIV K. Use per kg of the rabbit's weight 16 mg of the substance being examined dissolved in 5 ml of *water for injections*.

Sterility Complies with the *test for sterility*, Appendix XVI A.

Frangula Bark ☆

Frangula Bark is the dried bark of the stems and branches of *Rhamnus frangula* L. (*Frangula alnus* Miller). It contains not less than 6.0 per cent of glucofrangulins, calculated as glucofrangulin A.

Characteristics Odour, faint.

Macroscopical Curved or nearly flat fragments or single or double quilled pieces, 0.5 to 2 mm thick, of variable length and width. Outer surface greyish-brown, wrinkled longitudinally and covered with numerous greyish, transversely elongated lenticels. Inner surface, smooth, with fine, longitudinal striations, orange-brown to brownish-red, turning red when treated with alkali. Fracture, short in the outer part, fibrous in the inner part.

Microscopical Cork, brownish-red, composed of several layers of flattened cells, perforated by lenticels; cortex consisting of a few layers of collenchymatous cells and several layers of rounded or oval, pitted parenchyma; the young bark may show large, intercellular spaces filled with mucilage; calcium oxalate cluster crystals, about 15 mm in diameter and occasional starch granules, about 5 mm in diameter. Phloem with phloem fibres, 12 to 25 mm in diameter, in numerous groups forming tangential bands, with crystal sheaths of calcium oxalate prisms; parenchyma, containing calcium oxalate cluster crystals and occasional starch granules, medullary rays, one to three cells wide; when treated with a 0.5% w/v solution of *potassium hydroxide* the cells of the parenchyma and medullary rays turn bright red.

Identification A. Carry out the method for *thin-layer chromatography*, Appendix III A, using *silica gel G* as the coating substance and a mixture of 100 volumes of *ethyl acetate*, 17 volumes of *methanol* and 13 volumes of *water* as the mobile phase, but allowing the solvent front to ascend 10 cm above the line of application. Apply separately to the chromatoplate, as bands 20 mm long and not more than 3 mm wide, 10 µl of each of the following solutions. For solution (1) heat to boiling 0.5 g, in *No. 180 powder*, with 5 ml of *ethanol (70%)*, cool and centrifuge; decant the supernatant liquid immediately and use within 30 minutes. For solution (2) dissolve 20 mg of *barbaloin* in 10 ml of *ethanol (70%)*. After removal of the plate, allow the solvent to evaporate for 5 minutes at room temperature, then spray immediately with a freshly prepared 0.1% w/v solution of N,N-*dimethyl-p-nitroso-aniline* in *pyridine*, using about 10 ml for a plate 200 mm × 200 mm in size, and examine immediately; no greyish-blue bands appear (anthrones). Spray with a 5% w/v solution of *potassium hydroxide* in *ethanol (50%)*, heat at 100° to 105° for 15 minutes and examine immediately. The chromatogram obtained with solution (2) shows a reddish-brown band due to barbaloin (Rf value 0.4 to 0.5). The chromatogram obtained with solution (1) shows several bands, the most marked having Rf values of about 0.25 to 0.35 (glucofrangulins). A red band with an Rf value of about 0.10 to 0.15 should not be present. When examined under *ultra-violet light (365 nm)*, the chromatogram obtained with solution (1) shows no bands with an intense yellow or blue fluorescence (absence of other species of *Rhamnus*).

B. Heat 50 mg, in powder, with 25 ml of 2M *hydrochloric acid* on a water-bath for 15 minutes. Cool, transfer to a separating funnel, extract with 20 ml of *ether* and shake the ether layer with 10 ml of 5M *ammonia*. A reddish-purple colour is produced in the ammoniacal layer.

Foreign matter Not more than 1%, Appendix XI D, Test B.

Sulphated ash Not more than 8.0%, Appendix IX A, Method II. Use 1 g, in powder.

Assay Add 25 ml of *methanol (70%)* to 0.25 g, in *No. 180 powder*, in a round-bottomed flask fitted with a ground-glass neck, mix and weigh. Heat under a reflux condenser in a water-bath for 15 minutes. Cool, restore the original weight with *methanol (70%)* and filter. To 5 ml of the filtrate, in a separating funnel, add 50 ml of *water* and 0.1 ml of *hydrochloric acid* and shake with three 20-ml quantities of *ether*. Wash the combined ether layers with two 15-ml quantities of *water* and rinse the separating funnel with the washings. To the combined aqueous solution and washings add 5 ml of a 5% w/v solution of *sodium carbonate* and dilute to 100 ml with *water*. Transfer 40 ml to a round-bottomed flask fitted with a ground-glass neck, add 20 ml of a 20% w/v solution of *iron(III) chloride hexahydrate*, immerse in a water-bath so that the water level is above that of the liquid in the flask and heat under a reflux condenser for 20 minutes. Add 2 ml of *hydrochloric acid* and heat for a further 20 minutes, shaking frequently until the precipitate is dissolved. Allow to cool, transfer to a separating funnel, extract with three 25-ml quantities of *ether*, previously used to wash the flask, and wash the combined ether extracts with two 15-ml quantities of *water*. Dilute the ether extracts to 100 ml with *ether*. Evaporate 20 ml to dryness and dissolve the residue in 10 ml of a 0.5% w/v solution of *magnesium acetate* in *methanol*. Measure the *absorbance* of the solution at 515 nm, Appendix II B, using *methanol* in the reference cell. Calculate the content of glucofrangulins, expressed as glucofrangulin A, taking 192 as the value of A(1%, 1 cm) at 515 nm.

Storage Frangula Bark should be protected from light and moisture.

Action and use Stimulant laxative.

Powdered Frangula Bark

Powdered Frangula Bark is Frangula Bark in powder. It contains not less than 6.0 per cent of glucofrangulins, calculated as glucofrangulin A.

Characteristics Yellowish-brown. Diagnostic structures: numerous bundles of thick-walled fibres with crystal sheaths; reddish-brown fragments of cork; fragments of parenchyma containing calcium oxalate cluster crystals and occasional small starch granules; when treated with alkalis, the powder turns red; sclereids absent.

Identification Complies with the tests described under Frangula Bark.

Sulphated ash Not more than 8.0%, Appendix IX A, Method II. Use 1 g.

Assay Carry out the Assay described under Frangula Bark. Calculate the content of glucofrangulins, expressed as glucofrangulin A, taking 192 as the value of A(1%, 1 cm) at 515 nm.

Storage Powdered Frangula Bark should be protected from light and moisture.

Action and use Stimulant laxative.

Fructose ☆

C₆H₁₂O₆   180.2   57-48-7

Fructose is D-(-)-fructopyranose.

Characteristics A white, crystalline powder; odourless; taste, very sweet.

Solubility Soluble in 0.3 part of *water* and in 15 parts of *ethanol (96%)*.

Identification A. Carry out the method for *thin-layer chromatography*, Appendix III A, using *silica gel G* as the coating substance and a mixture of 50 volumes of *1,2-dichloroethane*, 25 volumes of *anhydrous glacial acetic acid*, 15 volumes of *methanol* and 10 volumes of *water*, accurately measured, as the mobile phase. Apply separately to the chromatoplate 2 μl of each of three solutions in *methanol (60%)* containing (1) 0.05% w/v of the substance being examined, (2) 0.05% w/v of *fructose EPCRS* and (3) 0.05% each of *fructose EPCRS*, *glucose EPCRS*, *lactose EPCRS* and *sucrose EPCRS*. Thoroughly dry the points of application before developing the chromatogram. After removal of the plate, dry it in a current of warm air and repeat the development using fresh mobile phase. After removal of the plate, dry it in a current of warm air and spray evenly with a 0.5% w/v solution of *thymol* in *ethanolic sulphuric acid (5%)* and heat at 130° for 10 minutes. The principal spot in the chromatogram obtained with solution (1) is similar in position, colour and size to that spot in the chromatogram obtained with solution (2). The test is not valid unless the chromatogram obtained with solution (3) shows four clearly separated principal spots.

B. To 10 ml of a 1% w/v solution add 3 ml of *potassium cupri-tartrate solution* and heat. A red precipitate is produced.

C. To 10 ml of a 1% w/v solution add 5 ml of *hydrochloric acid* and heat at 70°. A brown colour is produced.

D. Dissolve 5 g in sufficient *water* to produce 10 ml. To 0.5 ml of the solution add 0.2 g of *resorcinol* and 9 ml of *2M hydrochloric acid* and heat on a water-bath for 2 minutes. A red colour is produced.

Acidity or alkalinity Dissolve 6.0 g in 25 ml of *carbon dioxide-free water* and add 0.3 ml of *dilute phenolphthalein solution*. The solution is colourless and not more than 0.15 ml of *0.1M sodium hydroxide VS* is required to change the colour of the solution to pink.

Clarity and colour of solution Dissolve 5.0 g in sufficient *water* to produce 10 ml. The solution is *clear*, Appendix IV A, and, after diluting with an equal volume of *water*, is *colourless*, Appendix IV B, Method II.

Specific optical rotation Dissolve 10 g in 80 ml of *water*, add 0.2 ml of *6M ammonia*, allow to stand for 30 minutes and dilute to 100 ml with *water*. The *specific optical rotation* in the resulting solution is −91.0° to −93.5°, Appendix V F.

Barium To 10 ml of a 10.0% w/v solution in *distilled water* add 1 ml of *1M sulphuric acid*. Examine the solution immediately and after 1 hour. Any opalescence produced is not more intense than that in a mixture of 10 ml of the 10% w/v solution and 1 ml of *distilled water*.

Lead Complies with *limit test A for lead in sugars*, Appendix VII (0.5 ppm).

Foreign sugars Dissolve 5.0 g in sufficient *water* to produce 10 ml. To 1 ml of the solution add 9 ml of *ethanol (96%)*. Any opalescence produced is not more intense than that in a mixture of 1 ml of the initial solution and 9 ml of *water*.

5-Hydroxymethylfurfural and related compounds To 5 ml of a 10.0% w/v solution add 5 ml of *water*. The *absorbance* of the resulting solution at the maximum at 284 nm is not more than 0.32, Appendix II B.

Sulphated ash Not more than 0.1% when determined by the following method. Dissolve 5 g in 10 ml of *water*, add 2 ml of *sulphuric acid*, evaporate to dryness on a water-bath and ignite to constant weight.

Water Not more than 0.5%, Appendix IX C. Use 1 g.

Storage Fructose should be kept in a well-closed container.

Preparation

Fructose Intravenous Infusion

The title of the monograph in the European Pharmacopœia is Laevulose.

Frusemide ☆

C₁₂H₁₁ClN₂O₅S   330.7   54-31-9

Frusemide is 4-chloro-N-furfuryl-5-sulphamoyl-anthranilic acid. It contains not less than 98.5 per cent and not more than 101.0 per cent of C₁₂H₁₁ClN₂O₅S, calculated with reference to the dried substance.

Characteristics A white or almost white, crystalline powder. It melts at about 210°, with decomposition.

Solubility Practically insoluble in *water* and in *chloroform*; soluble in 75 parts of *ethanol (96%)*; soluble in *acetone*; slightly soluble in *ether*. It dissolves in dilute aqueous solutions of the alkali hydroxides.

Identification *Test A may be omitted if tests B and C are carried out. Tests B and C may be omitted if test A is carried out.*

A. The *infra-red absorption spectrum*, Appendix II A, is concordant with the spectrum of *furosemide EPCRS*.

B. The *light absorption*, Appendix II B, in the range 220 to 350 nm of a 0.0005% w/v solution in *0.1M sodium hydroxide* exhibits three maxima, at 228, 270 and 333 nm. The ratio of the *absorbance* at the maximum at 270 nm to that at the maximum at 228 nm is 0.52 to 0.57.

C. Dissolve 25 mg in 10 ml of *ethanol (96%)* and to 5 ml of the solution add 10 ml of *water*. To 0.2 ml of the resulting solution add 10 ml of *2M hydrochloric acid*, heat under a reflux condenser for 15 minutes, cool and add 18 ml of *1M sodium hydroxide* and 1 ml of a 0.5% w/v solution of *sodium nitrite*. Allow to stand for 3 minutes, add 2 ml of a 2.5% w/v solution of *sulphamic acid*, mix and add 1 ml of a 0.5% w/v solution of N-*(1-naphthyl)-ethylene-1,2-diamine dihydrochloride*. A violet-red colour is produced.

Heavy metals 1.0 g complies with *limit test C for heavy metals*, Appendix VII (20 ppm). Use 2 ml of *lead standard solution (10 ppm Pb)* to prepare the standard.

Chloride Shake 0.5 g with a mixture of 30 ml of *water* and 0.2 ml of *nitric acid* for 5 minutes, allow to stand for 15 minutes and filter. 15 ml of the filtrate complies with the *limit test for chlorides*, Appendix VII (200 ppm).

Sulphate Shake 1.0 g with a mixture of 30 ml of *water* and 0.2 ml of 5M *acetic acid* for 5 minutes, allow to stand for 15 minutes and filter. 15 ml of the filtrate complies with the *limit test for sulphates*, Appendix VII (300 ppm).

Free primary aromatic amines Dissolve 0.1 g in 25 ml of *methanol*. To 1 ml of the solution add 3 ml of *dimethyl-formamide*, 12 ml of *water* and 1 ml of 1M *hydrochloric acid*. Cool, add 1 ml of a 0.5% w/v solution of *sodium nitrite*, shake and allow to stand for 5 minutes. Add 1 ml of a 2.5% w/v solution of *sulphamic acid*, shake, allow to stand for 3 minutes, add 1 ml of a 0.5% w/v solution of N-*(1-naphthyl)ethylenediamine dihydrochloride* and dilute to 25 ml with *water*. Measure the *absorbance* of the resulting solution at the maximum at 530 nm, Appendix II B, using in the reference cell a solution prepared by treating 1 ml of *methanol* and 3 ml of *dimethylformamide* in the same manner. The absorbance is not more than 0.12.

Loss on drying When dried to constant weight at 100° to 105°, loses not more than 0.5% of its weight. Use 1 g.

Sulphated ash Not more than 0.1%, Appendix IX A, Method II. Use 1 g.

Assay Dissolve 0.25 g in 20 ml of *dimethylformamide*, add 0.2 ml of a 1% w/v solution of *bromothymol blue* in *dimethylformamide* and titrate with 0.1M *sodium hydroxide VS* until a blue colour is obtained. Repeat the operation without the substance being examined. The difference between the titrations represents the amount of sodium hydroxide required. Each ml of 0.1M *sodium hydroxide VS* is equivalent to 0.03307 g of $C_{12}H_{11}ClN_2O_5S$.

Storage Frusemide should be protected from light.

Preparations
Frusemide Injection
Frusemide Tablets

Action and use Diuretic.

The title of the monograph in the European Pharmacopœia is Furosemide.

Characteristics A yellow, crystalline powder; odourless or almost odourless.

Solubility Very slightly soluble in *water* and in *ethanol (96%)*; slightly soluble in *chloroform*; practically insoluble in *ether*.

Identification A. The *infra-red absorption spectrum*, Appendix II A, is concordant with the *reference spectrum* of furazolidone.
B. Dissolve 1 mg in 1 ml of *dimethylformamide* and add 0.05 ml of 1M *ethanolic potassium hydroxide*. A deep blue colour is produced.

Acidity or alkalinity Shake 1 g for 15 minutes with 100 ml of *carbon dioxide-free water* and filter. The pH of the filtrate is 4.5 to 7.0, Appendix V L.

Nitrofurfural diacetate Carry out in subdued light the method for *thin-layer chromatography*, Appendix III A, using *silica gel G* as the coating substance and a mixture of 95 volumes of *toluene* and 5 volumes of *1,4-dioxan* as the mobile phase. Apply separately to the chromatoplate 20 μl of solution (1) and 10 μl of solution (2). For solution (1) dissolve 50 mg of the substance being examined in 5 ml of *dimethylformamide* by heating on a water-bath for a few minutes, allow to cool and dilute to 10 ml with *acetone*. Solution (2) contains 0.010% w/v solution of *nitrofurfural diacetate BPCRS* in a mixture of equal volumes of *dimethylformamide* and *acetone*. After removal of the plate, heat it at 105° for 5 minutes and spray with a solution prepared by dissolving 0.75 g of *phenylhydrazine hydrochloride* in 10 ml of *ethanol (96%)*, diluting to 50 ml with *water*, adding *decolorising charcoal*, filtering and then adding 25 ml of *hydrochloric acid* and sufficient *water* to produce 200 ml. Any spot corresponding to nitrofurfural diacetate in the chromatogram obtained with solution (1) is not more intense than the spot in the chromatogram obtained with solution (2).

Loss on drying When dried to constant weight at 105°, loses not more than 0.5% of its weight. Use 1 g.

Sulphated ash Not more than 0.1%, Appendix IX A.

Assay Carry out the following procedure protected from light. To 80 mg add 150 ml of *dimethylformamide*, swirl to dissolve and add sufficient *water* to produce 500 ml. Dilute 5 ml to 100 ml with *water* and mix. Measure the *absorbance* of the resulting solution at the maximum at 367 nm, Appendix II B. Calculate the content of $C_8H_7N_3O_5$ taking 750 as the value of A(1%, 1 cm) at the maximum at 367 nm.

Storage Furazolidone should be protected from light.

Action and use Antibacterial; antifungal; antiprotozoal.

Furazolidone

$C_8H_7N_3O_5$ 225.2   *67-45-8*

Furazolidone is 3-(5-nitrofurfurylideneamino)-oxazolidin-2-one. It contains not less than 97.0 per cent and not more than 103.0 per cent of $C_8H_7N_3O_5$, calculated with reference to the dried substance.

Fusidic Acid

C$_{31}$H$_{48}$O$_6$,$\frac{1}{2}$H$_2$O   525.7   *6990-06-3*

Fusidic Acid is (17Z)-16β-acetoxy-3α,11α-dihydroxyfusida-17(20),24-dien-21-oic acid hemihydrate, an antimicrobial substance produced by the growth of certain strains of *Fusidium coccineum* (K. Tubaki). It contains not less than 97.5 per cent and not more than 100.5 per cent of C$_{31}$H$_{48}$O$_6$, calculated with reference to the anhydrous substance.

Characteristics A white, crystalline powder.

Solubility Practically insoluble in *water*; soluble in 5 parts of *ethanol (96%)*, in 4 parts of *chloroform* and in 60 parts of *ether*.

Identification A. The *infra-red absorption spectrum*, Appendix II A, is concordant with the *reference spectrum* of fusidic acid.
B. Carry out the method described under Related substances, applying separately to the chromatoplate 5 µl of each of two solutions in *ethanol (96%)* containing (1) 0.20% w/v of the substance being examined and (2) 0.24% w/v of *diethanolamine fusidate BPCRS*. The principal spot in the chromatogram obtained with solution (1) corresponds to that in the chromatogram obtained with solution (2).

Related substances Carry out the method for *thin-layer chromatography*, Appendix III A, using *silica gel G* as the coating substance and a mixture of 160 volumes of *chloroform*, 20 volumes of *glacial acetic acid*, 20 volumes of *cyclohexane* and 5 volumes of *methanol* as the mobile phase. Apply separately to the chromatoplate 5 µl of each of three solutions in *ethanol (96%)* containing (1) 2.0% w/v of the substance being examined, (2) 0.040% w/v of *diethanolamine fusidate BPCRS* and (3) 0.040% w/v of *3-ketofusidic acid BPCRS*. After removal of the plate, dry it at 110° for 10 minutes, spray with *ethanolic sulphuric acid (10%)*, dry at 110° for 10 minutes and examine under *ultra-violet light (365 nm)*. Any red *secondary spot* in the chromatogram obtained with solution (1) is not more intense than the principal spot in the chromatogram obtained with solution (2). Any yellow spot in the chromatogram obtained with solution (1) is not more intense than the principal spot in the chromatogram obtained with solution (3).

Sulphated ash Not more than 0.2%, Appendix IX A.

Water 1.4 to 2.0% w/w, Appendix IX C. Use 1.5 g.

Assay Dissolve 0.5 g in 10 ml of *ethanol (96%)* and titrate with 0.1M *sodium hydroxide VS* using *phenolphthalein solution* as indicator. Each ml of 0.1M *sodium hydroxide VS* is equivalent to 0.05167 g of C$_{31}$H$_{48}$O$_6$.

Storage Fusidic Acid should be kept in a well-closed container and protected from light.

Preparation
Fusidic Acid Oral Suspension
Action and use Antibacterial.

Gallamine Triethiodide ☆

C$_{30}$H$_{60}$I$_3$N$_3$O$_3$ 892   *65-29-2*

Gallamine Triethiodide is 2,2′,2″-(benzene-1,2,3-triyltrioxy)tris(tetraethylammonium) tri-iodide. It contains not less than 98.0 per cent and not more than 101.0 per cent of C$_{30}$H$_{60}$I$_3$N$_3$O$_3$, calculated with reference to the dried substance.

Characteristics A white or almost white powder; odourless; hygroscopic.

Solubility Soluble in 0.6 part of *water*; slightly soluble in *ethanol (96%)*; very slightly soluble in *chloroform*; practically insoluble in *ether*.

Identification Test A may be omitted if tests B, C and D are carried out. Tests B and C may be omitted if tests A and D are carried out.
A. The *infra-red absorption spectrum*, Appendix II A, is concordant with the spectrum of *gallamine triethiodide EPCRS*.
B. The *light absorption*, Appendix II B, in the range 220 to 350 nm of a 0.001% w/v solution in 0.01M *hydrochloric acid* exhibits a maximum only at 225 nm. The A(1%, 1 cm) at 225 nm is 500 to 550.
C. To 5 ml of a 2% w/v solution add 1 ml of *potassium mercuri-iodide solution*. A yellow precipitate is produced.
D. Acidify 2 ml of a 0.5% w/v solution with 0.2 ml of 2M *nitric acid*. The resulting solution yields *reaction A* characteristic of iodides, Appendix VI.

Acidity or alkalinity To 50 ml of *water* add 0.2 ml of *methyl red solution* and adjust the pH to 6 by adding either 0.01M *sulphuric acid* or 0.02M *sodium hydroxide* until the colour is orange-yellow. Add 1 g of the substance being examined and shake to dissolve. Not more than 0.2 ml of 0.01M *sulphuric acid VS* or 0.02M *sodium hydroxide VS* is required to restore the orange-yellow colour.

Clarity and colour of solution A 2.0% w/v solution is *clear*, Appendix IV A, and, when freshly prepared, not more intensely coloured than *reference solution Y$_7$*, Appendix IV B, Method II.

Related substances Carry out the method for *thin-layer chromatography*, Appendix III A, using *microcrystalline cellulose* as the coating substance (Avicel is suitable) and a mixture of 66 volumes of *butan-1-ol*, 17 volumes of *glacial acetic acid* and 17 volumes of *water* as the mobile phase, but allowing the solvent front to ascend 10 cm above the line of application. Apply separately to the chromatoplate 10 µl of each of two solutions of the substance being examined in *ethanol (96%)* containing (1) 0.50% w/v and (2) 0.0050% w/v. After removal of the plate, dry it in a current of warm air and spray with *dilute potassium iodoplatinate solution*. In the chromatogram obtained with solution (1) an elongated blue spot, which may appear to be double, is produced. Any *secondary spot* in the chromatogram obtained with solution (1) of higher Rf value than the principal spot is not more intense than the spot in the chromatogram obtained with solution (2).

Loss on drying When dried to constant weight at 100° to 105°, loses not more than 1.5% of its weight. Use 1 g.

Sulphated ash Not more than 0.1%, Appendix IX A, Method II. Use 1 g.

Assay Dissolve 0.27 g in a mixture of 40 ml of *acetone* and 15 ml of *mercury(II) acetate solution* and carry out Method I for *non-aqueous titration*, Appendix VIII A, determining the end-point potentiometrically. Each ml of 0.1M *perchloric acid VS* is equivalent to 0.02972 g of $C_{30}H_{60}I_3N_3O_3$.

Storage Gallamine Triethiodide should be kept in an airtight container and protected from light.

Preparation
Gallamine Injection

Action and use Skeletal muscle relaxant.

Gelatin ☆

Gelatin⋆ is a purified protein obtained either by partial acid hydrolysis (type A) or by partial alkaline hydrolysis (type B) of animal collagen. It may be a mixture of types A and B.

Characteristics Light amber to faintly yellow, translucent sheets, shreds, powder or granules; odour, slight. The isoelectric point of type A gelatin is between pH 6.3 and 9.2 and of type B gelatin is between pH 4.7 and 5.2. The moisture content of powdered or finely divided gelatin varies rapidly with the humidity of the atmosphere to which it is exposed.

Solubility Swells and softens when immersed in *water*, gradually absorbing from five to ten times its own weight; soluble in hot *water*, forming a jelly on cooling; practically insoluble in *ethanol (96%)*, in *chloroform* and in *ether*.

Identification A. Dissolve 1 g in sufficient *carbon dioxide-free water* at about 55° to produce 100 ml and maintain the solution (solution A) at this temperature until required for use. To 2 ml of solution A add 0.05 ml of *copper sulphate solution*, mix and add 0.5 ml of 2M *sodium hydroxide*. A violet colour is produced.

B. Add 10 ml of *water* to 0.5 g in a test-tube, allow to stand for 10 minutes, heat at 60° for 15 minutes, allow to stand upright at 0° for 6 hours and invert the test-tube. The contents do not immediately flow out.

Acidity or alkalinity pH of solution A, 3.8 to 7.6, Appendix V L.

Clarity and colour of solution Solution A prepared from either type A or type B Gelatin is not more opalescent than *reference suspension IV*, Appendix IV A; mixtures of type A and type B Gelatin may give opalescent solutions through the formation of coacervates. Solution A is not more intensely coloured than *reference solution Y_4*, Appendix IV B, Method II.

Arsenic To 1.0 g add a mixture of 10 ml of *water*, 2.5 ml of *sulphuric acid*, 2.5 ml of *nitric acid* and a slight excess of *bromine water*. Allow to stand for 30 minutes, boil under a reflux condenser for 1 hour and allow to cool. The

resulting solution complies with the *limit test for arsenic*, Appendix VII (1 ppm).

Heavy metals 2.0 g complies with *limit test C for heavy metals*, Appendix VII (50 ppm). Use 10 ml of *lead standard solution (10 ppm Pb)* to prepare the standard.

Peroxides Dissolve 1.0 g in 10 ml of *water* with the aid of heat and add 2 ml of *vanadium pentoxide solution*. Any pink colour produced is not more intense than that produced by adding 2 ml of *vanadium pentoxide solution* to a mixture of 1 ml of a 0.01% w/v solution of *hydrogen peroxide* and 9 ml of *water* (100 ppm H_2O_2).

Phenolic preservatives Carry out in subdued light the method for *thin-layer chromatography*, Appendix III A, using *silica gel GF254* as the coating substance and a mixture of 92 volumes of *toluene* and 8 volumes of *absolute ethanol* as the mobile phase, but allowing the solvent front to ascend 12 cm above the line of application. Apply separately to the chromatoplate 10 µl of each of the following solutions as bands (20 mm × 3 mm). For solution (1) add 20 ml of *methanol* and 2 ml of 9M *ammonia* to 1 g of the substance being examined and allow to stand for 20 hours; decant the clear supernatant liquid, evaporate to dryness and dissolve the residue in 0.5 ml of *methanol*. For solution (2) dissolve 2 mg of *1-naphthyl-amine* and 2 mg of *ethyl 4-hydroxybenzoate* or *methyl 4-hydroxybenzoate* or *propyl 4-hydroxybenzoate* in 10 ml of *methanol*. Solution (3) is a 0.1% w/v solution of *dansyl chloride* in *acetone*. Apply 10 µl of solution (3) to the dried starting bands obtained from solutions (1) and (2). Spray the three bands with a 5% w/v solution of *sodium tetraborate* and dry the plate at 60° for 15 minutes before development.

After removal of the plate, allow it to dry in air and examine immediately under *ultra-violet light (365 nm)*. The chromatogram obtained with solution (2) shows a strong yellow fluorescent band with an Rf value of 0.4 to 0.6 (5-dimethylaminonaphthalene-1-sulphonate). The chromatogram obtained with solution (3) shows bands of blue fluorescence at the line of application and near the solvent front. The chromatogram obtained with solution (1) does not show a band of yellow to orange or blue fluorescence in the middle of the chromatogram or bands of blue fluorescence with higher Rf values (amino-acid derivatives). Examine under *ultra-violet light (254 nm)*. The chromatogram obtained with solution (2) shows bands of fluorescence quenching with Rf values of 0.3 to 0.5 (4-hydroxybenzoates). The chromatogram obtained with solution (1) does not show bands of fluorescence quenching at these Rf values (4-hydroxybenzoates or pentachlorophenol).

Sulphur dioxide Not more than 200 ppm, Appendix IX B, Method II. Use 25 g and add to the flask using 100 ml of *water*.

Loss on drying When dried at 100° to 105°, loses not more than 15.0% of its weight. Use 1 g.

Ash Not more than 2.0%, Appendix IX J, Method II.

Microbial contamination† 1 g is free from *Escherichia coli*; 10 g is free from salmonellae, Appendix XVI B1.

Storage Gelatin should be kept in an airtight container.

Labelling The label states whether the material is suitable for the preparation of pessaries or suppositories and, if so, the Jelly strength.

Gelatin intended for the preparation of pessaries or suppositories complies with the following additional requirement.

Jelly strength 150 to 250 g expressed as the weight necessary to give a 4-mm depression in a jelly containing 6.67% w/w of the substance being examined, matured at 10°, using a plunger 12.7 mm in diameter.

Use a gelometer consisting of a cylindrical piston 12.6 to 12.8 mm in diameter with a plane pressure surface with a rounded edge 0.5 mm in radius attached to a device whereby the load exerted by the piston can be increased at a constant rate of 40 g per second and the vertical movement of the piston can be stopped within 0.025 seconds when it has descended 3.9 to 4.1 mm. Place 7.5 g of the substance being examined in a bottle 58 to 60 mm in internal diameter and 85 mm high, add 105 ml of *water*, cover the bottle with a watch-glass and allow to stand for 3 hours. Heat in a water-bath at 65° for 15 minutes, stirring gently with a glass rod and ensuring that the solution is uniform and that any condensed water on the inner walls of the bottle is incorporated. Allow to cool at room temperature for 15 minutes, transfer to a water-bath maintained at 9.9° to 10.1° and ensure that the base of the bottle is horizontal. Close the bottle with a rubber stopper and allow to stand for 16 to 18 hours. Immediately transfer the bottle to the gelometer and adjust the height of the bottle so that the piston just comes into contact with the surface of the gel without exerting any pressure. Increase the load on the piston at a rate of 40 g per second until it has descended 3.9 to 4.1 mm. The load, measured with a precision of ±0.5 g, exerted by the piston at that moment represents the jelly strength. Carry out three or more determinations and use the mean value.

*Gelatin described in this monograph is not necessarily suitable for preparations for parenteral use or for other special purposes.

†In certain states party to the Convention on the Elaboration of a European Pharmacopœia, Gelatin may be required to comply with a limit for a total viable aerobic count of 10^3 micro-organisms per gram, determined by plate count, Appendix XVI B2.

Gentamicin Sulphate ☆

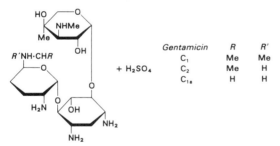

1405-41-0

Gentamicin	R	R'
C₁	Me	Me
C₂	Me	H
C₁ₐ	H	H

Gentamicin Sulphate is a mixture of the sulphates of antimicrobial substances produced by *Micromonospora purpurea*. The potency is not less than 590 Units per mg, calculated with reference to the anhydrous substance.

Characteristics A white or almost white powder.

Solubility Freely soluble in *water*; practically insoluble in *ethanol (96%)*, in *chloroform* and in *ether*.

Identification *Test A may be omitted if tests B, C and D are carried out. Tests B and C may be omitted if tests A and D are carried out.*

A. The *nuclear magnetic resonance spectrum* of a 20% w/v solution in *deuterium oxide*, Appendix II C, is concordant with that of a similar solution of *gentamicin sulphate EPCRS*. (Differences may be observed in the integrals of the peaks at about δ1.25, δ1.35, δ2.75 and δ2.95, due to differences in the proportions of the components.)

B. Dissolve 10 mg in 1 ml of *water* and add 5 ml of a 40% w/v solution of *sulphuric acid*. Heat on a water-bath for 100 minutes, cool and dilute to 25 ml with *water*. The *light absorption* of the resulting solution, Appendix II B, exhibits no maximum in the range 240 to 330 nm.

C. Carry out the method for *thin-layer chromatography*, Appendix III A, using *silica gel G* as the coating substance and as the mobile phase the lower layer obtained by shaking together equal volumes of 13.5M *ammonia*, *chloroform* and *methanol* and allowing to separate. Apply separately to the chromatoplate 10 μl of each of two solutions in *water* containing (1) 0.5% w/v of the substance being examined and (2) 0.5% w/v of *gentamicin sulphate EPCRS*. After removal of the plate, allow it to dry in air, spray with a solution prepared by dissolving 1 g of *ninhydrin* in 50 ml of *ethanol (96%)* and adding 10 ml of *glacial acetic acid* and heat at 110° for 5 minutes. The three principal spots in the chromatogram obtained with solution (1) are similar in position, colour and size to the three principal spots in the chromatogram obtained with solution (2).

D. Yields *reaction A* characteristic of sulphates, Appendix VI.

Acidity pH of a 4% w/v solution, 3.5 to 5.5, Appendix V L.

Clarity and colour of solution A 4.0% w/v solution is *clear*, Appendix IV A, and not more intensely coloured than degree 6 of the appropriate range of *reference solutions*, Appendix IV B, Method II.

Nuclear magnetic resonance Examine by *nuclear magnetic resonance spectrometry*, Appendix II C, using a 60-MHz spectrometer. Adjust the spectrometer controls as follows. Using the peak at about δ4.75 given by a 10% w/v solution of *magnesium sulphate* in *deuterium oxide*, adjust the phase control until the instrument is operating in the pure absorption mode. Carry out the remaining adjustments using as a reference solution a 20% w/v solution of *gentamicin sulphate EPCRS* in *deuterium oxide* that has been filtered into a nuclear magnetic resonance tube and freed from oxygen by slow bubbling of nitrogen. Set a scan speed of about 1 Hz per second. Record the height of the peak at about δ2.95 at successive radio-frequency settings. Employ the highest setting at which the height of the peak at about δ2.95 is not saturated. Further adjust the phase control, if necessary. Adjust the sensitivity control so that the peak at about δ2.95 is as near full-scale deflection as possible. Record the proton absorption spectrum.

Using a 20% w/v solution of the substance being examined in *deuterium oxide* that has been filtered into a nuclear magnetic resonance tube and freed from oxygen by slow bubbling of nitrogen, record the proton absorption spectrum three times on separate charts under the operating conditions defined above, if necessary after further adjustments of the phase and sensitivity controls. The ratio of the height of the peak at about δ2.75 to that of the peak at about δ2.95 is between 0.260 and 0.440, and the ratio of the height of the peak at about δ1.25 to that of the peak at about δ1.35 is between 0.200 and

0.260. The peak heights are measured with respect to a line drawn between the mean baseline between δ0 and δ0.5 and that between δ6.1 and δ6.6. The ratios are the arithmetic means of the values obtained from each spectrum.

Specific optical rotation In a 10% w/v solution, +107° to +121°, Appendix V F.

Sulphate 32.0 to 35.0% of SO_4, calculated with reference to the anhydrous substance, when determined by the following method. Dissolve 0.25 g in 100 ml of *water*, adjust the pH to 11 with 13.5M *ammonia* and add 10 ml of 0.1M *barium chloride VS*. Titrate with 0.1M *disodium edetate VS* using 0.5 mg of *metalphthalein* as indicator; when the colour of the solution begins to change add 50 ml of *ethanol (96%)* and continue the titration until the violet-blue colour disappears. Each ml of 0.1M *barium chloride VS* is equivalent to 0.009606 g of sulphate, SO_4.

Methanol Not more than 1.0% w/w when determined by the method for *gas chromatography*, Appendix III B, using three solutions in *water* containing (1) 0.25% v/v of *methanol* and 0.25% v/v of *propan-1-ol* (internal standard), (2) 25% w/w of the substance being examined and (3) 25% w/w of the substance being examined and 0.25% v/v of the internal standard.

The chromatographic procedure may be carried out using a glass column (1.5 m × 4 mm) packed with porous polymer beads (80 to 100 mesh) (Porapak Q is suitable) and maintained at a constant temperature in the range 120° to 140° with the inlet port temperature and the detector temperature at least 50° higher than the column temperature.

Calculate the percentage w/w of methanol taking 0.792 g as its weight per ml at 20°.

Sulphated ash Not more than 1.0%, Appendix IX A, Method II. Use 0.5 g.

Water Not more than 15.0% w/w, Appendix IX C. Use 0.3 g.

Assay Carry out the *biological assay of antibiotics*, Appendix XIV A. The precision of the assay is such that the fiducial limits of error are not less than 95% and not more than 105% of the estimated potency.

Storage Gentamicin Sulphate should be kept in a well-closed container. If it is intended for use in the manufacture of parenteral or ophthalmic dosage forms and is sterile, the container should be sterile, tamper-evident and sealed so as to exclude micro-organisms.

Labelling The label states (1) the number of Units per mg; (2) the date after which the material is not intended to be used; (3) the conditions under which it should be stored; (4) whether or not it is intended for use in the manufacture of parenteral or ophthalmic dosage forms; (5) whether or not it is sterile.

Preparations
Gentamicin Cream
Gentamicin Eye Drops
Gentamicin Ointment
Gentamicin Injection

Action and use Antibacterial.

Gentamicin Sulphate intended for use in the manufacture of a parenteral dosage form complies with the following additional requirements.

Abnormal toxicity Complies with the *test for abnormal toxicity*, Appendix XIV L. Use 1 mg dissolved in 0.5 ml of *saline solution*.

Pyrogens Complies with the *test for pyrogens*, Appendix XIV K. Use per kg of the rabbit's weight 2.5 ml of a solution in *water for injections* containing 8 mg per ml of the substance being examined.

Gentamicin Sulphate intended for use in the manufacture of parenteral or ophthalmic dosage forms without further sterilisation complies with the following additional requirement.

Sterility Complies with the *test for sterility*, Appendix XVI A.

Gentian ☆

Gentian consists of the dried underground organs of *Gentiana lutea* L.

Characteristics Odour, characteristic; taste, strong and persistently bitter.

Macroscopical Single or branched sub-cylindrical pieces up to and occasionally exceeding 200 mm long, usually 10 to 40 mm in diameter but occasionally up to 80 mm at the crown. Outer surface, greyish-brown, facture yellowish to reddish-yellow but not reddish-brown. Rhizome, frequently bearing a terminal bud and always encircled by closely arranged leaf scars; root, longitudinally wrinkled and bearing occasional rootlet scars. Both rhizome and root brittle when dry, breaking with a short fracture, but absorbing moisture readily to become flexible. Smoothed, transversely cut surface showing bark, occupying about one third of the radius, separated by well marked cambium from indistinctly radiate and mainly parenchymatous xylem.

Microscopical Cork cells, thin-walled, yellowish-brown occurring in four to six layers; phelloderm of several layers, the outer of collenchyma and the inner of tangentially elongated parenchyma. Small groups of sieve tissue embedded in phloem parenchyma; xylem, mainly parenchymatous with scattered vessels showing reticulate, spiral or annular thickening, occurring singly or in small groups and with small groups of interxylary phloem. Triarch primary xylem in root and a parenchymatous pith in the rhizome. Droplets of oil and numerous acicular crystals or slender prisms of calcium oxalate throughout parenchyma; starch, almost completely absent.

Identification Carry out the method for *thin-layer chromatography*, Appendix III A, using as the coating substance a suitable silica gel containing a fluorescent indicator with an optimal intensity at 254 nm (Merck silica gel 60 F254 is suitable) and a mixture of 70 volumes of *acetone*, 30 volumes of *chloroform* and 2 volumes of *water* as the mobile phase. Apply separately to the chromatoplate, as bands 30 mm × 8 mm in size, 50 μl of solution (1) and 10 μl of solution (2). For solution (1) add 50 ml of *methanol* to 2.00 g, in *No. 250 powder*, stir mechanically for 20 minutes, filter without allowing the solvent to evaporate and evaporate 25 ml of the filtrate to dryness at a temperature not exceeding 50° and at a pressure of 2 kPa. Dissolve the residue in sufficient *methanol* to produce 5 ml of a solution which may contain sediment. Solution (2) is a 0.50% w/v solution of *phenazone* in *methanol*. After removal of the plate, allow it to dry in air and examine under *ultra-violet light (254 nm)*. The chromatogram obtained with solution (1) shows quenching bands in the lower part and usually in the upper part. In the middle part of the chromatogram there is a quenching band at about the same Rf value as the quenching band in the chromatogram obtained with solution (2) (amarogentine). Mark the band due to phenazone, spray the plate with a freshly prepared 0.2% w/v solution of *fast red B salt* and allow to stand for 10 minutes; the band due to amarogentine is orange. Expose the plate to ammonia vapour; the colour of the band due to amarogentine changes to red. Other coloured bands are visible in the lower and upper parts of the chromatogram obtained with solution (1); in particular there may be a band, which is usually very intense, in the upper part having the same colour as the band due to amarogentine.

Related species of *Gentiana* Examine the chromatograms obtained in the test for Identification after exposure to ammonia vapour. The chromatogram obtained with solution (1) does not show violet bands immediately above the band due to amarogentine.

Bitterness value Not less than 10,000 when determined by comparison with *quinine hydrochloride* (bitterness value 200,000); the bitterness value is the reciprocal of the greatest dilution that still has a bitter taste. Place in successive tubes 4.2, 4.4, 4.6, 4.8, 5.0, 5.2, 5.4, 5.6 and 5.8 ml of a 0.0010% w/v solution of *quinine hydrochloride* and dilute the contents to 10.00 ml with *water*. To determine the dilution with the lowest concentration that still has a bitter taste take all 10 ml of the least concentrated solution into the mouth and pass it from side to side over the back of the tongue for 30 seconds. If the solution is not found to be bitter, spit it out and wait for 1 minute. Rinse the mouth with water and after 10 minutes use the next dilution in order of increasing concentration. Continue until the dilution of lowest concentration that is bitter has been identified. Calculate the correction factor, k, from the expression $5.00/n$ where n is the number of ml of the 0.00100% w/v solution of quinine hydrochloride in the dilution of lowest concentration that is bitter.

Prepare an extract of the substance being examined as follows. Add 1000 ml of boiling *water* to 1.00 g, in *No. 710 powder*, heat on a water-bath for 30 minutes, cool and dilute to 1000 ml with *water*. Shake vigorously and filter, discarding the first 20 ml of filtrate. Dilute $10/k$ ml of the filtrate to 100 ml with *water*. 10 ml of this dilution has a bitter taste.

Water-soluble extractive Not less than 33% when determined by the following method. To 5 g, in *No. 710 powder*, add 200 ml of boiling *water* and allow to stand for 10 minutes, shaking at intervals. Cool, dilute to 200 ml with *water* and filter. Evaporate 20 ml of the filtrate to dryness on a water-bath and dry the residue to constant weight at 100° to 105°.

Sulphated ash Not more than 5.0%, Appendix IX A, Method II. Use 1 g, in powder.

Storage Gentian should be kept in a well-closed container and protected from light.

Preparation
Compound Gentian Infusion

Action and use Bitter.

The title of the monograph in the European Pharmacopœia is Gentian Root.

Powdered Gentian

Powdered Gentian is Gentian in powder.

Characteristics Yellowish-brown to light brown. Diagnostic structures: a small number of lignified vessels with reticulate, spiral or annular thickening; small acicular crystals of calcium oxalate; droplets of oil; numerous parenchymatous cells with moderately thick walls, starch granules rare. Fibres and sclereids absent.

Identification; Related species of *Gentiana*; Bitterness value; Water-soluble extractive; Sulphated ash Complies with the requirements stated under Gentian.

Storage Powdered Gentian should be kept in a well-closed container and protected from light.

Action and use Bitter.

Ginger

Ginger is the rhizome of *Zingiber officinale* Roscoe, scraped or unscraped. It is known in commerce as unbleached ginger.

Characteristics Odour, agreeable and aromatic; taste, agreeable and pungent.

Macroscopical Rhizome laterally compressed, bearing short, flattened, obovate oblique branches on the upper side, each sometimes having a depressed scar at the apex; whole rhizomes about 5 to 10 cm long, 1.5 to 3 or 4 cm wide and 1 to 1.5 cm thick, sometimes split longitudinally. Scraped rhizome with buff external surface showing longitudinal striations and occasional loose fibres; outer surface of the unscraped rhizome varying from pale to dark brown and more or less covered with cork which shows conspicuous, narrow, longitudinal and transverse ridges; the cork readily exfoliates from the lateral surfaces but persists between the branches. Fracture, short and starchy, with projecting fibres. Smoothed transversely cut surface exhibiting a narrow cortex separated by an endodermis from a much wider stele; numerous, scattered, fibrovascular bundles; abundant scattered oleo-resin cells with yellow contents. The unscraped rhizome shows in addition an outer layer of dark brown cork.

Microscopical Starch abundant in the thin-walled ground tissue, as flattened, ovate to subrectangular, transversely striated, simple granules, each with the hilum in a projection towards one end, mostly up to about 50 μm long and up to about 25 μm wide and 7 μm thick. Oleo-resin cells, with suberised cell walls and yellow contents, numerous in the ground tissue. Pigment cells with dark, reddish-brown contents occurring either singly in the ground tissue or in axial rows accompanying the vascular bundles. Vessels with spiral or reticulate thickening in the scattered vascular bundles not yielding the *reaction* characteristic of lignin, Appendix VI. Irregularly shaped thin-walled fibres with delicate, transverse septa, yielding only slightly the *reaction* characteristic of lignin. In the unscraped drug varying amounts of cork, composed of thin-walled cells. Sclereids and calcium oxalate crystals absent.

Extractive soluble in ethanol (90%) Not less than 4.5%, Appendix XI B.

Ash Not more than 6.0%, Appendix XI J.

Water-soluble ash Not less than 1.7%, Appendix XI L.

Water-soluble extractive Not less than 10.0%,
Appendix XI C.

Storage Ginger should be kept in a well-closed container
and protected from light and moisture.

Action and use Flavour.

Powdered Ginger

Powdered Ginger is Ginger in powder.

Characteristics Light yellow (scraped) or yellowish-brown
(unscraped). Diagnostic structures: parenchymatous cells;
fibres; vessels, often accompanied by pigment cells; oleo-
resin in fragments or droplets, staining with *iodine
solution*; abundant starch. Fragments of cork, composed of
thin-walled, polygonal cells, from the unscraped drug.
Sclerenchymatous cells, trichomes and calcium oxalate,
absent.

**Extractive soluble in ethanol (90%); Ash; Water-soluble
ash; Water-soluble extractive** Complies with the
requirements stated under Ginger.

Storage Powdered Ginger should be kept in a well-closed
container and protected from light and moisture.

Preparation
Strong Ginger Tincture

Action and use Flavour.

Glibenclamide

$C_{23}H_{28}ClN_3O_5S$ 494.0   *10238-21-8*

Glibenclamide is 1-{4-[2-(5-chloro-2-methoxy-
benzamido)ethyl]benzenesulphonyl}-3-cyclo-
hexylurea. It contains not less than 99.0 per
cent and not more than 101.0 per cent of
$C_{23}H_{28}ClN_3O_5S$, calculated with reference to the
dried substance.

Characteristics A white or almost white, crystalline
powder; odourless or almost odourless.

Solubility Practically insoluble in *water* and in *ether*;
slightly soluble in *ethanol (96%)* and in *methanol*; sparingly
soluble in *chloroform*.

Identification A. The *infra-red absorption spectrum*,
Appendix II A, is concordant with the *reference spectrum* of
glibenclamide.
B. The *light absorption*, Appendix II B, in the range 230 to
350 nm of a 0.02% w/v solution in 0.01M *methanolic
hydrochloric acid* exhibits a maximum at 300 nm and a less
intense maximum at 275 nm. The *absorbance* at 300 nm is
about 1.26.
C. Boil 50 mg with 1 ml of 6M *sodium hydroxide*. The
fumes evolved as soon as the water has evaporated are
alkaline to *litmus paper* and have a pungent, amine-like
odour.
D. Mix 0.2 g with 0.25 g of *anhydrous sodium carbonate*
and 0.25 g of *potassium carbonate*. Ignite the mixture for

10 minutes, cool, add 10 ml of hot *water* to the residue,
stir for 1 minute and filter. The filtrate yields the *reactions*
characteristic of chlorides and of sulphates, Appendix VI.

Melting point 172° to 174°, Appendix V A.

Heavy metals Ignite 1.5 g gently until free from carbon.
Add to the residue 2 ml of *nitric acid* and 0.25 ml of
sulphuric acid. Heat until white fumes are evolved, ignite
at a temperature not exceeding 500°, add 2 ml of
hydrochloric acid to the residue and evaporate to dryness
on a water-bath. Add 10 ml of *water* and 0.1 ml of 6M
hydrochloric acid and heat on a water-bath for 2 minutes.
Cool and add sufficient *water* to produce 15 ml. 12 ml of
the resulting solution complies with *limit test A for heavy
metals*, Appendix VII (20 ppm). Use *lead standard solution
(2 ppm Pb)* to prepare the standard.

Related substances Carry out the method for *thin-layer
chromatography*, Appendix III A, using *silica gel GF254* as
the coating substance and a mixture of 45 volumes of
chloroform, 45 volumes of *cyclohexane*, 5 volumes of *ethanol
(96%)* and 5 volumes of *glacial acetic acid* as the mobile
phase. Apply separately to the chromatoplate 10 µl of each
of four solutions in a mixture of equal volumes of
methanol and *chloroform* containing (1) 2.0% w/v of the
substance being examined, (2) 0.0080% w/v of *4-[2-(5-
chloro-2-methoxybenzamido)ethyl]benzenesulphonamide
BPCRS*, (3) 0.0080% w/v of *methyl N-4-[2-(5-chloro-2-
methoxybenzamido)ethyl]benzenesulphonyl-N-methylcarbamate
BPCRS* and (4) 0.0040% w/v of the substance being
examined. After removal of the plate, allow it to dry in air
and examine under *ultra-violet light (254 nm)*. Any spots
corresponding to 4-[2-(5-chloro-2-methoxybenzamido)-
ethyl]benzenesulphonamide and methyl *N*-4-[2-(5-chloro-
2-methoxybenzamido)ethyl]benzenesulphonyl-*N*-methyl-
carbamate in the chromatogram obtained with solution (1)
are not more intense than the spots in the chromatograms
obtained with solutions (2) and (3) respectively. Any other
secondary spot in the chromatogram obtained with solution
(1) is not more intense than the spot in the chromatogram
obtained with solution (4).

Loss on drying When dried to constant weight at 105°,
loses not more than 1.0% of its weight. Use 1 g.

Sulphated ash Not more than 0.1%, Appendix IX A.

Assay Dissolve 0.5 g in 100 ml of hot *ethanol (96%)*
previously neutralised to *phenolphthalein solution*. Titrate
with 0.1M *sodium hydroxide VS* using *phenolphthalein
solution* as indicator and protecting against exposure to
atmospheric carbon dioxide. Each ml of 0.1M *sodium
hydroxide VS* is equivalent to 0.04940 g of $C_{23}H_{28}ClN_3O_5S$.

Preparation
Glibenclamide Tablets

Action and use Hypoglycaemic.

Glipizide

$C_{21}H_{27}N_5O_4S$ 445.5   *29064-61-9*

Glipizide is 1-cyclohexyl-3-{4-[2-(5-methyl-pyrazine-2-carboxamido)ethyl]benzene-sulphonyl}urea. It contains not less than 98.0 per cent and not more than 102.0 per cent of $C_{21}H_{27}N_5O_4S$, calculated with reference to the dried substance.

Characteristics A white or almost white, crystalline powder; odourless or almost odourless.

Solubility Practically insoluble in *water* and in *ethanol (96%)*; sparingly soluble in *acetone*; soluble in *chloroform*. It dissolves in dilute solutions of alkali hydroxides.

Identification A. The *infra-red absorption spectrum*, Appendix II A, is concordant with the *reference spectrum* of glipizide.

B. The *light absorption*, Appendix II B, in the range 210 to 350 nm of a 0.002% w/v solution in *methanol* exhibits maxima at 226 nm and 274 nm. The *absorbance* at 226 nm is about 1.1 and at 274 nm is about 0.5.

C. Dissolve 50 mg in 5 ml of *1,4-dioxan*, add 1 ml of a 0.5% w/v solution of *2,4-dinitrofluorobenzene* in *1,4-dioxan* and boil for 2 to 3 minutes. A bright yellow colour is produced.

Heavy metals 2.0 g complies with *limit test C for heavy metals*, Appendix VII (20 ppm). Use 4 ml of *lead standard solution (10 ppm Pb)* to prepare the standard.

Related substances Carry out the method for *thin-layer chromatography*, Appendix III A, using a silica gel GF254 precoated chromatoplate (Merck silica gel 60 F254 plates are suitable) and a mixture of 40 volumes of *dichloromethane*, 40 volumes of *carbon tetrachloride*, 20 volumes of *ethyl acetate* and 20 volumes of *anhydrous formic acid* as the mobile phase. Apply separately to the plate 10 µl of each the following solutions in a mixture of equal volumes of *methanol* and *chloroform*. Solutions (1), (2) and (3) contain 2.0% w/v, 0.010% w/v and 0.0040% w/v respectively of the substance being examined. Solution (4) contains 0.010% w/v of *4-[2-(5-methylpyrazine-2-carboxamido)-ethyl]benzenesulphonamide BPCRS*. After removal of the plate, allow it to dry in air and examine under *ultra-violet light (254 nm)*. Any spot corresponding to 4-[2-(5-methylpyrazine-2-carboxamido)ethyl]benzene-sulphonamide in the chromatogram obtained with solution (1) is not more intense than the spot in the chromatogram obtained with solution (4). Any other *secondary spot* is not more intense than the spot in the chromatogram obtained with solution (2) and not more than two such spots are more intense than the spot in the chromatogram obtained with solution (3).

Loss on drying When dried to constant weight at 100° to 105°, loses not more than 0.5% of its weight. Use 1 g.

Sulphated ash Not more than 0.2%, Appendix IX A.

Assay Dissolve 0.4 g in 50 ml of *dimethylformamide* and carry out Method II for *non-aqueous titration*,

Appendix VIII A, using 0.1M *lithium methoxide VS* as titrant and *quinaldine red solution* as indicator. Repeat the operation without the substance being examined. The difference between the titrations represents the amount of lithium methoxide required. Each ml of 0.1M *lithium methoxide VS* is equivalent to 0.04455 g of $C_{21}H_{27}N_5O_4S$.

Preparation
Glipizide Tablets

Action and use Hypoglycaemic.

Glucagon

16941-32-5

Glucagon is a polypeptide hormone, obtained from beef or pork pancreas, that increases the blood glucose concentration as the result of the rapid breakdown of liver glycogen. It is prepared in conditions designed to minimise microbial contamination.

Characteristics A white or almost white powder.

Solubility Practically insoluble in *water* and in most organic solvents. It dissolves in dilute solutions of alkali hydroxides and mineral acids.

Identification A. Causes a rise of blood glucose concentration when injected as directed under the Assay.

B. Dissolve 5 mg in 3.5 ml of 0.01M *hydrochloric acid*, add 1 ml of a 10% w/v solution of *urea* and 0.5 ml of *mixed phosphate buffer pH 6.8*; a white crystalline precipitate is produced. Warm to about 50° until a clear solution is produced and allow to stand for 24 hours at room temperature; rhombic, dodecahedral crystals, visible under a microscope, are produced.

Light absorption *Absorbance* of a 0.025% w/v solution in 0.01M *hydrochloric acid* at the maximum at 276 nm, 0.52 to 0.62, Appendix II B.

Zinc Not more than 0.15% of Zn when determined by the following method. Prepare a 0.1% w/v solution in 0.01M *hydrochloric acid* and determine by *atomic absorption spectrophotometry*, Appendix II D, measuring at 214 nm and using *zinc solution ASp*, diluted if necessary with *water*, for the standard solutions.

Nitrogen 16.0 to 18.5%, calculated with reference to the dried substance, when determined by Method V, Appendix VIII H. Use 1 to 3 mg.

Related peptides Carry out Method I for *polyacrylamide gel electrophoresis*, Appendix III F, using the following solutions. Solutions (1) to (5) contains 2, 4, 6, 8 and 10 milliUnits respectively of the Standard Preparation of glucagon in 50 µl of 0.01M *sodium hydroxide*. Solutions (6) and (7) contain 50 µg and 1 µg respectively of the substance being examined in 50 µl of 0.01M *sodium hydroxide*. After electrophoresis and staining, evaluate the gels on a cold light illuminator.

In the gel prepared with solution (7) the intensity of any band, other than the band due to bromophenol blue, that migrates between two and three times the distance of the principal band does not exceed that of the principal band in the gel prepared with solution (1). In the gel prepared with solution (6) the intensity of any band that migrates immediately ahead of the principal band does not exceed that of the principal band in the gel prepared with solution (5). The test is not valid unless a band can be detected in the gel prepared with solution (1) and a gradation is observed in the intensity of staining of the gels prepared with solutions (1) to (5).

Loss on drying When dried to constant weight at 105°, loses not more than 10% of its weight. Use 0.25 g.

Assay Carry out the *biological assay of glucagon*, Appendix XIV C13. The estimated potency is not less than 80% and not more than 125% of the stated potency. The fiducial limits of error are not less than 64% and not more than 156% of the stated potency.

Storage Glucagon should be kept in a well-closed glass or metal container and stored at a temperature of 2° to 8°.

Labelling The label states (1) the number of Units in the container; (2) the number of Units per mg; (3) the date after which the material is not intended to be used; (4) the conditions under which it should be stored.

Preparation
Glucagon Injection

Action and use Hyperglycaemic hormone.

Anhydrous Glucose ☆
Anhydrous Glucose for Parenteral Use

C₆H₁₂O₆   180.2   *50-99-7*

$C_6H_{12}O_6$ 180.2   *50-99-7*

Anhydrous Glucose★ is D–(+)-glucopyranose.

Characteristics A white, crystalline powder; odourless; taste, sweet.

Solubility Soluble in 1 part of *water*; sparingly soluble in *ethanol (96%)*.

Identification A. Complies with the test for Specific optical rotation.
B. Carry out the method for *thin-layer chromatography*, Appendix III A, using *silica gel G* as the coating substance and a mixture of 50 volumes of *1,2-dichloroethane*, 25 volumes of *anhydrous glacial acetic acid*, 15 volumes of *methanol* and 10 volumes of *water*, accurately measured, as the mobile phase. Apply separately to the chromatoplate 2 μl of each of three solutions in *methanol (60%)* containing (1) 0.05% w/v of the substance being examined, (2) 0.05% w/v of *glucose EPCRS* and (3) 0.05% w/v each of *fructose EPCRS*, *glucose EPCRS*, *lactose EPCRS* and *sucrose EPCRS*. Thoroughly dry the points of application before developing the chromatogram. After removal of the plate, dry it in a current of warm air and repeat the development with fresh mobile phase. After removal of the plate, dry it in a current of warm air, spray evenly with a 5% w/v solution of *thymol* in *ethanolic sulphuric acid (5%)* and heat at 130° for 10 minutes. The principal spot in the chromatogram obtained with solution (1) is similar in position, colour and size to that spot in the chromatogram obtained with solution (2). The test is not valid unless the chromatogram obtained with solution (3) shows four clearly separated principal spots.
C. Dissolve 0.1 g in 10 ml of *water*, add 3 ml of *potassium cupri-tartrate solution* and heat. A red precipitate is produced.

Acidity or alkalinity Dissolve 6 g in 25 ml of *carbon dioxide-free water* and add 0.3 ml of *dilute phenolphthalein solution*. The solution is colourless and not more than 0.15 ml of 0.1M *sodium hydroxide VS* is required to change the colour of the solution to pink.

Clarity, odour and colour of solution Dissolve 10.0 g in 15 ml of *water*. The solution is *clear*, Appendix IV A, odourless and not more intensely coloured than *reference solution BY₇*, Appendix IV B, Method II.

Specific optical rotation Dissolve 10 g in 80 ml of *water*, add 0.2 ml of 6M *ammonia*, allow to stand for 30 minutes and dilute to 100 ml with *water*. The *specific optical rotation* in the resulting solution is +52.5° to +53.3°, Appendix V F.

Arsenic 1.0 g complies with the *limit test for arsenic*, Appendix VII (1 ppm).

Barium To 10 ml of a 10.0% w/v solution in *distilled water* (solution A) add 1 ml of 1M *sulphuric acid*. Examine immediately and after 1 hour. Any opalescence in the solution is not more intense than that in a mixture of 10 ml of solution A and 1 ml of *water*.

Calcium 5 ml of solution A diluted to 15 ml with *distilled water* complies with the *limit test for calcium*, Appendix VII (200 ppm).

Lead Complies with *limit test A for lead in sugars*, Appendix VII (0.5 ppm).

Chloride 4 ml of solution A diluted to 15 ml with *water* complies with the *limit test for chlorides*, Appendix VII (125 ppm).

Sulphate 7.5 ml of solution A diluted to 15 ml with *distilled water* complies with the *limit test for sulphates*, Appendix VII (200 ppm).

Sulphite Dissolve 5 g in *water*, add 2 ml of 0.1M *sodium hydroxide* and dilute to 50 ml with *water*. To 10 ml of the solution add 1 ml of a 31% w/v solution of *hydrochloric acid*, 2 ml of *faded magenta solution* and 2 ml of a 0.5% v/v solution of *formaldehyde*. Allow to stand for 30 minutes and measure the *absorbance* at the maximum at 583 nm, Appendix II B. The absorbance is not more than that of a standard prepared in the following manner. To 3 ml of a 0.0076% w/v solution of *sodium metabisulphite* add 4 ml of 0.1M *sodium hydroxide* and dilute to 100 ml with *water*. Treat 10 ml of the resulting solution in the same manner as the test solution beginning at the words 'add 1 ml of a 31% w/v solution . . .'. Use in the reference cell for both measurements a solution prepared in the same manner using 10 ml of *water*.

Foreign sugars, soluble starch and dextrins Boil 1.0 g in 30 ml of *ethanol (90%)* to dissolve. The appearance of the solution does not change on cooling.

Sulphated ash Not more than 0.1% when determined by the following method. Dissolve 5 g in 5 ml of *water*, add 2 ml of *sulphuric acid*, evaporate to dryness and ignite to constant weight. If necessary, repeat the heating with the sulphuric acid.

Water Not more than 1.0% w/w, Appendix IX C. Use 0.5 g.

Storage Anhydrous Glucose should be kept in a well-closed container.

Preparations
Glucose Intravenous Infusion
Potassium Chloride and Glucose Intravenous Infusion

Potassium Chloride, Sodium Chloride and Glucose
  Intravenous Infusion
Sodium Chloride and Glucose Intravenous Infusion
Oral Rehydration Salts

The title of the monograph in the European
Pharmacopœia is Anhydrous Dextrose.

*In certain states party to the Convention on the Elaboration of a
European Pharmacopœia, Anhydrous Glucose intended for use in
large-volume preparations for parenteral use may be required to
comply with the *test for pyrogens*, Appendix XIV K, using per kg
of the rabbit's weight 10 ml of a solution containing 50 mg
per ml.

Glucose ☆
Dextrose Monohydrate for Parenteral Use; Glucose for
Parenteral Use

$C_6H_{12}O_6,H_2O$ 198.2   *5996-10-1*

Glucose★ is D-(+)-glucopyranose monohydrate.

Characteristics A white, crystalline powder; odourless.

Solubility Soluble in 1 part of *water*; sparingly soluble in
ethanol (96%).

**Identification; Acidity or alkalinity; Clarity, odour and
colour of solution; Specific optical rotation; Arsenic;
Barium; Calcium; Lead; Chloride; Sulphate; Sulphite;
Foreign sugars, soluble starch and dextrins; Sulphated
ash** Complies with the requirements stated under
Anhydrous Glucose.

Water 7.0 to 9.5%, Appendix IX C. Use 0.5 g.

Storage Glucose should be kept in a well-closed container.

Preparations
Glucose Intravenous Infusion
Potassium Chloride and Glucose Intravenous Infusion
Potassium Chloride, Sodium Chloride and Glucose
  Intravenous Infusion
Sodium Chloride and Glucose Intravenous Infusion
Oral Rehydration Salts

When Anhydrous Glucose is prescribed or demanded,
Anhydrous Glucose or an equivalent amount of Glucose
may be dispensed or supplied.

The title of the monograph in the European
Pharmacopœia is Dextrose Monohydrate.

*In certain states party to the Convention on the Elaboration of a
European Pharmacopœia, Glucose intended for use in large-
volume preparations for parenteral use may be required to
comply with the *test for pyrogens*, Appendix XIV K, using per kg
of the rabbit's weight 10 ml of a solution containing 55 mg
per ml.

Strong Glutaraldehyde Solution

CH₂·CHO
|
CH₂
|
CH₂·CHO

$C_5H_8O_2$ 100.1   *111-30-8 (anhydrous)*

Strong Glutaraldehyde Solution is an aqueous
solution of glutaraldehyde (pentanedial). It
contains not less than 47.0 per cent and not
more than 53.0 per cent w/w of glutaraldehyde,
$C_5H_8O_2$.

Characteristics A colourless or almost colourless solution.

Identification A. Heat 1 ml with 10 ml of a solution
containing 1 g of *hydroxylamine hydrochloride* and 2 g of
sodium acetate in *water* on a water-bath for 10 minutes,
allow to cool and filter. The *melting point* of the residue,
after washing with *water* and drying at 105°, is about 178°,
Appendix V A.

B. Add 0.05 ml to 2 ml of *ammoniacal silver nitrate solution*
and mix gently for a few minutes. Silver is deposited.

Acidity Dilute 10 ml with 10 ml of *carbon dioxide-free
water* and titrate with 0.1M *sodium hydroxide VS* using
bromothymol blue solution as indicator. Not more than
5.0 ml of 0.1M *sodium hydroxide VS* is required to change
the colour of the solution.

Clarity and colour of solution Dilute 1 volume with 4
volumes of *water*. The resulting solution is *clear*,
Appendix IV A, and not more intensely coloured than
reference solution B₆, Appendix IV B, Method I.

Weight per ml 1.126 to 1.134 g, Appendix V G.

Assay Dissolve 4 g in 100 ml of a 7% w/v solution of
hydroxylamine hydrochloride previously neutralised to
bromophenol blue solution with 1M *sodium hydroxide VS* and
allow to stand for 30 minutes. Add 20 ml of *petroleum
spirit (boiling range, 40° to 60°)* and titrate with 1M *sodium
hydroxide VS* until the colour of the aqueous phase
corresponds to that of a 7% w/v solution of *hydroxylamine
hydrochloride* previously neutralised to *bromophenol blue
solution* with 1M *sodium hydroxide VS*. Each ml of 1M
sodium hydroxide VS is equivalent to 0.05005 g of $C_5H_8O_2$.

Storage Strong Glutaraldehyde Solution should be kept in
a well-closed container and stored at a temperature not
exceeding 15°.

Preparation
Glutaraldehyde Solution

Action and use Used in treatment of warts.

Glutethimide

$C_{13}H_{15}NO_2$ 217.3   *77-21-4*

Glutethimide is 2-ethyl-2-phenylglutarimide. It
contains not less than 99.0 per cent and not
more than 100.5 per cent of $C_{13}H_{15}NO_2$, calculated with reference to the dried substance.

Characteristics Colourless crystals or a white powder;
odourless or almost odourless.

Solubility Practically insoluble in *water*; soluble in 5 parts
of *ethanol (96%)*, in less than 1 part of *chloroform* and in
12 parts of *ether*.

Identification A. The *light absorption*, Appendix II B, in
the range 230 to 350 nm of a 0.06% w/v solution in
absolute ethanol exhibits three maxima, at 252, 258 and
264 nm. The *absorbance* at 252 nm is about 1.0, at
258 nm, about 1.1 and at 264 nm, about 0.86.

B. Heat 1 g with 5 ml of 5M *sodium hydroxide* and 15 ml of
water on a water-bath for 30 minutes, cool and acidify to
litmus paper with 2M *hydrochloric acid*. The *melting point* of

the precipitate, after washing with *water* and drying at 100°, is about 159°, Appendix V A.

C. Shake 10 mg with 2 ml of *water*, 0.1 g of *hydroxylamine hydrochloride* and 1 ml of *5M sodium hydroxide*, allow to stand for 10 minutes and add 2 ml of *2M hydrochloric acid* and 1 ml of *iron(III) chloride test-solution*. A deep brownish-red colour is produced.

Melting point 85° to 88°, Appendix V A.

Related substances Carry out the method for *thin-layer chromatography*, Appendix III A, using *silica gel G* as the coating substance and a mixture of 90 volumes of *ethyl acetate*, 5 volumes of *methanol* and 5 volumes of *water* as the mobile phase. Apply separately to the chromatoplate 10 µl of each of two solutions of the substance being examined in *methanol* containing (1) 5.0% w/v and (2) 0.025% w/v. After removal of the plate, allow it to dry in air, place in a tank containing chlorine prepared by the addition of *hydrochloric acid* to a 5% w/v solution of *potassium permanganate* and allow to stand for 1 minute. Dry the plate in a current of warm air and spray with *potassium iodide and starch solution*. Any *secondary spot* in the chromatogram obtained with solution (1) is not more intense than the spot in the chromatogram obtained with solution (2).

Loss on drying When dried over *phosphorus pentoxide* at a pressure not exceeding 0.7 kPa for 24 hours, loses not more than 1.0% of its weight. Use 1 g.

Sulphated ash Not more than 0.1%, Appendix IX A.

Assay Boil 0.5 g with 10 ml of *0.5M ethanolic potassium hydroxide VS* under a reflux condenser on a water-bath for 1 hour, cool and titrate with *0.2M hydrochloric acid VS* using *phenolphthalein solution* as indicator. Repeat the operation without the substance being examined. The difference between the titrations represents the amount of alkali required. Each ml of *0.2M hydrochloric acid VS* is equivalent to 0.04345 g of $C_{13}H_{15}NO_2$.

Storage Glutethimide should be protected from light.

Action and use Hypnotic.

Glycerol ☆
Glycerin

```
CH₂OH
|
CHOH
|
CH₂OH
```

$C_3H_8O_3$ 92.1   *56-81-5*

Glycerol is propane-1,2,3-triol. It contains not less than 98.0 per cent and not more than 101.0 per cent of $C_3H_8O_3$, calculated with reference to the anhydrous substance.

Characteristics A clear, colourless or almost colourless, syrupy liquid; slippery to the touch; hygroscopic.

Solubility Miscible with *water* and with *ethanol (96%)*; slightly soluble in *acetone*; practically insoluble in *ether* and in fixed and essential oils.

Identification *Test A may be omitted if tests B, C and D are carried out. Tests B and C may be omitted if tests A and D are carried out.*

A. To 5 ml add 1 ml of *water* and mix carefully. The *infra-red absorption spectrum* of the resulting solution, Appendix II A, is concordant with the European Pharmacopœia reference spectrum of glycerol (85 per cent).

B. Mix 1 ml with 0.5 ml of *nitric acid* and superimpose 0.5 ml of a 10.6% w/v solution of *potassium dichromate*; a blue ring is produced at the interface of the two liquids. Allow to stand for 10 minutes; the blue colour does not diffuse into the lower layer.

C. Heat 1 ml with 2 g of *potassium hydrogen sulphate* in an evaporating dish. Irritant, lachrymatory vapours are evolved which blacken filter paper moistened with *alkaline potassium mercuri-iodide reagent*.

D. Complies with the test for Refractive index.

Acidity To 50 ml of a 50.0% w/v solution in *carbon dioxide-free water* (solution A) add 0.5 ml of *dilute phenolphthalein solution*. The solution is colourless and not more than 0.2 ml of *0.1M sodium hydroxide VS* is required to produce a pink colour. Reserve the final solution for the test for Ester.

Clarity and colour of solution Solution A is *clear*, Appendix IV A. Dilute 10 ml of solution A to 25 ml with *water*. The solution is *colourless*, Appendix IV B, Method II.

Refractive index 1.470 to 1.475, Appendix V E.

Heavy metals Dilute 6 ml of solution A to 15 ml with *water*. 12 ml of the resulting solution complies with *limit test A for heavy metals*, Appendix VII (5 ppm). Use *lead standard solution (1 ppm Pb)* to prepare the standard.

Chloride 1 ml of solution A diluted to 15 ml with *water* complies with the *limit test for chlorides*, Appendix VII (10 ppm). Use 1 ml of *chloride standard solution (5 ppm Cl)* diluted to 15 ml with *water* to prepare the standard.

Aldehydes and reducing substances To 7.5 ml of solution A in a glass-stoppered flask add 7.5 ml of *water* and 1 ml of *decolorised pararosaniline solution*, close the flask and allow to stand for 1 hour. Any colour produced is not more intense than that produced in a standard prepared at the same time and in the same manner but using 75 ml of *formaldehyde standard solution (5 ppm CH₂O)* in place of solution A. The test is not valid unless the standard solution is pink.

Ester Add *0.1M sodium hydroxide VS* to the solution reserved in the test for Acidity until a total of 10.0 ml has been added and boil under a reflux condenser for 5 minutes. Cool, add 0.5 ml of *dilute phenolphthalein solution* and titrate with *0.1M hydrochloric acid VS*. Not less than 8.0 ml of *0.1M hydrochloric acid VS* is required to decolorise the solution.

Halogenated compounds To 10 ml of solution A add 1 ml of *2M sodium hydroxide*, 5 ml of *water* and 50 mg of *Raney nickel catalyst*. Heat the mixture on a water-bath for 10 minutes, allow to cool and filter. Wash the flask and the filter with *water* until 25 ml of filtrate is obtained. To 5 ml of the filtrate add 4 ml of *ethanol (96%)*, 2.5 ml of *water*, 0.5 ml of *nitric acid* and 0.05 ml of *0.1M silver nitrate* and mix. After 2 minutes any opalescence produced is not more intense than that produced in a standard prepared at the same time by mixing 7.0 ml of *chloride standard solution (5 ppm Cl)*, 4 ml of *ethanol (96%)*, 0.5 ml of *water*, 0.5 ml of *nitric acid* and 0.05 ml of *0.1M silver nitrate* (35 ppm).

Sugars Heat 10 ml of solution A with 1 ml of *1M sulphuric acid* on a water-bath for 5 minutes. Add 2 ml of *2M* *sodium hydroxide (carbonate-free)* and 1 ml of 0.5M *copper(II) sulphate*; a clear blue solution is produced. Continue heating on the water-bath for 5 minutes; the solution remains blue and no precipitate is produced.

Sulphated ash Not more than 0.01%, Appendix IX A, Method II, after heating to boiling and igniting. Use 5 g.

Water Not more than 2.0%, Appendix IX C. Use 1.5 g.

Assay Thoroughly mix 0.1 g with 45 ml of *water*, add 25 ml of a 2.14% w/v solution of *sodium metaperiodate* and 1 ml of 1M *sulphuric acid VS* and allow to stand for 15 minutes. Add 5 ml of a 50% w/v solution of *ethane-1,2-diol* and titrate with 0.1M *sodium hydroxide VS* using 0.5 ml of *dilute phenolphthalein solution* as indicator. Repeat the procedure without the substance being examined. The difference between the titrations represents the amount of sodium hydroxide required. Each ml of 0.1M *sodium hydroxide VS* is equivalent to 0.00921 g of $C_3H_8O_3$.

Storage Glycerol should be kept in an airtight container.

Preparation

Glycerol Suppositories

Action and use Lubricant; laxative.

Glycerol (85 per cent) ☆

Glycerol (85 per cent) contains not less than 83.5 per cent w/w and not more than 88.5 per cent w/w of propane-1,2,3-triol, $C_3H_8O_3$.

Characteristics A clear, colourless or almost colourless, syrupy liquid; slippery to the touch; hygroscopic.

Solubility Miscible with *water* and with *ethanol (96%)*; slightly soluble in *acetone*; practically insoluble in *ether* and in fixed and essential oils.

Glycerol (85 per cent) complies with the requirements for Glycerol with the following modifications.

Identification A. The *infra-red absorption spectrum*, Appendix II A, is concordant with the European Pharmacopœia reference spectrum of glycerol (85 per cent).

Acidity; Clarity and colour of solution; Heavy metals; Chloride; Aldehydes and reducing substances; Halogenated compounds; Sugars Use as solution A a solution prepared by diluting 58.0 g of the substance being examined to 100.0 ml with *carbon dioxide-free water*.

Refractive index 1.449 to 1.455, Appendix V E.

Water 12.0 to 16.0%, Appendix IX C. Use 0.2 g.

Assay Carry out the Assay described under Glycerol.

Storage Glycerol (85 per cent) should be kept in an airtight container.

Glyceryl Monostearate 40-50 ☆

31566-31-1

Glyceryl Monostearate 40-50 is a mixture of monoacylglycerols, mostly stearoyl- and palmitoylglycerol, together with variable quantities of di- and triacylglycerols. It contains not less than 40.0 per cent and not more than 50.0 per cent of 1-monoacylglycerols, calculated as 2,3-dihydroxypropyl stearate, $C_{21}H_{42}O_4$, and not more than 6.0 per cent of free glycerol.

Characteristics A white or almost white, hard, waxy mass or unctuous powder or flakes.

Solubility Practically insoluble in *water*; soluble in *ether* and, at 60°, in *ethanol (96%)*.

Identification A. Heat 1 g with 2 g of *potassium hydrogen sulphate* in an evaporating dish. Irritant, lachrymatory vapours are evolved which darken filter paper moistened with *alkaline potassium mercuri-iodide reagent*.

B. Heat 2.5 g with 40 ml of *ethanolic potassium hydroxide solution* under a reflux condenser on a water-bath for 30 minutes. Add 30 ml of *water*, evaporate the ethanol, acidify the hot mixture with 15 ml of 2M *hydrochloric acid*, cool and extract with 50 ml of *ether*. Wash the ether layer with three 10-ml quantities of a 20% w/v solution of *sodium chloride*, dry the ether layer over *anhydrous sodium sulphate* and filter. Evaporate the solvent and dry the residue under reduced pressure. The *melting point* of the residue, after melting, introducing it into capillary tubes and allowing to stand for 24 hours in a desiccator, is not less than 53°, Appendix V A, Method IV.

C. The *melting point*, Appendix V A, Method IV, is 54° to 64°. Melt the substance being examined, introduce it into the capillary tubes and allow to stand for 24 hours in a desiccator.

Acid value Not more than 3.0, Appendix X B. Use 1 g.

Iodine value Not more than 3.0 (*iodine bromide method*), Appendix X E.

Saponification value 158 to 177, Appendix X G, Method II.

Sulphated ash Not more than 0.1%, Appendix IX A, Method II, using *sulphuric acid* in place of 1M sulphuric acid. Use 1 g.

Water Not more than 2.0%, Appendix IX C. Use 0.5 g and a mixture of 10 ml of *anhydrous methanol* and 10 ml of *chloroform*.

Assay *For free glycerol* Dissolve 0.4 g in 50 ml of *dichloromethane* in a ground-glass stoppered separating funnel, cool if necessary, add 25 ml of *water* and shake vigorously for 1 minute; add 0.2 ml of *glacial acetic acid*, if necessary, to break the emulsion. Repeat the extraction a further three times using 25-, 20- and 20-ml quantities of *water* and reserve the dichloromethane solution. Filter the combined aqueous extracts through a filter paper moistened with *water*, wash the filter with two 5-ml quantities of *water* and dilute the combined filtrate and washings to 100 ml with *water*. To 50 ml of the solution add 25 ml of *periodic—acetic acid solution*, shaking cautiously. Allow to stand for 30 minutes at 25° to 30° and add 100 ml of *water* and 12 ml of 1M *potassium iodide*. Titrate the liberated iodine with 0.1M *sodium thiosulphate VS* using 1 ml of *starch solution* as indicator. Repeat the determination using 50 ml of *water* in place of the 50 ml of solution being examined. The difference between the titrations represents the amount of sodium thiosulphate required. Each ml of 0.1M *sodium thiosulphate VS* is equivalent to 0.0023 g of glycerol.

For 1-monoacylglycerol Filter the dichloromethane solution reserved in the Assay for free glycerol through absorbent cotton. Wash the separating funnel and the filter with three 5-ml quantities of *dichloromethane*. Dilute the combined filtrate and washings to 100 ml with *dichloromethane* and carry out the Assay for free glycerol using 50 ml of the dichloromethane solution and beginning at the words 'add 25 ml of *periodic—acetic acid solution . . .*'. Each ml of 0.1M *sodium thiosulphate VS* is equivalent to 0.0179 g of 1-monoacylglycerols, calculated as $C_{21}H_{42}O_4$. The quantity of 0.1M *sodium thiosulphate VS* used in the assay is not less than 85% of the quantity of sodium thiosulphate used in the blank assay.

Storage Glyceryl Monostearate 40-50 should be kept in an airtight container and protected from light.

Action and use Pharmaceutical aid.

Self-emulsifying Glyceryl Monostearate

Self-emulsifying Monostearin; Self-emulsifying Mono- and Diglycerides of Food Fatty Acids

Self-emulsifying Glyceryl Monostearate is a mixture consisting principally of mono-, di- and triglycerides of stearic and palmitic acids and of minor proportions of other fatty acids; it may also contain free glycerol, free fatty acids and soap. It contains not less than 30.0 per cent of monoglycerides, calculated as $C_{21}H_{42}O_4$, not more than 7.0 per cent of free glycerol, calculated as $C_3H_8O_3$, and not more than 6.0 per cent of soap, calculated as sodium oleate, $C_{18}H_{33}NaO_2$, all calculated with reference to the anhydrous substance.

Characteristics A white to cream-coloured, hard, waxy solid; odour, faint and fatty.

Solubility Dispersible in hot *water*; soluble in hot *absolute ethanol*, in hot *liquid paraffin* and, subject to turbidity at concentrations below 20%, in hot vegetable oils.

Acid value Not more than 6, Appendix X B.

Iodine value Not more than 3 (*iodine monochloride method*), Appendix X E.

Alkalinity Shake 1 g with 20 ml of hot *carbon dioxide-free water* and allow to cool with continuous shaking. The pH of the aqueous layer is 8.0 to 10.0, Appendix V L.

Heavy metals 2.0 g complies with *limit test C for heavy metals*, Appendix VII (10 ppm). Use 2 ml of *lead standard solution (10 ppm Pb)* to prepare the standard.

Water Not more than 2.0% w/w, Appendix IX C. Use 0.5 g and a mixture of 10 ml of *anhydrous methanol* and 10 ml of anhydrous *chloroform*.

Assay *For free glycerol* Carry out the Assay for free glycerol described under Glyceryl Monostearate 40-50.

For monoglycerides Filter the chloroform solution reserved in the Assay for free glycerol through absorbent cotton. Wash the separating funnel and the filter with three 5-ml quantities of *chloroform*. Dilute the combined filtrate and washings to 100 ml with *chloroform* and carry out the Assay for free glycerol described under Glyceryl Monostearate 40-50 using 50 ml of the chloroform solution and beginning at the words 'add 25 ml of *periodic—acetic acid solution . . .*'. Each ml of 0.1M *sodium thiosulphate VS* is equivalent to 0.01793 g of monoglycerides, calculated as $C_{21}H_{42}O_4$. The quantity of 0.1M *sodium thiosulphate VS* used in the assay is not less

than 85% of the quantity of thiosulphate used in the blank assay.

For soap Add 10 g to a mixture of 60 ml of *acetone* and 0.15 ml of a 0.5% w/v solution of *bromophenol blue* in a mixture of 20 ml of *ethanol (20%)* and 80 ml of *water*, the solvent having been previously neutralised with 0.1M *hydrochloric acid VS* or 0.1M *sodium hydroxide VS*. Warm gently on a water-bath until solution is complete and titrate with 0.1M *hydrochloric acid VS* until the blue colour is discharged. Allow to stand for 20 minutes, warm until any solidified matter has redissolved and, if the blue colour reappears, continue the titration. Each ml of 0.1M *hydrochloric acid VS* is equivalent to 0.03045 g of $C_{18}H_{33}NaO_2$.

Action and use Pharmaceutical aid.

Concentrated Glyceryl Trinitrate Solution

Concentrated Glyceryl Trinitrate Solution is a solution of propane-1,2,3-triol trinitrate in Ethanol (96 per cent). It contains not less than 9.0 per cent w/v and not more than 11.0 per cent w/v of $C_3H_5N_3O_9$.

CAUTION Undiluted glyceryl trinitrate can be exploded by percussion or excessive heat. Appropriate precautions should be exercised and only exceedingly small amounts should be isolated.

Characteristics A clear, colourless to pale yellow solution, miscible with *acetone* and with *ether*.

Identification A. Carry out the procedure described under Related substances but using *toluene* as the mobile phase and the following solutions. For solution (1) dilute the solution being examined with *acetone* to contain 0.050% w/v of glyceryl trinitrate. For solution (2) extract one powdered *glyceryl trinitrate tablet 0.5 mg BPCRS* with 1 ml of *acetone* and centrifuge. The spot in the chromatogram obtained with solution (1) corresponds to that in the chromatogram obtained with solution (2).
B. To 1 ml add 200 ml of *ether*, evaporate 6 ml of the resulting solution to dryness and dissolve the residue in 0.2 ml of *sulphuric acid* containing a trace of *diphenylamine*. An intense blue colour is produced.

Weight per ml 0.830 to 0.850 g, Appendix V G.

Inorganic nitrates Carry out the method for *thin-layer chromatography*, Appendix III A, using *silica gel H* as the coating substance and a mixture of 60 volumes of *toluene*, 30 volumes of *acetone* and 15 volumes of *glacial acetic acid* as the mobile phase. Apply separately to the chromato-plate 5 µl of each of the following solutions. For solution (1) use the solution being examined. Solution (2) is a freshly prepared 0.10% w/v solution of *potassium nitrate* in *ethanol (90%)*. After removal of the plate, dry it in a stream of air and spray with *diphenylamine solution*. Any spot corresponding to nitrate in the chromatogram obtained with solution (1) is not more intense than the spot in the chromatogram obtained with solution (2).

Related substances Carry out the method for *thin-layer chromatography*, Appendix III A, using *silica gel G* as the coating substance and a mixture of 80 volumes of *toluene* and 20 volumes of *ethyl acetate* as the mobile phase. Apply separately to the chromatoplate 5 µl of each of the following solutions. For solution (1) use the solution being examined. For solution (2) dilute 1 volume of solution (1) to 100 volumes with *acetone*. After removal of the plate, dry it in a stream of air and spray with *diphenylamine solution*. Any *secondary spot* in the chromatogram obtained with solution (1) is not more intense than the spot in the chromatogram obtained with solution (2).

Assay Dilute 1 ml to 50 ml with a 90% v/v solution of *glacial acetic acid* and dilute 10 ml of this solution to 100 ml with the same solvent. To 1 ml of the resulting solution add 2 ml of *phenoldisulphonic acid solution*, mix and allow to stand for 15 minutes. Add 8 ml of *water*, mix well, allow to cool and add slowly, with swirling, 10 ml of 13.5M *ammonia*. Cool and dilute to 20 ml with *water*. Measure the *absorbance* of the resulting solution at 405 nm, Appendix II B, using in the reference cell 1 ml of a 90% v/v solution of *glacial acetic acid* treated in the same manner, beginning at the words 'add 2 ml of *phenoldisulphonic acid solution* . . .'. Dissolve 0.1335 g of *potassium nitrate* previously dried at 105° in sufficient *water* to produce 50 ml; to 10 ml add sufficient *glacial acetic acid* to produce 100 ml. Using 1 ml of this solution, repeat the procedure beginning at the words 'add 2 ml of *phenoldisulphonic acid solution* . . .'. Calculate the content of $C_3H_5N_3O_9$ from the values of the absorbances so obtained. Each ml of the potassium nitrate solution is equivalent to 0.2000 mg of $C_3H_5N_3O_9$.

Storage Concentrated Glyceryl Trinitrate Solution should be kept in a well-closed container, protected from light and stored at a temperature of 8° to 15°.

Preparation
Glyceryl Trinitrate Tablets

Action and use Vasodilator.

Glycine

H$_2$NCH$_2$·CO$_2$H

$C_2H_5NO_2$ 75.07   *56-40-6*

Glycine contains not less than 99.0 per cent and not more than 101.0 per cent of $C_2H_5NO_2$, calculated with reference to the dried substance.

Characteristics A white crystalline powder; odourless or almost odourless.

Solubility Soluble in 4 parts of *water*; very slightly soluble in *ethanol (96%)* and in *ether*.

Identification A. The *infra-red absorption spectrum*, Appendix II A, is concordant with the *reference spectrum* of glycine.
B. To 5 ml of a 10.0% w/v solution (solution A) add 0.25 ml of 2M *hydrochloric acid* and 1 ml of *sodium nitrite solution*. A gas is evolved vigorously.
C. To 2 ml of solution A add 1 ml of *iron(III) chloride test-solution*. A red colour is produced which is discharged by an excess of hydrochloric acid and is restored by an excess of ammonia.
D. To 2 ml of solution A add 0.05 ml of *liquefied phenol*, shake and add carefully without shaking 5 ml of *dilute sodium hypochlorite solution*. A blue colour is produced.

Acidity pH of a 5% w/v solution, 5.9 to 6.3, Appendix V L.

Ammonium compounds Dissolve 0.20 g in 70 ml of *water* in an ammonia-distillation apparatus, add 25 ml of *nitrogen-free sodium hydroxide solution* and distil into 2 ml of a saturated solution of *boric acid* until 50 ml is obtained. Add 2 ml of *ammonia-free sodium hydroxide solution* and 2 ml of *alkaline potassium mercuri-iodide reagent*. Any colour is not more intense than that produced by treating 70 ml of *water* containing 4 ml of *ammonia standard solution (10 ppm NH$_4$)* in the same manner, beginning at the words 'add 25 ml of . . .' (200 ppm).

Chloride 15 ml of a 5.0% w/v solution complies with the *limit test for chlorides*, Appendix VII (70 ppm).

Heavy metals 12 ml of solution A complies with *limit test A for heavy metals*, Appendix VII (10 ppm). Use *lead standard solution (1 ppm Pb)* to prepare the standard.

Readily carbonisable substances Dissolve 0.5 g in 5 ml of *sulphuric acid*. The solution is colourless.

Loss on drying When dried to constant weight at 105°, loses not more than 0.2% of its weight. Use 1 g.

Sulphated ash Not more than 0.1%, Appendix IX A.

Assay Carry out Method I for *non-aqueous titration*, Appendix VIII A, using 0.15 g and determining the end-point potentiometrically. Each ml of 0.1M *perchloric acid VS* is equivalent to 0.007507 g of $C_2H_5NO_2$.

Preparation
Glycine Irrigation Solution

Action and use Bladder irrigation during surgery.

Gonadorelin

Glu—His—Trp—Ser—Tyr—Gly—Leu—Arg—Pro—Gly—NH₂

$C_{55}H_{75}N_{17}O_{13}$ 1182   *33515-09-2*

Gonadorelin is a hypothalamic peptide that releases follicle stimulating hormone and luteinising hormone from the pituitary. It contains not less than 840 Units per mg, calculated with reference to the peptide content. It is obtained by synthesis and is available in the acetate or chloride form.

Characteristics A white to faintly yellowish-white powder.

Solubility Soluble in 25 parts of *water*, in 50 parts of *methanol* and in 25 parts of a 1% v/v solution of *glacial acetic acid*.

Identification A. Causes depletion of the ovarian ascorbic acid content of pseudo-pregnant rats when administered as directed in the Assay.
B. In tests A and B for Related peptides, the principal spot in the chromatogram obtained with solution (2) corresponds to that in the chromatogram obtained with solution (4).

Clarity and colour of solution A 1.0% w/v solution is *clear*, Appendix IV A, Method I, and not more intensely coloured than *reference solution Y$_5$*, Appendix IV B, Method II.

Light absorption *Absorbance* of a 0.01% w/v solution at the maximum at 278 nm, 0.55 to 0.59, Appendix II B, calculated with reference to the peptide content.

Specific optical rotation In a 1% w/v solution containing 1% v/v of *glacial acetic acid*, −54° to −63°, Appendix V F, calculated with reference to the peptide content.

Acetic acid Not more than 6.0% w/w when determined by the method for *gas chromatography*, Appendix III B, using solutions in *water* containing (1) 0.1% w/v of *glacial acetic acid* and 0.1% v/v of *1,4-dioxan* (internal standard), (2) 2.0% w/v of the substance being examined and (3) 2.0% w/v of the substance being examined and 0.1% v/v of the internal standard.

The chromatographic procedure may be carried out using a glass column (2 m × 2 mm) packed with porous polymer beads (100 to 120 mesh) (Porapak Q is suitable) and maintained at 150°.

Amino acids Carry out the method for *amino acid analysis*, Appendix III G, using 2.5 mg. Use 0.03% w/v of DL-*norleucine* (internal standard) and heat for 24 hours. Express the content of each amino acid in moles and calculate the relative proportions of the amino acids, taking that for arginine to be equivalent to 1. The values fall within the following limits: serine 0.7 to 1.0, glutamic acid 0.9 to 1.1, proline 0.8 to 1.2, glycine 1.8 to 2.2, leucine 0.9 to 1.1, tyrosine 0.9 to 1.1, histidine 0.9 to 1.1. Not more than traces of other amino acids are present in the hydrolysate.

Chloride 0.83 mg dissolved in 15 ml of *water* complies with the *limit test for chlorides*, Appendix VII (6%).

Peptide Not less than 87% of the peptide, $C_{55}H_{75}N_{17}O_{13}$, calculated with reference to the anhydrous substance, when determined by the following method. Carry out the method for *high-performance liquid chromatography*, Appendix III D, using two solutions in a mixture of 85 volumes of 0.1M *orthophosphoric acid* adjusted to pH 3.0 with *triethylamine* and 15 volumes of *acetonitrile* containing (1) 0.01% w/v of the substance being examined and (2) 0.01% w/v of *gonadorelin BPCRS*.

The chromatographic procedure may be carried out using (a) a stainless steel column (15 cm × 4.1 mm) packed with *stationary phase C* (5 μm) (Spherisorb ODS 1 is suitable), (b) as the mobile phase with a flow rate of 1 ml per minute a mixture of 0.1M *orthophosphoric acid*, adjusted to pH 3.0 with *triethylamine*, and *acetonitrile*, the mixture being adjusted so that the retention time of gonadorelin is about 10 minutes (a mixture of 75 volumes of *orthophosphoric acid* adjusted to pH 3.0 with *triethylamine* and 25 volumes of *acetonitrile* is usually suitable) and (c) a detection wavelength of 220 nm.

Calculate the content of $C_{55}H_{75}N_{17}O_{13}$ using the declared content of $C_{55}H_{75}N_{17}O_{13}$ in *gonadorelin BPCRS*. The result obtained is not valid unless the *column efficiency* is not less than 20,000 theoretical plates per metre.

Related peptides A. Carry out the method for *thin-layer chromatography*, Appendix III A, using *silica gel G* as the coating substance and a mixture of 60 volumes of *chloroform*, 45 volumes of *methanol*, 14 volumes of *water* and 6 volumes of *glacial acetic acid* as the mobile phase. Apply separately to the chromatoplate 10 μl of each of four solutions in *water* containing (1) 1.0% w/v of the substance being examined, (2) 0.1% w/v of the substance being examined, (3) 0.020% w/v of the substance being examined and (4) 0.1% w/v of *gonadorelin BPCRS*. After removal of the plate, allow it to dry in a stream of cold air for 5 minutes. Place the plate in a closed tank of chlorine gas, prepared by addition of *hydrochloric acid* to a 5% w/v solution of *potassium permanganate* in a container placed at the bottom of the tank, and allow to stand for 2 minutes. Dry in a current of cold air until a sprayed area of the plate below the line of application gives at most a very faint blue colour with 0.05 ml of a 0.5% w/v solution of *potassium iodide* in *starch mucilage*; avoid prolonged exposure to cold air. Spray the plate with a 0.5% w/v solution of *potassium iodide* in *starch mucilage*. Any *secondary spot* in the chromatogram obtained with solution (1) is not more intense than the spot in the chromatogram obtained with solution (3).

B. Complies with test A but using a mixture of 60 volumes of *chloroform*, 45 volumes of *methanol* and 20 volumes of 13.5M *ammonia* as the mobile phase.

Water Not more than 7% w/w when determined by the following method. Use dry glassware throughout; siliconised glassware may be used. Carry out the method for *gas chromatography*, Appendix III B, using the following solutions. For solution (1) dilute 50 μl of *anhydrous methanol* (internal standard) with sufficient *anhydrous propan-2-ol* to produce 100 ml. For solution (2) dissolve 4 mg of the substance being examined in 1 ml of *anhydrous propan-2-ol*. For solution (3) dissolve 4 mg of the substance being examined in 1 ml of solution (1). For solution (4) add 10 μl of *water* to 50 μl of solution (1).

The chromatographic procedure may be carried out using (a) a stainless steel column (1 m × 2 mm) packed with porous polymer beads (Chromosorb 102 is suitable) (60 to 80 mesh) and maintained at 120°, (b) helium as the carrier gas and (c) a thermal conductivity detector maintained at 150°.

From the chromatograms obtained and taking into account any water detectable in solution (1), calculate the percentage w/w of water taking 0.9972 g as its weight per ml at 20°.

Assay Carry out the *biological assay of gonadorelin*, Appendix XIV C6. The estimated potency is not less than 80% and not more than 125% of the stated potency. The fiducial limits of error are not less than 64% and not more than 156% of the stated potency.

Labelling The label states (1) the number of Units per mg; (2) the weight of the peptide in the container; (3) the date after which the material is not intended to be used; (4) the conditions under which it should be stored.

Preparation
Gonadorelin Injection

Action and use Gonadotrophin-releasing hormone.

Griseofulvin ☆

$C_{17}H_{17}ClO_6$ 352.8   *126-07-8*

Griseofulvin is (2*S*,4′*R*)-7-chloro-2′,4,6-trimethoxy-4′-methylspiro[benzofuran-2(3*H*),3′-cyclohexene]-3,6′-dione, produced by the growth of certain strains of *Penicillium griseofulvum* or obtained by any other means. It contains not less than 97.0 per cent and not more than 102.0 per cent of $C_{17}H_{17}ClO_6$, calculated with reference to the dried substance.

Characteristics A white to yellowish-white powder, the particles of which are generally up to 5 µm in maximum dimension, although larger particles, which may occasionally exceed 30 µm, may be present; almost odourless. It melts at about 220°.

Solubility Practically insoluble in *water*; slightly soluble in *ethanol (96%)* and in *methanol*; soluble in *chloroform*; freely soluble in *dimethylformamide* and in *1,1,2,2-tetrachloro-ethane*.

Identification A. The *infra-red absorption spectrum*, Appendix II A, is concordant with the spectrum of *griseofulvin EPCRS*.
B. Dissolve 5 mg in 1 ml of *sulphuric acid* and add 5 mg of powdered *potassium dichromate*. A red colour is produced.

Acidity Suspend 0.25 g in 20 ml of *ethanol (96%)* and titrate with 0.02M *sodium hydroxide VS* using *dilute phenolphthalein solution* as indicator. Not more than 1.0 ml of 0.02M *sodium hydroxide VS* is required to change the colour of the solution.

Clarity and colour of solution A 7.5% w/v solution in *dimethylformamide* is *clear*, Appendix IV A, and not more intensely coloured than *reference solution Y_4*, Appendix IV B, Method II.

Specific optical rotation In a 1% w/v solution in *dimethylformamide*, +354° to +364°, Appendix V F.

Matter soluble in petroleum spirit Not more than 0.2% when determined by the following method. Extract 1 g with 20 ml of *petroleum spirit (boiling range, 50° to 70°)* by boiling under a reflux condenser for 10 minutes, cool, filter, wash the filter with three 15-ml quantities of the petroleum spirit, evaporate the combined filtrate and washings to dryness and dry the residue at 100° to 105° for 1 hour.

Related substances Carry out the method for *gas chromatography*, Appendix III B, using three solutions in *acetone* containing (1) 1.0% w/v of the substance being examined and 0.020% w/v of *9,10-diphenylanthracene* (internal standard), (2) 1.0% w/v of the substance being examined and (3) 0.050% w/v of *griseofulvin EPCRS* and 0.020% w/v of the internal standard.

The chromatographic procedure may be carried out using a glass column (1 m × 4 mm) packed with *diatomaceous support* (125 to 180 mesh) (Chromosorb W is suitable) coated with 1% w/w of cyanopropyl methyl phenyl silicone fluid (OV-225 is suitable) and maintained at 250° with an inlet port temperature of 270° and a detector temperature of 300°. Continue the chromatography for three times the retention time of griseofulvin.

The chromatogram obtained with solution (2) shows a peak due to griseofulvin (retention time about 11 minutes) and may show a peak due to dechlorogriseofulvin (retention time about 0.6 times that of griseofulvin) and a peak due to dehydrogriseofulvin (retention time about 1.4 times that of griseofulvin). The ratio of the area of any peak corresponding to dechlorogriseofulvin to that of the peak due to the internal standard in the chromatogram obtained with solution (1) is less than 0.6 times the ratio of the area of the peak due to griseofulvin to that of the peak due to the internal standard in the chromatogram obtained with solution (3). The ratio of the area of any peak corresponding to dehydrogriseofulvin to that of the

peak due to the internal standard in the chromatogram obtained with solution (1) is less than 0.15 times the ratio of the area of the peak due to griseofulvin to that of the peak due to the internal standard in the chromatogram obtained with solution (3).

Loss on drying When dried to constant weight at 100° to 105°, loses not more than 1.0% of its weight. Use 1 g.

Sulphated ash Not more than 0.2%, Appendix IX A, Method II. Use 1 g.

Abnormal toxicity A suspension containing 0.1 g in 0.5 to 1 ml of *water* given by mouth to each of five mice does not cause the death of any of the mice within 48 hours.

Assay Dissolve 80 mg in sufficient *absolute ethanol* to produce 200 ml and dilute 2 ml to 100 ml with *absolute ethanol*. Measure the *absorbance* of the resulting solution at the maximum at 291 nm, Appendix II B. Calculate the content of $C_{17}H_{17}ClO_6$ taking 686 as the value of A(1%, 1 cm) at 291 nm.

Storage Griseofulvin should be kept in a well-closed container.

Preparation
Griseofulvin Tablets

Action and use Antifungal.

Guaiphenesin

OH
OCH$_2$·CH·CH$_2$OH
OMe

$C_{10}H_{14}O_4$ 198.2   *93-14-1*

Guaiphenesin is 3-(2-methoxyphenoxy)propane-1,2-diol. It contains not less than 99.0 per cent and not more than 100.5 per cent of $C_{10}H_{14}O_4$, calculated with reference to the dried substance.

Characteristics White crystals or crystalline aggregates; odourless or almost odourless.

Solubility Soluble in 33 parts of *water*, in 11 parts of *ethanol (96%)*, in 11 parts of *chloroform*, in 15 parts of *propane-1,2-diol* and, with warming, in 15 parts of *glycerol*; slightly soluble in *ether*.

Identification A. The *infra-red absorption spectrum*, Appendix II A, is concordant with the *reference spectrum* of guaiphenesin.
B. The *light absorption*, Appendix II B, in the range 230 to 350 nm of a 0.008% w/v solution exhibits a maximum only at 272 nm. The *absorbance* at 272 nm is about 0.96.
C. *Melting point*, about 82°, Appendix V A.

Acidity or alkalinity pH of a 2% w/v solution, 5.0 to 7.0, Appendix V L.

Clarity and colour of solution A 2.0% w/v solution is *clear*, Appendix IV A, and not more intensely coloured than either *reference solution BY_6* or *Y_6*, Appendix IV B, Method II.

Guaiacol Dissolve 0.4 g in *water* by warming, cool and dilute to 10 ml with the same solvent. Add 0.1 ml of a mixture of equal volumes of *iron(III) chloride solution* and *water*. After 5 minutes the colour of the resulting solution is not more intense than that of a mixture of 1.0 ml of *yellow primary solution*, 2.0 ml of *red primary solution* and 7.0 ml of 0.3M *hydrochloric acid*, Appendix IV B, Method II.

Related substances Carry out the method for *thin-layer chromatography*, Appendix III A, using *silica gel G* as the coating substance and a mixture of 80 volumes of *chloroform* and 20 volumes of *ethanol (96%)* as the mobile phase. Apply separately to the chromatoplate 10 μl of each of two solutions of the substance being examined in *chloroform* containing (1) 1.0% w/v and (2) 0.0050% w/v. After removal of the plate, allow it to dry in air and spray with a mixture of 1 volume of *formaldehyde solution* and 9 volumes of *sulphuric acid*. Any *secondary spot* in the chromatogram obtained with solution (1) is not more intense than the spot in the chromatogram obtained with solution (2).

Loss on drying When dried to constant weight over *phosphorus pentoxide* at a pressure not exceeding 0.7 kPa, loses not more than 0.5% of its weight. Use 1 g.

Sulphated ash Not more than 0.1%, Appendix IX A.

Assay Heat 2 g on a water-bath for 2 hours with 20 ml of a 15% v/v solution of *acetic anhydride* in *pyridine* taking care to avoid losses; cool, add 40 ml of *water* and titrate with 1M *sodium hydroxide VS* using a 1% w/v solution of *phenolphthalein* in *pyridine* as indicator. Repeat the titration without the substance being examined. The difference between the titrations represents the amount of acetic anhydride required. Each ml of 1M *sodium hydroxide VS* is equivalent to 0.09911 g of $C_{10}H_{14}O_4$.

Action and use Expectorant.

In some countries the material described in this monograph may be known as Guaifenesin.

Guanethidine Monosulphate ☆

$C_{10}H_{22}N_4,H_2SO_4$ 296.4   *645-43-2*

Guanethidine Monosulphate is 1-[2-(perhydro-azocin-1-yl)ethyl]guanidine sulphate (1:1). It contains not less than 99.0 per cent and not more than 101.0 per cent of $C_{10}H_{22}N_4,H_2SO_4$, calculated with reference to the dried substance.

Characteristics A colourless, crystalline powder; odourless. It melts at about 250°, with decomposition.

Solubility Soluble in 1.5 parts of *water*; practically insoluble in *ethanol (96%)*, in *chloroform* and in *ether*.

Identification A. Dissolve 25 mg in 5 ml of *water*, add 1 ml of 10M *sodium hydroxide*, 1 ml of *dilute 1-naphthol solution* and, dropwise with shaking, 0.5 ml of *dilute sodium hypochlorite solution*. A bright pink precipitate is produced which becomes violet-red on standing.
B. Dissolve 25 mg in 25 ml of *water* and add 20 ml of a 1% w/v solution of *2,4,6-trinitrophenol*. The *melting point* of

the precipitate, after washing with *water* and drying at 100° to 105°, is about 154°, Appendix V A, Method I.
C. Yields the *reactions* characteristic of sulphates, Appendix VI.

Acidity pH of a 2% w/v solution, 4.7 to 5.5, Appendix V L.

Colour of solution A 2.0% w/v solution in *carbon dioxide-free water* is not more intensely coloured than *reference solution GY₆*, Appendix IV B, Method II.

Heavy metals 2.0 g complies with *limit test C for heavy metals*, Appendix VII (10 ppm). Use 2 ml of *lead standard solution (10 ppm Pb)* to prepare the standard

Oxidisable substances Dissolve 1.0 g in 25 ml of *water* and add 25 ml of 2M *sodium hydroxide*. Allow to stand for 10 minutes, add 1 g of *potassium bromide* and 1 ml of 0.00833M *potassium bromate VS* and acidify with 30 ml of 2M *hydrochloric acid*. Mix and allow to stand for 5 minutes protected from light. Add 2 g of *potassium iodide*, shake, allow to stand for 2 minutes and titrate the liberated iodine with 0.05M *sodium thiosulphate VS* using *starch solution* as indicator. Not less than 0.3 ml of 0.05M *sodium thiosulphate VS* is required.

Loss on drying When dried to constant weight at 100° to 105°, loses not more than 0.5% of its weight. Use 1 g.

Sulphated ash Not more than 0.1%, Appendix IX A, Method II. Use 1 g.

Assay Dissolve 0.25 g in 30 ml of *anhydrous glacial acetic acid*, warming if necessary, add 15 ml of *acetic anhydride* and carry out Method I for *non-aqueous titration*, Appendix VIII A, using 0.1 ml of *brilliant green solution* as indicator and titrating until a yellowish-green colour is produced. Each ml of 0.1M *perchloric acid VS* is equivalent to 0.02964 g of $C_{10}H_{22}N_4,H_2SO_4$.

Storage Guanethidine Monosulphate should be kept in a well-closed container and protected from light.

Preparation
Guanethidine Tablets

Action and use Adrenergic neurone blocking agent.

Halibut-liver Oil

Halibut-liver Oil is the fixed oil extracted from the fresh, or suitably preserved, liver of the halibut species belonging to the genus *Hippoglossus* and refined. It contains in 1 g not less than 30,000 Units of vitamin A.

Characteristics A pale to golden-yellow liquid; odour and taste, fishy, but not rancid.

Solubility Practically insoluble in *ethanol (96%)*; miscible with *chloroform*, with *ether* and with *petroleum spirit (boiling range, 40° to 60°)*.

Acid value Not more than 2.0, Appendix X B.

Iodine value Not less than 112 (*pyridine bromide method*), Appendix X E.

Iodine value of glycerides 112 to 150 when determined by the following method. Isolate the unsaponifiable matter as described in Appendix X H, but using 1 g of the oil and evaporating the acetone, drying the residue at 80° in a current of nitrogen and omitting the final titration. Weigh the residue and immediately determine the *iodine value (pyridine bromide method)*, Appendix X E.

Calculate the iodine value of the glycerides from the expression $(100x - Sy)/(100 - S)$, where x is the iodine value of the oil, y is the iodine value of the unsaponifiable matter and S is the percentage of unsaponifiable matter in the oil.

Saponification value Not more than 180, Appendix X G.

Unsaponifiable matter Not less than 7.0%, Appendix X H.

Weight per ml 0.915 to 0.925 g, Appendix V G.

Assay Determine the content of vitamin A by the *assay of vitamin A*, Appendix VIII K.

Storage Halibut-liver Oil should be kept in a well-filled, well-closed container and protected from light.

Preparation
Halibut-liver Oil Capsules

Action and use Source of vitamin A.

Halibut-liver Oil may contain up to about 3000 Units of vitamin D activity per g. When a statement is made of the number of Units of vitamin D in Halibut-liver Oil, the Units enumerated should be the Units described under the *biological assay of antirachitic vitamin (vitamin D)*, Appendix XIV G.

Haloperidol

F—⟨◯⟩—CO·(CH₂)₃—N⟨◯⟩ OH ⟨◯⟩—Cl

$C_{21}H_{23}ClFNO_2$ 375.9   *52-86-8*

Haloperidol is 4-[4-(4-chlorophenyl)-4-hydroxy-piperidino]-4′-fluorobutyrophenone. It contains not less than 98.0 per cent and not more than 101.0 per cent of $C_{21}H_{23}ClFNO_2$, calculated with reference to the dried substance.

Characteristics A white to faintly yellowish, amorphous or crystalline powder.

Solubility Practically insoluble in *water*; soluble in 50 parts of *ethanol (96%)* and in 20 parts of *chloroform*; slightly soluble in *ether*.

Identification A. The *infra-red absorption spectrum*, Appendix II A, is concordant with the *reference spectrum* of haloperidol.
B. The *light absorption*, Appendix II B, in the range 230 to 350 nm of a 0.002% w/v solution in a mixture of 1 volume of 0.1M *hydrochloric acid* and 9 volumes of *methanol* exhibits a maximum only at 245 nm.
C. Burn 20 mg by the method for *oxygen-flask combustion*, Appendix VIII C, using 5 ml of 1.25M *sodium hydroxide* as the absorbing liquid. When the process is complete, dilute to 10 ml with *water* (solution A). Add 0.1 ml of solution A to a mixture of 0.1 ml of freshly prepared *alizarin red S solution* and 0.1 ml of *zirconyl nitrate solution*. The red colour changes to clear yellow.
D. Acidify 5 ml of solution A with 1M *sulphuric acid* and boil gently for 2 minutes. The resulting solution complies with *reaction A* characteristic of chlorides, Appendix VI.

Melting point 147° to 151°, Appendix V A.

Light absorption *Absorbance* of a 0.0015% w/v solution in a mixture of 1 volume of 0.1M *hydrochloric acid* and 9 volumes of *methanol* at the maximum at 245 nm, 0.49 to 0.53, Appendix II B.

Related substances Carry out the method for *thin-layer chromatography*, Appendix III A, using a silica gel precoated chromatoplate (Merck silica gel 60 plates are suitable) and a mixture of 80 volumes of *chloroform*, 10 volumes of *glacial acetic acid* and 10 volumes of *methanol* as the mobile phase. Apply separately to the plate 10 µl of each of three solutions of the substance being examined in *chloroform* containing (1) 1.0% w/v, (2) 0.010% w/v and (3) 0.0050% w/v. After removal of the plate, allow it to dry in air and spray with *dilute potassium iodobismuthate solution*. Any *secondary spot* in the chromatogram obtained with solution (1) is not more intense than the spot in the chromatogram obtained with solution (2) and not more than one such spot is more intense than the spot in the chromatogram obtained with solution (3).

Loss on drying When dried to constant weight at 60° at a pressure not exceeding 0.7 kPa, loses not more than 0.5% of its weight. Use 1 g.

Sulphated ash Not more than 0.1%, Appendix IX A, Method II. Use 1 g.

Assay Carry out Method I for *non-aqueous titration*, Appendix VIII A, using 0.3 g and determining the end-point potentiometrically. Each ml of 0.1M *perchloric acid VS* is equivalent to 0.03759 g of $C_{21}H_{23}ClFNO_2$.

Preparations
Haloperidol Oral Solution
Strong Haloperidol Oral Solution
Haloperidol Injection
Haloperidol Tablets

Action and use Antipsychotic.

Halothane ☆

CHBrCl·CF₃

$C_2HBrClF_3$ 197.4   *151-67-7*

Halothane is (*RS*)-2-bromo-2-chloro-1,1,1-trifluoroethane. It contains 0.01 per cent of Thymol.

Characteristics A clear, colourless, mobile, dense liquid; non-flammable.

Solubility Slightly soluble in *water*; miscible with *absolute ethanol*, with *chloroform*, with *ether* and with *trichloro-ethylene*.

Identification Test A may be omitted if tests B and C are carried out. Tests B and C may be omitted if test A is carried out.
A. The *infra-red absorption spectrum*, Appendix II A, is concordant with the European Pharmacopœia reference spectrum of halothane. Examine the substance as a gas.
B. To 0.1 ml add 2 ml of *2-methylpropan-2-ol*, 1 ml of *copper edetate solution*, 0.5 ml of 13.5M *ammonia*, 2 ml of *hydrogen peroxide solution (20 vol)* and 1.6 ml of *water* (solution A). Prepare a standard at the same time and in the same manner but omitting the substance being examined (solution B). Warm both solutions in a water-bath at 50° for 15 minutes, cool and add 0.3 ml of *glacial acetic acid* to each.

To 1 ml of each of solutions A and B add 0.5 ml of a mixture of equal volumes of freshly prepared *alizarin red S solution* and *zirconyl nitrate solution*. Solution A is yellow and solution B is red.

To 1 ml of each of solutions A and B add 1 ml of *neutral phthalate buffer pH 5.2*, 1 ml of *phenol red solution* diluted to 10 times its volume with *water* and 0.1 ml of a 2% w/v solution of *chloramine T*. Solution A is bluish-purple and solution B is yellow.

To 2 ml of each of solutions A and B add 0.5 ml of *sulphuric acid (25%)*, 0.5 ml of *acetone* and 0.2 ml of a 5% w/v solution of *potassium bromate* and shake. Warm the solutions in a water-bath at 50° for 2 minutes, cool and add 0.5 ml of a 50% v/v solution of *nitric acid* and 0.5 ml of 0.1M *silver nitrate*. Solution A is cloudy and a white precipitate is produced after a few minutes. Solution B remains clear.

C. Complies with the test for Distillation range.

Acidity or alkalinity Shake 20 ml with 20 ml of *carbon dioxide-free water* for 3 minutes. Separate the aqueous layer and add 0.2 ml of *bromocresol purple solution*. Not more than 0.1 ml of 0.01M *sodium hydroxide VS* or 0.6 ml of 0.01M *hydrochloric acid VS* is required to change the colour of the solution.

Distillation range Distils completely between 49.0° and 51.0°, 95% distilling within a range of 1.0°, Appendix V C.

Relative density 1.872 to 1.877, Appendix V G.

Halides Shake 10 ml with 20 ml of *carbon dioxide-free water* for 3 minutes. To 5 ml of the aqueous layer add 5 ml of *water*, 0.05 ml of *nitric acid* and 0.2 ml of 0.25M *silver nitrate*. The solution is not more opalescent than a mixture of 5 ml of the aqueous layer and 5 ml of *water*.

Free halogens To 10 ml of the aqueous layer prepared in the test for Halides add 1 ml of *potassium iodide and starch solution*. No blue colour is produced.

Thymol Use three dry 25-ml stoppered cylinders. Place in cylinder (1) 0.5 ml of the substance being examined, in cylinder (2) 0.5 ml of a 0.0225% w/v solution of *thymol* in *carbon tetrachloride* and in cylinder (3) 0.5 ml of a 0.015% w/v solution of *thymol* in *carbon tetrachloride*. To each cylinder add 5 ml of *carbon tetrachloride* and 5.0 ml of *titanium dioxide solution*, shake vigorously for 30 seconds and allow to separate. The intensity of the yellowish-brown colour of the lower layer in cylinder (1) is intermediate between those of the lower layers in cylinders (2) and (3) (0.008 to 0.012% w/w).

Volatile related compounds Carry out the method for *gas chromatography*, Appendix III B, using the following solutions. For solution (1) use the substance being examined. Solution (2) contains 0.0050% v/v of *1,1,2-trichlorotrifluoroethane* (internal standard) in the substance being examined.

The chromatographic procedure may be carried out using a column (2.75 m × 5 mm) packed with *pink diatomaceous support* (60 to 80 mesh) the first 1.8 m of which is coated with 30% w/w of polyethylene glycol 400 and the remainder with 30% w/w of *dinonyl phthalate* and maintained at 50°.

In the chromatogram obtained with solution (2) the sum of the areas of any *secondary peaks* is not greater than the area of the peak corresponding to the internal standard corrected, if necessary, for any impurity with the same retention time as the internal standard.

Non-volatile matter Evaporate 50 ml on a water-bath and dry the residue at 100° to 105° for 2 hours. The residue weighs not more than 1 mg (0.002% w/v).

Storage Halothane should be kept in a well-closed container, protected from light and stored at a temperature of 8° to 15°. The choice of material for the container should take into account the particular reactivity of Halothane with certain metals.

Action and use General anaesthetic.

Helium

He   4.003   7440-59-7

Helium is obtained from natural petroleum gas by liquefaction and rectification at low temperatures. It contains not less than 98.0 per cent v/v of He. For convenience in use it is compressed in metal cylinders.

Characteristics A colourless gas; odourless.

Solubility 1 volume, measured at 0° and 101.3 kPa, dissolves in 72.5 volumes of *water*.

Acidity or alkalinity, Oxidising substances and Reducing substances In the following tests place the reagent in a 100-ml cylinder about 20 cm high closed with a stopper fitted with an inlet tube and an outlet tube; the inlet tube has a bore not exceeding 0.5 mm and reaches to the bottom of the cylinder. Pass a volume equivalent to 2000 ml at 0° and 101.3 kPa through the reagent during 30 minutes.

ACIDITY OR ALKALINITY To 300 ml of *water* add 1 ml of *methyl red solution* and boil for 5 minutes. Transfer 100 ml of this solution to each of three similar cylinders labelled (1), (2) and (3). While the solutions are still warm add 0.10 ml of 0.01M *hydrochloric acid* to cylinder (1) and 0.20 ml to each of cylinders (2) and (3); close cylinders (1) and (3) and pass the gas through cylinder (2). The colour in cylinder (2) is not more intensely yellow than that in cylinder (1) and not more intensely pink than that in cylinder (3).

OXIDISING SUBSTANCES Pass the gas through a freshly prepared solution of 0.5 g of *soluble starch* and 0.5 g of *potassium iodide* in 100 ml of *water* containing 0.05 ml of *glacial acetic acid*. No colour is produced.

REDUCING SUBSTANCES Pass the gas through 100 ml of *water* containing 0.2 ml of 0.02M *potassium permanganate*. The colour and the intensity of the colour remain unchanged when compared with the untreated solution.

Carbonaceous compounds Pass a volume equivalent to 500 ml at 0° and 101.3 kPa over *activated copper oxide* heated to 600° and then through 100 ml of a 3% w/v solution of *barium hydroxide* at a rate not exceeding 4000 ml per hour. The turbidity produced is not greater than that produced by adding 1 ml of a 0.2% w/v solution of *sodium hydrogen carbonate* in freshly boiled and cooled *water* to 100 ml of a 3% w/v solution of *barium hydroxide*.

Relative density Not greater than 0.16 when determined in the following manner. Weigh a glass bulb with a capacity of about 100 ml, evacuate, fill with the sample and reweigh.

Assay Introduce into a small bulb about 1 ml of a suitable granular coconut shell charcoal in *coarse powder* for each 3 ml of sample to be examined. Place the bulb in liquid oxygen, evacuate, introduce a measured volume of the sample and pump off the unabsorbed gases. Not less than 98.0% of the volume taken is recovered.

Labelling The metal cylinder is painted brown and carries a label stating 'Helium'. In addition, 'Helium' or the symbol 'He' is stencilled in paint on the shoulder of the cylinder.

Action and use Used in treatment of respiratory embarrassment.

Heparin Calcium ☆

Heparin Calcium is a preparation containing the calcium salt of a sulphated glucosamino-glycan present in mammalian tissues. On complete hydrolysis D-glucosamine, D-glucuronic acid, L-iduronic acid, acetic acid and sulphuric acid are released. It has the characteristic property of delaying the clotting of freshly shed blood. Heparin Calcium intended for use in the manufacture of a parenteral dosage form contains not less than 150 Units per mg and Heparin Calcium not intended for use in the manufacture of a parenteral dosage form contains not less than 120 Units per mg, both calculated with reference to the dried substance.

Heparin Calcium may be prepared from the lungs of oxen or the intestinal mucosa of oxen, pigs or sheep. It is prepared in conditions designed to minimise microbial contamination.

Characteristics A white or almost white powder; moderately hygroscopic.

Solubility Soluble in less than 5 parts of *water*.

Identification A. It delays the clotting of freshly shed blood.
B. Carry out the method for *agarose-gel electrophoresis*, Appendix III F, using the following solutions. Solution (1) contains 0.25% w/v of the substance being examined in *water*. For solution (2) dilute 1 volume of *heparin sodium EPBRP* to 2 volumes with *water*. The ratio of the distance migrated by the principal band or bands in the gel obtained with solution (1) to the distance migrated by the principal band in the gel obtained with solution (2) is 0.9 to 1.1.
C. *Specific optical rotation*, determined in a 4% w/v solution, not less than +35°, Appendix V F.
D. Yields *reactions A and B* characteristic of calcium salts, Appendix VI.

Acidity or alkalinity pH of a 1% w/v solution, 5.5 to 8.0, Appendix V L.

Clarity and colour of solution A solution containing 5000 Units per ml is *clear*, Appendix IV A, and not more intensely coloured than degree *5* of the appropriate range of *reference solutions*, Appendix IV B, Method II.

Calcium 9.5 to 11.5%, calculated with reference to the dried substance, when determined by the *complexometric titration of calcium*, Appendix VIII D. Use 0.2 g.

Heavy metals 0.5 g complies with *limit test C for heavy metals*, Appendix VII (30 ppm). Use 1.5 ml of *lead standard solution (10 ppm Pb)* to prepare the standard.

Nitrogen Not more than 2.5%, calculated with reference to the dried substance, when determined by Method IV, Appendix VIII H. Use 0.1 g.

Protein Add 0.25 ml of a 20% w/v solution of *trichloroacetic acid* to 1 ml of a 1% w/v solution in *carbon dioxide-free water*. No precipitate or turbidity is produced.

Sulphur Not less than 10.0%, calculated with reference to the dried substance, when determined by Method I for *oxygen-flask combustion for sulphur*, Appendix VIII C, but using a flask with a nominal capacity of 1 litre. Use 25 mg.

Loss on drying When dried over *phosphorus pentoxide* at 60° at a pressure not exceeding 0.7 kPa for 3 hours, loses not more than 8.0% of its weight. Use 1 g.

Sulphated ash 32 to 40%, calculated with reference to the dried substance, Appendix IX A, Method II. Use 0.2 g.

Assay Carry out the *biological assay of heparin*, Appendix XIV D3. The estimated potency is not less than 90% and not more than 111% of the stated potency. The fiducial limits of error are not less than 80% and not more than 125% of the stated potency.

Storage Heparin Calcium should be kept in an airtight container. If the contents are intended for use in the manufacture of a parenteral dosage form, the container should be sterile and tamper-evident.

Labelling The label states (1) the number of Units in the container; (2) the number of Units per mg; (3) the name and quantity of any added substance; (4) the date after which the material is not intended to be used; (5) the conditions under which it should be stored; (6) whether or not it is intended for use in the manufacture of a parenteral dosage form; (7) the source of the material (lung or mucous).

Preparation
Heparin Injection

Action and use Anticoagulant.

Heparin Calcium intended for use in the manufacture of a parenteral dosage form complies with the following additional requirements.

Abnormal toxicity Complies with the *test for abnormal toxicity*, Appendix XIV L. Use a solution containing 200 Units in 0.5 ml of *water for injections* or *saline solution*.

Depressor substances Complies with the *test for depressor substances*, Appendix XIV M. Use per kg of the cat's weight 1.0 ml of a solution containing 5000 Units.

Pyrogens★ Complies with the *test for pyrogens*, Appendix XIV K. Use per kg of the rabbit's weight 1.0 ml of a solution in *water for injections* containing 2000 Units.

★In certain states party to the Convention on the Elaboration of a European Pharmacopœia, Heparin Calcium intended for use in the manufacture of a parenteral dosage form may not be required to comply with this test.

Heparin Sodium ☆

Heparin Sodium is a preparation containing the sodium salt of a sulphated glucosaminoglycan present in mammalian tissues. On complete hydrolysis D-glucosamine, D-glucuronic acid, L-iduronic acid, acetic acid and sulphuric acid are released. It has the characteristic property of delaying the clotting of freshly shed blood.

Heparin Sodium intended for use in the manufacture of a parenteral dosage form contains not less than 150 Units per mg and Heparin Sodium not intended for use in the manufacture of a parenteral dosage form contains not less than 120 Units per mg, both calculated with reference to the dried substance.

Heparin Sodium may be prepared from the lungs of oxen or the intestinal mucosa of oxen, pigs or sheep. It is prepared in conditions designed to minimise microbial contamination.

Characteristics A white or almost white powder; moderately hygroscopic.

Solubility Soluble in 2.5 parts of *water*.

Identification A. It delays the clotting of freshly shed blood.

B. Carry out the method for *agarose-gel electrophoresis*, Appendix III F, using the following solutions. Solution (1) contains 0.25% w/v of the substance being examined in *water*. For solution (2) dilute 1 volume of *heparin sodium EPBRP* to 2 volumes with *water*. The ratio of the distance migrated by the principal band or bands in the gel obtained with solution (1) to the distance migrated by the principal band in the gel obtained with solution (2) is 0.9 to 1.1.

C. *Specific optical rotation*, determined in a 4% w/v solution, not less than +35°, Appendix V F.

D. The residue obtained in the test for Sulphated ash yields *reaction A* characteristic of sodium salts, Appendix VI.

Acidity or alkalinity pH of a 1% w/v solution, 5.5 to 8.0, Appendix V L.

Clarity and colour of solution A solution containing 5000 Units per ml is *clear*, Appendix IV A, and not more intensely coloured than degree *5* of the appropriate range of *reference solutions*, Appendix IV B, Method II.

Heavy metals 0.5 g complies with *limit test C for heavy metals*, Appendix VII (30 ppm). Use 1.5 ml of *lead standard solution (10 ppm Pb)* to prepare the standard.

Nitrogen Not more than 2.5%, calculated with reference to the dried substance, when determined by Method IV, Appendix VIII H. Use 0.1 g.

Protein Add 0.25 ml of a 20% w/v solution of *trichloroacetic acid* to 1 ml of a 1% w/v solution in *carbon dioxide-free water*. No precipitate or turbidity is produced.

Sodium 9.5 to 12.5% of Na, calculated with reference to the dried substance, when determined by the following method. Prepare a 0.050% w/v solution in 0.1M *hydrochloric acid* containing 0.127% w/v of *caesium chloride*. Carry out the method for *atomic absorption spectrophotometry*, Appendix II D, measuring at 330.3 nm and using a sodium hollow-cathode lamp as the source of radiation and a flame of suitable composition (for example, 11 litres of air and 2 litres of acetylene per minute). Use dilutions of *sodium solution ASp* containing 25, 50 and 75 ppm of Na in a 0.127% w/v solution of *caesium chloride* in 0.1M *hydrochloric acid* as the standard solutions.

Sulphur Not less than 10.0%, calculated with reference to the dried substance, when determined by Method I for *oxygen-flask combustion for sulphur*, Appendix VIII C, but using a flask with a nominal capacity of 1 litre. Use 25 mg.

Loss on drying When dried over *phosphorus pentoxide* at 60° at a pressure not exceeding 0.7 kPa for 3 hours, loses not more than 8.0% of its weight. Use 1 g.

Sulphated ash 30 to 43%, calculated with reference to the dried substance, Appendix IX A, Method II. Use 0.2 g.

Assay Carry out the *biological assay of heparin*, Appendix XIV D3. The estimated potency is not less than 90% and not more than 111% of the stated potency. The fiducial limits of error are not less than 80% and not more than 125% of the stated potency.

Storage Heparin Sodium should be kept in an airtight container. If the contents are intended for use in the manufacture of a parenteral dosage form, the container should be sterile and tamper-evident.

Labelling The label states (1) the number of Units in the container; (2) the number of Units per mg; (3) the name and quantity of any added substance; (4) the date after which the material is not intended to be used; (5) the conditions under which it should be stored; (6) whether or not it is intended for use in the manufacture of a parenteral dosage form; (7) the source of the material (lung or mucous).

Preparation
Heparin Injection

Action and use Anticoagulant.

Heparin Sodium intended for use in the manufacture of a parenteral dosage form complies with the following additional requirements.

Abnormal toxicity Complies with the *test for abnormal toxicity*, Appendix XIV L. Use a solution containing 200 Units in 0.5 ml of *water for injections* or *saline solution*.

Depressor substances Complies with the *test for depressor substances*, Appendix XIV M. Use per kg of the cat's weight 1.0 ml of a solution containing 5000 Units.

Pyrogens* Complies with the *test for pyrogens*, Appendix XIV K. Use per kg of the rabbit's weight 1.0 ml of a solution in *water for injections* containing 2000 Units.

*In certain states party to the Convention on the Elaboration of a European Pharmacopœia, Heparin Sodium intended for use in the manufacture of a parenteral dosage form may not be required to comply with this test.

Hexachlorophane

C$_{13}$H$_6$Cl$_6$O$_2$ 406.9   *70-30-4*

Hexachlorophane is 2,2'-methylenebis(3,4,6-trichlorophenol). It contains not less than 98.0 per cent and not more than 100.5 per cent of C$_{13}$H$_6$Cl$_6$O$_2$, calculated with reference to the dried substance.

Characteristics A white or pale buff, crystalline powder; odourless or almost odourless.

Solubility Practically insoluble in *water*; soluble in 3.5 parts of *ethanol (96%)*, in less than 1 part of *acetone* and in less than 1 part of *ether*. It dissolves in dilute solutions of the alkali hydroxides.

Identification A. The *infra-red absorption spectrum*, Appendix II A, is concordant with the *reference spectrum* of hexachlorophane.

B. Heat 0.1 g in a dry tube. A colourless to amber liquid is produced which, on further heating, becomes green, blue and finally purple.

C. Dissolve 5 mg in 5 ml of *ethanol (96%)* and add 0.05 ml of *iron(III) chloride solution*. A transient purple colour is produced immediately.

D. Dissolve 0.1 g in 0.5 ml of *acetone*, add *titanium(III) chloride solution* and shake. A yellowish-orange oil separates which is soluble in *chloroform* and in *ether*.

E. *Melting point*, about 164°, Appendix V A.

Chloride Dissolve 5.0 g in 2 ml of *ethanol (96%)*, dilute to 25 ml with *water* and filter. 5 ml of the clear filtrate diluted to 15 ml with *water* complies with the *limit test for chlorides*, Appendix VII (500 ppm).

Related substances Carry out the method for *high-performance liquid chromatography*, Appendix III D, using solutions of the substance being examined in *methanol* containing (1) 0.020% w/v and (2) 1.0% w/v.

The chromatographic procedure may be carried out using (a) a stainless steel column (20 cm × 5 mm) packed with *stationary phase C* (10 μm) (Spherisorb ODS 1 is suitable), (b) a mixture of 100 volumes of *methanol*, 20 volumes of *water* and 1 volume of *glacial acetic acid* as the mobile phase with a flow rate of 2 ml per minute and (c) a detection wavelength of 300 nm.

In the chromatogram obtained with solution (2) the sum of the areas of any *secondary peaks* with a retention time not more than three times that of the principal peak is not greater than twice the area of the principal peak in the chromatogram obtained with solution (1) and not more than one such peak has an area greater than half of the area of the principal peak in the chromatogram obtained with solution (1).

Non-phenolic substances Dissolve 5 g in 38 ml of *methanol*, add 125 ml of 0.25M *sodium hydroxide* and extract with three 15-ml quantities of n-*pentane*, retaining any foamy interphase with the aqueous layer. Dry the combined extracts over *anhydrous sodium sulphate* and evaporate to dryness at a pressure of 2 kPa. The residue, when dried to constant weight at a pressure of 2 kPa, weighs not more than 37.5 mg.

Loss on drying When dried to constant weight at 105°, loses not more than 1.0% of its weight. Use 1 g.

Sulphated ash Not more than 0.1%, Appendix IX A.

Assay Dissolve 1 g in 25 ml of *ethanol (96%)* previously adjusted to pH 9.0 and titrate with 0.1M *sodium hydroxide VS* to pH 9.0 determining the end-point potentiometrically. Each ml of 0.1M *sodium hydroxide VS* is equivalent to 0.04069 g of $C_{13}H_6Cl_6O_2$.

Storage Hexachlorophane should be kept in a well-closed container and protected from light.

Preparation

Hexachlorophane Dusting Powder

Action and use Antiseptic.

In some countries the material described in this monograph may be known as Hexachlorophene.

Hexobarbitone ☆

$C_{12}H_{16}N_2O_3$ 236.3   56-29-1

Hexobarbitone is 5-cyclohexenyl-1,5-dimethyl-barbituric acid. It contains not less than 99.0 per cent and not more than 101.0 per cent of $C_{12}H_{16}N_2O_3$, calculated with reference to the dried substance.

Characteristics A white, crystalline powder; odourless.

Solubility Very slightly soluble in *water*; sparingly soluble in *ethanol (96%)* and in *ether*; freely soluble in *chloroform*. It dissolves in aqueous solutions of alkali hydroxides and carbonates and in aqueous ammonia.

Identification *Test A may be omitted if tests B, C and D are carried out. Tests B and C may be omitted if tests A and D are carried out.*

A. The *infra-red absorption spectrum*, Appendix II A, is concordant with the spectrum of *hexobarbital EPCRS*.

B. Complies with the test for *identification of barbiturates*, Appendix III A.

C. To 10 mg add 1.0 ml of a 1% w/v solution of *vanillin* in *ethanol (96%)* and 2 ml of a cooled mixture of 1 volume of *water* and 2 volumes of *sulphuric acid*. Shake and allow to stand for 5 minutes; a greenish-yellow colour is produced. Heat on a water-bath for 10 minutes; the colour changes to dark red.

D. Determine the *melting point*, Appendix V A, Method I, of the substance being examined. Mix equal parts of the substance being examined and *hexobarbital EPCRS* and determine the *melting point* of the mixture. The difference between the melting points (which are about 146°) is not greater than 2°.

Acidity Boil 1 g with 50 ml of *water* for 2 minutes, allow to cool and filter. To 10 ml of the filtrate add 0.15 ml of *methyl red solution*. The solution is orange-yellow and not more than 0.1 ml of 0.1M *sodium hydroxide VS* is required to produce a pure yellow colour.

Clarity and colour of solution A solution containing 1.0 g in a mixture of 4 ml of 2M *sodium hydroxide* and 6 ml of *carbon dioxide-free water* is clear, Appendix IV A, and not more intensely coloured than *reference solution* Y_6, Appendix IV B, Method II.

Related substances Complies with the test for *related substances in barbiturates*, Appendix III A.

Loss on drying When dried to constant weight at 100° to 105°, loses not more than 0.5% of its weight. Use 1 g.

Sulphated ash Not more than 0.1%, Appendix IX A, Method II. Use 1 g.

Assay Dissolve 0.2 g in 5 ml of *pyridine*, add 10 ml of *silver nitrate—pyridine reagent* and titrate with 0.1M *ethanolic sodium hydroxide VS*, using 0.5 ml of *thymolphthalein solution* as indicator, until a pure blue colour is produced. Repeat the operation without the substance being examined. The difference between the titrations represents the amount of sodium hydroxide required. Each ml of 0.1M *ethanolic sodium hydroxide VS* is equivalent to 0.02363 g of $C_{12}H_{16}N_2O_3$.

The title of the monograph in the European Pharmacopœia is Hexobarbital.

Hexylresorcinol

$C_{12}H_{18}O_2$ 194.3   *136-77-6*

Hexylresorcinol is 4-hexylresorcinol. It contains not less than 98.0 per cent and not more than 101.0 per cent of $C_{12}H_{18}O_2$.

Characteristics White or almost white needles, crystalline powder, plates or plate aggregates composed of needle masses; odour, pungent. Acquires a brownish-pink tint on exposure to light and air.

Solubility Very slightly soluble in *water*; freely soluble in *ethanol (96%)*, in *chloroform*, in *ether*, in *glycerol* and in fixed oils; practically insoluble in *petroleum spirit (boiling range, 40° to 60°)*.

Identification A. Dissolve 0.1 g in 10 ml of *ethanol (90%)* and add 0.2 ml of *iron(III) chloride test-solution*. A green colour is produced.
B. To 1 ml of a saturated solution add 1 ml of *nitric acid*. A light red colour is produced.
C. To 1 ml of a saturated solution add 1 ml of *bromine water*; a yellow, flocculent precipitate is produced. Add 2 ml of *5M ammonia*; the precipitate dissolves giving a yellow solution.

Melting point 66° to 68°, Appendix V A.

Acidity Dissolve 1 g in 50 ml of *ether* previously neutralised to *phenolphthalein solution*, add 50 ml of *carbon dioxide-free water* and titrate with 0.1M *sodium hydroxide VS* shaking vigorously after each addition. Not more than 0.80 ml of 0.1M *sodium hydroxide VS* is required to change the colour of the solution.

Sulphated ash Not more than 0.1%, Appendix IX A.

Assay Dissolve 1.2 g in sufficient *glacial acetic acid* to produce 100 ml. Transfer 10 ml to a glass-stoppered flask, add 50 ml of 0.05M *bromine VS* and 10 ml of *hydrochloric acid*, insert the stopper, allow to stand for 15 minutes, swirling occasionally, and allow to stand overnight protected from light. Add 10 ml of *potassium iodide solution* and titrate with 0.1M *sodium thiosulphate VS* until only a faint yellow colour remains. Add 0.2 ml of *starch mucilage* and 10 ml of *chloroform* and complete the titration, shaking vigorously. Repeat the operation without the substance being examined. The difference between the titrations represents the amount of bromine required. Each ml of 0.05M *bromine VS* is equivalent to 0.004857 g of $C_{12}H_{18}O_2$.

Storage Hexylresorcinol should be kept in a well-closed container and protected from light.

Action and use Anthelmintic.

Histamine Dihydrochloride ☆

$C_5H_9N_3,2HCl$ 184.1   *56-92-8*

Histamine Dihydrochloride is 2-(1*H*-imidazol-4-yl)ethylamine dihydrochloride. It contains not less than 98.5 per cent and not more than 101.0 per cent of $C_5H_9N_3,2HCl$, calculated with reference to the dried substance.

Characteristics A white, crystalline powder or colourless crystals; odourless; hygroscopic.

Solubility Very soluble in *water*; soluble in *ethanol (96%)*; practically insoluble in *chloroform* and in *ether*.

Identification *Test A may be omitted if tests B, C and D are carried out. Tests B and C may be omitted if tests A and D are carried out.*
A. The *infra-red absorption spectrum*, Appendix II A, is concordant with the spectrum of *histamine dihydrochloride EPCRS*. Examine as discs prepared using 1 mg of the substance being examined.
B. In the test for Histidine, the principal spot in the chromatogram obtained with solution (2) corresponds in position, colour and size to that in the chromatogram obtained with solution (3).
C. Dissolve 0.1 g in 7 ml of *water* and add 3 ml of a 20% w/v solution of *sodium hydroxide* (solution A). Dissolve 50 mg of *sulphanilic acid* in a mixture of 0.1 ml of *hydrochloric acid* and 10 ml of *water* and add 0.1 ml of *sodium nitrite solution* (solution B). Add solution B to solution A and mix. A red colour is produced.
D. Yields *reaction A* characteristic of chlorides, Appendix VI.

Acidity pH of a 5.0% w/v solution in *carbon dioxide-free water* prepared from *distilled water* (solution C), 2.85 to 3.60, Appendix V L.

Clarity and colour of solution Solution C is *clear*, Appendix IV A, and not more intensely coloured than *reference solution Y_7*, Appendix IV B, Method II.

Sulphate 3 ml of solution C diluted to 15 ml with *distilled water* complies with the *limit test for sulphates*, Appendix VII (0.1%).

Histidine Carry out the method for *thin-layer chromatography*, Appendix III A, using *silica gel G* as the coating substance and a mixture of 75 volumes of *acetonitrile*, 20 volumes of *water* and 5 volumes of 13.5M *ammonia* as the mobile phase. Apply separately to the chromatoplate 1 µl of each of solutions (1) to (4) and 2 µl of solution (5). Solutions (1) and (2) contain 5.0% w/v and 1.0% w/v respectively of the substance being examined in *water*. Solution (3) contains 1.0% w/v of *histamine dihydrochloride EPCRS* in *water*. Solution (4) contains 0.05% w/v of DL-*histidine monohydrochloride* in *water*. Solution (5) is a mixture of equal volumes of solutions (1) and (4). After removal of the plate, dry it in a current of air and repeat the development in the same direction. After removal of the plate, dry it in a current of air, spray with *ethanolic ninhydrin solution* and heat at 110° for 10 minutes. Any spot corresponding to histidine in the chromatogram obtained with solution (1) is not more intense than the spot in the chromatogram obtained with solution (4). The test is not valid unless the chromatogram obtained with solution (5) shows two clearly separated spots.

Loss on drying When dried to constant weight at 100° to 105°, loses not more than 0.5% of its weight. Use 0.2 g.

Sulphated ash Not more than 0.1%, Appendix IX A, Method II. Use 0.5 g.

Assay Dissolve 80 mg in 5 ml of *anhydrous formic acid*, add 20 ml of *anhydrous glacial acetic acid* and 6 ml of *mercury(II) acetate solution* and carry out Method I for *non-aqueous titration*, Appendix VIII A, determining the end-point potentiometrically. Repeat the operation without the substance being examined. The difference between the titrations represents the amount of perchloric acid required. Each ml of 0.1M *perchloric acid VS* is equivalent to 0.009203 g of $C_5H_9N_3,2HCl$.

Storage Histamine Dihydrochloride should be kept in a well-closed container and protected from light.

Histamine Phosphate ☆

$C_5H_9N_3,2H_3PO_4,H_2O$ 325.2   *51-74-1 (anhydrous)*

Histamine Phosphate is 2-(1*H*-imidazol-4-yl)ethylamine diphosphate monohydrate. It contains not less than 98.0 per cent and not more than 101.0 per cent of $C_5H_9N_3,2H_3PO_4$, calculated with reference to the anhydrous substance.

Characteristics Colourless, long prismatic crystals; odourless.

Solubility Freely soluble in *water*; slightly soluble in *ethanol (96%)*.

Identification *Test A may be omitted if tests B, C and D are carried out. Tests B and C may be omitted if tests A and D are carried out.*

A. The *infra-red absorption spectrum*, Appendix II A, is concordant with the spectrum of *histamine phosphate EPCRS*. Examine as discs prepared using 0.1 mg of the substance being examined.

B. In the test for Histidine, the principal spot in the chromatogram obtained with solution (2) corresponds in position, colour and size to that in the chromatogram obtained with solution (3).

C. Dissolve 0.1 g in 7 ml of *water* and add 3 ml of a 20% w/v solution of *sodium hydroxide* (solution A). Dissolve 50 mg of *sulphanilic acid* in a mixture of 0.1 ml of *hydrochloric acid* and 10 ml of *water* and add 0.1 ml of *sodium nitrite solution* (solution B). Add solution B to solution A and mix. A red colour is produced.

D. Yields *reaction A* characteristic of phosphates, Appendix VI.

Acidity pH of a 5.0% w/v solution in *carbon dioxide-free water* prepared from *distilled water* (solution C), 3.75 to 3.95, Appendix V L.

Clarity and colour of solution Solution C is *clear*, Appendix IV A, and not more intensely coloured than *reference solution BY_7*, Appendix IV B, Method II.

Sulphate 3 ml of solution C diluted to 15 ml with *distilled water* complies with the *limit test for sulphates*, Appendix VII (0.1%).

Histidine Carry out the method for *thin-layer chromatography*, Appendix III A, using *silica gel G* as the coating

substance and a mixture of 75 volumes of *acetonitrile*, 20 volumes of *water* and 5 volumes of 13.5M *ammonia* as the mobile phase. Apply separately to the chromatoplate 1 µl of each of solutions (1) to (4) and 2 µl of solution (5). Solutions (1) and (2) contain 5.0% w/v and 1.0% w/v respectively of the substance being examined in *water*. Solution (3) contains 1.0% w/v of *histamine phosphate EPCRS* in *water*. Solution (4) contains 0.05% w/v of DL-*histidine monohydrochloride* in *water*. Solution (5) is a mixture of equal volumes of solutions (1) and (4). After removal of the plate, dry it in a current of air and repeat the development in the same direction. After removal of the plate, dry it in a current of air, spray with *ethanolic ninhydrin solution* and heat at 110° for 10 minutes. Any spot corresponding to histidine in the chromatogram obtained with solution (1) is not more intense than the spot in the chromatogram obtained with solution (4). The test is not valid unless the chromatogram obtained with solution (5) shows two clearly separated spots.

Water 5.0 to 6.2% w/w, Appendix IX C. Use 0.3 g.

Assay Dissolve 0.14 g in 5 ml of *anhydrous formic acid*, add 20 ml of *anhydrous glacial acetic acid* and carry out Method I for *non-aqueous titration*, Appendix VIII A, determining the end-point potentiometrically. Repeat the operation without the substance being examined. The difference between the titrations represents the amount of perchloric acid required. Each ml of 0.1M *perchloric acid VS* is equivalent to 0.01536 g of $C_5H_9N_3,2H_3PO_4$.

Storage Histamine Phosphate should be kept in a well-closed container and protected from light.

Homatropine Hydrobromide ☆

$C_{16}H_{21}NO_3,HBr$ 356.3   *51-56-9*

Homatropine Hydrobromide is (1*R*,3*r*,5*S*)-3-mandeloyloxytropanium bromide. It contains not less than 99.0 per cent and not more than 101.0 per cent of $C_{16}H_{21}NO_3,HBr$, calculated with reference to the dried substance.

Characteristics Colourless crystals or a white, crystalline powder. It melts at about 215°, with decomposition.

Solubility Soluble in 6 parts of *water* and in 60 parts of *ethanol (96%)*; slightly soluble in *chloroform*; very slightly soluble in *ether*.

Identification *Test A may be omitted if tests B, C and D are carried out. Tests B and C may be omitted if tests A and D are carried out.*

A. The *infra-red absorption spectrum*, Appendix II A, is concordant with the spectrum of *homatropine hydrobromide EPCRS*.

B. Dissolve 50 mg in 1 ml of *water* and add 2 ml of 2M *acetic acid*. Heat, add 4 ml of a 1% w/v solution of *2,4,6-trinitrophenol* and allow to cool, shaking occasionally. The *melting point* of the crystals, after washing with two 3-ml quantities of iced *water* and drying at 100° to 105°, is 182° to 186°, Appendix V A, Method I.

C. Dissolve 10 mg in 1 ml of *water*, add a slight excess of 10M *ammonia* and shake with 5 ml of *chloroform*. Evaporate the chloroform layer to dryness on a water-bath and add 1.5 ml of a 2% w/v solution of *mercury(II) chloride* in *ethanol (60%)*. A yellow colour is produced which becomes red on warming.

D. Yields *reaction A* characteristic of bromides, Appendix VI.

Acidity pH of a 5% w/v solution, 5.0 to 6.5, Appendix V L.

Clarity and colour of solution A 5.0% w/v solution in *carbon dioxide-free water* is *clear*, Appendix IV A, and not more intensely coloured than *reference solution B₉*, Appendix IV B, Method II.

Related substances Carry out the method for *thin-layer chromatography*, Appendix III A, using *silica gel G* as the coating substance and a mixture of 134 volumes of *ethyl acetate*, 33 volumes of *anhydrous formic acid* and 33 volumes of *water* as the mobile phase. Apply separately to the chromatoplate 5 μl of each of two solutions of the substance being examined in *methanol (90%)* containing (1) 4.0% w/v and (2) 0.020% w/v. After removal of the plate, dry it at 100° to 105° until the odour of the solvent is no longer detectable, allow to cool and spray with *dilute potassium iodobismuthate solution* until spots appear. Any *secondary spot* in the chromatogram obtained with solution (1) is not more intense than the spot in the chromatogram obtained with solution (2).

Loss on drying When dried to constant weight at 100° to 105°, loses not more than 0.5% of its weight. Use 0.5 g.

Sulphated ash Not more than 0.1%, Appendix IX A, Method II. Use 0.5 g.

Assay Dissolve 0.3 g in 20 ml of *anhydrous glacial acetic acid*, add 7 ml of *mercury(II) acetate solution* and carry out Method I for *non-aqueous titration*, Appendix VIII A, determining the end-point potentiometrically. Each ml of 0.1M *perchloric acid VS* is equivalent to 0.03563 g of $C_{16}H_{21}NO_3,HBr$.

Storage Homatropine Hydrobromide should be kept in a well-closed container and protected from light.

Preparation
Homatropine Eye Drops

Action and use Mydriatic; cycloplegic.

Purified Honey

Purified Honey is obtained by purification of the honey from the comb of the bee, *Apis mellifera* L. and other species of *Apis*. The honey is extracted by centrifugation, pressure or other suitable procedure, melted at not more than 80° and allowed to stand; the impurities that rise to the surface are skimmed off and Water is added until the product complies with the requirement for Weight per ml.

Characteristics A thick, syrupy, translucent, pale yellow or yellowish-brown liquid; odour, pleasant and characteristic, becoming more pronounced but otherwise

unchanged when heated on a water-bath; taste, sweet and characteristic, varying according to the floral origin.

Optical rotation +0.6° to −3.0°, Appendix V F, measured in a 20% w/v solution containing 0.2% v/v of 13.5M *ammonia* after decolorising with *decolorising charcoal* if necessary.

Weight per ml 1.35 to 1.36 g, Appendix V G.

Chlorides 15 ml of a 1.00% w/v solution complies with the *limit test for chlorides*, Appendix VII (350 ppm).

Sulphates 15 ml of a 4.0% w/v solution complies with the *limit test for sulphates*, Appendix VII (240 ppm).

Ash Not more than 0.3%, Appendix XI J.

Action and use Demulcent; sweetening agent.

Hydralazine Hydrochloride

$C_8H_8N_4,HCl$ 196.6   *304-20-1*

Hydralazine Hydrochloride is phthalazin-1-yl-hydrazine hydrochloride. It contains not less than 98.5 per cent and not more than 101.0 per cent of $C_8H_8N_4,HCl$, calculated with reference to the dried substance.

Characteristics A white or almost white, crystalline powder; odourless or almost odourless.

Solubility Soluble in *water*; slightly soluble in *ethanol (96%)* and in *methanol*; practically insoluble in *chloroform* and in *ether*.

Identification A. The *infra-red absorption spectrum*, Appendix II A, is concordant with the *reference spectrum* of hydralazine hydrochloride.

B. The *light absorption*, Appendix II B, in the range 230 to 350 nm of a 0.002% w/v solution exhibits four maxima, at 240, 260, 305 and 315 nm. The *absorbance* at 240 nm is about 1.1, at 260 nm, about 1.1, at 305 nm, about 0.53 and at 315 nm, about 0.43.

C. Yields the *reactions* characteristic of chlorides, Appendix VI.

Acidity pH of a 2% w/v solution, 3.5 to 4.2, Appendix V L.

Clarity of solution A 2.0% w/v solution is not more than *slightly opalescent*, Appendix IV A.

Colour of solution A 2.0% w/v solution in 0.01M *hydrochloric acid* is not more intensely coloured than *reference solution GY₆*, Appendix IV B, Method II.

Heavy metals Moisten the residue obtained in the test for Sulphated ash with 2 ml of *hydrochloric acid*, evaporate to dryness and dissolve the residue in sufficient *water* to produce 20 ml. 12 ml of the resulting solution complies with *limit test A for heavy metals*, Appendix VII (20 ppm). Use *lead standard solution (2 ppm Pb)* to prepare the standard.

Hydrazine Carry out the method for *thin-layer chromatography*, Appendix III A, using a silica gel precoated chromatoplate (Merck silica gel 60 plates are suitable) and as the mobile phase the upper layer obtained by shaking together 80 volumes of *hexane*, 20 volumes of *ethyl acetate* and 20 volumes of 13.5M *ammonia* and allowing to separate. Apply separately to the chromatoplate 40 μl of each of the following solutions. For solution (1) add 1 ml of a 2% w/v solution of *salicylaldehyde* in *methanol* and 0.1 ml of *hydrochloric acid* to 2 ml of a 0.5% w/v solution of the substance being examined in 0.1M *methanolic hydrochloric acid*, centrifuge and use the supernatant liquid. Prepare solution (2) in the same manner, but using 2 ml of a 0.00025% w/v solution of *hydrazine sulphate* in 0.1M *methanolic hydrochloric acid* in place of the solution of the substance being examined. After removal of the plate, allow it to dry in air and spray with *dimethylaminobenzaldehyde solution*. Any spot corresponding to hydrazine in the chromatogram obtained with solution (1) is not more intense than the spot in the chromatogram obtained with solution (2).

Loss on drying When dried to constant weight over *phosphorus pentoxide* at a pressure not exceeding 0.7 kPa, loses not more than 0.5% of its weight. Use 1 g.

Sulphated ash Not more than 0.1%, Appendix IX A. Use 2.0 g.

Assay Dissolve 0.1 g in a mixture of 25 ml of *water* and 35 ml of *hydrochloric acid* and titrate with 0.025M *potassium iodate VS* determining the end-point potentiometrically using platinum and calomel electrodes. Each ml of 0.025M *potassium iodate VS* is equivalent to 0.004916 g of $C_8H_8N_4,HCl$.

Storage Hydralazine Hydrochloride should be kept in a well-closed container.

Preparations
Hydralazine Injection
Hydralazine Tablets

Action and use Vasodilator.

Hydrochloric Acid ☆

HCl   36.46   *7647-01-0*

Hydrochloric Acid contains not less than 35.0 per cent w/w and not more than 39.0 per cent w/w of HCl.

Characteristics A clear, colourless, fuming liquid; odour, pungent. It has a relative density of about 1.18.

Solubility Miscible with *water*.

Identification A. Yields the *reactions* characteristic of chlorides, Appendix VI.
B. Dilute with *water*; the solution is strongly acidic.

Clarity and colour of solution A solution of 2 ml in 8 ml of *water* is *clear*, Appendix IV A, and *colourless*, Appendix IV B, Method II.

Arsenic Dilute 4.2 ml to 10 ml with *water*. 1 ml of the resulting solution complies with the *limit test for arsenic*, Appendix VII (2 ppm).

Heavy metals Dissolve the residue obtained in the test for Residue on evaporation in 1 ml of 2M *hydrochloric acid* and dilute to 25 ml with *water*; dilute 5 ml of this solution to 20 ml with *water*. 12 ml of the resulting solution complies with *limit test A for heavy metals*, Appendix VII (2 ppm). Use *lead standard solution (2 ppm Pb)* to prepare the standard.

Free chlorine To 15 ml add 100 ml of *carbon dioxide-free water*, 1 ml of a 10% w/v solution of *potassium iodide* and 0.5 ml of *iodide-free starch solution*. Allow to stand in the dark for 2 minutes. Any blue colour disappears on the addition of 0.2 ml of 0.01M *sodium thiosulphate VS* (4 ppm).

Sulphate Mix 6.4 ml with 10 mg of *sodium hydrogen carbonate*, evaporate to dryness on a water-bath and dissolve the residue in 15 ml of *water*. The resulting solution complies with the *limit test for sulphates*, Appendix VII (20 ppm).

Residue on evaporation Not more than 0.01%. Use 100 g.

Assay Weigh 1.5 ml into a glass-stoppered flask containing 30 ml of *water* and titrate with 1M *sodium hydroxide VS* using *methyl red solution* as indicator. Each ml of 1M *sodium hydroxide VS* is equivalent to 0.03646 g of HCl.

Storage Hydrochloric Acid should be kept in a stoppered container of glass or other inert material and stored at a temperature not exceeding 30°.

Preparation
Dilute Hydrochloric Acid

The title of the monograph in the European Pharmacopœia is Concentrated Hydrochloric Acid.

Dilute Hydrochloric Acid ☆

Dilute Hydrochloric Acid contains 9.5 to 10.5 per cent w/w of HCl and is prepared by mixing 274 g of Hydrochloric Acid and 726 g of Purified Water.

Identification A. Yields the *reactions* characteristic of chlorides, Appendix VI.
B. The solution is strongly acidic.

Clarity and colour *Clear*, Appendix IV A, and *colourless*, Appendix IV B, Method II.

Arsenic Dilute 17 ml to 20 ml with *water*. 2 ml of the resulting solution complies with the *limit test for arsenic*, Appendix VII (0.5 ppm).

Heavy metals Dissolve the residue obtained in the test for Residue on evaporation in 1 ml of 2M *hydrochloric acid*, dilute to 25 ml with *water* and dilute 5 ml of this solution to 20 ml with *water*. 12 ml of the resulting solution complies with *limit test A for heavy metals*, Appendix VII (2 ppm). Use *lead standard solution (2 ppm Pb)* to prepare the standard.

Free chlorine To 60 ml add 50 ml of *carbon dioxide-free water*, 1 ml of a 10% w/v solution of *potassium iodide* and 0.5 ml of *iodide-free starch solution* and allow to stand in the dark for 2 minutes. Any blue colour produced disappears on the addition of 0.2 ml of 0.01M *sodium thiosulphate VS* (1 ppm).

Sulphate Mix 26 ml with 10 mg of *sodium hydrogen carbonate*, evaporate to dryness on a water-bath and dissolve the residue in 15 ml of *water*. The resulting solution complies with the *limit test for sulphates*, Appendix VII (5 ppm).

Residue on evaporation Not more than 0.01%. Use 100 g.

Assay To 6 g add 30 ml of *water*, mix and titrate with 1M *sodium hydroxide VS* using *methyl red solution* as indicator. Each ml of 1M *sodium hydroxide VS* is equivalent to 0.03646 g of HCl.

Storage Dilute Hydrochloric Acid should be kept in a stoppered container of glass or other inert material and stored at a temperature not exceeding 30°.

Hydrochlorothiazide ☆

C₇H₈ClN₃O₄S₂   297.7   58-93-5

Hydrochlorothiazide is 6-chloro-3,4-dihydro-2*H*-1,2,4-benzothiadiazine-7-sulphonamide 1,1-dioxide. It contains not less than 98.0 per cent and not more than 102.0 per cent of $C_7H_8ClN_3O_4S_2$, calculated with reference to the dried substance.

Characteristics A white or almost white, crystalline powder; odourless.

Solubility Very slightly soluble in *water*; sparingly soluble in *ethanol (96%)*; soluble in *acetone*. It dissolves in dilute solutions of alkali hydroxides.

Identification *Test A may be omitted if tests B, C and D are carried out. Tests B and D may be omitted if tests A and C are carried out.*

A. The *infra-red absorption spectrum*, Appendix II A, is concordant with the spectrum of *hydrochlorothiazide EPCRS*.

B. The *light absorption*, Appendix II B, of a 0.001% w/v solution in 0.01M *sodium hydroxide* in the range 250 to 300 nm exhibits a maximum at 273 nm; the A(1%, 1 cm) at the maximum is 500 to 540. The *light absorption* of a 0.005% w/v solution in 0.01M *sodium hydroxide* in the range 300 to 350 nm exhibits a maximum at 323 nm; the A(1%, 1 cm) at the maximum is 89 to 96.

C. Carry out the method for *thin-layer chromatography*, Appendix III A, using *silica gel GF254* as the coating substance and *ethyl acetate* as the mobile phase but allowing the solvent front to ascend 10 cm above the line of application. Apply separately to the chromatoplate 4 μl of each of two solutions in *acetone* containing (1) 0.50% w/v of the substance being examined and (2) 0.50% w/v of *hydrochlorothiazide EPCRS*. After removal of the plate, dry it in a current of air and examine under *ultra-violet light (254 nm)*. The principal spot in the chromatogram obtained with solution (1) is similar in position and size to that in the chromatogram obtained with solution (2).

D. Heat gently 1 mg with 2 ml of a freshly prepared 0.05% w/v solution of *chromotropic acid sodium salt* in a cooled mixture of 7 volumes of *water* and 13 volumes of *sulphuric acid*. A violet colour is produced.

Acidity or alkalinity Shake 0.5 g of the powdered substance being examined with 25 ml of *carbon dioxide-free water* for 2 minutes and filter. To 10 ml of the filtrate add 0.2 ml of 0.01M *sodium hydroxide VS* and 0.15 ml of *methyl red solution*. The solution is yellow and not more

than 0.4 ml of 0.01M *hydrochloric acid VS* is required to change the colour to red.

Chloride Dissolve 1.0 g in 25 ml of *acetone* and dilute to 30 ml with *water*. 15 ml of the resulting solution complies with the *limit test for chlorides*, Appendix VII (100 ppm). Use a mixture of 10 ml of *chloride standard solution (5 ppm Cl)* and 5 ml of a 15% v/v solution of *water* in *acetone* to prepare the standard.

Related substances Carry out the method for *thin-layer chromatography*, Appendix III A, using *silica gel G* as the coating substance and a mixture of 85 volumes of *ethyl acetate* and 15 volumes of *propan-2-ol* as the mobile phase but allowing the solvent front to ascend 10 cm above the line of application. Apply separately to the chromatoplate 5 μl of each of two solutions of the substance being examined in *acetone* containing (1) 2.0% w/v and (2) 0.010% w/v. After removal of the plate, dry it in a current of air until the odour of solvent is no longer detectable (about 10 minutes) and spray with *ethanolic sulphuric acid (10%)*; use about 10 ml for a plate 200 mm × 200 mm in size and spray in small portions, allowing the solvent to evaporate each time to avoid excessive wetting. Heat at 100° to 105° for 30 minutes and immediately place above but not in 10 ml of a saturated solution of *sodium nitrite* in a glass tank. Add 0.5 ml of *sulphuric acid* to the sodium nitrite solution and allow to stand in the closed tank for 15 minutes. Remove the plate, heat it in a ventilated oven at 40° for 15 minutes, spray with three 5-ml quantities of a freshly prepared 0.5% w/v solution of N-*(1-naphthyl)-ethylenediamine dihydrochloride* in *ethanol (96%)* and examine by transmitted light. Any *secondary spot* in the chromatogram obtained with solution (1) is not more intense than the spot in the chromatogram obtained with solution (2).

Loss on drying When dried to constant weight at 100° to 105°, loses not more than 0.5% of its weight. Use 1 g.

Sulphated ash Not more than 0.1%, Appendix IX A. Use 1 g.

Assay Dissolve 0.12 g in 50 ml of *anhydrous pyridine* and carry out Method II for *non-aqueous titration*, Appendix VIII A, using 0.1M *tetrabutylammonium hydroxide VS* as titrant and determining the end-point potentiometrically at the second inflection. Repeat the operation without the substance being examined. The difference between the titrations represents the amount of tetrabutylammonium hydroxide required. Each ml of 0.1M *tetrabutylammonium hydroxide VS* is equivalent to 0.01488 g of $C_7H_8ClN_3O_4S_2$.

Preparation
Hydrochlorothiazide Tablets

Action and use Diuretic.

Hydrocortisone ☆

$C_{21}H_{30}O_5$ 362.5   *50-23-7*

Hydrocortisone is 11β,17α,21-trihydroxypregn-4-ene-3,20-dione. It contains not less than 96.0 per cent and not more than 104.0 per cent of $C_{21}H_{30}O_5$, calculated with reference to the dried substance.

Characteristics A white or almost white, crystalline powder. It melts at about 214°, with decomposition.

Solubility Practically insoluble in *water*; soluble in 80 parts of *acetone* and in 40 parts of *ethanol* (96%); slightly soluble in *chloroform*; very slightly soluble in *ether*.

Identification *Tests A and B may be omitted if tests C and D are carried out. Tests C and D may be omitted if tests A and B are carried out.*
A. The *infra-red absorption spectrum*, Appendix II A, is concordant with the spectrum of *hydrocortisone EPCRS*. If the spectra are not concordant, dissolve the substances in the minimum volume of *acetone*, evaporate to dryness on a water-bath and prepare new spectra of the residues as halogen salt discs or as dispersions in *liquid paraffin*.
B. Carry out the method for *thin-layer chromatography*, Appendix III A, using *silica gel GF254* as the coating substance, a mixture of 77 volumes of *dichloromethane*, 15 volumes of *ether*, 8 volumes of *methanol* and 1.2 volumes of *water* as the first mobile phase and a mixture of 80 volumes of *ether*, 15 volumes of *toluene* and 5 volumes of *butan-1-ol* saturated with *water* as the second mobile phase. Apply separately to the chromatoplate 2 µl of each of two solutions in a mixture of 90 volumes of *chloroform* and 10 volumes of *methanol* containing (1) 0.25% w/v of the substance being examined and (2) 0.25% w/v of *hydrocortisone EPCRS* and develop the chromatograms successively with each mobile phase. After both developments have been carried out, allow the plate to dry in air and examine under *ultra-violet light (254 nm)*. The principal spot in the chromatogram obtained with solution (1) corresponds to that in the chromatogram obtained with solution (2). Spray with *ethanolic sulphuric acid (20%)*, heat at 120° for 10 minutes or until spots appear and allow to cool. Examine the chromatograms in daylight and under *ultra-violet light (365 nm)*. The principal spot in the chromatogram obtained with solution (1) is similar in colour in daylight, fluorescence under ultra-violet light (365 nm), position and size to the principal spot in the chromatogram obtained with solution (2).
C. Carry out the method for *thin-layer chromatography*, Appendix III A, using the coating substance prescribed in the test for Related substances, a mixture of 77 volumes of *dichloromethane*, 15 volumes of *ether*, 8 volumes of *methanol* and 1.2 volumes of *water* as the first mobile phase and a mixture of 80 volumes of *ether*, 15 volumes of *toluene* and 5 volumes of *butan-1-ol* saturated with *water* as the second mobile phase. Apply separately to the chromatoplate 5 µl of each of solutions (1) and (3) and 25 µl of each of solutions (2) and (4) applying the latter two

in small quantities in order to obtain small spots. For solution (1) dissolve 25 mg of the substance being examined in *methanol* and dilute to 5 ml with the same solvent (solution A). Dilute 2 ml of this solution to 10 ml with *chloroform*. For solution (2) transfer 0.4 ml of solution A to a stoppered-glass tube (100 mm × 20 mm) and evaporate the solvent in a stream of nitrogen with gentle heating. Add 2 ml of a 15% v/v solution of *glacial acetic acid* and 50 mg of *sodium bismuthate*. Stopper the tube and shake the suspension for 1 hour protected from light. Add 2 ml of a 15% v/v solution of *glacial acetic acid* and filter into a 50-ml separating funnel, washing the filter with two 5-ml quantities of *water*. Shake the clear filtrate with 10 ml of *dichloromethane*. Wash the organic layer with 5 ml of 1M *sodium hydroxide* and two 5-ml quantities of *water* and dry over *anhydrous sodium sulphate*. For solution (3) dissolve 25 mg of *hydrocortisone EPCRS* in *methanol* and dilute to 5 ml with the same solvent (solution B). Dilute 2 ml of this solution to 10 ml with *chloroform*. Prepare solution (4) in the same manner as solution (2), but using 0.4 ml of solution B in place of 0.4 ml of solution A. Develop the plate successively with each mobile phase.

After both developments have been carried out, allow the plate to dry in air and examine under *ultra-violet light (254 nm)*. The principal spots in the chromatograms obtained with solutions (1) and (2) correspond to those in the chromatograms obtained with solutions (3) and (4) respectively. Spray the plate with *ethanolic sulphuric acid (20%)* and heat at 120° for 10 minutes or until spots appear. Allow to cool and examine the plate in daylight and under *ultra-violet light (365 nm)*. The principal spot in each of the chromatograms obtained with solutions (1) and (2) is similar in colour in daylight, fluorescence under ultra-violet light (365 nm), position and size to the principal spots in the chromatograms obtained with solutions (3) and (4) respectively. The principal spots in the chromatograms obtained with solutions (2) and (4) have Rf values distinctly higher than those of the principal spots in the chromatograms obtained with solutions (1) and (3).
D. To 2 ml of a 0.1% w/v solution in *ethanol* (96%) add 2 ml of *sulphuric acid*; an intense yellow colour is produced with a green fluorescence which is particularly intense under ultra-violet light (365 nm). Add the solution to 10 ml of *water* and mix; the fluorescence under ultra-violet light does not disappear.

Light absorption Dissolve 5 mg in sufficient *ethanol (96%)* to produce 100 ml and dilute 1 ml to 50 ml with the same solvent. Measure the *absorbance* of the resulting solution at the maximum at 240 nm, Appendix II B. The A(1%, 1 cm) at the maximum at 240 nm is 430 to 460.

Specific optical rotation In a 1% w/v solution in *1,4-dioxan*, +150° to +156°, Appendix V F.

Related substances Carry out the method for *thin-layer chromatography*, Appendix III A, using as the coating substance a suitable silica gel containing a fluorescent indicator with an optimal intensity at 254 nm (Merck silica gel 60 F254 is suitable) and a mixture of 77 volumes of *dichloromethane*, 15 volumes of *ether*, 8 volumes of *methanol* and 1.2 volumes of *water* as the mobile phase. Apply separately to the chromatoplate 5 µl of each of the following solutions in a mixture of 9 volumes of *chloroform* and 1 volume of *methanol*. Solutions (1), (2) and (3) contain 1.0% w/v, 0.020% w/v and 0.010% w/v respectively of the substance being examined. Solution (4) contains 1.0% w/v each of the substance being examined and *prednisolone EPCRS*. Allow the plate to dry in air and examine under *ultra-violet light (254 nm)*. Any *secondary spot* in the chromatogram obtained with solution (1) is not more intense than the spot in the chromatogram obtained with solution (2) and not more than one such spot is more intense than the spot in the chromatogram obtained with solution (3). The test is not valid unless the chromatogram obtained with solution (4) shows two clearly separated principal spots.

Loss on drying When dried for 3 hours at 100° to 105°, loses not more than 1.0% of its weight. Use 0.5 g.

Assay Carry out the *tetrazolium assay of steroids*, Appendix VIII P, and calculate the content of $C_{21}H_{30}O_5$ from the *absorbance* obtained by repeating the operation using *hydrocortisone EPCRS* in place of the substance being examined.

Storage Hydrocortisone should be kept in a well-closed container and protected from light.

Preparations
Hydrocortisone Cream
Hydrocortisone Ointment
Hydrocortisone and Neomycin Cream
Hydrocortisone and Clioquinol Ointment

Action and use Corticosteroid.

Hydrocortisone Acetate ☆

$C_{23}H_{32}O_6$ 404.5   *50-03-3*

Hydrocortisone Acetate is 11β,17α,21-trihydroxypregn-4-ene-3,20-dione 21-acetate. It contains not less than 96.0 per cent and not more than 104.0 per cent of $C_{23}H_{32}O_6$, calculated with reference to the dried substance.

Characteristics A white or almost white, crystalline powder. It melts at about 220°, with decomposition.

Solubility Practically insoluble in *water*; slightly soluble in *ethanol (96%)* and in *chloroform*.

Identification *Tests A and B may be omitted if tests C, D and E are carried out. Tests C, D and E may be omitted if tests A and B are carried out.*
A. The *infra-red absorption spectrum*, Appendix II A, is concordant with the spectrum of *hydrocortisone acetate EPCRS*.
B. Examine the chromatograms obtained in the test for Related substances under *ultra-violet light (254 nm)*. The principal spot in the chromatogram obtained with solution (2) corresponds to that in the chromatogram obtained with solution (5). Spray the plate with *ethanolic sulphuric acid (20%)* and heat at 120° for 10 minutes or until the spots appear. Allow to cool and examine in daylight and under *ultra-violet light (365 nm)*. The principal spot in the

chromatogram obtained with solution (2) is similar in colour in daylight, fluorescence under ultra-violet light (365 nm), position and size to that in the chromatogram obtained with solution (5).
C. Carry out the method for *thin-layer chromatography*, Appendix III A, using *silica gel GF254* as the coating substance and a mixture of 77 volumes of *dichloromethane*, 15 volumes of *ether*, 8 volumes of *methanol* and 1.2 volumes of *water* as the mobile phase. Apply separately to the chromatoplate 5 µl of each of the following solutions. For solution (1) dissolve 25 mg of the substance being examined in *methanol* and dilute to 5 ml with the same solvent (solution A). Dilute 2 ml of this solution to 10 ml with *chloroform*. For solution (2) transfer 2 ml of solution A to a stoppered 15-ml glass tube, add 10 ml of *saturated methanolic potassium hydrogen carbonate solution* and immediately pass a stream of *nitrogen* briskly through the solution for 5 minutes. Stopper the tube, heat in a water-bath at 45° protected from light for 150 minutes and allow to cool. For solution (3) dissolve 25 mg of *hydrocortisone acetate EPCRS* in *methanol*, dilute to 5 ml with the same solvent (solution B) and dilute 2 ml of this solution to 10 ml with *chloroform*. Prepare solution (4) in the same manner as solution (2) but use 2 ml of solution B in place of 2 ml of solution A. After removal of the plate, allow it to dry in air and examine under *ultra-violet light (254 nm)*. The principal spots in each of the chromatograms obtained with solutions (1) and (2) correspond to those in the chromatograms obtained with solutions (3) and (4) respectively. Spray with *ethanolic sulphuric acid (20%)* and heat at 120° for 10 minutes or until spots are produced. Allow to cool, examine in daylight and under *ultra-violet light (365 nm)*. The principal spots in the chromatograms obtained with solutions (1) and (2) are similar in colour in daylight, fluorescence under ultra-violet light (365 nm), position and size to those in the chromatograms obtained with solutions (3) and (4) respectively. The principal spots in the chromatograms obtained with solutions (2) and (4) have Rf values distinctly lower than those of the principal spots in the chromatograms obtained with solutions (1) and (3).
D. Dissolve 2 mg in 2 ml of *ethanol (96%)*, add 2 ml of *sulphuric acid* and mix; an orange colour is produced with a green fluorescence which is particularly intense under ultra-violet light (365 nm). Add the solution to 10 ml of *water* and mix; the fluorescence under ultra-violet light (365 nm) does not disappear.
E. Yields the *reaction* characteristic of acetyl groups, Appendix VI.

Light absorption Dissolve 5 mg in sufficient *ethanol (96%)* to produce 100 ml and dilute 10 ml to 50 ml with the same solvent. Measure the *absorbance* of the resulting solution at the maximum at 240 nm, Appendix II B. The A(1%, 1 cm) at the maximum at 240 nm is 385 to 415.

Specific optical rotation In a 1% w/v solution in *1,4-dioxan*, +158° to +167°, Appendix V F.

Related substances Carry out the method for *thin-layer chromatography*, Appendix III A, using as the coating substance a suitable silica gel containing a fluorescent indicator with an optimal intensity at 254 nm (Merck silica gel 60 F254 is suitable) and a mixture of 77 volumes of *dichloromethane*, 15 volumes of *ether*, 8 volumes of *methanol* and 1.2 volumes of *water* as the mobile phase. Apply separately to the plate 5 µl of each of the following solutions in a mixture of 9 volumes of *chloroform* and 1 volume of *methanol*. Solutions (1), (2), (3) and (4) contain 1.0% w/v, 0.10% w/v, 0.020% w/v and 0.010% w/v respectively of the substance being examined. Solution (5) contains 0.10% w/v of *hydrocortisone acetate EPCRS*. Solution (6) contains 0.10% w/v each of the substance being examined and *cortisone acetate EPCRS*. After removal of the plate, allow it to dry in air and examine under *ultra-violet light (254 nm)*. Any *secondary spot* in the chromatogram obtained with solution (1) is not more intense than the spot in the chromatogram obtained with solution (3) and not more than one such spot is more intense than the spot in the chromatogram obtained with solution (4). The test is not valid unless the chromatogram obtained with solution (6) shows two clearly separated spots.

Loss on drying When dried at 100° to 105° for 3 hours, loses not more than 0.5% of its weight. Use 0.5 g.

Assay Carry out the *tetrazolium assay of steroids*, Appendix VIII P, and calculate the content of $C_{23}H_{32}O_6$ from the *absorbance* obtained by repeating the operation using *hydrocortisone acetate EPCRS* in place of the substance being examined.

Storage Hydrocortisone Acetate should be kept in a well-closed container and protected from light.

Preparations
Hydrocortisone Acetate Cream
Hydrocortisone Acetate Ointment
Hydrocortisone Acetate Injection
Hydrocortisone Acetate and Clioquinol Cream
Hydrocortisone and Neomycin Ear Drops
Hydrocortisone and Neomycin Eye Drops
Hydrocortisone and Neomycin Ointment

Action and use Corticosteroid.

Hydrocortisone Hydrogen Succinate

$C_{25}H_{34}O_8$ 462.5   *2203-97-6*

Hydrocortisone Hydrogen Succinate is 11β,17α, 21-trihydroxypregn-4-ene-3,20-dione 21-hydrogen succinate. It contains not less than 97.0 per cent and not more than 103.0 per cent of $C_{25}H_{34}O_8$, calculated with reference to the dried substance.

Characteristics A white or almost white, crystalline powder; odourless or almost odourless.

Solubility Practically insoluble in *water*; soluble in 25 parts of *sodium hydrogen carbonate solution*, in 40 parts of *ethanol (96%)* and in 7 parts of *absolute ethanol*. It dissolves in 5M *sodium hydroxide* with decomposition.

Identification A. The *infra-red absorption spectrum*, Appendix II A, is concordant with the *reference spectrum* of hydrocortisone hydrogen succinate.
B. Carry out the method for *thin-layer chromatography*, Appendix III A, using *silica gel G* as the coating substance

and a freshly prepared mixture of 60 volumes of *butan-1-ol*, 20 volumes of *acetic anhydride* and 20 volumes of *water* as the mobile phase. Apply separately to the chromatoplate 2 μl of each of the following solutions in *methanol*. Solution (1) contains 0.25% w/v of the substance being examined. Solution (2) contains 0.25% w/v of *hydrocortisone hydrogen succinate BPCRS*. Solution (3) is a mixture of equal volumes of solutions (1) and (2). After removal of the plate, allow it to dry in air, spray with *ethanolic sulphuric acid (20%)*, heat at 120° for 10 minutes, allow to cool and examine under *ultra-violet light (365 nm)*. The principal spot in the chromatogram obtained with solution (1) corresponds to that in the chromatogram obtained with solution (2). The principal spot in the chromatogram obtained with solution (3) appears as a single, compact spot.
C. Gently boil 25 mg with 10 ml of 2M *hydrochloric acid* for 10 minutes and evaporate to dryness on a water-bath. Add 5 ml of 5M *ammonia*, evaporate to dryness in a small dish and dry at 100° for 30 minutes. Mix the residue with 2.5 g of *zinc powder*, transfer to a test-tube, heat gently over a flame and expose the escaping vapours to a pine wood shaving, previously well-moistened with *hydrochloric acid*. The shaving becomes red to brownish-red.

Acidity Dissolve a quantity equivalent to 1 g of the dried substance in 20 ml of *absolute ethanol* previously neutralised to *phenolphthalein solution* and titrate with 0.1M *sodium hydroxide VS*. Not less than 20.9 ml and not more than 22.3 ml is required to change the colour of the solution.

Specific optical rotation In a 1% w/v solution in *absolute ethanol*, +147° to +153°, Appendix V F.

Related foreign steroids Carry out Method A for *related foreign steroids*, Appendix III A, using solutions in a mixture of equal volumes of *chloroform* and *methanol* containing (1) 1.5% w/v of the substance being examined, (2) 1.5% w/v of *hydrocortisone hydrogen succinate BPCRS* and (3) 0.030% w/v of each of *hydrocortisone EPCRS* and *hydrocortisone acetate EPCRS*. Any *secondary spot* in the chromatogram obtained with solution (1) is not more intense than the proximate spot in the chromatogram obtained with solution (3).

Loss on drying When dried to constant weight at 100° at a pressure not exceeding 0.7 kPa, loses not more than 5.0% of its weight. Use 1 g.

Sulphated ash Not more than 0.1%, Appendix IX A.

Assay Dissolve 15 mg in sufficient *absolute ethanol* to produce 100 ml, dilute 10 ml to 50 ml with *absolute ethanol* and measure the *absorbance* of the resulting solution at the maximum at 240 nm, Appendix II B. Calculate the content of $C_{25}H_{34}O_8$ taking 345 as the value of A(1%, 1 cm) at the maximum at about 240 nm.

Storage Hydrocortisone Hydrogen Succinate should be protected from light.

Preparation
Hydrocortisone Sodium Succinate Injection

Action and use Corticosteroid.

Hydrocortisone Sodium Phosphate

C_{21}H_{29}Na_2O_8P   486.4   *6000-74-4*

Hydrocortisone Sodium Phosphate is disodium 11β,17α-dihydroxy-3,20-dioxopregn-4-en-21-yl orthophosphate. It contains not less than 96.0 per cent and not more than 103.0 per cent of $C_{21}H_{29}Na_2O_8P$, calculated with reference to the anhydrous substance.

Characteristics A white or almost white powder; hygroscopic.

Solubility Soluble in 4 parts of *water*; practically insoluble in *absolute ethanol* and in *chloroform*.

Identification *Test A may be omitted if tests B, C and D are carried out. Tests B and C may be omitted if tests A and D are carried out.*

A. Dissolve 50 mg in 1 ml of *deuterium oxide* containing 0.1% w/v of *sodium 3-trimethylsilylpropanesulphonate*. The *nuclear magnetic resonance spectrum* of the resulting solution, Appendix II C, is concordant with that of a similar solution of *hydrocortisone sodium phosphate BPCRS*.

B. Carry out the method for *thin-layer chromatography*, Appendix III A, using *silica gel G* as the coating substance and a freshly prepared mixture of 60 volumes of *butan-1-ol*, 20 volumes of *acetic anhydride* and 20 volumes of *water* as the mobile phase. Apply separately to the chromatoplate 2 μl of each of the following solutions. Solution (1) contains 0.25% w/v of the substance being examined in *methanol*. Solution (2) contains 0.25% w/v of *hydrocortisone sodium phosphate BPCRS* in *methanol*. Solution (3) is a mixture of equal volumes of solutions (1) and (2). Solution (4) is a mixture of equal volumes of solution (1) and a 0.25% w/v solution of *betamethasone sodium phosphate BPCRS* in *methanol*. After removal of the plate, allow it to dry in air until the odour of solvent is no longer detectable, spray with *ethanolic sulphuric acid (20%)*, heat at 120° for 10 minutes and examine under *ultra-violet light (365 nm)*. The principal spot in the chromatogram obtained with solution (1) corresponds to that in the chromatogram obtained with solution (2). The principal spot in the chromatogram obtained with solution (3) appears as a single compact spot and the chromatogram obtained with solution (4) shows two principal spots with almost identical Rf values.

C. Dissolve 2 mg in 2 ml of *sulphuric acid*. A yellowish-green fluorescence is produced immediately (distinction from betamethasone sodium phosphate, dexamethasone sodium phosphate and prednisolone sodium phosphate).

D. Heat gently 40 mg with 2 ml of *sulphuric acid* until white fumes are evolved, add *nitric acid* dropwise until oxidation is complete and cool. Add 2 ml of *water*, heat until white fumes are again evolved, cool, add 10 ml of *water* and neutralise to *litmus paper* with 5M *ammonia*. The resulting solution yields *reactions A* and *C* characteristic of sodium salts and *reaction B* characteristic of phosphates, Appendix VI.

Alkalinity pH of a 0.5% w/v solution, 7.5 to 9.0, Appendix V L.

Specific optical rotation In a 1% w/v solution, +121° to +129°, Appendix V F.

Inorganic phosphate Dissolve 25 mg in 10 ml of *water*, add 4 ml of 1M *sulphuric acid*, 1 ml of a 10% w/v solution of *ammonium molybdate* and 2 ml of *methylaminophenol—sulphite reagent* and allow to stand for 15 minutes. Add sufficient *water* to produce 25 ml and allow to stand for a further 15 minutes. The *absorbance* of a 4-cm layer of the resulting solution at 730 nm, Appendix II B, is not more than that of a 4-cm layer of a solution prepared by treating 10 ml of a 0.0036% w/v solution of *potassium dihydrogen orthophosphate* in the same manner, beginning at the words 'add 4 ml . . .'.

Related substances Carry out the method for *thin-layer chromatography*, Appendix III A, using *silica gel GF254* as the coating substance and a mixture of 77 volumes of *dichloromethane*, 15 volumes of *ether*, 8 volumes of *methanol* and 1.2 volumes of *water* as the mobile phase. Apply separately to the chromatoplate 2 μl of each of three solutions in *methanol* containing (1) 1.0% w/v of the substance being examined, (2) 1.0% w/v of *hydrocortisone sodium phosphate BPCRS* and (3) 0.020% w/v of *hydrocortisone EPCRS*. After removal of the plate, allow it to dry in air for 5 minutes and examine under *ultra-violet light (254 nm)*. Any *secondary spot* in the chromatogram obtained with solution (1) is not more intense than the spot in the chromatogram obtained with solution (3).

Assay Dissolve 0.1 g in sufficient *water* to produce 200 ml. Dilute 5 ml to 100 ml with *water* and measure the *absorbance* of the resulting solution at the maximum at 248 nm, Appendix II B. Calculate the content of $C_{21}H_{29}Na_2O_8P$ taking 333 as the value of A(1%, 1 cm) at the maximum at 248 nm.

Storage Hydrocortisone Sodium Phosphate should be kept in a well-closed container and protected from light.

Preparation

Hydrocortisone Sodium Phosphate Injection

Action and use Corticosteroid.

Hydroflumethiazide

C_8H_8F_3N_3O_4S_2   331.3   *135-09-1*

Hydroflumethiazide is 3,4-dihydro-6-trifluoro-methyl-2*H*-1,2,4-benzothiadiazine-7-sulphonamide 1,1-dioxide. It contains not less than 98.0 per cent and not more than 102.0 per cent of $C_8H_8F_3N_3O_4S_2$, calculated with reference to the dried substance.

Characteristics White or almost white, glistening crystals or crystalline powder; odourless or almost odourless.

Solubility Practically insoluble in *water*; soluble in *ethanol (96%)*; practically insoluble in *chloroform* and in *ether*.

Identification A. The *infra-red absorption spectrum*, Appendix II A, is concordant with the *reference spectrum* of hydroflumethiazide.

B. Dissolve 10 mg in 10 ml of 0.1M *sodium hydroxide*, add sufficient *water* to produce 100 ml and dilute 10 ml to 50 ml with 0.01M *sodium hydroxide*. The *light absorption* of the resulting solution, Appendix II B, in the range 230 to 350 nm exhibits two maxima, at 274 nm and 333 nm. The *absorbance* at 274 nm is about 0.92 and at 333 nm is about 0.19.

C. Carry out the method for *thin-layer chromatography*, Appendix III A, using *silica gel GF254* as the coating substance and *ethyl acetate* as the mobile phase. Apply separately to the chromatoplate 5 μl of each of two solutions in *acetone* containing (1) 0.1% w/v of the substance being examined and (2) 0.1% w/v of *hydroflumethiazide BPCRS*. After removal of the plate, dry it in a current of air, examine under *ultra-violet light (254 nm)* and then reveal the spots by *Method I*. By both methods of visualisation the principal spot in the chromatogram obtained with solution (1) corresponds in colour and intensity to that in the chromatogram obtained with solution (2).

Related substances Carry out the method for *thin-layer chromatography*, Appendix III A, using *silica gel G* as the coating substance and *ethyl acetate* as the mobile phase. Apply separately to the chromatoplate 10 μl of each of two solutions of the substance being examined in *acetone* containing (1) 1.0% w/v and (2) 0.001% w/v. After removal of the plate, dry it in a current of air and reveal the spots by *Method I*. Any *secondary spot* in the chromatogram obtained with solution (1) is not more intense than the spot in the chromatogram obtained with solution (2).

Loss on drying When dried to constant weight at 105°, loses not more than 0.5% of its weight. Use 1 g.

Sulphated ash Not more than 0.1%, Appendix IX A.

Assay Dissolve 0.3 g in 50 ml of *anhydrous pyridine* and carry out Method II for *non-aqueous titration*, Appendix VIII A, using 0.1M *tetrabutylammonium hydroxide VS* as titrant and determining the end-point potentiometrically. Each ml of 0.1M *tetrabutylammonium hydroxide VS* is equivalent to 0.01656 g of $C_8H_8F_3N_3O_4S_2$.

Preparation
Hydroflumethiazide Tablets

Action and use Diuretic.

Hydrogen Peroxide Solution (30 per cent) ☆

7722-84-1

Hydrogen Peroxide Solution (30 per cent) contains not less than 29.0 per cent w/w and not more than 31.0 per cent w/w of H_2O_2 (34.01), corresponding to about 100 times its volume of available oxygen. It may contain a suitable stabilising agent.

Characteristics A clear, colourless liquid. It decomposes vigorously in contact with oxidisable organic matter and with certain metals and if allowed to become alkaline.

Identification A. To 1 ml add, cautiously, 0.1 ml of 2M *sodium hydroxide*. It decomposes with vigorous effervescence.

B. Shake 0.05 ml with 2 ml of 1M *sulphuric acid*, 2 ml of *ether* and 0.05 ml of *potassium chromate solution*. The ether layer is deep blue.

Acidity Dilute 10 ml with 100 ml of *water* and add 0.25 ml of *methyl red solution*. Not less than 0.05 ml and not more than 0.5 ml of 0.1M *sodium hydroxide VS* is required to change the colour of the solution.

Organic stabilisers Shake 20 ml with successive quantities of 10, 5 and 5 ml of *chloroform*. Evaporate the combined chloroform extracts at a temperature not exceeding 25° under reduced pressure and dry in a desiccator. Any residue weighs not more than 10 mg (500 ppm).

Non-volatile matter Place 10 ml in a platinum dish and allow to stand until effervescence has ceased, cooling if necessary. Evaporate the solution on a water-bath. Any residue, when dried at 100° to 105°, weighs not more than 20 mg (0.2% w/v).

Assay Dilute 1 g to 100 ml with *water*. To 10 ml of the resulting solution add 20 ml of 1M *sulphuric acid* and titrate with 0.02M *potassium permanganate VS*. Each ml of 0.02M *potassium permanganate VS* is equivalent to 0.001701 g of H_2O_2 or 0.56 ml of oxygen.

Storage Hydrogen Peroxide Solution (30 per cent) should be protected from light. If the solution does not contain a stabilising agent, it should be stored at a temperature not exceeding 15°.

Labelling The label states whether or not the solution contains a stabilising agent.

Hydrogen Peroxide Solution (27 per cent)

Hydrogen Peroxide Solution (27 per cent) contains not less than 26.0 per cent w/w and not more than 28.0 per cent w/w of H_2O_2 (34.01), corresponding to about 90 times its volume of available oxygen. It may contain a suitable stabilising agent.

Characteristics A clear, colourless liquid. It decomposes vigorously in contact with oxidisable organic matter and with certain metals and if allowed to become alkaline.

Identification; Acidity; Organic stabilisers; Non-volatile matter Complies with the requirements stated under Hydrogen Peroxide Solution (30 per cent).

Assay Carry out the Assay described under Hydrogen Peroxide Solution (30 per cent).

Storage Hydrogen Peroxide Solution (27 per cent) should be protected from light. If the solution does not contain a stabilising agent, it should be stored at a temperature not exceeding 15°.

Labelling The label on the container states whether or not the solution contains a stabilising agent.

Hydrogen Peroxide Solution (6 per cent)

Hydrogen Peroxide Solution

Hydrogen Peroxide Solution (6 per cent) is an aqueous solution of hydrogen peroxide containing not less than 5.0 per cent w/v and not more than 7.0 per cent w/v of H_2O_2 (34.01), corresponding to about 20 times its volume of available oxygen. It may contain a suitable stabilising agent.

Characteristics A clear, colourless liquid. It decomposes in contact with oxidisable organic matter and with certain metals and if allowed to become alkaline.

Identification; Non-volatile matter Complies with the requirements stated under Hydrogen Peroxide Solution (30 per cent).

Acidity Dilute 10 ml with 20 ml of *water* and add 0.25 ml of *methyl red solution*. Not less than 0.20 ml and not more than 1.0 ml of 0.1M *sodium hydroxide VS* is required to change the colour of the solution.

Organic stabilisers Shake 20 ml with successive quantities of 10, 5 and 5 ml of *chloroform*. Evaporate the combined chloroform extracts at a temperature not exceeding 25° at a pressure of 2 kPa and dry in a desiccator. Any residue weighs not more than 5 mg (250 ppm).

Assay Dilute 10 ml to 100 ml with *water*. To 10 ml of the resulting solution add 20 ml of 1M *sulphuric acid* and titrate with 0.02M *potassium permanganate VS*. Each ml of 0.02M *potassium permanganate VS* is equivalent to 0.001701 g of H_2O_2 or 0.56 ml of oxygen.

Storage Hydrogen Peroxide Solution (6 per cent) should be protected from light. If the solution does not contain a stabilising agent, it should be stored at a temperature not exceeding 15°. It should not be stored for long periods.

Labelling The label whether or not the solution contains a stabilising agent.

Action and use Antiseptic; deodorant.

When Hydrogen Peroxide is prescribed or demanded, Hydrogen Peroxide Solution (6 per cent) shall be dispensed or supplied.

Hydrogen Peroxide Solution (3 per cent) ☆

Dilute Hydrogen Peroxide Solution

Hydrogen Peroxide Solution (3 per cent) contains not less than 2.5 per cent w/w and not more than 3.5 per cent w/w of H_2O_2 (34.01), corresponding to about 10 times its volume of available oxygen. It may contain a suitable stabilising agent.

Characteristics A clear, colourless liquid. It decomposes in contact with oxidisable organic matter and with certain metals and if allowed to become alkaline.

Identification; Non-volatile matter Complies with the requirements stated under Hydrogen Peroxide Solution (30 per cent).

Acidity To 10 ml add 20 ml of *water* and 0.25 ml of *methyl red solution*. Not less than 0.05 ml and not more

than 1.0 ml of 0.1M *sodium hydroxide VS* is required to change the colour of the solution.

Organic stabilisers Shake 20 ml with successive quantities of 10, 5 and 5 ml of *chloroform*. Evaporate the combined chloroform extracts at a temperature not exceeding 25° under reduced pressure and dry in a desiccator. Any residue weighs not more than 5 mg (250 ppm).

Assay Dilute 10 g to 100 ml with *water*. To 10 ml of the resulting solution add 20 ml of 1M *sulphuric acid* and titrate with 0.02M *potassium permanganate VS*. Each ml of 0.02M *potassium permanganate VS* is equivalent to 0.001701 g of H_2O_2 or 0.56 ml of oxygen.

Storage Hydrogen Peroxide Solution (3 per cent) should be protected from light. If the solution does not contain a stabilising agent, it should be stored at a temperature not exceeding 15°. It should not be stored for long periods.

Labelling The label states whether or not the solution contains a stabilising agent.

Action and use Antiseptic; deodorant.

Hydrotalcite

$Al_2Mg_6(OH)_{16}CO_3,4H_2O$ 604.0   *12304-65-3*

Hydrotalcite is a hydrated form of an aluminium magnesium basic carbonate corresponding to the formula $Al_2Mg_6(OH)_{16}CO_3,4H_2O$. It contains not less than 14.4 per cent and not more than 19.4 per cent w/w of Al_2O_3, and not less than 34.0 per cent and not more than 46.0 per cent w/w of MgO. The ratio of the content of Al_2O_3 to the content of MgO is not less than 0.40 and not more than 0.45.

Characteristics A white or almost white, free-flowing, granular powder.

Solubility Practically insoluble in *water*. It dissolves in dilute mineral acids with slight effervescence.

Identification A. Dissolve 1.0 g in 20 ml of 2M *hydrochloric acid*. Effervescence occurs. Add 30 ml of *water*, boil, add 2M *ammonia* until just alkaline to *methyl red solution*, continue boiling for 2 minutes and filter, reserving the filtrate for test B. Wash the precipitate with 50 ml of a hot 2% w/v solution of *ammonium chloride* and dissolve in 15 ml of 2M *hydrochloric acid*. The resulting solution yields the *reactions* characteristic of aluminium salts, Appendix VI.
B. Dilute 1 ml of the filtrate obtained in test A to 10 ml with *water*. The resulting solution yields the *reactions* characteristic of magnesium salts, Appendix VI.

Alkalinity pH of a 4% w/v suspension in *carbon dioxide-free water*, 8.0 to 10.0, Appendix V L.

Neutralising capacity Mix 0.2 g with a small quantity of *water* to give a smooth paste and gradually add sufficient further quantities of *water* to produce 100 ml. Warm at 37°, add 100 ml of 0.1M *hydrochloric acid VS* previously heated to 37° and stir continuously for 1 hour using a paddle stirrer at a rate of about 200 revolutions per minute, maintaining the temperature at 37°, and titrate with 0.1M *sodium hydroxide VS* to pH 3.5. Subtract the volume of 0.1M *sodium hydroxide VS* from 100 ml to obtain the number of ml of 0.1M *hydrochloric acid VS* required for neutralisation. Not less than 260 ml of 0.1M *hydrochloric acid VS* is required to neutralise 1 g.

Arsenic Dissolve 0.33 g in 5 ml of 2M *hydrochloric acid*. The resulting solution complies with the *limit test for arsenic*, Appendix VII (3 ppm).

Heavy metals Dissolve 2.7 g in 20 ml of 2M *hydrochloric acid* and 10 ml of *water*, add 0.5 ml of *nitric acid* and boil for 30 seconds. Cool, add 2 g of *ammonium chloride* and 2 g of *ammonium thiocyanate* and extract with three 10-ml quantities of a mixture of equal volumes of *amyl alcohol* and *ether*. Add to the aqueous layer 0.1 ml of *dilute phenolphthalein solution* and 13.5M *ammonia* until a pink colour is produced. Cool, add *glacial acetic acid* until the solution is decolorised and add a further 5 ml of *glacial acetic acid*. Filter, if necessary, and dilute the solution to 40 ml with *water*. 12 ml of the resulting solution complies with *limit test A for heavy metals*, Appendix VII (30 ppm). Use *lead standard solution (2 ppm Pb)* to prepare the standard.

Sodium Not more than 0.1% of Na when determined by Method II for *atomic emission spectrophotometry*, Appendix II D. To prepare the test solution dissolve 0.1 g in 4 ml of 5M *hydrochloric acid*, dilute to 200 ml with *water* and measure at 589 nm. Use *sodium solution ASp*, diluted if necessary with 0.1M *hydrochloric acid*, for the standard solution.

Chloride Dissolve 0.18 g in 10 ml of 2M *nitric acid*, boil, allow to cool and dilute to 100 ml with *water*. To 10 ml add 5 ml of *water*. The resulting solution complies with the *limit test for chlorides*, Appendix VII (0.3%).

Sulphate Dissolve 0.14 g in 15 ml of 1M *hydrochloric acid* and dilute to 100 ml with *water*. 15 ml of the resulting solution complies with the *limit test for sulphates*, Appendix VII (0.7%).

Loss on ignition When ignited at 800°, loses 40.0 to 50.0% of its weight. Use 1 g.

Assay *For Al₂O₃* Dissolve 0.3 g in 2 ml of 7M *hydrochloric acid*, add 250 ml of *water* and 50 ml of 0.05M *disodium edetate VS* and neutralise with 1M *sodium hydroxide* using *methyl red solution* as indicator. Heat the solution on a water-bath for 30 minutes and allow to cool. Add 3 g of *hexamine* and titrate the excess of disodium edetate with 0.05M *lead(II) nitrate VS* using *xylenol orange solution* as indicator. Each ml of 0.05M *disodium edetate VS* is equivalent to 0.002549 g of Al₂O₃.

For MgO Dissolve 0.125 g in the minimum volume of 7M *hydrochloric acid*, add 30 ml of *water*, 1 g of *ammonium chloride*, 10 ml of *triethanolamine*, 150 ml of *water* and 5 ml of *ammonia buffer pH 10.9* and titrate immediately with 0.05M *disodium edetate VS* using *mordant black 11 solution* as indicator. Each ml of 0.05M *disodium edetate VS* is equivalent to 0.002015 g of MgO.

Preparation
Hydrotalcite Tablets

Action and use Antacid.

Hydroxocobalamin

$C_{62}H_{89}CoN_{13}O_{15}P$ 1346.3   *13422-51-0*

Hydroxocobalamin is $Co\alpha$-[α-(5,6-dimethyl-benzimidazolyl)]-$Co\beta$-hydroxocobamide. It occurs either as aquocobalamin chloride ($Co\alpha$-[α-(5,6-dimethylbenzimidazolyl)]-$Co\beta$-aquo-cobamide chloride), which contains not less than 96.0 per cent and not more than 102.0 per cent of $C_{62}H_{90}ClCoN_{13}O_{15}P$, or as aquo-cobalamin sulphate, which contains not less than 96.0 per cent and not more than 102.0 per cent of $C_{124}H_{180}Co_2N_{26}O_{34}P_2S$, both calculated with reference to the dried substance.

Characteristics Dark red crystals or crystalline powder; odourless or almost odourless. Some decomposition may occur on drying.

Solubility Soluble in *water*.

Identification A. Measure the *absorbance* of the solution used in the Assay at the maxima at 274, 351 and 525 nm, Appendix II B. The ratios of the absorbances at 274 nm and 525 nm to the absorbance at 351 nm are about 0.8 and about 0.3 respectively.

B. Fuse 1 mg with 50 mg of *potassium hydrogen sulphate*, cool, break up the mass, add 3 ml of *water* and boil until dissolved. Add 0.05 ml of *phenolphthalein solution* and sufficient 5M *sodium hydroxide* to produce a faint pink colour. Add 0.5 g of *sodium acetate*, 0.5 ml of 1M *acetic acid* and 0.5 ml of a 0.2% w/v solution of *nitroso R salt*; a red or orange-red colour is produced immediately. Add 0.5 ml of *hydrochloric acid* and boil for 1 minute; the red colour persists.

C. Yields the *reactions* characteristic of chlorides or of sulphates, Appendix VI.

Coloured impurities Not more than 5.0% when determined by the following method.

Carry out the following procedure protected from light. Shake together 500 ml of *water* and 500 ml of *butan-2-ol* and allow to stand overnight at 25° to 30°.

Carry out the method for *descending paper chromatography*, Appendix III E, using in the bottom of the tank the lower layer of the solvent mixture with the addition of 5 ml of 6M *acetic acid* and 0.5 g of *potassium cyanide* and, as the mobile phase, the upper layer with the addition of 5% v/v of *butan-2-ol* and 1% v/v of 6M *acetic acid*. Dissolve 2 mg of the substance being examined in

1 ml of *water*, add 0.05 ml of *hydrocyanic acid solution*, allow to stand for 15 minutes and apply all of the solution to the paper in successive bands along the pencil line on the paper, which should be 22.5 cm wide, leaving 2.5 cm clear at both ends, drying each application in a current of nitrogen without the aid of heat. Insert the paper in the tank and allow to stand for not less than 4 hours before development. Develop until the hydroxocobalamin has travelled about two-thirds of the length of the paper.

Cut out and discard the main hydroxocobalamin band from the dried paper, trim the remaining pieces of paper of any uncoloured zones at the top and bottom, fasten together the vertical edges of each of the two remaining strips and allow the cylinders so obtained to stand on filter paper moistened with *water* until the coloured material reaches the top edges. Remove the uncoloured paper, elute the coloured material by descending chromatography with the minimum quantity of *water*, combine the eluates, dilute to a suitable volume with *water*, filter through a sintered-glass filter and measure the *absorbance* of the filtrate at the maximum at 361 nm, Appendix II B, using in the reference cell the solution obtained by repeating the procedure without the substance being examined; make the cylinders from pieces of the paper of the same size and cut from the same positions as those used for the test solution. Calculate the content of coloured impurities taking 207 as the value of A(1%, 1 cm) at the maximum at 361 nm.

Other cobalamins Not more than 3.0% when determined by the following method.

Slurry 10 g of *diethylaminoethylcellulose* (Whatman DE-23 is suitable) with 150 ml of 0.5M *hydrochloric acid* for 1 hour, filter and wash with *water* until the pH of the washings is above 4.5. Slurry the diethylaminoethyl-cellulose with 150 ml of 0.5M *sodium hydroxide* for 1 hour, filter and wash with *water* until the pH of the washings is 7 to 7.5. Using 1000 ml of *water* transfer the slurry in portions to a glass column (22 cm × 1.2 cm) fitted with a sintered-glass disc and a tap. Allow to settle until the height of the absorbent is about 19 cm, wash with *water* until the pH of the effluent is constant and tamp down to a height of about 14.5 cm.

Prepare a second column in exactly the same manner but using *carboxymethylcellulose* (Whatman CM-23 is suitable) in place of the diethylaminoethylcellulose and reversing the order of the acid and alkali treatments. Tamp down the column to a height of about 10 cm.

Place a plug of glass wool on each column and allow to drain until only a small amount of water remains above the column. Support the columns so that the effluent from the diethylaminoethylcellulose column runs into the carboxymethylcellulose column.

Dissolve 50 mg of the substance being examined in 20 ml of *water* containing sufficient *hydrochloric acid* to give a pH below 4.0. Add the solution to the diethyl-aminoethylcellulose column and allow to run through both columns, discarding the first colourless effluent. Elute with *water* and collect 50 ml of the coloured effluent from the carboxymethylcellulose column. Measure the *absorbance* of the resulting solution at the maximum at 361 nm, Appendix II B. Calculate the content of other cobalamins taking 207 as the value of A(1%, 1 cm) at the maximum at 361 nm.

Acidic impurities Not more than 3.0% when determined by the following method carried out immediately after the test for Other cobalamins.

Elute the diethylaminoethylcellulose column used in the test for Other cobalamins with a 1% w/v solution of *sodium chloride* and collect 50 ml of the effluent. Measure the *absorbance* of the resulting solution at the maximum between 351 and 361 nm, Appendix II B. Calculate the content of acidic impurities taking 190 as the value of A(1%, 1 cm) at the maximum between 351 and 361 nm.

Loss on drying When dried to constant weight at 100° at a pressure not exceeding 0.7 kPa, loses 8.0 to 12.0% of its weight (aquocobalamin chloride) or 8.0 to 16.0% of its weight (aquocobalamin sulphate). Use 1 g.

Assay Carry out the following procedure protected from light. Dissolve 25 mg in sufficient of a solution containing 0.8% v/v of *glacial acetic acid* and 1.09% w/v of *sodium acetate* to produce 1000 ml and measure the *absorbance* of the resulting solution at the maximum at 351 nm, Appendix II B. Calculate the content of $C_{62}H_{90}ClCoN_{13}O_{15}P$ or of $C_{124}H_{180}Co_2N_{26}O_{34}P_2S$ taking 190 or 188 respectively as the value of A(1%, 1 cm) at the maximum at 351 nm.

Storage Hydroxocobalamin should be kept in a well-closed container, protected from light and stored at a temperature not exceeding 15°.

Labelling The label on the container states whether the contents are aquocobalamin chloride or aquocobalamin sulphate.

Preparation
Hydroxocobalamin Injection

Hydroxychloroquine Sulphate

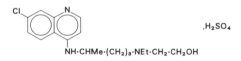

$C_{18}H_{26}ClN_3O,H_2SO_4$ 434.0   747-36-4

Hydroxychloroquine Sulphate is 2-{N-[4-(7-chloro-4-quinolylamino)pentyl]-N-ethylamino}-ethanol sulphate. It contains not less than 98.0 per cent and not more than 100.5 per cent of $C_{18}H_{26}ClN_3O,H_2SO_4$, calculated with reference to the dried substance.

Characteristics A white or almost white, crystalline powder; odourless or almost odourless.

Solubility Soluble in 5 parts of *water*; practically insoluble in *ethanol* (96%), in *chloroform* and in *ether*.

Identification A. Dissolve 0.1 g in 10 ml of *water*, add 2 ml of 2M *sodium hydroxide* and extract with two 20-ml quantities of *chloroform*. Wash the chloroform extracts with *water*, dry with *anhydrous sodium sulphate*, evaporate to dryness and dissolve the residue in 2 ml of *chloroform*. The *infra-red absorption spectrum* of the resulting solution, Appendix II A, is concordant with the *reference spectrum* of hydroxychloroquine.

B. The *light absorption*, Appendix II B, in the range 240 to 350 nm of a 0.002% w/v solution in 0.01M *hydrochloric acid* exhibits three maxima, at 257, 329 and 343 nm. The *absorbance* at 257 nm is about 0.78, at 329 nm, about 0.86 and at 343 nm, about 0.94.

C. Dissolve 0.2 g in 10 ml of *water*, add 30 ml of hot *trinitrophenol solution* and allow to cool. The *melting point* of the precipitate, after washing with 10 ml of *water*, is about 189°, Appendix V A.

D. Yields the *reactions* characteristic of sulphates, Appendix VI.

E. *Melting point*, about 240° or about 198°, Appendix V A.

Acidity pH of a 1% w/v solution, 3.5 to 5.5, Appendix V L.

Clarity and colour of solution A 10.0% w/v solution is not more than slightly turbid and not more than slightly yellow.

Lead Not more than 20 ppm when determined by the following method. Carefully heat 2.0 g for 10 minutes with 8 ml of *water* and 6 ml of *nitric acid* in a round-bottomed, long-necked flask. Cool, add 4 ml of *sulphuric acid* and heat until the mixture darkens. Continue heating, with the dropwise addition of *nitric acid*, until the liquid becomes colourless and white fumes of sulphur trioxide are produced. Add 3 ml of *water*, carefully evaporate until white fumes are again produced, cool and dilute to 18 ml with *water*. Add and dissolve 2 g of *citric acid*, make alkaline with 5M *ammonia* and add 1 ml of *potassium cyanide solution PbT*. Transfer to a separating funnel, add 10 ml of *dithizone solution*, shake vigorously and remove the lower layer. Repeat the extraction with two 5-ml quantities of *dithizone solution*. If, after the third extraction, the chloroform layer is bright red, continue the extraction with further 5-ml quantities of *dithizone solution* until the colour of the reagent no longer changes to bright red. Wash the combined chloroform solutions by shaking with 10 ml of *water* and then extract with two 10-ml quantities of 2M *hydrochloric acid*. Wash the combined acid solutions with 10 ml of *chloroform* and discard the chloroform. Transfer the solution to a *Nessler cylinder* and make alkaline with 5M *ammonia*. In a second *Nessler cylinder* mix 2 ml of 6M *acetic acid* with 20 ml of 2M *hydrochloric acid*, make alkaline with 5M *ammonia* and add 4 ml of *lead standard solution (10 ppm Pb)*.

Treat the contents of each cylinder as follows. Add 1 ml of *potassium cyanide solution PbT*; the solutions should not be more than faintly opalescent. If the colours of the solutions differ, equalise them by the addition of a few drops of a highly diluted solution of burnt sugar or other non-reactive substance. Dilute to 50 ml with *water*, add 0.1 ml of a solution prepared by dissolving 10 g of *sodium sulphide* in sufficient *water* to produce 100 ml and filtering and mix thoroughly. Compare the colours of the two solutions by a suitable method, such as by light reflected from a white tile through the Nessler cylinders. The colour of the solution in the first cylinder is not more intense than that of the solution in the second cylinder.

Chloride Dissolve 0.50 g in 50 ml of *water*. 15 ml of the resulting solution complies with the *limit test for chlorides*, Appendix VII (350 ppm).

Related substances Carry out the method for *thin-layer chromatography*, Appendix III A, using *silica gel GF254* as the coating substance and a mixture of 72 volumes of *methanol*, 25 volumes of *water* and 3 volumes of 13.5M *ammonia* as the mobile phase. Apply separately to the chromatoplate 2 μl of each of three solutions of the substance being examined in *water* containing (1) 5.0% w/v, (2) 0.050% w/v and (3) 0.025% w/v. After removal of the plate, allow it to dry in air and examine under *ultra-violet light (254 nm)*. Any *secondary spot* in the

chromatogram obtained with solution (1) is not more intense than the spot in the chromatogram obtained with solution (2) and not more than one such spot is more intense than the spot in the chromatogram obtained with solution (3).

Loss on drying When dried to constant weight at 105°, loses not more than 2.0% of its weight. Use 1 g.

Sulphated ash Not more than 0.2%, Appendix IX A.

Assay Dissolve 0.5 g in 10 ml of *water*, add 20 ml of 1M *sodium hydroxide* and extract with four 25-ml quantities of *chloroform*. Combine the chloroform extracts and evaporate to a volume of about 10 ml. Add 40 ml of *anhydrous glacial acetic acid* and carry out Method I for *non-aqueous titration*, Appendix VIII A, using *oracet blue B solution* as indicator. Each ml of 0.1M *perchloric acid VS* is equivalent to 0.02170 g of $C_{18}H_{26}ClN_3O,H_2SO_4$.

Storage Hydroxychloroquine Sulphate should be protected from light.

Preparation

Hydroxychloroquine Tablets

Action and use Antimalarial.

Hydroxyethylcellulose ☆

9004-62-0

Hydroxyethylcellulose is a cellulose having some of the hydroxyl groups in the form of the 2-hydroxyethyl ether. Various grades are available and are distinguished by appending a number indicative of the apparent viscosity in millipascal seconds of a 2 per cent w/v solution measured at 20°.

Characteristics A white, yellowish-white or greyish-white powder or granules; practically odourless; hygroscopic after drying.

Solubility Soluble in hot and cold *water* forming a colloidal solution; practically insoluble in *absolute ethanol*, in *acetone*, in *ether* and in *toluene*.

Identification A. Disperse a quantity containing the equivalent of 1.0 g of the dried substance in 50 ml of *carbon dioxide-free water*. After 10 minutes, dilute to 100 ml with the same solvent and stir until solution is complete (solution A). Heat 10 ml of solution A in a water-bath, with stirring. No precipitate or cloudiness is produced at temperatures above 50°.

B. To 10 ml of solution A add 0.3 ml of 2M *acetic acid* and 2.5 ml of a 10% w/v solution of *tannic acid*. A yellowish-white, flocculent precipitate is produced which dissolves in 6M *ammonia*.

C. Thoroughly mix 1 g with 2 g of finely powdered *manganese(II) sulphate* in a test-tube about 16 cm long. Impregnate a strip of filter paper with a freshly prepared mixture of 11 volumes of a 5% w/v solution of *sodium nitroprusside* and 1 volume of a 20% v/v solution of *diethanolamine*, adjusted to pH 9.8 with 1M *hydrochloric acid*. Insert the strip to a depth of 2 cm into the upper part of the tube, immerse the tube to a depth of 8 cm in a silicone oil-bath and heat at 190° to 200°. The filter paper becomes blue within 10 minutes. Carry out a blank test.

D. Without heating, completely dissolve 0.2 g in 15 ml of a 70% w/w solution of *sulphuric acid*, pour the solution, with stirring, into 100 ml of iced *water* and dilute to 250 ml with iced *water*. In a test-tube kept in ice, mix thoroughly 1 ml of the solution with 8 ml of *sulphuric acid*, added dropwise. Heat in a water-bath for exactly 3 minutes and cool immediately in ice. When the mixture is cool, carefully add 0.6 ml of a solution of 3 g of *ninhydrin* in 100 ml of a 4.55% w/v solution of *sodium metabisulphite*, mix well and allow to stand at 25°. A pink colour is produced immediately which does not become violet within 100 minutes.

E. Place 1 ml of solution A on a glass plate. After evaporation of the water a thin film is produced.

Acidity or alkalinity pH of solution A, 5.5 to 8.5, Appendix V L.

Clarity and colour of solution Solution A is not more opalescent than *reference suspension III*, Appendix IV A, and not more intensely coloured than *reference solution* Y_6, Appendix IV B, Method II.

Apparent viscosity 75 to 140% of the declared value when determined by the following method. To 50 ml of *water* add, with stirring, a quantity containing the equivalent of 2 g of the dried substance. Dilute to 100 ml with *water* and continue stirring until solution is complete. Determine the *viscosity*, Appendix V H, Method IV, at 20° using a shear rate of 10 s^{-1}. If necessary, use rates slightly below and slightly above 10 s^{-1} and interpolate.

Heavy metals 1.0 g complies with *limit test C for heavy metals*, Appendix VII (20 ppm). Use 2 ml of *lead standard solution (10 ppm Pb)* to prepare the standard.

Chloride Dilute 1 ml of solution A to 30 ml with *water*. 15 ml of the resulting solution complies with the *limit test for chlorides*, Appendix VII (1.0%).

Nitrate To 1 ml of solution A add 19 ml of *water*, 2 ml of 13.5M *ammonia*, 0.5 ml of a 1% w/v solution of *manganese(II) sulphate* and 1 ml of a 1% w/v solution of *sulphanilamide*. Add 0.1 g of *granulated zinc* and allow to stand for 30 minutes in ice, shaking occasionally. Filter through a sintered-glass filter (BS porosity No. 3). To 10 ml of the filtrate add 2.5 ml of *hydrochloric acid* and 0.5 ml of a 1% w/v solution of N-*(1-naphthyl)ethylene-diamine dihydrochloride* and allow to stand for 15 minutes. Any violet-red colour in the solution is not more intense than that in a standard prepared at the same time and in the same manner using 1 ml of *nitrate standard solution (10 ppm NO₃)* in place of solution A (0.1%).

Loss on drying When dried to constant weight at 100° to 105°, loses not more than 10.0% of its weight. Use 1 g.

Sulphated ash Not more than 4%, Appendix IX A, Method II. Use 1 g.

Storage Hydroxyethylcellulose should be kept in a well-closed container.

Labelling The label states the apparent viscosity in millipascal seconds of a 2% w/v solution.

Action and use Pharmaceutical aid.

Hydroxyethylmethylcellulose ☆

Hydroxyethylmethylcellulose is a cellulose having some of the hydroxyl groups in the form of the methyl ether and some in the form of the 2-hydroxyethyl ether. Various grades are available and are distinguished by appending a number indicative of the apparent viscosity in millipascal seconds of a 2 per cent w/v solution measured at 20°.

Characteristics A white, yellowish-white or greyish-white powder or granules; practically odourless; hygroscopic after drying.

Solubility Practically insoluble in hot *water*, in *absolute ethanol*, in *acetone*, in *ether* and in *toluene*. It dissolves in cold *water* forming a colloidal solution.

Identification A. Whilst stirring, introduce a quantity containing the equivalent of 1.0 g of the dried substance into 50 ml of *carbon dioxide-free water* heated to 90°. Allow to cool, dilute to 100 ml with *carbon dioxide-free water* and continue stirring until solution is complete (solution A). Heat 10 ml of solution A in a water-bath, with stirring. At temperatures above 50° the solution becomes cloudy or a flocculent precipitate is produced. On cooling the solution becomes clear again.

B. To 10 ml of solution A add 0.3 ml of 2M *acetic acid* and 2.5 ml of a 10% w/v solution of *tannic acid*. A yellowish-white, flocculent precipitate is produced which dissolves in 6M *ammonia*.

C. Mix thoroughly 1 g with 2 g of finely powdered *manganese(II) sulphate* in a test-tube about 16 cm long. Impregnate a strip of filter paper with a freshly prepared mixture of 11 volumes of a 5% w/v solution of *sodium nitroprusside* and 1 volume of a 20% v/v solution of *diethanolamine*, adjusted to pH 9.8 with 1M *hydrochloric acid*. Insert the strip to a depth of 2 cm into the upper part of the tube, immerse the tube to a depth of 8 cm in a silicone oil-bath and heat at 190° to 200°. The filter paper becomes blue within 10 minutes. Carry out a blank test.

D. Without heating, completely dissolve 0.2 g in 15 ml of a 70% w/w solution of *sulphuric acid*, pour the solution, with stirring, into 100 ml of iced *water* and dilute to 250 ml with iced *water*. In a test-tube kept in ice, mix thoroughly 1 ml of the solution with 8 ml of *sulphuric acid*, added dropwise. Heat in a water-bath for exactly 3 minutes and cool immediately in ice. When the mixture is cool carefully add 0.6 ml of a solution of 3 g of *ninhydrin* in 100 ml of a 4.55% w/v solution of *sodium metabisulphite*, mix well and allow to stand at 25°. A pink colour is produced immediately which does not become violet within 100 minutes.

E. Place 1 ml of solution A on a glass plate. After evaporation of the water a thin film is produced.

Acidity or alkalinity pH of solution A, 5.5 to 8.0, Appendix V L.

Clarity and colour of solution Solution A is not more opalescent than *reference suspension II*, Appendix IV A, and not more intensely coloured than *reference solution* Y_6, Appendix IV B, Method II.

Apparent viscosity 75 to 140% of the declared value when determined by the following method. To 50 ml of *water* heated to 90° add, with stirring, a quantity containing the equivalent of 2 g of the dried substance. Dilute to 100 ml with *water* and continue stirring until solution is complete. Determine the *viscosity*, Appendix V H, Method IV, at 20° using a shear rate of 10 s^{-1}. If necessary, use rates slightly below and slightly above 10 s^{-1} and interpolate.

Heavy metals 1.0 g complies with *limit test C for heavy metals*, Appendix VII (20 ppm). Use 2 ml of *lead standard solution (10 ppm Pb)* to prepare the standard.

Chloride Dilute 1 ml of solution A to 15 ml with *water*. The resulting solution complies with the *limit test for chlorides*, Appendix VII (0.5%).

Loss on drying When dried to constant weight at 100° to 105°, loses not more than 10.0% of its weight. Use 1 g.

Sulphated ash Not more than 1.0%, Appendix IX A, Method II. Use 1 g.

Storage Hydroxyethylmethylcellulose should be kept in a well-closed container.

Labelling The label states the apparent viscosity in millipascal seconds of a 2% w/v solution.

Action and use Pharmaceutical aid.

The title of the monograph in the European Pharmacopœia is Methylhydroxyethylcellulose.

Hydroxyprogesterone Hexanoate

$C_{27}H_{40}O_4$ 428.6   *630-56-8*

Hydroxyprogesterone Hexanoate is 3,20-dioxo-pregn-4-en-17α-yl hexanoate. It contains not less than 97.0 per cent and not more than 103.0 per cent of $C_{27}H_{40}O_4$, calculated with reference to the dried substance.

Characteristics A white or almost white crystalline powder; odourless or almost odourless.

Solubility Practically insoluble in *water*; soluble in 10 parts of *ethanol* (96%), in 0.4 part of *chloroform* and in 10 parts of *ether*. It dissolves in fixed oils and esters.

Identification A. The *infra-red absorption spectrum*, Appendix II A, is concordant with the *reference spectrum* of hydroxyprogesterone hexanoate.
B. Complies with the test for *identification of steroids*, Appendix III A, using *impregnating solvent II* and *mobile phase E*.
C. Dissolve 1 mg in 1 ml of *sulphuric acid* and allow to stand for 2 minutes. A faint yellow colour is produced which, on the addition of 0.5 ml of *water*, changes first to green, then to red and finally to reddish-violet with a blue fluorescence.
D. Heat 50 mg with 2 ml of 0.5M *ethanolic potassium hydroxide* in a water-bath for 5 minutes. Add 3 ml of *water*, evaporate the ethanol, add 2 ml of *sulphuric acid* (50%) and heat on a water-bath. The odour of hexanoic acid is produced.
E. Shake 1.5 g of *2,4-dinitrophenylhydrazine* with 90 ml of *methanol*, add 5 ml of *hydrochloric acid* and sufficient *methanol* to produce 100 ml and continue to shake until all the crystals have dissolved. To 5 ml of the solution add 50 mg of the substance being examined, heat under a reflux condenser for 5 minutes, shaking frequently, filter and wash the residue with two 5-ml quantities of cold *methanol*. The *melting point* of the residue, after recrystallisation from *ethyl acetate*, is about 173°, with decomposition, Appendix V A.

Acidity Dissolve 0.2 g in 25 ml of *absolute ethanol* previously neutralised to *bromothymol blue solution* and titrate immediately with 0.01M *sodium hydroxide VS* until a faint blue colour is produced. Not more than 1.0 ml of 0.01M *sodium hydroxide VS* is required.

Melting point 120° to 124°, Appendix V A.

Specific optical rotation In a 2% w/v solution in *1,4-dioxan*, +44° to +49°, Appendix V F.

Related foreign steroids Carry out the method for *thin-layer chromatography*, Appendix III A, using *silica gel HF254* as the coating substance and a mixture of equal volumes of *cyclohexane* and *ethyl acetate* as the mobile phase. Apply separately to the chromatoplate 10 μl of each of two solutions of the substance being examined in *chloroform* containing (1) 1.0% w/v and (2) 0.010% w/v. After removal of the plate, allow it to dry in air and examine under *ultra-violet light (254 nm)*. Any *secondary spot* in the chromatogram obtained with solution (1) is not more intense than the spot in the chromatogram obtained with solution (2).

Loss on drying When dried over *phosphorus pentoxide* at a pressure not exceeding 0.7 kPa for 24 hours, loses not more than 0.5% of its weight. Use 1 g.

Sulphated ash Not more than 0.1%, Appendix IX A.

Assay Dissolve 60 mg in sufficient *absolute ethanol* to produce 100 ml, dilute 5 ml to 250 ml with *absolute ethanol* and measure the *absorbance* of the resulting solution at the maximum at 240 nm, Appendix II B. Calculate the content of $C_{27}H_{40}O_4$ taking 395 as the value of A(1%, 1 cm) at the maximum at 240 nm.

Storage Hydroxyprogesterone Hexanoate should be protected from light.

Preparation
Hydroxyprogesterone Injection

Action and use Progestogen.

In some countries the material described in this monograph may be known as Hydroxyprogesterone Caproate.

Hydroxypropylcellulose ☆

9004-64-2

Hydroxypropylcellulose is a cellulose having some of the hydroxyl groups in the form of the 2-hydroxypropyl ether. Various grades are available and are distinguished by appending a number indicative of the apparent viscosity in millipascal seconds of a 2 per cent w/v solution measured at 20°.

Characteristics A white or yellowish-white powder; practically odourless; hygroscopic after drying.

Solubility Soluble in cold *water*, in *absolute ethanol*, in *methanol*, in *chloroform* and in *propane-1,2-diol* forming colloidal solutions; sparingly soluble or slightly soluble in *acetone* depending on the degree of substitution; very slightly soluble in *toluene*; practically insoluble in hot *water* and in *ethane-1,2-diol*. It dissolves in *glacial acetic acid* forming a colloidal solution.

Identification A. Whilst stirring, introduce a quantity containing the equivalent of 1.0 g of the dried substance into 50 ml of *carbon dioxide-free water* heated to 90°. Allow to cool, dilute to 100 ml with *carbon dioxide-free water* and continue stirring until solution is complete (solution A). Heat 10 ml of solution A on a water-bath, with stirring. At temperatures above 40° the solution becomes cloudy or a flocculent precipitate is formed. On cooling the solution becomes clear.

B. To 10 ml of solution A add 0.3 ml of 2M *acetic acid* and 2.5 ml of a 10% w/v solution of *tannic acid*. A yellowish-white, flocculent precipitate is produced which dissolves in 6M *ammonia*.

C. Mix thoroughly 1 g with 2 g of finely powdered *manganese(II) sulphate* in a test-tube about 16 cm long. Impregnate a strip of filter paper with a freshly prepared mixture of 11 volumes of a 5% w/v solution of *sodium nitroprusside* and 1 volume of a 20% v/v solution of *diethanolamine*, adjusted to pH 9.8 with 1M *hydrochloric acid*. Insert the strip to a depth of 2 cm into the upper part of the tube, immerse the tube to a depth of 8 cm in a silicone oil-bath and heat at 190° to 200°. The filter paper becomes blue within 10 minutes. Carry out a blank test.

D. Without heating, completely dissolve 0.2 g in 15 ml of a 70% w/w solution of *sulphuric acid*, pour the solution, with stirring, into 100 ml of iced *water* and dilute to 250 ml with iced *water*. In a test-tube kept in ice, mix thoroughly 1 ml of the solution with 8 ml of *sulphuric acid*, added dropwise. Heat in a water-bath for exactly 3 minutes and cool immediately in ice. When the mixture is cool, carefully add 0.6 ml of a solution containing 3 g of *ninhydrin* in 100 ml of a 4.55% w/v solution of *sodium metabisulphite*, mix well and allow to stand at 25°. A pink colour is produced immediately which becomes violet within 100 minutes.

E. Place 1 ml of solution A on a glass plate. After evaporation of the water a thin film is produced.

F. 0.2 g does not dissolve in 10 ml of *toluene*, but dissolves completely in 10 ml of *absolute ethanol*.

Acidity or alkalinity pH of solution A, 5.0 to 8.5, Appendix V L.

Clarity and colour of solution Solution A is not more opalescent than *reference suspension II*, Appendix IV A, and not more intensely coloured than *reference solution Y_6*, Appendix IV B, Method II.

Apparent viscosity 75 to 140% of the declared value when determined by the following method. To 50 ml of *water* heated to 90° add, with stirring, a quantity containing the equivalent of 2 g of the dried substance or, for a product of low viscosity use the quantity required to give the concentration indicated on the label. Allow to cool, dilute to 100 ml with *water* and continue stirring until solution is complete. Determine the *viscosity*, Appendix V H, Method IV, at 20° using a shear rate of 10 s^{-1}. If necessary, use rates slightly below and slightly above 10 s^{-1} and interpolate.

Heavy metals 1.0 g complies with *limit test C for heavy metals*, Appendix VII (20 ppm). Use 2 ml of *lead standard solution (10 ppm Pb)* to prepare the standard.

Chloride Dilute 1 ml of solution A to 15 ml with *water*. The resulting solution complies with the *limit test for chlorides*, Appendix VII (0.5%).

Loss on drying When dried to constant weight at 100° to 105°, loses not more than 7.0% of its weight. Use 1 g.

Sulphated ash Not more than 0.5%, Appendix IX A, Method II. Use 1 g.

Storage Hydroxypropylcellulose should be kept in a well-closed container.

Labelling The label states the apparent viscosity in millipascal seconds of a 2% w/v solution. For a product of low viscosity, the label states the concentration of the solution to be used and the apparent viscosity in millipascal seconds.

Action and use Pharmaceutical aid.

In some countries the material described in this monograph may be known as Hyprolose.

Hydroxyurea

$NH_2 \cdot CO \cdot NHOH$

$CH_4N_2O_2$ 76.05   *127-07-1*

Hydroxyurea contains not less than 98.0 per cent and not more than 100.5 per cent of $CH_4N_2O_2$, calculated with reference to the dried substance.

Characteristics A white to off-white crystalline powder; odourless or almost odourless; hygroscopic.

Solubility Freely soluble in *water* and in hot *ethanol (96%)*.

Identification A. The *infra-red absorption spectrum*, Appendix II A, is concordant with the *reference spectrum* of hydroxyurea.

B. In the test for Urea and related substances the principal spot in the chromatogram obtained with solution (3) corresponds to that in the chromatogram obtained with solution (4).

Heavy metals Moisten 2.0 g in a silica crucible with *sulphuric acid*, ignite gently and carry out *limit test C for heavy metals*, Appendix VII, beginning at the words 'Allow to cool . . .'. Use 3 ml of *lead standard solution (10 ppm Pb)* to prepare the standard (30 ppm).

Urea and related substances Carry out the method for *descending paper chromatography*, Appendix III E, using chromatographic paper (Whatman No 1 is suitable) impregnated with *citro-phosphate buffer pH 6.5* and as the mobile phase the upper layer obtained after shaking together equal volumes of *2-methylpropan-1-ol* and *water* and allowing the layers to separate; place the lower layer in the bottom of the tank. Apply separately to the dried paper 10 μl of each of four solutions in *water* containing (1) 10% w/v of the substance being examined, (2) 0.050% w/v of *urea*, (3) 1.0% w/v of the substance being examined and (4) 1.0% w/v of *hydroxyurea BPCRS*. Place the paper in the chromatographic chamber and after adding the mobile phase allow to develop for 24 hours. Remove the paper from the tank, allow it to dry in air and develop for a further 24 hours. After removal of the paper, allow it to dry in air, spray with *dimethylaminobenzaldehyde solution* and dry at 90° for 2 minutes. Any *secondary spot* in the chromatogram obtained with solution (1) is not more intense than the spot in the chromatogram obtained with solution (2).

Loss on drying When dried to constant weight at 60° at a pressure not exceeding 0.7 kPa, loses not more than 1.0% of its weight. Use 1 g.

Sulphated ash Not more than 0.2%, Appendix IX A.

Assay Dissolve 50 mg in sufficient *water* to produce 50 ml. To 2 ml add 5 ml of a 10% w/v solution of *sodium hydrogen carbonate*, mix and allow to stand for 15 minutes. Add 20 ml of 0.005M *iodine VS* and allow to stand for 5 minutes. Add 5 ml of a 20% w/v solution of *sodium dihydrogen orthophosphate*, mix, allow to stand until effervescence ceases and titrate with 0.01M *sodium thiosulphate VS* using *starch mucilage* as indicator. Repeat the procedure using 2 ml of *water* in place of the solution of the substance being examined and beginning at the words 'add 5 ml . . .'. Repeat the assay using *hydroxyurea BPCRS* in place of the substance being examined. Calculate the content of $CH_4N_2O_2$ using the declared content of $CH_4N_2O_2$ in *hydroxyurea BPCRS*.

Storage Hydroxyurea should be kept in a well-closed container and protected from moisture.

Preparation
Hydroxyurea Capsules

Action and use Cytotoxic.

In some countries the material described in this monograph may be known as Hydroxycarbamide.

Hyoscine Butylbromide
Scopolamine Butylbromide

$C_{21}H_{30}BrNO_4$　　440.4　　*149-64-4*

Hyoscine Butylbromide is (1*S*,3*s*,5*R*,6*R*,7*S*,8*s*)-6,7-epoxy-8-butyl-3-(*S*)-tropoyloxy]tropanium bromide. It contains not less than 98.0 per cent and not more than 101.0 per cent of $C_{21}H_{30}BrNO_4$, calculated with reference to the dried substance.

Characteristics A white or almost white, crystalline powder; odourless or almost odourless.

Solubility Soluble in 1 part of *water*, in 50 parts of *ethanol* (96%) and in 5 parts of *chloroform*.

Identification A. The *infra-red absorption spectrum*, Appendix II A, is concordant with the *reference spectrum* of hyoscine butylbromide.
B. The *light absorption*, Appendix II B, in the range 240 to 350 nm of a 0.15% w/v solution in 0.01M *hydrochloric acid* exhibits maxima at 252, 257 and 264 nm and a less well-defined maximum at about 247 nm. The *absorbance* at 252 nm is about 0.50, at 257 nm, about 0.67 and at 264 nm, about 0.50.
C. To 1 mg add 0.2 ml of *fuming nitric acid* and evaporate to dryness on a water-bath. Dissolve the residue in 2 ml of *acetone* and add 0.1 ml of a 3% w/v solution of *potassium hydroxide* in *methanol*. A violet colour is produced.
D. Yields *reaction B* characteristic of bromides, Appendix VI.

Acidity pH of a 10% w/v solution, 5.5 to 6.5, Appendix V L.

Specific optical rotation In a 10% w/v solution, −18° to −20°, Appendix V F.

Apo-compounds Ratio of the *absorbance* of a 0.1% w/v solution in 0.01M *hydrochloric acid* at the maximum at 247 nm to that at the maximum at 264 nm, not more than 0.94, Appendix II B.

Related substances Carry out the method for *thin-layer chromatography*, Appendix III A, using *microcrystalline cellulose* as the coating substance and, as the mobile phase, the upper layer obtained by shaking together 50 volumes of *butan-1-ol*, 25 volumes of *water* and 5 volumes of *anhydrous formic acid*. Apply separately to the chromatoplate 10 µl of each of three solutions in *methanol* (50%) containing (1) 2.0% w/v of the substance being examined, (2) 0.0020% w/v of *hyoscine hydrobromide BPCRS* and (3) 0.0040% w/v of the substance being examined. After removal of the plate, allow it to dry in air and spray with *dilute potassium iodobismuthate solution*. In the chromatogram obtained with solution (1) any spot corresponding to hyoscine hydrobromide is not more intense than the spot in the chromatogram obtained with solution (2) and any other *secondary spot* is not more intense than the spot in the chromatogram obtained with solution (3).

Loss on drying When dried to constant weight at 105°, loses not more than 2.5% of its weight. Use 1 g.

Sulphated ash Not more than 0.1%, Appendix IX A.

Assay Carry out Method I for *non-aqueous titration*, Appendix VIII A, using 0.3 g, 5 ml of *mercury(II) acetate solution* and *1-naphtholbenzein solution* as indicator. Each ml of 0.1M *perchloric acid VS* is equivalent to 0.04404 g of $C_{21}H_{30}BrNO_4$.

Storage Hyoscine Butylbromide should be kept in a well-closed container and protected from light.

Preparations
Hyoscine Butylbromide Injection
Hyoscine Butylbromide Tablets

Action and use Antispasmodic.

Hyoscine Hydrobromide ☆
Scopolamine Hydrobromide

$C_{17}H_{21}NO_4,HBr,3H_2O$　　438.3　　*6533-68-2*

Hyoscine Hydrobromide is (1*S*,3*s*,5*R*,6*R*,7*S*)-6,7-epoxytropan-3-yl (*S*)-tropate hydrobromide trihydrate. It contains not less than 99.0 per cent and not more than 101.0 per cent of $C_{17}H_{21}NO_4,HBr$, calculated with reference to the anhydrous substance.

Characteristics Colourless crystals or a white, crystalline powder; odourless; efflorescent. When dried over *phosphorus pentoxide* at a pressure of 2 to 3 kPa for 24 hours and then at 100° to 105° for 2 hours it melts at about 197°, with decomposition.

Solubility Soluble in 3.5 parts of *water* and in 30 parts of *ethanol (96%)*; practically insoluble in *chloroform* and in *ether*.

Identification *Test A may be omitted if tests B, C, D and E are carried out. Tests B, C and D may be omitted if tests A and E are carried out.*

A. The *infra-red absorption spectrum*, Appendix II A, is concordant with the spectrum of *hyoscine hydrobromide EPCRS*. If the spectra are not concordant, prepare new spectra by the following procedure. Dissolve 3 mg in 1 ml of *ethanol (96%)* and evaporate to dryness on a water-bath. Dissolve the residue in 0.5 ml of *chloroform* and add 0.2 g of *potassium bromide IR* and 15 ml of *ether*. Allow to stand for 5 minutes with frequent shaking, decant and dry the residue on a water-bath until the odour of the solvent is no longer detectable. Use the residue to prepare a new dispersion and dry it at 100° to 105° for 3 hours before recording the spectrum.

B. To 1 mg add 0.2 ml of *fuming nitric acid* and evaporate to dryness on a water-bath. Dissolve the residue in 2 ml of *acetone* and add 0.1 ml of a 3% w/v solution of *potassium hydroxide* in *methanol*. A violet colour is produced.

C. Dissolve 50 mg in 5 ml of *water* and add 5 ml of a 1% w/v solution of *2,4,6-trinitrophenol* dropwise with shaking. The *melting point* of the precipitate, after washing and drying at 100° to 105° for 2 hours, is 188° to 193°, Appendix V A, Method I.

D. Yields the *reaction* characteristic of alkaloids, Appendix VI.

E. Yields the *reactions* characteristic of bromides, Appendix VI.

Acidity pH of a 5% w/v solution, 4.0 to 5.5, Appendix V L.

Specific optical rotation In a 5% w/v solution in *carbon dioxide-free water*, −24° to −27°, Appendix V F.

Related substances and decomposition products Carry out the method for *thin-layer chromatography*, Appendix III A, using *silica gel G* as the coating substance and a mixture of 50 volumes of *chloroform*, 30 volumes of *acetone*, 10 volumes of *methanol* and 2 volumes of 13.5M *ammonia* as the mobile phase, but allowing the solvent front to ascend 10 cm above the line of application. Apply separately to the chromatoplate 10 µl of each of three solutions of the substance being examined in *methanol* containing (1) 2.0% w/v, (2) 0.020% w/v and (3) 0.010% w/v. After removal of the plate, dry it at 100° to 105° for 15 minutes, allow to cool and spray with *dilute potassium iodobismuthate solution* until spots appear. Any *secondary spot* in the chromatogram obtained with solution (1) is not more intense than the spot in the chromatogram obtained with solution (2) and not more than one such spot is more intense than the spot in the chromatogram obtained with solution (3). Disregard any yellow spot on the line of application.

Apohyoscine Dissolve 0.1 g in sufficient 0.01M *hydrochloric acid* to produce 100 ml and measure the *absorbance* at 245 nm, Appendix II B. The A(1%, 1 cm) is not more than 3.6 (about 0.5%).

Sulphated ash Not more than 0.1%, Appendix IX A, Method II. Use 1 g.

Water 10.0 to 13.0% w/w, Appendix IX C, Method I B. Use 0.2 g.

Assay Dissolve 0.4 g in 10 ml of *anhydrous glacial acetic acid*, warming if necessary. Cool the solution, add 20 ml of *1,4-dioxan* and carry out Method I for *non-aqueous titration*, Appendix VIII A, using 7 ml of *mercury(II) acetate solution* and determining the end-point potentiometrically. Each ml of 0.1M *perchloric acid VS* is equivalent to 0.03843 g of $C_{17}H_{21}NO_4,HBr$.

Storage Hyoscine Hydrobromide should be kept in a well-filled, airtight container of small capacity, protected from light and stored at a temperature not exceeding 15°.

Preparations
Hyoscine Eye Drops
Hyoscine Injection
Hyoscine Tablets

Action and use Antiemetic; mydriatic; cycloplegic.

Hyoscyamine Sulphate ☆

$(C_{17}H_{23}NO_3)_2,H_2SO_4,2H_2O$ 713 6835-16-1

Hyoscyamine Sulphate is (1*R*,3*r*,5*S*)-tropan-3-yl (*S*)-tropate sulphate dihydrate. It contains not less than 98.0 per cent and not more than 100.5 per cent of $(C_{17}H_{23}NO_3)_2,H_2SO_4$, calculated with reference to the anhydrous substance.

Characteristics A white, crystalline powder or colourless needles. It melts at about 203° with decomposition.

Solubility Very soluble in *water*; sparingly soluble to soluble in *ethanol (96%)*; practically insoluble in *chloroform* and in *ether*.

Identification *Tests A and B may be omitted if tests C, D and E are carried out. Tests C and D may be omitted if tests A, B and E are carried out.*

A. The *infra-red absorption spectrum*, Appendix II A, is concordant with the spectrum of *hyoscyamine sulphate EPCRS*.

B. Complies with the test for Specific optical rotation.

C. To 1 mg add 0.2 ml of *fuming nitric acid* and evaporate to dryness on a water-bath. Dissolve the residue in 2 ml of *acetone* and add 0.2 ml of a 3% w/v solution of *potassium hydroxide* in *methanol*. A violet colour is produced.

D. Heat 0.5 ml of a 5% w/v solution with 2 ml of 2M *acetic acid*. To the hot solution add 4 ml of a 1% w/v solution of *2,4,6-trinitrophenol* and allow to cool, shaking occasionally. Collect the crystals, wash with two 3-ml quantities of iced *water* and dry at 100° to 105°. The *melting point* of the dried crystals is 164° to 168°, Appendix V A, Method I.

E. Yields *reaction A* characteristic of sulphates, Appendix VI.

Acidity pH of a 2% w/v solution, 4.5 to 6.2, Appendix V L.

Colour of solution A 5.0% w/v solution is not more intensely coloured than *reference solution BY₆*, Appendix IV B, Method II.

Specific optical rotation In a 5% w/v solution, $-24°$ to $-29°$, Appendix V F.

Related substances Carry out the method for *thin-layer chromatography*, Appendix III A, using *silica gel G* as the coating substance and a mixture of 85 volumes of *chloroform* and 15 volumes of *methanol* as the mobile phase. Place 10 ml of 13.5M *ammonia* in a container in the chromatography tank and allow the tank to become saturated with the vapours of both the mobile phase and the ammonia. Apply separately to the chromatoplate 2 µl of each of two solutions of the substance being examined in *methanol* containing (1) 10.0% w/v and (2) 0.050% w/v. After removal of the plate, dry it at 100° to 105° for 15 minutes, allow to cool and spray with *dilute potassium iodobismuthate solution* until spots appear. Any *secondary spot* in the chromatogram obtained with solution (1) is not more intense than the spot in the chromatogram obtained with solution (2).

Apo-atropine Dissolve 0.1 g in sufficient 0.01M *hydrochloric acid* to produce 100 ml. The A(1%, 1 cm) of the resulting solution, Appendix II B, at 245 nm is not more than 4.0 (about 0.5%).

Sulphated ash Not more than 0.1%, Appendix IX A, Method II. Use 1 g.

Water 2.0 to 5.5% w/w, Appendix IX C. Use 0.5 g.

Assay Dissolve 0.5 g in 25 ml of *anhydrous glacial acetic acid* and carry out Method I for *non-aqueous titration*, Appendix VIII A, determining the end-point potentiometrically. Each ml of 0.1M *perchloric acid VS* is equivalent to 0.06770 g of $(C_{17}H_{23}NO_3)_2,H_2SO_4$.

Storage Hyoscyamine Sulphate should be kept in an airtight container and protected from light.

Action and use Parasympatholytic.

Hyoscyamus Leaf ☆

Hyoscyamus Leaf consists of the dried leaf or the dried leaf, flowering tops and occasionally fruits of *Hyoscyamus niger* L. It contains not less than 0.05 per cent of total alkaloids, calculated as hyoscyamine and with reference to the material dried at 100° to 105°. The alkaloids consist of those of the hyoscyamine—atropine group together with hyoscine in varying proportions.

Characteristics Odour, nauseous and disagreeable.

Macroscopical Leaves: yellowish-green to brownish-green, brittle and frequently broken. Lamina up to 25 cm long, ovate-lanceolate to triangular-ovate with an acute apex; base cordate on sessile leaves and acute on petiolate leaves. Margin irregularly dentately lobed with large triangular lobes, leaves densely pubescent and sticky on both surfaces, especially on the midrib and main veins.

Midrib broad and conspicuous; secondary veins arising at a wide angle and terminating in the apices of the lobes. Flowering tops: densely pubescent, in compact flattened masses, the flowers being crowded together and arising in the axils of large bracts. Stems: hollow and subcylindrical. Flowers: gamosepalous calyx, broadly campanulate with five triangular cuspidate lobes; corolla five-lobed, shortly funnel-shaped, yellowish. Fruit: pyxis, about 1.5 cm long when mature, enclosed in the persistent calyx, containing numerous brownish-grey seeds with a wavy, reticulated testa.

Microscopical Leaf: epidermal cells with wavy anticlinal walls and smooth cuticle; numerous multicellular, uniseriate covering trichomes and glandular trichomes with thin, smooth walls; numerous glandular trichomes with long, multicellular stalks or short, unicellular stalks and with clavate bicellular or multicellular heads. Stomata *anisocytic*, more frequent on the lower epidermis. Midrib showing an open arc of vascular bundles with isolated groups of intraxylary phloem; dorsiventral mesophyll with single layer of palisade cells under which is a row of cells each containing single or twinned calcium oxalate prisms, 5 to 20 µm long, or occasional cluster crystals; epidermal cells of the corolla with wavy, anticlinal walls and well-marked infoldings.

Identification A. Shake 1 g, in powder, with 10 ml of 0.05M *sulphuric acid* for 2 minutes, filter, add 1 ml of 13.5M *ammonia* and 5 ml of *water* to the filtrate, extract cautiously with 15 ml of *chloroform* to avoid the formation of an emulsion, dry the chloroform layer over *anhydrous sodium sulphate* and filter. Evaporate the chloroform in a porcelain dish, add 0.5 ml of *fuming nitric acid* and evaporate to dryness on a water-bath. Add 10 ml of *acetone* and, dropwise, a 3% w/v solution of *potassium hydroxide* in *ethanol (96%)*. A violet colour is produced.

B. Carry out the method for *thin-layer chromatography*, Appendix III A, using *silica gel G* as the coating substance and a mixture of 90 volumes of *acetone*, 7 volumes of *water* and 3 volumes of 13.5M *ammonia* as the mobile phase, but allowing the solvent front to ascend 10 cm above the line of application. Apply separately to a chromatoplate 200 mm × 200 mm in size, as bands 20 mm × 3 mm, 1 cm apart, 10 µl and 20 µl of each of the following solutions. For solution (1) add 20 ml of 0.05M *sulphuric acid* to 2 g of the leaf, in *No. 180 powder*, shake for 15 minutes, filter and wash the filter with 0.05M *sulphuric acid* until 25 ml of filtrate is obtained; add 1 ml of 13.5M *ammonia* to the filtrate, extract with two 10-ml quantities of *peroxide-free ether*, separate the ether layer, by centrifugation if necessary, dry the combined extracts over *anhydrous sodium sulphate*, filter, evaporate to dryness on a water-bath and dissolve the residue in 0.5 ml of *methanol*. For solution (2) dissolve 50 mg of *hyoscyamine sulphate* in 9 ml of *methanol* (solution A) and dissolve 15 mg of *hyoscine hydrobromide* in 10 ml of *methanol* (solution B); mix 3.8 ml of solution A with 4.2 ml of solution B and dilute to 10 ml with *methanol*.

After removal of the plate, dry it at 100° to 105° for 15 minutes, allow to cool and spray with 10 ml of *modified potassium iodobismuthate solution* until the bands become visible as orange or brown on a yellow background. The bands in the chromatograms obtained with solution (1) are similar to those in the chromatograms obtained with solution (2) with regard to their Rf values (hyoscyamine in the lower third of the chromatogram; hyoscine in the upper third) and their colour and are at least equal in size. Faint secondary bands may appear, particularly in the middle of the chromatogram obtained with 20 µl of solution (1) or near the line of application in the chromatogram obtained with 10 µl of solution (1). Spray the plate with a freshly prepared 10% w/v solution of *sodium nitrite* until transparent and examine after 15 minutes. The colours due to hyoscyamine in the chromatograms change from brown to reddish-brown, but not to greyish-blue (atropine); any secondary bands are no longer visible.

Foreign matter Not more than 2.5% of stem with a diameter exceeding 7 mm, Appendix XI D, Test B.

Acid-insoluble ash Not more than 12.0%, Appendix XI K, Method II.

Assay Reduce 100 g, selected from a well-mixed sample, to *No. 180 powder* and determine the moisture content of 2 g by drying to constant weight at 100° to 105°. Moisten 40 g with a mixture of 8 ml of 10M *ammonia*, 10 ml of *ethanol (96%)* and 30 ml of *peroxide-free ether* and mix thoroughly. Transfer the mixture to a small percolator with the aid of the extracting mixture if necessary, allow to macerate for 4 hours and then percolate with a mixture of 1 volume of *chloroform* and 3 volumes of *peroxide-free ether* until *complete extraction* of the alkaloids is effected. Concentrate the percolate to about 50 ml by distillation on a water-bath and transfer to a separating funnel with the aid of *peroxide-free ether*. Add a quantity of *peroxide-free ether* at least 2.1 times the volume of the percolate to produce a liquid considerably less dense than water. Extract the solution with not less than three 20-ml quantities of 0.25M *sulphuric acid*, separating the layers by centrifugation if necessary, and transfer each acid extract to a second separating funnel. Make the combined acid extracts alkaline with 10M *ammonia* and extract with three 30-ml quantities of *chloroform*. Combine the chloroform extracts, add 4 g of *anhydrous sodium sulphate* and allow to stand for 30 minutes, shaking occasionally. Decant the chloroform and wash the sodium sulphate with three 10-ml quantities of *chloroform*. Evaporate the combined chloroform extracts and washings to dryness on a water-bath and heat the residue at 100° to 105° for 15 minutes. Dissolve the residue in several ml of *chloroform*, add 20 ml of 0.01M *sulphuric acid VS*, remove the chloroform by evaporation on a water-bath and titrate the excess of acid with 0.02M *sodium hydroxide VS* using *methyl red solution* as indicator. Each ml of 0.01M *sulphuric acid VS* is equivalent to 0.005788 g of total alkaloids, calculated as hyoscyamine.

Storage Hyoscyamus Leaf should be kept in an airtight container and protected from light.

Preparations
Prepared Hyoscyamus
Hyoscyamus Dry Extract

Action and use Antispasmodic.

Powdered Hyosycamus Leaf

Powdered Hyoscyamus Leaf is Hyoscyamus Leaf in powder. It contains not less than 0.05 per cent of total alkaloids, calculated as hyoscyamine and with reference to the material dried at 100° to 105°. The alkaloids consist of those of the hyoscyamine—atropine group together with hyoscine in varying proportions.

Characteristics Yellowish-green to greyish-green; odour that of the unground drug. Diagnostic structures: fragments of leaf lamina with wavy-walled epidermal cells and numerous *anisocytic* stomata, abundant smooth-walled glandular trichomes, frequently fragmented, and fewer covering trichomes; fragments of parenchyma with cells containing single or twinned prisms of calcium oxalate; occasional reticulately-thickened vessels from the stem; epidermis of the corolla with wavy, infolded walls; subspherical pollen grains, 35 to 55 µm in diameter; numerous isolated calcium oxalate prisms and occasional clusters and microsphenoidal crystals.

Identification Complies with the tests for Identification described under Hyoscyamus Leaf.

Acid-insoluble ash Not more than 12.0%, Appendix XI K.

Assay Carry out the Assay described under Hyoscyamus Leaf.

Storage Powdered Hyoscyamus Leaf should be kept in an airtight container and protected from light.

Action and use Antispasmodic.

Prepared Hyosycamus ☆

Prepared Hyoscyamus is Hyoscyamus Leaf in *No. 180 powder* adjusted, if necessary, by the addition of Lactose or hyoscyamus leaf powder of lower alkaloidal content to contain 0.05 to 0.07 per cent of total alkaloids, calculated as hyoscyamine and with reference to the material dried at 100° to 105°.

Characteristics Grey to greyish-green powder. Diagnostic structures as described under Hyoscyamus Leaf; additionally, when mounted in *glycerol (85%)*, crystals of lactose may be seen.

Identification Complies with the tests for Identification described under Hyoscyamus Leaf.

Acid-insoluble ash Not more than 12.0%, Appendix XI K, Method II.

Loss on drying When dried to constant weight at 100° to 105°, loses not more than 5.0% of its weight. Use 1 g.

Assay Carry out the Assay described under Hyoscyamus Leaf.

Storage Prepared Hyoscyamus should be kept in an airtight container and protected from light.

Hypromellose ☆

9004-65-3

Hypromellose is a cellulose having some of the hydroxyl groups in the form of the methyl ether and some in the form of the 2-hydroxypropyl ether. Various grades are available and are distinguished by appending a number indicative of the apparent viscosity in millipascal seconds of a 2 per cent w/v solution measured at 20°.

Characteristics A white, yellowish-white or greyish-white powder or granules; practically odourless; hygroscopic after drying.

Solubility Practically insoluble in hot *water*, in *absolute ethanol*, in *acetone*, in *ether* and in *toluene*. It dissolves in cold *water* forming a colloidal solution.

Identification A. Whilst stirring, introduce a quantity containing the equivalent of 1.0 g of the dried substance into 50 ml of *carbon dioxide-free water* heated to 90°. Allow to cool, dilute to 100 ml with the same solvent and continue stirring until solution is complete (solution A). Heat 10 ml of solution A in a water-bath, with stirring. At temperatures above 50° the solution becomes cloudy or a flocculent precipitate is produced. On cooling the solution becomes clear.
B. To 10 ml of solution A add 0.3 ml of 2M *acetic acid* and 2.5 ml of a 10% w/v solution of *tannic acid*. A yellowish-white, flocculent precipitate is produced which dissolves in 6M *ammonia*.
C. Mix thoroughly 1 g with 2 g of *manganese(II) sulphate* in a test-tube about 16 cm long. Impregnate a strip of filter paper with a freshly prepared mixture of 11 volumes of a 5% w/v solution of *sodium nitroprusside* and 1 volume of a 20% v/v solution of *diethanolamine*, adjusted to pH 9.8 with 1M *hydrochloric acid*. Insert the strip to a depth of 2 cm into the upper part of the tube, immerse the tube to a depth of 8 cm in a silicone oil-bath and heat at 190° to 200°. The filter paper becomes blue within 10 minutes. Carry out a blank test.
D. Without heating, completely dissolve 0.2 g in 15 ml of a 70% w/w solution of *sulphuric acid*, pour the solution, with stirring, into 100 ml of iced *water* and dilute to 250 ml with iced *water*. In a test-tube kept in ice, mix thoroughly 1 ml of the solution with 8 ml of *sulphuric acid*, added dropwise. Heat in a water-bath for exactly 3 minutes and cool immediately in ice. When the mixture is cool, carefully add 0.6 ml of a solution of 3 g of *ninhydrin* in 100 ml of a 4.55% w/v solution of *sodium metabisulphite*, mix well and allow to stand at 25°. A pink colour is produced immediately that changes to violet within 100 minutes.
E. Place 1 ml of solution A on a glass plate. After evaporation of the water a thin film is produced.

Acidity or alkalinity pH of solution A, 5.5 to 8.0, Appendix V L.

Clarity and colour of solution Solution A is not more opalescent than *reference suspension II*, Appendix IV A, and not more intensely coloured than *reference solution Y₆*, Appendix IV B, Method II.

Apparent viscosity 75 to 140% of the declared value when determined by the following method. To 50 ml of *water* heated to 90° add, with stirring, a quantity containing the equivalent of 2 g of the dried substance. Allow to cool, dilute to 100 ml with *water* and continue stirring until solution is complete. Determine the *viscosity*, Appendix V H, Method IV, at 20° using a shear rate of 10 s⁻¹. If necessary, use rates slightly below and slightly above 10 s⁻¹ and interpolate.

Heavy metals 1.0 g complies with *limit test C for heavy metals*, Appendix VII (20 ppm). Use 2 ml of *lead standard solution (10 ppm Pb)* to prepare the standard.

Chloride 1 ml of solution A diluted to 15 ml with *water* complies with the *limit test for chlorides*, Appendix VII (0.5%).

Loss on drying When dried to constant weight at 100° to 105°, loses not more than 10.0% of its weight. Use 1 g.

Sulphated ash Not more than 1.0%, Appendix IX A, Method II. Use 1 g.

Storage Hypromellose should be kept in a well-closed container.

Labelling The label states the apparent viscosity in millipascal seconds of a 2% w/v solution.

Action and use Used in treatment of tear deficiency.

The title of the monograph in the European Pharmacopœia is Methylhydroxypropylcellulose.

Hypromellose Phthalate ☆

Hypromellose Phthalate is a cellulose having some of the hydroxyl groups in the form of the methyl ether, some in the form of the 2-hydroxypropyl ether and some in the form of the phthalyl ester. It contains not less than 20.0 per cent and not more than 35.0 per cent of phthaloyl groups ($C_8H_5O_3$), calculated with reference to the dried substance.

Characteristics White to slightly off-white, free-flowing flakes or a granular powder; odourless or with a slight acidic odour.

Solubility Practically insoluble in *water* and in *absolute ethanol*; very slightly soluble in *acetone* and in *toluene*; soluble in a mixture of equal volumes of *acetone* and *methanol* and in a mixture of equal volumes of *dichloromethane* and *methanol*.

Identification A. Mix thoroughly 1 g with 2 g of *manganese(II) sulphate* in a test-tube about 16 cm long. Impregnate a strip of filter paper with a freshly prepared mixture of 11 volumes of a 5% w/v solution of *sodium nitroprusside* and 1 volume of a 20% v/v solution of *diethanolamine*, adjusted to pH 9.8 with 1M *hydrochloric acid*. Insert the strip to a depth of 2 cm into the upper part of the tube, immerse the tube to a depth of 8 cm in a silicone oil-bath and heat at 190° to 200°. The filter paper becomes blue within 10 minutes. Carry out a blank test.
B. Without heating, completely dissolve 0.2 g in 15 ml of a 70% w/w solution of *sulphuric acid*, pour the solution, with stirring, into 100 ml of iced *water* and dilute to 250 ml with iced *water*. In a test-tube kept in ice, mix thoroughly 1 ml of the solution with 8 ml of *sulphuric acid*, added dropwise. Heat on a water-bath for exactly 3 minutes and cool immediately in ice. When the mixture is cool, add carefully 0.6 ml of a solution containing 3 g of *ninhydrin* in 100 ml of a 4.55% w/v solution of *sodium metabisulphite*, mix well and allow to stand at 25°. A pink colour is produced immediately that changes to violet within 100 minutes.
C. Gently boil 0.5 g with 5 ml of 2M *sodium hydroxide* and 50 ml of *water* for 15 minutes, cool and filter. To the filtrate add 5 ml of 2M *hydrochloric acid*, evaporate the solution to dryness on a water-bath and dry the residue at 100° to 105°. To 0.1 g of the residue in a dry boiling-tube add 0.1 g of *resorcinol* and 3 ml of *sulphuric acid* and heat gently (below 180°) over a small flame until the liquid becomes dark brown. Cool, pour the mixture into 150 ml of *water* and make strongly alkaline by adding 20 ml of

10M *sodium hydroxide*. A yellow colour with an intense green fluorescence is produced.

Clarity and colour of solution A 15.0% w/v solution in a mixture of equal volumes of *dichloromethane* and *methanol* (solution A) is not more opalescent than *reference suspension II*, Appendix IV A, and not more intensely coloured than *reference solution Y₅*, Appendix IV B, Method II.

Appearance of a film Allow 1 ml of solution A to flow over a glass plate and dry. A thin, colourless, transparent, glossy film is produced.

Solubility of a film Immerse a glass tube (15 cm × 1.5 cm) to a depth of 3 cm in solution A, the immersed end being covered with a piece of absorbent gauze held in place by adhesive tape. Remove the tube, fix in a vertical position and allow the solution to drain. Leave the resulting film to dry at 20° in an atmosphere with a relative humidity not exceeding 60%. Repeat this procedure twice more. Pour 2 ml of a 0.15% w/v solution of *methylene blue* into the tube and immerse the closed end of the tube in 0.1M *hydrochloric acid* to a depth of 1 cm at 37° for 3 hours; the acid is not blue. Remove the tube, rinse the outside with *water*, immerse it in *citro-phosphate buffer pH 6.8* at 37° for 20 minutes; the buffer solution is blue.

Free acid Not more than 2%, calculated as phthalic acid, $C_8H_6O_4$, with reference to the dried substance. To 1.5 g, finely powdered, in a separating funnel add 50 ml of a mixture of 3 volumes of *absolute ethanol* and 2 volumes of *dichloromethane*. After dissolution, add 75 ml of *water*, mix thoroughly, add 100 ml of *hexane*, shake well and allow to separate. Collect the aqueous layer. Add 50 ml of *water* to the funnel, shake, allow to separate and combine the aqueous extracts. Titrate the combined extracts with 0.1M *sodium hydroxide VS* using *dilute phenolphthalein solution* as indicator. Repeat the operation without the substance being examined. The difference between the titrations represents the amount of sodium hydroxide required. Each ml of 0.1M *sodium hydroxide VS* is equivalent to 0.0083 g of free acid, calculated as $C_8H_6O_4$.

Heavy metals 2.0 g complies with *limit test C for heavy metals*, Appendix VII (10 ppm). Use 2 ml of *lead standard solution (10 ppm Pb)* to prepare the standard.

Loss on drying When dried at 100° to 105° for 2 hours, loses not more than 5.0% of its weight. Use 1 g.

Sulphated ash Not more than 0.1%, Appendix IX A, Method II. Use 1 g.

Assay Dissolve 1 g (*w* g calculated with reference to the dried substance) in 50 ml of a mixture of 2 volumes of *absolute ethanol*, 2 volumes of *acetone* and 1 volume of *water*. Titrate with 0.1M *sodium hydroxide VS*, using *dilute phenolphthalein solution* as indicator, until a faint pink colour is obtained (*c* ml). Repeat the procedure without the substance being examined (*d* ml). Calculate the percentage content of phthaloyl groups, $C_8H_5O_3$, from the expression $[1.49(c - d)/w] - 1.795S$ where S is the percentage content of free acid.

Action and use Used in treatment of tear deficiency.

The title of the monograph in the European Pharmacopœia is Methylhydroxypropylcellulose Phthalate.

Ibuprofen

'Bu—⟨○⟩—CHMe·CO₂H

$C_{13}H_{18}O_2$ 206.3   *15687-27-1*

Ibuprofen is 2-(4-isobutylphenyl)propionic acid. It contains not less than 98.5 per cent and not more than 100.5 per cent of $C_{13}H_{18}O_2$, calculated with reference to the dried substance.

Characteristics White or almost white powder or crystals; odour, characteristic.

Solubility Practically insoluble in *water*; soluble in 1.5 parts of *ethanol (96%)* and of *acetone*, in 1 part of *chloroform* and in 2 parts of *ether*. It dissolves in aqueous solutions of alkali hydroxides and carbonates.

Identification A. The *infra-red absorption spectrum*, Appendix II A, is concordant with the *reference spectrum* of ibuprofen.

B. The *light absorption*, Appendix II B, in the range 220 to 350 nm of a 0.025% w/v solution in 0.1M *sodium hydroxide* exhibits two maxima, at 264 nm and 273 nm, and a less well-defined maximum at 259 nm. The *absorbance* at 264 nm is about 0.93 and at 273 nm is about 0.78.

Melting point 75.0° to 77.5°, Appendix V A.

Related substances Carry out the method for *high-performance liquid chromatography*, Appendix III D, using solutions of the substance being examined in *acetonitrile* containing (1) 0.005% w/v, (2) 0.5% w/v and (3) 0.0015% w/v.

The chromatographic procedure may be carried out using (a) a stainless steel column (15 cm × 3.9 mm) packed with *stationary phase C* (5 μm) (Resolve C18 is suitable), (b) a mixture of 660 volumes of *water*, 340 volumes of *acetonitrile* and 0.5 volume of *orthophosphoric acid* as the mobile phase with a flow rate of 2 ml per minute and (c) a detection wavelength of 214 nm.

In the chromatogram obtained with solution (2) the area of any *secondary peak* is not greater than the area of the peak obtained with solution (1), not more than one such peak has an area greater than that of the peak obtained with solution (3) and the sum of the areas of the *secondary peaks* is not greater than one and a half times the area of the peak in the chromatogram obtained with solution (1). The method is not valid unless the *column efficiency* is at least 50,000 theoretical plates per metre.

Heavy metals 12 ml of a 10.0% w/v solution in *methanol* complies with *limit test A for heavy metals*, Appendix VII (10 ppm). Use 10 ml of a solution obtained by diluting 5 ml of *lead standard solution (20 ppm Pb)* to 100 ml with *methanol* to prepare the standard.

Loss on drying When dried to constant weight over *phosphorus pentoxide* at a pressure not exceeding 0.7 kPa, loses not more than 0.5% of its weight. Use 1 g.

Sulphated ash Not more than 0.1%, Appendix IX A.

Assay Dissolve 0.5 g in 100 ml of *ethanol (96%)* previously neutralised to *phenolphthalein solution* and titrate with 0.1M *sodium hydroxide VS* using *phenolphthalein solution* as indicator. Each ml of 0.1M *sodium hydroxide VS* is equivalent to 0.02063 g of $C_{13}H_{18}O_2$.

Preparation
Ibuprofen Tablets

Action and use Anti-inflammatory; analgesic.

Ichthammol

Ammonium Ichthosulphonate

8029-68-3

Ichthammol consists mainly of the ammonium salts of the sulphonic acids of an oily substance prepared from a bituminous schist or shale, together with ammonium sulphate and water. It contains not less than 10.5 per cent w/w of organically combined sulphur, calculated with reference to the dried substance, and not more than 25.0 per cent of the total sulphur is in the form of sulphates.

Characteristics An almost black, viscid liquid; odour, strong and characteristic.

Solubility Soluble in *water*; partly soluble in *ethanol (96%)* and in *ether*.

Identification A. When warmed with an equal volume of 5M *sodium hydroxide* ammonia is evolved.

B. 1 g dissolves in 50 ml of *water*, forming a clear, dark brown solution. On addition of *hydrochloric acid* a dark resinous mass is precipitated.

Solubility in glycerol 1 ml dissolves completely in 9 ml of *glycerol* and remains in solution for not less than 24 hours.

Loss on drying When dried to constant weight at 105°, loses not more than 50.0% of its weight. Use 1 g.

Sulphated ash Not more than 0.3%, Appendix IX A.

Assay *For organically combined sulphur* Mix 0.5 g with 4 g of *anhydrous sodium carbonate* and 3 ml of *chloroform* in a porcelain crucible of about 50-ml capacity, warm and stir until all the chloroform has evaporated. Add 10 g of coarsely powdered *copper(II) nitrate*, mix thoroughly and heat the mixture very gently using a small flame. When the initial reaction has subsided, increase the temperature slightly until most of the material has blackened. Cool, place the crucible in a large beaker, add 20 ml of *hydrochloric acid* and, when the reaction has ceased, add 100 ml of *water* and boil until all the copper oxide has dissolved. Filter the solution, dilute with 400 ml of *water*, heat to boiling and add 20 ml of *barium chloride solution*. Allow to stand for 2 hours, filter, wash with *water*, dry and ignite at a temperature of about 600° until, after further ignition, two successive weighings do not differ by more than 0.2% of the weight of the residue. Each g of residue is equivalent to 0.1374 g of total sulphur.

Calculate the percentage of total sulphur and subtract the percentage of sulphur in the form of sulphates.

For sulphur in the form of sulphates Dissolve 2 g in 100 ml of *water*, add 2 g of *copper(II) chloride* dissolved in 80 ml of *water* and sufficient *water* to produce 200 ml, shake well and filter. Heat 100 ml of the filtrate almost to boiling, add 1 ml of *hydrochloric acid* and 5 ml of *barium chloride solution* dropwise and heat on a water-bath. Filter, wash the precipitate with *water*, dry and ignite at a temperature of about 600° until, after further ignition, two successive weighings do not differ by more than 0.2% of the weight of the residue. Each g of residue is equivalent to 0.1374 g of sulphur present in the form of sulphates. Calculate the percentage of total sulphur in the form of sulphates.

Preparation

Zinc and Ichthammol Cream

Action and use Used in treatment of psoriasis.

Idoxuridine

$C_9H_{11}IN_2O_5$ 354.1   *54-42-2*

Idoxuridine is 5-iodo-2'-deoxyuridine. It contains not less than 97.0 per cent and not more than 103.0 per cent of $C_9H_{11}IN_2O_5$, calculated with reference to the dried substance.

Characteristics Colourless crystals or a white, crystalline powder; odourless or almost odourless.

Solubility Slightly soluble in *water* and in *ethanol (96%)*; practically insoluble in *chloroform* and in *ether*.

Identification A. The *infra-red absorption spectrum*, Appendix II A, is concordant with the *reference spectrum* of idoxuridine.

B. The *light absorption*, Appendix II B, in the range 230 to 350 nm of a 0.006% w/v solution in 0.01M *sodium hydroxide* exhibits a maximum only at 279 nm. The *absorbance* at 279 nm is about 0.95.

C. On heating, vapours of iodine are evolved.

Specific optical rotation In a 1% w/v solution in 1M *sodium hydroxide*, +28° to +32°, Appendix V F.

Inorganic iodide Dissolve 0.25 g in a mixture of 25 ml of *water* and 2.5 ml of 1M *sodium hydroxide*, add 10 ml of 1M *hydrochloric acid* and sufficient *water* to produce 50 ml, mix and filter. To 25 ml of the filtrate add 2.5 ml of *hydrogen peroxide solution (20 vol)* and extract with 10 ml of *chloroform*. Any pink colour produced in the chloroform layer is not more intense than that produced by treating 0.275 mg of *potassium iodide* in the same manner.

2'-Deoxyuridine and 5-iodouracil Carry out the method for *high-performance liquid chromatography*, Appendix III D, using three solutions containing (1) 0.00040% w/v of *2'-deoxyuridine*, 0.00040% w/v of *5-iodouracil* and 0.00010% w/v of *sulphanilamide* (internal standard), (2) 0.080% w/v of the substance being examined and (3) 0.080% w/v of the substance being examined and 0.00010% w/v of the internal standard.

The chromatographic conditions described under the Assay may be used but using a mixture of 96 volumes of *water* and 4 volumes of *methanol* as the mobile phase. The order of elution of peaks following the internal standard is deoxyuridine, iodouracil and idoxuridine.

In the chromatogram obtained with solution (3), the ratios of the areas of any peaks corresponding to 2'-deoxy-uridine and 5-iodouracil to the area of the peak due to sulphanilamide are not greater than the ratios of the areas of the corresponding peaks in the chromatogram obtained with solution (1).

Loss on drying When dried at 60° at a pressure not exceeding 0.7 kPa for 2 hours, loses not more than 1.0% of its weight. Use 1 g.

Sulphated ash Not more than 0.1%, Appendix IX A.

Assay Prepare a solution containing 0.12 g of *sulpha-thiazole* (internal standard) in 10 ml of *ethanol (96%)* with warming if necessary and dilute to 100 ml with *water* (solution A). Shake 0.1 g of the substance being examined with 50 ml of *water* until dissolved and add sufficient *water* to produce 100 ml (solution B). Carry out the method for *high-performance liquid chromatography*, Appendix III D, using the following solutions. For solution (1) shake 0.1 g of *idoxuridine BPCRS* with 50 ml of *water* until dissolved and then dilute to 100 ml with *water*; to 15 ml of this solution add 2 ml of solution A and dilute to 20 ml with *water*. For solution (2) add 2 ml of a 10% v/v solution of *ethanol (96%)* to 15 ml of solution B and dilute to 20 ml with *water*. For solution (3) add 2 ml of solution A to 15 ml of solution B and dilute to 20 ml with *water*.

The chromatographic procedure may be carried out using (a) a stainless steel column (30 cm × 4 mm) packed with *stationary phase C* (10 μm) (μBondapak C18 is suitable), (b) a mixture of 87 volumes of *water* and 13 volumes of *methanol* as the mobile phase with a flow rate of 1.7 ml per minute and (c) a detection wavelength of 254 nm.

Calculate the content of $C_9H_{11}IN_2O_5$ using the declared content of $C_9H_{11}IN_2O_5$ in *idoxuridine BPCRS*.

Storage Idoxuridine should be kept in a well-closed container and protected from light.

Preparation
Idoxuridine Eye Drops

Action and use Antiviral.

Imipramine Hydrochloride ☆

$C_{19}H_{24}N_2$,HCl   316.9   *113-52-0*

Imipramine Hydrochloride is 3-(10,11-dihydro-5*H*-dibenz[*b,f*]azepin-5-yl)propyldimethylamine hydrochloride. It contains not less than 98.5 per cent and not more than 101.0 per cent of $C_{19}H_{24}N_2$,HCl, calculated with reference to the dried substance.

Characteristics A white or slightly yellow, crystalline powder; almost odourless.

Solubility Soluble in 2 parts of *water* and in 1.5 parts of *ethanol (96%)*; freely soluble in *chloroform*; practically insoluble in *ether*.

Identification *Test A may be omitted if tests B, C, D, E and F are carried out. Tests B, C and D may be omitted if tests A, E and F are carried out.*

A. The *infra-red absorption spectrum*, Appendix II A, is concordant with the spectrum of *imipramine hydrochloride EPCRS*.

B. The *light absorption*, Appendix II B, in the range 230 to 350 nm of a 0.002% w/v solution in 0.01M *hydrochloric acid* exhibits a maximum only at 251 nm and a shoulder at 270 nm. The A(1%, 1 cm) at 251 nm is about 260.

C. Dissolve 5 mg in 2 ml of *nitric acid*. An intense blue colour is produced.

D. Dissolve 50 mg in 3 ml of *water* and add 0.05 ml of a 2.5% w/v solution of *quinhydrone* in *methanol*. No red colour is produced within 15 minutes.

E. 20 mg yields *reaction A* characteristic of chlorides, Appendix VI.

F. *Melting point*, about 172°, Appendix V A, Method I.

Acidity To 3.0 g add 20 ml of *carbon dioxide-free water*, dissolve rapidly by shaking and triturating with a glass rod and dilute to 30 ml with the same solvent (solution A). The pH of the resulting solution, measured immediately after preparation, is 3.6 to 5.0, Appendix V L.

Clarity and colour of solution Solution A is *clear*, Appendix IV A. Immediately after preparation dilute solution A with an equal volume of *water*. The resulting solution is not more intensely coloured than *reference solution BY₆*, Appendix IV B, Method I.

Heavy metals 2.0 g complies with *limit test C for heavy metals*, Appendix VII (20 ppm). Use 4 ml of *lead standard solution (10 ppm Pb)* to prepare the standard.

Related substances Carry out the method for *thin-layer chromatography*, Appendix III A, using *silica gel G* as the coating substance and a mixture of 55 volumes of *ethyl acetate*, 35 volumes of *glacial acetic acid*, 5 volumes of *hydrochloric acid* and 5 volumes of *water* as the mobile phase but allowing the solvent front to ascend 12 cm above the line of application. Apply separately to the chromatoplate 10 μl of each of three solutions in *methanol* prepared immediately before use and containing (1) 2.5% w/v of the substance being examined, (2) 0.0050% w/v of the substance being examined and (3) 0.0050% w/v of *iminodibenzyl*. After removal of the plate, allow the solvent to evaporate for 5 minutes at ambient temperature, spray with a 0.5% w/v solution of *potassium dichromate* in *sulphuric acid (20%)* and examine immediately. In the chromatogram obtained with solution (1) any spot corresponding to iminodibenzyl is not more intense than the spot in the chromatogram obtained with solution (3) and any other *secondary spot* is not more intense than the spot in the chromatogram obtained with solution (2).

Loss on drying When dried to constant weight at 100° to 105°, loses not more than 0.5% of its weight. Use 1 g.

Sulphated ash Not more than 0.1%, Appendix IX A, Method II. Use 1 g.

Assay Dissolve 0.3 g in 50 ml of *chloroform* and carry out Method I for *non-aqueous titration*, Appendix VIII A, adding 10 ml of *mercury(II) acetate solution* and using 0.5 ml of *metanil yellow solution* as indicator. Each ml of 0.1M *perchloric acid VS* is equivalent to 0.03169 g of $C_{19}H_{24}N_2$,HCl.

Storage Imipramine Hydrochloride should be kept in a well-closed container and protected from light.

Preparation
Imipramine Tablets

Action and use Antidepressant.

Indomethacin ☆

C₁₉H₁₆ClNO₄   357.8   53-86-1

$C_{19}H_{16}ClNO_4$ 357.8   53-86-1

Indomethacin is 1-(4-chlorobenzoyl)-5-methoxy-2-methylindol-3-ylacetic acid. It contains not less than 98.5 per cent and not more than 100.5 per cent of $C_{19}H_{16}ClNO_4$, calculated with reference to the dried substance.

Characteristics A white to yellow, crystalline powder; odourless or almost odourless.

Solubility Practically insoluble in *water*; soluble in 50 parts of *ethanol (96%)*, in 30 parts of *chloroform* and in 45 parts of *ether*.

Identification *Test A may be omitted if tests B, C, D and E are carried out. Tests B, C and D may be omitted if tests A and E are carried out.*

A. The *infra-red absorption spectrum*, Appendix II A, is concordant with the spectrum of *indometacin EPCRS*.

B. The *light absorption*, Appendix II B, in the range 300 to 350 nm of a 0.0025% w/v solution in a mixture of 1 volume of 1M *hydrochloric acid* and 9 volumes of *methanol* exhibits a maximum only at 318 nm. The A(1%, 1 cm) at 318 nm is 170 to 190.

C. Dissolve 0.1 g in 10 ml of *ethanol (96%)*, heating gently if necessary. To 0.1 ml add 2 ml of a freshly prepared mixture of 1 volume of a 25% w/v solution of *hydroxylamine hydrochloride* and 3 volumes of 2M *sodium hydroxide*. Add 2 ml of 2M *hydrochloric acid* and 1 ml of a 1.3% w/v solution of *iron(III) chloride hexahydrate* and mix. A violet-pink colour is produced.

D. Dissolve 0.1 g in 10 ml of *ethanol (96%)*, heating gently if necessary. To 0.5 ml add 0.5 ml of a 2% w/v solution prepared without heating of *4-dimethylamino-benzaldehyde* in a 55% v/v solution of *hydrochloric acid*; a precipitate is produced which redissolves on shaking. Heat on a water-bath; a bluish-green colour is produced. Continue to heat for 5 minutes and then cool for 2 minutes in ice; a precipitate is produced and the colour changes to pale greyish-green. Add 3 ml of *ethanol (96%)*; the resulting solution is clear and violet-pink.

E. *Melting point*, 158° to 162°, Appendix V A, Method I.

Heavy metals 2.0 g complies with *limit test C for heavy metals*, Appendix VII (20 ppm). Use 4 ml of *lead standard solution (10 ppm Pb)* to prepare the standard.

Related substances Carry out the method for *thin-layer chromatography*, Appendix III A, using a suspension of *silica gel HF254* in a 4.68% w/v solution of *sodium dihydrogen orthophosphate* to coat the plate and a mixture of 70 volumes of *ether* and 30 volumes of *petroleum spirit (boiling range, 50° to 70°)* as the mobile phase. Apply separately to the chromatoplate 10 µl of each of two solutions of the substance being examined in *methanol* prepared immediately before use containing (1) 2.0% w/v and (2) 0.010% w/v. After removal of the plate, allow it to dry in air and examine under *ultra-violet light (254 nm)*. Any *secondary spot* in the chromatogram obtained with solution (1) is not more intense than the spot in the chromatogram obtained with solution (2).

Loss on drying When dried to constant weight at 100° to 105°, loses not more than 0.5% of its weight. Use 1 g.

Sulphated ash Not more than 0.1%, Appendix IX A, Method II. Use 1 g.

Assay Dissolve 0.45 g in 75 ml of *acetone* through which *nitrogen* free from carbon dioxide has previously been passed for a few minutes. Maintaining a constant stream of the nitrogen through the solution titrate with carbonate-free 0.1M *sodium hydroxide VS* using 0.2 ml of *dilute phenolphthalein solution* as indicator. Repeat the operation without the substance being examined. The difference between the titrations represents the amount of sodium hydroxide required. Each ml of 0.1M *sodium hydroxide VS* is equivalent to 0.03578 g of $C_{19}H_{16}ClNO_4$.

Storage Indomethacin should be kept in a well-closed container and protected from light.

Preparations
Indomethacin Capsules
Indomethacin Suppositories

Action and use Anti-inflammatory; analgesic.

The title of the monograph in the European Pharmacopœia is Indometacin.

Inositol Nicotinate

C₄₂H₃₀N₆O₁₂   810.7   6556-11-2

$C_{42}H_{30}N_6O_{12}$ 810.7   6556-11-2

Inositol Nicotinate is *meso*-inositol hexanicotinate. It contains not less than 98.0 per cent and not more than 101.0 per cent of $C_{42}H_{30}N_6O_{12}$, calculated with reference to the dried substance.

Characteristics A white or almost white powder; odourless or almost odourless.

Solubility Practically insoluble in *water*, in *ethanol (96%)*, in *acetone* and in *ether*; sparingly soluble in *chloroform*. It dissolves in dilute mineral acids.

Identification A. The *infra-red absorption spectrum*, Appendix II A, is concordant with the *reference spectrum* of inositol nicotinate.

B. Dissolve 50 mg in 1M *hydrochloric acid* and dilute to 100 ml with the same solvent. Dilute 5 ml of this solution to 100 ml with *water*. The *light absorption* of the resulting solution, Appendix II B, in the range 230 to 350 nm exhibits a maximum only at 261 nm. The *absorbance* at 261 nm is about 0.88.

C. Heat a small quantity with four times its weight of *anhydrous sodium carbonate*. Pyridine, recognisable by its odour, is evolved.

Clarity and colour of solution A 5.0% w/v solution in 0.5M *sulphuric acid* is *clear*, Appendix IV A, and not more intensely coloured than *reference solution BY₆*, Appendix IV B, Method II.

Heavy metals 4.0 g complies with *limit test C for heavy metals*, Appendix VII (10 ppm). Use 4 ml of *lead standard solution (10 ppm Pb)* to prepare the standard.

Chloride Dissolve 0.14 g in a sufficient quantity of 2M *nitric acid* and dilute to 16 ml with *water*. The resulting solution complies with the *limit test for chlorides*, Appendix VII, beginning at the words 'and immediately add . . .' (350 ppm).

Free nicotinic acid To 1 g add 75 ml of *water*, shake for 15 minutes and titrate with 0.02M *sodium hydroxide VS* using *phenolphthalein solution* as indicator. Not more than 0.8 ml of 0.02M *sodium hydroxide VS* is required to produce the first pink colour.

Related substances Carry out the method for *thin-layer chromatography*, Appendix III A, using a chromatoplate 200 mm × 200 mm in size and *silica gel GF254* as the coating substance. For the first separation use a mixture of 90 volumes of *chloroform* and 10 volumes of *methanol* as the mobile phase. Apply to the bottom right-hand corner of the plate 5 μl of solution (1) containing 5.0% w/v of the substance being examined in a mixture of 9 volumes of *chloroform* and 1 volume of *methanol* and develop over a path of 12 cm. After removal of the plate, allow it to dry in air and turn the plate through 90° in a clockwise direction. Apply separately to the bottom right-hand corner of the plate, and to the right of the solvent front, 5 μl of each of two solutions of the substance being examined in a mixture of 9 volumes of *chloroform* and 1 volume of *methanol* containing (2) 0.075% w/v and (3) 0.050% w/v. For the second separation use a mixture of 50 volumes of *ethyl acetate* and 5 volumes each of *glacial acetic acid*, *ethanol (96%)* and *water* as the mobile phase. After removal of the plate, allow it to dry in air and examine under *ultra-violet light (254 nm)*. In the chromatogram obtained with solution (1) any *secondary spot* is not more intense than the spot in the chromatogram obtained with solution (2) and not more than one such spot is more intense than the spot in the chromatogram obtained with solution (3).

Acetone Prepare a 0.020% v/v solution of *butan-2-one* (internal standard) in *dimethylformamide* (solution A). Carry out the method for *gas chromatography*, Appendix III B, using the following solutions. Solution (1) contains 0.020% v/v of *acetone* in solution A. For solution (2) add 5 ml of *dimethylformamide* to 0.20 g of the substance being examined contained in a suitable vessel, stopper securely, suspend in a water-bath until solution is complete and allow to cool. Prepare solution (3) in the same manner as solution (2) but using 5 ml of solution A in place of the dimethylformamide.

The chromatographic procedure may be carried out using a glass column (1.5 m × 4 mm) packed with *acid-washed, silanised diatomaceous support* coated with 10% w/w of polyethylene glycol 1000 and maintained at 60°.

In the chromatogram obtained with solution (3) the ratio of the area of any peak corresponding to acetone to the area of the peak due to the internal standard is not greater than the corresponding ratio in the chromatogram obtained with solution (1).

Loss on drying When dried to constant weight at 105°, loses not more than 0.5% of its weight. Use 1 g.

Sulphated ash Not more than 0.1%, Appendix IX A.

Assay Carry out Method I for *non-aqueous titration*, Appendix VIII A, using 0.2 g and *1-naphtholbenzein solution* as indicator. Each ml of 0.1M *perchloric acid VS* is equivalent to 0.01351 g of $C_{42}H_{30}N_6O_{12}$.

Storage Inositol Nicotinate should be kept in a well-closed container.

Preparation
Inositol Nicotinate Tablets

Action and use Vasodilator.

Insulin ☆

Insulin is the natural antidiabetic hormone of the pancreas of either the pig or the ox, appropriately purified. It is prepared in conditions designed to minimise microbial contamination.

Insulin contains not less than 26 Units per mg calculated with reference to the dried material.

Characteristics A white or almost white powder.

Solubility Practically insoluble in *water*, in *ethanol (96%)*, in *chloroform* and in *ether*. It dissolves in dilute solutions of mineral acids and, with degradation, in solutions of alkali hydroxides.

Identification A. Causes a fall in blood glucose when injected as directed in the Assay.
B. In the test for Related proteins the principal band in the gel obtained with solution (6) corresponds in position to the principal band in the gel obtained with solution (5).
C. Carry out the method for *high-performance liquid chromatography*, Appendix III D, injecting 50 μl of each of two solutions in 0.05M *hydrochloric acid* containing (1) 0.05% w/v of the substance being examined and (2) 0.05% w/v of *insulin EPBRP*.

The chromatographic procedure may be carried out using (a) a stainless steel column (25 cm × 4.6 mm) packed with *stationary phase C* (5 μm) (Ultrasphere ODS is suitable) and maintained at 45°, (b) *acetonitrile—phosphate solution* as the mobile phase with a flow rate of 1 ml per minute and (c) a detection wavelength of 280 nm.

In the chromatogram obtained with solution (2) the two largest peaks are due to beef insulin (eluting first) and pork insulin respectively. The principal peak in the chromatogram obtained with solution (1) corresponds in position to one or other of the two largest peaks in the chromatogram obtained with solution (2) in accordance with the animal source stated on the label. The test is not valid unless the *symmetry factors* of the principal peaks are between 0.8 and 2.0 and the *column efficiency*, determined using the principal peak in the chromatogram obtained with solution (2), is not less than 1000 theoretical plates per metre.

Light absorption *Absorbance* of a 0.05% w/v solution in 0.01M *hydrochloric acid* at the maximum at 276 nm, 0.48 to 0.56, Appendix II B.

Related proteins Carry out Method II for *polyacrylamide-gel electrophoresis*, Appendix III F, using five solutions of *insulin EPBRP* in 0.1 ml of *sample application buffer* containing (1) 0.50 μg, (2) 1.0 μg, (3) 3.0 μg, (4) 5.0 μg and (5) 100 μg and two solutions of the substance being examined in 0.1 ml of *sample application buffer* containing (6) 100 μg and (7) 500 μg. Apply each solution to a tube of the gel. After electrophoresis and staining, evaluate the gels on a cold-light illuminator.

In the gel prepared with solution (6) any band corresponding in position to the faster of the two bands behind the principal band in the gel prepared with solution (5) (arginyl insulin and insulin ethyl ester) is not more intense than the principal band in the gel prepared with solution (3). In the gel prepared with solution (7) any band corresponding in position to the slower of the two bands behind the principal band in the gel prepared with solution (5) (proinsulin) is not more intense than the principal band in the gel prepared with solution (1).

The test is not valid unless a band can be detected in the gel prepared with solution (1) and a gradation is observed in the intensity of staining of the gels prepared with solutions (1) to (4).

Proteins of higher molecular weight Carry out the method for *size-exclusion chromatography*, Appendix III C, equilibrating the column with 1M *acetic acid* and applying, per square centimetre of column cross-sectional area, 0.4 ml of a 5% w/v solution of the substance being examined in 1M *acetic acid*.

The chromatographic procedure may be carried out using (a) a column not less than 60 cm long and not less than 9 mm in internal diameter packed with a cross-linked dextran suitable for fractionation of proteins in the range of molecular weights from 1500 to 30,000 (Sephadex G-50-SF is suitable), (b) 1M *acetic acid* as the mobile phase with a flow rate of 7 ml per square centimetre of column cross-sectional area per hour and (c) a detection wavelength of 276 nm.

The sum of the areas of any peaks eluting before the principal peak is not greater than 1% of the total area of the peaks in the chromatogram.

Zinc Not more than 0.6% of Zn, calculated with reference to the dried substance, when determined by the following method. Prepare a 0.2% w/v solution in 0.01M *hydrochloric acid*. Dilute, if necessary, to a suitable concentration (for example 0.4 to 1.6 ppm of Zn) with 0.01M *hydrochloric acid*. Carry out the method for *atomic absorption spectrophotometry*, Appendix II D, measuring at 213.9 nm and using a zinc hollow-cathode lamp as the source of radiation and an air—acetylene flame of suitable composition (for example, 11 litres of air and 2 litres of acetylene per minute). Use freshly prepared dilutions in 0.01M *hydrochloric acid* of *zinc solution ASp* containing 0.10, 0.40, 0.80, 1.00, 1.20 and 1.60 ppm of Zn as the standard solutions.

Nitrogen 14.5 to 16.5%, calculated with reference to the dried substance, when determined by Method IV, Appendix VIII H. Use 12 to 20 mg.

Loss on drying When dried over *phosphorus pentoxide* at 105° at a pressure of 1.5 to 2.5 kPa for 24 hours, loses not more than 10.0% of its weight. Use 0.2 g.

Sulphated ash Not more than 2.0%, calculated with reference to the dried substance, Appendix IX A, Method II. Use 0.2 g.

Assay Carry out the *biological assay of insulin*, Appendix XIV C10. The estimated potency is not less than 90% and not more than 111% of the stated potency. The fiducial limits of error are not less than 80% and not more than 125% of the stated potency.

Storage Insulin should be kept in an airtight container, protected from light and stored at a temperature not exceeding −20°.

Labelling The label states (1) the number of Units in the container; (2) the number of Units per mg; (3) the animal source of the insulin; (4) the conditions under which the material should be stored; (5) the date after which it is not intended to be used.

Human Insulin

$C_{257}H_{383}N_{65}O_{77}S_6$ 5807.6   *11061-68-0*

Human Insulin is a protein having the normal structure of the natural antidiabetic hormone produced by the human pancreas. It is produced either by the enzymatic modification of insulin obtained from the pancreas of the pig or by a procedure based on recombinant deoxyribonucleic acid (DNA) technology in micro-organisms followed, in either case, by appropriate purification. When Human Insulin is prepared using recombinant DNA technology, production is based on an approved host-vector system. Human Insulin is prepared in conditions designed to minimise microbial contamination.

Human Insulin contains not less than 26 Units per mg calculated with reference to the dried material.

Characteristics A white or almost white powder.

Solubility Practically insoluble in *water*, in *ethanol (96%)*, in *chloroform* and in *ether*. It dissolves in dilute solutions of mineral acids and, with degradation, in solutions of alkali hydroxides.

Identification A. Causes a fall in blood glucose when injected as directed in the Assay.
B. In the test for Related proteins the principal band in the gel obtained with solution (6) corresponds in position to the principal band in the gel obtained with solution (5).
C. Carry out the method for *high-performance liquid chromatography*, Appendix III D, injecting 50 µl of each of three solutions in 0.05M *hydrochloric acid* containing (1) 0.05% w/v of the substance being examined, (2) 0.05% w/v of *human insulin BPCRS* and (3) 0.05% w/v of *human insulin BPCRS* and 0.05% w/v of *insulin EPBRP*.

The chromatographic procedure may be carried out using (a) a stainless steel column (25 cm × 4.6 mm) packed with *stationary phase C* (5 µm) (Ultrasphere ODS is suitable) and maintained at 45°, (b) *acetonitrile—phosphate solution* as the mobile phase with a flow rate of 1 ml per minute and (c) a detection wavelength of 280 nm.

The principal peak in the chromatogram obtained with solution (1) corresponds in position to the principal peak in the chromatogram obtained with solution (2). The test is not valid unless the *symmetry factors* of the principal peaks are between 0.8 and 2.0 and the *column efficiency*, determined using the principal peak in the chromatogram obtained with solution (2), is not less than 4000 theoretical plates per metre, and the peak in the chromatogram obtained with solution (3) corresponding to the principal peak in the chromatogram obtained with solution (2) is clearly separated from the four additional peaks in the chromatogram.

Light absorption *Absorbance* of a 0.05% w/v solution in 0.01M *hydrochloric acid* at the maximum at 276 nm, 0.48 to 0.56, Appendix II B.

Related proteins Carry out Method II for *polyacrylamide-gel electrophoresis*, Appendix III F, using five solutions of *insulin EPBRP* in 0.1 ml of *sample application buffer* containing (1) 0.50 µg, (2) 1.0 µg, (3) 3.0 µg, (4) 5.0 µg and (5) 100 µg and two solutions of the substance being examined in 0.1 ml of *sample application buffer* containing (6) 100 µg and (7) 500 µg. Apply each solution to a tube of the gel. After electrophoresis and staining, evaluate the gels on a cold-light illuminator.

In the gel prepared with solution (6) any band corresponding in position to the faster of the two bands behind the principal band in the gel prepared with solution (5) (arginyl insulin and insulin ethyl ester) is not more intense than the principal band in the gel prepared with solution (3). In the gel prepared with solution (7) any band corresponding in position to the slower of the two bands behind the principal band in the gel prepared with solution (5) (proinsulin) is not more intense than the principal band in the gel prepared with solution (1).

The test is not valid unless a band can be detected in the gel prepared with solution (1) and a gradation is observed in the intensity of staining of the gels prepared with solutions (1) to (4).

Proteins of higher molecular weight Carry out the method for *size-exclusion chromatography*, Appendix III C, equilibrating the column with 1M *acetic acid* and applying, per square centimetre of column cross-sectional area, 0.4 ml of a 5% w/v solution of the substance being examined in 1M *acetic acid*.

The chromatographic procedure may be carried out using (a) a column not less than 60 cm long and not less than 9 mm in internal diameter packed with a cross-linked dextran suitable for fractionation of proteins in the range of molecular weights from 1500 to 30,000 (Sephadex G-50-SF is suitable), (b) 1M *acetic acid* as the mobile phase with a flow rate of 7 ml per square centimetre of column cross-sectional area per hour and (c) a detection wavelength of 276 nm.

The sum of the areas of any peaks eluting before the principal peak is not greater than 1% of the total area of the peaks in the chromatogram.

Zinc Not more than 1.0% of Zn, calculated with reference to the dried substance, when determined by the following method. Prepare a 0.2% w/v solution in 0.01M *hydrochloric acid*. Dilute, if necessary, to a suitable concentration (for example 0.4 to 1.6 ppm of Zn) with 0.01M *hydrochloric acid*. Carry out the method for *atomic absorption spectrophotometry*, Appendix II D, measuring at 213.9 nm and using a zinc hollow-cathode lamp as the source of radiation and an air—acetylene flame of suitable composition (for example, 11 litres of air and 2 litres of acetylene per minute). Use freshly prepared dilutions in 0.01M *hydrochloric acid* of *zinc solution ASp* containing 0.10, 0.40, 0.80, 1.00, 1.20 and 1.60 ppm of Zn as the standard solutions.

Nitrogen 14.5 to 16.5%, calculated with reference to dried substance, when determined by Appendix VIII H, Method IV. Use 12 to 20 mg.

Loss on drying When dried over *phosphorus pentoxide* at 105° at a pressure of 2 kPa for 24 hours, loses not more than 10.0% of its weight. Use 0.2 g.

Sulphated ash Not more than 2.0%, calculated with reference to the dried substance, Appendix IX A, Method II. Use 0.2 g.

Assay Carry out the *biological assay of human insulin*, Appendix XIV C11. The estimated potency is not less than 90% and not more than 111% of the stated potency. The fiducial limits of error are not less than 80% and not more than 125% of the stated potency.

Storage Human Insulin should be kept in an airtight container, protected from light and stored at a temperature not exceeding −20°.

Labelling The label states (1) the number of Units in the container; (2) the number of Units per mg; (3) the approved code in lower case letters indicative of the method of production; (4) the conditions under which the material should be stored; (5) the date after which it is not intended to be used.

Inulin

Inulin consists of polysaccharide granules obtained from the tubers of *Dahlia variabilis*, *Helianthus tuberosus* and other genera of the family Compositae.

Characteristics A white, amorphous, granular powder; odourless or almost odourless; hygroscopic.

Microscopical When mounted in *absolute ethanol*, appears as large, very irregular, angular masses, whole or fragmented, with occasional smaller, spherical to ovoid particles.

Solubility Slightly soluble in *water*; freely soluble in hot *water*; slightly soluble in organic solvents.

Identification A. Carry out the method for *thin-layer chromatography*, Appendix III A, using a suspension of *silica gel G* in a 0.3% w/v solution of *sodium acetate* to coat the chromatoplate, but spreading a layer 0.5 mm thick. Use a mixture of 70 volumes of *glacial acetic acid*, 60 volumes of *chloroform* and 10 volumes of *water* as the mobile phase. Apply separately to the plate 1 µl of each of three solutions in *water* containing (1) 2.5% w/v of the substance being examined, prepared using heat, (2) 2.5% w/v of the substance being examined and 10% w/v of *oxalic acid*, prepared by boiling for 10 minutes and cooling, and (3) 2.5% w/v of *D-fructose* and 0.1% w/v of *D-glucose monohydrate*. Develop the chromatograms in a continuous elution tank for about 4 hours. After removal of the plate, evaporate the solvent in a current of warm air and spray with a solution in *acetone* containing 1% v/v of *diphenylamine*, 1% v/v of *aniline* and 1% v/v of *ortho-phosphoric acid* and heat for 10 minutes at 130°. The two principal spots in the chromatogram obtained with solution (2) correspond to those in the chromatogram obtained with solution (3). The spot in the chromatogram obtained with solution (1) remains on the line of application.

B. Dissolve 10 mg in 2 ml of hot *water*, add 3 ml of a 0.15% w/v solution of *resorcinol* in *ethanol (96%)* followed by 3 ml of *hydrochloric acid*, mix and heat at 80°. A red colour is produced.

C. Boil 5 ml of a 10% w/v solution for 2 minutes with 0.5 ml of *hydrochloric acid*, cool and neutralise to *litmus paper* with 5M *sodium hydroxide*. Add 0.5 ml of *potassium cupri-tartrate solution* and heat. A red precipitate is produced.

Acidity Dissolve 5 g in 50 ml of freshly boiled *water* and titrate with 0.1M *sodium hydroxide VS* using *phenolphthalein solution* as indicator. Not more than 0.20 ml is required to change the colour of the solution to pink.

Clarity and colour of solution A 10.0% w/v solution in hot *water* is *clear*, Appendix IV A, Method I, and *colourless*, Appendix IV B, Method I.

Specific optical rotation In a 2% w/v solution, prepared using heat, $-36.5°$ to $-40.5°$, Appendix V F.

Arsenic 1.0 g dissolved in 25 ml of hot *water* complies with the *limit test for arsenic*, Appendix VII (1 ppm).

Calcium Dissolve 1.0 g in 10 ml of hot *water*, place the solution in a water-bath at 40°, add 0.5 ml of a 2.5% w/v solution of *ammonium oxalate* and allow to stand for 15 minutes. Any turbidity produced is not greater than that obtained by treating 10 ml of a 0.010% w/v solution of *calcium chloride* in the same manner (270 ppm).

Lead 2.5 g dissolved in 20 ml of hot *water* complies with *limit test B for lead in sugars*, Appendix VII (2 ppm).

Chloride Dissolve 2.0 g in hot *water*, cool and dilute to 100 ml with *water*. 15 ml of the resulting solution complies with the *limit test for chlorides*, Appendix VII (170 ppm).

Oxalate Dissolve 1.0 g in 10 ml of hot *water*, place the solution in a water-bath at 40°, add 0.5 ml of a 7% w/v solution of *calcium chloride* and allow to stand for 15 minutes. Any turbidity produced is not greater than that obtained by treating 10 ml of a 0.003% w/v solution of *oxalic acid* in the same manner.

Sulphate Dissolve 2.3 g in 20 ml of hot *water*, cool, add 2 ml of 2M *hydrochloric acid* and dilute to 45 ml with *water*. The solution complies with the *limit test for sulphates*, Appendix VII (200 ppm).

Reducing sugars Heat 10 ml of *potassium cupri-tartrate solution* and titrate with a 10% w/v solution of the substance being examined, adding a few ml at a time and boiling for 10 to 15 seconds between each addition. When the solution becomes greenish-yellow, add 0.25 ml of a 1% w/v solution of *methylene blue* and continue the titration until the solution becomes orange. Repeat the operation using a 0.20% w/v solution of *D-fructose* in place of the solution of the substance being examined. The volume of the fructose solution required is not greater than that of the solution of the substance being examined.

Loss on drying When dried to constant weight at 105°, loses not more than 10.0% of its weight. Use 1 g.

Sulphated ash Not more than 0.1%, Appendix IX A.

Preparation
Inulin Injection

Action and use Used for the measurement of glomerular filtration rate.

Iodine ☆

I$_2$ 253.8   7553-56-2

Iodine contains not less than 99.5 per cent and not more than 100.5 per cent of I$_2$.

Characteristics Brittle plates or small crystals, greyish-violet with a metallic sheen; odour, irritant. It volatilises slowly at room temperature.

Solubility Very slightly soluble in *water*; soluble in 8 parts of *ethanol (96%)* and in 30 parts of *chloroform*; slightly soluble in *glycerol*; very soluble in concentrated solutions of iodides.

Identification A. When heated gently in a test-tube, a violet vapour is evolved and a bluish-black crystalline sublimate is produced.

B. A saturated solution yields a blue colour in the presence of *starch solution*, which disappears when the solution is boiled and reappears when it is cooled.

Chloride and bromide Triturate 3.0 g with 20 ml of *water*, filter, wash the filter, dilute the filtrate to 30 ml with *water* and add 1 g of *zinc powder*. When the solution is decolorised, filter and wash the filter with sufficient *water* to produce 40 ml of filtrate (solution A). To 10 ml of solution A add 3 ml of 10M *ammonia* and 6 ml of 0.1M *silver nitrate*, filter, wash the filter with *water* and dilute to 20 ml with *water*. To 10 ml of the filtrate add 1.5 ml of *nitric acid*. After 1 minute any opalescence produced is not more intense than that produced in a solution prepared at the same time by mixing 10.75 ml of *water*, 0.25 ml of 0.01M *hydrochloric acid VS*, 0.2 ml of 2M *nitric acid* and 0.3 ml of 0.1M *silver nitrate* (250 ppm).

Non-volatile matter Heat 1 g in a porcelain dish on a water-bath until the iodine has volatilised and dry at 100° to 105°. The residue weighs not more than 1 mg.

Assay Add 0.2 g to a flask containing 1 g of *potassium iodide* and 2 ml of *water* and add 1 ml of 2M *acetic acid*, dissolve and dilute to 50 ml with *water*. Titrate with 0.1M *sodium thiosulphate VS* using *starch solution* as indicator. Each ml of 0.1M *sodium thiosulphate VS* is equivalent to 0.01269 g of I.

Storage Iodine should be kept in a glass-stoppered container.

Preparations
Aqueous Iodine Oral Solution
Weak Iodine Solution

Action and use Antiseptic; antithyroid.

Iopanoic Acid

CH$_2$·CHEt·CO$_2$H

NH$_2$

C$_{11}$H$_{12}$I$_3$NO$_2$ 571.0   96-83-3

Iopanoic Acid is 2-(3-amino-2,4,6-tri-iodobenzyl)butyric acid. It contains not less than 98.5 per cent and not more than 101.0 per cent of C$_{11}$H$_{12}$I$_3$NO$_2$, calculated with reference to the dried substance.

Characteristics A white to cream powder; odourless or almost odourless.

Solubility Practically insoluble in *water*; soluble in 25 parts of *ethanol (96%)*; soluble in *acetone*. It dissolves in aqueous solutions of the alkali hydroxides.

Identification A. The *infra-red absorption spectrum*, Appendix II A, is concordant with the *reference spectrum* of iopanoic acid.

B. Heat 50 mg strongly. Violet vapours of iodine are evolved.

C. *Melting point*, about 155°, Appendix V A.

Inorganic iodide Dissolve 0.80 g in the minimum quantity of 0.2M *sodium hydroxide*, dilute to 10 ml with *water*, add sufficient 2M *nitric acid* dropwise to ensure complete precipitation of the iodinated acid and add 3 ml in excess. Filter, wash the precipitate with 5 ml of *water*, add to the filtrate 1 ml of *hydrogen peroxide solution (100 vol)* and 1 ml of *chloroform* and shake. Any purple colour in the chloroform is not more intense than that obtained by adding 2 ml of *iodide standard solution (20 ppm I)* to a mixture of 3 ml of 2M *nitric acid* and sufficient *water* to equal the volume of the test solution, adding 1 ml of *hydrogen peroxide solution (100 vol)* and 1 ml of *chloroform* and shaking (50 ppm).

Loss on drying When dried at 105° for 1 hour, loses not more than 0.5% of its weight. Use 1 g.

Sulphated ash Not more than 0.1%, Appendix IX A.

Assay Mix 0.4 g with 12 ml of 5M *sodium hydroxide* and 20 ml of *water*, add 1 g of *zinc powder* and boil under a reflux condenser for 30 minutes. Cool, rinse the condenser with 30 ml of *water*, filter through absorbent cotton and wash the flask and filter with two 20-ml quantities of *water*. To the combined filtrate and washings add 80 ml of *hydrochloric acid*, cool and titrate with 0.05M *potassium iodate VS* until the dark brown solution becomes light brown. Add 5 ml of *chloroform* and continue the titration, shaking well after each addition, until the chloroform becomes colourless. Each ml of 0.05M *potassium iodate VS* is equivalent to 0.01903 g of $C_{11}H_{12}I_3NO_2$.

Storage Iopanoic Acid should be protected from light.

Preparation
Iopanoic Acid Tablets

Action and use Radio-opaque substance used in cholecystography.

Iothalamic Acid

$C_{11}H_9I_3N_2O_4$ 613.9   2276-90-6

Iothalamic Acid is 5-acetamido-2,4,6-tri-iodo-*N*-methylisophthalamic acid. It contains not less than 99.0 per cent and not more than 101.0 per cent of $C_{11}H_9I_3N_2O_4$, calculated with reference to the dried substance.

Characteristics A white powder; odourless or almost odourless.

Solubility Slightly soluble in *water* and in *ethanol (96%)*; practically insoluble in *chloroform*; very soluble in solutions of *sodium hydroxide*.

Identification A. Dissolve 0.1 g in the minimum volume of 1M *sodium hydroxide*, dilute to 10 ml with *water* and acidify with 1M *hydrochloric acid*. Filter, wash the precipitate with *water* and dry at 105°. The *infra-red*

absorption spectrum of the residue, Appendix II A, is concordant with the *reference spectrum* of iothalamic acid.

B. Heat 50 mg. Violet vapours of iodine are evolved.

C. Heat 0.5 g with 2 ml of *ethanol (96%)* and 1 ml of *sulphuric acid*. Ethyl acetate, recognisable by its odour, is produced.

Free amine Keep the solutions in ice, protected from light, and cool the reagents to about 5° before use. Shake 0.50 g with 15 ml of *water* in a 50-ml graduated flask, cool in ice, add 1 ml of 1M *sodium hydroxide* and shake. Add 5 ml of a freshly prepared 0.5% w/v solution of *sodium nitrite* followed immediately by 12 ml of 1M *hydrochloric acid*, swirl gently and allow to stand. Exactly 2 minutes after the addition of the acid add 10 ml of a 2% w/v solution of *ammonium sulphamate*, allow to stand for 5 minutes, shaking frequently, and add 0.15 ml of a 10% w/v solution of *1-naphthol* in *ethanol (96%)*. Mix, allow to stand for 1 minute and add 3.5 ml of a solution prepared by dissolving 6.75 g of *ammonium chloride* in 30 ml of *water* and adding 57 ml of 13.5M *ammonia* and sufficient *water* to produce 100 ml. Mix, add sufficient *water* to produce 50 ml and within 20 minutes measure the *absorbance* of the resulting solution at the maximum at 485 nm, Appendix II B, using in the reference cell a solution prepared by treating 15 ml of *water* in the same manner. The absorbance is not more than 0.15.

Hydrazo compound Suspend 5.0 g in 25 ml of *water*, add sufficient 5M *sodium hydroxide* to effect solution and adjust the pH to between 8.0 and 9.0 with 0.1M *sodium hydroxide* or 1M *acetic acid*. Cool to 20° and add *iodine solution* dropwise until the solution turns *starch—iodide paper* blue. The solution does not become brown or reddish-brown.

Inorganic iodide Dissolve 0.80 g in the minimum quantity of 0.2M *sodium hydroxide*, dilute to 10 ml with *water*, add sufficient 2M *nitric acid* dropwise to ensure complete precipitation of the iodinated acid and add 3 ml in excess. Filter, wash the precipitate with 5 ml of *water*, add to the filtrate 1 ml of *hydrogen peroxide solution (100 vol)* and 1 ml of *chloroform* and shake. Any purple colour in the chloroform is not more intense than that obtained by adding 2 ml of *iodide standard solution (20 ppm I)* to a mixture of 3 ml of 2M *nitric acid* and sufficient *water* to equal the volume of the test solution, adding 1 ml of *hydrogen peroxide solution (100 vol)* and 1 ml of *chloroform* and shaking (50 ppm).

Loss on drying When dried to constant weight at 105°, loses not more than 0.5% of its weight. Use 1 g.

Sulphated ash Not more than 0.1%, Appendix IX A.

Assay Mix 0.4 g with 12 ml of 5M *sodium hydroxide* and 20 ml of *water*, add 1 g of *zinc powder* and boil under a reflux condenser for 30 minutes. Cool, rinse the condenser with 30 ml of *water*, filter through absorbent cotton and wash the flask and filter with two 20-ml quantities of *water*. To the combined filtrate and washings add 80 ml of *hydrochloric acid*, cool and titrate with 0.05M *potassium iodate VS* until the dark brown solution becomes light brown. Add 5 ml of *chloroform* and continue the titration, shaking well after each addition, until the chloroform becomes colourless. Each ml of 0.05M *potassium iodate VS* is equivalent to 0.02046 g of $C_{11}H_9I_3N_2O_4$.

Storage Iothalamic Acid should be protected from light.

Preparations
Meglumine Iothalamate Injection
Sodium Iothalamate Injection

In some countries the material described in this monograph may be known as Iotalamic Acid.

Ipecacuanha ☆

Ipecacuanha consists of the underground organs of *Cephaelis ipecacuanha* (Brot.) A Rich, known in commerce as Matto Grosso Ipecacuanha, or of *Cephaelis acuminata* Karsten, known in commerce as Costa Rica Ipecacuanha, or of a mixture of both species. It contains not less than 2.0 per cent of total alkaloids of ipecacuanha, calculated as emetine and with reference to the material dried at 100° to 105°.

Characteristics Odour, slight.

Cephaelis ipecacuanha

Macroscopical Root: somewhat tortuous pieces, seldom more than 15 cm long or 6 mm thick; from dark brick red to very dark brown; closely annulated externally, ridges rounded and completely encircling the root; fracture, short in the bark and splintery in the wood, the smoothed, transversely cut surface showing a wide, greyish bark and a small uniformly dense wood. Rhizome: short lengths usually attached to roots, cylindrical, up to 2 mm in diameter, finely wrinkled longitudinally and with pith occupying approximately one sixth of the whole diameter.

Microscopical Root: in transverse section, consisting of a narrow, brown cork layer of thin-walled polyhedral, tabular cells and a wide, parenchymatous band of phelloderm; phloem present as a narrow, unlignified band; xylem dense, consisting mainly of narrow tracheids intermixed with a smaller proportion of vessels, both with numerous bordered pits in their lateral walls, the vessel elements having simple, circular perforations. Cells of the phelloderm and medullary rays containing abundant starch consisting of simple granules and two- to eight-compound granules, the individual granules, oval, rounded or roughly hemispherical, seldom being more than 15 µm in diameter. Crystal cells, each containing a bundle of raphides, 30 to 80 µm long present in the parenchymatous regions. Rhizome: in transverse section through an internode, exhibiting several layers of thin-walled cork; somewhat collenchymatous cortex; pericycle containing groups of large, distinctly pitted sclereids, a narrow ring of phloem and a wide ring of xylem surrounding a pith composed of thin-walled, pitted, parenchymatous cells.

Cephaelis acuminata

In general resembles the root of *Cephaelis ipecacuanha*, but differs in the following particulars: often up to 9 mm thick; external surface greyish-brown or reddish-brown with transverse ridges at intervals of about 1 to 3 mm, the ridges about 0.5 to 1 mm wide, extending about half way round the circumference and fading at the extremities into the general surface level; individual starch granules up to 22 µm in diameter.

Identification Carry out the method for *thin-layer chromatography*, Appendix III A, using *silica gel G* as the coating substance and a mixture of 186 volumes of *chloroform*, 13 volumes of *methanol* and 1 volume of 13.5M *ammonia* as the mobile phase, but allowing the solvent front to ascend 10 cm above the line of application. Apply separately to the chromatoplate, as bands 20 mm × 3 mm, 10 µl of each of the following solutions. For solution (1) add 0.05 ml of 13.5M *ammonia* and 5 ml of *chloroform* to 0.1 g, in *No. 180 powder*, in a small test-tube, stir vigorously with a glass rod, allow to stand for 30 minutes and filter. For solution (2) dilute 1 ml of solution (1) to 25 ml with *chloroform*. For solution (3) dissolve 5 mg of *emetine dihydrochloride* and 6 mg of *cephaeline dihydrochloride* in sufficient *methanol* to produce 20 ml.

After removal of the plate, allow it to dry in air until the odour of solvent is no longer detectable, spray with a 0.5% w/v solution of *iodine* in *chloroform* using about 10 ml for a plate 200 mm × 200 mm in size and heat at 60° for 10 minutes. The chromatograms exhibit a lemon yellow band at about the mid point corresponding to emetine and below it a light brown band corresponding to cephaeline. Examine under *ultra-violet light (365 nm)*. The bands corresponding to emetine and cephaeline show an intense yellow fluorescence and a light blue fluorescence respectively. The chromatogram obtained with solution (1) also shows very small bands due to secondary alkaloids. The chromatogram obtained with solution (2) shows only two bands corresponding to bands in the chromatogram obtained with solution (3).

With *C. acuminata* the principal bands in the chromatogram obtained with solution (1) are similar in position, size and fluorescence to those in the chromatogram obtained with solution (3). With *C. ipecacuanha*, the band corresponding to cephaeline in the chromatogram obtained with solution (1) is much smaller than the band due to cephaeline in the chromatogram obtained with solution (3).

Foreign matter Not more than 1.0%, Appendix XI D, Test B.

Acid-insoluble ash Not more than 3.0%, Appendix XI K, Method II.

Sulphated ash Not more than 6.0%, Appendix IX A, Method II. Use 1 g, in powder.

Assay To 7.5 g, in *No. 180 powder*, in a dry flask add 100 ml of *ether* and shake for 5 minutes. Add 5 ml of 6M *ammonia*, shake frequently for 1 hour, add 5 ml of *water*, shake vigorously and decant the ether layer into a dry flask through a plug of absorbent cotton. Wash the residue in the flask with two 25-ml quantities of *ether*, decanting each portion through the same plug of absorbent cotton. Combine the ether solutions and remove most of the ether by distillation and the remainder by gently warming in a current of air. Dissolve the residue in 2 ml of *ethanol (90%)*, evaporate the ethanol and heat at 100° for 5 minutes. Dissolve the residue in 5 ml of previously neutralised *ethanol (90%)* by warming on a water-bath, add 15 ml of 0.1M *hydrochloric acid VS* and titrate the excess of acid with 0.1M *sodium hydroxide VS* using 0.5 ml of *methyl red—methylene blue solution* as indicator. Each ml of 0.1M *hydrochloric acid VS* is equivalent to 0.02403 g of total alkaloids, calculated as emetine.

Storage Ipecacuanha should be kept in a well-closed container and protected from light.

Preparation

Ipecacuanha Liquid Extract

Action and use Expectorant; emetic.

The title of the monograph in the European Pharmacopœia is Ipecacuanha Root.

When Ipecacuanha or Ipecacuanha Root is prescribed, Prepared Ipecacuanha shall be dispensed.

Powdered Ipecacuanha

Powdered Ipecacuanha is Ipecacuanha in powder. It contains not less than 2.0 per cent of total alkaloids of ipecacuanha, calculated as emetine and with reference to the material dried at 100° to 105°.

Characteristics Light grey to yellowish-brown. Diagnostic structures: cork cells; starch granules, simple or two- to eight-compound, individual granules up to 15 μm (*C. ipecacuanha*) or 22 μm (*C. acuminata*) in diameter; raphides of calcium oxalate up to 80 μm in length, in bundles or scattered throughout the powder; fragments of tracheids and vessels (10 to 20 μm in diameter) with bordered pits; larger vessels and sclereids from the rhizome.

Identification; Acid-insoluble ash; Sulphated ash Complies with the requirements stated under Ipecacuanha.

Assay Carry out the Assay described under Ipecacuanha. Each ml of 0.1M *hydrochloric acid VS* is equivalent to 0.02403 g of total alkaloids, calculated as emetine.

Storage Powdered Ipecacuanha should be kept in a well-closed container and protected from light.

Action and use Expectorant; emetic.

When Powdered Ipecacuanha is prescribed, Prepared Ipecacuanha shall be dispensed.

Prepared Ipecacuanha ☆

Prepared Ipecacuanha is Ipecacuanha in *No. 180 powder*, adjusted if necessary by the addition of Lactose or an ipecacuanha powder of a lower alkaloidal content to contain 1.9 to 2.1 per cent of total alkaloids, calculated as emetine and with reference to the dried material.

Characteristics A light grey to yellowish-brown powder; odour, slight.

Microscopical Exhibits the characters described under Powdered Ipecacuanha and, when mounted in *glycerol (85%)*, crystals of lactose may be present.

Identification; Acid-insoluble ash; Sulphated ash Complies with the requirements stated under Ipecacuanha.

Loss on drying When dried to constant weight at 100° to 105°, loses not more than 5.0% of its weight. Use 1 g.

Assay Carry out the Assay described under Ipecacuanha. Each ml of 0.1M *hydrochloric acid VS* is equivalent to 0.02403 g of total alkaloids, calculated as emetine.

Storage Prepared Ipecacuanha should be kept in a well-closed container and protected from light.

Action and use Expectorant; emetic.

Isoniazid ☆

$C_6H_7N_3O$ 137.1   *54-85-3*

Isoniazid is isonicotinohydrazide. It contains not less than 99.0 per cent and not more than 101.0 per cent of $C_6H_7N_3O$, calculated with reference to the dried substance.

Characteristics Colourless crystals or a white, crystalline powder; odourless.

Solubility Soluble in 8 parts of *water*; sparingly soluble in *ethanol (96%)*; slightly soluble in *chloroform*; very slightly soluble in *ether*.

Identification *Test A may be omitted if tests B and C are carried out. Test B may be omitted if tests A and C are carried out.*

A. The *infra-red absorption spectrum*, Appendix II A, is concordant with the spectrum of *isoniazid EPCRS*.

B. Dissolve 0.1 g in 2 ml of *water*, add a warm solution of 0.1 g of *vanillin* in 10 ml of *water*, allow to stand and scratch the inside of the test-tube with a glass rod. A yellow precipitate is produced. The *melting point* of the precipitate, after recrystallisation from 5 ml of *ethanol (70%)* and drying at 100° to 105°, is 226° to 231°, Appendix V A, Method I.

C. *Melting point*, 170° to 174°, Appendix V A, Method I.

Acidity or alkalinity pH of a 5% w/v solution, 6.0 to 8.0, Appendix V L.

Clarity and colour of solution A 5.0% w/v solution in *carbon dioxide-free water* is *clear*, Appendix IV A, and not more intensely coloured than *reference solution BY₇*, Appendix IV B, Method II.

Heavy metals 2.0 g complies with *limit test C for heavy metals*, Appendix VII (10 ppm). Use 2 ml of *lead standard solution (10 ppm Pb)* to prepare the standard.

Hydrazine and related substances Carry out the method for *thin-layer chromatography*, Appendix III A, using *silica gel GF254* as the coating substance and a mixture of 50 volumes of *ethyl acetate*, 20 volumes of *acetone*, 20 volumes of *methanol* and 10 volumes of *water* as the mobile phase. Apply separately to the chromatoplate 5 μl of each of the following solutions. For solution (1) dissolve 1.0 g of the substance being examined in a mixture of equal volumes of *acetone* and *water* and dilute to 10 ml with the same solvent. For solution (2) dissolve 50 mg of *hydrazine sulphate* in 50 ml of *water* and dilute to 100 ml with *acetone*; to 10 ml of this solution add 0.2 ml of solution (1) and dilute to 100 ml with a mixture of equal volumes of *acetone* and *water*. After removal of the plate, allow it to dry in air and examine under *ultra-violet light (254 nm)*. Any *secondary spot* in the chromatogram obtained with solution (1) is not more intense than the spot in the chromatogram obtained with solution (2). Spray with *dimethylaminobenzaldehyde solution* and examine in daylight. The additional spot in the chromatogram obtained with solution (2) is more intense than any corresponding spot in the chromatogram obtained with solution (1).

Loss on drying When dried to constant weight at 100° to 105°, loses not more than 0.5% of its weight. Use 1 g.

Sulphated ash Not more than 0.1%, Appendix IX A, Method II. Use 1 g.

Assay Dissolve 0.25 g in sufficient *water* to produce 100 ml. To 20 ml of the resulting solution add 100 ml of *water*, 20 ml of *hydrochloric acid* and 0.2 g of *potassium bromide* and titrate slowly with continuous shaking with 0.0167M *potassium bromate VS* using 0.05 ml of *methyl red solution* as indicator. Each ml of 0.0167M *potassium bromate VS* is equivalent to 0.003429 g of $C_6H_7N_3O$.

Preparations
Isoniazid Injection
Isoniazid Tablets

Action and use Antituberculous.

Isoprenaline Hydrochloride

$C_{11}H_{17}NO_3,HCl$ 247.7   *51-39-6*

Isoprenaline Hydrochloride is 1-(3,4-dihydroxy-phenyl)-2-isopropylaminoethanol hydrochloride. It contains not less than 98.0 per cent and not more than 101.5 per cent of $C_{11}H_{17}NO_3,HCl$, calculated with reference to the dried substance.

Characteristics A white or almost white, crystalline powder; odourless or almost odourless. Gradually darkens on exposure to air and light; aqueous solutions become pink to brownish-pink on standing exposed to air and almost immediately when made alkaline.

Solubility Very soluble in *water*; soluble in 55 parts of *ethanol (96%)*; insoluble in *chloroform* and in *ether*.

Identification A. The *infra-red absorption spectrum*, Appendix II A, is concordant with the *reference spectrum* of isoprenaline hydrochloride.
B. The *light absorption*, Appendix II B, in the range 240 to 350 nm of a 0.01% w/v solution exhibits a maximum only at 280 nm. The *absorbance* at 280 nm is about 1.0.
C. To 2 ml of a 1% w/v solution add 0.1 ml of *iron(III) chloride test-solution*. An emerald-green colour is produced which, on the gradual addition of *sodium hydrogen carbonate solution*, changes first to blue and then to red.
D. Yields the *reactions* characteristic of chlorides, Appendix VI.

Melting point 166° to 170°, Appendix V A.

Sulphate Dissolve 0.50 g in 100 ml of *water*. 15 ml of the resulting solution complies with the *limit test for sulphates*, Appendix VII (0.2%).

Phenones *Absorbance* of a 0.2% w/v solution in 0.005M *sulphuric acid* at 310 nm, not more than 0.15, Appendix II B.

Loss on drying When dried over *phosphorus pentoxide* at a pressure not exceeding 0.7 kPa for 4 hours, loses not more than 1.0% of its weight. Use 1 g.

Sulphated ash Not more than 0.1%, Appendix IX A.

Assay Carry out Method I for *non-aqueous titration*, Appendix VIII A, using 0.5 g dissolved in *anhydrous glacial acetic acid* with the aid of the minimum of heat and *crystal violet solution* as indicator. Each ml of 0.1M *perchloric acid VS* is equivalent to 0.02477 g of $C_{11}H_{17}NO_3,HCl$.

Storage Isoprenaline Hydrochloride should be kept in a well-closed container and protected from light.

Preparation Isoprenaline Injection

Action and use Sympathomimetic; beta-adrenoceptor agonist.

Isoprenaline Sulphate ☆

$(C_{11}H_{17}NO_3)_2,H_2SO_4,2H_2O$ 556.6   *6700-39-6*

Isoprenaline Sulphate is 1-(3,4-dihydroxy-phenyl)-2-isopropylaminoethanol sulphate dihydrate. It contains not less than 98.0 per cent and not more than 102.0 per cent of $(C_{11}H_{17}NO_3)_2,H_2SO_4$, calculated with reference to the anhydrous substance.

Characteristics A white or almost white, crystalline powder. It melts at about 128°, with decomposition.

Solubility Soluble in 4 parts of *water*; slightly soluble in *ethanol (96%)*; practically insoluble in *chloroform* and in *ether*.

Identification *Test A may be omitted if tests B, C and D are carried out. Tests B and C may be omitted if tests A and D are carried out.*
A. Dissolve 0.5 g in 1.5 ml of *water*, add 3.5 ml of *propan-2-ol*, scratch the walls of the container with a glass rod to initiate crystallisation, collect the crystals and dry over *phosphorus pentoxide* at 60° at a pressure of 1.5 to 2.5 kPa. The *infra-red absorption spectrum* of the crystals, Appendix II A, is concordant with the spectrum of *isoprenaline sulphate EPCRS* that has been treated in the same manner.
B. To 1 ml of a 1% w/v solution add 0.05 ml of a 10.5% w/v solution of *iron(III) chloride hexahydrate*; a green colour is produced. Add, dropwise, *sodium hydrogen carbonate solution*; the colour changes to blue and then to red.
C. To 10 ml of a 1% w/v solution in *carbon dioxide-free water* add 0.25 ml of 0.25M *silver nitrate*. A shining, greyish, fine precipitate is produced within 10 minutes and the solution becomes pink.
D. A 10% w/v solution in *carbon dioxide-free water* yields the *reactions* characteristic of sulphates, Appendix VI.

Acidity pH of a freshly prepared 5% w/v solution, 4.3 to 5.5, Appendix V L.

Clarity and colour of solution A freshly prepared 10.0% w/v solution in *carbon dioxide-free water* is *clear*, Appendix IV A, and not more intensely coloured than *reference solution* Y_6, Appendix IV B, Method II.

Phenones *Absorbance* of a 0.2% w/v solution in 0.005M *sulphuric acid* at 310 nm, not more than 0.20, Appendix II B.

Sulphated ash Not more than 0.1%, Appendix IX A, Method II. Use 1 g.

Water 5.0 to 7.5% w/w, Appendix IX C. Use 0.2 g.

Assay Dissolve 0.4 g in 20 ml of *anhydrous glacial acetic acid*, warming gently if necessary, and add 20 ml of

4-methylpentan-2-one. Carry out Method I for *non-aqueous titration*, Appendix VIII A, determining the end-point potentiometrically. Each ml of 0.1M *perchloric acid VS* is equivalent to 0.05206 g of $(C_{11}H_{17}NO_3)_2,H_2SO_4$.

Storage Isoprenaline Sulphate should be kept in a well-closed container and protected from light.

Action and use Sympathomimetic; beta-adrenoceptor agonist.

Isopropyl Alcohol

CH₃·CH·CH₃
|
OH

C_3H_8O 60.10   *67-63-0*

Isopropyl Alcohol is propan-2-ol.

Characteristics A clear, colourless liquid; odour, characteristic and spirituous; flammable.

Solubility Miscible with *water*, with *chloroform* and with *ether*.

Identification A. Mix 1 ml of a 10% v/v solution with 2 ml of *mercury(II) sulphate solution* and heat just to boiling. A white or yellowish-white precipitate is produced.
B. Gently heat 1 ml with 4 ml of *potassium dichromate solution* and 1 ml of *sulphuric acid*. Acetone, recognisable by its odour, is evolved.

Acidity or alkalinity Gently boil 25 ml for 5 minutes with 25 ml of *carbon dioxide-free water* and cool, taking precautions to exclude carbon dioxide. Not more than 0.06 ml of 0.1M *sodium hydroxide VS* is required to make the resulting solution alkaline to *phenolphthalein solution*.

Distillation range Not less than 95.0% v/v distils between 81° and 83°, Appendix V C.

Refractive index 1.377 to 1.378, Appendix V E.

Weight per ml 0.784 to 0.786 g, Appendix V G.

Aldehydes and ketones Mix in a cylinder 25 ml with 25 ml of *water* and 50 ml of *hydroxylamine solution*, allow to stand for 5 minutes and titrate with 0.1M *sodium hydroxide VS* until the colour is concordant with that of 50 ml of *hydroxylamine solution* contained in a similar cylinder, each being viewed down the axis of the cylinder. Not more than 2.0 ml of 0.1M *sodium hydroxide VS* is required.

Benzene Record second-derivative ultra-violet absorption spectra of the following solutions using a path-length of up to 4 cm in the range 230 to 300 nm. Solution (1) is the substance being examined. Solution (2) contains 0.00020% v/v of *benzene* in the substance being examined.

An ultra-violet spectrophotometer capable of operation in the second-derivative mode or any other appropriate means of producing second-derivative spectra may be used.

In the spectrum obtained with solution (2) measure the amplitude (Y_2) as shown in Fig. 1. Measure any corresponding amplitude (Y_1) in the spectrum obtained with solution (1). The value of Y_1 is not greater than $Y_2 - Y_1$ (2 ppm).

The test is not valid unless the amplitude in the spectrum obtained with solution (2) is more than eight times the average peak-to-peak noise in the range 280 to 300 nm.

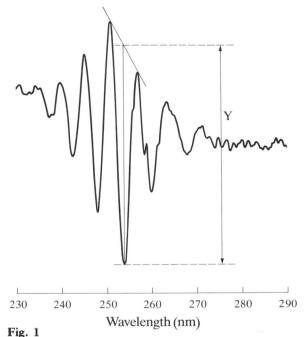

Fig. 1
Typical second-derivative ultra-violet absorption spectrum of isopropyl alcohol containing about 2 ppm of benzene.

Non-volatile matter When evaporated and dried at 105°, leaves not more than 0.0016% w/v of residue.

Water-insoluble matter Mix 1 volume with 19 volumes of *water*. No opalescence is produced.

Water Not more than 0.50% w/w, Appendix IX C. Use 5 g.

Storage Isopropyl Alcohol should be kept in a well-closed container.

Isopropyl Myristate

CH₃·(CH₂)₁₂·CO·OCHMe₂

$C_{17}H_{34}O_2$ 270.5   *110-27-0*

Isopropyl Myristate consists of the isopropyl ester of myristic acid, the chief component of which is tetradecanoic acid.

Characteristics A colourless mobile liquid; odourless or almost odourless.

Solubility Immiscible with *water* and with *glycerol*; soluble in 3 parts of *absolute ethanol*; miscible with liquid hydrocarbons and with fixed oils.

Identification A. The *infra-red absorption spectrum*, Appendix II A, is concordant with the *reference spectrum* of isopropyl myristate.
B. Carry out the method for *gas chromatography*, Appendix III B, using the following solutions. For solution (1) boil 0.2 g with 25 ml of 5M *sodium hydroxide* under a reflux condenser for 2 hours, distil 10 ml and use the distillate. Solution (2) is *propan-2-ol*.

The chromatographic conditions described under the test for Related substances may be used but maintaining the column temperature at 60°.

The principal peak in the chromatogram obtained with solution (1) has the same retention time as the peak in the chromatogram obtained with solution (2).

Acid value Not more than 0.5, Appendix X B.

Iodine value Not more than 1.0 (*iodine monochloride method*), Appendix X E.

Ester value Not less than 205, Appendix X C, but using 1.1 g of the substance being examined and 20 ml of *ethanolic potassium hydroxide* in the determination of the *saponification value*.

Refractive index 1.434 to 1.437, Appendix V E.

Relative density 0.850 to 0.855, Appendix V G.

Related substances Carry out the method for *gas chromatography*, Appendix III B, using solutions in *chloroform* containing (1) 0.25% w/v of the substance being examined and 0.25% v/v of *dimethyl phthalate* (internal standard), (2) 5.0% w/v of the substance being examined and (3) 5.0% w/v of the substance being examined and 0.25% v/v of the internal standard.

The chromatographic procedure may be carried out using a glass column (1.5 m × 4 mm) packed with *acid-washed diatomaceous support* (80 to 100 mesh) coated with 10% w/w of polyethylene glycol (Carbowax 20M is suitable) and maintained at 190°.

In the chromatogram obtained with solution (3) the ratio of the sum of the areas of any *secondary peaks* to the area of the peak due to the internal standard is not greater than twice the ratio of the area of the peak due to isopropyl myristate to that of the peak due to the internal standard in the chromatogram obtained with solution (1).

Action and use Pharmaceutical aid.

Diluted Isosorbide Dinitrate

Diluted Sorbide Nitrate

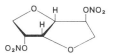

$C_6H_8N_2O_8$ 236.1   87-33-2

Diluted Isosorbide Dinitrate is a dry mixture of 1,4:3,6-dianhydro-D-glucitol 2,5-dinitrate with Lactose, Mannitol or other suitable inert diluent. It may contain up to 1 per cent of a suitable stabiliser. It contains not less than 95.0 per cent and not more than 105.0 per cent of the content of isosorbide dinitrate stated on the label and usually contains 20 per cent to 50 per cent of isosorbide dinitrate.

CAUTION Undiluted isosorbide dinitrate can be exploded by percussion or excessive heat. Appropriate precautions should be exercised and only exceedingly small amounts should be isolated.

Characteristics A fine, white, crystalline powder; odourless or almost odourless.

Solubility Undiluted isosorbide dinitrate is very slightly soluble in *water*, sparingly soluble in *ethanol (96%)*, very soluble in *acetone* and freely soluble in *chloroform*.

Identification A. Shake a quantity containing 50 mg of isosorbide dinitrate with 15 ml of *acetone* for 2 minutes. Filter, evaporate the filtrate to dryness at a temperature not exceeding 35° and dry the residue over *phosphorus pentoxide* at a pressure of 0.7 kPa for 16 hours. The *infra-red absorption spectrum* of the residue, Appendix II A, is concordant with the *reference spectrum* of isosorbide dinitrate.

B. Carry out the method for *thin-layer chromatography*, Appendix III A, using *silica gel G* as the coating substance and *toluene* as the mobile phase. Apply separately to the chromatoplate 20 μl of each of the following solutions. For solution (1) extract a quantity containing 2 mg of isosorbide dinitrate with 1 ml of *ether* and centrifuge. Prepare solution (2) in the same manner but using *diluted isosorbide dinitrate BPCRS* in place of the substance being examined. After removal of the plate, dry it in a current of air, spray with a 1% w/v solution of *diphenylamine* in *methanol* and irradiate for 15 minutes with *ultra-violet light (254 and 365 nm)*. The principal spot in the chromatogram obtained with solution (1) corresponds to that in the chromatogram obtained with solution (2).

C. Extract a quantity containing 10 mg of isosorbide dinitrate with 10 ml of *ether* and filter. Evaporate the resulting solution to dryness at a temperature not exceeding 35° and dissolve the residue in 0.15 ml of *sulphuric acid (50%)* containing a trace of *diphenylamine*. An intense blue colour is produced.

Inorganic nitrates Carry out the method for *thin-layer chromatography*, Appendix III A, using *silica gel H* as the coating substance and a mixture of 60 volumes of *toluene*, 30 volumes of *acetone* and 15 volumes of *glacial acetic acid* as the mobile phase. Apply separately to the chromatoplate 5 μl of each of the following solutions. Solution (1) is a solution of the substance being examined in *ethanol (96%)* containing the equivalent of 2.5% w/v of isosorbide dinitrate. Solution (2) is a freshly prepared 0.10% w/v solution of *potassium nitrate* in *ethanol (90%)*. After removal of the plate dry it in a stream of air and spray with *diphenylamine solution*. Any spot corresponding to potassium nitrate in the chromatogram obtained with solution (1) is not more intense than the spot in the chromatogram obtained with solution (2).

Related substances Carry out the method for *thin-layer chromatography*, Appendix III A, using *silica gel G* as the coating substance and a mixture of 80 volumes of *toluene* and 20 volumes of *ethyl acetate* as the mobile phase. Apply separately to the chromatoplate 20 μl of each of the following two solutions. For solution (1) shake a quantity of the substance being examined containing 0.2 g of isosorbide dinitrate with 5 ml of *acetone* and filter. For solution (2) dilute 1 volume of solution (1) to 200 volumes with *acetone*. After removal of the plate, dry it in a current of air and spray with *diphenylamine solution*. Any *secondary spot* in the chromatogram obtained with solution (1) is not more intense than the spot in the chromatogram obtained with solution (2).

Loss on drying When dried over *phosphorus pentoxide* at a pressure not exceeding 0.7 kPa for 16 hours, loses not more than 1.0% of its weight. Use 1 g.

Assay Shake a quantity containing 25 mg of isosorbide dinitrate with 15 ml of *glacial acetic acid* for 15 minutes, add sufficient *glacial acetic acid* to produce 25 ml and filter. To 1 ml of the filtrate add 2 ml of *phenoldisulphonic acid solution*, allow to stand for 15 minutes, add 50 ml of *water*, make alkaline with 13.5M *ammonia*, cool and add sufficient *water* to produce 100 ml. Measure the *absorbance* of the resulting solution at 405 nm, Appendix II B, using in the reference cell 1 ml of *glacial acetic acid* treated in the same manner, beginning at the words 'add 2 ml of *phenoldisulphonic acid solution . . .*'. Dissolve 0.2 g of *potassium nitrate*, previously dried at 105°, in 5 ml of *water* and add sufficient *glacial acetic acid* to produce 25 ml. To

5 ml add sufficient *glacial acetic acid* to produce 50 ml. Using 1 ml of this solution repeat the assay beginning at the words 'add 2 ml of *phenoldisulphonic acid solution . . .*'. Calculate the content of $C_6H_8N_2O_8$ from the absorbances so obtained. Each ml of the potassium nitrate solution is equivalent to 0.000934 g of $C_6H_8N_2O_8$.

Storage Diluted Isosorbide Dinitrate should be kept in a well-closed container, protected from light and stored at a temperature not exceeding 15°.

Labelling The label states the percentage content of isosorbide dinitrate, $C_6H_8N_2O_8$.

Preparation
Isosorbide Dinitrate Tablets

Action and use Vasodilator.

Isoxsuprine Hydrochloride

$C_{18}H_{23}NO_3,HCl$ 337.8   579-56-6

Isoxsuprine Hydrochloride is (1*SR*,2*RS*)-1-(4-hydroxyphenyl)-2-[(2*RS*)-1-methyl-2-phenoxy-ethylamino]propan-1-ol hydrochloride. It contains not less than 98.5 per cent and not more than 101.0 per cent of $C_{18}H_{23}NO_3,HCl$, calculated with reference to the dried substance.

Characteristics A white or almost white, crystalline powder; odourless or almost odourless.

Solubility Slightly soluble in *water* and in *ethanol (96%)*; practically insoluble in *chloroform* and in *ether*.

Identification A. The *infra-red absorption spectrum*, Appendix II A, is concordant with the *reference spectrum* of isoxsuprine hydrochloride. If the spectra are not concordant dissolve 50 mg in 2 ml of *methanol*, add 15 ml of *dichloromethane*, evaporate to dryness and prepare a new spectrum.

B. The *light absorption*, Appendix II B, in the range 230 to 350 nm of a 0.01% w/v solution in 0.1M *hydrochloric acid* exhibits two maxima, at 269 nm and 274 nm. The *absorbance* at 269 nm is about 0.73 and at 274 nm is about 0.72.

C. Dissolve 10 mg in 1 ml of *water* and add 0.05 ml of *copper sulphate solution* and 1 ml of 5M *sodium hydroxide*; a blue colour is produced. Add 1 ml of *ether* and shake; the ether layer remains colourless.

D. Yields the *reactions* characteristic of chlorides, Appendix VI.

Acidity pH of a 1% w/v solution, prepared with gentle warming if necessary, 4.5 to 6.0, Appendix V L.

Phenones *Absorbance* of a 0.01% w/v solution at 310 nm, not more than 0.20, Appendix II B.

Related substances Carry out the method for *gas chromatography*, Appendix III B, using the following freshly prepared solutions. For solution (1) add 0.5 ml of N-*trimethylsilylimidazole* to 10 mg of the substance being examined and heat at 65° for 10 minutes. Allow to cool and add 2 ml of a 0.5% w/v solution of *hexacosane*

(internal standard) in 2,2,4-*trimethylpentane* and 2 ml of *water*. Shake well, allow to separate and dilute 1 ml of the upper layer to 50 ml with 2,2,4-*trimethylpentane*. For solution (2) add 0.5 ml of N-*trimethylsilylimidazole* to 10 mg of the substance being examined and heat at 65° for 10 minutes. Allow to cool and add 2 ml of 2,2,4-*trimethyl-pentane* and 2 ml of *water*. Shake well, allow to separate and use the upper layer. Prepare solution (3) in the same manner as solution (2) but add 2 ml of a 0.01% w/v solution of the internal standard in 2,2,4-*trimethylpentane* in place of the 2 ml of 2,2,4-trimethylpentane.

The chromatographic procedure may be carried out using a glass column (1.5 m × 4 mm) packed with *acid-washed, silanised diatomaceous support* (100 to 120 mesh) coated with 3% w/w of dimethyl silicone gum (SE-30 is suitable) and maintained at 215°.

In the chromatogram obtained with solution (3) the ratio of the sum of the areas of any *secondary peaks* to the area of the peak due to the internal standard is not greater than the ratio of the area of the peak due to the trimethylsilyl derivative of isoxsuprine to that of the internal standard in the chromatogram obtained with solution (1).

The *column efficiency*, determined using the peak due to the internal standard in the chromatogram obtained with solution (1), should be not less than 2000 theoretical plates per metre.

Loss on drying When dried to constant weight at 105°, loses not more than 0.5% of its weight. Use 1 g.

Sulphated ash Not more than 0.1%, Appendix IX A.

Assay Carry out Method I for *non-aqueous titration*, Appendix VIII A, using 0.6 g and *1-naphtholbenzein solution* as indicator. Each ml of 0.1M *perchloric acid VS* is equivalent to 0.03378 g of $C_{18}H_{23}NO_3,HCl$.

Storage Isoxsuprine Hydrochloride should be kept in a well-closed container.

Preparations
Isoxsuprine Injection
Isoxsuprine Tablets

Action and use Vasodilator; uterine relaxant.

Ispaghula Husk

Ispaghula Husk consists of the epidermis and the collapsed adjacent layers removed from the dried ripe seeds of *Plantago ovata* Forssk.

Characteristics

Macroscopical Pale buff, brittle flakes, more or less lanceolate, up to 2 mm long and 1 mm wide at the centre, much broken into smaller fragments; many of the flakes have a small, brownish, oval spot, about 0.8 to 1.0 mm long, in the centre; the material swells rapidly in water, forming a stiff mucilage.

Microscopical Mounted in *cresol*, the particles are transparent and angular, the edges straight or curved and sometimes rolled. They are composed of polygonal prismatic cells with four to six straight or slightly curved walls; the cells vary in size in different parts of the seed-coat, from about 25 to 60 μm at the summit of the seed, that is, near and over the brown spot, to 25 to 100 μm for the remainder of the epidermis except at the edges of the seed, where the cells are smaller, about 45 to 70 μm.

When mounted in *ethanol (96%)* and irrigated with *water*, the mucilage in the outer part of the epidermal cells swells rapidly and goes into solution, while the two inner layers of mucilage are more resistant and swell to form rounded papillae. When mounted in 0.005M *iodine*, occasional simple and two- to four-compound starch granules, about 2 to 10 μm, can be seen in some of the cells. Occasional fragments of thick-walled, reddish-brown endosperm, cells with pitted walls and elongated fragments of grey embryo may be present.

Loss on drying When dried at 105° for 5 hours, loses not more than 12.0% of its weight. Use 1 g.

Ash Not more than 4.5%, Appendix XI J.

Swelling power Transfer 1 g to a 100-ml stoppered cylinder containing 90 ml of *water*, shake well for 30 seconds and allow to stand for 24 hours, shaking gently on three occasions during this period. Add sufficient *water* to produce 100 ml, mix gently for 30 seconds, avoiding the entrainment of air, allow to stand for 5 hours and measure the volume of mucilage. Repeat the determination three times. The average of the four determinations is not less than 40 ml.

Action and use Antidiarrhoeal; bulk-forming laxative.

Kanamycin Acid Sulphate ☆

Kanamycin Acid Sulphate is a form of kanamycin sulphate prepared by adding Sulphuric Acid to a solution of Kanamycin Sulphate and drying by a suitable method. The potency is not less than 670 Units per mg, calculated with reference to the dried substance.

Characteristics A white or almost white powder; odourless or almost odourless; hygroscopic.

Solubility Soluble in 1 part of *water*; practically insoluble in *ethanol (96%)*, in *acetone*, in *chloroform* and in *ether*.

Identification A. Complies with test A for Identification described under Kanamycin Sulphate.
B. Dissolve 0.5 g in 10 ml of *water*, add 10 ml of a 1% w/v solution of *2,4,6-trinitrophenol*, if necessary initiate crystallisation by scratching the wall of the container with a glass rod, allow to stand and filter. The *melting point* of the crystals, after washing with 20 ml of *water* and drying at 100°, is about 235°, with decomposition, Appendix V A, Method I.
C. Dissolve 50 mg in 2 ml of *water*, add 1 ml of a 1% w/v solution of *ninhydrin* and heat for a few minutes on a water-bath. A violet colour is produced.
D. Yields the *reactions* characteristic of sulphates, Appendix VI.

Acidity or alkalinity pH of a 1% w/v solution, 5.5 to 7.5, Appendix V L.

Specific optical rotation In a 1% w/v solution in *carbon dioxide-free water*, +103° to +115°, Appendix V F.

Kanamycin B Complies with the test described under Kanamycin Sulphate, using as solution (1) a 0.55% w/v solution of the substance being examined.

Sulphate 23.0 to 26.0% of SO_4, calculated with reference to the dried substance, when determined by the following method. Dissolve 0.175 g in 100 ml of *water* and adjust the pH of the solution to 11 using 13.5M *ammonia*. Add 10 ml of 0.1M *barium chloride VS* and 0.5 mg of *metalphthalein* and titrate with 0.1M *disodium edetate VS*; when the colour of the solution begins to change, add 50 ml of *ethanol (96%)* and continue the titration until the violet-blue colour disappears. Each ml of 0.1M *barium chloride VS* is equivalent to 0.009606 g of SO_4.

Loss on drying When dried at 60° at a pressure not exceeding 0.7 kPa for 3 hours, loses not more than 5.0% of its weight. Use 1 g.

Sulphated ash Not more than 0.5%, Appendix IX A, Method II. Use 1 g.

Assay Carry out the *biological assay of antibiotics*, Appendix XIV A. The precision of the assay is such that the fiducial limits of error are not less than 95% and not more than 105% of the estimated potency.

Storage Kanamycin Acid Sulphate should be kept in a well-closed container. If the material is intended for use in the manufacture of a parenteral dosage form, the container should be sterile and sealed so as to exclude micro-organisms.

Labelling The label states (1) the number of Units per mg; (2) the date after which the material is not intended to be used; (3) the conditions under which it should be stored; (4) whether or not it is intended for use in the manufacture of a parenteral dosage form.

Preparation
Kanamycin Injection

Action and use Antibacterial.

Kanamycin Acid Sulphate intended for use in the manufacture of a parenteral dosage form complies with the following additional requirements.

Abnormal toxicity Complies with the *test for abnormal toxicity*, Appendix XIV L. Use 0.5 ml of a solution in *water for injections* containing 2 mg per ml.

Depressor substances Complies with the *test for depressor substances*, Appendix XIV M. Use per kg of the cat's weight 1 ml of a solution containing 4 mg per ml.

Pyrogens Complies with the *test for pyrogens*, Appendix XIV K. Use per kg of the rabbit's weight 1 ml of a solution in *water for injections* containing 10 mg per ml.

Sterility Complies with the *test for sterility*, Appendix XVI A.

Kanamycin Sulphate ☆

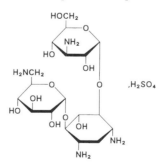

$C_{18}H_{36}N_4O_{11},H_2SO_4,H_2O$ 601   *25389-94-0 (anhydrous)*

Kanamycin Sulphate is the monohydrate of 6-*O*-(3-amino-3-deoxy-α-D-glucopyranosyl)-4-*O*-(6-amino-6-deoxy-α-D-glucopyranosyl)-2-deoxy-streptamine sulphate, an antimicrobial substance produced by the growth of certain strains of *Streptomyces kanamyceticus*. The potency is not less than 750 Units per mg, calculated with reference to the dried substance.

Characteristics A white or almost white, crystalline powder; odourless or almost odourless.

Solubility Soluble in 8 parts of *water*; practically insoluble in *ethanol (96%)*, in *acetone*, in *chloroform* and in *ether*.

Identification A. Carry out the method for *thin-layer chromatography*, Appendix III A, using a chromatoplate coated with a 0.75-mm layer of the following mixture. Mix 0.3 g of *carbomer* (Carbopol 934 is suitable) with 240 ml of *water* and allow to stand, with moderate shaking, for 1 hour; adjust to pH 7 by the gradual addition, with continuous shaking, of 2M *sodium hydroxide* and add 30 g of *silica gel H*. Heat the plate at 110° for 1 hour, allow to cool and use immediately. Use a 7% w/v solution of *potassium dihydrogen orthophosphate* as the mobile phase and allow the solvent front to ascend 12 cm above the line of application. Apply separately to the plate 10 μl of each of three solutions in *water* containing (1) 0.1% w/v of the substance being examined, (2) 0.1% w/v of *kanamycin monosulphate EPCRS* and (3) 0.1% w/v each of *kanamycin monosulphate EPCRS*, *neomycin sulphate EPCRS* and *streptomycin sulphate EPCRS*. After removal of the plate, dry it in a current of warm air, spray with a mixture of equal volumes of a 0.2% w/v solution of *naphthalene-1,3-diol* in *ethanol (96%)* and a 46% w/v solution of *sulphuric acid* and heat at 150° for 5 to 10 minutes. The principal spot in the chromatogram obtained with solution (1) is similar in position, colour and size to that in the chromatogram obtained with solution (2). The test is not valid unless the chromatogram obtained with solution (3) shows three clearly separated principal spots.

B. Dissolve 0.5 g in 10 ml of *water*, add 10 ml of a 1% w/v solution of *2,4,6-trinitrophenol*, if necessary initiate crystallisation by scratching the wall of the container with a glass rod, allow to stand and filter. The *melting point* of the crystals, after washing with 20 ml of *water* and drying at 100°, is about 235°, with decomposition, Appendix V A, Method I.

C. Dissolve 50 mg in 2 ml of *water*, add 1 ml of a 1% w/v solution of *ninhydrin* and heat for a few minutes on a water-bath. A violet colour is produced.

D. Yields the *reactions* characteristic of sulphates, Appendix VI.

Acidity or alkalinity pH of a 1% w/v solution, 6.5 to 8.5, Appendix V L.

Specific optical rotation In a 1% w/v solution in *carbon dioxide-free water*, +112° to +123°, Appendix V F.

Kanamycin B Carry out the method for *thin-layer chromatography*, Appendix III A, using a chromatoplate prepared immediately before use as described under test A for Identification. Use a 7% w/v solution of *potassium dihydrogen orthophosphate* as the mobile phase and allow the solvent front to ascend 12 cm above the line of application. Apply separately to the plate 4 μl of each of two solutions in *water* containing (1) 0.50% w/v of the substance being examined and (2) 0.020% w/v of *kanamycin B sulphate EPCRS*. After removal of the plate, dry it in a current of warm air, spray with *ninhydrin and stannous chloride reagent* and heat at 110° for 15 minutes. Any spot corresponding to kanamycin B in the chromatogram obtained with solution (1) is not more intense than the spot in the chromatogram obtained with solution (2).

Sulphate 15.0 to 17.0% of SO$_4$, calculated with reference to the dried substance, when determined by the following method. Dissolve 0.25 g in 100 ml of *water* and adjust the pH of the solution to 11 using 13.5M *ammonia*. Add 10 ml of 0.1M *barium chloride VS* and 0.5 mg of *metalphthalein* and titrate with 0.1M *disodium edetate VS*; when the colour of the solution begins to change, add 50 ml of *ethanol (96%)* and continue the titration until the violet-blue colour disappears. Each ml of 0.1M *barium chloride VS* is equivalent to 0.009606 g of SO$_4$.

Loss on drying When dried at 60° at a pressure not exceeding 0.7 kPa for 3 hours, loses not more than 1.5% of its weight. Use 1 g.

Sulphated ash Not more than 0.5%, Appendix IX A, Method II. Use 1 g.

Assay Carry out the *biological assay of antibiotics*, Appendix XIV A. The precision of the assay is such that the fiducial limits of error are not less than 95% and not more than 105% of the estimated potency.

Storage Kanamycin Sulphate should be kept in a well-closed container. If the contents are intended for use in the manufacture of a parenteral dosage form, the container should be sterile and sealed so as to exclude micro-organisms.

Labelling The label states (1) the number of Units per mg; (2) the date after which the material is not intended to be used; (3) the conditions under which it should be stored; (4) whether or not the material is intended for use in the manufacture of a parenteral dosage form.

Preparation
Kanamycin Injection

Action and use Antibacterial.

Kanamycin Sulphate intended for use in the manufacture of a parenteral dosage form complies with the following additional requirements.

Abnormal toxicity Complies with the *test for abnormal toxicity*, Appendix XIV L, using 0.5 ml of a solution in *water for injections* containing 2 mg per ml.

Depressor substances Complies with the *test for depressor substances*, Appendix XIV M. Use per kg of the cat's weight 1 ml of a solution containing 4 mg per ml.

Pyrogens Complies with the *test for pyrogens*, Appendix XIV K. Use per kg of the rabbit's weight 1 ml of a solution in *water for injections* containing 10 mg per ml.

Sterility Complies with the *test for sterility*, Appendix XVI A.

The title of the monograph in the European Pharmacopœia is Kanamycin Monosulphate.

Heavy Kaolin ☆

Heavy Kaolin★ is a purified, natural, hydrated aluminium silicate of variable composition.

Characteristics A fine, white or greyish-white powder; unctuous.

Solubility Practically insoluble in *water* and in organic solvents.

Identification A. To 0.5 g in a metal crucible add 1 g of *potassium nitrate* and 3 g of *anhydrous sodium carbonate*, heat until the mixture has melted and cool. To the residue add 20 ml of boiling *water*, mix, filter, wash the residue with 50 ml of *water* and discard the filtrate and washings. To the residue add 1 ml of *hydrochloric acid* and 5 ml of *water* and filter. To the filtrate add 3 ml of 2M *ammonium chloride*. A gelatinous, white precipitate is produced.
B. To 100 ml of a 1% w/v solution of *sodium dodecyl sulphate* in a graduated cylinder add 2.0 g in 0.1-g portions at intervals of 2 minutes, allowing each portion to settle before adding the next, and allow to stand for 2 hours. The apparent volume of the sediment is not greater than 5 ml.
C. 0.25 g yields the *reaction* characteristic of silicates, Appendix VI.

Acidity or alkalinity To 1 g add 20 ml of *carbon dioxide-free water*, shake for 2 minutes and filter. To 10 ml of the filtrate add 0.1 ml of *dilute phenolphthalein solution*. The solution is colourless and not more than 0.25 ml of 0.01M *sodium hydroxide VS* is required to change the colour of the solution.

Calcium Shake 4.0 g with a mixture of 34 ml of *distilled water* and 6 ml of 5.4M *acetic acid* for 1 minute and filter (solution A). 4 ml of solution A diluted to 15 ml with *distilled water* complies with the *limit test for calcium*, Appendix VII (250 ppm).

Heavy metals Boil 5.0 g with a mixture of 7.5 ml of 2M *hydrochloric acid* and 27.5 ml of *water* for 5 minutes, filter, wash the residue with *water* and dilute the combined filtrate and washings to 50 ml with *water* (solution B). To 5 ml of solution B add 5 ml of *water*, 10 ml of *hydrochloric acid* and 25 ml of *4-methylpentan-2-one*, shake for 2 minutes, allow the layers to separate and evaporate the aqueous layer to dryness on a water-bath. Dissolve the residue in 1 ml of 5.4M *acetic acid*, dilute to 25 ml with *water* and filter. 12 ml of the filtrate complies with *limit test A for heavy metals*, Appendix VII (50 ppm). Use *lead standard solution (1 ppm Pb)* to prepare the standard.

Chloride 2 ml of solution A diluted to 15 ml with *water* complies with the *limit test for chlorides*, Appendix VII (250 ppm).

Sulphate 1.5 ml of solution A diluted to 15 ml with *water* complies with the *limit test for sulphates*, Appendix VII (0.1%).

Acid-soluble substances To 10 ml of solution B add 1.5 ml of 1M *sulphuric acid*, evaporate to dryness on a water-bath, ignite and weigh. The residue weighs not more than 10 mg (1%).

Readily carbonisable substances Heat 0.3 g to redness in a calcination tube. The residue is only slightly more coloured than the original substance.

Adsorption power In a glass-stoppered test-tube shake 1.0 g with 10 ml of a 0.37% w/v solution of *methylene blue* for 2 minutes and allow to settle. Centrifuge and dilute 1 ml of the solution to 100 ml with *water*. The solution is not more intensely coloured than a 0.0030% w/v solution of *methylene blue*.

Swelling power Triturate 2 g with 2 ml of *water*. The mixture does not flow.

Labelling The label states whether or not the material is intended for internal use.

Preparation
Kaolin Poultice

When Kaolin is prescribed or demanded, Light Kaolin shall be dispensed or supplied, unless it is ascertained that Light Kaolin (Natural) is required.

Heavy Kaolin intended for internal use complies with the requirements stated above with the following modification.
Heavy metals Boil 5.0 g with a mixture of 7.5 ml of 2M *hydrochloric acid* and 27.5 ml of *water* for 5 minutes, filter, wash the residue with *water* and dilute the combined filtrate and washings to 50 ml with *water* (solution B). To 10 ml of solution B add 10 ml of *water*, 20 ml of *hydrochloric acid* and 25 ml of *4-methylpentan-2-one*, shake for 2 minutes, allow the layers to separate and evaporate the aqueous layer to dryness on a water-bath. Dissolve the residue in 1 ml of 5.4M *acetic acid*, dilute to 25 ml with *water* and filter. 12 ml of the filtrate complies with *limit test A for heavy metals*, Appendix VII (25 ppm). Use *lead standard solution (1 ppm Pb)* to prepare the standard.

*In certain states party to the Convention on the Elaboration of a European Pharmacopœia, Heavy Kaolin may be required to comply with a limit for total viable aerobic count of 10^2 micro-organisms per gram, determined by plate count, Appendix XVI B2.

Light Kaolin

Light Kaolin is a native hydrated aluminium silicate, freed from most of its impurities by elutriation and dried. It contains a suitable dispersing agent.

Characteristics A light, white powder free from gritty particles; odourless or almost odourless; unctuous.

Solubility Practically insoluble in *water* and in mineral acids.

Identification A. Fuse 1 g with 2 g of *anhydrous sodium carbonate*, warm the residue with 10 ml of *water*, filter, wash the filter with 5 ml of *water* and reserve the residue. To the combined filtrate and washings add 3 ml of *hydrochloric acid*. A gelatinous precipitate is produced.
B. Dissolve the residue reserved in test A in 10 ml of 2M *hydrochloric acid*. The solution yields *reaction B* characteristic of aluminium salts, Appendix VI.
C. Triturate 2 g with 2 ml of *water*. The resulting mixture flows.

Coarse particles Transfer 5 g to a stoppered cylinder (about 16 cm × 35 mm), add 60 ml of a 1% w/v solution of *sodium pyrophosphate*, shake thoroughly and allow to stand for 5 minutes. Using a pipette, withdraw 50 ml from a point about 5 cm below the surface of the liquid. To the remaining liquid add 50 ml of *water*, shake, allow to stand for 5 minutes and withdraw 50 ml in the same manner as before. Repeat the operation until a total of 400 ml of suspension has been withdrawn under the prescribed conditions. Transfer the remainder to an evaporating dish and evaporate to dryness on a water-bath. The residue, after drying at 105°, weighs not more than 25 mg.

Fine particles Disperse 5 g in 250 ml of *water* by shaking vigorously for 2 minutes in a stoppered flask, pour immediately into a glass cylinder 5 cm in diameter and transfer 20 ml to a glass dish using a pipette. Evaporate to dryness and dry to constant weight at 105°. Allow the remainder of the suspension to stand for 4 hours at 20° and withdraw a second 20-ml portion using a pipette with its tip exactly 5 cm below the surface and without disturbing the sediment. Transfer the second portion to a glass dish, evaporate to dryness and dry to constant weight at 105°. The weight of the residue from the second portion is not less than 70% of the weight of the residue from the first portion.

Arsenic 0.50 g dispersed in 25 ml of *water* complies with the *limit test for arsenic*, Appendix VII (2 ppm).

Heavy metals Heat 6.0 g for 15 minutes under a reflux condenser on a water-bath with a mixture of 70 ml of *water* and 10 ml of *hydrochloric acid* and filter. To 40 ml of the filtrate add 0.5 ml of *nitric acid* and evaporate to low bulk. Add 20 ml of *water*, 2 g of *ammonium chloride* and 2 g of *ammonium thiocyanate* and extract with two 10-ml quantities of a mixture of equal volumes of *amyl alcohol* and *ether*. To the aqueous layer add 2 g of *citric acid* and sufficient *water* to produce 60 ml. 12 ml of the resulting solution complies with *limit test A for heavy metals*, Appendix VII (20 ppm). Use *lead standard solution (1 ppm Pb)* to prepare the standard.

Chloride Boil 1.0 g with 80 ml of *water* and 20 ml of 2M *nitric acid* under a reflux condenser for 5 minutes, cool and filter. 15 ml of the filtrate complies with the *limit test for chlorides*, Appendix VII (330 ppm).

Loss on drying When dried to constant weight at 105°, loses not more than 1.5% of its weight. Use 1 g.

Loss on ignition When ignited at red heat, loses not more than 15.0% of its weight.

Soluble matter Boil 2 g with 100 ml of 0.2M *hydrochloric acid* under a reflux condenser for 5 minutes, cool, filter and evaporate 50 ml of the filtrate to dryness. The residue, after ignition at about 600° for 30 minutes, weighs not more than 10 mg.

Preparations
Kaolin Mixture
Kaolin and Morphine Mixture

Action and use Antidiarrhoeal.

When Kaolin or Light Kaolin is prescribed or demanded, Light Kaolin shall be dispensed or supplied unless it is ascertained that Light Kaolin (Natural) is required.

Light Kaolin (Natural)

Light Kaolin (Natural) is a native hydrated aluminium silicate, freed from most of its impurities by elutriation and dried. It does not contain a dispersing agent.

Characteristics A light, white powder free from gritty particles; odourless or almost odourless; unctuous.

Solubility Practically insoluble in *water* and in mineral acids.

Identification A. Fuse 1 g with 2 g of *anhydrous sodium carbonate*, warm the residue with 10 ml of *water*, filter, wash the filter with 5 ml of *water* and reserve the residue. To the combined filtrate and washings add 3 ml of *hydrochloric acid*. A gelatinous precipitate is produced.
B. Dissolve the residue reserved in test A in 10 ml of 2M *hydrochloric acid*. The solution yields *reaction B* characteristic of aluminium salts, Appendix VI.

C. Triturate 2 g with 2 ml of *water*. The resulting mixture does not flow.

Coarse particles; Arsenic; Heavy metals; Chloride; Loss on drying; Loss on ignition; Soluble matter Complies with the requirements stated under Light Kaolin.

Fine particles Disperse 5 g in 250 ml of *water* containing 50 mg of *sodium pyrophosphate* by shaking vigorously for 2 minutes in a stoppered flask, pour immediately into a glass cylinder 5 cm in diameter and transfer 20 ml to a glass dish using a pipette. Evaporate to dryness and dry to constant weight at 105°. Allow the remainder of the suspension to stand for 4 hours at 20° and withdraw a second 20-ml portion using a pipette with its tip exactly 5 cm below the surface and without disturbing the sediment. Transfer the second portion to a glass dish, evaporate to dryness and dry to constant weight at 105°. The weight of the residue from the second portion is not less than 70% of the weight of the residue from the first portion.

Preparations
Kaolin Mixture
Kaolin and Morphine Mixture

Action and use Antidiarrhoeal.

When Kaolin or Light Kaolin is prescribed or demanded, Light Kaolin shall be dispensed or supplied unless it is ascertained that Light Kaolin (Natural) is required.

Ketoprofen

$C_{16}H_{14}O_3$ 254.3   *22071-15-4*

Ketoprofen is 2-(3-benzoylphenyl)propionic acid. It contains not less than 98.5 per cent and not more than 100.5 per cent of $C_{16}H_{14}O_3$, calculated with reference to the dried substance.

Characteristics A white or almost white, crystalline powder; odourless or almost odourless.

Solubility Practically insoluble in *water*; freely soluble in *ethanol (96%)*, in *chloroform* and in *ether*.

Identification A. The *infra-red absorption spectrum*, Appendix II A, is concordant with the *reference spectrum* of ketoprofen.
B. The *light absorption*, Appendix II B, in the range 230 to 350 nm of a 0.002% w/v solution in *methanol (75%)* exhibits a maximum only at 258 nm. The *absorbance* at the maximum at 258 nm is about 1.3.

Melting point 93° to 96°, Appendix V A.

Related substances Carry out the method for *thin-layer chromatography*, Appendix III A, using *silica gel GF254* as the coating substance and a mixture of 70 volumes of *toluene*, 30 volumes of *di-isopropyl ether* and 1 volume of *formic acid* as the mobile phase. Apply separately and rapidly to the chromatoplate 5 µl of each of three solutions of the substance being examined in *acetone* containing (1) 10.0% w/v, (2) 0.050% w/v and (3) 0.020% w/v and develop the chromatograms within 10 minutes of applying the first spot. After removal of the plate, allow it to dry in air and examine under *ultra-violet light (254 nm)*. Any *secondary spot* in the chromatogram obtained with solution (1) is not more intense than the spot in the chromatogram obtained with solution (2) and not more than three such spots are more intense than the spot in the chromatogram obtained with solution (3).

Loss on drying When dried to constant weight at 60° at a pressure not exceeding 0.7 kPa, loses not more than 0.5% of its weight. Use 1 g.

Sulphated ash Not more than 0.1%, Appendix IX A.

Assay Dissolve 0.5 g in 25 ml of *ethanol (96%)* previously neutralised to *phenolphthalein solution*, add 25 ml of *water* and titrate with 0.1M *sodium hydroxide VS* using *phenolphthalein solution* as indicator. Each ml of 0.1M *sodium hydroxide VS* is equivalent to 0.02543 g of $C_{16}H_{14}O_3$.

Preparation
Ketoprofen Capsules

Action and use Anti-inflammatory; analgesic.

Labetalol Hydrochloride

$C_{19}H_{24}N_2O_3,HCl$ 364.9   *32780-64-6*

Labetalol Hydrochloride is *all-rac*-2-hydroxy-5-[1-hydroxy-2-(1-methyl-3-phenylpropylamino)-ethyl]benzamide hydrochloride. It contains not less than 98.5 per cent and not more than 101.0 per cent of $C_{19}H_{24}N_2O_3,HCl$, calculated with reference to the dried substance.

Characteristics A white or almost white powder or granules.

Solubility Soluble in 60 parts of *water* and in 60 parts of *ethanol (96%)*; practically insoluble in *chloroform* and in *ether*.

Identification A. The *infra-red absorption spectrum*, Appendix II A, is concordant with the *reference spectrum* of labetalol hydrochloride.
B. The *light absorption*, Appendix II B, in the range 230 to 350 nm of a 0.01% w/v solution in 0.1M *hydrochloric acid* exhibits a maximum only at 302 nm. The *absorbance* at 302 nm is about 0.86.
C. Dissolve 10 mg in 5 ml of *water* and add 1 ml of *iron(III) chloride test-solution*. A purple colour is produced.
D. Yields the *reactions* characteristic of chlorides, Appendix VI.

Acidity pH of a 1% w/v solution, 4.0 to 5.0, Appendix V L.

Clarity and colour of solution A 1.0% w/v solution is *clear*, Appendix IV A, and not more intensely coloured than *reference solution Y_6*, Appendix IV B, Method II.

Heavy metals 2.0 g complies with *limit test C for heavy metals*, Appendix VII (20 ppm). Use 2 ml of *lead standard solution (20 ppm Pb)* to prepare the standard.

Racemate ratio Carry out the method for *gas chromatography*, Appendix III B, using a solution prepared in the following manner. Dissolve 2 mg of the substance

being examined in 1 ml of a 1.2% w/v solution of *1-butane-boronic acid* in *anhydrous pyridine* and allow to stand for 20 minutes.

The chromatographic procedure may be carried out using a glass column (1.5 m × 4 mm) packed with *acid-washed, silanised diatomaceous support* (100 to 120 mesh) coated with 3% w/w of phenyl methyl silicone fluid (50% phenyl) (OV-17 is suitable) and maintained at 295°.

Two peaks due to the two racemates appear in the chromatogram. Adjust the sensitivity of the instrument so that in the chromatogram obtained, the height of the taller of the racemate peaks is about 80% of full-scale deflection. The area of each peak is not less than 45% and not more than 55% of the sum of the areas of the two peaks. The test is not valid unless the height of the trough separating the racemate peaks is less than 5% of full-scale deflection.

Related substances Carry out the method for *thin-layer chromatography*, Appendix III A, using *silica gel GF254* as the coating substance and a mixture of 75 volumes of *dichloromethane*, 25 volumes of *methanol* and 5 volumes of 13.5M *ammonia* as the mobile phase. Apply separately to the chromatoplate 5 µl of each of three solutions of the substance being examined in *methanol* containing (1) 8.0% w/v, (2) 0.080% w/v and (3) 0.040% w/v. After removal of the plate, dry it in a stream of warm air, heat at 105° for 30 minutes, cool and examine under *ultra-violet light (254 nm)*. Any *secondary spot* in the chromatogram obtained with solution (1) is not more intense than the spot in the chromatogram obtained with solution (2) and not more than one such spot is more intense than the spot in the chromatogram obtained with solution (3).

Loss on drying When dried to constant weight at 100° at a pressure not exceeding 0.7 kPa, loses not more than 1.0% of its weight. Use 1 g.

Sulphated ash Not more than 0.1%, Appendix IX A.

Assay Carry out Method I for *non-aqueous titration*, Appendix VIII A, using 1 g, 20 ml of *mercury(II) acetate solution* and *oracet blue B solution* as indicator. Each ml of 0.1M *perchloric acid VS* is equivalent to 0.03649 g of $C_{19}H_{24}N_2O_3,HCl$.

Storage Labetalol Hydrochloride should be kept in a well-closed container.

Preparations
Labetalol Injection
Labetalol Tablets

Action and use Combined alpha- and beta-adrenoceptor antagonist.

Lactic Acid ☆

$C_3H_6O_3$ 90.08   *50-21-5*

Lactic Acid★ consists of a mixture of 2-hydroxy-propionic acid, its condensation products, such as lactoyl-lactic acid and other polylactic acids, and water. The equilibrium between lactic acid and polylactic acids depends on concentration and temperature.

Lactic Acid is usually in the form of the racemate ((RS)-lactic acid), but in some cases the (+)-(S)-isomer is predominant. Lactic Acid contains the equivalent of not less than 88.0 per cent w/w and not more than 92.0 per cent w/w of $C_3H_6O_3$.

Characteristics A colourless or slightly yellow, viscous liquid.

Solubility Miscible with *water*, with *ethanol (96%)* and with *ether*.

Identification A. Yields *reactions A* and *B* characteristic of lactates, Appendix VI.
B. *Relative density*, 1.20 to 1.21, Appendix V G.
C. A 10% w/v solution is strongly acidic.

Colour Not more intensely coloured than *reference solution* Y_6, Appendix IV B, Method II.

Calcium Dissolve 5.0 g in 42 ml of 1M *sodium hydroxide* and dilute to 50 ml with *distilled water* (solution A). 5 ml of solution A diluted to 15 ml with *distilled water* complies with the *limit test for calcium*, Appendix VII (200 ppm).

Heavy metals 12 ml of solution A complies with *limit test A for heavy metals*, Appendix VII (10 ppm). Use *lead standard solution (1 ppm Pb)* to prepare the standard.

Sulphate 7.5 ml of solution A diluted to 15 ml with *distilled water* complies with the *limit test for sulphates*, Appendix VII (200 ppm).

Citric, oxalic and phosphoric acids To 5 ml of solution A add 6M *ammonia* until slightly alkaline. Add 1 ml of 0.5M *calcium chloride* and heat on a water-bath for 5 minutes. Both before and after heating, any opalescence in the solution is not more intense than that in a mixture of 5 ml of solution A and 1 ml of *water*.

Ether-insoluble substances Dissolve 1.0 g in 25 ml of *ether*. The solution is not more opalescent than 25 ml of *ether*.

Methanol and methyl esters Place 2.0 g in a round-bottomed flask and add 10 ml of *water*. Cool in ice, add cautiously 30 ml of a 30% w/v solution of *potassium hydroxide* and cool in ice for a further 10 to 15 minutes. Steam distil the mixture into a 10-ml graduated cylinder containing 1 ml of *ethanol (96%)*, collecting a volume of at least 9.5 ml and dilute to 10.0 ml with *water*. To 1.0 ml of the distillate add 5 ml of *potassium permanganate—orthophosphoric acid reagent* and mix. After 15 minutes add 2 ml of *oxalic acid—sulphuric acid reagent*, stir with a glass rod until the solution is colourless and then add 5 ml of *decolorised magenta solution*. After 2 hours any colour in the solution is not more intense than that of a solution obtained by treating 1 ml of a reference solution containing 0.1 mg of *methanol* and 0.1 ml of *absolute ethanol* at the same time and in the same manner beginning at the words 'add 5 ml of *potassium permanganate—orthophosphoric acid reagent . . .*' (500 ppm of methanol).

Reducing substances Acidify 1 ml of solution A with 1 ml of 1M *hydrochloric acid*, heat to boiling, allow to cool, add 1.5 ml of 1M *sodium hydroxide* and 2 ml of *potassium cupri-tartrate solution* and heat to boiling again. No red or green precipitate is produced.

Volatile fatty acids Cautiously heat 5 g in a glass-stoppered flask at 50° for 10 minutes. No unpleasant odour resembling that of the lower fatty acids is detectable immediately after opening the flask.

Sulphated ash Not more than 0.1%, Appendix IX A, Method II. Use 1 g.

Assay To 1 g add 10 ml of *water* and 20 ml of 1M *sodium hydroxide VS*, stopper the flask and allow to stand for 30 minutes. Add 0.5 ml of *dilute phenolphthalein solution* and titrate with 1M *hydrochloric acid VS*. Each ml of 1M *sodium hydroxide VS* is equivalent to 0.0901 g of $C_3H_6O_3$.

Storage Lactic Acid should be kept in a well-closed container.

Preparations
Sodium Lactate Intravenous Infusion
Compound Sodium Lactate Intravenous Infusion
Lactic Acid Pessaries

*In certain states party to the convention on the Elaboration of a European Pharmacopœia, Lactic Acid intended for use in large-volume preparations for parenteral use may be required to comply with the *test for pyrogens*, Appendix XIV K, using per kg of the rabbit's weight 10 ml of a solution prepared in the following manner. To a quantity containing the equivalent of 3.46 g of $C_3H_6O_3$ add 38.4 ml of 1M *sodium hydroxide*, prepared using *water for injections*, and 100 ml of *water for injections*, boil for 5 minutes, cool and dilute to 250 ml with the same solvent.

Lactose ☆

$C_{12}H_{22}O_{11},H_2O$ 360.3   *10039-26-6*

Lactose* is *O*-β-D-galactopyranosyl-(1→4)-α-D-glucopyranose monohydrate.

Characteristics A white or almost white, crystalline powder; odourless.

Solubility Slowly soluble in 6 parts of *water*; practically insoluble in *ethanol (96%)*.

Identification A. Carry out the method for *thin-layer chromatography*, Appendix III A, using *silica gel G* as the coating substance and a mixture of 50 volumes of *1,2-dichloroethane*, 25 volumes of *anhydrous glacial acetic acid*, 15 volumes of *methanol* and 10 volumes of *water*, measured accurately, as the mobile phase. Apply separately to the chromatoplate 2 μl of each of three solutions in *methanol (60%)* containing (1) 0.05% w/v of the substance being examined, (2) 0.05% w/v of *lactose EPCRS* and (3) 0.05% w/v each of *fructose EPCRS*, *glucose EPCRS*, *lactose EPCRS* and *sucrose EPCRS*. Dry the points of application thoroughly before developing the chromatogram. After removal of the plate, dry it in a current of warm air and repeat the development after renewing the mobile phase. After removal of the plate, dry it in a current of warm air, spray with a 0.5% w/v solution of *thymol* in *ethanolic sulphuric acid (5%)* and heat at 130° for 10 minutes. The principal spot in the chromatogram obtained with solution (1) is similar in position, colour and size to the spot in the chromatogram obtained with solution (2). The test is not valid unless the chromatogram obtained with solution (3) shows four clearly separated principal spots.

B. To 10 ml of a 1% w/v solution add 3 ml of *potassium cupri-tartrate solution* and heat. A red precipitate is produced.

C. Heat 5 ml of a 5% w/v solution with 5 ml of 9M *ammonia* on a water-bath at 80° for 10 minutes. A red colour is produced.

Acidity or alkalinity Dissolve 6 g in 25 ml of *carbon dioxide-free water* by boiling, cool and add 0.3 ml of *dilute phenolphthalein solution*. The solution is colourless and not more than 0.4 ml of 0.1M *sodium hydroxide VS* is required to change the colour of the solution to pink.

Clarity, colour and odour of solution Dissolve 1.0 g in *water* by heating to 50°, dilute to 10 ml with *water* and allow to cool. The solution is *clear*, Appendix IV A, not more intensely coloured than *reference solution BY₇*, Appendix IV B, Method II, and odourless.

Specific optical rotation Dissolve 10 g in 80 ml of *water* by heating to 50° and allow to cool. Add 0.2 ml of 6M *ammonia*, allow to stand for 30 minutes and dilute to 100 ml with *water*. The *specific optical rotation* in the resulting solution is +54.4° to +55.9°, Appendix V F.

Lead Complies with *limit test A for lead in sugars*, Appendix VII (0.5 ppm). Use a solution prepared by dissolving 20.0 g in sufficient 1M *acetic acid* to produce 200 ml.

Proteins and light-absorbing impurities Measure the *light absorption* of a 1% w/v solution, Appendix II B, in the range 210 to 300 nm. The *absorbance* is not more than 0.25 in the range 210 to 220 nm and is not more than 0.07 in the range 270 to 300 nm.

Sulphated ash Not more than 0.1% w/w when determined in the following manner. To 1.0 g add 1 ml of *sulphuric acid*, evaporate to dryness on a water-bath and ignite to constant weight.

Water 4.5 to 5.5%, Appendix IX C. Use 0.5 g.

Storage Lactose should be kept in a well-closed container.

*Lactose described in this monograph is not necessarily suitable for use in the manufacture of a parenteral preparation or for other special purposes.

In certain states party to the Convention on the Elaboration of a European Pharmacopœia, Lactose may be required to comply either with the test for *Escherichia coli*, Appendix XVI B1, or with a limit for total viable aerobic count of 10² micro-organisms per gram, determined by plate count, Appendix XVI B2, or with both of these tests.

Lactulose Solution

Lactulose Solution is an aqueous solution of lactulose (4-*O*-β-D-galactopyranosyl-D-fructose) and lesser amounts of other sugars including lactose, galactose, tagatose and epilactose. It contains not less than 62.0 per cent w/v and not more than 74.0 per cent w/v of lactulose, $C_{12}H_{22}O_{11}$. It may contain an antimicrobial preservative.

Characteristics A colourless to brownish-yellow, clear or not more than slightly opalescent solution.

Identification A. In the test for Related substances the principal spot in the chromatogram obtained with solution (1) corresponds to that in the chromatogram obtained with solution (2).

B. Heat 1.5 ml with 10 ml of *water* and 5 ml of *potassium cupri-tartrate solution*. A red precipitate is produced.

Clarity and colour of solution Dilute 1 volume of the solution with 2 volumes of *water*. The resulting solution is *clear*, Appendix IV A, and not more intensely coloured than *reference solution BY₄*, Appendix IV B, Method I.

Heavy metals 2.0 g complies with *limit test C for heavy metals*, Appendix VII (20 ppm). Use 4 ml of *lead standard solution (10 ppm)* to prepare the standard.

Sulphite Dissolve 5 g in 40 ml of *water*, add 2.0 ml of 0.1M *sodium hydroxide VS* and dilute to 100 ml with *water*. To 10 ml of the solution add 1 ml of 8.4M *hydrochloric acid*, 2 ml of *faded magenta solution* and 2 ml of a 0.5% v/v aqueous dilution of *formaldehyde solution*. Allow to stand for 30 minutes and measure the *absorbance* of the resulting solution at the maximum at 583 nm, Appendix II B, using in the reference cell a solution prepared by treating 10 ml of *water* in the same manner beginning at the words 'add 1 ml of 8.4M *hydrochloric acid* . . .'. The absorbance is not more than that of a solution prepared using 10 ml of *sulphite standard solution (1.5 ppm SO₂)* and beginning at the words 'add 1 ml of 8.4M *hydrochloric acid* . . .' (30 ppm).

Fructose Carry out the following procedures using enzymes and associated reagents suitable for the determination of fructose together with a suitable β-galactosidase (a combination of Boehringer Mannheim assay kit 139106 and β-galactosidase 150797 is suitable)*.

Dilute a quantity of the solution with *water* to obtain a solution containing 0.5% w/v of lactulose. Transfer 0.200 ml to a stoppered 1-cm cuvette, add 3.0 ml of triethanolamine buffer solution with co-enzymes (flask 1 in Boehringer Mannheim assay kit 139106 diluted with 80 ml of *water*), 20 μl of hexokinase and glucose-6-phosphate dehydrogenase reagent and mix. Allow to stand for 10 minutes and measure the *absorbance* of the resulting solution at the maximum at 340 nm, Appendix II B. Add 20 μl of phosphoglucose isomerase reagent, mix, allow to stand for 10 minutes and again measure the *absorbance* at 340 nm. The difference between the absorbances is less than that obtained by repeating the operation using a 0.0050% w/v solution of *D-fructose* in place of the diluted solution being examined.

Total sugars *Refractive index*, Appendix V E, not more than 1.475 (72.0% w/w).

Related substances Carry out the method for *thin-layer chromatography*, Appendix III A, using a silica gel precoated chromatoplate (Merck silica gel 60 plates are suitable) and a mixture of 55 volumes of *ethyl acetate*, 20 volumes of *methanol*, 15 volumes of a 5% w/v solution of *boric acid* and 10 volumes of *glacial acetic acid* as the mobile phase. Apply separately to the plate 2 μl of each of six solutions containing (1) 2.0% w/v of lactulose, prepared by dilution of the solution being examined with *water*, (2) 2.0% w/v of *lactulose BPCRS*, (3) 0.44% w/v of *D-galactose*, (4) 0.24% w/v of *lactose*, (5) 0.16% w/v of *lactose* and (6) 0.080% w/v of *D-tagatose*. After removal of the plate, dry it at 110° for 5 minutes, allow to cool and spray with a 0.1% w/v solution of *naphthalene-1,3-diol* in *ethanolic sulphuric acid (10%)*. Heat at 110° for 5 minutes. In the chromatogram obtained with solution (1) any spots corresponding to D-galactose, lactose and D-tagatose are not more intense than the spots in the chromatograms obtained with solutions (3), (4) and (6) respectively and any other *secondary spot* is not more intense than the spot in the chromatogram obtained with solution (5). Disregard any blue spot with an Rf value of about 0.6.

Sulphated ash Not more than 0.2%, Appendix IX A. Use 2.5 g.

Assay Carry out the following procedures using enzymes and associated reagents suitable for the determination of fructose, together with a suitable β-galactosidase (a combination of Boehringer Mannheim assay kit 139106 and β-galactosidase 150797 is suitable)*.

Dilute a weighed quantity of the solution with *water* to obtain a solution containing 0.5% w/v of lactulose and dilute 5 ml of the resulting solution to 100 ml with *phosphate buffer pH 7.3*. Transfer 0.2 ml to a stoppered 1-cm cuvette and add 30 μl of β-galactosidase reagent. Stopper the cuvette, mix and heat at 37° for 2 hours. Add 3.0 ml of triethanolamine buffer solution with co-enzymes (flask 1 in Boehringer Mannheim assay kit 139106, diluted with 80 ml of *water*), 20 μl of hexokinase and glucose-6-phosphate dehydrogenase reagent and mix. Allow to stand for 10 minutes and measure the *absorbance* of the resulting solution at the maximum at 340 nm, Appendix II B. Add 20 μl of phosphoglucose isomerase reagent mix, allow to stand for 10 minutes and again measure the *absorbance* at 340 nm. From the difference between the absorbances, calculate the content of $C_{12}H_{22}O_{11}$ by repeating the operation using a 0.5% w/v solution of *lactulose BPCRS* and beginning at the words 'dilute 5 ml of the resulting solution . . .'. Determine the *weight per ml*, Appendix V G, and calculate the percentage of $C_{12}H_{22}O_{11}$, weight in volume.

Storage Lactulose Solution should be stored at a temperature not exceeding 20°.

Action and use Osmotic laxative.

*If a combination of enzymes and reagents other than that referred to above is used, it may be necessary to modify the volumes and conditions stated.

Lanatoside C ☆

$C_{49}H_{76}O_{20}$ 985.1   *17575-22-3*

Lanatoside C is 3-[(*O*-β-D-glucopyranosyl-(1→4)-*O*-3-acetyl-2,6-dideoxy-β-D-*ribo*-hexopyranosyl-(1→4)-*O*-2,6-dideoxy-β-D-*ribo*-hexopyranosyl-(1→4)-*O*-2,6-dideoxy-β-D-*ribo*-hexopyranosyl)oxy]-12,14-dihydroxy-3β,5β,12β-card-20(22)-enolide. It contains not less than

97.0 per cent and not more than 103.0 per cent of $C_{49}H_{76}O_{20}$, calculated with reference to the dried substance.

Characteristics A white or slightly yellowish, crystalline or finely crystalline powder; hygroscopic. It loses water in an atmosphere of low relative density.

Solubility Practically insoluble in *water*, in *chloroform* and in *ether*; soluble in 20 parts of *methanol*.

Identification *Test A may be omitted if tests B, C and D are carried out. Tests B, C and D may be omitted if test A is carried out.*

A. The *infra-red absorption spectrum*, Appendix II A, is concordant with the spectrum of *lanatoside C EPCRS*. Examine the substances as dispersions prepared by dissolving 1 mg in 0.3 ml of *methanol* and triturating with 0.4 g of dry, finely powdered *potassium bromide IR* until the mixture is uniform and completely dry. When comparing the spectra special attention should be given to the presence of a distinct maximum at 1260 cm⁻¹ and to the intensity of the maximum at 1740 cm⁻¹.

B. In the test for Related substances, the principal band in the chromatogram obtained with solution (2) is similar in position, colour and size to that in the chromatogram obtained with solution (3).

C. Suspend 0.5 mg in 0.2 ml of *ethanol (60%)* and add 0.1 ml of a 2% w/v solution of *3,5-dinitrobenzoic acid* in *ethanol (96%)* and 0.1 ml of 1.25M *sodium hydroxide*. The suspension becomes violet.

D. Dissolve 5 mg in 5 ml of *glacial acetic acid*, add 0.05 ml of *iron(III) chloride test-solution*, add 2 ml of *sulphuric acid* so as to form a subjacent layer and allow to stand. A brown but not reddish ring is produced at the interface and a greenish-yellow colour, which changes to bluish-green, diffuses from it into the upper layer.

Clarity and colour of solution A 2.0% w/v solution in *methanol* is *clear*, Appendix IV A, and not more intensely coloured than *reference solutions Y_7 or BY_7*, Appendix IV B, Method II.

Specific optical rotation In a 2% w/v solution in *methanol*, +32.0° to +35.5°, Appendix V F.

Related substances Carry out the method for *thin-layer chromatography*, Appendix III A, using *silica gel G* as the coating substance and a mixture of 60 volumes of *toluene*, 30 volumes of *ethanol (96%)*, 20 volumes of *dichloromethane* and 1 volume of *water* as the mobile phase. Apply separately to the chromatoplate as 10-mm bands 5 μl of each of six solutions in *methanol* containing (1) 2.0% w/v of the substance being examined, (2) 0.2% w/v of the substance being examined, (3) 0.2% w/v of *lanatoside C EPCRS*, (4) 0.030% w/v of *lanatoside C EPCRS*, (5) 0.020% w/v of *lanatoside C EPCRS* and (6) 0.010% w/v of *lanatoside C EPCRS*. After development of the plate dry it in a current of cool air and carry out a second development in the same direction. After removal of the plate, dry it in a current of cool air for 5 minutes, spray with *ethanolic sulphuric acid (5%)* and heat at 140° for 15 minutes. Examine in daylight. In the chromatogram obtained with solution (1) any *secondary band* is not more intense than the band in the chromatogram obtained with solution (4), not more than three such bands are more intense than the band in the chromatogram obtained with solution (5) and not more than one of these bands is more intense than the band in the chromatogram obtained with solution (6).

Loss on drying When dried to constant weight over *phosphorus pentoxide* at 100° to 105° at a pressure of 1.5 to 2.5 kPa, loses not more than 7.5% of its weight. Use 0.5 g.

Sulphated ash Not more than 0.1%, Appendix IX A, Method II. Use the residue from the test for Loss on drying.

Assay Carry out the following procedure protected from light. Dissolve 50 mg in sufficient *ethanol (96%)* to produce 50 ml and dilute 5 ml to 100 ml with the same solvent. To 5 ml of this solution add 3 ml of *alkaline trinitrophenol solution* and allow to stand in a water-bath at 19° to 21° for 40 minutes. Measure the *absorbance* of the resulting solution at the maximum at 484 nm, Appendix II B, using in the reference cell a mixture of 5 ml of *ethanol (96%)* and 3 ml of *alkaline trinitrophenol solution* prepared at the same time. Calculate the content of $C_{49}H_{76}O_{20}$ from the *absorbance* obtained by simultaneously carrying out the operation using *lanatoside C EPCRS* in place of the substance being examined.

Storage Lanatoside C should be kept in an airtight, glass container, protected from light and stored at a temperature not exceeding 10°.

Action and use Cardiac glycoside.

Lemon Oil

Lemon Oil is obtained by expression from the outer part of the fresh pericarp of the ripe or nearly ripe fruit of *Citrus limon* (L.) Burm. f.

Characteristics A pale yellow or greenish-yellow liquid, visibly free from water; odour, that of lemon.

Optical rotation +57° to +65°, Appendix V F.

Refractive index 1.474 to 1.476, Appendix V E.

Solubility in ethanol Soluble with opalescence, at 20°, in 12 volumes of *ethanol (90%)*, Appendix X M. Miscible in all proportions with *absolute ethanol*.

Weight per ml 0.850 to 0.856 g, Appendix V G.

Residue on evaporation 2.0 to 3.0% when determined by the method for *residue on evaporation of volatile oils*, Appendix X M. Use 1 g and heat for 4 hours.

Content of aldehydes Not less than 3.5% w/w, calculated as citral, $C_{10}H_{16}O$. Carry out the method for the *determination of aldehydes*, Appendix X K, using 10 g, omitting the *toluene* and using a volume, not less than 7 ml, of *hydroxylamine solution in ethanol (60%)* that exceeds by 1 to 2 ml the volume of 0.5M *potassium hydroxide in ethanol (60%) VS* required. Each ml of 0.5M *potassium hydroxide in ethanol (60%) VS* is equivalent to 0.07673 g of $C_{10}H_{16}O$.

Storage Lemon Oil should be kept in a well-filled, well-closed container, protected from light and stored at a temperature not exceeding 25°.

Action and use Flavour.

Terpeneless Lemon Oil

Terpeneless Lemon Oil may be prepared by concentrating Lemon Oil under reduced pressure until most of the terpenes have been removed or by solvent partition.

Characteristics A clear, colourless or pale yellow liquid, visibly free from water; odour and taste, those of lemon.

Optical rotation −5° to +2°, Appendix V F.

Refractive index 1.475 to 1.485, Appendix V E.

Solubility in ethanol Soluble, at 20°, in 1 volume of *ethanol (80%)*, Appendix X M.

Weight per ml 0.880 to 0.895 g, Appendix V G.

Content of aldehydes Not less than 40% w/w, calculated as citral, $C_{10}H_{16}O$. Carry out the method for *determination of aldehydes*, Appendix X K, using 1 g, omitting the *toluene* and using a volume, not less than 7 ml, of *hydroxylamine solution in ethanol (60%)* that exceeds by 1 to 2 ml the volume of 0.5M *potassium hydroxide in ethanol (60%) VS* required. Each ml of 0.5M *potassium hydroxide in ethanol (60%) VS* is equivalent to 0.07673 g of $C_{10}H_{16}O$.

Storage Terpeneless Lemon Oil should be kept in a well-filled, well-closed container, protected from light and stored at a temperature not exceeding 25°.

Preparations
Lemon Spirit
Compound Orange Spirit

Action and use Flavour

Dried Lemon Peel

Dried Lemon Peel is the dried outer part of the pericarp of the ripe, or nearly ripe, fruit of *Citrus limon* (L.) Burm. f.

Characteristics Odour, aromatic; taste, aromatic and bitter.

Macroscopical In strips or pieces; outer surface yellow and somewhat rough from the presence of numerous minute pits, each corresponding to an oil gland; inner surface with only a small remnant of white, spongy pericarp. Fracture short.

Microscopical Epidermis of small polyhedral cells. Tissue subjacent to the epidermis parenchymatous, many of the cells containing prismatic crystals of calcium oxalate. Numerous large oil glands and small vascular strands embedded in the parenchyma.

Volatile oil Not less than 2.5% v/w, Appendix XI E. Use 20 g, crushed under *water*, and distil for 3 hours.

Levamisole Hydrochloride

C₁₁H₁₂N₂S,HCl   240.8   *16595-80-5*

Levamisole Hydrochloride is (S)-2,3,5,6-tetrahydro-6-phenylimidazo[2,1-*b*]thiazole hydrochloride. It contains not less than 98.5 per cent and not more than 101.0 per cent of C₁₁H₁₂N₂S,HCl, calculated with reference to the dried substance.

Characteristics A white to pale cream, crystalline powder; odourless or almost odourless.

Solubility Soluble in 2 parts of *water* and in 5 parts of *methanol*; practically insoluble in *ether*.

Identification A. Dissolve 0.5 g in 20 ml of *water* and add 6 ml of 1M *sodium hydroxide*. Extract with 20 ml of *dichloromethane*, discard the aqueous layer and wash the dichloromethane layer with 10 ml of *water*. Shake with *anhydrous sodium sulphate*, filter, evaporate the dichloromethane at room temperature and dry at a pressure of 2 kPa at a temperature not exceeding 40°. The *infra-red absorption spectrum* of the residue, Appendix II A, is concordant with the *reference spectrum* of levamisole.
B. *Melting point* of the residue obtained in test A, about 59°, Appendix V A.
C. A 5% w/v solution is laevorotatory and yields *reaction A* characteristic of chlorides, Appendix VI.

Light absorption *Absorbance* of a 0.1% w/v solution in 0.2M *methanolic hydrochloric acid* at 310 nm, not more than 0.20, Appendix II B.

Specific optical rotation In a freshly prepared, filtered 5% w/v solution, not less than −121.5°, Appendix V F.

2,3-Dihydro-6-phenylimidazo[2,1-*b*]thiazole hydrochloride Carry out the method for *thin-layer chromatography*, Appendix III A, using *silica gel G* as the coating substance and a mixture of 90 volumes of *toluene*, 16 volumes of *methanol* and 8 volumes of *glacial acetic acid* as the mobile phase. Apply separately to the chromatoplate 10 μl of each of two solutions in *methanol* containing (1) 5.0% w/v of the substance being examined and (2) 0.025% w/v of *2,3-dihydro-6-phenylimidazo[2,1-b]thiazole hydrochloride BPCRS*. After removal of the plate, allow it to dry in air and spray with *potassium iodoplatinate solution*. Any spot corresponding to 2,3-dihydro-6-phenylimidazo[2,1-*b*]thiazole hydrochloride in the chromatogram obtained with solution (1) is not more intense than the spot in the chromatogram obtained with solution (2).

Loss on drying When dried to constant weight at 105°, loses not more than 0.5% of its weight. Use 1 g.

Sulphated ash Not more than 0.1%, Appendix IX A.

Assay Carry out Method I for *non-aqueous titration*, Appendix VIII A, using 0.5 g and *1-naphtholbenzein solution* as indicator. Each ml of 0.1M *perchloric acid VS* is equivalent to 0.02408 g of C₁₁H₁₂N₂S,HCl.

Action and use Anthelmintic.

Levodopa ☆
L-Dopa

C₉H₁₁NO₄   197.2   *59-92-7*

Levodopa is 3-(3,4-dihydroxyphenyl)-L-alanine. It contains not less than 99.0 per cent and not more than 101.0 per cent of C₉H₁₁NO₄, calculated with reference to the dried substance.

Characteristics A white or slightly cream, crystalline powder; odourless.

Solubility Slightly soluble in *water*; practically insoluble in *ethanol* (96%), in *chloroform* and in *ether*; freely soluble in 1M *hydrochloric acid* but sparingly soluble in 0.1M *hydrochloric acid*.

Identification *Test A may be omitted if tests B, C and D are carried out. Tests B, C and D may be omitted if test A is carried out.*
A. The *infra-red absorption spectrum*, Appendix II A, is concordant with the spectrum of *levodopa EPCRS*.
B. Dissolve 2 mg in 2 ml of *water* and add 0.2 ml of 0.05M *iron(III) chloride hexahydrate*. A green colour is produced which changes to bluish-violet on the addition of 0.1 g of *hexamine*.
C. Dissolve 5 mg in a mixture of 5 ml of 1M *hydrochloric acid* and 5 ml of *water*. Add 0.1 ml of *sodium nitrite solution* containing 10% w/v of *ammonium molybdate*. A yellow colour is produced which changes to red on the addition of 10M *sodium hydroxide*.
D. Mix 5 mg with 1 ml of *water*, 1 ml of *pyridine* and 5 mg of *4-nitrobenzoyl chloride* and allow to stand for 3 minutes; a violet colour is produced which changes to pale yellow on boiling. Add, whilst shaking, 0.2 ml of 1M *sodium carbonate*; the violet colour reappears.

Acidity or alkalinity pH of a suspension prepared by shaking 0.1 g with 10 ml of *water* for 15 minutes, 4.5 to 7.0, Appendix V L.

Colour of solution A 4.0% w/v solution in 1M *hydrochloric acid* is not more intensely coloured than *reference solution BY₆*, Appendix IV B, Method II.

Light absorption Dissolve 30 mg in sufficient 0.1M *hydrochloric acid* to produce 100 ml and dilute 10 ml to 100 ml with 0.1M *hydrochloric acid*. The *light absorption* of the resulting solution, Appendix II B, in the range 230 to 350 nm exhibits a maximum only at 280 nm. The A(1%, 1 cm) at the maximum at 280 nm is 137 to 147.

Optical rotation −1.27° to −1.34°, Appendix V F, determined in a solution prepared in the following manner. Dissolve a quantity equivalent to 0.20 g of the dried substance and 5 g of *hexamine* in 10 ml of 1M *hydrochloric acid*, add sufficient 1M *hydrochloric acid* to produce 25 ml and allow to stand for 3 hours, protected from light.

Heavy metals 2.0 g complies with *limit test C for heavy metals*, Appendix VII (10 ppm). Use 2 ml of *lead standard solution (10 ppm Pb)* to prepare the standard.

Related substances Carry out the method for *thin-layer chromatography*, Appendix III A, using *cellulose* as the coating substance and a mixture of 50 volumes of *butan-*

1-ol, 25 volumes of *glacial acetic acid* and 25 volumes of *water* as the mobile phase. Apply separately to the chromatoplate, as bands 20 mm long, 10 μl of each of solutions (1) and (2) and 20 μl of solution (3), prepared immediately before use. Solution (1) contains 1.0% w/v of the substance being examined in a mixture of equal volumes of *anhydrous formic acid* and *methanol*. For solution (2) dilute 1 volume of solution (1) to 200 volumes with *methanol*. Solution (3) is a mixture of equal volumes of solution (1) and a solution prepared by dissolving 30 mg of *L-tyrosine* in 1 ml of *anhydrous formic acid* and diluting to 100 ml with *methanol*. After removal of the plate, allow it to dry in warm air, spray with a freshly prepared mixture of equal volumes of a 10% w/v solution of *iron(III) chloride hexahydrate* and a 5% w/v solution of *potassium hexacyanoferrate(III)* and examine the plate immediately. Any *secondary band* in the chromatogram obtained with solution (1) is not more intense than the band in the chromatogram obtained with solution (2). The test is not valid unless the chromatogram obtained with solution (3) shows a distinct band, at a higher Rf value than the principal band, which is more intense than the band in the chromatogram obtained with solution (2).

Loss on drying When dried to constant weight at 100° to 105°, loses not more than 1.0% of its weight. Use 0.5 g.

Sulphated ash Not more than 0.1%, Appendix IX A, Method II. Use 1 g.

Assay Dissolve 0.18 g, heating if necessary, in 5 ml of *anhydrous formic acid* and add 25 ml of *anhydrous glacial acetic acid* and 25 ml of *1,4-dioxan*. Carry out Method I for *non-aqueous titration*, Appendix VIII A, using 0.1 ml of *crystal violet solution* as indicator and titrating until a green colour is produced. Each ml of 0.1M *perchloric acid VS* is equivalent to 0.01972 g of $C_9H_{11}NO_4$.

Storage Levodopa should be kept in a well-closed container and protected from light.

Preparations
Levodopa Capsules
Levodopa Tablets
Levodopa and Carbidopa Tablets

Action and use Used in treatment of Parkinson's disease.

Levonorgestrel

$C_{21}H_{28}O_2$ 312.5   *797-63-7*

Levonorgestrel is (−)-13β-ethyl-17β-hydroxy-18,19-dinor-17α-pregn-4-en-20-yn-3-one. It contains not less than 98.0 per cent and not more than 101.0 per cent of $C_{21}H_{28}O_2$, calculated with reference to the dried substance.

Characteristics A white or almost white, crystalline powder; odourless or almost odourless.

Solubility Practically insoluble in *water*; slightly soluble in *ethanol (96%)*, in *acetone* and in *ether*; soluble in 45 parts of *chloroform*.

Identification A. The *infra-red absorption spectrum*, Appendix II A, is concordant with the *reference spectrum* of levonorgestrel.

B. The *light absorption*, Appendix II B, in the range 220 to 350 nm of a 0.001% w/v solution in *methanol* exhibits a maximum only at 240 nm. The *absorbance* at 240 nm is about 0.54.

C. Dissolve 2 mg in 0.3 ml of a 0.5% w/v solution of *1,3-dinitrobenzene* in *ethanol (96%)* and add 0.1 ml of *benzalkonium chloride solution*. Mix and add 2 ml of 5M *ammonia*. A pink colour is immediately produced.

D. *Melting point*, about 237°, Appendix V A.

Specific optical rotation In a 2% w/v solution in *chloroform*, −30° to −35°, Appendix V F.

Related substances Carry out the method for *thin-layer chromatography*, Appendix III A, using *silica gel G* as the coating substance and a mixture of 96 volumes of *chloroform* and 4 volumes of *absolute ethanol* as the mobile phase. Apply separately to the chromatoplate 5 μl of each of three solutions of the substance being examined in *chloroform* containing (1) 2.0% w/v, (2) 0.010% w/v and (3) 0.0040% w/v. After removal of the plate, allow it to dry in air and spray with *phosphomolybdic acid solution*. Any *secondary spot* in the chromatogram obtained with solution (1) is not more intense than the spot in the chromatogram obtained with solution (2) and not more than two such spots are more intense than the spot in the chromatogram obtained with solution (3).

Loss on drying When dried to constant weight at 105°, loses not more than 0.5% of its weight. Use 1 g.

Sulphated ash Not more than 0.1%, Appendix IX A.

Assay Dissolve 0.3 g in 40 ml of *tetrahydrofuran*, add 15 ml of a 10% w/v solution of *silver nitrate* and titrate with 0.1M *sodium hydroxide VS* determining the end-point potentiometrically. Repeat the operation without the substance being examined. The difference between the titrations represents the amount of sodium hydroxide required. Each ml of 0.1M *sodium hydroxide* is equivalent to 0.03125 g of $C_{21}H_{28}O_2$.

Storage Levonorgestrel should be kept in a well-closed container and stored at a temperature not exceeding 15°.

Action and use Progestogen.

Levorphanol Tartrate

$C_{17}H_{23}NO,C_4H_6O_6,2H_2O$ 443.5   *6700-40-9*

Levorphanol Tartrate is (−)-3-hydroxy-*N*-methylmorphinan hydrogen tartrate dihydrate. It contains not less than 98.5 per cent and not more than 101.0 per cent of $C_{17}H_{23}NO,C_4H_6O_6$, calculated with reference to the dried substance.

Characteristics A white, crystalline powder; odourless or almost odourless.

Solubility Soluble in 45 parts of *water* and in 50 parts of *ether*; slightly soluble in *ethanol* (96%).

Identification A. Dissolve 0.1 g in 5 ml of *water*, warming if necessary, and add 0.2M *ammonia* dropwise until no further precipitation occurs. Filter, wash the residue with 5 ml of *water* and dry at 60° at a pressure not exceeding 0.7 kPa for 1 hour. The *infra-red absorption spectrum* of the residue, Appendix II A, is concordant with the *reference spectrum* of levorphanol.

B. The *light absorption*, Appendix II B, in the range 230 to 350 nm of a 0.02% w/v solution exhibits a maximum only at 279 nm. The *absorbance* at 279 nm is about 0.92.

C. Yields *reaction B* characteristic of tartrates, Appendix VI.

D. *Melting point*, about 116°, Appendix V A.

Acidity pH of a 0.2% w/v solution, 3.4 to 4.0, Appendix V L.

Specific optical rotation of the base −73° to −77°, determined by measuring the *optical rotation*, Appendix V F, of the chloroform extract obtained in the Assay and calculating the *specific optical rotation* from the content of levorphanol, $C_{17}H_{23}NO$, indicated by the titration taking each ml of 0.05M *perchloric acid VS* as equivalent to 0.01287 g of $C_{17}H_{23}NO$.

Loss on drying When dried to constant weight at 105°, loses 7.0 to 9.0% of its weight. Use 1 g.

Sulphated ash Not more than 0.1%, Appendix IX A.

Assay Dissolve 1.4 g in 50 ml of hot *water*, add 10 ml of *sodium carbonate solution*, cool and extract with successive quantities of 25, 10 and 10 ml of *chloroform*. Wash each extract with the same two 10-ml quantities of *water*, filter into a dry flask and dilute the combined extracts, which must be clear and free from droplets of water, to 50 ml with *chloroform*. To 10 ml add 10 ml of *anhydrous glacial acetic acid* and carry out the method for *non-aqueous titration*, Appendix VIII A, using 0.05M *perchloric acid VS* and 0.15 ml of *oracet blue B solution* as indicator. Each ml of 0.05M *perchloric acid VS* is equivalent to 0.02037 g of $C_{17}H_{23}NO,C_4H_6O_6$.

Storage Levorphanol Tartrate should be kept in a well-closed container.

Preparations
Levorphanol Injection
Levorphanol Tablets

Action and use Narcotic analgesic.

Lignocaine Hydrochloride ☆

$C_{14}H_{22}N_2O,HCl,H_2O$ 288.8   *6108-05-0*

Lignocaine Hydrochloride is 2-diethylamino-aceto-2′,6′-xylidide hydrochloride monohydrate. It contains not less than 99.0 per cent and not more than 101.0 per cent of $C_{14}H_{22}N_2O,HCl$, calculated with reference to the anhydrous substance.

Characteristics A white, crystalline powder; odourless or almost odourless.

Solubility Soluble in 0.7 part of *water* and in 1.5 parts of *ethanol* (96%); soluble in *chloroform*; practically insoluble in *ether*.

Identification *Test A may be omitted if tests B, C, D, E and F are carried out. Tests B, C and D may be omitted if tests A, E and F are carried out.*

A. The *infra-red absorption spectrum*, Appendix II A, is concordant with the spectrum of *lidocaine hydrochloride EPCRS*.

B. To 5 mg add 0.5 ml of *fuming nitric acid*, evaporate to dryness on a water-bath, cool, dissolve the residue in 5 ml of *acetone* and add 1 ml of 0.1M *ethanolic potassium hydroxide*. A green colour is produced.

C. To 5 ml of a 5% w/v solution add 5 ml of *water* and make alkaline with 2M *sodium hydroxide*. Filter, wash the precipitate with *water*, dissolve half of the precipitate in 1 ml of *ethanol* (96%) and add 0.5 ml of a 10% w/v solution of *cobalt(II) nitrate*. A bluish-green precipitate is produced.

D. Dissolve 0.2 g in 10 ml of *water* and add 10 ml of a 1% w/v solution of *2,4,6-trinitrophenol*. The *melting point* of the precipitate, after washing with *water* and drying, is about 230°, Appendix V A, Method I.

E. Yields *reaction A* characteristic of chlorides, Appendix VI.

F. *Melting point*, 74° to 79°, determined without previous drying, Appendix V A, Method I.

Acidity pH of a 0.5% w/v solution, 4.0 to 5.5, Appendix V L.

Clarity and colour of solution A 5.0% w/v solution in *carbon dioxide-free water* is *clear*, Appendix IV A, and *colourless*, Appendix IV B, Method II.

Heavy metals Dissolve 1.0 g in sufficient *water* to produce 25 ml and carry out *limit test E for heavy metals*, Appendix VII, using 10 ml of the filtrate obtained in the first filtration. Use 2 ml of *lead standard solution (1 ppm Pb)* to prepare the standard (5 ppm).

2,6-Dimethylaniline To 2 ml of a 2.5% w/v solution of the substance being examined in *methanol* (solution A), add 1 ml of a 1% w/v solution of *4-dimethylaminobenzaldehyde* in *methanol* and 2 ml of *glacial acetic acid* and allow to stand for 10 minutes at room temperature. The yellow colour produced is more intense than that obtained by repeating the operation using 2 ml of *methanol* in place of solution A and less intense than the colour produced using a mixture of 1 ml of a solution of *2,6-dimethylaniline* in *methanol* containing 5 µg per ml and 1 ml of *methanol* in place of solution A (100 ppm).

Sulphated ash Not more than 0.1%, Appendix IX A, Method II. Use 1 g.

Water 5.5 to 7.0% w/w, Appendix IX C. Use 0.25 g.

Assay Dissolve 0.25 g in 30 ml of *anhydrous glacial acetic acid*, add 6 ml of *mercury(II) acetate solution* and carry out Method I for *non-aqueous titration*, Appendix VIII A, using 0.05 ml of *crystal violet solution* as indicator. Each ml of 0.1M *perchloric acid VS* is equivalent to 0.02708 g of $C_{14}H_{22}N_2O,HCl$.

Storage Lignocaine Hydrochloride should be kept in a well-closed container and protected from light.

Preparations
Lignocaine Gel
Lignocaine Injection
Lignocaine and Chlorhexidine Gel
Lignocaine and Adrenaline Injection

Action and use Local anaesthetic; anti-arrhythmic.

The title of the monograph in the European Pharmacopœia is Lidocaine Hydrochloride.

Lincomycin Hydrochloride

$C_{18}H_{34}N_2O_6S,HCl,H_2O$ 461.0   7179-49-9

Lincomycin Hydrochloride is the monohydrate of methyl 6-amino-6,8-dideoxy-N-[(2S,4R)-1-methyl-4-propylprolyl]-1-thio-α-D-*erythro*-D-*galacto*-octopyranoside hydrochloride, an antimicrobial substance produced by *Streptomyces lincolnensis* var. *lincolnensis* or by any other means. It contains not less than 90.0 per cent and not more than 100.5 per cent of lincomycin hydrochloride, $C_{18}H_{34}N_2O_6S,HCl$, calculated with reference to the anhydrous substance.

Characteristics A white or almost white, crystalline powder.

Solubility Soluble in 2 parts of *water*, in 40 parts of *ethanol (96%)* and in 20 parts of *dimethylformamide*; very slightly soluble in *acetone*; practically insoluble in *chloroform* and in *ether*.

Identification A. The *infra-red absorption spectrum*, Appendix II A, is concordant with the *reference spectrum* of lincomycin hydrochloride.
B. A 1% w/v solution yields *reaction A* characteristic of chlorides, Appendix VI.

Acidity pH of a 10% w/v solution, 3.0 to 5.5, Appendix V L.

Specific optical rotation In a 4% w/v solution, +135° to +150°, Appendix V F.

Lincomycin B Examine solution (3) as described under the Assay but increasing the sensitivity by eight to ten times whilst recording the peak derived from lincomycin B, which is eluted immediately before that derived from lincomycin. The area of the peak derived from lincomycin B, when corrected for the sensitivity factor, is not more than 5% of the area of the peak derived from lincomycin.

Sulphated ash Not more than 0.5%, Appendix IX A.

Water 3.0 to 6.0% w/w, Appendix IX C. Use 0.5 g.

Assay Carry out the method for *gas chromatography*, Appendix III B, using the following solutions. For solution (1) add 1 ml of a 1% w/v solution of *tetraphenylcyclopentadienone* (internal standard) in *dimethylformamide* and 0.4 ml of a mixture of 9 volumes

of N,O-*bis(trimethylsilyl)acetamide* and 1 volume of *trimethylchlorosilane* to 1 ml of a 1% w/v solution of *lincomycin hydrochloride BPCRS* in *dimethylformamide*, mix and allow to stand for 15 minutes. For solution (2) add 1 ml of *dimethylformamide* and 0.4 ml of a mixture of 9 volumes of N,O-*bis(trimethylsilyl)acetamide* and 1 volume of *trimethylchlorosilane* to 1 ml of a 1% w/v solution of the substance being examined in *dimethylformamide*, mix and allow to stand for 15 minutes. Prepare solution (3) in the same manner as solution (1) but using 1 ml of a 1% w/v solution of the substance being examined in place of the solution of *lincomycin hydrochloride BPCRS*.

The chromatographic procedure may be carried out using a glass column (1.5 m × 3 mm) packed with *silanised diatomaceous support* (100 to 120 mesh) coated with 3% w/w of dimethyl silicone gum (SE-30 is suitable) and maintained at 260° with a detector temperature of 260° to 290°.

Calculate the content of $C_{18}H_{34}N_2O_6S,HCl$ using the declared content of $C_{18}H_{34}N_2O_6S,HCl$ in *lincomycin hydrochloride BPCRS*.

Storage Lincomycin Hydrochloride should be kept in a well-closed container and stored at a temperature not exceeding 30°. If it is intended for use in the manufacture of a parenteral dosage form, the container should be sterile and sealed so as to exclude micro-organisms.

Labelling The label states (1) the date after which the material is not intended to be used; (2) the conditions under which it should be stored; (3) whether or not it is intended for use in the manufacture of a parenteral dosage form.

Preparations
Lincomycin Capsules
Lincomycin Injection

Action and use Antibacterial.

Lincomycin Hydrochloride intended for use in the manufacture of a parenteral dosage form complies with the following additional requirements.

Pyrogens Complies with the *test for pyrogens*, Appendix XIV K. Use per kg of the rabbit's weight 1 ml of a solution in *sodium chloride injection* containing 0.6 mg per ml.

Sterility When intended for use in the manufacture of a parenteral dosage form without further sterilisation, complies with the *test for sterility*, Appendix XVI A.

Lindane

Gamma Benzene Hexachloride

$C_6H_6Cl_6$ 290.8   58-89-9

Lindane is 1α,2α,3β,4α,5α,6β-hexachlorocyclohexane. It contains not less than 99.0 per cent and not more than 100.5 per cent of $C_6H_6Cl_6$.

Characteristics A white, crystalline powder; odour, slight.

Solubility Practically insoluble in *water*; soluble in 19 parts of *absolute ethanol*, in 2 parts of *acetone* and in 5.5 parts of *ether*.

Identification To 1 ml of a 0.5% w/v solution in *ethanol (96%)* in a stoppered cylinder add 3 ml of *ethanol (96%)* and 1 ml of *ethanolic potassium hydroxide solution* and allow to stand for 10 minutes. The solution yields *reaction A* characteristic of chlorides, Appendix VI.

Acidity Dissolve 10 g in 25 ml of *acetone*, warming if necessary, add 75 ml of *water* and titrate with 0.02M *sodium hydroxide VS* using *methyl red solution* as indicator. Repeat the operation without the substance being examined. The difference between the titrations is not more than 13.7 ml.

Crystallising point Not lower than 112.0°, Appendix V B, but melting a sufficient quantity in the inner test-tube by immersion in an oil-bath at about 120°. A suitable cooling liquid is liquid paraffin or glycerol which should be maintained at 102° to 107° throughout.

Alpha benzene hexachloride Carry out the method for *gas chromatography*, Appendix III B, using the following solutions. Solution (1) contains 0.010% w/v of *alpha benzene hexachloride CRS* in a 0.0040% w/v solution of *hexacosane* (internal standard) in *chloroform*. Solution (2) contains 1.0% w/v of the substance being examined in *chloroform*. Solution (3) contains 1.0% w/v of the substance being examined in a 0.0040% w/v solution of *hexacosane* in *chloroform*.

The chromatographic procedure may be carried out using (a) a glass column (1.5 m × 4 mm) packed with *acid-washed, silanised diatomaceous support* (80 to 100 mesh) coated with 3% w/w of cyanopropylmethyl phenyl methyl silicone fluid (OV-225 is suitable) and maintained at 200°.

In the chromatogram obtained with solution (3) the ratio of the area of any peak corresponding to alpha benzene hexachloride to the area of the peak due to the internal standard is not greater than the corresponding ratio in the chromatogram obtained with solution (1).

Loss on drying When dried to constant weight over *phosphorus pentoxide* at a pressure not exceeding 0.7 kPa, loses not more than 0.1% of its weight. Use 1 g.

Sulphated ash Not more than 0.1%, Appendix IX A.

Assay To 0.4 g add 25 ml of *ethanol (96%)* and warm on a water-bath until dissolved. Cool, add 10 ml of 1M *ethanolic potassium hydroxide VS*, swirl gently and allow to stand for 10 minutes. Dilute to 150 ml with *water*, neutralise with 2M *nitric acid* and add 10 ml in excess, followed by 50 ml of 0.1M *silver nitrate VS*. Filter, wash the residue with *water* and titrate the combined filtrate and washings with 0.1M *ammonium thiocyanate VS* using *ammonium iron(III) sulphate solution* as indicator. Each ml of 0.1M *silver nitrate VS* is equivalent to 0.009694 g of $C_6H_6Cl_6$.

Preparations
Lindane Application
Lindane Cream

Action and use Topical parasiticide.

Linseed ☆

Linseed consists of the dried, ripe seeds of *Linum usitatissimum* L.

Characteristics Odour and taste, not rancid.

Macroscopical Seeds, flattened, elongated ovoid, 4 to 6 mm long, 2 to 3 mm wide and 1.5 to 2 mm thick; one end rounded and at the other end an oblique point near which the hilum appears as a slight depression. Testa, dark reddish-brown, smooth and glossy but when viewed with a lens the surface is seen to be minutely pitted. Inside the testa there is a narrow, whitish endosperm and an embryo composed of two large, flattened, yellowish and oily cotyledons; the radicle points towards the hilum.

Microscopical Testa composed of an epidermis of isodiametric cells with mucilaginous outer walls and suberised inner walls; within this an area of collenchymatous cells followed by a single layer of longitudinally elongated sclereids, each 120 to 190 μm long and 12 to 15 μm wide, with thickened and pitted walls; next is a hyaline layer composed of thin-walled parenchyma and an inner epidermis formed of a layer of flattened polygonal cells each containing a mass of orange-brown pigment. Endosperm and cotyledons, composed of polygonal parenchymatous cells with slightly thickened walls, containing aleurone grains up to 20 μm in diameter and globules of fixed oil; starch absent.

Swelling index Not less than 4 for the whole drug and not less than 4.5 for the substance in *No. 710 powder*, Appendix XI M.

Foreign matter Not more than 1.5%, Appendix XI D, Test B.

Sulphated ash Not more than 6.0%, Appendix IX A, Method II. Use 1 g, in powder.

Storage Linseed should be kept in a well-closed container and protected from light.

Action and use Demulcent.

Powdered Linseed

Powdered Linseed is Linseed in powder.

Characteristics Yellowish-brown; odour, characteristic; greasy to the touch. Diagnostic structures; fragments of outer epidermal cells of the testa filled with mucilage; sub-epidermal collenchymatous layer seen in surface view as round cells with distinct triangular intercellular spaces, often associated with groups of elongated sclereids with pitted walls; thin-walled pitted cells of the hyaline layer often remaining attached to the elongated sclereids and crossing them at right angles; pigmented cells of the inner epidermis of the testa; parenchyma of the endosperm and cotyledons containing aleurone grains and fixed oil. Starch granules, absent.

Swelling index Not less than 4.5, Appendix XI M. Use the substance in *moderately coarse powder*.

Sulphated ash Not more than 6.0%, Appendix IX A, Method II. Use 1 g.

Storage Powdered Linseed should be kept in a well-closed container and protected from light.

Action and use Demulcent.

Liothyronine Sodium

$C_{15}H_{11}I_3NNaO_4$　　673.0　　55-06-1

Liothyronine Sodium is sodium O^4-(4-hydroxy-3-iodophenyl)-3,5-di-iodo-L-tyrosinate. It contains organically combined iodine equivalent to not less than 95.0 per cent and not more than 101.0 per cent of $C_{15}H_{11}I_3NNaO_4$, calculated with reference to the dried substance.

Characteristics A white to buff solid; odourless or almost odourless.

Solubility Practically insoluble in *water*, in *chloroform* and in *ether*; slightly soluble in *ethanol (96%)*. It dissolves in solutions of alkali hydroxides.

Identification A. *Absorbance* of a 0.015% w/v solution in 0.1M *sodium hydroxide* at the maximum at 319 nm, about 0.99, Appendix II B.
B. Dissolve 5 mg in 2 ml of *ethanol (50%)* containing 0.05 ml of *hydrochloric acid*, add 0.05 ml of a 10% w/v solution of *sodium nitrite* and boil; a yellow colour is produced. Cool and make alkaline with 5M *ammonia*; the solution becomes red.
C. Moisten with *sulphuric acid* and ignite. When moistened with *hydrochloric acid* and introduced on a platinum wire into a flame, the residue imparts a yellow colour to the flame.

Colour of solution A solution of 0.10 g in a mixture of 2 ml of 1M *hydrochloric acid* and 8 ml of *ethanol (96%)* is not more than pale brown in colour.

Specific optical rotation In a 2% w/v solution in a mixture of 1 volume of 1M *hydrochloric acid* and 4 volumes of *ethanol (96%)*, +18.0° to +22.0°, Appendix V F.

Sodium 2.9 to 4.0%, calculated with reference to the dried substance, when determined by the following method. Moisten 1 g with *sulphuric acid* in a silica dish and ignite gently, taking precautions to avoid loss of sodium iodide by volatilisation. Allow to cool, again moisten with *sulphuric acid* and ignite. Each g of residue is equivalent to 0.3238 g of sodium. Correct the result for the amount of sodium equivalent to the chloride found in the test for Chloride taking each ml of 0.05M *silver nitrate VS* to be equivalent to 0.001149 g of Na.

Chloride Not more than 1.2%, calculated with reference to the dried substance, when determined by the following method. Dissolve 0.50 g in 5 ml of 1M *sodium hydroxide* and 90 ml of *water*, add 15 ml of 2M *nitric acid* and titrate with 0.05M *silver nitrate VS*, determining the end-point potentiometrically. Each ml of 0.05M *silver nitrate VS* is equivalent to 0.001773 g of Cl.

Inorganic iodide Dissolve 0.25 g in a mixture of 25 ml of *water* and 2.5 ml of 1M *sodium hydroxide*, add 10 ml of 1M *hydrochloric acid* and sufficient *water* to produce 50 ml, mix and filter. To 25 ml of the filtrate add 2.5 ml of *hydrogen peroxide solution (20 vol)* and extract with 10 ml of *chloroform*. Any pink colour produced in the chloroform layer is not more intense than that produced by treating 0.275 mg of *potassium iodide* in the same manner.

Di-iodo-L-thyronine and thyroxine sodium Shake together 50 volumes of *amyl alcohol*, 50 volumes of *2-methylbutan-2-ol*, 3 volumes of 13.5M *ammonia* and 30 volumes of *water* and allow to separate. Transfer the lower layer to the bottom of an airtight chamber maintained at 25° and the upper layer to a central trough. Describe a circle 3.8 cm in diameter about the centre of a piece of chromatographic paper (Whatman 3MM is suitable) 36 cm in diameter. Place on one point of the circumference of the circle 20 µl of a 1.0% w/v solution of the substance being examined in a mixture of 5 volumes of 13.5M *ammonia* and 70 volumes of *ethanol (96%)* (solution 1). Place on another point of the circumference 20 µl of a solution in the same solvent mixture containing 0.050% w/v of the substance being examined, 0.050% w/v of *levothyroxine sodium EPCRS* and 0.020% w/v of *3,5-di-iodo-L-thyronine* (solution 2). Insert a cotton wick through a hole in the centre of the circle, place the paper horizontally in the chamber and allow to stand for 4 hours. Adjust the paper so that the wick dips into the liquid in the central trough and allow elution to proceed until the solvent front has travelled about 15 cm. After removal of the paper, allow it to dry in air, immerse in a 0.25% w/v solution of *ninhydrin* in *acetone* containing 1% v/v of *glacial acetic acid* and allow to dry in air for 2 hours. The chromatogram obtained with solution (2) exhibits three spots corresponding to thyroxine, liothyronine and di-iodothyronine in order of increasing Rf values. The spots corresponding to thyroxine and di-iodothyronine in the chromatogram obtained with solution (1) are not more intense than the spots due to thyroxine and di-iodothyronine respectively in the chromatogram obtained with solution (2).

Loss on drying When dried to constant weight at 105°, loses not more than 4.0% of its weight. Use 1 g.

Assay Carry out the method for *oxygen-flask combustion (for iodine)*, Appendix VIII C, using 25 mg. Each ml of 0.02M *sodium thiosulphate VS* is equivalent to 0.7480 mg of $C_{15}H_{11}I_3NNaO_4$.

Storage Liothyronine Sodium should be kept in a well-closed container and protected from light.

Preparation
Liothyronine Tablets

Action and use Thyroid hormone.

Liquorice ☆

Liquorice consists of the dried, unpeeled roots and stolons of *Glycyrrhiza glabra* L. It contains not less than 4.0 per cent of glycyrrhizinic acid.

Characteristics Odour, characteristic and slightly aromatic. Taste, very sweet, faintly astringent; the bark is not bitter.

Macroscopical Root with few branches, up to 1 m long and 0.5 to 3 cm in diameter. Bark, brownish-grey to brown with longitudinal striations, bearing traces of lateral roots. Stolon, cylindrical, 1 to 2 cm in diameter and up to several metres long, but may be cut into lengths of 10 to 15 cm, similar in external appearance to the root but with occasional small buds. Fracture of the root and stolon, granular and fibrous. Cork layer, thin; secondary phloem region, wide, light yellow with radial striations; xylem, compact, yellow, with radiate structure. The stolon has a central pith which is absent from the root.

Microscopical Cork and phelloderm narrow. Phloem consisting mainly of bundles of thick-walled, yellow fibres 700 to 1200 μm long and 10 to 20 μm wide surrounded by cells each containing a prism of calcium oxalate, 10 to 35 μm long and 2 to 5 μm wide, alternating in the external layers with areas of strongly hyaline keratenchyma; normal sieve tissue near the cambium. Xylem of radial rows of tracheids and vessels alternating with bundles of partially lignified fibres with crystal sheaths similar to those of the secondary phloem; vessels 30 to 150 μm in diameter with walls 5 to 10 μm thick having numerous bordered pits with slit-shaped openings, associated with lignified xylem parenchyma. Medullary rays, two to five cells wide. Parenchymatous cells throughout containing simple, round or oval starch granules 2 to 20 μm, mostly 5 to 12 μm, in diameter; parenchymatous pith present only in the stolon.

Identification A. Carry out the method for *thin-layer chromatography*, Appendix III A, using *silica gel GF254* as the coating substance and as the mobile phase the upper layer, even if turbid, of a mixture of 60 volumes of *ethyl acetate*, 27 volumes of 1M *ammonia* and 13 volumes of *absolute ethanol*, shaken together and allowed to stand for 5 minutes. Prepare the following solutions. For solution (1) shake 1.0 g, in *No. 180 powder*, with 20 ml of *chloroform* for 15 minutes, filter and reserve the extracted powder for the preparation of solution (2). Evaporate the filtrate to dryness and dissolve the residue in 2 ml of a mixture of equal volumes of *chloroform* and *methanol*. For solution (2) add to the extracted powder 30 ml of 0.5M *sulphuric acid* and heat under a reflux condenser for 1 hour, allow to cool and extract with two 20-ml quantities of *chloroform*; dry the combined chloroform extracts with *anhydrous sodium sulphate*, filter, evaporate to dryness and dissolve the residue in 2 ml of a mixture of equal volumes of *chloroform* and *methanol*. For solution (3) dissolve 10 mg of *glycyrrhetic acid* in 2 ml of a mixture of equal volumes of *chloroform* and *methanol*. Apply separately to the chromatoplate in three bands, each 20 mm long and not more than 3 mm wide, 10 μl of solutions (1) and (2) and 20 μl of solution (3).

After removal of the plate, allow it to dry in air for 5 minutes and examine under *ultra-violet light (254 nm)*. The chromatogram obtained with solution (3) exhibits a band corresponding to β-glycyrrhetic acid with an Rf value of about 0.1. The chromatogram obtained with solution (2) exhibits a corresponding band but this is not seen in the chromatogram obtained with solution (1). Spray the plate with *anisaldehyde solution* using about 10 ml for a plate 200 mm × 200 mm in size, heat at 100° to 105° for 10 minutes and examine in daylight. The β-glycyrrhetic acid bands become bluish-violet. One or two bands with an Rf value of about 0.6, visible in daylight before spraying, become orange-yellow and several other bluish-violet bands appear in the chromatograms obtained with solutions (1) and (2). The band corresponding to β-glycyrrhetic acid in the chromatogram obtained with solution (2) is at least equal in size to the band in the chromatogram obtained with solution (3).

B. Mix a small quantity, in powder, with 0.05 ml of *sulphuric acid*. The powder particles become orange-yellow and some fragments change, more slowly, to pinkish-red.

Water-soluble extractive Not less than 20% when determined by the following method. Mix 2.5 g, in *No.*

180 powder, with 50 ml of *water* and allow to stand for 2 hours, shaking frequently. Filter, evaporate a quantity of the filtrate equivalent to 0.5 g of the powder to dryness on a water-bath and dry the residue at 100° to 105°.

Acid-insoluble ash Not more than 2.0%, Appendix XI K, Method II.

Sulphated ash Not more than 10.0%, Appendix IX A, Method II. Use 1 g, in powder.

Assay Carry out the method for *thin-layer chromatography*, Appendix III A, using *silica gel GF254* as the coating substance and as the mobile phase the upper layer, even if turbid, of a mixture of 60 volumes of *ethyl acetate*, 27 volumes of 1M *ammonia* and 13 volumes of *absolute ethanol*, shaken together and allowed to stand for 5 minutes. Apply separately to the chromatoplate two 60-μl quantities of each of the following solutions as bands 20 mm long and not more than 3 mm wide, but ensuring that part of the plate remains free from the solutions being examined. For solution (1) mix 1 g, in *No. 180 powder*, with 25 ml of 1M *hydrochloric acid* and 2.5 ml of *1,4-dioxan*. Heat under a reflux condenser in a water-bath for 2 hours, allow to cool, filter through a hardened filter paper 9 cm in diameter and discard the filtrate. Rinse the flask and filter with five 20-ml quantities of *water* and discard the rinsings. Dry the flask and filter at 105° for 20 minutes, transfer the filter paper to the flask and add 50 ml of *chloroform*. Boil under a reflux condenser in a water-bath for 5 minutes and filter the warm chloroform solution through a hardened filter paper 9 cm in diameter. Repeat the extraction with two 25-ml quantities of *chloroform*, using the same filter each time. Transfer the filter paper to the flask, extract with 25 ml of *chloroform* and filter through another hardened filter paper 9 cm in diameter. Evaporate the combined filtrates to dryness, dissolve the residue in a mixture of equal volumes of *chloroform* and *methanol* and transfer to a 10-ml graduated flask. Rinse with two 10-ml quantities of *chloroform* and evaporate the rinsings until 2 ml remains. Transfer this solution to the graduated flask and dilute to 10 ml with a mixture of equal volumes of *chloroform* and *methanol*. For solution (2) mix 50 mg of *glycyrrhizinic acid EPCRS* with 25 ml of 1M *hydrochloric acid* and 2.5 ml of *1,4-dioxan* and proceed as described for solution (1) beginning at the words 'Heat under a reflux condenser . . .'.

After removal of the plate, allow it to dry in air, examine under *ultra-violet light (254 nm)* and mark the areas corresponding to β-glycyrrhetic acid in all four chromatograms. Carefully scrape off the coating substance from the marked areas and treat each separately in the following manner. Shake with 5 ml of *absolute ethanol* for 15 minutes and filter through a small sintered-glass filter (BS porosity No. 4). Rinse the filter with *absolute ethanol* and dilute the filtrate to 10 ml with the same solvent. Measure the *absorbance* of each of the four solutions at 250 nm, Appendix II B, using in the reference cell a solution prepared by treating in the same manner an area of the coating substance corresponding in position and size to the marked areas of β-glycyrrhetic acid but taken from the part of the plate that has remained free from the solutions being examined. Calculate the content of glycyrrhizinic acid from the absorbances of solutions (1) and (2) and the declared content of glycyrrhizinic acid in *glycyrrhizinic acid EPCRS*.

Storage Liquorice should be kept in an airtight container and protected from light.

Preparations
Liquorice Liquid Extract
Deglycyrrhizinised Liquorice Extract

Action and use Flavour.

The title of the monograph in the European Pharmacopœia is Liquorice Root.

Powdered Liquorice

Powdered Liquorice is Liquorice in powder. It contains not less than 4.0 per cent of glycyrrhizinic acid.

Characteristics Light yellow and faintly greyish. Diagnostic structures: fragments of fibres accompanied by crystal sheaths; fragments of vessels with thick walls and numerous bordered pits; fragments of cork and isolated prisms of calcium oxalate; starch abundant.

Identification; water-soluble extractive; Acid-insoluble ash; Sulphated ash Complies with the requirements stated under Liquorice.

Assay Carry out the Assay described under Liquorice.

Storage Powdered Liquorice should be kept in an airtight container and protected from light.

Action and use Flavour.

Lithium Carbonate ☆

Li_2CO_3 73.9   *554-13-2*

Lithium Carbonate contains not less than 98.5 per cent and not more than 100.5 per cent of Li_2CO_3.

Characteristics A white powder.

Solubility Slightly soluble in *water*; practically insoluble in *ethanol (96%)*.

Identification A. When moistened with *hydrochloric acid*, imparts a red colour to a non-luminous flame.
B. Dissolve 0.2 g in 1 ml of *hydrochloric acid* and evaporate to dryness on a water-bath. The residue is soluble in 3 ml of *ethanol (96%)*.
C. Yields *reaction A* characteristic of carbonates, Appendix VI.

Clarity and colour of solution Suspend 10.0 g in 30 ml of *distilled water* and dissolve by adding 22 ml of *nitric acid*. Neutralise with 2M *sodium hydroxide* and dilute to 100 ml with *distilled water* (solution A). The solution is *clear*, Appendix IV A, and *colourless*, Appendix IV B, Method II.

Arsenic 0.50 g complies with the *limit test for arsenic*, Appendix VII (2 ppm).

Calcium 5 ml of solution B diluted to 15 ml with *distilled water* complies with the *limit test for calcium*, Appendix VII (200 ppm).

Heavy metals 12 ml of solution A complies with *limit test A for heavy metals*, Appendix VII (20 ppm). Use *lead standard solution (2 ppm Pb)* to prepare the standard.

Iron 5 ml of solution A diluted to 10 ml with *water* complies with the *limit test for iron*, Appendix VII (20 ppm).

Magnesium Dilute 1 ml of solution A to 15 ml with *water*. 10 ml of the resulting solution complies with the *limit test for magnesium*, Appendix VII (150 ppm).

Potassium Not more than 300 ppm when determined by the following method. Dissolve 1.0 g in 10 ml of 7M *hydrochloric acid*, add sufficient *water* to produce 50 ml and determine by *atomic emission spectrophotometry*, Appendix II D, measuring at 766.5 nm and using *potassium solution ASp*, suitably diluted with *water*, for the standard solution.

Sodium Not more than 300 ppm when determined by the following method. Dissolve 1.0 g in 10 ml of 7M *hydrochloric acid*, add sufficient *water* to produce 50 ml and determine by *atomic emission spectrophotometry*, Appendix II D, measuring at 589.0 nm and using *sodium solution ASp*, suitably diluted with *water*, for the standard solution.

Chloride 2.5 ml of solution A diluted to 15 ml with *water* complies with the *limit test for chlorides*, Appendix VII (200 ppm).

Sulphate Disperse 1.25 g in 5 ml of *distilled water* and dissolve by adding 5 ml of 7M *hydrochloric acid*. Boil for 2 minutes, cool, neutralise with 2M *sodium hydroxide* and dilute to 25 ml with *distilled water*. The resulting solution complies with the *limit test for sulphates*, Appendix VII (200 ppm).

Assay Dissolve 0.5 g in 25 ml of 1M *hydrochloric acid VS* and titrate with 1M *sodium hydroxide VS* using *methyl orange solution* as indicator. Each ml of 1M *hydrochloric acid VS* is equivalent to 0.03695 g of Li_2CO_3.

Preparation
Lithium Carbonate Tablets

Action and use Prophylaxis of affective disorders.

Lobelia
Lobelia Herb

Lobelia consists of the dried aerial parts of *Lobelia inflata* L. It contains not less than 0.25 per cent of total alkaloids, calculated as lobeline, $C_{22}H_{27}NO_2$.

Characteristics Odour, slight and somewhat irritating.

Macroscopical Stems green, often with a purplish tint, smooth and cylindrical, hairy and winged in the upper part, channelled, angled and nearly glabrous below; trichomes up to about 1.2 mm in length; alternate leaves or leaf scars present, phyllotaxis of 1:3. Leaves pale green, broadly ovate to ovate-lanceolate and varying from about 3 to 8 cm in length, margin irregularly toothed, lamina bearing scattered, bristly trichomes, especially on the veins of the lower surface. Inflorescence of racemes of about six to twenty flowers arising in the axils of the upper leaves; bracts foliaceous; pedicels slender, about 3 to 5 mm long; flowers hermaphrodite and zygomorphic, about 7 mm long; calyx superior with five sepals, subulate, about 2.5 mm long; corolla epigynous, tubular, about 4 mm long, bilabiate, upper lip of two lanceolate segments between which the corolla tube is split down to the base, lower lip of three, spreading, triangular-ovate lobes, pale violet-blue; androecium of five epigynous stamens with syngynesious anthers, each anther having an apical tuft of trichomes; gynoecium of two carpels, ovary inferior, bilocular, ovules numerous, placentation axile, stigma bifid and surrounded by the anther tube. Fruit an inflated, ovoid or ellipsoidal bilocular capsule, dehiscing by apical pores and containing when ripe numerous brown, ovoid, reticulate seeds, about 0.5 to 0.7 mm long and about 0.3 mm wide.

Microscopical Leaf: epidermal cells of adaxial surface with straight walls, papillose, cuticle striated; cells of abaxial surface with wavy and beaded anticlinal walls; stomata *anomocytic*, on abaxial surface only; trichomes conical, unicellular or rarely two-celled, with thin, warty walls and usually about 300 μm but sometimes as much as 1.2 mm long; palisade ratio usually about 4 to 4.3, up to 5.3; mesophyll with many cells containing abundant fat crystals in the form of slender prisms 10 to 15 μm long and 2 μm thick, often arranged in small fan-shaped groups of five or six; on warming the crystals are replaced by droplets of oil; laticiferous vessels anastomosing. Stem: epidermis and trichomes as in leaf; cuticle striated; anastomosing laticiferous vessels also present; pith with lignified and pitted parenchyma. Pollen grains spherical, about 24 to 30 μm in diameter, extine smooth or faintly pitted, with three pores. Pericarp with irregular, pitted sclereids. Seed: epidermal cells about 100 μm by 25 μm, elongated polygonal, with highly refractive, lignified anticlinal walls.

Acid-insoluble ash Not more than 5.0%, Appendix XI K.

Foreign matter Not more than 2.0%, Appendix XI D.

Stems Not more than 60%.

Assay Add 10 g, in *No. 125 powder*, to 10 g of ignited sand, transfer to a stoppered flask and add 75 ml of a mixture of 4 volumes of *ether* and 1 volume of *ethanol (96%)*, shake well, allow to stand for 15 minutes, add 5 ml of 5M *ammonia* and allow to stand for 1 hour, shaking frequently. Transfer the mixture to a small percolator containing an absorbent cotton plug, allow the liquid to flow into a separating funnel and, when the liquid ceases to flow, pack firmly and continue the percolation, first with 25 ml of the ether—ethanol mixture and then with *ether* until *complete extraction* of the alkaloids is effected. To the percolate add 30 ml of 0.5M *sulphuric acid*, shake well, allow to separate and transfer the lower layer to another separating funnel. Repeat the extraction with a mixture of 25 ml of 0.25M *sulphuric acid* and 5 ml of *ethanol (96%)*, remove the lower layer and repeat the extraction with three or more successive 20-ml quantities of the acid—ethanol mixture until *complete extraction* of the alkaloids is effected. Wash the mixed acid solutions with successive quantities of 10, 5 and 3 ml of *chloroform*, washing each chloroform solution with the same 20 ml of 0.25M *sulphuric acid* contained in another separating funnel, discard the chloroform, transfer the acidic liquid from the second to the first separating funnel, neutralise to *litmus paper* with 5M *ammonia* and add a further 5 ml in excess. Extract with successive quantities of *chloroform* until *complete extraction* of the alkaloids is effected, wash each chloroform solution separately with the same 5 ml of *water* and filter through a 7-cm filter paper into a flask. Wash the filter thoroughly with *chloroform*, collect the washings in the flask and warm to evaporate the chloroform until about 2 ml remains. Add 2 ml of *absolute ethanol* and continue the evaporation, using a gentle current of air to complete the process; repeat with two further quantities of *absolute ethanol* and dry the residue for 1 hour at 80°. Add to the

residue 2 ml of *ethanol (96%)*, warm until dissolved, add 10 ml of 0.01M *sulphuric acid VS*, cool and titrate the excess of acid with 0.02M *sodium hydroxide VS* using *methyl red solution* as indicator. Each ml of 0.01M *sulphuric acid VS* is equivalent to 0.006749 g of total alkaloids calculated as $C_{22}H_{27}NO_2$.

Action and use Respiratory stimulant.

Powdered Lobelia

Powdered Lobelia is Lobelia in powder. It contains not less than 0.25 per cent of total alkaloids, calculated as lobeline, $C_{22}H_{27}NO_2$.

Characteristics Dull greenish-yellow. Diagnostic structures: fragments of the leaf lamina showing papillose cells of the upper epidermis or sinuous-walled cells of the lower epidermis with *anomocytic* stomata; numerous large, conical, unicellular trichomes; lignified parenchyma and laticiferous tissue of the stem; conspicuous large, thickened, polygonal cells of the epidermis of the testa; unevenly thickened sclereids from the pericarp; occasional spherical pollen grains with three distinct pores and furrows. Calcium oxalate crystals absent.

Acid-insoluble ash Not more than 5.0 per cent, Appendix XI K.

Assay Carry out the Assay described under Lobelia. Each ml of 0.01M *sulphuric acid VS* is equivalent to 0.06749 g of total alkaloids calculated as $C_{22}H_{27}NO_2$.

Action and use Respiratory stimulant.

Lomustine

$C_9H_{16}ClN_3O_2$ 233.7   *13010-47-4*

Lomustine is 1-(2-chloroethyl)-3-cyclohexyl-1-nitrosourea. It contains not less than 98.5 per cent and not more than 100.5 per cent of $C_9H_{16}ClN_3O_2$, calculated with reference to the dried substance.

Characteristics A yellow, crystalline powder.

Solubility Practically insoluble in *water*; soluble in *ethanol (96%)*; freely soluble in *acetone* and in *chloroform*.

Identification A. The *infra-red absorption spectrum*, Appendix II A, is concordant with the *reference spectrum* of lomustine.
B. Carry out the test in subdued light and prepare the solution immediately before use. The *light absorption*, Appendix II B, in the range 200 to 350 nm of a 0.0020% w/v solution in *ethanol (96%)* exhibits a maximum at 230 nm. The *absorbance* at 230 nm is about 0.52.
C. Dissolve 25 mg in 1 ml of *methanol*, add 0.1 ml of 1M *sodium hydroxide* and 2 ml of *water* and acidify by adding, dropwise, 1M *nitric acid*. The resulting solution yields *reaction A* characteristic of chlorides, Appendix VI.

Melting point 88° to 90°, Appendix V A.

Chloride Carry out the following procedure, except the final comparison, in subdued light. Dissolve 0.24 g in 4 ml of *methanol* and add 20 ml of *water*, allow to stand for 20 minutes and filter. To 10 ml of the filtrate add 5 ml of *methanol*. The resulting solution complies with the *limit test for chlorides*, Appendix VII, replacing the 5 ml of water in the standard solution with 5 ml of *methanol* (500 ppm).

Related substances A. Carry out in subdued light the method for *thin-layer chromatography*, Appendix III A, using a silica gel precoated chromatoplate (Merck silica gel 60 plates are suitable) and a mixture of 80 volumes of *toluene* and 20 volumes of *glacial acetic acid* as the mobile phase. Apply separately to the plate 4 µl of each of three freshly prepared solutions of the substance being examined in *methanol* containing (1) 2.5% w/v, (2) 0.010% w/v and (3) 0.0050% w/v. After removal of the plate, heat it at 110° for 1 hour, place the hot plate in a closed tank containing chlorine, produced by adding *hydrochloric acid* to a 5% w/v solution of *potassium permanganate* contained in a beaker placed at the bottom of the tank, and allow to stand for 2 minutes. Dry in a current of cold air until an area of the plate below the line of application produces at most a very faint blue colour with 0.05 ml of a 0.5% w/v solution of *potassium iodide* in *starch mucilage*; avoid prolonged exposure to cold air. Spray the plate with a 0.5% w/v solution of *potassium iodide* in *starch mucilage*. Any *secondary spot* in the chromatogram obtained with solution (1) is not more intense than the spot in the chromatogram obtained with solution (2) and not more than one such spot is more intense than the spot in the chromatogram obtained with solution (3).

B. Carry out in subdued light the method for *high-performance liquid chromatography*, Appendix III D, using two freshly prepared solutions of the substance being examined in *methanol* containing (1) 0.025% w/v and (2) 2.5% w/v.

The chromatographic procedure may be carried out using (a) a stainless steel column (20 cm × 4 mm) packed with *stationary phase C* (10 µm) (Nucleosil C18 is suitable), (b) a mixture of equal volumes of *methanol* and *water* as the mobile phase with a flow rate of 2 ml per minute and (c) a detection wavelength of 230 nm.

In the chromatogram obtained with solution (2) the sum of the areas of any *secondary peaks* is not greater than the area of the peak in the chromatogram obtained with solution (1).

Loss on drying When dried over *phosphorus pentoxide* at a pressure not exceeding 0.7 kPa for 24 hours, loses not more than 1.0% of its weight. Use 1 g.

Assay To 0.2 g add 20 ml of a 20% w/v solution of *potassium hydroxide* and boil under a reflux condenser for 2 hours. Add 75 ml of *water* and 4 ml of *nitric acid*, cool and titrate with 0.05M *silver nitrate VS* determining the end-point potentiometrically. Repeat the operation without the substance being examined. The difference between the titrations represents the amount of silver nitrate required. Each ml of 0.05M *silver nitrate VS* is equivalent to 0.01168 g of $C_9H_{16}ClN_3O_2$.

Preparation
Lomustine Capsules

Action and use Cytotoxic.

Lorazepam

$C_{15}H_{10}Cl_2N_2O_2$ 321.2   *846-49-1*

Lorazepam is 7-chloro-5-(2-chlorophenyl)-1,3-dihydro-3-hydroxy-1,4-benzodiazepin-2-one. It contains not less than 98.5 per cent and not more than 101.0 per cent of $C_{15}H_{10}Cl_2N_2O_2$, calculated with reference to the dried substance.

Characteristics A white or almost white, crystalline powder; odourless or almost odourless.

Solubility Practically insoluble in *water*; sparingly soluble in *ethanol* (96%); slightly soluble in *chloroform*.

Identification A. The *infra-red absorption spectrum*, Appendix II A, is concordant with the *reference spectrum* of lorazepam.
B. The *light absorption*, Appendix II B, in the range 210 to 350 nm of a 0.001% w/v solution in *ethanol* (96%) exhibits two maxima, at 230 nm and 316 nm. The *absorbance* at 230 nm is about 1.1.

Related substances Carry out the method for *thin-layer chromatography*, Appendix III A, using a silica gel F254 precoated chromatoplate (Merck silica gel 60 F254 plates are suitable) and a mixture of 100 volumes of *chloroform* and 10 volumes of *methanol* as the mobile phase. Apply separately to the plate 20 µl of each of three solutions of the substance being examined in *acetone* containing (1) 0.50% w/v, (2) 0.0010% w/v and (3) 0.00050% w/v. After removal of the plate, allow it to dry in air and examine under *ultra-violet light (254 nm)*. Any *secondary spot* in the chromatogram obtained with solution (1) is not more intense than the spot in the chromatogram obtained with solution (2) and not more than one such spot is more intense than the spot in the chromatogram obtained with solution (3).

Loss on drying When dried to constant weight at 105° at a pressure not exceeding 0.7 kPa, loses not more than 0.5% of its weight. Use 1 g.

Sulphated ash Not more than 0.1%, Appendix IX A.

Assay Dissolve 0.5 g in a mixture of 5 ml of *anhydrous glacial acetic acid* and 45 ml of *acetic anhydride* and carry out Method I for *non-aqueous titration*, Appendix VIII A, determining the end-point potentiometrically. Each ml of 0.1M *perchloric acid VS* is equivalent to 0.03212 g of $C_{15}H_{10}Cl_2N_2O_2$.

Storage Lorazepam should be kept in a well-closed container and protected from light.

Preparation
Lorazepam Tablets

Action and use Anxiolytic.

Lymecycline

992-21-2

Lymecycline is a water-soluble combination of tetracycline, lysine and formaldehyde. The potency is not less than 900 Units per mg, calculated with reference to the anhydrous substance.

Characteristics A yellow powder; very hygroscopic.

Solubility Soluble in less than 1 part of *water*; slightly soluble in *ethanol (96%)*; practically insoluble in *acetone*, in *chloroform* and in *ether*.

Identification A. Carry out the method for *thin-layer chromatography* using *ethyl acetate* saturated with 0.1M *disodium edetate* previously adjusted to pH 7 with 5M *ammonia* as the mobile phase and a chromatoplate prepared as follows. Boil 50 g of *kieselguhr G* with a mixture of 250 ml of *hydrochloric acid* and 250 ml of *water* for 10 minutes, filter and wash the filter with *water* until the washings are alkaline to *congo red solution*. Dry the residue at 105° and slurry 25 g with a mixture of 2.5 ml of a 20% v/v solution of *polyethylene glycol 400* in *glycerol* and 47.5 ml of 0.1M *disodium edetate* previously adjusted to pH 7 with 5M *ammonia*. After spreading the plate, allow it to dry at room temperature until the surface acquires a uniform matt appearance (usually after 1 to 2 hours) and place in a tank the atmosphere of which has been allowed to equilibrate with a saturated solution of *ammonium chloride* for at least 24 hours. Allow the plate to remain in the tank for 24 hours and use immediately after removal.

Apply separately to the plate 1 μl of each of two freshly prepared solutions in *methanol* containing (1) 0.05% w/v of the substance being examined and (2) 0.05% w/v of *lymecycline BPCRS*. After removal of the plate, allow to dry in air, expose to the vapour of 13.5M *ammonia* and examine under *ultra-violet light (365 nm)*. The principal spot in the chromatogram obtained with solution (1) corresponds to that in the chromatogram obtained with solution (2).

B. To 0.5 mg add 2 ml of *sulphuric acid*. A purplish-red colour is produced.

C. Dissolve 50 mg in 5 ml of *water*, add 50 mg of *ninhydrin*, boil and add 15 ml of *water*. A bluish-violet colour is produced.

D. Dissolve 0.2 g in 5 ml of *water*, add 0.3 ml of *orthophosphoric acid* and distil. To 1 ml of the distillate add 10 ml of *chromotropic acid solution*. A violet colour is produced.

Alkalinity pH of a 1% w/v solution, 7.8 to 8.1, Appendix V L.

Light absorption To 10 ml of a 0.01% w/v solution in 0.01M *hydrochloric acid* add 75 ml of *water* and 5 ml of 5M *sodium hydroxide*, add sufficient *water* to produce 100 ml and mix immediately. The *absorbance* of the resulting solution at the maximum at 380 nm, when measured exactly 6 minutes after the addition of the sodium hydroxide solution, is 0.27 to 0.31, Appendix II B.

Specific optical rotation In a 0.5% w/v solution, −180° to −210°, Appendix V F.

Light-absorbing impurities The *absorbance* of a 0.25% w/v solution in 0.01M *hydrochloric acid* at 430 nm, when measured within 1 hour of preparing the solution, is not more than 0.50, Appendix II B.

Free tetracycline To 0.5 g add 50 ml of *butyl acetate* and allow to stand for 1 hour at 25°. Filter and extract the filtrate with two 25-ml quantities of 0.1M *hydrochloric acid*. Combine the extracts, add sufficient 0.1M *hydrochloric acid* to produce 50 ml and dilute 10 ml of this solution to 100 ml with 0.1M *hydrochloric acid*. The *absorbance* of the resulting solution at 355 nm is not more than 0.64, Appendix II B.

Related substances Carry out the method for *thin-layer chromatography*, Appendix III A, using the coating and method of equilibrating the chromatoplate described under test A for Identification. Use as the mobile phase the solution obtained by shaking 5 ml of 0.1M *disodium edetate*, previously adjusted to pH 7 with 5M *ammonia*, with 200 ml of a mixture consisting of 3 volumes of *acetone*, 1 volume of *chloroform* and 1 volume of *ethyl acetate*, the emulsion being removed by filtering through absorbent cotton. Apply separately to the plate 1 μl of each of the following solutions. For solution (1) add 5 ml of *water* and 1 ml of a 4% w/v solution of *sodium metabisulphite* to 0.125 g of the substance being examined and allow to stand for 16 hours at room temperature, without stirring. Add sufficient 0.1M *hydrochloric acid* to produce 10 ml and filter if necessary. Solutions (2) to (5) are freshly prepared solutions in *methanol* containing (2) 0.0050% w/v of *anhydrotetracycline hydrochloride EPCRS*, (3) 0.0050% w/v of *4-epianhydrotetracycline hydrochloride EPCRS*, (4) 0.020% w/v of *chlortetracycline hydrochloride EPCRS* and (5) 0.050% w/v of *epitetracycline EPCRS*. After removal of the plate, allow it to dry in air, expose to the vapour of 13.5M *ammonia* and examine under *ultra-violet light (365 nm)*. Any *secondary spot* in the chromatogram obtained with solution (1) is not more intense than the corresponding spot in the chromatograms obtained with solutions (2) to (5).

Water Not more than 5.0% w/w, Appendix IX C. Use 0.5 g.

Assay Carry out the *biological assay of antibiotics*, Appendix XIV A. The precision of the assay is such that the fiducial limits of error are not less than 95% and not more than 105% of the estimated potency.

Storage Lymecycline should be kept in a well-closed container, protected from light and stored at a temperature not exceeding 25°. If the contents are intended for use in the manufacture of a parenteral dosage form, the container should be sterile and sealed so as to exclude micro-organisms.

Labelling The label states (1) the number of Units per mg; (2) the date after which the material is not intended to be used; (3) the conditions under which it should be stored; (4) whether or not it is intended for use in the manufacture of a parenteral dosage form.

Preparation

Lymecycline Capsules

Action and use Antibacterial.

135 mg of Lymecycline is equivalent to approximately 100 mg of tetracycline.

Lymecycline intended for use in the manufacture of a parenteral dosage form complies with the following additional requirements.

Depressor substances Complies with the *test for depressor substances*, Appendix XIV M. Use per kg of the cat's weight 1 ml of a solution in *saline solution* or in *water for injections* containing 3000 Units per ml.

Pyrogens Complies with the *test for pyrogens*, Appendix XIV K. Use per kg of the rabbit's weight 1 ml of *water for injections* containing 1000 Units per ml.

Sterility When intended for use in the manufacture of a parenteral dosage form without further sterilisation, complies with the *test for sterility*, Appendix XVI A.

Lynoestrenol

$C_{20}H_{28}O$ 284.4   52-76-6

Lynoestrenol is 19-nor-17α-pregn-4-en-20-yn-17β-ol. It contains not less than 97.0 per cent and not more than 102.0 per cent of $C_{20}H_{28}O$, calculated with reference to the dried substance.

Characteristics A white or almost white, crystalline powder; odourless or almost odourless.

Solubility Practically insoluble in *water*; soluble in 15 parts of *ethanol (96%)*, in 15 parts of *absolute ethanol*, in 12 parts of *acetone*, in 8 parts of *chloroform* and in 12 parts of *ether*.

Identification A. The *infra-red absorption spectrum*, Appendix II A, is concordant with the *reference spectrum* of lynoestrenol.
B. The *light absorption*, Appendix II B, of a 1% w/v solution in *methanol* exhibits no maximum in the range 230 to 350 nm.
C. Carry out the method for *thin-layer chromatography*, Appendix III A, using *silica gel G* as the coating substance and a mixture of 80 volumes of *heptane* and 20 volumes of *acetone* as the mobile phase but allowing the solvent front to ascend 10 cm above the line of application. Apply separately to the chromatoplate 2 µl of each of the following solutions. Solution (1) contains 0.25% w/v of the substance being examined in a mixture of 9 volumes of *chloroform* and 1 volume of *methanol*. Solution (2) contains 0.25% w/v of *lynoestrenol BPCRS* in the same solvent. Solution (3) is a mixture of equal volumes of solutions (1) and (2). After removal of the plate, heat it at 105° for 10 minutes, spray with *ethanolic sulphuric acid (20%)*, heat at 105° for a further 10 minutes, allow to cool and examine in daylight and under *ultra-violet light (365 nm)*. The principal spot in the chromatogram obtained with solution (1) corresponds to that in the chromatogram obtained with solution (2) and the principal spot in the chromatogram obtained with solution (3) appears as a single, compact spot.
D. Dissolve 1 mg in 1 ml of *sulphuric acid*; an orange colour is produced. Add 4 ml of *water* followed by 6 ml of *sulphuric acid*; the solution exhibits a greenish-yellow fluorescence when examined under ultra-violet light (254 nm).

Melting point 160° to 164°, Appendix V A.

Specific optical rotation In a 5% w/v solution in *1,4-dioxan*, −8° to −12°, Appendix V F.

Related substances Carry out the method for *thin-layer chromatography*, Appendix III A, using *silica gel G* as the coating substance and a mixture of 80 volumes of n-*heptane* and 20 volumes of *acetone* as the mobile phase. Apply separately to the chromatoplate 10 µl of each of three solutions of the substance being examined in *chloroform* containing (1) 2.0% w/v, (2) 0.020% w/v and (3) 0.010% w/v. After removal of the plate, allow it to dry in air, spray with a freshly prepared 5% w/v solution of *phosphomolybdic acid* in *ethanol (96%)* and heat at 120° for 15 minutes. Any *secondary spot* in the chromatogram obtained with solution (1) is not more intense than the spot in the chromatogram obtained with solution (2) and not more than one such spot is more intense than the spot in the chromatogram obtained with solution (3).

Loss on drying When dried to constant weight at 105°, loses not more than 0.5% of its weight. Use 1 g.

Sulphated ash Not more than 0.1%, Appendix IX A.

Assay Dissolve 0.2 g in 40 ml of *tetrahydrofuran*, add 10 ml of a 10% w/v solution of *silver nitrate* and titrate with 0.1M *sodium hydroxide VS*, determining the end-point potentiometrically. Repeat the operation without the substance being examined. The difference between the titrations represents the amount of sodium hydroxide required. Each ml of 0.1M *sodium hydroxide VS* is equivalent to 0.02844 g of $C_{20}H_{28}O$.

Storage Lynoestrenol should be kept in a well-closed container and protected from light.

Action and use Progestogen.

In some countries the material described in this monograph may be known as Lynestrenol.

Macrogol 300
Polyethylene Glycol 300

25322-68-3

Macrogol 300 is a mixture of the poly-condensation products of ethylene oxide and water obtained under controlled conditions. It is represented by the formula $CH_2(OH)\cdot(CH_2\cdot O\cdot CH_2)_m\cdot CH_2OH$, where m is 5 or 6.

Characteristics A clear, colourless, viscous liquid; odour, faint and characteristic.

Solubility Miscible with *water*, with *ethanol (96%)* and with glycols; practically insoluble in *ether*.

Acidity or alkalinity pH of a 5% w/v solution, 4.0 to 7.0, Appendix V L.

Colour of solution A 50% w/v solution is not more intensely coloured than *reference solution BY_6*, Appendix IV B, Method I.

Hydroxyl value 356 to 394, Appendix X D. Use 0.75 g.

Refractive index 1.462 to 1.466, Appendix V E.

Viscosity At 25°, 59 to 73 mm^2 s^{-1}, Appendix V H, Method I, using a size-E U-tube viscometer.

Weight per ml 1.120 to 1.130 g, Appendix V G.

Ethylene oxide Place 200 g in a 1000-ml round-bottomed flask provided with an air-inlet tube reaching almost to the bottom and a thermometer and connected in series to three absorption vessels, each containing 50 ml of a 45% w/v solution of *magnesium bromide* in 0.01M *sulphuric acid VS*. Maintain the flask at 60° and pass a current of air through the liquid at a rate of about 300 ml per minute.

After 2 hours, disconnect the absorption vessels and titrate the contents separately with 0.02M *sodium hydroxide VS* using *bromocresol green solution* as indicator, until the solution becomes blue. Repeat the titration using 50 ml of the magnesium bromide solution. The difference between the volume of 0.02M *sodium hydroxide VS* required in the blank titration and one-third of the total volume required by the contents of the absorption vessels is not more than 1.5 ml.

Sulphated ash Not more than 0.1% w/w, Appendix IX A.

Water Not more than 1.0% w/w, Appendix IX C. Use 2.5 g.

Action and use Pharmaceutical aid.

Macrogol 1540
Polyethylene Glycol 1540

25322-68-3

Macrogol 1540 is a mixture of the polycondensation products of ethylene oxide and water obtained under controlled conditions. It is represented by the formula $CH_2(OH) \cdot (CH_2 \cdot O \cdot CH_2)_m \cdot CH_2OH$, where m is 28 to 36.

Characteristics A creamy-white, soft, wax-like solid; odour, faint and characteristic.

Solubility Freely soluble in *water* and in *chloroform*; sparingly soluble in *absolute ethanol*; practically insoluble in *ether*.

Acidity or alkalinity pH of a 5% w/v solution, 4.0 to 7.0, Appendix V L.

Colour of solution A 25% w/v solution is not more intensely coloured than *reference solution BY_6*, Appendix IV B, Method I.

Hydroxyl value 70 to 86, Appendix X D. Use 5 g.

Freezing point 42° to 46°, Appendix V B.

Viscosity At 100°, 25 to 32 mm² s⁻¹, Appendix V H, Method I, using a size-D U-tube viscometer.

Sulphated ash Not more than 0.1%, Appendix IX A.

Action and use Pharmaceutical aid.

Macrogol 4000
Polyethylene Glycol 4000

25322-68-3

Macrogol 4000 is a mixture of the polycondensation products of ethylene oxide and water obtained under controlled conditions. It is represented by the formula $CH_2(OH) \cdot (CH_2 \cdot O \cdot CH_2)_m \cdot CH_2OH$, where m is 69 to 84.

Characteristics A creamy-white, hard, wax-like solid, powder or flakes; odour, faint and characteristic.

Solubility Soluble in 3 parts of *water*, in 2 parts of *ethanol* (96%) and in 2 parts of *chloroform*; practically insoluble in *ether*.

Acidity or alkalinity pH of a 5% w/v solution, 4.5 to 7.5, Appendix V L.

Colour of solution A 20.0% w/v solution is not more intensely coloured than *reference solution BY_6*, Appendix IV B, Method I.

Hydroxyl value 30 to 36, Appendix X D. Use 20 g.

Freezing point 53° to 56°, Appendix V B.

Viscosity At 100°, 76 to 110 mm² s⁻¹, Appendix V H, Method I, using a size-E U-tube viscometer.

Sulphated ash Not more than 0.1%, Appendix IX A.

Action and use Pharmaceutical aid.

Magnesium Acetate

$C_4H_6MgO_4,4H_2O$ 214.5   *142-72-3*

Magnesium Acetate contains not less than 98.0 per cent and not more than 100.5 per cent of $C_4H_6MgO_4,4H_2O$.

Characteristics Colourless crystals or a white, crystalline powder; odourless or almost odourless.

Solubility Soluble in 1.5 parts of *water* and in 4 parts of *ethanol (96%)*.

Identification Yields the *reactions* characteristic of magnesium salts and of acetates, Appendix VI.

Alkalinity pH of a 5% w/v solution, 7.5 to 8.5, Appendix V L.

Aluminium Dissolve 4.0 g in 100 ml of *water* and add 10 ml of *acetate buffer pH 6.0*. The resulting solution complies with the *limit test for aluminium*, Appendix VII (1 ppm).

Calcium 1.0 g dissolved in sufficient *water* to produce 15 ml complies with the *limit test for calcium*, Appendix VII (100 ppm).

Heavy metals Dissolve 1.0 g in 20 ml of *water*. 12 ml of the resulting solution complies with *limit test A for heavy metals*, Appendix VII (40 ppm). Use *lead standard solution (2 ppm Pb)* to prepare the standard.

Potassium Not more than 0.1% of K when determined by *atomic emission spectrophotometry*, Appendix II D, Method II, using a 0.5% w/v solution and measuring at 766.7 nm. Use *potassium solution ASp*, suitably diluted with *water*, for the standard solution.

Sodium Not more than 0.5% of Na when determined by *atomic emission spectrophotometry*, Appendix II D, Method II, using a 1.0% w/v solution and measuring at 589.0 nm. Use *sodium solution ASp*, suitably diluted with *water*, for the standard solution.

Chloride Dissolve 1.0 g in 100 ml of *water*. 15 ml of the resulting solution complies with the *limit test for chlorides*, Appendix VII (330 ppm).

Nitrate Dissolve 1.0 g in 10 ml of *water*, add 5 mg of *sodium chloride*, 0.05 ml of *indigo carmine solution* and, with stirring, 10 ml of *nitrogen-free sulphuric acid*. A blue colour is produced which persists for at least 10 minutes.

Sulphate 0.25 g complies with the *limit test for sulphates*, Appendix VII (600 ppm).

Readily oxidisable substances Dissolve 2.0 g in 100 ml of boiling water, add 6 ml of 5M *sulphuric acid* and 0.3 ml of 0.02M *potassium permanganate*, mix and boil gently for 5 minutes. The pink colour is not completely discharged.

Assay Carry out the *complexometric titration of magnesium*, Appendix VIII D, using 0.5 g. Each ml of 0.1M *disodium edetate VS* is equivalent to 0.02145 g of $C_4H_6MgO_4,4H_2O$.

Storage Magnesium Acetate should be kept in a well-closed container.

Action and use Used in solutions for haemodialysis and peritoneal dialysis.

Heavy Magnesium Carbonate ☆

546-93-0

Heavy Magnesium Carbonate is a hydrated basic magnesium carbonate. It contains the equivalent of not less than 40.0 per cent and not more than 45.0 per cent of MgO.

Characteristics A white powder; odourless. 15 g occupies a volume of about 30 ml.

Solubility Practically insoluble in *water*. It dissolves in dilute acids with strong effervescence.

Identification A. Dissolve 15 mg in 2 ml of 2M *nitric acid* and neutralise with 2M *sodium hydroxide*. The resulting solution yields *reaction A* characteristic of magnesium salts, Appendix VI.

B. Yields *reaction A* characteristic of carbonates, Appendix VI.

Colour of solution Dissolve 5.0 g in 100 ml of 2M *acetic acid*. When effervescence has ceased, boil for 2 minutes, cool and dilute to 100 ml with 2M *acetic acid*, filtering, if necessary, through a previously ignited and tared porcelain or silica crucible of suitable porosity to give a clear filtrate (solution A). Reserve any residue for the test for Substances insoluble in acetic acid. The solution is not more intensely coloured than *reference solution B_4*, Appendix IV B, Method II.

Arsenic 10 ml of solution A complies with the *limit test for arsenic*, Appendix VII (2 ppm).

Calcium Dilute 2.6 ml of solution A to 150 ml with *distilled water*. 15 ml of the resulting solution complies with the *limit test for calcium*, Appendix VII (0.75%).

Heavy metals To 20 ml of solution A add 15 ml of 7M *hydrochloric acid* and shake with 25 ml of *4-methylpentan-2-one* for 2 minutes. Separate the layers, evaporate the aqueous layer to dryness, dissolve the residue in 1 ml of 5M *acetic acid* and dilute to 20 ml with *water*. 12 ml of the resulting solution complies with *limit test A for heavy metals*, Appendix VII (20 ppm). Use *lead standard solution (1 ppm Pb)* to prepare the standard.

Iron Dissolve 0.1 g in 3 ml of 2M *hydrochloric acid* and dilute to 10 ml with *water*. 2.5 ml of the resulting solution diluted to 10 ml with *water* complies with the *limit test for iron*, Appendix VII (400 ppm).

Chloride 1.5 ml of solution A diluted to 15 ml with *distilled water* complies with the *limit test for chlorides*, Appendix VII (0.07%).

Sulphate 0.5 ml of solution A diluted to 15 ml with *distilled water* complies with the *limit test for sulphates*, Appendix VII (0.6%).

Soluble substances Mix 2 g with 100 ml of *water*, boil for 5 minutes, filter whilst hot through a sintered-glass filter (BS porosity No. 3), allow to cool and dilute to 100 ml with *water*. Evaporate 50 ml of the filtrate to dryness. The residue, when dried at 100° to 105°, weighs not more than 10 mg (1.0%).

Substances insoluble in acetic acid Any residue obtained during the preparation of solution A, when washed, dried and ignited at 600°, weighs not more than 2.5 mg (0.05%).

Assay Dissolve 0.15 g in 20 ml of *water* to which has been added 2 ml of 2M *hydrochloric acid* and carry out the *complexometric titration of magnesium*, Appendix VIII D. Each ml of 0.1M *disodium edetate VS* is equivalent to 0.004030 g of MgO.

Action and use Antacid; osmotic laxative.

Light Magnesium Carbonate ☆

546-93-0

Light Magnesium Carbonate is a hydrated basic magnesium carbonate. It contains the equivalent of not less than 40.0 per cent and not more than 45.0 per cent of MgO.

Characteristics A white powder; odourless. 15 g occupies a volume of about 180 ml.

Solubility Practically insoluble in *water*. It dissolves in dilute acids with strong effervescence.

Identification; Colour of solution; Arsenic; Calcium; Heavy metals; Iron; Chloride; Soluble substances; Substances insoluble in acetic acid Complies with the requirements stated under Heavy Magnesium Carbonate.

Sulphate 1 ml of solution A diluted to 15 ml with *distilled water* complies with the *limit test for sulphates*, Appendix VII (0.3%).

Assay Dissolve 0.15 g in 20 ml of *water* to which has been added 2 ml of 2M *hydrochloric acid* and carry out the *complexometric titration of magnesium*, Appendix VIII D. Each ml of 0.1M *disodium edetate VS* is equivalent to 0.004030 g of MgO.

Preparation
Aromatic Magnesium Carbonate Mixture

Action and use Antacid; osmotic laxative.

Magnesium Chloride ☆

$MgCl_2,6H_2O$ 203.3   *7791-18-6*

Magnesium Chloride* contains not less than 98.0 per cent and not more than 101.0 per cent of $MgCl_2,6H_2O$.

Characteristics Colourless crystals; hygroscopic.

Solubility Soluble in 1 part of *water* and in 2 parts of *ethanol (96%)*.

Identification Yields *reaction A* characteristic of magnesium salts and *reaction A* characteristic of chlorides, Appendix VI.

Acidity or alkalinity To 5 ml of a 10.0% w/v solution in *carbon dioxide-free water* prepared from *distilled water* (solution A) add 0.05 ml of *phenol red solution*. Not more than 0.3 ml of either 0.01M *hydrochloric acid VS* or 0.01M *sodium hydroxide VS* is required to change the colour of the solution.

Clarity and colour of solution Solution A is *clear*, Appendix IV A, and *colourless*, Appendix IV B, Method II.

Arsenic 0.50 g complies with the *limit test for arsenic*, Appendix VII (2 ppm).

Calcium Dilute 1 ml of solution A to 15 ml with *distilled water*. The resulting solution complies with the *limit test for calcium*, Appendix VII (0.1%).

Heavy metals 12 ml of solution A complies with *limit test A for heavy metals*, Appendix VII (10 ppm). Use *lead standard solution (1 ppm Pb)* to prepare the standard.

Iron 10 ml of solution A complies with the *limit test for iron*, Appendix VII (10 ppm).

Sulphate 15 ml of solution A complies with the *limit test for sulphates*, Appendix VII (100 ppm).

Assay Dissolve 0.3 g in 50 ml of *water* and carry out the *complexometric titration of magnesium*, Appendix VIII D. Each ml of 0.1M *disodium edetate VS* is equivalent to 0.02033 g of $MgCl_2,6H_2O$.

Storage Magnesium Chloride should be kept in an airtight container.

Action and use Used in treatment of electrolyte deficiency.

*The magnesium chloride described in this monograph is not necessarily suitable for the preparation of dialysis solutions.

Magnesium Hydroxide ☆

$Mg(OH)_2$ 58.32   *1309-42-8*

Magnesium Hydroxide contains not less than 95.0 per cent and not more than 100.5 per cent of $Mg(OH)_2$.

Characteristics A white, fine, amorphous powder; odourless.

Solubility Practically insoluble in *water* yielding a solution which is alkaline to *phenolphthalein*. It dissolves in dilute acids.

Identification Dissolve 15 mg in 2 ml of 2M *nitric acid* and neutralise with 2M *sodium hydroxide*. The resulting solution yields *reaction A* characteristic of magnesium salts, Appendix VI.

Colour of solution Dissolve 5.0 g in a mixture of 50 ml of 6M *acetic acid* and 50 ml of *distilled water*. Not more than a slight effervescence is produced. Boil for 2 minutes, cool and dilute to 100 ml with 2M *acetic acid*. Filter, if necessary, through a previously ignited and tared porcelain or silica crucible of a suitable porosity to give a clear filtrate (solution A). Reserve any residue for the test for Substances insoluble in acetic acid. Solution A is not more intensely coloured than *reference solution B_3*, Appendix IV B, Method II.

Arsenic 5 ml of solution A complies with the *limit test for arsenic*, Appendix VII (4 ppm).

Calcium Dilute 1.3 ml of solution A to 150 ml with *distilled water*. 15 ml of the resulting solution complies with the *limit test for calcium*, Appendix VII (1.5%).

Heavy metals Dissolve 1.0 g in 15 ml of 7M *hydrochloric acid* and shake with 25 ml of *4-methylpentan-2-one* for 2 minutes. Separate the layers, evaporate the aqueous layer to dryness and dissolve the residue in 15 ml of *water*. 12 ml of the resulting solution complies with *limit test A for heavy metals*, Appendix VII (30 ppm). Use *lead standard solution (2 ppm Pb)* to prepare the standard.

Iron Dissolve 0.15 g in 5 ml of 2M *hydrochloric acid* and dilute to 10 ml with *water*. 1 ml of the resulting solution diluted to 10 ml with *water* complies with the *limit test for iron*, Appendix VII (0.07%).

Chloride 1 ml of solution A diluted to 15 ml with *water* complies with the *limit test for chlorides*, Appendix VII (0.1%).

Sulphate 0.6 ml of solution A diluted to 15 ml with *distilled water* complies with the *limit test for sulphates*, Appendix VII (0.5%).

Soluble substances Mix 2 g with 100 ml of *water* and boil for 5 minutes. Filter whilst hot through a sintered-glass filter (BS porosity No. 3), allow to cool and dilute to 100 ml with *water*. Evaporate 50 ml of the solution to dryness. The residue, when dried to constant weight at 100° to 105°, weighs not more than 20 mg (2.0%).

Substances insoluble in acetic acid Any residue obtained during the preparation of solution A when washed with *water*, dried and ignited at 600°, weighs not more than 5 mg (0.1%).

Loss on ignition When heated progressively to 900° and then ignited to constant weight, loses 30.0 to 32.5% of its weight. Use 0.5 g.

Assay Dissolve 0.1 g in 2 ml of 2M *hydrochloric acid* and carry out the *complexometric titration of magnesium*, Appendix VIII D. Each ml of 0.1M *disodium edetate VS* is equivalent to 0.005832 g of $Mg(OH)_2$.

Storage Magnesium Hydroxide should be kept in a well-closed container.

Action and use Antacid; osmotic laxative.

Heavy Magnesium Oxide ☆

MgO   40.30   *1309-48-4*

Heavy Magnesium Oxide contains not less than 98.0 per cent and not more than 100.5 per cent of MgO, calculated with reference to the substance ignited at 900°.

Characteristics A fine, white powder; odourless. 15 g occupies a volume of about 30 ml.

Solubility Practically insoluble in *water* yielding a solution which is alkaline to *phenolphthalein*. It dissolves in dilute acids with at most slight effervescence.

Identification Dissolve 15 mg in 2 ml of 2M *nitric acid* and neutralise with 2M *sodium hydroxide*. The resulting solution yields *reaction A* characteristic of magnesium salts, Appendix VI.

Colour of solution Dissolve 5.0 g in a mixture of 70 ml of 6M *acetic acid* and 30 ml of *distilled water*, boil for 2 minutes, cool and dilute to 100 ml with 2M *acetic acid*. Filter, if necessary, through a previously ignited and tared porcelain or silica crucible of suitable porosity to give a clear filtrate (solution A). Reserve any residue for the test for Substances insoluble in acetic acid. Solution A is not more intensely coloured than *reference solution B_3*, Appendix IV B, Method II.

Arsenic 5 ml of solution A complies with the *limit test for arsenic*, Appendix VII (4 ppm).

Calcium Dilute 1.3 ml of solution A to 150 ml with *distilled water*. 15 ml of the resulting solution complies with the *limit test for calcium*, Appendix VII (1.5%).

Heavy metals To 20 ml of solution A add 15 ml of 7M *hydrochloric acid* and shake with 25 ml of *4-methylpentan-2-one* for 2 minutes. Separate the layers, evaporate the aqueous layer to dryness, dissolve the residue in 1 ml of 6M *acetic acid* and dilute to 30 ml with *water*. 12 ml of the resulting solution complies with *limit test A for heavy metals*, Appendix VII (30 ppm). Use *lead standard solution (1 ppm Pb)* to prepare the standard.

Iron Dissolve 0.15 g in 5 ml of 2M *hydrochloric acid* and dilute to 10 ml with *water*. 1 ml of the resulting solution diluted to 10 ml with *water* complies with the *limit test for iron*, Appendix VII (0.07%).

Chloride 1 ml of solution A diluted to 15 ml with *water* complies with the *limit test for chlorides*, Appendix VII (0.1%).

Sulphate 0.3 ml of solution A diluted to 15 ml with *distilled water* complies with the *limit test for sulphates*, Appendix VII (1.0%).

Soluble substances Mix 2 g with 100 ml of *water* and boil for 5 minutes. Filter whilst hot through a sintered-glass filter (BS porosity No. 3), allow to cool and dilute to 100 ml with *water*. Evaporate 50 ml of the solution to dryness. The residue, when dried to constant weight at 100° to 105°, weighs not more than 20 mg (2.0%).

Substances insoluble in acetic acid Any residue obtained during the preparation of solution A, when washed with *water*, dried and ignited at 600°, weighs not more than 5 mg (0.1%).

Loss on ignition When ignited at 900°, loses not more than 8.0% of its weight. Use 1 g.

Assay Dissolve 0.7 g in 20 ml of 2M *hydrochloric acid* and dilute to 100 ml with *water*. Using 10 ml of the solution carry out the *complexometric titration of magnesium*, Appendix VIII D. Each ml of 0.1M *disodium edetate VS* is equivalent to 0.004030 g of MgO.

Storage Heavy Magnesium Oxide should be kept in a well-closed container.

Action and use Antacid.

Light Magnesium Oxide ☆
Light Magnesia

MgO   40.30   *1309-48-4*

Light Magnesium Oxide contains not less than 98.0 per cent of MgO, calculated with reference to the substance ignited at 900°.

Characteristics A white, fine, amorphous powder; odourless. 20 g occupies a volume of about 150 ml.

Solubility Practically insoluble in *water* yielding a solution which is alkaline to *phenolphthalein*. It dissolves in dilute acids with at most slight effervescence.

Identification; Arsenic; Calcium; Heavy metals; Sulphate; Soluble substances; Substances insoluble in acetic acid; Loss on ignition Complies with the requirements stated under Heavy Magnesium Oxide using, where necessary, solution A prepared in the test for colour of solution.

Colour of solution Dissolve 5.0 g in a mixture of 70 ml of 6M *acetic acid* and 30 ml of *distilled water*, boil for 2 minutes, cool and dilute to 100 ml with 2M *acetic acid*, filtering if necessary through a previously ignited and

tared porcelain or silica crucible of a suitable porosity to yield a clear filtrate (solution A). Solution A is not more intensely coloured than *reference solution B_2*, Appendix IV B, Method II.

Iron Dissolve 50 mg in 5 ml of 2M *hydrochloric acid* and dilute to 10 ml with *water*. 2 ml of the resulting solution complies with *limit test B for iron*, Appendix VII (0.1%).

Chloride 0.7 ml of solution A diluted to 15 ml with *water* complies with the *limit test for chlorides*, Appendix VII (0.15%).

Assay Dissolve 0.7 g in 20 ml of 2M *hydrochloric acid* and dilute to 100 ml with *water*. Using 10 ml of the solution carry out the *complexometric titration of magnesium*, Appendix VIII D. Each ml of 0.1M *disodium edetate VS* is equivalent to 0.004030 g of MgO.

Storage Light Magnesium Oxide should be kept in a well-closed container.

Preparation
Magnesium Hydroxide Mixture

Action and use Antacid; osmotic laxative.

Magnesium Stearate ☆

Magnesium Stearate consists mainly of magnesium stearate, $(C_{17}H_{35}CO_2)_2Mg$, with variable proportions of magnesium palmitate, $(C_{15}H_{31}CO_2)_2Mg$, and magnesium oleate, $(C_{17}H_{33}CO_2)_2Mg$. It contains not less than 3.8 per cent and not more than 5.0 per cent of Mg, calculated with reference to the dried substance.

Characteristics A very fine, light, white powder; odourless or with a very faint odour of stearic acid; unctuous.

Solubility Practically insoluble in *water*, in *absolute ethanol* and in *ether*.

Identification A. To 5.0 g add 50 ml of *ether*, 20 ml of 2M *nitric acid* and 20 ml of *distilled water* and heat under a reflux condenser until dissolution is complete. Allow to cool, separate the aqueous layer and shake the ether layer with two 4-ml quantities of *distilled water*. Combine the aqueous layers, wash with 15 ml of *ether* and dilute to 50 ml with *distilled water* (solution A). Evaporate the ether layer to dryness and dry the residue at 100° to 105°. The *freezing point* of the residue is not lower than 53°, Appendix V B.

B. 1 ml of solution A yields *reaction A* characteristic of magnesium salts, Appendix VI.

Acidity or alkalinity Mix 1 g with 20 ml of *carbon dioxide-free water*, boil for 1 minute, shaking continuously, cool and filter. To 10 ml of the filtrate add 0.05 ml of *bromothymol blue solution*. Not more than 0.05 ml of 0.1M *hydrochloric acid VS* or 0.1M *sodium hydroxide VS* is required to change the colour of the solution.

Colour of solution Solution A is not more intensely coloured than *reference solution Y_6*, Appendix IV B, Method II.

Acid value of the fatty acids 195 to 210, Appendix X B, using 0.2 g of the residue obtained in test A for Identification dissolved in 25 ml of the prescribed mixture of solvents.

Clarity and colour of solution of the fatty acids Dissolve 0.5 g of the residue obtained in test A for Identification in 10 ml of *chloroform*. The solution is *clear*, Appendix IV A, and not more intensely coloured than *reference solution Y₅*, Appendix IV B, Method II.

Heavy metals 1.0 g complies with *limit test D for heavy metals*, Appendix VII (20 ppm). Use 2 ml of *lead standard solution (10 ppm Pb)* to prepare the standard.

Chloride 2 ml of solution A diluted to 15 ml with *water* complies with the *limit test for chlorides*, Appendix VII (250 ppm).

Sulphate 0.3 ml of solution A diluted to 15 ml with *distilled water* complies with the *limit test for sulphates*, Appendix VII (0.5%).

Loss on drying When dried to constant weight at 100° to 105°, loses not more than 6.0% of its weight. Use 1 g.

Assay To 0.75 g add 25 ml of *butan-1-ol*, 25 ml of *absolute ethanol*, 5 ml of 13.5M *ammonia*, 3 ml of *ammonia buffer pH 10.0*, 30 ml of 0.1M *disodium edetate VS* and 15 mg of *mordant black 11 mixture*, heat to 45° to 50° and titrate with 0.1M *zinc sulphate VS* until the colour changes from blue to violet. Repeat the operation without the substance being examined. The difference between the titrations represents the amount of disodium edetate required. Each ml of 0.1M *disodium edetate VS* is equivalent to 0.002431 g of Mg.

Action and use Pharmaceutical aid.

Magnesium Sulphate ☆
Epsom Salts

$MgSO_4,7H_2O$ 246.5   *10034-99-8*

Magnesium Sulphate contains not less than 99.0 per cent and not more than 100.5 per cent of $MgSO_4$, calculated with reference to the dried substance.

Characteristics Brilliant, colourless crystals or a white, crystalline powder; odourless.

Solubility Soluble in 1.5 parts of *water*; very soluble in boiling *water*; practically insoluble in *ethanol (96%)*.

Identification Yields *reaction A* characteristic of magnesium salts and the *reactions* characteristic of sulphates, Appendix VI.

Acidity or alkalinity To 10 ml of a 10.0% w/v solution (solution A) add 0.05 ml of *phenol red solution*. Not more than 0.2 ml of either 0.01M *hydrochloric acid VS* or 0.01M *sodium hydroxide VS* is required to change the colour of the solution.

Clarity and colour of solution Solution A is *clear*, Appendix IV A, and *colourless*, Appendix IV B, Method II.

Arsenic 0.50 g complies with the *limit test for arsenic*, Appendix VII (2 ppm).

Heavy metals 12 ml of solution A complies with *limit test A for heavy metals*, Appendix VII (10 ppm). Use *lead standard solution (1 ppm Pb)* to prepare the standard.

Iron 5 ml of solution A diluted to 10 ml with *water* complies with the *limit test for iron*, Appendix VII (20 ppm).

Chloride 1.7 ml of solution A diluted to 15 ml with *water* complies with the *limit test for chlorides*, Appendix VII (300 ppm).

Loss on drying When dried at 110° to 120° for 1 hour and then at 400° to constant weight, loses 48.0 to 52.0% of its weight. Use 0.5 g.

Assay Dissolve 0.45 g in 100 ml of *water* and carry out the *complexometric titration of magnesium*, Appendix VIII D. Each ml of 0.1M *disodium edetate VS* is equivalent to 0.01204 g of $MgSO_4$.

Preparation
Magnesium Sulphate Mixture

Action and use Osmotic laxative.

Dried Magnesium Sulphate
Dried Epsom Salts

Dried Magnesium Sulphate may be prepared by drying magnesium sulphate at 100° until it has lost approximately 25 per cent of its weight. It contains not less than 62.0 per cent and not more than 70.0 per cent of $MgSO_4$.

Characteristics A white powder; odourless or almost odourless.

Solubility Soluble in 2 parts of *water*; more rapidly soluble in hot *water*.

Identification Yields the *reactions* characteristic of magnesium salts and of sulphates, Appendix VI.

Acidity or alkalinity To 10 ml of a 7.5% w/v solution in *carbon dioxide-free water* add 0.05 ml of *phenol red solution*. Not more than 0.2 ml of either 0.01M *hydrochloric acid VS* or 0.01M *sodium hydroxide VS* is required to change the colour of the solution.

Arsenic 0.33 g dissolved in 25 ml of *water* complies with the *limit test for arsenic*, Appendix VII (3 ppm).

Heavy metals Dissolve 1.3 g in 20 ml of *water* and add 1 g of *ammonium chloride*. 12 ml of the resulting solution complies with *limit test A for heavy metals*, Appendix VII (15 ppm). Use *lead standard solution (1 ppm Pb)* to prepare the standard.

Iron 0.33 g dissolved in 10 ml of *water* complies with the *limit test for iron*, Appendix VII (16 ppm).

Chloride 0.13 g dissolved in 15 ml of *water* complies with the *limit test for chlorides*, Appendix VII (500 ppm).

Insoluble matter 7.5 g dissolves in 20 ml of *water*, producing a solution which may be slightly turbid at first, but becomes clear in a few minutes.

Assay Dissolve 0.3 g in 50 ml of *water* and carry out the *complexometric titration of magnesium*, Appendix VIII D. Each ml of 0.1M *disodium edetate VS* is equivalent to 0.01204 g of $MgSO_4$.

Storage Dried Magnesium Sulphate should be kept in a well-closed container.

Preparation
Magnesium Sulphate Paste

Magnesium Trisilicate ☆

Magnesium Trisilicate Powder; Magnesium Trisilicate
Oral Powder

Magnesium Trisilicate is a hydrated magnesium
silicate of the approximate composition 2MgO,
3SiO$_2$, containing water of crystallisation.
It contains not less than the equivalent of
29.0 per cent of MgO and not less than the
equivalent of 65.0 per cent of SiO$_2$, both
calculated with reference to the substance
ignited at 900°.

Characteristics A white powder.

Solubility Practically insoluble in *water* and in *ethanol
(96%)*.

Identification A. To 2.0 g add a mixture of 4 ml of *nitric
acid* and 4 ml of *distilled water* and heat to boiling,
shaking frequently. Add 12 ml of *distilled water*, allow to
cool, filter or centrifuge to obtain a clear solution and
dilute the filtrate to 20 ml with *distilled water* (solution A).
Solution A, after neutralisation with 2M *sodium hydroxide*,
yields *reaction A* characteristic of magnesium salts,
Appendix VI.
B. 0.25 g yields the *reaction* characteristic of silicates,
Appendix VI.

Alkalinity In a tared 200-ml conical flask on a water-bath
heat 10 g with 100 g of *water* for 30 minutes, allow to cool
and restore the initial weight with *water*. Allow to stand,
filter and reserve the filtrate. To 10 ml of the clear filtrate
add 0.1 ml of *dilute phenolphthalein solution*. Not more
than 1.0 ml of 0.1M *hydrochloric acid VS* is required to
change the colour of the solution.

Arsenic 2.5 ml of solution A complies with the *limit test
for arsenic*, Appendix VII (4 ppm).

Heavy metals Neutralise 7.5 ml of solution A with 6M
ammonia using *metanil yellow solution* as external indicator,
dilute to 15 ml with *water* and filter if necessary. 12 ml of
the resulting solution complies with *limit test A for heavy
metals*, Appendix VII (40 ppm). Use *lead standard solution
(2 ppm Pb)* to prepare the standard.

Chloride 0.5 ml of solution A diluted to 15 ml with *water*
complies with the *limit test for chlorides*, Appendix VII
(500 ppm). Use a mixture of 5 ml of *chloride standard
solution (5 ppm Cl)* and 10 ml of *water* to prepare the
standard.

Sulphate 0.3 ml of solution A diluted to 15 ml with
distilled water complies with the *limit test for sulphates*,
Appendix VII (0.5%).

Acid absorption Not less than 100 ml of 0.1M *hydrochloric
acid VS* per g when determined by the following method.
Suspend 0.25 g in 0.1M *hydrochloric acid VS*, dilute to
100 ml with the same reagent and allow to stand for 2
hours in a water-bath at 36.5° to 37.5°, shaking frequently.
After cooling add 0.1 ml of *bromophenol blue solution* to
20 ml of the supernatant liquid and titrate with 0.1M
sodium hydroxide VS until a blue colour is produced.

Soluble salts In a tared platinum dish evaporate to
dryness on a water-bath 20 ml of the filtrate reserved in
the test for Alkalinity. The residue, ignited to constant
weight at 900°, weighs not more than 30 mg (1.5%).

Loss on ignition When ignited at 900°, loses 17 to 34% of
its weight. Use 0.5 g.

Assay *For MgO* To 1 g add 35 ml of *hydrochloric acid* and
60 ml of *water* and heat on a water-bath for 15 minutes.
Allow to cool, filter, wash the residue with *water* and
dilute the combined filtrate and washings to 250 ml with
water. Neutralise 50 ml with 10M *sodium hydroxide* (about
8 ml) and carry out the *complexometric titration of
magnesium*, Appendix VIII D. Each ml of 0.1M *disodium
edetate VS* is equivalent to 0.004030 g of MgO.

For SiO$_2$ To 0.7 g add 10 ml of 1M *sulphuric acid* and
10 ml of *water* and heat for 1.5 hours on a water-bath,
shaking frequently and replacing the evaporated water.
Allow to cool, decant onto an ashless filter paper 7 cm in
diameter, wash the precipitate by decantation with three
5-ml quantities of hot *water*, transfer it to the filter paper
and wash it with hot *water* until 1 ml of the filtrate
remains clear on the addition of 2 ml of 0.25M *barium
chloride* and 0.05 ml of 2M *hydrochloric acid*. Ignite the
filter paper and its contents in a tared platinum crucible at
900° to constant weight. The residue is SiO$_2$.

Storage Magnesium Trisilicate should be kept in a well-
closed container.

Preparations
Magnesium Trisilicate Mixture
Compound Magnesium Trisilicate Oral Powder
Compound Magnesium Trisilicate Tablets

Action and use Antacid.

Pregelatinised Maize Starch

Pregelatinised Maize Starch is prepared by
heating an aqueous slurry of Maize Starch and
removing the water from the resulting paste. It
contains no added substances but it may be
modified to render it compressible and to
improve its flow characteristics.

Characteristics A white to pale cream-coloured powder;
odourless or almost odourless. It disperses in cold *water*.

Microscopical Irregular, translucent, cream-coloured flakes
with a reticulated surface and numerous fragmented
flakes; very occasional starch grains with a well-marked
cross when viewed under polarised light.

Identification Disperse 0.5 g in 2 ml of *water* without
heating; a gel is produced. Add 0.05 ml of *iodine solution*;
a dark blue colour is produced.

Acidity or alkalinity pH of a 5% w/v dispersion in *water*,
4.5 to 7.0, Appendix V L.

Protein Not more than 0.5% w/w when determined by the
following method. Carry out Method I for the
determination of nitrogen, Appendix VIII H, using 5 g and
30 ml of *nitrogen-free sulphuric acid*. Calculate the content
of protein by multiplying the percentage of nitrogen in the
substance being examined by 6.25.

Loss on drying When dried to constant weight at 105°,
loses not more than 15.0% of its weight. Use 1 g.

Sulphated ash Not more than 0.5%, Appendix IX A.

Microbial contamination 1.0 g is free from *Escherichia
coli*, Appendix XVI B1.

Action and use Pharmaceutical aid.

Sterilisable Maize Starch

Sterilisable Maize Starch is prepared by treating maize starch by chemical and physical means so that it does not gelatinise on exposure to moisture. It contains magnesium oxide, in a proportion not greater than 2.2 per cent.

Characteristics A white, free-flowing powder; odourless or almost odourless.

Identification A. When boiled with 15 times its weight of *water* and cooled, a translucent viscous fluid or jelly is not produced. On the subsequent addition of *iodine solution* a purplish-blue or deep blue colour is produced.
B. Ignite 1 g, dissolve the residue in 5 ml of 2M *hydrochloric acid*, add a slight excess of 5M *ammonia* and 0.2 ml of *ammonium carbonate solution*, boil, filter, cool and add a 10% w/v solution of *diammonium hydrogen orthophosphate*. A white crystalline precipitate is produced.
C. When examined under a microscope, exhibits polyhedral or rounded granules about 5 to 30 μm, usually 10 to 20 μm, in diameter and having in the centre a distinct cavity or a two- to five-rayed cleft.

Alkalinity pH of a 10% w/v suspension, 9.5 to 10.8, Appendix V L.

Sedimentation Boil 100 ml of a 10% w/v suspension in *water* for 20 minutes, cool, transfer to a 100-ml graduated cylinder having the 100-ml graduation mark between 13 and 16 cm from the 10-ml graduation mark, replace the water lost by evaporation and allow to stand for 24 hours. The upper level of the starch is not below the 45-ml and not above the 75-ml graduation mark.

Chloride Fuse 0.30 g with 0.2 g of *anhydrous sodium carbonate* and 0.2 g of *potassium nitrate*, dissolve the residue in *water*, filter if necessary, neutralise to *litmus paper* by the dropwise addition of *nitric acid*, add 3 ml of 2M *nitric acid* and dilute to 135 ml with *water*. 15 ml of the resulting solution complies with the *limit test for chlorides*, Appendix VII (0.15%).

Sulphate To 0.30 g add 3 ml of *nitric acid* and 0.1 ml of *bromine* and allow to stand for 1 hour. Warm on a water-bath to remove the bromine, fuse the residue with 0.5 g of *anhydrous sodium carbonate* and 0.5 g of *potassium nitrate*, dissolve the residue in *water*, filter if necessary, neutralise to *litmus paper* by the dropwise addition of *hydrochloric acid*, add 10 ml of 2M *hydrochloric acid* and dilute to 60 ml with *water*. 15 ml of the resulting solution complies with the *limit test for sulphates*, Appendix VII (0.2%).

Formaldehyde Mix 1.0 g with 10 ml of a solution prepared by dissolving 2.72 g of *sodium acetate* in 60 ml of *water* and adding 22 ml of 1M *hydrochloric acid* and sufficient *water* to produce 100 ml. Adjust the pH to between 1.7 and 2.0 by the addition of 0.5M *hydrochloric acid*, add 5 ml of a freshly prepared 1% w/v solution of *phenylhydrazine hydrochloride* and allow to stand for 20 minutes. Filter rapidly, wash the residue with *water* and add to the combined filtrate and washings 1.25 ml of a 5% w/v solution of *potassium hexacyanoferrate(III)*. Allow to stand for 1 minute and add 5 ml of *hydrochloric acid* and sufficient *water* to produce 250 ml. The colour of the resulting solution is not more intense than that of a solution obtained by treating 1 ml of a solution containing 0.010% w/v of formaldehyde, CH_2O, in the same manner.

Magnesium oxide Dilute the combined filtrate and washings obtained in the test for Acid-insoluble ash with sufficient *water* to produce 100 ml. To 20 ml add 0.5 ml of a 10% w/v solution of *potassium cyanide* and 10 ml of *ammonia buffer pH 10.9*. Titrate with 0.05M *disodium edetate VS* using *mordant black 11 mixture* as indicator. Not more than 10.9 ml of 0.05M *disodium edetate VS* is required.

Acid-insoluble ash Not more than 0.3%, Appendix XI K. Reserve the filtrate and washings for the test for Magnesium oxide.

Ash Not more than 3.5%, Appendix XI J. Use 5 g.

Loss on drying When dried to constant weight at 105°, loses not more than 15.0% of its weight. Use 1 g.

Labelling The label states that care should be taken to avoid the use of excessive amounts of the powder on surgeons' gloves.

Action and use Lubricant for surgeons' gloves.

When Absorbable Dusting Powder is demanded, Sterilisable Maize Starch shall be supplied.

Maleic Acid ☆

HCCO₂H
‖
HCCO₂H

$C_4H_4O_4$ 116.1   *110-16-7*

Maleic Acid is (Z)-butenedioic acid. It contains not less than 99.0 per cent and not more than 101.0 per cent of $C_4H_4O_4$, calculated with reference to the anhydrous substance.

Characteristics A white, crystalline powder; odourless.

Solubility Soluble in 1.5 parts of *water* and in 2 parts of *ethanol (96%)*; sparingly soluble in *ether*.

Identification A. In the test for Fumaric acid, the principal spot in the chromatogram obtained with solution (2) is similar in position and size to that in the chromatogram obtained with solution (3).
B. To 0.3 ml of a 1% w/v solution add a solution of 10 mg of *resorcinol* in 3 ml of *sulphuric acid* and heat on a water-bath for 15 minutes; no colour is produced. To 3 ml of the 1% w/v solution add 1 ml of *bromine water*, heat on a water-bath to remove the bromine, heat to boiling and cool. To 0.2 ml of this solution add a solution of 10 mg of *resorcinol* in 3 ml of *sulphuric acid* and heat on a water-bath for 15 minutes; a violet-pink colour is produced.
C. The pH of a 5% w/v solution is less than 2, Appendix V L.

Clarity and colour of solution A 10.0% w/v solution is *clear*, Appendix IV A, and not more intensely coloured than *reference solution Y₇*, Appendix IV B, Method II.

Heavy metals 1.0 g complies with *limit test D for heavy metals*, Appendix VII (10 ppm). Use 1 ml of *lead standard solution (10 ppm Pb)* to prepare the standard.

Iron To 10 ml of a 10.0% w/v solution add 2 ml of 2M *hydrochloric acid* and 0.05 ml of *bromine water*. After 5 minutes pass a current of air through the solution to remove the excess of bromine, add 3 ml of a 9.7% w/v solution of *potassium thiocyanate*, shake and allow to stand for 5 minutes. Any red colour produced is not more intense than that of a standard solution prepared at the same time and in the same manner using a mixture of 5 ml of *iron standard solution (1 ppm Fe)*, 1 ml of 2M *hydrochloric acid*, 6 ml of *water* and 0.05 ml of *bromine water* (5 ppm).

Fumaric acid Carry out the method for *thin-layer chromatography*, Appendix III A, using *silica gel GF254* as the coating substance and a mixture of 44 volumes of *heptane*, 32 volumes of *butan-1-ol*, 16 volumes of *chloroform* and 12 volumes of *anhydrous formic acid* as the mobile phase but carrying out the chromatography in an unsaturated tank and allowing the solvent front to ascend 10 cm above the line of application. Apply separately to the chromatoplate 5 µl of each of solutions (1) to (4) and 10 µl of solution (5). Solutions (1) and (2) contain 10.0% w/v and 0.20% w/v respectively of the substance being examined in *acetone*. Solution (3) contains 0.20% w/v of *maleic acid EPCRS* in *acetone*. Solution (4) contains 0.15% w/v of *fumaric acid EPCRS* in *acetone*. Solution (5) is a mixture of equal volumes of solutions (3) and (4). After removal of the plate, dry it at 100° for 15 minutes and examine under *ultra-violet light (254 nm)*. Any spot corresponding to fumaric acid in the chromatogram obtained with solution (1) is not more intense than the spot in the chromatogram obtained with solution (4). The test is not valid unless the chromatogram obtained with solution (5) shows two clearly separated principal spots.

Sulphated ash Not more than 0.1%, Appendix IX A, Method II. Use 1 g.

Water Not more than 2.0% w/w, Appendix IX C. Use 1 g.

Assay Dissolve 0.5 g in 50 ml of *water* and titrate with 1M *sodium hydroxide VS* using 0.5 ml of *phenolphthalein solution* as indicator. Each ml of 1M *sodium hydroxide VS* is equivalent to 0.05804 g of $C_4H_4O_4$.

Storage Maleic Acid should be kept in a well-closed, glass container and protected from light.

Manganese Sulphate

$MnSO_4,4H_2O$ 223.1   *7785-87-7*

Manganese Sulphate is manganese(II) sulphate tetrahydrate. It contains not less than 98.0 per cent and not more than 100.5 per cent of $MnSO_4$, calculated with reference to the substance ignited at 450° to 500°.

Characteristics Pale pink crystals or crystalline powder; odourless or almost odourless.

Solubility Soluble in 1 part of *water*; practically insoluble in *ethanol (96%)*.

Identification A. Dissolve 0.5 g in 10 ml of *water* and add 1 ml of *sodium sulphide solution*. A pink precipitate is produced which is soluble in 6M *acetic acid*.
B. To 0.1 g add 2 g of *lead(IV) oxide* and 5 ml of *nitric acid*, boil gently for a few minutes, add 100 ml of *water* and filter. A purple solution is produced.
C. Yields the *reactions* characteristic of sulphates, Appendix VI.

Arsenic 0.25 g complies with the *limit test for arsenic*, Appendix VII (4 ppm).

Heavy metals Dissolve 0.50 g in 50 ml of *water*, add 1 ml of 1M *acetic acid* and pass *hydrogen sulphide* through the

solution for 20 seconds. The colour produced within 2 minutes is not more intense than that obtained by treating 10 ml of *lead standard solution (2 ppm Pb)* diluted to 50 ml in the same manner (40 ppm).

Iron Dissolve 1.0 g in 10 ml of *water* and add 2 ml of 1M *hydrochloric acid* and, dropwise, 0.05M *potassium permanganate* until a permanent pink colour is produced. Add 5 ml of a 10% w/v solution of *ammonium thiocyanate* and 20 ml of a mixture of equal volumes of *amyl alcohol* and *amyl acetate*, shake well and allow to separate. Any colour in the upper layer is not more intense than that obtained by treating 2 ml of *iron standard solution (20 ppm Fe)* diluted to 10 ml in the same manner (40 ppm).

Zinc Dissolve 2.0 g in 10 ml of *water*, add 3 ml of 1M *hydrochloric acid* and 0.3 ml of a freshly prepared 3% w/v solution of *potassium hexacyanoferrate(II)*, mix and allow to stand for 15 minutes. Any turbidity produced is not more intense than that obtained by treating 10 ml of *zinc standard solution (100 ppm Zn)* in the same manner (500 ppm).

Chloride 15 ml of a 1.0% w/v solution complies with the *limit test for chlorides*, Appendix VII (330 ppm).

Loss on ignition When ignited to constant weight at 450° to 500°, loses 31.0 to 34.0% of its weight.

Assay Dissolve 0.15 g in 40 ml of *water*, add 8 ml of freshly boiled and cooled *nitric acid*, cool, add 1.5 g of *sodium bismuthate* and shake for 2 minutes. Add 25 ml of a mixture of 3 volumes of *nitric acid* and 97 volumes of *water*, filter, wash the residue with 40 ml of the mixture, collecting the filtrate and washings in 50 ml of 0.1M *ammonium iron(II) sulphate VS*, and titrate immediately with 0.05M *potassium permanganate VS*. Repeat the operation without the substance being examined. The difference between the titrations represents the amount of ammonium iron(II) sulphate required. Each ml of 0.1M *ammonium iron(II) sulphate VS* is equivalent to 0.003020 g of $MnSO_4$.

Mannitol

```
    CH₂OH
    |
HOCH
    |
HOCH
    |
  HCOH
    |
  HCOH
    |
    CH₂OH
```

$C_6H_{14}O_6$ 182.2   *69-65-8*

Mannitol is D-mannitol. It contains not less than 98.0 per cent and not more than 102.0 per cent of $C_6H_{14}O_6$, calculated with reference to the dried substance.

Characteristics A white, crystalline powder; odourless or almost odourless.

Solubility Soluble in 6 parts of *water*; slightly soluble in *ethanol (96%)*; practically insoluble in *ether*.

Identification A. To 1 ml of a saturated solution add 0.5 ml of *iron(III) chloride test-solution* and then 0.25 ml of 5M *sodium hydroxide* and shake well. A clear solution is produced which remains clear on the further addition of 5M *sodium hydroxide*.

B. To 0.5 g add 3 ml of *acetic anhydride* and 1 ml of *pyridine*. Heat in boiling water, shaking frequently, for 15 minutes or until solution is complete and heat for a further 5 minutes. Allow to cool, add 20 ml of *water*, allow to stand for 5 minutes and collect the precipitate on a sintered-glass filter. The *melting point* of the precipitate, after recrystallisation from *ether*, is about 123°, Appendix V A.

Acidity Dissolve 5 g in 50 ml of *carbon dioxide-free water*. Not more than 0.3 ml of 0.02M *sodium hydroxide VS* is required for neutralisation using *phenolphthalein solution* as indicator.

Melting point 165° to 168°, Appendix V A.

Specific optical rotation To 5 g add 6.4 g of *sodium tetraborate* and sufficient *water* to produce about 45 ml, allow to stand for 1 hour, shaking occasionally, and dilute to 50 ml with *water*. The *specific optical rotation* in the resulting solution is +23° to +24°, Appendix V F.

Arsenic 0.50 g complies with the *limit test for arsenic*, Appendix VII (2 ppm).

Chloride 0.70 g complies with the *limit test for chlorides*, Appendix VII (70 ppm).

Sulphate 1.25 g complies with the *limit test for sulphates*, Appendix VII (120 ppm).

Absence of reducing sugars Dissolve 0.20 g in 2 ml of *water*, add 5 ml of *potassium cupri-tartrate solution* and heat in a water-bath for 5 minutes. Not more than a very slight precipitate is produced.

Loss on drying When dried to constant weight at 105°, loses not more than 0.5% of its weight. Use 1 g.

Sulphated ash Not more than 0.1%, Appendix IX A.

Assay Dissolve 0.4 g in sufficient *water* to produce 100 ml. Transfer 10 ml to a stoppered flask, add 20 ml of 0.1M *sodium metaperiodate* and 2 ml of 1M *sulphuric acid* and heat on a water-bath for 15 minutes. Cool, add 3 g of *sodium hydrogen carbonate* and 25 ml of 0.1M *sodium arsenite VS*, mix, add 5 ml of a 20% w/v solution of *potassium iodide*, allow to stand for 15 minutes and titrate with 0.05M *iodine VS* until the first trace of yellow colour appears. Repeat the operation without the substance being examined. The difference between the titrations represents the amount of iodine required. Each ml of 0.05M *iodine VS* is equivalent to 0.001822 g of $C_6H_{14}O_6$.

Preparation
Mannitol Intravenous Infusion

Matricaria Flowers ☆

Matricaria Flowers are the dried flower-heads of *Matricaria recutita* L. (*Chamomilla recutita* (L.) Rauschert).

Characteristics Odour, pleasant and aromatic; taste, slightly bitter.

Macroscopical Capitulum, when spread out, 10 to 17 mm in diameter, consisting of a receptacle, an involucre, 12 to 20 marginal ligulate florets and numerous central tubular florets; pedicel, 10 to 20 mm long, sometimes present. Receptacle hollow, 6 to 8 mm in diameter, hemispherical or conical, without paleae. Involucre consisting of 12 to 17 obovate to lanceolate bracts, about 2 mm × 0.5 mm, arranged in one to three rows with brownish-grey scarious margins. Ligulate florets white, up to 10 mm × 2 mm; base of corolla consisting of a light yellow tube, about 1.5 mm long, extending to an elongated oval, white ligule without a well-marked margin, with four veins converging in pairs towards three terminal teeth. Tubular florets, about 2.5 mm long, with yellow, five-toothed corolla broadening at the apex. Stamens syngenesious, with the filaments joined to the lower part of the corolla. Dark brown, oval to globular, inferior ovary at base of tubular and ligulate florets.

Microscopical Epidermal cells of the receptacle polygonal or rectangular in surface view, radially arranged at point of flower attachment. Underlying spongy tissue beneath, crossed by collateral radial vascular bundles, sometimes accompanied by fibres and several schizogenous secretory ducts. Involucral bracts, showing scarious margin with single layer of radially elongated cells; central part made up of chlorophyll-containing tissue covered with elongated epidermal cells with sinuous lateral walls, stomata and compositous glandular trichomes, and vascular bundles surrounded by numerous elongated, pitted sclereids with fairly large lumen. Corolla of ligulate and tubular florets in surface view showing isodiametric or elongated cells with more or less wavy walls and a few compositous glandular trichomes, the outer epidermis of ligulate florets consisting of papillose cells with cuticular striations radiating from their tips. In the mesophyll, very small cluster crystals of calcium oxalate sometimes present. Connective stamens with pitted and thickened cellular walls. Rounded to triangular pollen grains, diameter about 30 μm, with three pores and spiny exine. Ovaries of ligulate and tubular florets showing at the base a sclerous ring consisting of a single row of cells; the epidermis of the ovary composed of elongated cells with sinuous walls between which occur compositous glandular trichomes in longitudinal files alternating with elongated groups of scalariform cells containing mucilage, bursting easily to release the swollen mucilage. Numerous very small cluster crystals of calcium oxalate occur in the ovary.

Identification A. To 0.1 ml of solution (1) used in test B add 2.5 ml of a solution prepared by dissolving 0.25 g of *4-dimethylaminobenzaldehyde* in a mixture of 45 ml of 5M *acetic acid*, 5 ml of *orthophosphoric acid* and 45 ml of *water*. Heat on a water-bath for 5 minutes, allow to cool, add 5 ml of *petroleum spirit (boiling range, 60° to 80°)* and shake. The aqueous layer is distinctly greenish-blue to blue.

B. Carry out the method for *thin-layer chromatography*, Appendix III A, using *silica gel GF254* as the coating substance and *chloroform* as the mobile phase, but allowing the solvent front to ascend 10 cm above the line of application. Apply separately to the chromatoplate, as bands 20 mm × 3 mm, 10 μl of each of the following solutions. For solution (1) coarsely powder 1 g of the substance being examined in a porcelain mortar, transfer to a tube 15 cm × 15 mm, lightly tamp with a glass rod, rinse the mortar and pestle with two 10-ml quantities of *dichloromethane* and pour the solutions successively into the tube. Collect 15 ml of the percolate in a flask with a long, narrow neck, evaporate the solvent on a water-bath and dissolve the residue in 0.5 ml of *toluene*. For solution (2) dissolve 10 mg of d-*borneol*, 20 mg of d-*bornyl acetate* and 4 mg of *guaiazulene* in *toluene* and dilute to 10 ml with the same solvent. After removal of the plate, allow it to dry in air and examine under *ultra-violet light (254 nm)*. The chromatogram obtained with solution (1) shows a number of quenching areas, the largest of which has the same Rf value as the band due to *d*-bornyl acetate in the chromatogram obtained with solution (2) (enyne-dicycloether); there is also a band near the line of application (matricin). Spray the plate with *anisaldehyde solution*, using 10 ml for a plate 200 mm × 200 mm in size, heat at 100° to 105° for 5 to 10 minutes and examine in daylight while heating. The chromatogram obtained with solution (2) shows in the lower third a yellowish-brown band which becomes greyish-violet after a few hours (*d*-borneol), in the middle part a brownish-yellow to grey band (*d*-bornyl acetate) and in the upper third a blue band (guaiazulene). The chromatogram obtained with solution (1) shows a blue band near the line of application (matricin), several reddish-violet bands with Rf values between those of *d*-borneol and *d*-bornyl acetate (one of which is due to bisabolol), a brownish band with an Rf value similar to that of *d*-bornyl acetate (enyne-dicycloether) and red bands with Rf values similar to that of guaiazulene (terpenes). Other bands appear in the middle and lower parts of the chromatogram.

Broken flowers Not more than 25% passes through a sieve with a nominal mesh aperture of 710 μm.

Volatile oil Not less than 0.4% v/w of blue, volatile oil, Appendix XI E, using a 1000-ml flask, 300 ml of *water* as the distillation liquid and 0.50 ml of *xylene* in the graduated tube. Use 30 g and distil at a rate of 3 to 4 ml per minute for 4 hours.

Sulphated ash Not more than 13.0%, Appendix IX A, Method II. Use 1 g.

Storage Matricaria Flowers should be kept in a well-closed container and protected from light.

The title of the monograph in the European Pharmacopœia is Matricaria Flower.

Mebeverine Hydrochloride

CO·O·CH$_2$·(CH$_2$)$_2$·CH$_2$·NCH·CH$_2$ Me, Et

OMe, OMe, OMe, .HCl

C$_{25}$H$_{35}$NO$_5$,HCl   466.0   *2753-45-9*

Mebeverine Hydrochloride is 4-[ethyl(4-methoxy-α-methylphenethyl)amino]butyl veratrate hydrochloride. It contains not less than 99.0 per cent and not more than 101.0 per cent of C$_{25}$H$_{35}$NO$_5$,HCl, calculated with reference to the dried substance.

Characteristics A white or almost white, crystalline powder.

Solubility Very soluble in *water*; freely soluble in *ethanol* (96%); practically insoluble in *ether*.

Identification A. The *infra-red absorption spectrum*, Appendix II A, is concordant with the *reference spectrum* of mebeverine hydrochloride.

B. The *light absorption*, Appendix II B, in the range 230 to 350 nm of a 0.003% w/v solution in 0.1M *hydrochloric acid* exhibits a maximum at 263 nm and a less well-defined maximum at 292 nm. The *absorbance* at 263 nm is about 0.79 and at 292 nm is about 0.41.

C. Dissolve 25 mg in 2 ml of *water*, acidify with 2M *nitric acid* and centrifuge. The supernatant liquid yields *reaction A* characteristic of chlorides, Appendix VI, beginning at the words 'add 0.4 ml of . . .'.

D. *Melting point*, about 135°, Appendix V A.

Acidity pH of a 2% w/v solution, 4.5 to 6.5, Appendix V L.

Ether-soluble extractive Dissolve 40 mg in 25 ml of 2M *hydrochloric acid* and shake with 50 ml of *ether* for 1 minute. Wash the ether layer with three 25-ml quantities of *water*, evaporate the ether to dryness using a rotary evaporator and dissolve the residue in sufficient *methanol* to produce 20 ml. The *absorbance* of the resulting solution at 260 nm is not more than 0.23, Appendix II B.

Non-tertiary amine Dissolve 0.5 g in 5 ml of *pyridine*, add 5 ml of *copper chloride—pyridine reagent* and heat at 50° for 30 minutes. Cool, add sufficient *acetone* to produce 50 ml and measure the *absorbance* of the resulting solution at 405 nm, Appendix II B, using in the reference cell a solution obtained by treating 5 ml of *pyridine* in the same manner. The absorbance is not more than that obtained by repeating the test using 5 ml of a 0.0060% w/v solution of *di*-n-*butylamine* in *pyridine* and beginning at the words 'add 5 ml of *copper chloride—pyridine reagent* . . .'.

Related substances Carry out the method for *thin-layer chromatography*, Appendix III A, using a silica gel F254 precoated chromatoplate (Merck silica gel 60 F254 plates are suitable) and a mixture of 50 volumes of *absolute ethanol*, 50 volumes of *chloroform* and 1 volume of 18M *ammonia* as the mobile phase. Apply separately to the plate 10 μl of each of three solutions in *acetone* containing (1) 2.0% w/v of the substance being examined, (2) 0.010% w/v of the substance being examined and (3) 0.0020% w/v of *veratric acid*. After removal of the plate, allow it to dry in air and examine under *ultra-violet light (254 nm)*. Expose the plate to iodine vapour for 1 hour. When viewed under ultra-violet light any spot corresponding to veratric acid in the chromatogram obtained with solution (1) is not more intense than the spot in the chromatogram obtained with solution (3). Using both methods of visualisation any other *secondary* spot in the chromatogram obtained with solution (1) is not more intense than the spot in the chromatogram obtained with solution (2).

Loss on drying When dried at 105° for 1 hour, loses not more than 0.5% of its weight. Use 1 g.

Sulphated ash Not more than 0.1%, Appendix IX A.

Assay Carry out Method I for *non-aqueous titration*, Appendix VIII A, using 0.4 g and 7 ml of *mercury(II) acetate solution* and determining the end-point potentiometrically. Each ml of 0.1M *perchloric acid VS* is equivalent to 0.04660 g of C$_{25}$H$_{35}$NO$_5$,HCl.

Storage Mebeverine Hydrochloride should be kept in an airtight container, protected from light and stored at a temperature not exceeding 30°.

Preparation
Mebeverine Tablets

Action and use Antispasmodic.

Meclozine Hydrochloride

$C_{25}H_{27}ClN_2,2HCl$ 463.9   *1104-22-9*

Meclozine Hydrochloride is 1-(4-chloro-benzhydryl)-4-(3-methylbenzyl)piperazine dihydrochloride. It contains not less than 98.0 per cent and not more than 101.0 per cent of $C_{25}H_{27}ClN_2,2HCl$, calculated with reference to the anhydrous substance.

Characteristics A white or almost white, crystalline powder; odourless or almost odourless.

Solubility Slightly soluble in *water*; soluble in 25 parts of *ethanol (96%)* and in 5 parts of *chloroform*.

Identification A. The *infra-red absorption spectrum*, Appendix II A, is concordant with the *reference spectrum* of meclozine hydrochloride. If the spectra are not concordant dry the substance being examined at 60° at a pressure of 2 kPa for 3 hours, dissolve the residue in *chloroform IR* and prepare a new spectrum.
B. The *light absorption*, Appendix II B, in the range 220 to 350 nm of a 0.003% w/v solution in *ethanol (96%)* exhibits a maximum only at 230 nm. The *absorbance* at 230 nm is about 0.99.
C. Yields the *reactions* characteristic of chlorides, Appendix VI.

N-(3-Methylbenzyl)piperazine Carry out the method for *thin-layer chromatography*, Appendix III A, using *silica gel G* as the coating substance and a mixture of 75 volumes of *cyclohexane*, 15 volumes of *toluene* and 10 volumes of *diethylamine* as the mobile phase. Apply separately to the chromatoplate 10 μl of each of the following solutions. Solution (1) contains 10.0% w/v of the substance being examined in a mixture of equal volumes of *chloroform* and *methanol*. Solution (2) contains 0.050% w/v of N-(*3-methyl-benzyl)piperazine BPCRS* in *methanol*. After removal of the plate, dry it at 100° for 30 minutes and spray with a mixture of equal volumes of *acetone* and a mixture of 1 volume of a 10% w/v solution of *sodium hydroxide*, 1 volume of a 10% w/v solution of *sodium nitroprusside*, 1 volume of a 10% w/v solution of *potassium hexacyano-ferrate(III)* and 3 volumes of *water*. Any spot corresponding to *N*-(3-methylbenzyl)piperazine in the chromatogram obtained with solution (1) is not more intense than the spot in the chromatogram obtained with solution (2).

Sulphated ash Not more than 0.1%, Appendix IX A.

Water Not more than 5.0% w/w, Appendix IX C. Use 0.5 g.

Assay Carry out Method I for *non-aqueous titration*, Appendix VIII A, using 0.4 g, adding 5 ml of *acetic anhydride* to the solvent and using *oracet blue B solution* as indicator. Each ml of 0.1M *perchloric acid VS* is equivalent to 0.02319 g of $C_{25}H_{27}ClN_2,2HCl$.

Storage Meclozine Hydrochloride should be kept in a well-closed container.

Preparation
Meclozine Tablets

Action and use Anti-emetic.

Medazepam

$C_{16}H_{15}ClN_2$ 270.8   *2898-12-6*

Medazepam is 7-chloro-2,3-dihydro-1-methyl-5-phenyl-1*H*-1,4-benzodiazepine. It contains not less than 98.5 per cent and not more than 101.0 per cent of $C_{16}H_{15}ClN_2$, calculated with reference to the dried substance.

Characteristics A yellowish, crystalline powder; odourless or almost odourless.

Solubility Practically insoluble in *water*; soluble in 8 parts of *ethanol (96%)*, in 1 part of *chloroform* and in 5 parts of *ether*.

Identification A. The *infra-red absorption spectrum*, Appendix II A, is concordant with the *reference spectrum* of medazepam.
B. The *light absorption*, Appendix II B, in the range 230 to 320 nm of a 0.001% w/v solution in 0.1M *hydrochloric acid* exhibits a maximum only at 254 nm. The *absorbance* at 254 nm is about 0.86.
C. The *light absorption*, Appendix II B, in the range 360 to 550 nm of a 0.004% w/v solution in 0.1M *hydrochloric acid* exhibits a maximum only at 458 nm. The *absorbance* at 458 nm is about 0.64.

Melting point 101° to 104°, Appendix V A.

Related substances Carry out the method for *thin-layer chromatography*, Appendix III A, using a precoated silica gel F254 chromatoplate (Merck silica gel 60 F254 plates are suitable) and a mixture of 75 volumes of *chloroform* and 25 volumes of *ethyl acetate* as the mobile phase. Apply separately to the plate 20 μl of each of two solutions of the substance being examined in *ethyl acetate* containing (1) 2.5% w/v and (2) 0.0035% w/v. After removal of the plate, allow it to dry in air and examine under *ultra-violet light (254 nm)*. Any *secondary spot* in the chromatogram obtained with solution (1) is not more intense than the spot in the chromatogram obtained with solution (2).

Loss on drying When dried over *phosphorus pentoxide* at 80° at a pressure not exceeding 0.7 kPa for 4 hours, loses not more than 0.5% of its weight. Use 1 g.

Sulphated ash Not more than 0.1%, Appendix IX A.

Assay Dissolve 0.25 g in 75 ml of *acetic anhydride* and carry out Method I for *non-aqueous titration*, Appendix VIII A, determining the end-point potentiometrically. Each ml of 0.1M *perchloric acid VS* is equivalent to 0.02708 g of $C_{16}H_{15}ClN_2$.

Preparation
Medazepam Capsules

Action and use Anxiolytic.

Medroxyprogesterone Acetate

C₂₄H₃₄O₄   386.5   *71-58-9*

Medroxyprogesterone Acetate is 6α-methyl-3,20-dioxopregn-4-en-17α-yl acetate. It contains not less than 97.0 per cent and not more than 103.0 per cent of $C_{24}H_{34}O_4$, calculated with reference to the dried substance.

Characteristics A white or almost white, crystalline powder; odourless or almost odourless.

Solubility Practically insoluble in *water*; slightly soluble in *ethanol (96%)*, in *ether* and in *methanol*; soluble in 50 parts of *acetone*, in 10 parts of *chloroform* and in 60 parts of *1,4-dioxan*.

Identification A. The *infra-red absorption spectrum*, Appendix II A, is concordant with the *reference spectrum* of medroxyprogesterone acetate.
B. Complies with the test for *identification of steroids*, Appendix III A, using *impregnating solvent II* and *mobile phase E*.
C. Yields the *reaction* characteristic of acetyl groups, Appendix VI.
D. *Melting point*, about 204°, Appendix V A.

Specific optical rotation In a 1% w/v solution in *1,4-dioxan*, +45° to +51°, Appendix V F.

Related substances Carry out the method for *thin-layer chromatography*, Appendix III A, using *kieselguhr G* as the coating substance. Impregnate the dry chromatoplate by placing it in a tank containing a shallow layer of a mixture of 90 volumes of *acetone* and 10 volumes of *propane-1,2-diol*, allowing the solvent to ascend to the top, removing the plate from the tank and allowing the solvent to evaporate; use within 2 hours, with the flow of the mobile phase in the direction in which impregnation was carried out. Use a mixture of equal volumes of *cyclohexane* and *petroleum spirit (boiling range, 40° to 60°)* as the mobile phase. Apply separately to the plate 5 μl of each of three solutions of the substance being examined in *chloroform* containing (1) 0.50% w/v, (2) 0.015% w/v and (3) 0.0050% w/v. After removal of the plate, allow the solvent to evaporate and heat at 120° for 30 minutes. Spray with a 20% w/v solution of *toluene-p-sulphonic acid* in *ethanol (96%)*, heat at 120° for 10 minutes and expose to iodine vapour for 10 minutes. Any *secondary spot* in the chromatogram obtained with solution (1) is not more intense than the spot in the chromatogram obtained with solution (2) and not more than one such spot is more intense than the spot in the chromatogram obtained with solution (3).

Loss on drying When dried at 105° for 3 hours, loses not more than 0.5% of its weight. Use 1 g.

Sulphated ash Not more than 0.1%, Appendix IX A.

Assay Dissolve 0.1 g in sufficient *ethanol (96%)* to produce 100 ml, dilute 1 ml to 100 ml with *ethanol (96%)* and measure the *absorbance* of the resulting solution at the maximum at 241 nm, Appendix II B. Calculate the content of $C_{24}H_{34}O_4$ taking 426 as the value of A(1%, 1 cm) at the maximum at 241 nm.

Storage Medroxyprogesterone Acetate should be kept in a well-closed container and protected from light.

Action and use Progestogen.

Mefenamic Acid

C₁₅H₁₅NO₂   241.3   *61-68-7*

Mefenamic Acid is *N*-2,3-xylylanthranilic acid. It contains not less than 99.0 per cent and not more than 100.5 per cent of $C_{15}H_{15}NO_2$, calculated with reference to the dried substance.

Characteristics A white to greyish-white, microcrystalline powder; odourless or almost odourless.

Solubility Practically insoluble in *water*; slightly soluble in *ethanol (96%)* and in *chloroform*; sparingly soluble in *ether*.

Identification A. The *infra-red absorption spectrum*, Appendix II A, is concordant with the *reference spectrum* of mefenamic acid. If the spectra are not concordant dissolve a sufficient quantity in the minimum volume of *ethanol (96%)*, evaporate to dryness and prepare a new spectrum of the residue.
B. Dissolve 25 mg in 15 ml of *chloroform* and examine under ultra-violet light (254 nm); the solution exhibits a strong greenish-yellow fluorescence. Carefully add 0.5 ml of *trichloroacetic acid* dropwise and examine under ultra-violet light (254 nm); the solution does not exhibit fluorescence.
C. Dissolve 5 mg in 2 ml of *sulphuric acid* and add 0.05 ml of 0.0167M *potassium dichromate*. An intense blue colour is produced immediately, fading rapidly to brownish-green.

Light absorption *Absorbance* of a 0.002% w/v solution in a mixture of 1 volume of 1M *hydrochloric acid* and 99 volumes of *methanol* at the maximum at 279 nm, 0.69 to 0.74 and at the maximum at 350 nm, 0.56 to 0.60, Appendix II B.

Copper Moisten 1.0 g with *sulphuric acid* and ignite until all the carbon is removed. Add 10 ml of 1M *sulphuric acid* to the residue and allow to stand for 10 minutes. Transfer to a separating funnel using 20 ml of *water* and add 10 ml of a solution containing 20% w/v of *diammonium hydrogen citrate* and 5% w/v of *disodium edetate*. Add 0.2 ml of *thymol blue solution* and neutralise with 5M *ammonia*. Add 10 ml of *sodium diethyldithiocarbamate solution* and 15 ml of *carbon tetrachloride*, shake and allow to separate. The yellow colour of the carbon tetrachloride layer is not more intense than that produced by treating 2 ml of *copper standard solution (10 ppm Cu)* in the same manner, beginning at the words 'Transfer to a separating funnel using . . .'.

Related substances Carry out the method for *thin-layer chromatography*, Appendix III A, using *silica gel GF254* as the coating substance and a mixture of 90 volumes of *toluene*, 25 volumes of *1,4-dioxan* and 1 volume of *glacial acetic acid* as the mobile phase. Apply separately to the chromatoplate 20 µl of each of two solutions of the substance being examined in a mixture of 3 volumes of *chloroform* and 1 volume of *methanol* containing (1) 2.5% w/v and (2) 0.0050% w/v. After removal of the plate, allow it to dry in air, expose to iodine vapour for 5 minutes and examine under *ultra-violet light (254 nm)*. Any *secondary spot* in the chromatogram obtained with solution (1) is not more intense than the spot in the chromatogram obtained with solution (2).

2,3-Dimethylaniline Not more than 100 ppm when determined by the following method. Into two flat-bottomed tubes place separately (1) 2 ml of a 2.5% w/v solution of the substance being examined in a mixture of 3 volumes of *chloroform* and 1 volume of *methanol* and (2) a mixture of 1 ml of a 0.0005% w/v solution of *2,3-dimethyl-aniline* in *methanol* and 1 ml of *chloroform*. To each tube add 1 ml of a freshly prepared 1% w/v solution of *4-dimethylaminobenzaldehyde* in *methanol* and 2 ml of *glacial acetic acid* and allow to stand for 10 minutes. The yellow colour in tube (1) is not more intense than that in tube (2).

Loss on drying When dried to constant weight at 105°, loses not more than 0.5% of its weight. Use 1 g.

Sulphated ash Not more than 0.1%, Appendix IX A.

Assay Dissolve 0.6 g in 100 ml of warm *absolute ethanol* previously neutralised to *phenol red solution* and titrate with 0.1M *sodium hydroxide VS* using *phenol red solution* as indicator. Each ml of 0.1M *sodium hydroxide VS* is equivalent to 0.02413 g of $C_{15}H_{15}NO_2$.

Storage Mefenamic Acid should be kept in a well-closed container.

Preparation
Mefenamic Acid Capsules

Action and use Anti-inflammatory; analgesic.

Megestrol Acetate

$C_{24}H_{32}O_4$ 384.5   *595-33-5*

Megestrol Acetate is 6-methyl-3,20-dioxo-pregna-4,6-dien-17α-yl acetate. It contains not less than 97.0 per cent and not more than 103.0 per cent of $C_{24}H_{32}O_4$, calculated with reference to the dried substance.

Characteristics A white to creamy-white, crystalline powder; odourless or almost odourless.

Solubility Practically insoluble in *water*; soluble in 55 parts of *ethanol (96%)* and in 0.8 part of *chloroform*; slightly soluble in *ether* and fixed oils.

Identification A. The *infra-red absorption spectrum*, Appendix II A, is concordant with the *reference spectrum* of megestrol acetate.

B. Complies with the test for *identification of steroids*, Appendix III A, using *impregnating solvent II* and *mobile phase D*.

C. Yields the *reaction* characteristic of acetyl groups, Appendix VI.

D. *Melting point*, about 217°, Appendix V A.

Light absorption The *light absorption*, Appendix II B, in the range 230 to 350 nm of the solution obtained in the Assay exhibits a maximum only at 287 nm. The ratio of the *absorbance* at 240 nm to that at the maximum at 287 nm is not more than 0.17.

Specific optical rotation In a 5% w/v solution in *chloroform*, +9° to +12°, Appendix V F.

Related foreign steroids Carry out the method for *thin-layer chromatography*, Appendix III A, using *silica gel G* as the coating substance and a mixture of 92 volumes of *1,2-dichloroethane*, 8 volumes of *methanol* and 0.5 volume of *water* as the mobile phase. Apply separately to the chromatoplate 1 µl of each of two solutions in a mixture of 9 volumes of *chloroform* and 1 volume of *methanol* containing (1) 5.0% w/v of the substance being examined and (2) 0.025% w/v of *megestrol BPCRS*. After removal of the plate, allow it to dry in air until the odour of the solvent is no longer detectable, spray with *ethanolic sulphuric acid (20%)*, heat at 110° for 10 minutes and examine under *ultra-violet light (365 nm)*. Any *secondary spot* in the chromatogram obtained with solution (1) is not more intense than the spot in the chromatogram obtained with solution (2).

Loss on drying When dried to constant weight at 105°, loses not more than 0.5% of its weight. Use 1 g.

Sulphated ash Not more than 0.1%, Appendix IX A.

Assay Dissolve 10 mg in sufficient *absolute ethanol* to produce 100 ml, dilute 5 ml to 50 ml with *absolute ethanol* and measure the *absorbance* of the resulting solution at the maximum at 287 nm, Appendix II B. Calculate the content of $C_{24}H_{32}O_4$ taking 630 as the value of A(1%, 1 cm) at the maximum at 287 nm.

Storage Megestrol Acetate should be protected from light.

Action and use Progestogen.

Meglumine

$C_7H_{17}NO_5$ 195.2   *6284-40-8*

Meglumine is 1-deoxy-1-methylamino-D-glucitol. It contains not less than 99.0 per cent and not more than 100.5 per cent of $C_7H_{17}NO_5$, calculated with reference to the dried substance.

Characteristics A white, microcrystalline powder; odour, slight.

Solubility Soluble in 1 part of *water*; slightly soluble in *ethanol (96%)*; practically insoluble in *chloroform* and in *ether*.

Identification A. Dissolve 0.2 g in 2 ml of *water* and neutralise with 0.5M *sulphuric acid* using 0.05 ml of *methyl red solution* as indicator. To 1 ml of the solution add 2 ml of a freshly prepared mixture of 1 ml of *acetaldehyde* and 10 ml of a 1% w/v solution of *sodium nitroprusside* and then 2 ml of *sodium carbonate solution*. A blue colour is produced slowly.
B. To the remainder of the solution used in test A add 0.5 ml of 0.1M *sodium hydroxide* and 0.5 g of *boric acid*. The solution becomes distinctly acidic.

Melting point 128° to 131°, Appendix V A.

Specific optical rotation In a 10% w/v solution, −16.0° to −17.0°, Appendix V F.

Reducing sugars Dissolve 0.25 g in 5 ml of *water*, add 5 ml of *potassium cupri-tartrate solution*, boil for 1 minute and filter. No red colour is visible on the filter.

Loss on drying When dried to constant weight at 105°, loses not more than 1.0% of its weight. Use 1 g.

Sulphated ash Not more than 0.1%, Appendix IX A.

Assay Dissolve 0.8 g in 20 ml of *water* and titrate with 0.05M *sulphuric acid VS* using *methyl red—methylene blue solution* as indicator. Each ml of 0.05M *sulphuric acid VS* is equivalent to 0.01952 g of $C_7H_{17}NO_5$.

Meglumine intended for use in the manufacture of a parenteral dosage form complies with the following additional requirement.

Pyrogens Complies with the *test for pyrogens*, Appendix XIV K. Use 0.6 g per kg of the rabbit's weight dissolved in not more than 5 ml of *water for injections*.

Melphalan

$(ClCH_2 \cdot CH_2)_2N$—⟨benzene ring⟩—CH_2—$\underset{\underset{H}{|}}{\overset{\overset{NH_2}{|}}{C}}$—$CO_2H$

$C_{13}H_{18}Cl_2N_2O_2$　　305.2　　*148-82-3*

Melphalan is 4-bis(2-chloroethyl)amino-L-phenylalanine. It contains not less than 93.0 per cent and not more than 100.5 per cent of $C_{13}H_{18}Cl_2N_2O_2$, calculated with reference to the dried substance.

Characteristics A white or almost white powder; odourless or almost odourless.

Solubility Practically insoluble in *water*, in *chloroform* and in *ether*; slightly soluble in *methanol*. It dissolves in dilute mineral acids.

Identification A. The *light absorption*, Appendix II B, in the range 230 to 350 nm of a 0.001% w/v solution in *methanol* exhibits a maximum at 260 nm and a less well-defined maximum at 301 nm.
B. Dissolve 20 mg in 50 ml of *methanol* with the aid of gentle heat, add 1 ml of a 5% w/v solution of *4-(4-nitrobenzyl)pyridine* in *acetone* and evaporate to dryness. Dissolve the residue in 1 ml of hot *methanol* and add 0.1 ml of 13.5M *ammonia*. A red colour is produced.
C. Heat 0.1 g with 10 ml of 0.1M *sodium hydroxide* for 10 minutes on a water-bath. The resulting solution, after acidification with 2M *nitric acid*, yields *reaction A* characteristic of chlorides, Appendix VI.
D. A 0.5% w/v solution in *methanol* is laevorotatory.

E. *Melting point*, about 177°, with decomposition, Appendix V A.

Ionisable chlorine Dissolve 0.4 g in a mixture of 75 ml of *water* and 2 ml of *nitric acid*, allow to stand for 2 minutes and titrate with 0.1M *silver nitrate VS* determining the end-point potentiometrically. Not more than 0.8 ml is required.

Loss on drying When dried at 100° at a pressure not exceeding 0.7 kPa for 2 hours, loses not more than 7.0% of its weight. Use 1 g.

Sulphated ash Not more than 0.3%, Appendix IX A.

Assay To 0.4 g add 20 ml of a 20% w/v solution of *potassium hydroxide*, heat on a water-bath for 2 hours, replacing water lost by evaporation, and cool. Add 75 ml of *water* and 4 ml of *nitric acid*, cool and titrate with 0.1M *silver nitrate VS* determining the end-point potentiometrically. Subtract the volume of 0.1M *silver nitrate VS* used in the test for Ionisable chlorine. Each ml of 0.1M *silver nitrate VS* represented by the difference is equivalent to 0.01526 g of $C_{13}H_{18}Cl_2N_2O_2$.

Storage Melphalan should be kept in a well-closed container, protected from light and stored at a temperature not exceeding 25°.

Preparations
Melphalan Injection
Melphalan Tablets

Action and use Cytotoxic.

Menadiol Sodium Phosphate

⟨naphthalene structure with substituents: $OP(ONa)_2$ with O at position 1, Me at position 2, $OP(ONa)_2$ with O at position 4⟩

$C_{11}H_8Na_4O_8P_2,6H_2O$　　530.2　　*6700-42-1*

Menadiol Sodium Phosphate is tetrasodium 2-methylnaphthalene-1,4-diyl di(orthophosphate) hexahydrate. It contains not less than 98.0 per cent and not more than 100.5 per cent of $C_{11}H_8Na_4O_8P_2$, calculated with reference to the anhydrous substance.

Characteristics A white to pink, crystalline powder; odour, characteristic; hygroscopic.

Solubility Soluble in less than 1 part of *water*; practically insoluble in *ethanol (96%)*.

Identification A. The *infra-red absorption spectrum*, Appendix II A, is concordant with the *reference spectrum* of menadiol sodium phosphate.
B. To 10 ml of a 2% w/v solution add 10 ml of 1M *sulphuric acid*, 10 ml of 0.1M *cerium(IV) sulphate* and 1 ml of *hydrogen peroxide solution (20 vol)* and extract with two 10-ml quantities of *chloroform*. Evaporate the combined chloroform extracts to dryness on a water-bath and dry the residue at 40° at a pressure not exceeding 0.7 kPa. The *infra-red absorption spectrum* of the residue, Appendix II A, is concordant with the *reference spectrum* of menadione.

C. Dissolve 40 mg in 2 ml of *water*, heat gently with 2 ml of *sulphuric acid* until white fumes are evolved, add *nitric acid* dropwise until digestion is complete and cool. Add 2 ml of *water*, heat until white fumes are evolved again, cool, add a further 10 ml of *water* and neutralise to *litmus paper* with 5M *ammonia*. The solution yields *reaction A* characteristic of sodium salts and *reaction B* characteristic of phosphates, Appendix VI.

E. *Melting point* of the residue obtained in test B, about 105°, Appendix V A, Method I.

Inorganic phosphate Dissolve 25 mg in 10 ml of *water*, add 4 ml of 1M *sulphuric acid*, 1 ml of a 10% w/v solution of *ammonium molybdate* and 2 ml of *methylaminophenyl— sulphite reagent* and allow to stand for 15 minutes. The *absorbance* of the solution at 730 nm, Appendix II B, is not more than the *absorbance* of a solution prepared in the same manner but using 10 ml of a 0.0025% w/v solution of *potassium dihydrogen orthophosphate* in place of the solution of the substance being examined (0.7%).

Total phosphate Dissolve 85 mg in 50 ml of *glacial acetic acid*, add 5 ml of *mercury(II) acetate solution* and carry out Method I for *non-aqueous titration*, Appendix VIII A, determining the end-point potentiometrically. Not less than 7.7 ml and not more than 8.3 ml of 0.1M *perchloric acid VS* is required.

Related substances Carry out in subdued light the method for *thin-layer chromatography*, Appendix III A, using *silica gel GF254* as the coating substance and a mixture of 50 volumes of *propan-1-ol*, 50 volumes of a 2% w/v solution of *ammonium chloride*, 5 volumes of *butan-1-ol* and 1.5 volumes of *diethylamine* as the mobile phase. Apply separately to the chromatoplate 5 µl of each of three solutions in *methanol (50%)* containing (1) 4.0 w/v of the substance being examined, (2) 0.020% w/v of the substance being examined and (3) 0.0080% w/v of *2-methyl-1,4-naphthoquinone*. After removal of the plate, allow it to dry in air and examine under *ultra-violet light (254 nm)*. Any *secondary spot* in the chromatogram obtained with solution (1) is not more intense than the spot in the chromatogram obtained with solution (3). Examine the plate under *ultra-violet light (365 nm)*. Any *secondary spot* in the chromatogram obtained with solution (1) is not more intense than the spot in the chromatogram obtained with solution (2).

Water 19.0 to 21.5% w/w, Appendix IX A. Use 0.25 g.

Assay Dissolve 0.1 g in 25 ml of *water*, add 25 ml of *glacial acetic acid* and 25 ml of 3M *hydrochloric acid* and titrate with 0.02M *cerium(IV) sulphate VS* using platinum and calomel electrodes and determining the end-point potentiometrically. Each ml of 0.02M *cerium(IV) sulphate VS* is equivalent to 0.004221 g of $C_{11}H_8Na_4O_8P_2$.

Preparation
Menadiol Phosphate Tablets

Action and use Prevention of vitamin K deficiency.

Menadione ☆
Menaphthone

$C_{11}H_8O_2$ 172.2   58-27-5

Menadione is 2-methyl-1,4-naphthoquinone. It contains not less than 98.5 per cent and not more than 101.0 per cent of $C_{11}H_8O_2$, calculated with reference to the dried substance.

Characteristics A pale yellow, crystalline powder.

Solubility Practically insoluble in *water*; sparingly soluble in *ethanol (96%)* and in *methanol*; soluble in *ether*; freely soluble in *chloroform* and in *toluene*. It decomposes on exposure to light.

Identification *Test A may be omitted if tests B, C and D are carried out. Tests B and C may be omitted if tests A and D are carried out.*

A. The *infra-red absorption spectrum*, Appendix II A, is concordant with the spectrum of *menadione EPCRS*.

B. Dissolve 1 mg in 5 ml of *ethanol (96%)* and add 2 ml of *ammonia* and 0.2 ml of *ethyl cyanoacetate*. An intense bluish-violet colour is produced which disappears on the addition of 2 ml of *hydrochloric acid*.

C. Dissolve 10 mg in 1 ml of *ethanol (96%)*, add 1 ml of *hydrochloric acid* and heat in a water-bath. A red colour is produced.

D. *Melting point*, 105° to 108°, Appendix V A, Method I.

Related substances Carry out in subdued light the method for *thin-layer chromatography*, Appendix III A, using *silica gel GF254* as the coating substance and a mixture of 90 volumes of *cyclohexane*, 5 volumes of *1,2-dichloroethane*, 2 volumes of *acetone* and 1 volume of *nitromethane* as the mobile phase. Apply separately to the chromatoplate 5 µl of each of two solutions of the substance being examined in *acetone* containing (1) 2.0% w/v and (2) 0.01% w/v. After removal of the plate, dry it in a stream of hot air and repeat the development and drying twice. Examine the plate under *ultra-violet light (254 nm)*. Any *secondary spot* in the chromatogram obtained with solution (1) is not more intense than the spot in the chromatogram obtained with solution (2).

Loss on drying When dried over *phosphorus pentoxide* at a pressure of 2 to 3 kPa for 4 hours, loses not more than 0.5% of its weight. Use 1 g.

Sulphated ash Not more than 0.1%, Appendix IX A, Method II. Use 1 g.

Assay Dissolve 0.15 g in 15 ml of *glacial acetic acid* in a flask with a stopper fitted with a valve, add 15 ml of 2M *hydrochloric acid* and 1 g of *granulated zinc*, close the flask and allow to stand in the dark for 60 minutes, shaking occasionally. Filter the solution through absorbent cotton and wash the filter with three 10-ml quantities of *carbon dioxide-free water*, adding the washings to the filtrate. Add 1 ml of *ferroin sulphate solution* and immediately titrate the combined filtrate and washings with 0.1M *ammonium cerium(IV) nitrate VS*. Each ml of 0.1M *ammonium cerium(IV) nitrate VS* is equivalent to 0.00861 g of $C_{11}H_8O_2$.

Storage Menadione should be kept in a well-closed container and protected from light.

Action and use Synthetic vitamin K analogue.

Menotrophin ☆

9002-68-0

Menotrophin is a dry, sterile preparation containing glycoprotein gonadotrophins of pituitary origin obtained from urine of post-menopausal women. It has follicle stimulating and luteinising activities. It may be prepared by a suitable fractionation procedure followed by ion-exchange chromatography. The purified material thus obtained is sterilised by *Filtration* and is dried under reduced pressure. It contains not less than 40 Units of follicle stimulating hormone activity per mg. The ratio of Units of luteinising hormone (interstitial cell-stimulating hormone) to Units of follicle-stimulating hormone is approximately 1.

Characteristics An almost white or slightly yellow powder.

Solubility Soluble in *water*.

Identification Causes enlargement of the ovaries of immature female rats and increases the weight of the seminal vesicles and prostate gland of immature male rats when administered as directed in the Assay.

Water Not more than 5% w/w when determined by the method for *gas chromatography*, Appendix III B, using throughout dry glassware which may be siliconised and the following solutions. For solution (1) dilute 15 μl of *anhydrous methanol* (internal standard) with sufficient *anhydrous propan-2-ol* to produce 100 ml. For solution (2) dissolve 4 mg of the substance being examined in 0.5 ml of *anhydrous propan-2-ol*. For solution (3) dissolve 4 mg of the substance being examined in 0.5 ml of solution (1). For solution (4) add 10 μl of *water* to 50 ml of solution (1).

The chromatographic procedure may be carried out using a stainless-steel column (1 m × 2 mm) packed with porous polymer beads (60 to 80 mesh) (Chromosorb 102 is suitable), maintained at 120°, helium as the carrier gas and a thermal conductivity detector, maintained at 150°.

From the chromatograms obtained and taking into account any water detectable in solution (1), calculate the percentage w/w of water taking 0.9972 g as its weight per ml at 20°.

Assay Carry out the *biological assay of menotrophin*, Appendix XIV C4. For each component, the estimated potency is not less than 80% and not more than 125% of the stated potency. The fiducial limits of error are not less than 64% and not more than 156% of the stated potency.

Storage Menotrophin should be kept in an airtight container, protected from light and stored at a temperature not exceeding 25°. Under these conditions it may be expected to retain its potency for not less than 3 years.

If the contents are intended for use in the manufacture of a parenteral dosage form, the container should be sterile and sealed so as to exclude micro-organisms.

Labelling The label states (1) the number of Units of follicle stimulating hormone activity and the number of Units of luteinising hormone activity in the container; (2) the number of Units of follicle stimulating hormone activity per mg and the number of Units of luteinising hormone activity per mg; (3) the date after which the material is not intended to be used; (4) the conditions under which it should be stored; (5) whether or not it is intended for use in the manufacture of a parenteral dosage form.

Preparation
Menotrophin Injection

Action and use Gonadotrophic hormone.

Menotrophin intended for use in the manufacture of a parenteral dosage form complies with the following additional requirements.

Abnormal toxicity Complies with the *test for abnormal toxicity*, Appendix XIV L, the injection occupying not more than 60 seconds. Use a quantity containing 50 Units of follicle stimulating hormone activity dissolved in 0.5 ml of *sodium chloride injection*.

Pyrogens Complies with the *test for pyrogens*, Appendix XIV K. Use per kg of the rabbit's weight 1 ml of a solution in *sodium chloride injection* containing 5 Units of follicle stimulating hormone activity per ml.

Sterility Complies with the *test for sterility*, Appendix XVI A.

Menthol

$C_{10}H_{20}O$ 156.3   *1490-04-6*

Menthol is natural laevo-menthol, obtained from the volatile oils of various species of *Mentha*, or synthetic laevo-menthol or racemic menthol.

Characteristics Colourless, acicular or prismatic crystals; odour, penetrating, resembling that of peppermint.

Solubility Very soluble in *ethanol (96%)*, in *chloroform* and in *ether*; freely soluble in *liquid paraffin* and in volatile oils.

Identification Dissolve 10 mg in 1 ml of *sulphuric acid* and add 1 ml of a 1% w/v solution of *vanillin* in *sulphuric acid*; an orange-yellow colour is produced. Add 1 ml of *water*; the colour changes to violet (distinction from thymol).

Acidity or alkalinity A 5.0% w/v solution in *ethanol (96%)* is neutral to *litmus solution*.

Freezing point For racemic menthol, 27° to 28°; on prolonged stirring the temperature rises to 30° to 32°, Appendix V B.

Melting point For natural or synthetic laevo-menthol, 41° to 44°, Appendix V A.

Specific optical rotation For natural or synthetic laevo-menthol when determined in a 10% w/v solution in *ethanol (96%)*, −49° to −50°, Appendix V F.

Non-volatile matter When heated on a water-bath in an open dish and dried at 105°, leaves not more than 0.05% of residue. Use 5 g.

Storage Menthol should be kept in a well-closed container and stored at a temperature not exceeding 25°.

Preparation
Menthol and Benzoin Inhalation

Meprobamate ☆

$$CH_2 \cdot OCO \cdot NH_2$$
$$MeCPr^n$$
$$CH_2 \cdot OCO \cdot NH_2$$

$C_9H_{18}N_2O_4$ 218.3   57-53-4

Meprobamate is 2-methyl-2-propyltrimethylene dicarbamate. It contains not less than 97.0 per cent and not more than 100.5 per cent of $C_9H_{18}N_2O_4$, calculated with reference to the dried substance.

Characteristics A white or almost white, crystalline or amorphous powder.

Solubility Slightly soluble in *water* and in *ether*; soluble in 7 parts of *ethanol (96%)*.

Identification *Test A may be omitted if tests B, C and D are carried out. Tests B and C may be omitted if tests A and D are carried out.*

A. The *infra-red absorption spectrum*, Appendix II A, is concordant with the spectrum of *meprobamate EPCRS*.
B. Dissolve 0.2 g in 15 ml of 0.5M *ethanolic potassium hydroxide* and boil under a reflux condenser for 15 minutes. Add 0.5 ml of *glacial acetic acid* and 1 ml of a 5% w/v solution of *cobalt(II) nitrate* in *absolute ethanol*. A deep blue colour is produced.
C. To 0.5 g add 1 ml of *acetic anhydride* and 0.05 ml of *sulphuric acid*, mix and allow to stand for 30 minutes, shaking frequently. Pour the clear solution dropwise into 50 ml of *water*, mix and allow to stand. Initiate crystallisation by scratching the walls of the flask with a glass rod and filter. The *melting point* of the precipitate, after washing with *water* and drying at 60°, is 124° to 128°, Appendix V A, Method I.
D. *Melting point*, 104° to 108°, Appendix V A, Method I.

Clarity and colour of solution A 5.0% w/v solution in *absolute ethanol* is *clear*, Appendix IV A, and *colourless*, Appendix IV B, Method II.

Heavy metals Dissolve 2.0 g in a mixture of 3 volumes of *water* and 17 volumes of *acetone* and dilute to 20 ml with the same solvent mixture. 12 ml of the resulting solution complies with *limit test B for heavy metals*, Appendix VII (10 ppm). Use *lead standard solution (1 ppm Pb)* to prepare the standard.

Related substances Carry out the method for *thin-layer chromatography*, Appendix III A, using *silica gel G* as the coating substance and a mixture of 70 volumes of *hexane*, 30 volumes of *acetone* and 10 volumes of *pyridine* as the mobile phase. Apply separately to the chromatoplate 5 µl of each of two solutions of the substance being examined in *ethanol (96%)* containing (1) 2% w/v and (2) 0.02% w/v. After removal of the plate, heat it at 120° for 30 minutes, allow to cool, spray with a 0.5% w/v solution of *vanillin* in

ethanolic sulphuric acid (80%) and heat at 100° to 105° for 30 minutes. Any *secondary spot* in the chromatogram obtained with solution (1) is not more intense than the spot in the chromatogram obtained with solution (2).

Loss on drying When dried to constant weight over *phosphorus pentoxide* at 60° at a pressure of 1.5 to 2.5 kPa, loses not more than 0.5% of its weight. Use 1 g.

Sulphated ash Not more than 0.1%, Appendix IX A, Method II. Use 1 g.

Assay To 0.3 g add 15 ml of *sulphuric acid (25%)* and boil under a reflux condenser for 3 hours. Cool, add 60 ml of 5M *sodium hydroxide*, distil and collect the distillate in 40 ml of a 4% w/v solution of *boric acid* until the total volume in the receiver is about 110 ml. Titrate with 0.1M *hydrochloric acid VS* using *methyl red—methylene blue solution* as indicator. Repeat the operation without the substance being examined. The difference between the titrations represents the amount of hydrochloric acid required. Each ml of 0.1M *hydrochloric acid VS* is equivalent to 0.01091 g of $C_9H_{18}N_2O_4$.

Action and use Anxiolytic.

Mepyramine Maleate ☆

$$CH_2 \cdot CH_2 \cdot NMe_2$$

(structure) N, pyridine ring, CH_2, benzene ring OMe . $\begin{array}{c} HCCO_2H \\ \| \\ HCCO_2H \end{array}$

$C_{17}H_{23}N_3O,C_4H_4O_4$ 401.5   59-33-6

Mepyramine Maleate is 2-(*N-p*-anisyl-*N*-2-pyridylamino)ethyldimethylamine hydrogen maleate. It contains not less than 99.0 per cent and not more than 101.0 per cent of $C_{17}H_{23}N_3O,C_4H_4O_4$, calculated with reference to the dried substance.

Characteristics A white or slightly yellowish, crystalline powder; odourless or almost odourless.

Solubility Soluble in 0.5 part of *water*, in 2.5 parts of *ethanol (96%)* and in 1.5 parts of *chloroform*; very slightly soluble in *ether*.

Identification *Test A may be omitted if tests B, C, D and E are carried out. Tests B, C and D may be omitted if tests A and E are carried out.*

A. The *infra-red absorption spectrum*, Appendix II A, is concordant with the spectrum of *mepyramine maleate EPCRS*. Use 5% w/v solutions in *dichloromethane* and a 0.1-mm path length.
B. The *light absorption*, Appendix II B, in the range 220 to 350 nm of a 0.001% w/v solution in 0.01M *hydrochloric acid* exhibits two maxima, at 239 nm and 316 nm. The A(1%, 1 cm) at 239 nm is 431 to 477 and the A(1%, 1 cm) at 316 nm is 196 to 220.
C. In the test for Related substances, the principal spot in the chromatogram obtained with solution (2) is similar in position and size to that in the chromatogram obtained with solution (4).
D. Triturate 0.1 g with 3 ml of *water*, add 1 ml of 10M *sodium hydroxide* and shake with three 5-ml quantities of *ether*. To 0.1 ml of the aqueous layer add a solution of 10 mg of *resorcinol* in 3 ml of *sulphuric acid*; no colour is

produced on heating for 15 minutes on a water-bath. Heat the remainder of the aqueous layer on a water-bath for 15 minutes with 1 ml of *bromine water*, heat to boiling, cool and to 0.2 ml add a solution of 10 mg of *resorcinol* in 3 ml of *sulphuric acid*; a violet-pink colour is produced on heating for 15 minutes on a water-bath.

E. *Melting point*, 99° to 103°, Appendix V A, Method I.

Acidity pH of a 2% w/v solution, 4.9 to 5.2, Appendix V L.

Clarity and colour of solution A 4.0% w/v solution in *carbon dioxide-free water* is *clear*, Appendix IV A, and not more intensely coloured than *reference solution* Y_6, Appendix IV B, Method II.

Heavy metals 1.0 g complies with *limit test D for heavy metals*, Appendix VII (20 ppm). Use 2 ml of *lead standard solution (10 ppm Pb)* to prepare the standard.

Chloride 2.5 ml of a 20% w/v solution diluted to 15 ml with *water* complies with the *limit test for chlorides*, Appendix VII (100 ppm).

Related substances Carry out the method for *thin-layer chromatography*, Appendix III A, using *silica gel GF254* as the coating substance and a mixture of 100 volumes of *ethyl acetate* and 2 volumes of *diethylamine* as the mobile phase. Apply separately to the chromatoplate 5 µl of each of six solutions in *chloroform* prepared immediately before use containing (1) 4% w/v of the substance being examined, (2) 0.4% w/v of the substance being examined, (3) 4% w/v of *mepyramine maleate EPCRS*, (4) 0.4% w/v of *mepyramine maleate EPCRS*, (5) 0.008% w/v of *mepyramine maleate EPCRS* and (6) 0.004% w/v of *mepyramine maleate EPCRS*. After removal of the plate, allow it to dry in air and examine under *ultra-violet light (254 nm)*. Any *secondary spot* in the chromatogram obtained with solution (1) is not more intense than the spot in the chromatogram obtained with solution (5). The test is not valid unless the Rf values of the principal spots in the chromatograms obtained with solutions (1) and (3) are not less than 0.2 and unless the spot in the chromatogram obtained with solution (6) is clearly visible. Disregard the spot due to maleic acid on the line of application.

Loss on drying When dried to constant weight at 80°, loses not more than 0.25% of its weight. Use 1 g.

Sulphated ash Not more than 0.1%, Appendix IX A, Method II. Use the residue obtained in the test for Loss on drying.

Assay Dissolve 0.15 g in 40 ml of *anhydrous glacial acetic acid* and carry out Method I for *non-aqueous titration*, Appendix VIII A, determining the end-point potentiometrically. Each ml of 0.1M *perchloric acid VS* is equivalent to 0.02007 g of $C_{17}H_{23}N_3O,C_4H_4O_4$.

Storage Mepyramine Maleate should be kept in a well-closed container and protected from light.

Preparation
Mepyramine Tablets

Action and use Anti-emetic.

Mercaptopurine ☆

$C_5H_4N_4S,H_2O$ 170.2   *6112-76-1*

Mercaptopurine is purine-6-thiol monohydrate. It contains not less than 98.5 per cent and not more than 101.0 per cent of $C_5H_4N_4S$, calculated with reference to the anhydrous substance.

Characteristics A yellow, crystalline powder; odourless.

Solubility Practically insoluble in *water* and in *ether*; slightly soluble in *ethanol (96%)*. It dissolves in solutions of alkali hydroxides.

Identification A. Dissolve 20 mg in 5 ml of *dimethyl sulphoxide* and add sufficient 0.1M *hydrochloric acid* to produce 100 ml. Dilute 5 ml to 200 ml with 0.1M *hydrochloric acid*. The *light absorption* of the resulting solution, Appendix II B, in the range 230 to 350 nm exhibits a maximum only at 325 nm.

B. Dissolve 20 mg in 20 ml of *ethanol (96%)* heated to 60° and add 1 ml of a saturated solution of *mercury(II) acetate* in *ethanol (96%)*. A white precipitate is produced.

C. Dissolve 20 mg in 20 ml of *ethanol (96%)* heated to 60° and add 1 ml of a 1% w/v solution of *lead(II) acetate* in *ethanol (96%)*. A yellow precipitate is produced.

Hypoxanthine Carry out the method for *thin-layer chromatography*, Appendix III A, using *silica gel GF254* as the coating substance and a mixture of 90 volumes of *acetone*, 7 volumes of *water* and 3 volumes of 13.5M *ammonia* as the mobile phase, but allowing the solvent front to ascend 10 cm above the line of application. Apply separately to the chromatoplate 5 µl of each of the following solutions. For solution (1) dissolve 50 mg of the substance being examined in 1 ml of *dimethyl sulphoxide* and dilute to 10 ml with *methanol*. For solution (2) dissolve 10 mg of *hypoxanthine* in 10 ml of *dimethyl sulphoxide* and dilute to 100 ml with *methanol*. After removal of the plate, allow it to dry in air and examine under *ultra-violet light (254 nm)*. Any spot corresponding to hypoxanthine in the chromatogram obtained with solution (1) is not more intense than the spot in the chromatogram obtained with solution (2).

Sulphated ash Not more than 0.1%, Appendix IX A, Method II. Use 1 g.

Water 10.0 to 12.0% w/w, Appendix IX C. Use 0.25 g.

Assay Dissolve 0.1 g in 50 ml of *dimethylformamide* and carry out Method II for *non-aqueous titration*, Appendix VIII A, using 0.1M *tetrabutylammonium hydroxide VS* as titrant and determining the end-point potentiometrically. Each ml of 0.1M *tetrabutylammonium hydroxide VS* is equivalent to 0.01522 g of $C_5H_4N_4S$.

Storage Mercaptopurine should be kept in a well-closed container and protected from light.

Preparation
Mercaptopurine Tablets

Action and use Cytotoxic.

Mestranol ☆

C₂₁H₂₆O₂   310.4   72-33-3

Mestranol is 3-methoxy-19-nor-17α-pregna-1,3,5(10)-trien-20-yn-17β-ol. It contains not less than 98.0 per cent and not more than 102.0 per cent of $C_{21}H_{26}O_2$, calculated with reference to the dried substance.

Characteristics A white or almost white, crystalline powder.

Solubility Practically insoluble in *water*; soluble in 44 parts of *ethanol (96%)*, in 23 parts of *acetone*, in 4.5 parts of *chloroform*, in 12 parts of *1,4-dioxan* and in 23 parts of *ether*.

Identification *Test A may be omitted if tests B, C and D are carried out. Tests B, C and D may be omitted if test A is carried out.*
A. The *infra-red absorption spectrum*, Appendix II A, is concordant with the spectrum of *mestranol EPCRS*.
B. In the test for Related substances the principal spot in the chromatogram obtained with solution (2) corresponds to that in the chromatogram obtained with solution (5).
C. Dissolve 5 mg in 1 ml of *sulphuric acid*; a red colour is produced which appears greenish-yellow under ultra-violet light (365 nm). Add the solution to 10 ml of water and mix; the solution becomes pink and on standing a pink to violet precipitate is produced.
D. *Melting point*, 150° to 154°, Appendix V A, Method I.

Light absorption Dissolve 25 mg in sufficient *ethanol (96%)* to produce 25 ml and dilute 10 ml of the solution to 100 ml with *ethanol (96%)*. The *light absorption* of the resulting solution, Appendix II B, in the range 260 to 310 nm exhibits two maxima, at 279 nm and 288 nm, and a minimum at 286 nm. The A(1%, 1 cm) at 279 is 62 to 68 and at 288 nm is 59 to 64.

Specific optical rotation In a 1% w/v solution in *anhydrous pyridine*, −20° to −24°, Appendix V F.

Related substances Carry out the method for *thin-layer chromatography*, Appendix III A, using *silica gel G* as the coating substance and a mixture of 90 volumes of *toluene* and 10 volumes of *ethanol (96%)* as the mobile phase. Apply separately to the chromatoplate 5 μl of each of the following solutions in *chloroform*. Solutions (1) to (4) contain 1.0%, 0.10%, 0.010% and 0.0050% w/v respectively of the substance being examined. Solution (5) contains 0.10% w/v of *mestranol EPCRS*. After removal of the plate, allow it to dry in air, heat it at 110° for 10 minutes and spray with *ethanolic sulphuric acid (20%)*. Heat again at 110° for 10 minutes and examine in daylight and under *ultra-violet light (365 nm)*. Any *secondary spot* in the chromatogram obtained with solution (1) is not more intense than the spot in the chromatogram obtained with solution (3) and not more than one such spot is more intense than the spot in the chromatogram obtained with solution (4).

Loss on drying When dried at 100° to 105° for 3 hours, loses not more than 1.0% of its weight. Use 0.5 g.

Assay Dissolve 0.2 g in 40 ml of *tetrahydrofuran*, add 5 ml of a 10% w/v solution of *silver nitrate* and titrate with 0.1M *sodium hydroxide VS* determining the end-point potentiometrically. Repeat the operation without the substance being examined. The difference between the titrations represents the amount of sodium hydroxide required. Each ml of 0.1M *sodium hydroxide VS* is equivalent to 0.03104 g of $C_{21}H_{26}O_2$.

Storage Mestranol should be kept in a well-closed container and protected from light.

Action and use Oestrogen.

Metaraminol Tartrate

C₉H₁₃NO₂,C₄H₆O₆   317.3   17171-57-2

Metaraminol Tartrate is (−)-2-amino-1-(3-hydroxyphenyl)propan-1-ol hydrogen tartrate. It contains not less than 99.0 per cent and not more than 101.0 per cent of $C_9H_{13}NO_2,C_4H_6O_6$, calculated with reference to the dried substance.

Characteristics A white, crystalline powder; odourless or almost odourless.

Solubility Soluble in 3 parts of *water* and in 100 parts of *ethanol (96%)*; practically insoluble in *chloroform* and in *ether*.

Identification A. The *light absorption*, Appendix II B, in the range 230 to 350 nm of a 0.02% w/v solution exhibits a maximum only at 272 nm. The *absorbance* at 272 nm is about 1.2.
B. In the test for Related substances the principal spot in the chromatogram obtained with solution (2) corresponds to that in the chromatogram obtained with solution (4).
C. A 10% w/v solution is slightly laevorotatory.
D. To 0.5 ml of a 0.05% w/v solution add 0.5 ml of *lithium and sodium molybdotungstophosphate solution* and 5 ml of *sodium carbonate solution* and allow to stand for 5 minutes. An intense blue colour is produced.
E. To 4 ml of a 0.05% w/v solution add 5 ml of *borate buffer pH 9.6* and 1 ml of a freshly prepared 0.5% w/v solution of *sodium 1,2-naphthaquinone-4-sulphonate* and allow to stand for 1 minute. Add 0.2 ml of a 2% v/v solution of *benzalkonium chloride solution* and 5 ml of *toluene* and shake. A mauve colour is immediately produced in the toluene layer (distinction from phenylephrine).

Acidity pH of a 5% w/v solution, 3.2 to 3.5, Appendix V L.

Phenones *Absorbance* of a 0.2% w/v solution at 310 nm, not more than 0.2, Appendix II B.

Related substances Carry out in subdued light the method for *thin-layer chromatography*, Appendix III A, using a silica gel precoated chromatoplate (Merck silica gel 60 plates are suitable) and a mixture of 80 volumes of *chloroform*, 80 volumes of *methanol* and 10 volumes of 13.5M *ammonia* as the mobile phase. Apply separately to the plate 10 µl of each of the following solutions in *methanol*. Solutions (1), (2) and (3) are solutions of the substance being examined containing (1) 1.0% w/v, (2) 0.050% w/v and (3) 0.0050% w/v. Solution (4) contains 0.050% w/v of *metaraminol tartrate BPCRS*. After removal of the plate, allow it to dry in air and spray with a solution prepared in the following manner. Mix 25 ml of a 0.45% w/v solution of *sulphanilic acid* in 1M *hydrochloric acid* with 1.5 ml of a 5% w/v solution of *sodium nitrite*, allow to stand for 5 minutes and mix cautiously with 25 ml of 2M *sodium carbonate*. Any *secondary spot* in the chromatogram obtained with solution (1) is not more intense than the spot in the chromatogram obtained with solution (3).

Loss on drying When dried to constant weight at 105°, loses not more than 0.5% of its weight. Use 1 g.

Sulphated ash Not more than 0.1%, Appendix IX A.

Assay Carry out Method I for *non-aqueous titration*, Appendix VIII A, using 0.6 g and *crystal violet solution* as indicator. Each ml of 0.1M *perchloric acid VS* is equivalent to 0.03173 g of $C_9H_{13}NO_2,C_4H_6O_6$.

Storage Metaraminol Tartrate should be kept in a well-closed container.

Preparation
Metaraminol Injection

Action and use Sympathomimetic.

Metformin Hydrochloride

$$\begin{array}{cc} NH & NH \\ \parallel & \parallel \\ Me_2NCNH \cdot CNH_2 & ,HCl \end{array}$$

$C_4H_{11}N_5,HCl$ 165.6   *1115-70-4*

Metformin Hydrochloride is 1,1-dimethyl-biguanide hydrochloride. It contains not less than 98.5 per cent and not more than 101.0 per cent of $C_4H_{11}N_5,HCl$, calculated with reference to the dried substance.

Characteristics A white, crystalline powder; odourless or almost odourless; hygroscopic.

Solubility Soluble in 2 parts of *water*; slightly soluble in *ethanol* (96%); practically insoluble in *chloroform* and in *ether*.

Identification A. The *infra-red absorption spectrum*, Appendix II A, is concordant with the *reference spectrum* of metformin hydrochloride.
B. Dissolve 25 mg in 5 ml of *water*, add 1.5 ml of 5M *sodium hydroxide*, 1 ml of *1-naphthol solution* and, dropwise with shaking, 0.5 ml of *dilute sodium hypochlorite solution*. An orange-red colour is produced which darkens on standing.
C. Dissolve 10 mg in 10 ml of *water* and add 10 ml of a solution prepared by mixing equal volumes of a 10% w/v solution of *sodium nitroprusside*, a 10% w/v solution of *potassium hexacyanoferrate(III)* and a 10% w/v solution of *sodium hydroxide* and allowing to stand for 20 minutes. A red colour is produced within 3 minutes.
D. Yields *reaction A* characteristic of chlorides, Appendix VI.
E. *Melting point*, about 225°, Appendix V A.

Heavy metals A 10.0% w/v solution complies with *limit test A for heavy metals*, Appendix VII (20 ppm). Use *lead standard solution (2 ppm Pb)* to prepare the standard.

Related substances Carry out the method for *high-performance liquid chromatography*, Appendix III D, using three solutions in *water* containing (1) 0.0010% w/v of the substance being examined, (2) 1.0% w/v of the substance being examined and (3) 0.00020% w/v of *dicyandiamide*.

The chromatographic procedure may be carried out using (a) a stainless steel column (30 cm × 4 mm) packed with *stationary phase C* (10 µm) (µBondapak C18 is suitable), (b) 0.005M *sodium pentanesulphonate*, adjusted to pH 3.5 using a 1% v/v solution of *orthophosphoric acid*, as the mobile phase with a flow rate of 1 ml per minute and (c) a detection wavelength of 218 nm.

In the chromatogram obtained with solution (2) the area of any peak corresponding to dicyandiamide is not greater than the area of the peak obtained with solution (3) and the area of any other *secondary peak* is not greater than the area of the peak obtained with solution (1).

Loss on drying When dried to constant weight at 105°, loses not more than 0.5% of its weight. Use 1 g.

Sulphated ash Not more than 0.1%, Appendix IX A.

Assay Carry out Method I for *non-aqueous titration*, Appendix VIII A, using 0.25 g and 20 ml of *mercury(II) acetate solution* and determining the end-point potentiometrically. Each ml of 0.1M *perchloric acid VS* is equivalent to 0.008281 g of $C_4H_{11}N_5,HCl$.

Storage Metformin Hydrochloride should be kept in a well-closed container.

Preparation
Metformin Tablets

Action and use Hypoglycaemic.

Methadone Hydrochloride ☆

$$\begin{array}{c} CH_2 \cdot CH_3 \\ CO \\ C-CH_2 \cdot CHMe \cdot NMe_2 \quad ,HCl \end{array}$$

$C_{21}H_{27}NO,HCl$ 345.9   *1095-90-5*

Methadone Hydrochloride is dimethyl(1-methyl-4-oxo-3,3-diphenylhexyl)amine hydrochloride. It contains not less than 99.0 per cent and not more than 101.0 per cent of $C_{21}H_{27}NO,HCl$, calculated with reference to the dried substance.

Characteristics A white, crystalline powder.

Solubility Soluble in *water*; freely soluble in *ethanol* (96%) and in *chloroform*; practically insoluble in *ether*.

Identification *Test A may be omitted if tests B, C, D and E are carried out. Tests C and E may be omitted if tests A, B and D are carried out.*
A. The *infra-red absorption spectrum*, Appendix II A, is concordant with the European Pharmacopœia reference spectrum of methadone hydrochloride.
B. *Optical rotation* of a 2-dm layer of a 5% w/v solution in *carbon dioxide-free water*, −0.05° to +0.05°, Appendix V F.

C. To 2.0 ml of a 5% w/v solution of *carbon dioxide-free water* add 1 ml of 0.1M *hydrochloric acid* and 6 ml of 1M *ammonium thiocyanate*. A white precipitate is produced which becomes crystalline on stirring for a few minutes. The *melting point* of the precipitate, after drying at 100° to 105°, is 143° to 148°, Appendix V A, Method I.

D. Dissolve 50 mg in 5 ml of *carbon dioxide-free water*, add 1 ml of 6M *ammonia*, mix, allow to stand for 5 minutes and filter. The filtrate yields *reaction A* characteristic of chlorides, Appendix VI.

E. *Melting point*, 233° to 236°, Appendix V A, Method I.

Acidity or alkalinity To 10 ml of a 2.0% w/v solution in *carbon dioxide-free water* add 0.2 ml of *methyl red solution* and 0.2 ml of 0.01M *sodium hydroxide*; the solution is yellow. Add 0.4 ml of 0.01M *hydrochloric acid*; the solution is red.

Clarity and colour of solution A 5.0% w/v solution in *carbon dioxide-free water* is *clear*, Appendix IV A, and *colourless*, Appendix IV B, Method II.

Related substances Carry out the method for *thin-layer chromatography*, Appendix III A, using *silica gel G* as the coating substance and a mixture of 60 volumes of *ethanol (96%)*, 30 volumes of *glacial acetic acid* and 10 volumes of *water* as the mobile phase. Apply separately to the chromatoplate 10 µl of each of two solutions of the substance being examined in *ethanol (96%)* containing (1) 5.0% w/v and (2) 0.0050% w/v. After removal of the plate, allow it to dry in air and spray with *dilute potassium iodobismuthate solution*. Any *secondary spot* in the chromatogram obtained with solution (1) is not more intense than the spot in the chromatogram obtained with solution (2).

Loss on drying When dried to constant weight at 100° to 105°, loses not more than 0.5% of its weight. Use 1 g.

Sulphated ash Not more than 0.1%, Appendix IX A, Method II. Use 1 g.

Assay Dissolve 0.3 g in 50 ml of *anhydrous glacial acetic acid*, add 5 ml of *mercury(II) acetate solution* and carry out Method I for *non-aqueous titration*, Appendix VIII A, using *crystal violet solution* as indicator. Each ml of 0.1M *perchloric acid VS* is equivalent to 0.03459 g of $C_{21}H_{27}NO,HCl$.

Preparations
Methadone Linctus
Methadone Injection
Methadone Tablets

Storage Methadone Hydrochloride should be kept in a well-closed container and protected from light.

Action and use Narcotic analgesic.

Methaqualone ☆

$C_{16}H_{14}N_2O$ 250.3   72-44-6

Methaqualone is 2-methyl-3-*o*-tolylquinazolin-4-one. It contains not less than 99.0 per cent and not more than 101.0 per cent of $C_{16}H_{14}N_2O$, calculated with reference to the dried substance.

Characteristics A white or almost white, crystalline powder; odourless.

Solubility Very slightly soluble in *water*; soluble in 12 parts of *ethanol (96%)*, in 1 part of *chloroform* and in 50 parts of *ether*.

Identification *Test A may be omitted if tests B, C and D are carried out. Tests B and C may be omitted if tests A and D are carried out.*

A. The *infra-red absorption spectrum*, Appendix II A, is concordant with the European Pharmacopœia reference spectrum of methaqualone.

B. Dissolve 50 mg in 0.1M *hydrochloric acid*, warming if necessary, and add sufficient 0.1M *hydrochloric acid* to produce 100 ml. Dilute 1 ml to 100 ml with 0.1M *hydrochloric acid*. The *light absorption* of the resulting solution, Appendix II B, in the range 220 to 300 nm exhibits two maxima, at 235 nm and 270 nm. The A(1%, 1 cm) at 235 nm is 1270 to 1390 and the A (1%, 1 cm) at 270 nm is 315 to 345.

C. Dissolve 10 mg in 2 ml of *ethanol (96%)*. Add 1 ml of *dimethylaminobenzaldehyde solution* and heat on a water-bath for 5 minutes. A reddish-orange colour is produced.

D. *Melting point*, 114° to 117°, Appendix V A, Method I.

Acidity Shake 0.6 g with 30 ml of *carbon dioxide-free water* for 5 minutes, filter and to 10 ml of the filtrate add 0.1 ml of *dilute phenolphthalein solution*. Not more than 0.2 ml of 0.01M *sodium hydroxide VS* is required to change the colour of the solution.

Clarity and colour of solution A 4.0% w/v solution in *methanol* is *clear*, Appendix IV A, and not more intensely coloured than *reference solution BY₇*, Appendix IV B, Method II.

Heavy metals 1.0 g complies with *limit test C for heavy metals*, Appendix VII (20 ppm). Use 2 ml of *lead standard solution (10 ppm Pb)* to prepare the standard.

Anthranilic acid Dissolve 1.00 g in a mixture of 3 volumes of *ethanol (96%)* and 1 volume of *water* and dilute to 50 ml with the same solvent. Add 5 ml of 2M *hydrochloric acid*, cool in ice for 5 minutes, add 0.1 ml of *sodium nitrite solution*, again cool in ice for 5 minutes, add 1.5 ml of a freshly prepared 1% w/v solution of *sulphamic acid* and shake until the solution is colourless. Add 2.5 ml of a freshly prepared 0.2% w/v solution of N-(1-naphthyl)-ethylenediamine dihydrochloride and allow to stand for 150 minutes. The resulting solution is not more intensely coloured than a solution prepared at the same time by treating in the same manner 50 ml of a 0.00004% w/v solution of *anthranilic acid* in a mixture of 3 volumes of *ethanol (96%)* and 1 volume of *water*, beginning at the words 'Add 5 ml of 2M *hydrochloric acid* . . .'. Examine the solutions as described in Appendix IV B, Method II (20 ppm).

o-**Toluidine** Dissolve 0.50 g in *acetone* and dilute to 10 ml with the same solvent (test solution). Dissolve 50 mg of freshly distilled o-*toluidine* in 5 ml of *acetone* and dilute to 100 ml with 2M *hydrochloric acid*; dilute 10 ml to 100 ml with 2M *hydrochloric acid* and dilute 0.1 ml of this solution to 10 ml with *acetone* (reference solution). To each of the test solution and the reference solution simultaneously add 5 ml of *water*, cool in ice for 5 minutes, add 0.1 ml of *sodium nitrite solution*, again cool in ice for 5 minutes, add 10 ml of a freshly prepared 0.2% w/v solution of *2-naphthol* in 2M *sodium hydroxide* and examine as described in Appendix IV B, Method II. The colour resulting from the test solution is not more intense than that resulting from the reference solution (10 ppm).

Loss on drying When dried to constant weight at 100° to 105°, loses not more than 1.0% of its weight. Use 1 g.

Sulphated ash Not more than 0.1%, Appendix IX A, Method II. Use 1 g.

Assay Carry out Method I for *non-aqueous titration*, Appendix VIII A, using 0.2 g and determining the end-point potentiometrically. Each ml of 0.1M *perchloric acid VS* is equivalent to 0.02503 g of $C_{16}H_{14}N_2O$.

Storage Methaqualone should be kept in a well-closed container and protected from light.

Action and use Hypnotic.

Methoserpidine

$C_{33}H_{40}N_2O_9$ 608.7   *865-04-3*

Methoserpidine is methyl 11-demethoxy-10-methoxy-*O*-(3,4,5-trimethoxybenzoyl)reserpate. It contains not less than 98.5 per cent and not more than 101.5 per cent of $C_{33}H_{40}N_2O_9$, calculated with reference to the dried substance.

Characteristics A cream, microcrystalline powder; odourless or almost odourless; hygroscopic.

Solubility Practically insoluble in *water*; soluble in 60 parts of *ethanol (96%)*, in 5 parts of *chloroform* and in 8 parts of *1,4-dioxan*.

Identification A. The *light absorption*, Appendix II B, in the range 230 to 350 nm of a 0.002% w/v solution in *absolute ethanol* exhibits a maximum at 273 nm and less well-defined maxima at 295 nm and 308 nm. The *absorbance* at 273 nm is about 0.60.
B. Dissolve 10 mg in 5 ml of *glacial acetic acid*, add 10 mg of *xanthydrol* and 0.05 ml of *hydrochloric acid* and allow to stand for 1 hour. A blue colour is produced (distinction from reserpine).
C. To 1 mg add 0.2 ml of a freshly prepared 1% w/v solution of *vanillin* in *hydrochloric acid*. A blue colour is produced in about 1 minute (distinction from reserpine).
D. Mix 0.5 mg with 5 mg of *4-dimethylaminobenzaldehyde* and 0.2 ml of *glacial acetic acid* and add 0.2 ml of *sulphuric acid*; a green colour is produced. Add 1 ml of *glacial acetic acid*; the colour changes to red.
E. *Melting point*, about 171°, with decomposition, Appendix V A.

Specific optical rotation In a 1% w/v solution in *1,4-dioxan*, −144° to −154°, Appendix V F.

Related substances Carry out the method for *thin-layer chromatography*, Appendix III A, using a silica gel F254 precoated chromatoplate (Merck silica gel 60 F254 plates are suitable) and a mixture of 90 volumes of *chloroform*, 10

volumes of *methanol* and 1 volume of *water* as the mobile phase. Apply separately to the plate 5 µl of each of two solutions in *chloroform* containing (1) 2.0% w/v of the substance being examined and (2) 0.010% w/v of *3,4,5-trimethoxybenzoic acid*. After removal of the plate, allow it to dry in air and examine under *ultra-violet light (254 nm)*. Any *secondary spot* in the chromatogram obtained with solution (1) is not more intense than the spot in the chromatogram obtained with solution (2).

Loss on drying When dried at 60° at a pressure not exceeding 0.7 kPa for 2 hours, loses not more than 2.0% of its weight. Use 1 g.

Sulphated ash Not more than 0.2%, Appendix IX A.

Assay Carry out Method I for *non-aqueous titration*, Appendix VIII A, using 0.74 g and *1-naphtholbenzein solution* as indicator. Each ml of 0.1M *perchloric acid VS* is equivalent to 0.06087 g of $C_{33}H_{40}N_2O_9$.

Storage Methoserpidine should be kept in a well-closed container and protected from light. It darkens on exposure to light.

Preparation
Methoserpidine Tablets

Action and use Antihypertensive.

Methotrexate ☆

$C_{20}H_{22}N_8O_5$ 454.4   *59-05-2*

Methotrexate is 4-amino-4-deoxy-10-methyl-pteroyl-L-glutamic acid. It contains not less than 97.0 per cent and not more than 102.0 per cent of $C_{20}H_{22}N_8O_5$, calculated with reference to the anhydrous substance.

Characteristics A yellow or orange, crystalline powder.

Solubility Practically insoluble in *water*, in *ethanol (96%)*, in *chloroform*, in *1,2-dichloroethane* and in *ether*. It dissolves in solutions of mineral acids and in dilute solutions of alkali hydroxides and carbonates.

Identification A. The *infra-red absorption spectrum*, Appendix II A, is concordant with the spectrum of *methotrexate EPCRS*.
B. The *light absorption*, Appendix II B, in the range 230 to 380 nm of a 0.001% w/v solution in 0.1M *sodium hydroxide* exhibits three maxima, at 258, 303 and 371 nm. The ratio of the *absorbance* at the maximum at 303 nm to that at the maximum at 371 nm is 2.8 to 3.3.

Specific optical rotation In a 1% w/v solution in a 1.4% w/v solution of *sodium carbonate*, +19° to +24°, Appendix V F.

Sulphated ash Not more than 0.1%, Appendix IX A, Method II. Use 1 g.

Water Not more than 12.0% w/w, Appendix IX C. Use 0.25 g.

Assay Carry out the method for *high-performance liquid chromatography*, Appendix III D, using a fixed-volume loop injector and 20 μl of each of the following solutions. For solution (1) dissolve 25 mg of *methotrexate EPCRS* in 250 ml of the mobile phase. For solution (2) dissolve 25 mg of the substance being examined in 250 ml of the mobile phase. For solution (3) dissolve 25 mg of the substance being examined and 25 mg of *folic acid* in 250 ml of the mobile phase.

The chromatographic procedure may be carried out using (a) a stainless steel column (10 cm × 6 mm) packed with *stationary phase C* (5 μm) (Nucleosil C18 is suitable) in *acetonitrile*, (b) a mixture of 92 volumes of *phosphate buffer pH 6.0* and 8 volumes of *acetonitrile* as the mobile phase with a flow rate of 1.4 ml per minute and (c) a detection wavelength of 303 nm.

Determine the content of $C_{20}H_{22}N_8O_5$ using the declared content of $C_{20}H_{22}N_8O_5$ in *methotrexate EPCRS*.

The chromatography is not valid unless the relative standard deviation of the areas of the peaks due to methotrexate in the chromatograms obtained by injecting 20 μl of solution (3) six times is not more than 2.0% and the *resolution factor* between the peaks due to methotrexate and folic acid is not less than 5.0.

Storage Methotrexate should be kept in an airtight container and protected from light.

Preparations
Methotrexate Injection
Methotrexate Tablets

Action and use Cytotoxic.

Methotrimeprazine Hydrochloride ☆

$C_{19}H_{24}N_2OS,HCl$ 364.9   *4185-80-2*

Methotrimeprazine Hydrochloride is (*R*)-3-(2-methoxyphenothiazin-10-yl)-2-methylpropyl-dimethylamine hydrochloride. It contains not less than 98.5 per cent and not more than 101.0 per cent of $C_{19}H_{24}N_2OS,HCl$, calculated with reference to the dried substance.

Characteristics A white or very slightly yellow, crystalline powder; slightly hygroscopic. It deteriorates on exposure to air and light. It exists in two forms, one melting at about 142° and one at about 162°.

Solubility Freely soluble in *water*, in *ethanol (96%)* and in *chloroform*; practically insoluble in *ether*.

Identification A. Carry out the following procedure in subdued light. Dissolve 50 mg in sufficient *water* to produce 500 ml and dilute 10 ml to 100 ml with *water*. The *light absorption*, Appendix II B, in the range 230 to 340 nm of the resulting solution, measured immediately after preparation, exhibits two maxima, at 250 nm and at 302 nm. The A(1%, 1 cm) at the maximum at 250 nm is 640 to 700.
B. Complies with the test for *identification of phenothiazines*, Appendix III A.

C. To 0.2 g add 5 ml of *water* and 0.5 ml of 10M *sodium hydroxide* and shake vigorously with two 10-ml quantities of *ether*. Dry the combined ether layers over *anhydrous sodium sulphate*, evaporate the solvent, dry the residue at 100° to 105° for 15 minutes and allow to crystallise in ice. If necessary, initiate crystallisation by scratching the wall of the container with a glass rod. The *melting point* of the crystals, after drying at 60° for 2 hours, is 122° to 128°, Appendix V A, Method I.
D. Yields *reaction B* characteristic of chlorides, Appendix VI.

Acidity or alkalinity To 10 ml of a 10% w/v solution add 0.1 ml of *bromocresol green solution*. Not more than 0.5 ml of 0.01M *sodium hydroxide VS* or not more than 1.0 ml of 0.01M *hydrochloric acid VS* is required to change the colour of the solution.

Specific optical rotation In a 10% w/v solution in *carbon dioxide-free water*, +9.5° to +11.5°, Appendix V F.

Related substances Complies with the test for *related substances in phenothiazines*, Appendix III A, using *mobile phase A* but allowing the solvent front to ascend 15 cm above the line of application.

Loss on drying When dried at 100° to 105° for 3 hours, loses not more than 1.0% of its weight. Use 1 g.

Sulphated ash Not more than 0.1%, Appendix IX A, Method II. Use 1 g.

Assay Dissolve 0.3 g in 5 ml of *water*, add 50 ml of *propan-2-ol* and titrate with 0.1M *sodium hydroxide VS* determining the end-point potentiometrically. Each ml of 0.1M *sodium hydroxide VS* is equivalent to 0.03649 g of $C_{19}H_{24}N_2OS,HCl$.

Storage Methotrimeprazine Hydrochloride should be kept in an airtight container and protected from light.

Action and use Antipsychotic.

The title of the monograph in the European Pharmacopœia is Levomepromazine Hydrochloride.

Methoxamine Hydrochloride

$C_{11}H_{17}NO_3,HCl$ 247.7   *61-16-5*

Methoxamine Hydrochloride is 2-amino-1-(2,5-dimethoxyphenyl)propan-1-ol hydrochloride. It contains not less than 99.0 per cent and not more than 101.0 per cent of $C_{11}H_{17}NO_3,HCl$, calculated with reference to the dried substance.

Characteristics Colourless crystals or white, plate-like crystals or a white, crystalline powder; odourless or almost odourless.

Solubility Soluble in 2.5 parts of *water* and in 12 parts of *ethanol (96%)*; very slightly soluble in *chloroform* and in *ether*.

Identification A. The *infra-red absorption spectrum*, Appendix II A, is concordant with the *reference spectrum* of methoxamine hydrochloride.

B. The *light absorption*, Appendix II B, in the range 230 to 350 nm of a 0.006% w/v solution exhibits a maximum only at 290 nm. The *absorbance* at 290 nm is about 0.80.

C. Dissolve 20 mg in 2 ml of *water*, add 5 ml of *diazotised nitroaniline solution* and 1 ml of *sodium carbonate solution*, allow to stand for 2 minutes and add 1 ml of 1M *sodium hydroxide*. A deep red colour is produced which is extractable with *butan-1-ol*.

D. Yields the *reactions* characteristic of chlorides, Appendix VI.

E. *Melting point*, about 214°, Appendix V A.

Acidity pH of a 2% w/v solution, 4.0 to 6.0, Appendix V L.

Related substances Carry out the method for *thin-layer chromatography*, Appendix III A, using *silica gel GF254* as the coating substance and a mixture of 86 volumes of *chloroform*, 12 volumes of *methanol* and 2 volumes of 13.5M *ammonia* as the mobile phase. Apply separately to the chromatoplate 5 μl of each of three solutions in *methanol* containing (1) 2.0% w/v of the substance being examined, (2) 0.010% w/v of *2,5-dimethoxybenzaldehyde* and (3) 0.020% w/v of the substance being examined. After removal of the plate, allow it to dry in air and examine under *ultra-violet light (365 nm)*. Any spot corresponding to 2,5-dimethoxybenzaldehyde in the chromatogram obtained with solution (1) is not more intense than the spot in the chromatogram obtained with solution (2). Spray the plate with a 0.3% w/v solution of *ninhydrin* in *butan-1-ol* containing 3% v/v of *glacial acetic acid* and heat at 105° for 5 minutes. Any other *secondary spot* in the chromatogram obtained with solution (1) is not more intense than the spot in the chromatogram obtained with solution (3).

Loss on drying When dried at 105° for 2 hours, loses not more than 0.5% of its weight. Use 1 g.

Sulphated ash Not more than 0.1%, Appendix IX A.

Assay Carry out Method I for *non-aqueous titration*, Appendix VIII A, using 0.5 g and *1-naphtholbenzein solution* as indicator. Each ml of 0.1M *perchloric acid VS* is equivalent to 0.02477 g of $C_{11}H_{17}NO_3,HCl$.

Preparation
Methoxamine Injection

Action and use Sympathomimetic.

Methyl Hydroxybenzoate ☆
Methylparaben

$C_8H_8O_3$ 152.1   *99-76-3*

Methyl Hydroxybenzoate is methyl 4-hydroxybenzoate. It contains not less than 99.0 per cent and not more than 101.0 per cent of $C_8H_8O_3$, calculated with reference to the dried substance.

Characteristics Colourless crystals or a white, crystalline powder.

Solubility Very slightly soluble in *water*; freely soluble in *ethanol (96%)*, in *methanol* and in *ether*.

Identification A. The *light absorption*, Appendix II B, in the range 230 to 280 nm of a 0.0005% w/v solution in *ethanol (96%)* exhibits a maximum only at 258 nm.

B. Dissolve 0.1 g in 2 ml of *ethanol (96%)*, boil and add 0.5 ml of *mercury—nitric acid solution*. A precipitate is produced and the supernatant liquid becomes red.

C. *Melting point*, 125° to 128°, Appendix V A, Method I.

Acidity Dissolve 0.2 g in 5 ml of *ethanol (96%)*, add 5 ml of *carbon dioxide-free water* and 0.1 ml of *bromocresol green solution*. Not more than 0.1 ml of 0.1M *sodium hydroxide VS* is required to change the colour of the solution.

Clarity and colour of solution Dissolve 1.0 g in 10 ml of *ethanol (96%)*. The solution is *clear*, Appendix IV A, and not more intensely coloured than *reference solution BY₆*, Appendix IV B, Method II.

Loss on drying When dried over *phosphorus pentoxide* at 80° at a pressure of 1.5 to 2.5 kPa for 2 hours, loses not more than 0.5% of its weight. Use 1 g.

Sulphated ash Not more than 0.1%, Appendix IX A, Method II. Use 1 g.

Assay To 80 mg add 25 ml of 2M *sodium hydroxide* and boil gently under a reflux condenser for 30 minutes. Cool and add 25 ml of 0.0333M *potassium bromate VS*, 5 ml of a 12.5% w/v solution of *potassium bromide* and 40 ml of *glacial acetic acid*, cool in ice, add 10 ml of *hydrochloric acid*, immediately stopper the flask and allow to stand for 15 minutes. Add 15 ml of 1M *potassium iodide*, mix and titrate the liberated iodine with 0.1M *sodium thiosulphate VS* using 2 ml of *starch solution*, added towards the end of the titration, as indicator. Repeat the operation without the substance being examined. The difference between the titrations represents the amount of potassium bromate required. The volume of 0.0333M *potassium bromate VS* used is equivalent to half of the volume of 0.1M *sodium thiosulphate VS* required for the titration. Each ml of 0.0333M *potassium bromate VS* is equivalent to 0.005072 g of $C_8H_8O_3$.

Action and use Antimicrobial preservative.

The title of the monograph in the European Pharmacopœia is Methyl Parahydroxybenzoate.

Methyl Nicotinate

$C_7H_7NO_2$ 137.1   *93-60-7*

Methyl Nicotinate is methyl pyridine-3-carboxylate. It contains not less than 99.0 per cent and not more than 101.0 per cent of $C_7H_7NO_2$, calculated with reference to the anhydrous substance.

Characteristics White or almost white, crystals or crystalline powder; odour, characteristic.

Solubility Soluble in 0.7 part of *water* and of *ethanol (96%)*, in 0.4 part of *chloroform* and in 1 part of *ether*.

Identification A. The *infra-red absorption spectrum*, Appendix II A, is concordant with the *reference spectrum* of methyl nicotinate.

B. The *light absorption*, Appendix II B, in the range 230 to 350 nm of a 0.002% w/v solution exhibits a maximum only at 264 nm. The *absorbance* at 264 nm is about 0.46.

C. To 2 ml of a 0.1% w/v solution add 6 ml of *cyanogen bromide solution* and 1 ml of a 2.5% v/v solution of *aniline*. A golden yellow colour is produced.

Melting point 40° to 42°, Appendix V A.

Related substances Carry out the method for *thin-layer chromatography*, Appendix III A, using *silica gel GF254* as the coating substance and a mixture of 48 volumes of *chloroform*, 45 volumes of *ethanol (96%)* and 8 volumes of *water* as the mobile phase. Apply separately to the chromatoplate 10 µl of each of two solutions of the substance being examined in *methanol* containing (1) 5.0% w/v and (2) 0.025% w/v. After removal of the plate, allow it to dry in air and examine under *ultra-violet light (254 nm)*. Any *secondary spot* in the chromatogram obtained with solution (1) is not more intense than the spot in the chromatogram obtained with solution (2).

Water Not more than 0.5% w/w, Appendix IX C. Use 2 g.

Sulphated ash Not more than 0.1%, Appendix IX A.

Assay Carry out Method I for *non-aqueous titration*, Appendix VIII A, using 0.3 g and determining the end-point potentiometrically. Each ml of 0.1M *perchloric acid VS* is equivalent to 0.01371 g of $C_7H_7NO_2$.

Storage Methyl Nicotinate should be kept in a well-closed container.

Action and use Vasodilator.

Methyl Salicylate ☆

CO₂Me / OH

$C_8H_8O_3$ 152.1   *119-36-8*

Methyl Salicylate contains not less than 99.0 per cent and not more than 100.5 per cent of $C_8H_8O_3$.

Characteristics A colourless or pale yellow liquid; odour, strong, persistent, characteristic and aromatic.

Solubility Very slightly soluble in *water*; miscible with *ethanol (96%)*, with *chloroform* and with fixed and volatile oils.

Identification A. To 10 ml of a saturated aqueous solution add 0.05 ml of *iron(III) chloride test-solution*. A violet colour is produced.

B. Heat 0.25 ml with 2 ml of 2M *sodium hydroxide* on a water-bath for 5 minutes and add 3 ml of 1M *sulphuric acid*. Filter the precipitate and wash with *water*. The *melting point*, after drying at 100° to 105°, is 156° to 161°, Appendix V A, Method I.

Acidity Dissolve 5 g in a mixture of 50 ml of *ethanol (96%)* and 0.2 ml of *bromocresol green solution* previously neutralised to a blue colour by the addition of 0.1M *sodium hydroxide VS*. Not more than 0.4 ml of 0.1M *sodium hydroxide VS* is required to restore the colour.

Clarity and colour of solution To 2.0 ml add 10 ml of *ethanol (96%)*. The resulting solution is *clear*,

Appendix IV A, and not more intensely coloured than *reference solution Y_7*, Appendix IV B, Method II.

Refractive index 1.535 to 1.538, Appendix V E.

Relative density 1.180 to 1.186, Appendix V G.

Assay Dissolve 0.5 g in 25 ml of *ethanol (96%)*, add 0.05 ml of *phenol red solution* and neutralise with 0.1M *sodium hydroxide VS*. Add 50 ml of 0.1M *sodium hydroxide VS* and heat under a reflux condenser on a water-bath for 30 minutes. Cool and titrate with 0.1M *hydrochloric acid VS*. Repeat the operation without the substance being examined. The difference between the titrations represents the amount of sodium hydroxide used in the saponification. Each ml of 0.1M *sodium hydroxide VS* is equivalent to 0.01521 g of $C_8H_8O_3$.

Storage Methyl Salicylate should be kept in a well-closed container and protected from light.

Preparations
Methyl Salicylate Liniment
Methyl Salicylate Ointment

Action and use Counter-irritant.

When Oil of Wintergreen, Wintergreen or Wintergreen Oil is prescribed or demanded, Methyl Salicylate shall be dispensed or supplied, unless it is ascertained that Methyl Salicylate Liniment is required.

Industrial Methylated Spirit
Industrial Methylated Spirits; IMS

Industrial Methylated Spirit is a mixture of nineteen volumes of ethanol of an appropriate strength with one volume of approved wood naphtha and is Industrial Methylated Spirit of the quality known either as '66 OP' or as '74 OP'.

Characteristics A colourless, clear, mobile and volatile liquid, boiling at about 78°; odour, spirituous and of wood naphtha.

Identification Mix 0.1 ml with 0.05 ml of an 11% w/w solution of *orthophosphoric acid* and 0.25 ml of *potassium permanganate solution*. After 1 minute add a few mg of *sodium metabisulphite* and shake until the mixture is decolorised. Add 1.5 ml of a 50% v/v solution of *sulphuric acid* and a few mg of finely powdered *chromotropic acid sodium salt*, shake well and heat on a water-bath for 5 minutes. A deep violet colour is produced.

Acidity or alkalinity 25 ml requires not more than 0.2 ml of 0.1M *sodium hydroxide VS* to produce a pink colour with *phenolphthalein solution* and not more than 1.0 ml of 0.1M *hydrochloric acid VS* to produce a red colour with *methyl red solution*.

Clarity of solution Dilute 5.0 ml to 100 ml with *water*. The solution is *clear*, Appendix IV A, Method I.

Density For '66 OP' grade, not greater than 811.6 kg m⁻³ and for '74 OP' grade, not greater than 792.8 kg m⁻³, Appendix V G.

Aldehydes To 5.0 ml add 5 ml of *water* and 1 ml of *decolorised magenta solution* and allow to stand for 30 minutes. Any colour produced is not more intense than that obtained by treating in the same manner 5 ml of a 0.005% w/v solution of redistilled *acetaldehyde* in *aldehyde-free ethanol (96%)* (50 ppm).

Non-volatile matter When evaporated and dried at 105°, leaves not more than 0.01% w/v of residue.

Industrial Methylated Spirit (Ketone-free)

Industrial Methylated Spirit (Ketone-free) is a mixture of nineteen volumes of ethanol of an appropriate strength with one volume of approved wood naphtha and is Industrial Methylated Spirit of the quality known either as '66 OP' or as '74 OP', substantially free from ketones.

Characteristics; Identification; Acidity or alkalinity; Clarity of solution; Density; Aldehydes; Non-volatile matter Complies with the requirements stated under Industrial Methylated Spirit.

Ketones Dilute 5 ml to 10 ml with *water*, add 1 ml of a 1.0% w/v solution of *2-nitrobenzaldehyde* in *ethanol (50%)* followed by 1 ml of a 15% w/v solution of *sodium hydroxide* in *water* and allow to stand for 15 minutes. Any colour produced is not more intense than that produced by treating in the same manner 10 ml of a 0.025% v/v solution of *acetone* in *ethanol (50%)* (500 ppm).

Methylcellulose ☆

9004-67-5

Methylcellulose is a cellulose having some of the hydroxyl groups in the form of the methyl ether. Various grades are available and are distinguished by appending a number indicative of the apparent viscosity in millipascal seconds of a 2 per cent w/v solution measured at 20°.

Characteristics A white, yellowish-white or greyish-white powder or granules; practically odourless; hygroscopic after drying.

Solubility Practically insoluble in hot *water*, in *absolute ethanol*, in *acetone*, in *ether* and in *toluene*. It forms a colloidal solution in cold *water*.

Identification A. Whilst stirring, introduce a quantity containing the equivalent of 1.0 g of the dried substance into 50 ml of *carbon dioxide-free water* heated to 90°. Allow to cool, dilute to 100 ml with the same solvent and continue stirring until solution is complete (solution A). Heat 10 ml of solution A in a water-bath, with stirring. At temperatures above 50° the solution becomes cloudy or a flocculent precipitate is produced. The solution becomes clear on cooling.
B. To 10 ml of solution A add 0.3 ml of 2M *acetic acid* and 2.5 ml of a 10% w/v solution of *tannic acid*. A yellowish-white, flocculent precipitate is produced which dissolves in 6M *ammonia*.
C. Mix thoroughly 1 g with 2 g of finely powdered *manganese(II) sulphate* in a test-tube about 16 cm long. Impregnate a strip of filter paper with a freshly prepared mixture of 1 volume of a 20% v/v solution of *diethanolamine* and 11 volumes of a 5% w/v solution of *sodium nitroprusside*, adjusted to pH 9.8 with 1M *hydrochloric acid*. Insert the strip to a depth of 2 cm into the upper part of the tube, immerse the tube to a depth of 8 cm in a silicone oil-bath and heat at 190° to 200°. The filter paper does not become blue within 10 minutes. Carry out a blank test.

D. Without heating, completely dissolve 0.2 g in 15 ml of a 70% w/w solution of *sulphuric acid*, pour the solution, with stirring, into 100 ml of iced *water* and dilute to 250 ml with iced *water*. In a test-tube kept in ice, mix thoroughly 1 ml of the solution with 8 ml of *sulphuric acid*, added dropwise. Heat in a water-bath for exactly 3 minutes and cool immediately in ice. When the mixture is cool, carefully add 0.6 ml of a solution of 3 g of *ninhydrin* in 100 ml of a 4.55% w/v solution of *sodium metabisulphite*, mix well and allow to stand at 25°. A pink colour is produced immediately which does not become violet within 100 minutes.
E. Place 1 ml of solution A on a glass plate. After evaporation of the water a thin film is produced.

Acidity or alkalinity pH of solution A, 5.5 to 8.0, Appendix V L.

Clarity and colour of solution Solution A is not more opalescent than *reference suspension II*, Appendix IV A, and not more intensely coloured than *reference solution Y_6*, Appendix IV B, Method II.

Apparent viscosity 75 to 140% of the declared value when determined by the following method. To 50 ml of *water* heated to 90° add, with stirring, a quantity containing the equivalent of 2 g of the dried substance. Allow to cool, dilute to 100 ml with *water* and continue stirring until solution is complete. Determine the *viscosity*, Appendix V H, Method IV, at 20°, using a shear rate of 10 s^{-1}. If necessary, use rates slightly below and slightly above 10 s^{-1} and interpolate.

Heavy metals 1.0 g complies with *limit test C for heavy metals*, Appendix VII (20 ppm). Use 2 ml of *lead standard solution (10 ppm Pb)* to prepare the standard.

Chloride 1 ml of solution A diluted to 15 ml with *water* complies with the *limit test for chlorides*, Appendix VII (0.5%).

Loss on drying When dried to constant weight at 100° to 105°, loses not more than 10.0% of its weight. Use 1 g.

Sulphated ash Not more than 1.0%, Appendix IX A, Method II. Use 1 g.

Storage Methylcellulose should be kept in a well-closed container.

Labelling The label states the apparent viscosity in millipascal seconds of a 2% w/v solution.

Preparation
Methylcellulose Granules

Action and use Bulk-forming laxative; pharmaceutical aid.

Methyldopa ☆

$C_{10}H_{13}NO_4,1\frac{1}{2}H_2O$ 238.2   *41372-08-1*

Methyldopa is of 3-(3,4-dihydroxyphenyl)-2-methyl-L-alanine sesquihydrate. It contains not less than 98.5 per cent and not more than 101.0 per cent of $C_{10}H_{13}NO_4$, calculated with reference to the anhydrous substance.

Characteristics A white to yellowish-white, crystalline powder or colourless or almost colourless crystals.

Solubility Slightly soluble in *water* and in *ethanol (96%)*; practically insoluble in *chloroform* and in *ether*. It dissolves in dilute mineral acids.

Identification *Test A may be omitted if tests B, C and D are carried out. Tests B, C and D may be omitted if test A is carried out.*

A. The *infra-red absorption spectrum*, Appendix II A, is concordant with the spectrum of *methyldopa EPCRS*.

B. Dissolve 2 mg in 2 ml of *water* and add 0.2 ml of 0.05M *iron(III) chloride hexahydrate*. A green colour is produced which changes to bluish-violet on the addition of 0.1 g of *hexamine*.

C. Dissolve 5 mg in a mixture of 5 ml of 1M *hydrochloric acid* and 5 ml of *water* and add 0.1 ml of *sodium nitrite solution* containing 10% w/v of *ammonium molybdate*. A yellow colour is produced which changes to brownish-red on the addition of 10M *sodium hydroxide*.

D. To 5 mg add 1 ml of *water*, 1 ml of *pyridine* and 5 mg *4-nitrobenzoyl chloride*, heat to boiling and add, whilst shaking, 0.2 ml of 1M *sodium carbonate*. An orange or amber colour is produced.

Acidity Dissolve 1 g in 100 ml of *carbon dioxide-free water* with the aid of heat and add 0.1 ml of *methyl red solution*. Not more than 0.5 ml of 0.1M *sodium hydroxide VS* is required to produce a pure yellow colour.

Colour of solution A 4.0% w/v solution in 1M *hydrochloric acid* is not more intensely coloured than either *reference solution BY$_6$* or *B$_6$*, Appendix IV B, Method II.

Light absorption Dissolve 40 mg in sufficient 0.1M *hydrochloric acid* to produce 100 ml and dilute 10 ml to 100 ml with 0.1M *hydrochloric acid*. The *light absorption*, Appendix II B, in the range 230 to 350 nm exhibits a maximum only at 280 nm. The A(1%, 1 cm) at 280 nm is 122 to 137.

Optical rotation −1.10° to −1.23°, Appendix V F, in a solution prepared by dissolving a quantity containing the equivalent of 2.2 g of the dried substance in 25 ml of *aluminium chloride solution* and diluting to 50 ml with the same solvent.

Heavy metals 1.0 g complies with *limit test C for heavy metals*, Appendix VII (20 ppm). Use 2 ml of *lead standard solution (10 ppm Pb)* to prepare the standard.

3-Methoxy compound and related substances Carry out the method for *thin-layer chromatography*, Appendix III A, using *cellulose* as the coating substance and a mixture of 65 volumes of *butan-1-ol*, 25 volumes of *water* and 15 volumes of *glacial acetic acid* as the mobile phase, but allowing the solvent front to ascend 10 cm above the line of application. Apply separately to the chromatoplate 10 μl of each of solutions (1) and (2) and 20 μl of solution (3). Solution (1) contains 1.0% w/v of the substance being examined in a mixture of 4 volumes of 7M *hydrochloric acid* and 96 volumes of *methanol*. Solution (2) contains 0.0050% w/v of *methoxymethyldopa EPCRS* in *methanol*. Solution (3) is a mixture of equal volumes of solutions (1) and (2). After removal of the plate, dry it immediately in a current of warm air and spray with a mixture of 1 volume of a 5% w/v solution of *sodium nitrite* and 9 volumes of a 0.3% w/v solution of *4-nitroaniline* in a mixture of 80 volumes of *hydrochloric acid* and 20 volumes of *water*. Dry immediately in a current of warm air and spray with a 20% w/v solution of *sodium carbonate*. Any

secondary spot in the chromatogram obtained with solution (1) is not more intense than the spot in the chromatogram obtained with solution (2). The test is not valid unless the chromatogram obtained with solution (3) shows a spot corresponding to methyldopa clearly separated from the principal spot.

Sulphated ash Not more than 0.1%, Appendix IX A, Method II. Use 1 g.

Water 10.0 to 13.0% w/v, Appendix IX C. Use 0.2 g.

Assay Dissolve 0.2 g in a mixture of 15 ml of *anhydrous formic acid*, 30 ml of *anhydrous glacial acetic acid* and 30 ml of *1,4-dioxan* and carry out Method I for *non-aqueous titration*, Appendix VIII A, using 0.1 ml of *crystal violet solution* as indicator and titrating until a green colour is produced. Each ml of 0.1M *perchloric acid VS* is equivalent to 0.02112 g of C$_{10}$H$_{13}$NO$_4$.

Storage Methyldopa should be kept in a well-closed container and protected from light.

Preparation
Methyldopa Tablets

Action and use Antihypertensive.

Methyldopate Hydrochloride

C$_{12}$H$_{17}$NO$_4$,HCl   275.7   2508-79-4

Methyldopate Hydrochloride is ethyl 3-(3,4-dihydroxyphenyl)-2-methyl-L-alaninate hydrochloride. It contains not less than 98.5 per cent and not more than 101.0 per cent of C$_{12}$H$_{17}$NO$_4$,HCl, calculated with reference to the dried substance.

Characteristics A white or almost white, crystalline powder; odourless or almost odourless.

Solubility Soluble in 1 part of *water*, in 3 parts of *ethanol (96%)* and in 2 parts of *methanol*; slightly soluble in *chloroform*; practically insoluble in *ether*.

Identification A. The *infra-red absorption spectrum*, Appendix II A, is concordant with the *reference spectrum* of methyldopate hydrochloride.

B. The *light absorption*, Appendix II B, in the range 230 to 350 nm of a 0.008% w/v solution in 0.1M *hydrochloric acid* exhibits a maximum only at 280 nm. The *absorbance* at 280 nm is about 0.80.

C. Carry out the method for *thin-layer chromatography*, Appendix III A, using *microcrystalline cellulose* as the coating substance and a mixture of 50 volumes of *butan-1-ol*, 25 volumes of *glacial acetic acid* and 25 volumes of *water* as the mobile phase. Apply separately to the chromatoplate 5 μl of each of two solutions in 1M *hydrochloric acid* containing (1) 1% w/v of the substance being examined and (2) 1% w/v of *methyldopate hydrochloride BPCRS*. After removal of the plate, dry it in a current of warm air and spray with a freshly prepared solution of equal volumes of a 10% w/v solution of *iron(III) chloride hexahydrate* and a 5% w/v solution of *potassium hexacyanoferrate(III)*. The principal spot in the chromatogram obtained with solution (1) corresponds to that in the chromatogram obtained with solution (2).

D. Yields *reaction A* characteristic of chlorides, Appendix VI.

Acidity pH of a 1% w/v solution, 3.0 to 5.0, Appendix V L.

Specific optical rotation In a 4% w/v solution in 0.1M *hydrochloric acid* and determined at 405 nm, −13.5° to −14.9°, Appendix V F.

Related substances Carry out the method for *thin-layer chromatography*, Appendix III A, using *silica gel GF254* as the coating substance and a mixture of equal volumes of *acetone, butan-1-ol, glacial acetic acid, toluene* and *water* as the mobile phase, but allowing the solvent front to ascend 12 cm above the line of application. Apply separately to the chromatoplate 2 μl of each of three solutions in *methanol* containing (1) 10.0% w/v of the substance being examined, (2) 0.25% w/v of *methyldopa BPCRS* and (3) 0.040% w/v of *methyldopa BPCRS*. After removal of the plate, allow it to dry in air, heat at 105° for 10 minutes and examine under *ultra-violet light (254 nm)*. Expose the plate to iodine vapour for 10 minutes and examine again. Using both methods of visualisation, any spot corresponding to methyldopa in the chromatogram obtained with solution (1) is not more intense than the spot in the chromatogram obtained with solution (2) and any other *secondary spot* is not more intense than the spot in the chromatogram obtained with solution (3).

Loss on drying When dried to constant weight at 105° at a pressure not exceeding 0.7 kPa, loses not more than 0.5% of its weight. Use 1 g.

Sulphated ash Not more than 0.1%, Appendix IX A.

Assay Carry out Method I for *non-aqueous titration*, Appendix VIII A, using 0.5 g and determining the end-point potentiometrically. Each ml of 0.1M *perchloric acid VS* is equivalent to 0.02757 g of $C_{12}H_{17}NO_4,HCl$.

Storage Methyldopate Hydrochloride should be protected from light.

Preparation
Methyldopate Injection

Action and use Antihypertensive.

Methylphenobarbitone ☆

$C_{13}H_{14}N_2O_3$ 246.3   *113-38-8*

Methylphenobarbitone is 5-ethyl-1-methyl-5-phenylbarbituric acid. It contains not less than 99.0 per cent and not more than 102.0 per cent of $C_{13}H_{14}N_2O_3$, calculated with reference to the dried substance.

Characteristics Colourless crystals or a white, crystalline powder; odourless.

Solubility Practically insoluble in *water*; very slightly soluble in *absolute ethanol*; slightly soluble in *chloroform*

and in *ether*. It dissolves in aqueous solutions of alkali hydroxides and carbonates and in aqueous ammonia.

Identification *Test A may be omitted if tests B, C and D are carried out. Tests B and C may be omitted if tests A and D are carried out.*

A. The *infra-red absorption spectrum*, Appendix II A, is concordant with the spectrum of *methylphenobarbital EPCRS*.

B. Carry out the test for Related substances but allow the solvent front to ascend 18 cm above the line of application and apply to the chromatoplate 10 μl of each of two solutions in *chloroform* containing (1) 0.1% w/v of the substance being examined and (2) 0.1% w/v of *methylphenobarbital EPCRS*. After removal of the plate, examine immediately under *ultra-violet light (254 nm)*. The principal spot in the chromatogram obtained with solution (1) is similar in position and size to that in the chromatogram obtained with solution (2).

C. To 10 mg add 0.2 ml of *sulphuric acid* and 0.1 ml of *nitric acid* and heat on a water-bath for 10 minutes. Cool in ice and add 5 ml of *water* and 5 ml of 5M *sodium hydroxide*. Add 5 ml of *acetone*, shake and allow to stand. A dark red colour is produced in the upper layer.

D. Determine the *melting points*, Appendix V A, Method I, of the substance being examined and of a mixture of equal parts of the substance being examined and *methylphenobarbital EPCRS*. The difference between the melting points, which are about 178°, is not greater than 2°.

Acidity Boil 1 g with 50 ml of *water* for 2 minutes, allow to cool and filter. To 10 ml of the filtrate add 0.15 ml of *methyl red solution*. The solution is orange-yellow and not more than 0.1 ml of 0.1M *sodium hydroxide VS* is required to change the colour to a pure yellow.

Clarity and colour of solution Dissolve 1.0 g in 4 ml of 2M *sodium hydroxide* and 6 ml of *water*, with gentle heating. The solution is *clear*, Appendix IV A, and not more intensely coloured than *reference solution* Y_6, Appendix IV B, Method II.

Related substances Complies with the test for *related substances in barbiturates*, Appendix III A, but using as solution (2) a 0.01% w/v solution of *phenobarbital EPCRS* in *chloroform*.

Loss on drying When dried to constant weight at 100° to 105°, loses not more than 0.5% of its weight. Use 1 g.

Sulphated ash Not more than 0.1%, Appendix IX A, Method II. Use 1 g.

Assay Dissolve 0.2 g in 5 ml of *pyridine*, add 10 ml of *silver nitrate—pyridine reagent* and titrate with 0.1M *ethanolic sodium hydroxide VS*, using 0.5 ml of *thymolphthalein solution* as indicator, until a pure blue colour is obtained. Repeat the operation without the substance being examined. The difference between the titrations represents the amount of sodium hydroxide required. Each ml of 0.1M *ethanolic sodium hydroxide VS* is equivalent to 0.02463 g of $C_{13}H_{14}N_2O_3$.

Action and use Anticonvulsant.

The title of the monograph in the European Pharmacopœia is Methylphenobarbital.

Methylprednisolone

$C_{22}H_{30}O_5$ 374.5   *83-43-2*

Methylprednisolone is 11β,17α,21-trihydroxy-6α-methylpregna-1,4-diene-3,20-dione. It contains not less than 96.0 per cent and not more than 104.0 per cent of $C_{22}H_{30}O_5$, calculated with reference to the dried substance.

Characteristics A white or almost white, crystalline powder; odourless or almost odourless.

Solubility Practically insoluble in *water*; slightly soluble in *absolute ethanol* and in *chloroform*.

Identification A. The *infra-red absorption spectrum*, Appendix II A, is concordant with the *reference spectrum* of methylprednisolone. If the spectra are not concordant dissolve a sufficient quantity in the minimum volume of *chloroform IR*, evaporate to dryness and prepare a new spectrum of the residue.
B. Complies with the test for *identification of steroids*, Appendix III A, using *impregnating solvent I* and *mobile phase A*.
C. *Melting point*, about 243°, with decomposition, Appendix V A.

Light absorption *Absorbance* of a 0.001% w/v solution in *absolute ethanol* at the maximum at 240 nm, 0.39 to 0.41, Appendix II B. The ratio of the absorbance at the maximum at 240 nm to that at 263 nm is 1.50 to 1.70.

Specific optical rotation In a 1% w/v solution in *1,4-dioxan*, +79° to +86°, Appendix V F.

Related foreign steroids Complies with the test for *related foreign steroids*, Appendix III A, Method A.

Loss on drying When dried to constant weight at 105°, loses not more than 0.5% of its weight. Use 1 g.

Sulphated ash Not more than 0.1%, Appendix IX A.

Assay Carry out the *tetrazolium assay of steroids*, Appendix VIII P, using a quantity dissolved in sufficient *aldehyde-free absolute ethanol* to produce a solution containing between 390 and 410 µg in 10 ml. Calculate the content of $C_{22}H_{30}O_5$ from the *absorbance* obtained by repeating the operation using *methylprednisolone BPCRS* in place of the substance being examined.

Storage Methylprednisolone should be protected from light.

Preparation
Methylprednisolone Tablets

Action and use Corticosteroid.

Methylprednisolone Acetate

$C_{24}H_{32}O_6$ 416.5   *53-36-1*

Methylprednisolone Acetate is 11β,17α,21-trihydroxy-6α-methylpregna-1,4-diene-3,20-dione 21-acetate. It contains not less than 96.0 per cent and not more than 104.0 per cent of $C_{24}H_{32}O_6$, calculated with reference to the dried substance.

Characteristics A white or almost white, crystalline powder; odourless or almost odourless.

Solubility Practically insoluble in *water*; slightly soluble in *absolute ethanol*; very slightly soluble in *ether*.

Identification A. The *infra-red absorption spectrum*, Appendix II A, is concordant with the *reference spectrum* of methylprednisolone acetate.
B. Complies with the test for *identification of steroids*, Appendix III A, using *impregnating solvent I* and *mobile phase A*.

Light absorption *Absorbance* of a 0.001% w/v solution in *absolute ethanol* at the maximum at 240 nm, 0.34 to 0.37, Appendix II B. The ratio of the absorbance at the maximum at 240 nm to that at 263 nm is 1.50 to 1.70.

Specific optical rotation In a 1% w/v solution in *1,4-dioxan*, +97° to +105°, Appendix V F.

Related foreign steroids Complies with the test for *related foreign steroids*, Appendix III A, Method A.

Loss on drying When dried to constant weight at 105°, loses not more than 1.0% of its weight. Use 1 g.

Sulphated ash Not more than 0.2%, Appendix IX A.

Assay Dissolve 0.1 g in sufficient *absolute ethanol* to produce 200 ml, dilute 5 ml to 250 ml with *absolute ethanol* and mix. To 20 ml of the resulting solution add 2.0 ml of a 0.5% w/v solution of *tetrazolium blue* in *absolute ethanol*, mix, add 2.0 ml of a mixture of 1 volume of *tetramethylammonium hydroxide solution* and 9 volumes of *absolute ethanol*, mix and allow to stand in the dark for 90 minutes. Immediately measure the *absorbance* of the resulting solution at the maximum at 525 nm, Appendix II B, using in the reference cell 20 ml of *absolute ethanol* treated in the same manner. Calculate the content of $C_{24}H_{32}O_6$ from the *absorbance* obtained by carrying out the procedure at the same time using 0.1 g of *methylprednisolone acetate BPCRS* in place of the substance being examined.

Storage Methylprednisolone Acetate should be kept in a well-closed container and protected from light.

Preparation
Methylprednisolone Acetate Injection

Action and use Corticosteroid.

Methyltestosterone ☆

$C_{20}H_{30}O_2$ 302.5   *58-18-4*

Methyltestosterone is 17β-hydroxy-17α-methylandrost-4-en-3-one. It contains not less than 97.0 per cent and not more than 103.0 per cent of $C_{20}H_{30}O_2$, calculated with reference to the dried substance.

Characteristics A white or slightly yellowish-white, crystalline powder.

Solubility Practically insoluble in *water*; soluble in 5 parts of *ethanol (96%)* and in 10 parts of *acetone*; freely soluble in *chloroform* and in *1,4-dioxan*; slightly soluble in *ether*.

Identification *Test A may be omitted if tests B and C are carried out. Tests B and C may be omitted if test A is carried out.*
A. The *infra-red absorption spectrum*, Appendix II A, is concordant with the spectrum of *methyltestosterone EPCRS*.
B. After examination of the chromatograms obtained in the test for Related substances spray the chromatoplate with a saturated solution of *potassium dichromate* in *sulphuric acid (70%)* and examine immediately in daylight. The principal spot in the chromatogram obtained with solution (1) is similar in position, colour and size to that in the chromatogram obtained with solution (4).
C. *Melting point*, 162° to 168°, Appendix V A, Method I.

Specific optical rotation In a 1% w/v solution in *ethanol (96%)*, +79° to +85°, Appendix V F.

Related substances Carry out the method for *thin-layer chromatography*, Appendix II A, using as the coating substance a suitable silica gel containing a fluorescent indicator with an optimal intensity at 254 nm (Merck silica gel 60 F254 is suitable) and a mixture of 70 volumes of *butyl acetate*, 30 volumes of *petroleum spirit (boiling range, 50° to 70°)* and 1 volume of *glacial acetic acid* as the mobile phase. Apply separately to the chromatoplate 5 μl of each of the following five solutions in a mixture of 9 volumes of *chloroform* and 1 volume of *methanol*. Solutions (1), (2) and (3) contain 2.0% w/v, 0.020% w/v and 0.010% w/v respectively of the substance being examined. Solution (4) contains 2.0% w/v of *methyltestosterone EPCRS*. Solution (5) contains 0.10% w/v each of *methyltestosterone EPCRS* and *testosterone EPCRS*. After removal of the plate, allow it to dry in air and examine under *ultra-violet light (254 nm)*. Any *secondary spot* in the chromatogram obtained with solution (1) is not more intense than the spot in the chromatogram obtained with solution (2) and not more than one such spot is more intense than the spot in the chromatogram obtained with solution (3). The test is not valid unless the chromatogram obtained with solution (5) shows two clearly separated principal spots.

Loss on drying When dried at 100° to 105° for 2 hours, loses not more than 2.0% of its weight. Use 0.5 g.

Assay Dissolve 50 mg in sufficient *ethanol (96%)* to produce 50 ml, dilute 10 ml to 100 ml with the same solvent, further dilute 10 ml to 100 ml and measure the *absorbance* of the resulting solution at the maximum at 241 nm, Appendix II B. Calculate the content of $C_{20}H_{30}O_2$ taking 540 as the value of A(1%, 1 cm) at the maximum at 241 nm.

Storage Methyltestosterone should be kept in a well-closed container protected from light.

Action and use Androgen; anabolic steroid.

Methyprylone

$C_{10}H_{17}NO_2$ 183.3   *125-64-4*

Methyprylone is 3,3-diethyl-5-methylpiperidine-2,4-dione. It contains not less than 98.5 per cent and not more than 101.0 per cent of $C_{10}H_{17}NO_2$, calculated with reference to the dried substance.

Characteristics A white or almost white, crystalline powder; odour, slight and characteristic.

Solubility Soluble in 14 parts of *water*, in 0.7 part of *ethanol (96%)*, in 0.6 part of *chloroform* and in 3.5 parts of *ether*.

Identification A. The *infra-red absorption spectrum*, Appendix II A, is concordant with the *reference spectrum* of methyprylone.
B. Add 50 mg to a mixture of 5 ml of *water* and 2 ml of 1M *sodium hydroxide*, mix and add 0.5 ml of *potassium hexacyanoferrate(III) solution*. The solution exhibits a green fluorescence under ultra-violet light.

Melting point 74° to 77°, Appendix V A.

Light absorption *Absorbance* of a 0.15% w/v solution in *propan-1-ol* at the maximum at 296 nm, not more than 0.37, Appendix II B.

Related substances Carry out the method for *gas chromatography*, Appendix III B, using three solutions in *dichloromethane* containing (1) 0.010% w/v of the substance being examined and 0.02% w/v of *triphenylmethane* (internal standard), (2) 2.0% w/v of the substance being examined and (3) 2.0% w/v of the substance being examined and 0.02% w/v of the internal standard.

The chromatographic procedure may be carried out using a glass column (1.5 m × 4 mm) packed with *acid-washed, silanised diatomaceous support* (80 to 100 mesh) coated with 8% w/w of butane-1,4-diol succinate and maintained at 190°.

In the chromatogram obtained with solution (3) the ratio of the area of any *secondary peak* to the area of the peak due to the internal standard is not greater than the ratio of the area of the peak due to methyprylone to that of the peak due to the internal standard in the chromatogram obtained with solution (1). The sum of any such ratios calculated for solution (3) is not greater than twice the ratio calculated for solution (1).

Loss on drying When dried to constant weight at 50° at a pressure not exceeding 0.7 kPa, loses not more than 0.5% of its weight. Use 1 g.

Sulphated ash Not more than 0.1%, Appendix IX A.

Assay Dissolve 0.15 g in 40 ml of *water*, add 12.5 ml of 5M *sodium hydroxide* and titrate with 0.1M *alkaline potassium hexacyanoferrate(III) VS*. Use platinum and calomel electrodes and a direct-reading millivoltmeter as the indicator system and add the titrant rapidly to within about 1 ml of the calculated end-point and then dropwise until the rise of potential in the first minute after the addition of one drop suddenly falls to less than 20 mV. Each ml of 0.1M *alkaline potassium hexacyanoferrate(III) VS* is equivalent to 0.009163 g of $C_{10}H_{17}NO_2$.

Storage Methyprylone should be kept in a well-closed container and protected from light.

Preparation

Methyprylone Tablets

Action and use Sedative; hypnotic.

In some countries the material described in this monograph may be known as Methyprylon.

Methysergide Maleate

$C_{21}H_{27}N_3O_2,C_4H_4O_4$ 469.5   *129-49-7*

Methysergide Maleate is *N*-[1-(hydroxymethyl)propyl]-1-methyl-D-lysergamide hydrogen maleate. It contains not less than 98.0 per cent and not more than 101.0 per cent of $C_{21}H_{27}N_3O_2,C_4H_4O_4$, calculated with reference to the dried substance.

Characteristics A white or almost white, crystalline powder which may have a yellow or pink tinge; odourless or almost odourless.

Solubility Slightly soluble in *water* and in *methanol*; practically insoluble in *chloroform* and in *ether*.

Identification A. The *infra-red absorption spectrum*, Appendix II A, is concordant with the *reference spectrum* of methysergide maleate.

B. In the test for Related substances, the principal spot in the chromatogram obtained with solution (1) corresponds to that in the chromatogram obtained with solution (8).

C. Dissolve 1 mg in 1 ml of *ethanol (96%)* and add 1 ml of *dilute dimethylaminobenzaldehyde solution*. A brownish-red to violet colour is produced.

Acidity pH of a 0.2% w/v solution, 3.7 to 4.7, Appendix V L.

Specific optical rotation In a 0.25% w/v solution, +35.0° to +45.0°, Appendix V F.

Related substances Carry out in subdued light the method for *thin-layer chromatography*, Appendix III A, using a suspension of *silica gel G* in 0.1M *sodium hydroxide* to prepare the chromatoplate and a mixture of 90 volumes of *chloroform* and 10 volumes of *methanol* as the mobile phase. Apply separately to the plate 5 µl of each of the

following solutions. Solution (1) contains 2.0% w/v of the substance being examined in a mixture of 1 volume of 13.5M *ammonia* and 100 volumes of *methanol*. Solutions (2), (3), (4), (5), (6), (7) and (8) contain 0.0050% w/v, 0.010% w/v, 0.015% w/v, 0.020% w/v, 0.030% w/v, 0.040% w/v and 2.0% w/v respectively of *methysergide maleate BPCRS* in a mixture of 1 volume of 13.5M *ammonia* and 100 volumes of *methanol*. After removal of the plate, allow it to dry in air and examine under *ultra-violet light (365 nm)*. Assess the intensities of any *secondary spots* in the chromatogram obtained with solution (1) by reference to the spots in the chromatograms obtained with solutions (2) to (7), making allowance for area in assessing the intensities of spots of different Rf values and disregarding any spots less intense than the spot in the chromatogram obtained with solution (2). The total of the intensities so assessed does not exceed 2%.

Loss on drying When dried to constant weight at 120° at a pressure not exceeding 0.7 kPa, loses not more than 7.0% of its weight. Use 1 g.

Assay Carry out Method I for *non-aqueous titration*, Appendix VIII A, using 0.4 g and *1-naphtholbenzein solution* as indicator. Each ml of 0.1M *perchloric acid VS* is equivalent to 0.04695 g of $C_{21}H_{27}N_3O_2,C_4H_4O_4$.

Storage Methysergide Maleate should be kept in a well-closed container, protected from light and stored at a temperature of 2° to 8°.

Preparation

Methysergide Tablets

Action and use Prophylaxis of migraine.

Metoclopramide Hydrochloride

$C_{14}H_{22}ClN_3O_2,HCl,H_2O$ 354.3   *34143-57-6*

Metoclopramide Hydrochloride is 4-amino-5-chloro-*N*-(2-diethylaminoethyl)-2-methoxy-benzamide hydrochloride monohydrate. It contains not less than 98.0 per cent and not more than 101.0 per cent of $C_{14}H_{22}ClN_3O_2,HCl$, calculated with reference to the anhydrous substance.

Characteristics A white or almost white, crystalline powder; odourless or almost odourless.

Solubility Soluble in 0.7 part of *water*, in 3 parts of *ethanol (96%)* and in 55 parts of *chloroform*; practically insoluble in *ether*.

Identification A. The *infra-red absorption spectrum*, Appendix II A, is concordant with the *reference spectrum* of metoclopramide hydrochloride.

B. The *light absorption*, Appendix II B, in the range 230 to 350 nm of a 0.002% w/v solution in 0.01M *hydrochloric acid* exhibits two maxima, at 273 nm and 309 nm. The *absorbance* at 273 nm is about 0.79 and at 309 nm is about 0.69.

C. Dissolve 50 mg in 5 ml of *water* and add 5 ml of a 1% w/v solution of *4-dimethylaminobenzaldehyde* in 1M *hydrochloric acid*. A yellowish-orange colour is produced.

D. Yields *reaction A* characteristic of chlorides, Appendix VI.

Acidity pH of a 10% w/v solution, 4.5 to 6.5, Appendix V L.

Related substances Carry out the method for *thin-layer chromatography*, Appendix III A, using *silica gel GF254* as the coating substance and a mixture of 95 volumes of *butan-1-ol* and 5 volumes of 13.5M *ammonia* as the mobile phase. Apply separately to the chromatoplate 5 µl of each of two solutions of the substance being examined in *methanol* containing (1) 5.0% w/v and (2) 0.050% w/v. After removal of the plate, allow it to dry in air and examine under *ultra-violet light (254 nm)*. Any *secondary spot* in the chromatogram obtained with solution (1) is not more intense than the spot in the chromatogram obtained with solution (2).

Sulphated ash Not more than 0.1%, Appendix IX A.

Water 4.5 to 5.5% w/w, Appendix IX C. Use 0.5 g.

Assay To 0.3 g add 10 ml of *mercury(II) acetate solution* and 2 ml of *acetic anhydride*. Allow to stand in a stoppered flask for 3 hours, add 80 ml of *anhydrous glacial acetic acid* and titrate with 0.1M *perchloric acid VS* determining the end-point potentiometrically. Each ml of 0.1M *perchloric acid VS* is equivalent to 0.03363 g of $C_{14}H_{22}ClN_3O_2,HCl$.

Storage Metoclopramide Hydrochloride should be protected from light.

Preparations
Metoclopramide Injection
Metoclopramide Tablets

Action and use Antispasmodic; antiemetic.

Metronidazole

CH₂·CH₂OH structure

$C_6H_9N_3O_3$ 171.2   *443-48-1*

Metronidazole is 2-(2-methyl-5-nitroimidazol-1-yl)ethanol. It contains not less than 99.0 per cent and not more than 101.0 per cent of $C_6H_9N_3O_3$, calculated with reference to the dried substance.

Characteristics A white or creamy-white, crystalline powder; odourless or almost odourless.

Solubility Slightly soluble in *water*, in *ethanol (96%)*, in *chloroform* and in *ether*.

Identification A. The *infra-red absorption spectrum*, Appendix II A, is concordant with the *reference spectrum* of metronidazole.
B. The *light absorption*, Appendix II B, in the range 230 to 350 nm of a 0.002% w/v solution in 0.1M *hydrochloric acid* exhibits a maximum only at 277 nm. The *absorbance* at 277 nm is about 0.76.
C. Dissolve 0.1 g in 4 ml of 0.5M *sulphuric acid*, add 10 ml of *trinitrophenol solution* and allow to stand. The *melting point* of the precipitate, after washing with *water* and drying at 105°, is about 150°, Appendix V A.
D. Heat 10 mg in a water-bath with 10 mg of *zinc powder*, 1 ml of *water* and 0.25 ml of *hydrochloric acid* for 5

minutes, cool in ice, add 0.5 ml of *sodium nitrite solution* and remove the excess of nitrite with *sulphamic acid*. Add 0.5 ml of the product to a mixture of 0.5 ml of *2-naphthol solution* and 2 ml of 5M *sodium hydroxide*. An orange-red colour is produced.

Melting point 159° to 162°, Appendix V A.

Related substances Carry out the method for *thin-layer chromatography*, Appendix III A, using a silica gel F254 precoated chromatoplate (Merck silica gel 60 F254 plates are suitable) and a mixture of 80 volumes of *chloroform*, 20 volumes of *dimethylformamide* and 5 volumes of a 90% v/v solution of *formic acid* as the mobile phase. Apply separately to the plate 20 µl of each of three solutions in a mixture of equal volumes of *chloroform* and *methanol* containing (1) 4.0% w/v of the substance being examined, (2) 0.020% w/v of *2-methyl-5-nitroimidazole* and (3) 0.0080% w/v of *2-methyl-5-nitroimidazole*. After removal of the plate, allow the solvent to evaporate and examine under *ultra-violet light (254 nm)*. In the chromatogram obtained with solution (1) any spot corresponding to 2-methyl-5-nitroimidazole is not more intense than the spot in the chromatogram obtained with solution (2), any other *secondary spot* is not more intense than the spot in the chromatogram obtained with solution (2) and not more than two such spots are more intense than the spot in the chromatogram obtained with solution (3).

Loss on drying When dried to constant weight at 105°, loses not more than 0.5% of its weight. Use 1 g.

Sulphated ash Not more than 0.1%, Appendix IX A.

Assay Carry out Method I for *non-aqueous titration*, Appendix VIII A, using 0.45 g dissolved in 10 ml of *anhydrous glacial acetic acid* and *1-naphtholbenzein solution* as indicator. Each ml of 0.1M *perchloric acid VS* is equivalent to 0.01712 g of $C_6H_9N_3O_3$.

Preparations
Metronidazole Suppositories
Metronidazole Tablets

Action and use Antibacterial.

Metyrapone

CMe₂·CO structure

$C_{14}H_{14}N_2O$ 226.3   *54-36-4*

Metyrapone is 2-methyl-1,2-di(3-pyridyl)-propan-1-one. It contains not less than 97.0 per cent and not more than 103.0 per cent of $C_{14}H_{14}N_2O$, calculated with reference to the dried substance.

Characteristics A white to light amber, crystalline powder; odour, characteristic.

Solubility Soluble in 100 parts of *water*, in 3 parts of *ethanol (96%)* and in 3 parts of *chloroform*. It dissolves in dilute mineral acids.

Identification A. The *infra-red absorption spectrum*, Appendix II A, is concordant with *reference spectrum 1* of metyrapone.
B. The *light absorption*, Appendix II B, in the range 230 to 350 nm of a 0.002% w/v solution in 0.1M *hydrochloric acid*

exhibits a maximum only at 260 nm. The *absorbance* at 260 nm is about 1.0.

C. To 5 ml of a 1% w/v solution in 1M *sulphuric acid* add 0.2 ml of *potassium mercuri-iodide solution*. A cream precipitate is produced.

Melting point 50° to 53°, Appendix V A.

Related substances Carry out in subdued light the method for *thin-layer chromatography*, Appendix III A, using *silica gel GF254* as the coating substance and a mixture of 90 volumes of *propan-2-ol*, 5 volumes of 13.5M *ammonia* and 5 volumes of *water* as the mobile phase. Apply separately to the chromatoplate 10 μl of each of two solutions of the substance being examined in *chloroform* containing (1) 5.0% w/v and (2) 0.010% w/v. After removal of the plate, allow it to dry in air and examine under *ultra-violet light (254 nm)*. Any *secondary spot* in the chromatogram obtained with solution (1) is not more intense than the spot in the chromatogram obtained with solution (2).

Loss on drying When dried over *phosphorus pentoxide* at a pressure not exceeding 0.7 kPa for 6 hours, loses not more than 0.5% of its weight. Use 1 g.

Sulphated ash Not more than 0.1%, Appendix IX A.

Assay Carry out the following procedure protected from light. Dissolve 0.1 g in sufficient 0.1M *hydrochloric acid* to produce 100 ml. Dilute 5 ml to 50 ml with 0.1M *hydrochloric acid* and dilute 5 ml of this solution to 50 ml with 0.1M *hydrochloric acid*. Measure the *absorbance* of the resulting solution at the maximum at 260 nm, Appendix II B. Calculate the content of $C_{14}H_{14}N_2O$ taking 500 as the value of A(1%, 1 cm) at the maximum at 260 nm.

Storage Metyrapone should be protected from light.

Preparation

Metyrapone Capsules

Action and use Diagnostic agent for pituitary function.

Mexenone

Me—◯—CO—◯—OMe
　　　　　　　HO

$C_{15}H_{14}O_3$　　242.3　　*1641-17-4*

Mexenone is 2-hydroxy-4-methoxy-4'-methyl-benzophenone. It contains not less than 97.0 per cent and not more than 103.0 per cent of $C_{15}H_{14}O_3$, calculated with reference to the dried substance.

Characteristics A pale yellow, crystalline powder; odourless or almost odourless.

Solubility Practically insoluble in *water*; soluble in 70 parts of *ethanol (96%)* and in 7 parts of *acetone*.

Identification A. The *infra-red absorption spectrum*, Appendix II A, is concordant with the *reference spectrum* of mexenone.

B. The *light absorption*, Appendix II B, in the range 230 to 350 nm of a 0.0015% w/v solution in *methanol* exhibits three maxima, at 243, 287 and 325 nm. The *absorbance* at

243 nm is about 0.53, at 287 nm, about 0.90 and at 325 nm, about 0.66.

C. In the test for Related substances, the principal spot in the chromatogram obtained with solution (2) corresponds to the spot in the chromatogram obtained with solution (4).

Melting point 99° to 102°, Appendix V A.

Iron Ignite 1.0 g with 1 g of *anhydrous sodium carbonate*, cool, dissolve the residue in 5 ml of *hydrochloric acid* and dilute to 40 ml with *water*. 10 ml of the solution complies with the *limit test for iron*, Appendix VII (40 ppm).

Related substances Carry out the method for *thin-layer chromatography*, Appendix III A, using *silica gel GF254* as the coating substance and a mixture of 100 volumes of *toluene* and 10 volumes of *butan-2-one* as the mobile phase. Apply separately to the chromatoplate 5 μl of each of four solutions in *butan-2-one* containing (1) 10% w/v of the substance being examined, (2) 0.20% w/v of the substance being examined, (3) 0.10% w/v of the substance being examined and (4) 0.20% w/v of *mexenone BPCRS*. After removal of the plate, allow it to dry in air and examine under *ultra-violet light (254 nm)*. Any *secondary spot* in the chromatogram obtained with solution (1) is not more intense than the spot in the chromatogram obtained with solution (3).

Loss on drying When dried to constant weight at 60° at a pressure not exceeding 3.5 kPa, loses not more than 0.5% of its weight. Use 1 g.

Sulphated ash Not more than 0.1%, Appendix IX A.

Assay Dissolve 80 mg in sufficient *methanol* to produce 100 ml. Dilute 10 ml of the solution to 100 ml with *methanol* and further dilute 10 ml of this solution to 100 ml with *methanol*. Measure the *absorbance* of the resulting solution at the maximum at 287 nm, Appendix II B, and calculate the content of $C_{15}H_{14}O_3$ taking 640 as the value of A(1%, 1 cm) at the maximum at 287 nm.

Action and use Topical sun-screening substance.

Mexiletine Hydrochloride

　　Me
　　　　Me
◯—OCH₂·CH·NH₂　,HCl
　　Me

$C_{11}H_{17}NO,HCl$　　215.7　　*5370-01-4*

Mexiletine Hydrochloride is 1-methyl-2-(2,6-xylyloxy)ethylamine hydrochloride. It contains not less than 99.0 per cent and not more than 101.0 per cent of $C_{11}H_{17}NO,HCl$, calculated with reference to the anhydrous substance.

Characteristics A white or almost white, crystalline powder; odourless or almost odourless.

Solubility Freely soluble in *water* and in *methanol*; sparingly soluble in *chloroform*; practically insoluble in *ether*.

Identification A. The *light absorption*, Appendix II B, in the range 230 to 350 nm of a 0.04% w/v solution in 0.01M *hydrochloric acid* exhibits a maximum at 260 nm. The *absorbance* at 260 nm is about 0.46.

B. In the test for Related substances, the principal spot in the chromatogram obtained with solution (2) corresponds to that in the chromatogram obtained with solution (4).

C. Dissolve 0.1 g in 3 ml of 0.02M *hydrochloric acid* and add a few crystals of *sodium nitrite*. Nitrogen is evolved and a yellow colour may be produced slowly.

D. A 1% w/v solution yields *reaction A* characteristic of chlorides, Appendix VI.

Acidity pH of a 10% w/v solution, 4.0 to 5.5, Appendix V L.

Clarity and colour of solution A 5.0% w/v solution is *clear*, Appendix IV A, and *colourless*, Appendix IV B, Method II.

Heavy metals 2.0 g complies with *limit test C for heavy metals*, Appendix VII (10 ppm). Use 2 ml of *lead standard solution (10 ppm Pb)* to prepare the standard.

2,6-Dimethylphenol Carry out the procedure described under Related substances applying 10 μl of each of two solutions in *methanol* containing (1) 5.0% w/v of the substance being examined and (2) 0.010% w/v of *2,6-dimethylphenol*. After removal of the plate, allow it to dry in air, spray with a 0.1% w/v solution of *fast blue B salt* in *methanol*, dry at about 90° and then spray with 3M *methanolic potassium hydroxide*. Any spot corresponding to 2,6-dimethylphenol in the chromatogram obtained with solution (1) is not more intense than the spot in the chromatogram obtained with solution (2).

Related substances Carry out the method for *thin-layer chromatography*, Appendix III A, using *silica gel G* as the coating substance and a mixture of 85 volumes of *chloroform*, 14 volumes of *methanol* and 1 volume of 18M *ammonia* as the mobile phase. Apply separately to the chromatoplate 10 μl of each of the following solutions. Solutions (1), (2) and (3) are solutions of the substance being examined in *methanol* containing (1) 5.0% w/v, (2) 0.20% w/v and (3) 0.025% w/v. Solution (4) contains 0.20% w/v of *mexiletine hydrochloride BPCRS* in *methanol*. After removal of the plate, allow it to dry in air, spray with *ninhydrin solution* and heat at 110° for 15 minutes. Any *secondary spot* in the chromatogram obtained with solution (1) is not more intense than the spot in the chromatogram obtained with solution (3).

Sulphated ash Not more than 0.1%, Appendix IX A.

Water Not more than 0.5% w/v, Appendix IX C. Use 5 g.

Assay Carry out Method I for *non-aqueous titration*, Appendix VIII A, using 0.3 g and 10 ml of *mercury(II) acetate solution* and determining the end-point potentiometrically. Each ml of 0.1M *perchloric acid VS* is equivalent to 0.02157 g of $C_{11}H_{17}NO,HCl$.

Preparations
Mexiletine Capsules
Mexiletine Injection

Action and use Anti-arrhythmic.

Mianserin Hydrochloride

$C_{18}H_{20}N_2,HCl$ 300.8   *21535-47-7*

Mianserin Hydrochloride is 1,2,3,4,10,14b-hexahydro-2-methyldibenzo[*c,f*]pyrazino[1,2-*a*]-azepine hydrochloride. It contains not less than 98.5 per cent and not more than 101.0 per cent of $C_{18}H_{20}N_2,HCl$, calculated with reference to the dried substance.

Characteristics White or almost white crystals or crystalline powder; odourless or almost odourless.

Solubility Soluble in 50 parts of *water*, in 100 parts of *ethanol (96%)* and in 20 parts of *chloroform*.

Identification A. The *infra-red absorption spectrum*, Appendix II A, is concordant with the *reference spectrum* of mianserin hydrochloride. If the spectra are not concordant, dissolve a sufficient quantity in the minimum volume of *methanol*, evaporate to dryness and prepare a new spectrum of the residue.

B. The *light absorption*, Appendix II B, in the range 230 to 350 nm of a 0.017% w/v solution exhibits a maximum only at 279 nm. The *absorbance* at 279 nm is about 1.1.

C. Yields the *reactions* characteristic of chlorides, Appendix VI.

Acidity pH of a 1% w/v solution, 4.0 to 5.5, Appendix V L.

Related substances Carry out the method for *thin-layer chromatography*, Appendix III A, using *silica gel G* as the coating substance and a mixture of 90 volumes of *dichloromethane* and 10 volumes of *methanol* as the mobile phase. Apply separately to the chromatoplate 5 μl of each of three solutions of the substance being examined in a mixture of 4 volumes of *methanol* and 1 volume of 13.5M *ammonia* containing (1) 2.0% w/v, (2) 0.010% w/v and (3) 0.0020% w/v. After removal of the plate, allow it to dry in a current of cold air for 5 minutes and then expose to iodine vapour for 20 minutes. Any *secondary spot* in the chromatogram obtained with solution (1) is not more intense than the spot in the chromatogram obtained with solution (2) and not more than one such spot is more intense than the spot in the chromatogram obtained with solution (3).

Loss on drying When dried to constant weight at 105° at a pressure not exceeding 0.7 kPa, loses not more than 0.5% of its weight. Use 1 g.

Sulphated ash Not more than 0.1%, Appendix IX A.

Assay Carry out Method I for *non-aqueous titration*, Appendix VIII A, using 0.25 g and 7 ml of *mercury(II) acetate solution* and determining the end-point potentiometrically. Each ml of 0.1M *perchloric acid VS* is equivalent to 0.03008 g of $C_{18}H_{20}N_2,HCl$.

Storage Mianserin Hydrochloride should be kept in a well-closed container and protected from light.

Preparation
Mianserin Tablets

Action and use Antidepressant.

Miconazole Nitrate ☆

$C_{18}H_{14}Cl_4N_2O,HNO_3$ 479.1   *22832-87-7*

Miconazole Nitrate is 1-[2,4-dichloro-β-(2,4-dichlorobenzyloxy)phenethyl]imidazole nitrate. It contains not less than 98.5 per cent and not more than 101.5 per cent of $C_{18}H_{14}Cl_4N_2O,HNO_3$, calculated with reference to the dried substance.

Characteristics A white or almost white, crystalline or microcrystalline powder.

Solubility Very slightly soluble in *water* and in *ether*; slightly soluble in *ethanol (96%)* and in *chloroform*.

Identification *Test A may be omitted if tests B, C, D and E are carried out. Tests B, C and D may be omitted if tests A and E are carried out.*
A. The *infra-red absorption spectrum*, Appendix II A, is concordant with the spectrum of *miconazole nitrate EPCRS*.
B. Dissolve 40 mg in a mixture of 10 ml of *0.1M hydrochloric acid* and 50 ml of *propan-2-ol* and dilute to 100 ml with *propan-2-ol*. The *light absorption* of the resulting solution, Appendix II B, in the range 250 to 300 nm exhibits maxima at 264, 272 and 280 nm. The ratio of the *absorbance* at the maximum at 272 nm to that at the maximum at 280 nm is 1.18 to 1.22.
C. In the test for Related substances, the principal spot in the chromatogram obtained with solution (2) is similar in position and size to the principal spot in the chromatogram obtained with solution (3) when examined under *ultra-violet light (254 nm)* before exposure to iodine vapour.
D. Yields the *reaction* characteristic of nitrates, Appendix VI.
E. *Melting point*, 178° to 184°, Appendix V A, Method I.

Clarity and colour of solution A 1% w/v solution in *methanol* is *clear*, Appendix IV A, and not more intensely coloured than *reference solution* Y_7, Appendix IV B, Method II.

Related substances Carry out the method for *thin-layer chromatography*, Appendix III A, using *silica gel GF254* as the coating substance and a mixture of 60 volumes of n-*hexane*, 30 volumes of *chloroform*, 10 volumes of *methanol* and 1 volume of *13.5M ammonia* as the mobile phase. Apply separately to the chromatoplate 10 µl of each of four solutions in a mixture of 1 volume of *13.5M ammonia* and 9 volumes of *methanol* containing (1) 5.0% w/v of the substance being examined, (2) 0.5% w/v of the substance being examined, (3) 0.5% w/v of *miconazole nitrate EPCRS* and (4) 0.0125% w/v of *miconazole nitrate EPCRS*. After removal of the plate, allow it to dry in a current of air for 15 minutes and examine under *ultra-violet light (254 nm)*. Any *secondary spot* in the chromatogram obtained with solution (1) is not more intense than the spot in the chromatogram obtained with solution (4). Expose the plate to iodine vapour until a brown spot appears in the chromatogram obtained with solution (4) and examine immediately in daylight. Any *secondary spot* in the chromatogram obtained with solution (1) is not more intense than the spot in the chromatogram obtained with solution (4).

Loss on drying When dried to constant weight at 100° to 105° for 2 hours, loses not more than 0.5% of its weight. Use 1 g.

Sulphated ash Not more than 0.1%, Appendix IX A, Method II. Use 1 g.

Assay Dissolve 0.35 g in 75 ml of *anhydrous glacial acetic acid*, with gentle heating if necessary, and carry out Method I for *non-aqueous titration*, Appendix VIII A, determining the end-point potentiometrically. Repeat the operation without the substance being examined. The difference between the titrations represents the amount of perchloric acid required. Each ml of *0.1M perchloric acid VS* is equivalent to 0.04791 g of $C_{18}H_{14}Cl_4N_2O,HNO_3$.

Storage Miconazole Nitrate should be kept in a well-closed container and protected from light.

Preparation
Miconazole Cream

Action and use Antifungal.

Minocycline Hydrochloride

$C_{23}H_{27}N_3O_7,HCl,H_2O$ 511.9   *13614-98-7*

Minocycline Hydrochloride is (4S,4aS,5aR, 12aS)-4,7-bis(dimethylamino)-1,4,4a,5,5a,6, 11,12a-octahydro-3,10,12,12a-tetrahydroxy-1,11-dioxonaphthacene-2-carboxamide hydrochloride monohydrate. It contains not less than 96.0 per cent and not more than 102.5 per cent of $C_{23}H_{27}N_3O_7,HCl$, calculated with reference to the anhydrous substance.

Characteristics A yellow, crystalline powder.

Solubility Soluble in *water*; slightly soluble in *ethanol (96%)*; practically insoluble in *chloroform* and in *ether*. It dissolves in aqueous solutions of alkali hydroxides and carbonates.

Identification A. Complies with the test for *identification of tetracyclines*, Appendix III A, but using a mixture of 75 volumes of *ethyl acetate*, 15 volumes of *acetone* and 5 volumes of *water* as the mobile phase and allowing the solvent front to ascend 10 cm above the line of application. Apply separately to the chromatoplate 2 µl of each of three solutions in *0.01M hydrochloric acid* containing (1) 0.1% w/v of the substance being examined and 0.05% w/v each of *chlortetracycline hydrochloride EPCRS* and *oxytetracycline hydrochloride EPCRS*, (2) 0.05% w/v each of *chlortetracycline hydrochloride EPCRS* and *oxytetracycline hydrochloride EPCRS* and (3) 0.05% w/v each of *chlortetracycline hydrochloride EPCRS*, *minocycline hydrochloride BPCRS* and *oxytetracycline hydrochloride EPCRS*. The test is not valid unless the chromatogram obtained with solution (3) shows three clearly separated principal spots.

B. In the Assay, the principal peak in the chromatogram obtained with solution (2) has the same retention time as the principal peak in the chromatogram obtained with solution (1).

C. Yields the *reactions* characteristic of chlorides, Appendix VI.

Acidity pH of a 1% w/v solution, 3.5 to 4.5, Appendix V L.

Heavy metals Ignite 0.6 g with 0.2 ml of *sulphuric acid*, dissolve the residue in 0.5 ml of *hydrochloric acid*, evaporate to dryness, dissolve the residue in 2 ml of *water*, neutralise to *phenolphthalein solution* with 2M *sodium hydroxide* and dilute to 15 ml with *water*. 12 ml of the resulting solution complies with *limit test A for heavy metals*, Appendix VII (50 ppm). Use *lead standard solution (2 ppm Pb)* to prepare the standard.

Light-absorbing impurities *Absorbance* of a 1% w/v solution at 560 nm, measured within 1 hour of preparing the solution, not more than 0.06, Appendix II B.

Related substances Carry out the method for *high-performance liquid chromatography*, Appendix III D, using the following freshly prepared solutions. Solutions (1), (2) and (3) are solutions of the substance being examined in the mobile phase containing 0.00050% w/v, 0.00035% w/v and 0.025% w/v respectively. For solution (4) heat 5 ml of a 0.20% w/v solution of *minocycline hydrochloride BPCRS* on a water-bath for 60 minutes, evaporate to dryness and dissolve the residue in sufficient of the mobile phase to produce 25 ml.

The chromatographic procedure may be carried out using (a) a stainless steel column (20 cm × 4.6 mm) packed with *stationary phase C* (5 μm) (Nucleosil C8 is suitable), (b) as the mobile phase with a flow rate of 1 ml per minute a mixture of 50 volumes of 0.2M *ammonium oxalate*, 27 volumes of *dimethylformamide* and 25 volumes of 0.01M *disodium edetate*, adjusted to a pH of 6.2 to 7.0 by the addition of 0.4M *tetrabutylammonium hydroxide* (pH 7.0 is suitable with a Nucleosil C8 column), and (c) a detection wavelength of 280 nm. Allow the chromatography to proceed for 1.5 times the retention time of the principal peak of the substance being examined. After use, the apparatus should be flushed thoroughly with *water*.

In the chromatogram obtained with solution (3), the area of any peak with a retention time about 0.9 times that of the principal peak is not greater than the area of the peak in the chromatogram obtained with solution (2) and the sum of the areas of any other *secondary peaks* is not greater than the area of the peak in the chromatogram obtained with solution (1).

The test is not valid unless the *resolution factor* between the two principal peaks in the chromatogram obtained with solution (4) is not less than 2.0.

Sulphated ash Not more than 0.5%, Appendix IX A, Method II. Use 1 g.

Water 4.3% to 8.0% w/w, Appendix IX C. Use 0.5 g.

Assay Carry out the method for *high-performance liquid chromatography*, Appendix III D, using two freshly prepared solutions in the mobile phase containing (1) 0.0125% w/v of *minocycline hydrochloride BPCRS* and (2) 0.0125% w/v of the substance being examined.

The chromatographic procedure may be carried out using the conditions described in the test for Related substances.

Calculate the content of $C_{23}H_{27}N_3O_7$,HCl using the declared content of $C_{23}H_{27}N_3O_7$,HCl in *minocycline hydrochloride BPCRS*.

The *column efficiency*, determined using the peak in the chromatogram obtained with solution (1), should be not less than 15,000 theoretical plates per metre.

Labelling The label states (1) the date after which the material is not intended to be used; (2) the conditions under which it should be stored.

Preparation
Minocycline Tablets

Dementholised Mint Oil

Dementholised Mint Oil is obtained by steam distillation, followed by partial dementholisation and processing, from the flowering tops of *Mentha arvensis* L. var. *piperascens* Holmes. Brazilian oil contains not less than 3.0 per cent w/w and not more than 10.0 per cent w/w of esters, calculated as menthyl acetate, $C_{12}H_{22}O_2$, and not less than 35.0 per cent w/w and not more than 55.0 per cent w/w of free alcohols, calculated as menthol, $C_{10}H_{20}O$. Chinese oil contains not less than 3.0 per cent w/w and not more than 8.0 per cent w/w of esters, calculated as menthyl acetate, $C_{12}H_{22}O_2$, and not less than 41.0 per cent w/w and not more than 58.0 per cent w/w of free alcohols, calculated as menthol, $C_{10}H_{20}O$.

Characteristics A clear, colourless to pale yellow liquid, visibly free from water; odour, characteristic.

Identification Carry out the method for *thin-layer chromatography*, Appendix III A, using *silica gel G* as the coating substance and a mixture of 95 volumes of *toluene* and 5 volumes of *ethyl acetate* as the mobile phase. Apply separately to the chromatoplate, as bands 20 mm long and not more than 3 mm wide, 20 μl of each of three solutions in *toluene* containing (1) 1% v/v of the oil being examined, (2) 0.5% w/v of *menthol*, 0.2% v/v of *cineole*, 0.1% w/v of *thymol* and 0.1% v/v of *menthyl acetate* and (3) 0.1% v/v of *cineole*, 0.1% w/v of *thymol* and 0.1% w/v of *carvone*. After removal of the plate, allow it to dry in air, spray with *anisaldehyde solution*, using 10 ml for a plate 200 mm × 200 mm in size, and heat at 105° for 5 minutes. The chromatogram obtained with solution (2) shows, in order of increasing Rf values, a blue band due to menthol, a brown band due to cineole, a pink band due to thymol and a blue band due to menthyl acetate. In the chromatogram obtained with solution (1) the bands corresponding to menthol and menthyl acetate are prominent. There is no pink band corresponding to thymol but a pink band corresponding to carvone is present. In addition a blue band with an Rf value slightly higher that that of menthol and an orange band with an Rf value slightly lower than that of menthyl acetate may be present. In the chromatogram obtained with solution (3) three distinct bands are obtained.

Acidity To 2 g add 0.25 ml of *phenolphthalein solution* and titrate with 0.1M *ethanolic potassium hydroxide VS*. Not more than 1.2 ml is required to change the colour of the solution.

Optical rotation Brazilian oil, $-22°$ to $-29°$; Chinese oil, $-17°$ to $-24°$, Appendix V F.

Refractive index Brazilian oil, 1.456 to 1.463; Chinese oil, 1.458 to 1.466, Appendix V E.

Solubility in ethanol Soluble, at 20°, in 4 volumes of *ethanol (70%)*, Appendix X M; the solution may become cloudy when diluted.

Weight per ml 0.889 to 0.900 g, Appendix V G.

Cineole:limonene ratio Carry out the method for *gas chromatography*, Appendix III B, using three solutions in *ethyl acetate* containing (1) 0.35% w/v of *cineole*, 0.25% w/v of *limonene* and 0.5% w/v of *nonan-5-one* (internal standard), (2) 10.0% w/v of the oil and (3) 10.0% w/v of the oil and 0.50% w/v of the internal standard.

The chromatographic procedure may be carried out using a glass column (2.0 m × 4 mm) packed with *acid-washed, silanised diatomaceous support* (80 to 100 mesh) coated with 15% w/w of cyanopropylmethyl phenyl methyl silicone fluid (OV-225 is suitable) and maintained at 115°.

In the chromatograms obtained with solutions (1) and (3) measure the heights of the peaks due to limonene, cineole and the internal standard and calculate the percentages of limonene and cineole in the oil. The ratio of the cineole content to the limonene content is less than 1.0.

Assay *For esters* Carry out the method for the *determination of esters*, Appendix VIII L, using 5 g. Each ml of 0.5M *ethanolic potassium hydroxide VS* is equivalent to 0.09915 g of menthyl acetate, $C_{12}H_{22}O_2$.

For free alcohols Mix 10 ml with 20 ml of *acetic anhydride* in a round-bottomed flask and add 2 g of freshly fused *anhydrous sodium acetate*. Attach the flask to an air-cooled reflux condenser not less than 75 cm in length and boil gently for 2 hours. Allow to cool, add 50 ml of *water* through the condenser and heat on a water-bath for 15 minutes, shaking frequently. Cool and transfer the contents of the flask to a separating funnel, discarding the lower layer. Wash the acetylated oil successively with 50 ml of a saturated solution of *sodium chloride*, 50 ml of a saturated solution of *sodium chloride* containing 1 g of *anhydrous sodium carbonate* in solution and 50 ml of a saturated solution of *sodium chloride*; at each washing shake vigorously and allow complete separation to take place before discarding the lower layer. Finally shake gently with 20 ml of *water*, separate the oil, shake with 3 g of *anhydrous sodium sulphate* until clear and filter. Carry out the method for the *determination of esters*, Appendix VIII L, but adding 50 ml of 0.5M *ethanolic potassium hydroxide*. From the results obtained determine the ester value of the acetylated oil (*b*) using the expression 28.05*v/w*, where *v* is the volume of 0.5M ethanolic potassium hydroxide required and *w* is the weight of oil taken. Similarly determine the ester value of the original oil (*a*) from the results obtained in the Assay for esters.

Calculate the percentage of free alcohols, as menthol, from the expression $[156.3(b - a)] / [0.42(1335 - b)]$.

Storage Dementholised Mint Oil should be kept in a well-filled, well-closed container, protected from light and stored at a temperature not exceeding 25°.

Labelling The label states whether the oil is Brazilian oil or Chinese oil.

Action and use Flavour.

Mitobronitol

$$CH_2Br$$
$$HOCH$$
$$HOCH$$
$$HCOH$$
$$HCOH$$
$$CH_2Br$$

$C_6H_{12}Br_2O_4$ 308.0   *488-41-5*

Mitobronitol is 1,6-dibromo-1,6-dideoxy-D-mannitol. It contains not less than 98.5 per cent and not more than 101.0 per cent of $C_6H_{12}Br_2O_4$ calculated with reference to the dried substance.

Characteristics A white or almost white, crystalline solid.

Solubility Slightly soluble in *water*, in *ethanol (96%)* and in *acetone*; practically insoluble in *chloroform*.

Identification A. The *infra-red absorption spectrum*, Appendix II A, is concordant with the *reference spectrum* of mitobronitol.

B. Dissolve 0.1 g in 10 ml of 1M *sodium hydroxide*, boil, cool, acidify with 2M *nitric acid* and add 1 ml of *silver nitrate solution*. A pale yellow, curdy precipitate is produced.

C. Dissolve 20 mg in 2 ml of a mixture of 1 volume of *periodic acid solution* and 24 volumes of *water*. Add 1 ml of 0.25M *barium chloride* and shake well. A white, flocculent precipitate is produced.

Acidity Shake 2 g with 50 ml of *carbon dioxide-free water* for 15 minutes and filter. 40 ml of the filtrate requires not more than 0.3 ml of 0.02M *sodium hydroxide VS* for neutralisation using *phenolphthalein solution* as indicator.

Clarity and colour of solution A 4.0% w/v solution in *dimethylformamide* is *clear*, Appendix IV A, and *colourless*, Appendix IV B, Method I.

Heavy metals 1.0 g complies with *limit test C for heavy metals*, Appendix VII (20 ppm). Use 2 ml of *lead standard solution (10 ppm Pb)* to prepare the standard.

Ionic halide Shake 0.20 g with 30 ml of *water* for 5 minutes and filter. 15 ml of the filtrate complies with the *limit test for chlorides*, Appendix VII (500 ppm, calculated as Cl).

Loss on drying When dried at 105° for 2 hours, loses not more than 1.0% of its weight. Use 1 g.

Sulphated ash Not more than 0.2%, Appendix IX A.

Assay Dissolve 0.2 g in 20 ml of 1M *sodium hydroxide* by heating gently, cool, add 25 ml of 0.1M *silver nitrate VS* and acidify with 5 ml of 5M *nitric acid*. Add 2 ml of *ammonium iron(III) sulphate solution* and titrate the excess of silver nitrate with 0.1M *ammonium thiocyanate VS*. Each ml of 0.1M *silver nitrate VS* is equivalent to 0.01540 g of $C_6H_{12}Br_2O_4$.

Storage Mitobronitol should be kept in a well-closed container and protected from light.

Preparation
Mitobronitol Tablets

Action and use Cytotoxic.

Monosulfiram

Et₂N·CS·S·CS·NEt₂

$C_{10}H_{20}N_2S_3$ 264.5   95-05-6

Monosulfiram is tetraethylthiuram mono-sulphide. It contains not less than 98.0 per cent and not more than 101.0 per cent of $C_{10}H_{20}N_2S_3$, calculated with reference to the anhydrous substance.

Characteristics A yellow or yellowish-brown solid; odour, sulphurous.

Solubility Practically insoluble in *water*, in acids and in alkalis; freely soluble in organic solvents.

Identification A. The *light absorption*, Appendix II B, in the range 230 to 350 nm of a 0.002% w/v solution in *methanol* exhibits a well-defined maximum only at 281 nm. The *absorbance* at 281 nm is about 1.3.

B. Dissolve 0.1 g in a mixture of 0.15 ml of a 1% w/v solution of *copper(II) sulphate* and 5 ml of *ethanol (96%)*, evaporate on a water-bath and dissolve the residue in *chloroform*. A deep yellowish-brown colour is produced.

C. Boil 0.1 g with 2M *hydrochloric acid*. Fumes are evolved which turn *lead acetate paper* black.

Freezing point 28.5° to 32.0°, Appendix V B.

Related substances Carry out in subdued light the method for *thin-layer chromatography*, Appendix III A, using *silica gel GF254* as the coating substance and a mixture of 70 volumes of *hexane* and 30 volumes of *butyl acetate* as the mobile phase. Apply separately to the chromatoplate 5 μl of each of three solutions in *ethyl acetate* containing (1) 2.5% w/v of the substance being examined, (2) 0.125% w/v of *disulfiram BPCRS* and (3) 0.050% w/v of the substance being examined. After removal of the plate, allow it to dry in air and examine under *ultra-violet light (254 nm)*. In the chromatogram obtained with solution (1) any spot corresponding to disulfiram is not more intense than the spot in the chromatogram obtained with solution (2) and any other *secondary spot* is not more intense than the spot in the chromatogram obtained with solution (3).

Sulphated ash Not more than 0.1%, Appendix IX A.

Water Not more than 1.0% w/w, Appendix IX C, Method I B. Use 1 g.

Assay Carry out Method I for the *determination of nitrogen*, Appendix VIII H, using 0.35 g and 8 ml of *nitrogen-free sulphuric acid*. Each ml of 0.05M *sulphuric acid VS* is equivalent to 0.01322 g of $C_{10}H_{20}N_2S_3$.

Storage Monosulfiram should be stored at a temperature of 8° to 15° and protected from light.

Preparation

Monosulfiram Solution

Action and use Parasiticide used topically in treatment of scabies.

In some countries the material described in this monograph may be known as Sulfiram.

Morphine Hydrochloride ☆

$C_{17}H_{19}NO_3,HCl,3H_2O$ 375.9   52-26-6 *(anhydrous)*

Morphine Hydrochloride is the trihydrate of the hydrochloride of an alkaloid, 7,8-dide-hydro-4,5-epoxy-17-methylmorphinan-3,6-diol, which may be obtained from opium. It contains not less than 98.0 per cent and not more than 101.0 per cent of $C_{17}H_{19}NO_3,HCl$, calculated with reference to the dried substance.

Characteristics Colourless, silky crystals, cubical masses or a white or almost white, crystalline powder.

Solubility Soluble in 24 parts of *water* and in 10 parts of boiling *ethanol (90%)*; practically insoluble in *chloroform* and in *ether*. Soluble at 15° in 100 parts of *ethanol (96%)* and at 10° in 50 parts of *ethanol (96%)*.

Identification A. The *light absorption*, Appendix II B, in the range 250 to 350 nm of a 0.02% w/v solution exhibits a maximum only at 285 nm. The A(1%, 1 cm) at 285 nm is about 41.

B. The *light absorption*, Appendix II B, in the range 265 to 350 nm of a 0.02% w/v solution in 0.1M *sodium hydroxide* exhibits a maximum only at 298 nm. The A(1%, 1 cm) at 298 nm is about 70.

C. To 1 mg, in powder, in a porcelain dish add 0.5 ml of *sulphuric acid* containing 0.05 ml of *formaldehyde solution*. A purple colour is produced which turns to violet.

D. Dissolve 5 mg in 5 ml of *water*, add 0.15 ml of a freshly prepared 1% w/v solution of *potassium hexacyanoferrate(III)* and 0.05 ml of a 10.5% w/v solution of *iron(III) chloride hexahydrate*. A blue colour is produced immediately.

E. Dissolve 5 mg in 5 ml of *water*, add 1 ml of *hydrogen peroxide solution (10 vol)*, 1 ml of 6M *ammonia* and 0.05 ml of a 4% w/v solution of *copper(II) sulphate*. A red colour is produced.

F. Yields the *reaction* characteristic of alkaloids and *reaction A* characteristic of chlorides, Appendix VI.

Acidity or alkalinity To 10 ml of a 2% w/v solution add 0.05 ml of *methyl red solution*. Not more than 0.2 ml of either 0.02M *sodium hydroxide* or 0.02M *hydrochloric acid* is required to change the colour of the solution.

Clarity and colour of solution A 2.0% w/v solution is *clear*, Appendix IV A, and not more intensely coloured than *reference solution Y₆* or *BY₆*, Appendix IV B, Method II.

Specific optical rotation In a 2% w/v solution, −110° to −115°, Appendix V F.

Meconate To 10 ml of a 2% w/v solution add 1 ml of *hydrochloric acid* and 0.1 ml of a 10.5% w/v solution of *iron(III) chloride hexahydrate*. The *absorbance* at 480 nm is not more than 0.05, Appendix II B, using in the reference cell a solution prepared at the same time and in the same manner but using 10 ml of *water* in place of the solution of the substance being examined (0.2%).

Related substances Carry out the method for *thin-layer chromatography*, Appendix III A, using *silica gel G* as the coating substance and a mixture of 35 volumes of *ethanol (70%)*, 35 volumes of *toluene*, 32.5 volumes of *acetone* and 2.5 volumes of 13.5M *ammonia* as the mobile phase. Apply separately to the chromatoplate 10 µl of each of the following solutions. For solution (1) dissolve 0.1 g of the substance being examined in sufficient of a mixture of equal volumes of *ethanol (96%)* and *water* to produce 10 ml. For solution (2) dissolve 50 mg of *codeine phosphate* in 5 ml of solution (1) and dilute 0.1 ml of the resulting solution to 10 ml with a mixture of equal volumes of *ethanol (96%)* and *water*. After removal of the plate, dry it in a current of air, spray with *acetic potassium iodo-bismuthate solution*, dry for 15 minutes in a current of air and spray with *hydrogen peroxide solution (10 vol)*. The spot due to codeine is bluish-grey and the spot due to morphine is pinkish. In the chromatogram obtained with solution (1) any spot corresponding to codeine is not more intense than the spot due to codeine in the chromatogram obtained with solution (2) and any other *secondary spot* is not more intense than the spot due to morphine in the chromatogram obtained with solution (2). The test is not valid unless the chromatogram obtained with solution (2) shows a spot due to codeine clearly separated from the principal spot.

Loss on drying When dried to constant weight at 130°, loses 12.0 to 15.0% of its weight. Use 0.5 g.

Sulphated ash Not more than 0.1%, Appendix IX A, Method II. Use the residue obtained in the test for Loss on drying.

Assay Dissolve 0.35 g in 30 ml of *anhydrous glacial acetic acid*, heating if necessary. Cool and carry out Method I for *non-aqueous titration*, Appendix VIII A, using 6 ml of *mercury(II) acetate solution* and *crystal violet solution* as indicator. Each ml of 0.1M *perchloric acid VS* is equivalent to 0.03218 g of $C_{17}H_{19}NO_3,HCl$.

Storage Morphine Hydrochloride should be kept in a well-closed container and protected from light.

Action and use Narcotic analgesic.

Morphine Sulphate

$(C_{17}H_{19}NO_3)_2,H_2SO_4,5H_2O$ 758.8   *6211-15-0*

Morphine Sulphate is the pentahydrate of the sulphate of an alkaloid, 7,8-didehydro-4,5-epoxy-17-methylmorphinan-3,6-diol, which may be obtained from opium. It contains not less than 98.0 per cent and not more than 101.0 per cent of $(C_{17}H_{19}NO_3)_2,H_2SO_4$, calculated with reference to the dried substance.

Characteristics White, acicular crystals or cubical masses or a white crystalline powder; odourless or almost odourless.

Solubility Soluble in 21 parts of *water*; very slightly soluble in *ethanol (96%)*; practically insoluble in *chloroform* and in *ether*.

Identification A. The *light absorption*, Appendix II B, in the range 230 to 350 nm of a 0.015% w/v solution exhibits a maximum only at 285 nm. The *absorbance* at 285 nm is about 0.65.

B. The *light absorption*, Appendix II B, in the range 230 to 350 nm of a 0.015% w/v solution in 0.1M *sodium hydroxide*

exhibits a maximum only at 298 nm. The *absorbance* at 298 nm is about 1.1.

C. Add a few mg of the solid, in powder, to 1 ml of *sulphuric acid* containing 0.05 ml of *formaldehyde solution*. A purple colour is produced.

D. Dissolve 5 mg in 5 ml of *water* and add 0.15 ml of *potassium hexacyanoferrate(III) solution* and 0.05 ml of *iron(III) chloride test-solution*. A bluish-green colour is produced immediately, which changes rapidly to blue.

E. Yields the *reactions* characteristic of sulphates, Appendix VI.

Acidity Dissolve 0.2 g in 10 ml of freshly boiled and cooled *water* and titrate with 0.02M *sodium hydroxide VS* using *methyl red solution* as indicator. Not more than 0.2 ml is required to change the colour of the solution.

Other alkaloids Not more than 1.5%, calculated with reference to the dried substance, when determined by the following method. Transfer 0.5 g to a separating funnel, add 15 ml of *water*, 5 ml of 1M *sodium hydroxide* and 10 ml of *chloroform*, shake, allow to separate and transfer the chloroform solution to another separating funnel. Repeat the extraction with two 10-ml quantities of *chloroform*. Wash the mixed chloroform solutions with 10 ml of 0.1M *sodium hydroxide* and then with two 5-ml quantities of *water*, evaporate to dryness on a water-bath and dry the residue to constant weight at 105°.

Loss on drying When dried at 145° for 1 hour, loses 9.0 to 12.0% of its weight. Use 1 g.

Sulphated ash Not more than 0.1%, Appendix IX A.

Assay Carry out Method I for *non-aqueous titration*, Appendix VIII A, using 0.5 g and determining the end-point potentiometrically. Each ml of 0.1M *perchloric acid VS* is equivalent to 0.06688 g of $(C_{17}H_{19}NO_3)_2,H_2SO_4$.

Storage Morphine Sulphate should be kept in a well-closed container and protected from light.

Preparations
Morphine Sulphate Injection
Morphine Tablets
Morphine and Atropine Injection

Action and use Narcotic analgesic.

Mustine Hydrochloride
Nitrogen Mustard

$(ClCH_2 \cdot CH_2)_2NMe$ .HCl

$C_5H_{11}Cl_2N,HCl$ 192.5   *55-86-7*

Mustine Hydrochloride is bis(2-chloroethyl)-methylamine hydrochloride. It contains not less than 98.0 per cent and not more than 101.0 per cent of $C_5H_{11}Cl_2N,HCl$.

Characteristics A white or almost white crystalline powder or mass; hygroscopic; vesicant.

Solubility Very soluble in *water*.

Identification A. Dissolve 50 mg in 5 ml of *water* and add 1 ml of 5M *sodium hydroxide*. Oily globules are produced which dissolve on warming.

B. Dissolve 50 mg in 5 ml of *water* and add 0.02 ml of *potassium mercuri-iodide solution*. A cream precipitate is produced.

C. *Melting point*, about 108°, Appendix V A.

Assay To 0.2 g add 15 ml of 1M *ethanolic potassium hydroxide* and 15 ml of *water* and boil under a reflux condenser for 2 hours. Evaporate the solution to half its volume on a water-bath, dilute to 150 ml with *water*, add 3 ml of *nitric acid* and 50 ml of 0.1M *silver nitrate VS*, shake vigorously and filter. Wash the residue with *water* and titrate the excess of silver nitrate in the combined filtrate and washings with 0.1M *ammonium thiocyanate VS* using 1 ml of *ammonium iron(III) sulphate solution* as indicator. Each ml of 0.1M *silver nitrate VS* is equivalent to 0.006418 g of $C_5H_{11}Cl_2N,HCl$.

Storage Mustine Hydrochloride should be kept in a well-closed container and stored at a temperature of 8° to 15°.

Labelling The label states that the contents of the container are strongly vesicant.

Preparation
Mustine Injection

Action and use Cytotoxic.

In some countries the material described in this monograph may be known as Chlormethine Hydrochloride.

Nalidixic Acid

$C_{12}H_{12}N_2O_3$ 232.2   *389-08-2*

Nalidixic Acid is 1-ethyl-7-methyl-4-oxo-1,8-naphthyridine-3-carboxylic acid. It contains not less than 98.0 per cent and not more than 102.0 per cent of $C_{12}H_{12}N_2O_3$, calculated with reference to the dried substance.

Characteristics An almost white or very pale yellow, crystalline powder; odourless or almost odourless.

Solubility Practically insoluble in *water*; slightly soluble in *ethanol (96%)*; soluble in 35 parts of *chloroform*; slightly soluble in aqueous solutions of alkali hydroxides.

Identification A. The *infra-red absorption spectrum*, Appendix II A, is concordant with the *reference spectrum* of nalidixic acid.
B. The *light absorption*, Appendix II B, in the range 230 to 350 nm of a 0.0008% w/v solution in 0.1M *sodium hydroxide* exhibits two maxima, at 258 nm and 334 nm. The *absorbance* at 258 nm is about 0.90 and at 334 nm is about 0.39.
C. *Melting point*, about 228°, Appendix V A.

Related substances Carry out the method for *thin-layer chromatography*, Appendix III A, using *silica gel GF254* as the coating substance and a mixture of 70 volumes of *ethanol (96%)*, 20 volumes of *chloroform* and 10 volumes of 5M *ammonia* as the mobile phase. Apply separately to the chromatoplate 10 μl of each of two solutions of the substance being examined in *chloroform* containing (1) 2.0% w/v and (2) 0.010% w/v. After removal of the plate, allow it to dry in air and examine under *ultra-violet light (254 nm)*. Any *secondary spot* in the chromatogram

obtained with solution (1) is not more intense than the spot in the chromatogram obtained with solution (2).

Loss on drying When dried to constant weight at 105°, loses not more than 0.5% of its weight. Use 1 g.

Sulphated ash Not more than 0.2%, Appendix IX A.

Assay Dissolve 0.15 g in 25 ml of *dimethylformamide* and carry out Method II for *non-aqueous titration*, Appendix VIII A, using 0.1M *tetrabutylammonium hydroxide VS* as titrant and a 0.2% w/v solution of *thymolphthalein* in *methanol* as indicator. Each ml of 0.1M *tetrabutylammonium hydroxide VS* is equivalent to 0.02322 g of $C_{12}H_{12}N_2O_3$.

Storage Nalidixic Acid should be kept in a well-closed container and protected from light.

Preparations
Nalidixic Acid Oral Suspension
Nalidixic Acid Tablets

Action and use Antibacterial.

Nandrolone Decanoate

$C_{28}H_{44}O_3$ 428.7   *360-70-3*

Nandrolone Decanoate is 3-oxo-estr-4-en-17β-yl decanoate. It contains not less than 97.0 per cent and not more than 103.0 per cent of $C_{28}H_{44}O_3$, calculated with reference to the dried substance.

Characteristics A white to creamy-white, crystalline powder; odour, faint and characteristic.

Solubility Practically insoluble in *water*; soluble in 1 part of *ethanol (96%)*; freely soluble in *chloroform*, in *ether*, in fixed oils and in esters.

Identification A. The *infra-red absorption spectrum*, Appendix II A, is concordant with the *reference spectrum* of nandrolone decanoate.
B. Carry out the method for *thin-layer chromatography*, Appendix III A, using *silica gel G* as the coating substance and a mixture of 80 volumes of *heptane* and 20 volumes of *acetone* as the mobile phase but allowing the solvent front to ascend 10 cm above the line of application. Apply separately to the chromatoplate 2 μl of each of the following solutions. Solution (1) contains 0.5% w/v of the substance being examined in *carbon tetrachloride*. Solution (2) is a mixture of 1 volume of *nandrolone decanoate solution BPCRS* and 9 volumes of *carbon tetrachloride*. Solution (3) is a mixture of equal volumes of solutions (1) and (2). After removal of the plate, heat it at 105° for 10 minutes, spray with *ethanolic sulphuric acid (20%)*, heat at 105° for a further 10 minutes, allow to cool and examine in daylight and under *ultra-violet light (365 nm)*. The principal spot in the chromatogram obtained with solution (1) corresponds to that in the the chromatogram obtained with solution (2). The principal spot in the chromatogram obtained with solution (3) appears as a single, compact spot.

C. Dissolve 25 mg in 1 ml of *methanol*, add 2 ml of *semicarbazide acetate solution*, heat under a reflux condenser for 30 minutes and cool. The *melting point* of the precipitate, after recrystallisation from *ethanol (90%)*, is about 175°, Appendix V A.

D. *Melting point*, about 35°, Appendix V A.

Specific optical rotation In a 2% w/v solution in *1,4-dioxan*, +32° to +36°, Appendix V A.

Related substances Carry out the method for *thin-layer chromatography*, Appendix III A, using *silica gel GF254* as the coating substance and a mixture of 70 volumes of *heptane* and 30 volumes of *acetone* as the mobile phase. Apply separately to the chromatoplate 5 μl of each of three solutions in *chloroform* containing (1) 1.0% w/v of the substance being examined, (2) 0.0050% w/v of the substance being examined and (3) 0.010% w/v of *nandrolone BPCRS*. After removal of the plate, allow it to dry in air and examine under *ultra-violet light (254 nm)*. In the chromatogram obtained with solution (1) any spot corresponding to nandrolone is not more intense than the spot in the chromatogram obtained with solution (3) and any other *secondary spot* is not more intense than the spot in the chromatogram obtained with solution (2).

Loss on drying When dried over *phosphorus pentoxide* at a pressure not exceeding 0.7 kPa for 4 hours, loses not more than 0.5% of its weight. Use 1 g.

Sulphated ash Not more than 0.1%, Appendix IX A.

Assay Dissolve 10 mg in sufficient *absolute ethanol* to produce 100 ml, dilute 5 ml to 50 ml with *absolute ethanol* and measure the *absorbance* of the resulting solution at the maximum at 240 nm, Appendix II B. Calculate the content of $C_{28}H_{44}O_3$ taking 407 as the value of A(1%, 1 cm) at the maximum at 240 nm.

Storage Nandrolone Decanoate should be stored under nitrogen at a temperature of 2° to 8° and protected from light.

Preparation
Nandrolone Decanoate Injection

Action and use Anabolic steroid.

Nandrolone Phenylpropionate

$C_{27}H_{34}O_3$ 406.6   *62-90-8*

Nandrolone Phenylpropionate is 3-oxo-estr-4-en-17β-yl 3-phenylpropionate. It contains not less than 97.0 per cent and not more than 103.0 per cent of $C_{27}H_{34}O_3$, calculated with reference to the dried substance.

Characteristics A white to creamy-white, crystalline powder; odour, characteristic.

Solubility Practically insoluble in *water*; soluble in 20 parts of *ethanol (96%)*.

Identification A. The *infra-red absorption spectrum*, Appendix II A, is concordant with the *reference spectrum* of nandrolone phenylpropionate.

B. Complies with the test for *identification of steroids*, Appendix III A, using *impregnating solvent III* and *mobile phase F*.

C. Dissolve 25 mg in 1 ml of *methanol*, add 2 ml of *semicarbazide acetate solution*, heat under a reflux condenser for 30 minutes and cool. The *melting point* of the precipitate, after recrystallisation from *ethanol (90%)*, is about 182°, Appendix V A.

Melting point 95° to 99°, Appendix V A.

Specific optical rotation In a 1% w/v solution in *1,4-dioxan*, +48° to +51°, Appendix V F.

Related substances Carry out the method for *thin-layer chromatography*, Appendix III A, using *silica gel GF254* as the coating substance and a mixture of 70 volumes of *heptane* and 30 volumes of *acetone* as the mobile phase. Apply separately to the chromatoplate 5 μl of each of three solutions in *chloroform* containing (1) 1.0% w/v of the substance being examined, (2) 0.0050% w/v of the substance being examined and (3) 0.010% w/v of *nandrolone BPCRS*. After removal of the plate, allow it to dry in air and examine under *ultra-violet light (254 nm)*. In the chromatogram obtained with solution (1) any spot corresponding to nandrolone is not more intense than the spot in the chromatogram obtained with solution (3) and any other *secondary spot* is not more intense than the spot in the chromatogram obtained with solution (2).

Loss on drying When dried over *phosphorus pentoxide* at a pressure not exceeding 0.7 kPa for 4 hours, loses not more than 0.5% of its weight. Use 1.0 g.

Sulphated ash Not more than 0.1%, Appendix IX A.

Assay Dissolve 10 mg in sufficient *absolute ethanol* to produce 100 ml, dilute 5 ml to 50 ml with *absolute ethanol* and measure the *absorbance* of the resulting solution at the maximum at 240 nm, Appendix II B. Calculate the content of $C_{27}H_{34}O_3$ taking 430 as the value of A(1%, 1 cm) at the maximum at 240 nm.

Storage Nandrolone Phenylpropionate should be protected from light.

Preparation
Nandrolone Phenylpropionate Injection

Action and use Anabolic steroid.

Naphazoline Nitrate ☆

$C_{14}H_{14}N_2,HNO_3$ 273.3   *5144-52-5*

Naphazoline Nitrate is 2-(1-naphthylmethyl)-2-imidazoline nitrate. It contains not less than 99.0 per cent and not more than 101.0 per cent of $C_{14}H_{14}N_2,HNO_3$, calculated with reference to the dried substance.

Characteristics A white or almost white, crystalline powder; odourless or almost odourless.

Solubility Soluble in 36 parts of *water* and in 16 parts of *ethanol (96%)*; very slightly soluble in *chloroform*; practically insoluble in *ether*.

Identification *Test A may be omitted if tests B, C, D and E are carried out. Tests B and C may be omitted if tests A, D and E are carried out.*

A. The *infra-red absorption spectrum*, Appendix II A, is concordant with the spectrum of *naphazoline nitrate EPCRS*.

B. The *light absorption*, Appendix II B, in the range 230 to 350 nm of a 0.002% w/v solution in *0.01M hydrochloric acid* exhibits four maxima, at 270, 280, 287 and 291 nm. The A(1%, 1 cm) at 270 nm is about 215, at 280 nm, about 250, at 287 nm, about 175 and at 291 nm, about 170.

C. Dissolve 0.5 mg in 1 ml of *methanol*, add 0.5 ml of a freshly prepared 5% w/v solution of *sodium nitroprusside* and 0.5 ml of a 2% w/v solution of *sodium hydroxide*, allow to stand for 10 minutes and add 1 ml of an 8% w/v solution of *sodium hydrogen carbonate*. A violet colour is produced.

D. Dissolve 10 mg in 5 ml of *water*, add 0.20 g of *magnesium oxide*, shake mechanically for 30 minutes, add 10 ml of *chloroform* and shake vigorously. Allow to stand, separate the chloroform, filter and evaporate the aqueous layer to dryness. The residue yields the *reactions* characteristic of nitrates, Appendix VI.

E. *Melting point*, 167° to 170°, Appendix V A, Method I.

Acidity pH of a 1% w/v solution, 5.0 to 6.5, Appendix V L.

Clarity and colour of solution A 1.0% w/v solution in *carbon dioxide-free water* is *clear*, Appendix IV A, and *colourless*, Appendix IV B, Method II.

Chloride A 1.0% w/v solution in *carbon dioxide-free water* complies with the *limit test for chlorides*, Appendix VII (330 ppm).

N-(Naphthylacetyl)ethylenediamine Carry out the method for *thin-layer chromatography*, Appendix III A, using *silica gel G* as the coating substance and a mixture of 100 volumes of *methanol* and 1.5 volumes of *13.5M ammonia* as the mobile phase. Apply separately to the chromatoplate 10 μl of each of two solutions in *methanol* containing (1) 2.0% w/v of the substance being examined and (2) 2.0% w/v of *naphazoline nitrate EPCRS* and 0.010% w/v of *naphthylacetylethylenediamine hydrochloride EPCRS*. After removal of the plate, dry it at 100° to 105°, spray with a 0.5% w/v solution of *ninhydrin* in *methanol* and heat at 100° to 105° for 10 minutes. The spot due to N-(naphthylacetyl)ethylenediamine in the chromatogram obtained with solution (2) is more intense than any corresponding spot in the chromatogram obtained with solution (1). The test is not valid unless the chromatogram obtained with solution (2) shows a spot due to N-(naphthylacetyl)ethylenediamine clearly separated from the principal spot.

Loss on drying When dried to constant weight at 100° to 105°, loses not more than 0.5% of its weight. Use 1 g.

Sulphated ash Not more than 0.1%, Appendix IX A, Method II. Use 1 g.

Assay Dissolve 0.2 g in 30 ml of *anhydrous glacial acetic acid* and carry out Method I for *non-aqueous titration*, Appendix VIII A, determining the end-point potentiometrically. Each ml of *0.1M perchloric acid VS* is equivalent to 0.02733 g of $C_{14}H_{14}N_2,HNO_3$.

Storage Naphazoline Nitrate should be kept in a well-closed container and protected from light.

Action and use Sympathomimetic.

Naproxen

$C_{14}H_{14}O_3$ 230.3   *22204-53-1*

Naproxen is (+)-2-(6-methoxy-2-naphthyl)-propionic acid. It contains not less than 98.5 per cent and not more than 100.5 per cent of $C_{14}H_{14}O_3$, calculated with reference to the dried substance.

Characteristics A white or almost white, crystalline powder; odourless or almost odourless.

Solubility Practically insoluble in *water*; soluble in 25 parts of *ethanol* (96%), in 20 parts of *methanol*, in 15 parts of *chloroform* and in 40 parts of *ether*.

Identification A. The *infra-red absorption spectrum*, Appendix II A, is concordant with the *reference spectrum* of naproxen.

B. The *light absorption*, Appendix II B, in the range 230 to 350 nm of a 0.004% w/v solution in *methanol* exhibits four maxima, at 262, 271, 316 and 331 nm. The *absorbance* at 262 nm is about 0.91, at 271 nm, about 0.92, at 316 nm, about 0.26 and at 331 nm, about 0.30.

C. *Melting point*, about 156°, Appendix V A, Method I.

Specific optical rotation In a 4% w/v solution in *chloroform*, +63.0° to +68.5°, Appendix V F.

Heavy metals Dissolve the residue obtained in the test for Sulphated ash in 15 ml of *methanol*. 12 ml of the solution complies with *limit test A for heavy metals*, Appendix VII (20 ppm). Use *lead standard solution (2 ppm Pb)* to prepare the standard.

Related substances Carry out the method for *thin-layer chromatography*, Appendix III A, using *silica gel GF254* as the coating substance and a mixture of 90 volumes of *toluene*, 9 volumes of *tetrahydrofuran* and 3 volumes of *glacial acetic acid* as the mobile phase. Apply separately to the chromatoplate 10 μl of each of two solutions of the substance being examined in *methanol* containing (1) 2.0% w/v and (2) 0.010% w/v. After removal of the plate, allow it to dry in air and examine under *ultra-violet light (254 nm)*. Any *secondary spot* in the chromatogram obtained with solution (1) is not more intense than the spot in the chromatogram obtained with solution (2).

Residual organic bases Dissolve 3.5 g in 100 ml of *dichloromethane* and extract with three 10-ml quantities of *0.1M hydrochloric acid*. Wash the combined aqueous extracts with two 10-ml quantities of *dichloromethane* and to 20 ml of the aqueous layer add 5 ml of a 30% w/v solution of *sodium chloride*, 15 ml of *butan-1-ol* and 1 ml of a 5% w/v solution of *copper(II) chloride*. Shake for 30 seconds, add 3 ml of *6M sodium hydroxide*, shake for a further 30 seconds and centrifuge. To 10 ml of the butanol layer add 3 ml of *methanol* and mix. Measure the *absorbance* of the resulting solution at 274 nm, Appendix II B, using in the reference cell a solution prepared in the same manner but omitting the substance being examined. The absorbance is not more than 0.20.

Loss on drying When dried at 105° for 3 hours, loses not more than 0.5% of its weight. Use 1 g.

Sulphated ash Not more than 0.1%, Appendix IX A. Use 1.5 g and ignite at about 600°.

Assay Dissolve 0.5 g in a mixture of 75 ml of *methanol* and 25 ml of *water* and titrate with carbonate-free 0.1M *sodium hydroxide VS* using *phenolphthalein solution* as indicator. Each ml of 0.1M *sodium hydroxide VS* is equivalent to 0.02303 g of $C_{14}H_{14}O_3$.

Storage Naproxen should be kept in a well-closed container and protected from light.

Preparations
Naproxen Oral Suspension
Naproxen Suppositories
Naproxen Tablets

Action and use Anti-inflammatory; analgesic.

Neomycin Sulphate ☆

1405-10-3

Neomycin Sulphate is a mixture of the sulphates of substances produced by the growth of certain selected strains of *Streptomyces fradiae*. The potency is not less than 680 Units per mg, calculated with reference to the dried substance.

Characteristics A white or yellowish-white powder; almost odourless; hygroscopic.

Solubility Readily soluble in 3 parts of *water* and slowly soluble in 1 part of *water*; very slightly soluble in *ethanol* (96%); practically insoluble in *acetone*, in *chloroform* and in *ether*.

Identification A. Carry out the method for *thin-layer chromatography*, Appendix III A, using a chromatoplate prepared immediately before use as described in the test for Neamine and a 10% w/v solution of *potassium dihydrogen orthophosphate* as the mobile phase. Apply separately to the plate 10 µl of each of three solutions in *water* containing (1) 0.1% w/v of the substance being examined, (2) 0.1% w/v of *neomycin sulphate EPCRS* and (3) 0.1% w/v each of *kanamycin monosulphate EPCRS, neomycin sulphate EPCRS* and *streptomycin sulphate EPCRS*. Allow the solvent front to ascend 15 cm above the line of application but if a precoated plate is used allow the solvent front to reach the top of the plate. After removal of the plate, dry it in a current of warm air, spray with a mixture of equal volumes of a 46% w/v solution of *sulphuric acid* and a 0.2% w/v solution of *naphthalene-1,3-diol* in *ethanol* (96%) and heat at 150° for 5 to 10 minutes. The principal spot in the chromatogram obtained with solution (1) is similar in position, colour and size to that in the chromatogram obtained with solution (2). The test is not valid unless the chromatogram obtained with solution (3) shows three clearly separated principal spots.
B. Dissolve 10 mg in 5 ml of *water*, add 0.1 ml of *pyridine* and 2 ml of a 0.1% w/v solution of *ninhydrin* and heat in a water-bath at 65° to 70° for 10 minutes. An intense violet colour is produced.
C. Yields *reaction A* characteristic of sulphates, Appendix VI.

Acidity or alkalinity pH of a 1% w/v solution, 5.0 to 7.5, Appendix V L.

Specific optical rotation In a 10 w/v solution, +53.5° to +59.0°, Appendix V F.

Sulphate 27.0 to 31.0% of SO_4, calculated with reference to the dried substance, when determined by the following method. Dissolve 0.25 g in 100 ml of *water*, adjust to pH 11 with 13.5M *ammonia* and add 10 ml of 0.1M *barium chloride VS*. Titrate with 0.1M *disodium edetate VS* using 0.5 mg of *metalphthalein* as indicator; add 50 ml of *ethanol* (96%) when the colour of the solution begins to change and continue the titration until the violet-blue colour disappears. Each ml of 0.1M *barium chloride VS* is equivalent to 0.009606 g of sulphate, SO_4.

Neamine Carry out the method for *thin-layer chromatography*, Appendix III A, using a 10% w/v solution of *potassium dihydrogen orthophosphate* as the mobile phase and a chromatoplate prepared as follows. Mix 0.3 g of *carbomer* (Carbopol 934 is suitable) with 240 ml of *water*, allow to stand for 1 hour with moderate shaking, adjust to pH 7 by the gradual addition, with constant shaking, of 2M *sodium hydroxide* and add 30 g of *silica gel H*. Spread a uniform layer of the suspension 0.75 mm thick, heat at 110° for 1 hour, allow to cool and use the plate immediately. Apply separately to the plate 10 µl of each of two solutions in *water* containing (1) 0.25% w/v of the substance being examined and (2) 0.005% w/v of *neamine EPCRS*. Allow the solvent front to ascend 15 cm above the line of application but if a precoated plate is used allow the solvent front to reach the top of the plate. After removal of the plate, dry it in a current of warm air, spray with *ninhydrin and stannous chloride reagent* and heat at 110° for 15 minutes. Any spot corresponding to neamine in the chromatogram obtained with solution (1) is not more intense than the spot in the chromatogram obtained with solution (2).

Neomycin C Use a chromatographic column (40 cm × 6 mm), maintained at a constant uniform temperature (±1°) between 10° and 20° and provided with a suitable means of passing the mobile phase down the column at a constant rate. Introduce into the column, to within 1 cm of the top, successive portions of a suspension of an anion-exchange resin (Bio-Rad AG1-X2 is suitable) in *water* and wash the column with *water* for 90 minutes. Apply to the surface of the resin 0.1 ml of a 1% w/v solution of the substance being examined in *water* and use *water* adjusted to pH 7.5 with 0.01M *sodium hydroxide* as the mobile phase with a flow rate of 1 ml per minute. Collect the eluate in 1-ml fractions. Add 2 ml of *ninhydrin reagent* to each fraction, heat in a water-bath for 15 minutes, allow to cool and measure the *absorbance* at 570 nm, Appendix II B, using in the reference cell 1 ml of *water* treated in the same manner. If the absorbance is more than 0.6, dilute the contents of the tube by the addition of 6 ml of a mixture of equal volumes of *ethanol* (96%) and *water* and repeat the measurement. Plot a graph from the results obtained, correcting the absorbances for dilution if necessary, and determine the areas of the peaks corresponding to neomycin B and neomycin C.

Neamine is eluted first from the column, showing as a single peak or as a partly-resolved double peak, followed by neomycin C and then neomycin B. The area of the peak corresponding to neomycin C is 3 to 15% of the sum of the areas of the peaks corresponding to neomycin B and neomycin C. The test is not valid unless the *resolution factor* between the peaks corresponding to neomycin B and neomycin C is greater than 1.4.

Loss on drying When dried over *phosphorus pentoxide* at 60° at a pressure not exceeding 0.7 kPa for 3 hours, loses not more than 8.0% of its weight. Use 1 g.

Sulphated ash Not more than 1.0%, Appendix IX A, Method II. Use 1 g.

Assay Carry out the *biological assay of antibiotics*, Appendix XIV A. The precision of the assay is such that the fiducial limits of error are not less than 95% and not more than 105% of the estimated potency.

Storage Neomycin Sulphate should be kept in a well-closed container, protected from light and stored at a temperature not exceeding 30°.

Labelling The label states (1) the number of Units per mg; (2) the conditions under which the material should be stored.

Preparations
Neomycin Eye Drops
Neomycin Eye Ointment
Neomycin Oral Solution
Neomycin Tablets
Hydrocortisone and Neomycin Cream
Hydrocortisone and Neomycin Ear Drops
Hydrocortisone and Neomycin Eye Drops
Hydrocortisone and Neomycin Eye Ointment
Hydrocortisone and Neomycin Ointment

Action and use Antibacterial.

When neomycin is prescribed or demanded, Neomycin Sulphate shall be dispensed or supplied.

Neostigmine Bromide ☆

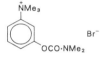

$C_{12}H_{19}BrN_2O_2$ 303.2   *114-80-7*

Neostigmine Bromide is 3-(dimethylcarbamoyloxy)trimethylanilinium bromide. It contains not less than 98.5 per cent and not more than 101.0 per cent of $C_{12}H_{19}BrN_2O_2$, calculated with reference to the dried substance.

Characteristics Colourless crystals or a white, crystalline powder; odourless; hygroscopic.

Solubility Soluble in 0.5 part of *water* and in 8 parts of *ethanol* (96%); freely soluble in *chloroform*; practically insoluble in *ether*.

Identification *Test A may be omitted if tests B, C, D and E are carried out. Tests B, C and D may be omitted if tests A and E are carried out.*

A. The *infra-red absorption spectrum*, Appendix II A, is concordant with the spectrum of *neostigmine bromide EPCRS*.

B. The *light absorption*, Appendix II B, in the range 230 to 350 nm of a 0.02% w/v solution in 0.5M *sulphuric acid* exhibits two maxima, at 260 nm and 266 nm. The A(1%, 1 cm) at 260 nm is about 16 and the A(1%, 1 cm) at 266 nm is about 14.

C. Warm 50 mg with 1 ml of 2M *sodium hydroxide*. The odour of dimethylamine is produced slowly.

D. Warm 50 mg with a mixture of 0.4 g of *potassium hydroxide* and 2 ml of *ethanol* (96%) on a water-bath for 3 minutes, replacing the evaporated ethanol. Cool, add 2 ml

of *water* and 2 ml of *dilute diazobenzenesulphonic acid solution*. An orange-red colour is produced.

E. Yields the *reactions* characteristic of bromides, Appendix VI.

Clarity and colour of solution A 5.0% w/v solution is *clear*, Appendix IV A, and *colourless*, Appendix IV B, Method II.

Sulphate A 5.0% w/v solution complies with the *limit test for sulphates*, Appendix VII (200 ppm).

3-Hydroxytrimethylanilinium bromide Dissolve 50 mg in a mixture of 1 ml of *sodium carbonate solution* and 9 ml of *water*. The *absorbance* of the resulting solution at 294 nm, measured immediately after preparation, is not more than 0.25, Appendix II B.

Loss on drying When dried to constant weight at 100° to 105°, loses not more than 1.0% of its weight. Use 1 g.

Sulphated ash Not more than 0.1%, Appendix IX A, Method II. Use 1 g.

Assay Dissolve 0.25 g in 10 ml of *anhydrous glacial acetic acid*, add 5 ml of *acetic anhydride* and carry out Method I for *non-aqueous titration*, Appendix VIII A, using 7 ml of *mercury(II) acetate solution* and 0.05 ml of *crystal violet solution* as indicator. Each ml of 0.1M *perchloric acid VS* is equivalent to 0.03032 g of $C_{12}H_{19}BrN_2O_2$.

Storage Neostigmine Bromide should be kept in a well-closed container and protected from light.

Preparation
Neostigmine Tablets

Action and use Anticholinesterase.

Neostigmine Methylsulphate

$C_{13}H_{22}N_2O_6S$ 334.4   *51-60-5*

Neostigmine Methylsulphate is 3-(dimethylcarbamoyloxy)trimethylanilinium methyl sulphate. It contains not less than 98.5 per cent and not more than 100.5 per cent of $C_{13}H_{22}N_2O_6S$, calculated with reference to the dried substance.

Characteristics Colourless crystals or a white, crystalline powder; odourless or almost odourless.

Solubility Soluble in 0.5 part of *water* and in 6 parts of *ethanol* (96%).

Identification A. The *infra-red absorption spectrum*, Appendix II A, is concordant with the *reference spectrum* of neostigmine methylsulphate.

B. The *light absorption*, Appendix II B, in the range 230 to 350 nm of a 0.04% w/v solution exhibits two maxima, at 260 nm and 266 nm. The *absorbance* at 260 nm is about 0.56 and at 266 nm is about 0.48.

C. To 0.1 ml of a 1% w/v solution add 0.5 ml of 5M *sodium hydroxide* and evaporate to dryness on a water-bath. Heat rapidly on an oil-bath to about 250° and maintain this temperature for about 30 seconds. Cool, dissolve the residue in 1 ml of *water*, cool in ice and add 1 ml of *diazobenzenesulphonic acid solution*. An orange-red colour is produced.

D. Mix 20 mg with 0.5 g of *sodium carbonate* and fuse in a small crucible. Boil the fused mass with 10 ml of *water* until disintegrated and filter. Add 0.2 ml of *bromine water* to the filtrate, heat to boiling, acidify with *hydrochloric acid* and expel the excess of bromine by boiling. The resulting solution yields the *reactions* characteristic of sulphates, Appendix VI.

Acidity Dissolve 0.2 g in 20 ml of *carbon dioxide-free water* and titrate to pH 7.0 with 0.02M *sodium hydroxide VS* (carbonate-free). Not more than 0.2 ml is required.

Melting point 144° to 149°, Appendix V A.

Light absorption Dissolve 50 mg in a mixture of 1 ml of *sodium carbonate solution* and 9 ml of *water*. The *absorbance* of the resulting solution at 294 nm is not more than 0.15, Appendix II B.

Chloride To 10 ml of a 2.0% w/v solution add 1 ml of 2M *nitric acid* and 1 ml of *silver nitrate solution*. No opalescence is produced immediately.

Sulphate 0.25 g complies with the *limit test for sulphates*, Appendix VII (600 ppm).

Related substances Carry out the method for *thin-layer chromatography*, Appendix III A, using *silica gel G* as the coating substance and a mixture of 67 volumes of *water*, 30 volumes of *methanol* and 3 volumes of *diethylamine* as the mobile phase. Apply separately to the chromatoplate 10 μl of each of two solutions of the substance being examined in *water* containing (1) 2.0% w/v and (2) 0.010% w/v. After removal of the plate, dry it in a current of warm air, spray with *diazotised nitroaniline solution* and then with 0.1M *sodium hydroxide*. Dry the plate in a current of warm air and spray with *dilute potassium iodobismuthate solution*. Any *secondary spot* in the chromatogram obtained with solution (1) is not more intense than the spot in the chromatogram obtained with solution (2).

Loss on drying When dried to constant weight at 105°, loses not more than 1.0% of its weight. Use 1 g.

Sulphated ash Not more than 0.1%, Appendix IX A.

Assay Dissolve 0.15 g in 20 ml of *water*, transfer to a semi-micro ammonia-distillation apparatus and add 20 ml of a 50% w/v solution of *sodium hydroxide*. Pass steam through the mixture, collect the distillate in 50 ml of 0.01M *sulphuric acid VS* until the total volume is about 200 ml and titrate the excess of acid with 0.02M *sodium hydroxide VS* using *methyl red solution* as indicator. Repeat the operation without the substance being examined. The difference between the titrations represents the amount of acid required to neutralise the dimethylamine produced. Each ml of 0.01M *sulphuric acid VS* is equivalent to 0.006688 g of $C_{13}H_{22}N_2O_6S$.

Storage Neostigmine Methylsulphate should be kept in a well-closed container and protected from light.

Preparation
Neostigmine Injection

Action and use Anticholinesterase.

Niclosamide

$C_{13}H_8Cl_2N_2O_4$ 327.1   *50-65-7*

Niclosamide is 2′,5-dichloro-4′-nitrosalicyl-anilide. It contains not less than 98.0 per cent and not more than 101.0 per cent of $C_{13}H_8Cl_2N_2O_4$, calculated with reference to the dried substance.

Characteristics A cream powder; odourless or almost odourless.

Solubility Practically insoluble in *water*; slightly soluble in *ethanol (96%)*; very slightly soluble in *chloroform* and in *ether*.

Identification A. The *infra-red absorption spectrum*, Appendix II A, is concordant with the *reference spectrum* of niclosamide. If the spectra are not concordant heat a sufficient quantity at 120° for 1 hour, cool and prepare a new spectrum of the residue.

B. Burn 20 mg by the method for *oxygen-flask combustion*, Appendix VIII C, using 5 ml of 2M *sodium hydroxide* as the absorbing liquid. The resulting solution yields a white precipitate with *silver nitrate solution* which is insoluble in 2M *nitric acid* but soluble in 5M *ammonia*.

C. Heat 50 mg with 5 ml of 1M *hydrochloric acid* and 0.1 g of *zinc powder* in a water-bath for 10 minutes, cool and filter. To the filtrate add 0.5 ml of a 1% w/v solution of *sodium nitrite* and allow to stand for 10 minutes. Add 2 ml of a 2% w/v solution of *ammonium sulphamate*, shake, allow to stand for 10 minutes and add 2 ml of a 0.5% w/v solution of *N-(1-naphthyl)ethylenediamine dihydrochloride*. A deep red colour is produced.

2-Chloro-4-nitroaniline Boil 0.10 g with 20 ml of *methanol* for 2 minutes, cool, add sufficient 1M *hydrochloric acid* to produce 50 ml and filter. To 10 ml of the filtrate add 0.5 ml of a 0.5% w/v solution of *sodium nitrite* and allow to stand for 10 minutes. Add 1 ml of a 2% w/v solution of *ammonium sulphamate*, shake, allow to stand for 10 minutes and add 1 ml of a 0.5% w/v solution of *N-(1-naphthyl)ethylenediamine dihydrochloride*. Any colour produced is not more intense than that produced by treating 20 ml of a solution in *methanol* containing 0.5 μg of *2-chloro-4-nitroaniline* per ml in the same manner and at the same time, beginning at the words 'add sufficient 1M *hydrochloric acid . . .*'.

5-Chlorosalicylic acid Boil 0.50 g with 10 ml of *water* for 2 minutes, cool, filter and add to the filtrate 0.2 ml of *iron(III) chloride test-solution*. No red or violet colour is produced.

Loss on drying. When dried to constant weight at 105°, loses not more than 0.5% of its weight. Use 1 g.

Sulphated ash Not more than 0.1%, Appendix IX A.

Assay Dissolve 0.3 g in 60 ml of *dimethylformamide* and carry out Method II for *non-aqueous titration*, Appendix VIII A, using 0.1M *tetrabutylammonium hydroxide VS* as titrant and determining the end-point potentiometrically. Each ml of 0.1M *tetrabutylammonium hydroxide VS* is equivalent to 0.03271 g of $C_{13}H_8Cl_2N_2O_4$.

Storage Niclosamide should be protected from light.

Preparation
Niclosamide Tablets

Action and use Anthelmintic.

Nicotinamide ☆

Niacinamide

C₆H₆N₂O   122.1   *98-92-0*

Nicotinamide is pyridine-3-carboxamide. It contains not less than 99.0 per cent and not more than 101.0 per cent of $C_6H_6N_2O$, calculated with reference to the dried substance.

Characteristics Colourless crystals or a white, crystalline powder; odour, faint and characteristic.

Solubility Soluble in 1 part of *water* and in 1.5 parts of *ethanol (96%)*; slightly soluble in *chloroform* and in *ether*.

Identification *Test A may be omitted if tests B, C and D are carried out. Tests B and C may be omitted if tests A and D are carried out.*
A. The *infra-red absorption spectrum*, Appendix II A, is concordant with the spectrum of *nicotinamide EPCRS*.
B. Boil 0.1 g with 1 ml of *2M sodium hydroxide*. Ammonia, recognisable by its odour, is evolved.
C. To 2 ml of a 0.1% w/v solution add 2 ml of *cyanogen bromide solution* followed by 3 ml of a 2.5% w/v solution of *aniline* and shake. A yellow colour is produced.
D. *Melting point*, 128° to 131°, Appendix V A, Method I.

Acidity or alkalinity pH of a 5% w/v solution, 6.0 to 7.5, Appendix V L.

Clarity and colour of solution A 5.0% w/v solution is *clear*, Appendix IV A, and not more intensely coloured than *reference solution BY₇*, Appendix IV B, Method II.

Heavy metals Dissolve 2.5 g in sufficient *water* to produce 50 ml and dilute 10 ml of the solution to 15 ml with *water*. 12 ml of the resulting solution complies with *limit test A for heavy metals*, Appendix VII (30 ppm). Use *lead standard solution (1 ppm Pb)* to prepare the standard.

Related substances Carry out the method for *thin-layer chromatography*, Appendix III A, using *silica gel GF254* as the coating substance and a mixture of 48 volumes of *chloroform*, 45 volumes of *absolute ethanol* and 4 volumes of *water* as the mobile phase but allowing the solvent front to ascend 10 cm above the line of application. Apply separately to the chromatoplate 5 μl of each of two solutions of the substance being examined in *ethanol (50%)* containing (1) 8% w/v and (2) 0.020% w/v. After removal of the plate, allow it to dry in air and examine under *ultra-violet light (254 nm)*. Any *secondary spot* in the chromatogram obtained with solution (1) is not more intense than the spot in the chromatogram obtained with solution (2).

Loss on drying When dried over *phosphorus pentoxide* at a pressure not exceeding 2.7 kPa for 18 hours, loses not more than 0.5% of its weight. Use 0.5 g.

Sulphated Ash Not more than 0.1%, Appendix IX A, Method II. Use 1 g.

Assay Dissolve 0.25 g in 20 ml of *anhydrous glacial acetic acid*, warming slightly if necessary. Add 5 ml of *acetic anhydride* and carry out Method I for *non-aqueous titration*, Appendix VIII A, using *crystal violet solution* as indicator and titrating until the colour changes to greenish-blue. Each ml of 0.1M *perchloric acid VS* is equivalent to 0.01221 g of $C_6H_6N_2O$.

Storage Nicotinamide should be kept in a well-closed container.

Preparation
Nicotinamide Tablets

Action and use Component of vitamin B.

Nicotinic Acid ☆

C₆H₅NO₂   123.1   *59-67-6*

Nicotinic Acid is pyridine-3-carboxylic acid. It contains not less than 99.5 per cent and not more than 100.5 per cent of $C_6H_5NO_2$, calculated with reference to the dried substance.

Characteristics A white, crystalline powder.

Solubility Soluble in boiling *water* and in boiling *ethanol (96%)*; sparingly soluble in *water*; very slightly soluble in *chloroform*; practically insoluble in *ether*. It dissolves in dilute aqueous solutions of alkali hydroxides and carbonates.

Identification *Test A may be omitted if tests B and C are carried out. Test B may be omitted if tests A and C are carried out.*
A. The *infra-red absorption spectrum*, Appendix II A, is concordant with the spectrum of *nicotinic acid EPCRS*.
B. To 2 ml of a 0.1% w/v solution add 2 ml of *cyanogen bromide solution* and 3 ml of a 2.5% w/v solution of *aniline* and shake. A yellow colour is produced.
C. *Melting point*, 234° to 240°, Appendix V A, Method I.

Heavy metals 1.0 g complies with *limit test C for heavy metals*, Appendix VII (20 ppm). Use 2 ml of *lead standard solution (10 ppm Pb)* to prepare the standard.

Chloride Dissolve 0.25 g in *water* by heating on a water-bath and dilute to 15 ml with *water*. The solution complies with the *limit test for chlorides*, Appendix VII (200 ppm).

Related substances Carry out the method for *thin-layer chromatography*, Appendix III A, using *silica gel GF254* as the coating substance and a mixture of 85 volumes of *propan-1-ol*, 10 volumes of *anhydrous formic acid* and 5 volumes of *water* as the mobile phase. Apply separately to the chromatoplate 5 μl of each of two solutions of the substance being examined in *water* containing (1) 2.0% w/v and (2) 0.01% w/v. If necessary in the preparation of solution (1) warm slightly to effect dissolution. After removal of the plate, dry it at 100° to 105° for 10 minutes and examine under *ultra-violet light (254 nm)*. Any *secondary spot* in the chromatogram obtained with solution (1) is not more intense than the spot in the chromatogram obtained with solution (2).

Loss on drying When dried at 100° to 105° for 1 hour, loses not more than 1.0% of its weight. Use 1 g.

Sulphated ash Not more than 0.1%, Appendix IX A, Method II. Use 1 g.

Assay Dissolve 0.25 g in 50 ml of *water* and titrate with 0.1M *sodium hydroxide VS* using 0.25 ml of *dilute phenolphthalein solution* as indicator. Repeat the operation without the substance being examined. The difference between the titrations represents the amount of sodium hydroxide required. Each ml of 0.1M *sodium hydroxide VS* is equivalent to 0.01231 g of $C_6H_5NO_2$.

Storage Nicotinic Acid should be protected from light.

Preparation
Nicotinic Acid Tablets

Action and use Component of vitamin B.

Nicotinyl Alcohol Tartrate

$C_6H_7NO,C_4H_6O_6$ 259.2   *6164-87-0*

Nicotinyl Alcohol Tartrate is 3-pyridylmethanol hydrogen tartrate. It contains not less than 98.5 per cent and not more than 101.5 per cent of $C_6H_7NO,C_4H_6O_6$, calculated with reference to the dried substance.

Characteristics A white or almost white crystalline powder; odourless or almost odourless.

Solubility Freely soluble in *water*; slightly soluble in *ethanol (96%)*; practically insoluble in *chloroform* and in *ether*.

Identification A. The *light absorption*, Appendix II B, in the range 230 to 350 nm of a 0.004% w/v solution in 0.1M *hydrochloric acid* exhibits a maximum only at 261 nm. The *absorbance* at 261 nm is about 0.84.

B. In the test for Related substances, the principal spot in the chromatogram obtained with solution (2) corresponds to that in the chromatogram obtained with solution (4).

C. Yields *reactions A* and *B* characteristic of tartrates, Appendix VI.

Acidity pH of a 5% w/v solution, 2.8 to 3.7, Appendix V L.

Clarity and colour of solution A 5.0% w/v solution is *clear*, Appendix IV A, and not more intensely coloured than *reference solution Y5*, Appendix IV B, Method II.

Melting point 146° to 150°, Appendix V A.

Heavy metals Dissolve the residue obtained in the test for Sulphated ash in 1 ml of 2M *hydrochloric acid* and dilute to 20 ml with *water*. 12 ml of the solution complies with *limit test A for heavy metals*, Appendix VII (20 ppm). Use *lead standard solution (2 ppm)* to prepare the standard.

Nicotinaldehyde Mix 10 ml of a 10% w/v solution of the substance being examined with 10 ml of a 1.0% w/v solution of *phenylhydrazine hydrochloride* in 3.6M *orthophosphoric acid*, dilute to 50 ml with *water* and allow to

stand for 30 minutes. Measure the *absorbance* of the solution at the maximum at 370 nm, Appendix II B, using in the reference cell a 0.20% w/v solution of *phenylhydrazine hydrochloride* in 0.72M *orthophosphoric acid*. The absorbance is not more than that of a solution prepared by treating 10 ml of a 0.0010% w/v solution of *pyridine-3-carboxaldehyde* in the same manner.

Related substances Carry out the method for *thin-layer chromatography*, Appendix III A, using *silica gel GF254* as the coating substance and a mixture of 50 volumes of *dichloromethane*, 30 volumes of *1,4-dioxan*, 16 volumes of *methanol* and 4 volumes of 13.5M *ammonia* as the mobile phase. Apply separately to the chromatoplate 5 μl of each of four solutions in 0.1M *ammonia* containing (1) 25% w/v of the substance being examined, (2) 0.050% w/v of the substance being examined, (3) 0.050% w/v of *3-picolylamine* and (4) 0.050% w/v of *nicotinyl alcohol tartrate BPCRS*. After removal of the plate, allow it to dry in air and examine under *ultra-violet light (254 nm)*. Spray with a 2% w/v solution of *2,4,6-trinitrochlorobenzene* in *absolute ethanol*, dry in a current of air and spray with a 5% w/v solution of *sodium carbonate*. Any spot corresponding to 3-picolylamine in the chromatogram obtained with solution (1) is not more intense than the spot in the chromatogram obtained with solution (3). Any other *secondary spot* in the chromatogram obtained with solution (1) is not more intense than the spot in the chromatogram obtained with solution (2). Disregard any spot due to tartaric acid on the line of application.

Loss on drying When dried at 105° for 3 hours, loses not more than 1.0% of its weight. Use 1 g.

Sulphated ash Not more than 0.1%, Appendix IX A. Use 2.0 g.

Assay Carry out Method I for *non-aqueous titration*, Appendix VIII A, using 0.25 g and determining the end-point potentiometrically. Each ml of 0.1M *perchloric acid VS* is equivalent to 0.02592 g of $C_6H_7NO,C_4H_6O_6$.

Preparation
Nicotinyl Alcohol Tablets

Action and use Vasodilator.

Nicoumalone

$C_{19}H_{15}NO_6$ 353.3   *152-72-7*

Nicoumalone is 4-hydroxy-3-(1-*p*-nitrophenyl-3-oxobutyl)coumarin. It contains not less than 98.5 per cent and not more than 100.5 per cent of $C_{19}H_{15}NO_6$, calculated with reference to the dried substance.

Characteristics An almost white to buff powder; odourless or almost odourless.

Solubility Practically insoluble in *water* and in *ether*; slightly soluble in *ethanol (96%)* and in *chloroform*. It dissolves in aqueous solutions of the alkali hydroxides.

Identification A. The *infra-red absorption spectrum*, Appendix II A, is concordant with the *reference spectrum* of nicoumalone. If the spectra are not concordant, dissolve 0.1 g of the substance being examined in 10 ml of *acetone* and add *water* dropwise until the solution becomes turbid. Heat on a water-bath until the solution is clear and allow to stand. Filter, wash the crystals with a mixture of equal volumes of *acetone* and *water* and dry at 100° at a pressure of 2 kPa for 30 minutes. Prepare a new spectrum of the residue.

B. The *light absorption*, Appendix II B, in the range 230 to 350 nm a 0.002% w/v solution in a mixture of 1 volume of 1M *hydrochloric acid* and 9 volumes of *methanol* exhibits two maxima, at 283 nm and 306 nm. The *absorbance* at 283 nm is about 1.3 and at 306 nm is about 1.0.

C. Heat 50 mg with 2.5 ml of *glacial acetic acid*, 0.5 ml of *hydrochloric acid* and 0.2 g of *zinc powder* on a water-bath for 5 minutes, cool and filter. To the filtrate add 0.05 ml of *sodium nitrite solution* and add the mixture to 10 ml of a 1% w/v solution of *2-naphthol* containing 3 ml of 5M *sodium hydroxide*. A bright red precipitate is produced.

D. *Melting point*, about 198°, Appendix V A.

Clarity and colour of solution A. A 2.0% w/v solution in *acetone* is *clear*, Appendix IV A.

B. The *absorbance* of a 4-cm layer of a 2.0% w/v solution in *acetone* at 460 nm is not more than 0.12, Appendix II B.

C. A 2.0% w/v solution in 5M *sodium hydroxide* is *clear*, Appendix IV A, and yellow.

Light absorption *Absorbance* of a 0.001% w/v solution in a mixture of 1 volume of 1M *hydrochloric acid* and 9 volumes of *methanol* at the maximum at 306 nm, 0.50 to 0.54, Appendix II B.

Related substances Carry out the method for *thin-layer chromatography*, Appendix III A, using *silica gel GF254* as the coating substance and a mixture of 50 volumes of *chloroform*, 50 volumes of *cyclohexane* and 20 volumes of *glacial acetic acid* as the mobile phase. Apply separately to the chromatoplate 20 μl of each of two solutions of the substance being examined in *acetone* containing (1) 2.0% w/v and (2) 0.0020% w/v. After removal of the plate, allow it to dry in air and immediately examine under *ultra-violet light (254 nm)*. Any *secondary spot* in the chromatogram obtained with solution (1) is not more intense than the spot in the chromatogram obtained with solution (2).

Loss on drying When dried to constant weight at 105°, loses not more than 0.5% of its weight. Use 1 g.

Sulphated ash Not more than 0.1%, Appendix IX A.

Assay Dissolve 0.6 g in 50 ml of *acetone* and titrate with 0.1M *sodium hydroxide VS* using *bromothymol blue solution* as indicator. Repeat the operation without the substance being examined. The difference between the titrations represents the amount of sodium hydroxide required. Each ml of 0.1M *sodium hydroxide VS* is equivalent to 0.03533 g of $C_{19}H_{15}NO_6$.

Preparation

Nicoumalone Tablets

Action and use Anticoagulant.

In some countries the material described in this monograph may be known as Acenocoumarol.

Nikethamide ☆

$C_{10}H_{14}N_2O$　　178.2　　59-26-7

Nikethamide is *N,N*-diethylpyridine-3-carboxamide. It contains not less than 99.0 per cent and not more than 101.0 per cent of $C_{10}H_{14}N_2O$, calculated with reference to the anhydrous substance.

Characteristics A colourless or slightly yellowish, oily liquid or crystalline mass; odour, slight and characteristic.

Solubility Miscible with *water*, with *ethanol (96%)*, with *chloroform* and with *ether*.

Identification *Test A may be omitted if tests B, C and D are carried out. Tests C and D may be omitted if tests A and B are carried out.*

A. The *infra-red absorption spectrum*, Appendix II A, is concordant with the spectrum of *nikethamide EPCRS*.

B. The *light absorption*, Appendix II B, in the range 230 to 350 nm of a 2-cm layer of a 0.0015% w/v solution in 0.01M *hydrochloric acid* exhibits a maximum only at 263 nm. The A(1%, 1 cm) at the maximum at 263 nm is about 285.

C. Heat 0.1 g with 1 ml of 2M *sodium hydroxide*. Diethylamine, recognisable by its odour, is evolved progressively; the fumes turn *litmus paper* blue.

D. To 2 ml of a 0.1% w/v solution add 2 ml of *cyanogen bromide solution* and 3 ml of a 2.5% w/v solution of *aniline* and shake. A yellow colour is produced.

Acidity or alkalinity pH of a 25% w/v solution, 6.0 to 7.8, Appendix V L.

Clarity and colour Nikethamide, in liquid form or liquefied by heating gently, is *clear*, Appendix IV A, and not more intensely coloured than *reference solution Y_5*, Appendix IV B, Method II.

Refractive index 1.524 to 1.526, Appendix V E.

Heavy metals A 10.0% w/v solution complies with *limit test A for heavy metals*, Appendix VII (10 ppm). Use *lead standard solution (1 ppm Pb)* to prepare the standard.

Related substances Carry out the method for *thin-layer chromatography*, Appendix III A, using *silica gel GF254* as the coating substance and a mixture of 75 volumes of *chloroform* and 25 volumes of *propan-1-ol* as the mobile phase. Apply separately to the chromatoplate 10 μl of each of three solutions in *methanol* containing (1) 4% w/v of the substance being examined, (2) 0.04% w/v of *ethylnicotinamide EPCRS* and (3) 0.004% w/v of *ethylnicotinamide EPCRS*. After removal of the plate, allow it to dry in air and examine under *ultra-violet light (254 nm)*. Any spot corresponding to ethylnicotinamide in the chromatogram obtained with solution (1) is not more intense than the spot in the chromatogram obtained with solution (2) and any other *secondary spot* is not more intense than the spot in the chromatogram obtained with solution (3).

Sulphated ash Not more than 0.1%, Appendix IX A, Method II. Use 1 g.

Water Not more than 0.3% w/w, Appendix IX C. Use 2 g.

Assay Dissolve 0.15 g in a mixture of 20 ml of *anhydrous glacial acetic acid* and 5 ml of *acetic anhydride* and carry out Method I for *non-aqueous titration*, Appendix VIII A, determining the end-point potentiometrically. Each ml of 0.1M *perchloric acid VS* is equivalent to 0.01782 g of $C_{10}H_{14}N_2O$.

Preparation
Nikethamide Injection

Action and use Respiratory stimulant.

Nitrazepam ☆

$C_{15}H_{11}N_3O_3$ 281.3   146-22-5

Nitrazepam is 1,3-dihydro-7-nitro-5-phenyl-2*H*-1,4-benzodiazepin-2-one. It contains not less than 99.0 per cent and not more than 101.0 per cent of $C_{15}H_{11}N_3O_3$, calculated with reference to the dried substance.

Characteristics A yellow, crystalline powder.

Solubility Practically insoluble in *water*; slightly soluble in *ethanol (96%)* and in *ether*; sparingly soluble in *chloroform*.

Identification *Test A may be omitted if tests B, C, D and E are carried out. Tests B, C and D may be omitted if tests A and E are carried out.*
A. The *infra-red absorption spectrum*, Appendix II A, is concordant with the spectrum of *nitrazepam EPCRS*.
B. Carry out the following procedure protected from light. The *light absorption*, Appendix II B, in the range 230 to 350 nm of a 0.0005% w/v solution in a 0.5% w/v solution of *sulphuric acid* in *methanol*, examined immediately after preparation, exhibits a maximum at 280 nm. The A(1%, 1 cm) at the maximum at 280 nm is 890 to 950.
C. Dissolve 20 mg in a mixture of 5 ml of *hydrochloric acid* and 10 ml of *water*. Boil for 5 minutes, cool and add 2 ml of a 0.1% w/v solution of *sodium nitrite*. Allow to stand for 1 minute, add 1 ml of a 0.5% w/v solution of *sulphamic acid*, mix, allow to stand for 1 minute and add 1 ml of a 0.1% w/v solution of N-*(1-naphthyl)ethylenediamine dihydrochloride*. A red colour is produced.
D. Dissolve 10 mg in 1 ml of *methanol*, warming if necessary, and add 0.05 ml of 2M *sodium hydroxide*. An intense yellow colour is produced.
E. *Melting point*, 226° to 230°, Appendix V A, Method I.

Heavy metals 1.0 g complies with *limit test D for heavy metals*, Appendix VII (20 ppm). Use 2 ml of *lead standard solution (10 ppm Pb)* to prepare the standard.

Related substances Carry out the method for *thin-layer chromatography*, Appendix III A, protected from light, using *silica gel GF254* as the coating substance and a mixture of 85 volumes of *nitromethane* and 15 volumes of *ethyl acetate* as the mobile phase but allowing the solvent front to ascend 12 cm above the line of application. Apply separately to the chromatoplate 10 μl of each of four solutions in *acetone* containing (1) 2.0% w/v of the substance being examined, prepared immediately before use, (2) 0.0020% w/v of *2-amino-5-nitrobenzophenone*, (3) 0.0020% w/v of *3-amino-6-nitro-4-phenyl-2-quinolone*

EPCRS and (4) 0.0020% w/v of the substance being examined. After removal of the plate, allow it to dry in air and examine under *ultra-violet light (254 nm)*. Any spots corresponding to 2-amino-5-nitrobenzophenone and 3-amino-6-nitro-4-phenyl-2-quinolone in the chromatogram obtained with solution (1) are not more intense than the spots in the chromatograms obtained with solutions (2) and (3) respectively and any other *secondary spot* in the chromatogram obtained with solution (1) is not more intense than the spot in the chromatogram obtained with solution (4).

Loss on drying When dried at 100° to 105° for 4 hours, loses not more than 0.5% of its weight. Use 1 g.

Sulphated ash Not more than 0.1%, Appendix IX A, Method II. Use 1 g.

Assay Dissolve 0.25 g in 25 ml of *acetic anhydride* and carry out Method I for *non-aqueous titration*, Appendix VIII A, determining the end-point potentiometrically. Each ml of 0.1M *perchloric acid VS* is equivalent to 0.02813 g of $C_{15}H_{11}N_3O_3$.

Storage Nitrazepam should be kept in a well-closed container and protected from light.

Preparations
Nitrazepam Capsules
Nitrazepam Tablets

Action and use Hypnotic.

Nitric Acid

HNO_3 63.01   7697-37-2

Nitric Acid contains not less than 69.0 per cent and not more than 71.0 per cent of HNO_3.

Characteristics A clear, colourless or almost colourless, fuming liquid.

Identification A. It is strongly acidic, even when freely diluted.
B. Dilute 1 ml to 10 ml with *water*. The resulting solution yields the *reactions* characteristic of nitrates, Appendix VI.

Weight per ml About 1.41 g, Appendix V G.

Arsenic Heat 1.0 g in a porcelain dish with 2 ml of *sulphuric acid* until white fumes are evolved, cool, add 2 ml of *water* and again heat until white fumes are evolved. Cool and dilute to 25 ml with *water*. The resulting solution complies with the *limit test for arsenic*, Appendix VII (1 ppm).

Copper and zinc To 1.0 ml add 20 ml of *water* and a slight excess of 5M *ammonia*; no blue colour is produced. Pass *hydrogen sulphide* through the solution; no precipitate is produced.

Iron 0.1 ml diluted to 10 ml with *water* complies with the *limit test for iron*, Appendix VII (80 ppm).

Lead Not more than 2 ppm when determined by the following procedure and using the following solutions. For solution (1) use 7.0 g of the substance being examined and for solution (2) mix 2.0 g with 1 ml of *lead standard solution (10 ppm Pb)*. Make solutions (1) and (2) alkaline by the cautious addition of 5M *ammonia* and to each add 1 ml of *potassium cyanide solution PbT*. The solutions should be not more than faintly opalescent. If the colours of the solutions differ, equalise by the addition of about 0.2 ml of a highly diluted solution of burnt sugar or other non-reactive substance. Dilute each solution to 50 ml with *water*, add 0.1 ml of a 10% w/v solution of *sodium sulphide* to each and mix thoroughly. The colour produced in solution (1) is not more intense than that produced in solution (2) when viewed against a white background.

Chloride Neutralise 0.5 ml to *litmus paper* with 5M *ammonia*. The resulting solution diluted to 15 ml with *water* complies with the *limit test for chlorides*, Appendix VII (70 ppm).

Sulphate To 4.4 ml add 20 mg of *sodium hydrogen carbonate*, evaporate to dryness on a water-bath and dissolve the residue in sufficient *water* to produce 150 ml. 15 ml of the resulting solution complies with the *limit test for sulphates*, Appendix VII (240 ppm).

Sulphated ash Not more than 0.01% w/w, Appendix IX A. Use 1 g.

Assay To 4 g add 40 ml of *water* and titrate with 1M *sodium hydroxide VS* using *methyl orange solution* as indicator. Each ml of 1M *sodium hydroxide VS* is equivalent to 0.06301 g of HNO_3.

Nitrofurantoin ☆

$C_8H_6N_4O_5$ 238.2   *67-20-9*

Nitrofurantoin is 1-(5-nitrofurfurylidene-amino)imidazolidine-2,4-dione. It contains not less than 98.0 per cent and not more than 102.0 per cent of $C_8H_6N_4O_5$, calculated with reference to the dried substance.

Characteristics A yellow, crystalline powder or crystals; odourless or almost odourless.

Solubility Very slightly soluble in *water* and in *ethanol* (96%); soluble in 16 parts of *dimethylformamide*.

Identification A. Carry out the following test in subdued light. The *light absorption*, Appendix II B, in the range 220 to 400 nm of the solution prepared as directed in the Assay exhibits two maxima, at 266 nm and 367 nm. The ratio of the *absorbance* at 367 nm to that at 266 nm is 1.36 to 1.42.

B. To 1 ml of a 0.1% w/v solution in *dimethylformamide* add 0.1 ml of 0.5M *ethanolic potassium hydroxide*. A brown colour is produced.

Related substances Carry out the method for *thin-layer chromatography*, Appendix III A, using *silica gel HF254* as the coating substance and a mixture of 90 volumes of *nitromethane* and 10 volumes of *methanol* as the mobile phase. Apply separately to the chromatoplate 10 µl of each of the following solutions. For solution (1) dissolve 0.25 g of the substance being examined in the minimum volume of *dimethylformamide* and dilute to 10 ml with *acetone*. For solution (2) dilute 1 volume of solution (1) to 100 volumes with *acetone*. After removal of the plate, allow it to dry in air, heat at 100° to 105° for 5 minutes and examine under *ultra-violet light (254 nm)*. Spray with *strong phenyl-hydrazine hydrochloride solution* and heat the plate at 100° to 105° for a further 10 minutes. By both methods of

visualisation, any *secondary spot* in the chromatogram obtained with solution (1) is not more intense than the spot in the chromatogram obtained with solution (2).

Loss on drying When dried to constant weight at 100° to 105°, loses not more than 1.0% of its weight. Use 1 g.

Sulphated ash Not more than 0.1%, Appendix IX A, Method II. Use 1 g.

Assay Carry out the following procedure in subdued light. Dissolve 0.12 g in 50 ml of *dimethylformamide*, add sufficient *water* to produce 1000 ml, mix and dilute 5 ml to 100 ml with a solution containing 1.8% w/v of *sodium acetate* and 0.14% v/v of *glacial acetic acid*. Measure the *absorbance* of the resulting solution at the maximum at 367 nm, Appendix II B, using the sodium acetate—acetic acid solution in the reference cell. Calculate the content of $C_8H_6N_4O_5$ taking 765 as the value of A(1%, 1 cm) at the maximum at 367 nm.

Storage Nitrofurantoin should be kept in a well-closed container, protected from light and stored at a temperature not exceeding 25°.

Preparations
Nitrofurantoin Oral Suspension
Nitrofurantoin Tablets

Action and use Antibacterial.

Nitrofurazone

$C_6H_6N_4O_4$ 198.1   *59-87-0*

Nitrofurazone is 5-nitro-2-furaldehyde semi-carbazone. It contains not less than 97.0 per cent and not more than 103.0 per cent of $C_6H_6N_4O_4$, calculated with reference to the dried substance.

Characteristics A yellow to brownish-yellow, crystalline powder; odourless or almost odourless.

Solubility Very slightly soluble in *water*; slightly soluble in *ethanol* (96%).

Identification A. The *infra-red absorption spectrum*, Appendix II A, is concordant with the *reference spectrum* of nitrofurazone.

B. Dissolve 1 mg in 1 ml of *dimethylformamide* and add 0.05 ml of 1M *ethanolic potassium hydroxide*. A ruby-red colour is produced.

Acidity or alkalinity To 1 g add 100 ml of *carbon dioxide-free water*, shake and filter. The pH of the filtrate is 5.0 to 7.0, Appendix V L.

Related substances Carry out in subdued light the method for *thin-layer chromatography*, Appendix III A, using *silica gel G* as the coating substance and a mixture of 95 volumes of *toluene* and 5 volumes of *1,4-dioxan* as the mobile phase. Apply separately to the chromatoplate 10 µl of each of three solutions in a mixture of equal volumes of *acetone* and *dimethylformamide* containing (1) 1.0% w/v of the substance being examined, (2) 0.0020% w/v of *5-nitrofurfurylidene azine BPCRS* and (3) 0.010% w/v of *nitrofurfural diacetate BPCRS*. After removal of the plate, heat it at 105° for 5 minutes and spray with *strong* *phenylhydrazine hydrochloride solution.* In the chromatogram obtained with solution (1) any spots corresponding to 5-nitrofurfurylidene azine and nitrofurfural diacetate are not more intense than the spots in the chromatograms obtained with solutions (2) and (3) respectively.

Loss on drying When dried to constant weight at 105°, loses not more than 0.5% of its weight. Use 1 g.

Sulphated ash Not more than 0.1%, Appendix IX A.

Assay Carry out the following procedure in subdued light. To 60 mg add 20 ml of *dimethylformamide*, swirl to dissolve and add sufficient *water* to produce 500 ml. Dilute 5 ml to 100 ml with *water* and mix. Measure the *absorbance* of the resulting solution at the maximum at 375 nm, Appendix II B. Calculate the content of $C_6H_6N_4O_4$ taking 822 as the value of A(1%, 1 cm) at the maximum at 375 nm.

Storage Nitrofurazone should be kept in a well-closed container and protected from light.

Action and use Antibacterial.

In some countries the material described in this monograph may be known as Nitrofural.

Nitrous Oxide ☆

N₂O   44.01   *10024-97-2*

Nitrous Oxide contains not less than 98.0 per cent v/v of N₂O in the gaseous phase.

The test for Carbon monoxide should be carried out on the first portion of gas drawn from the cylinder and that for Nitric oxide and nitrogen dioxide immediately thereafter. The cylinder from which the gas is taken should be kept at room temperature for not less than 6 hours before carrying out the following tests. In all the tests the cylinder is kept in the vertical position with the outlet valve uppermost when delivering the gas. The gas should be passed at a steady rate of 4 litres per hour unless otherwise stated.

Characteristics A colourless gas; odourless.

Solubility At 20° and at a pressure of 101.3 kPa, 1 volume of gas dissolves in about 1.5 volumes of *water*.

Identification A. The *infra-red absorption spectrum*, Appendix II A, is concordant with the European Pharmacopœia reference spectrum of nitrous oxide.
B. A glowing splinter of wood bursts into flame on contact with the gas.
C. Shake with *alkaline pyrogallol solution.* The gas being examined is not absorbed and the solution does not become brown.

Acidity or alkalinity Use a hermetically-closed, flat-bottomed, glass cylinder with dimensions such that 50 ml of liquid reaches a height of 12 to 14 cm, fitted with an outlet tube and with an inlet tube with an orifice of 1 mm in internal diameter reaching to within 2 mm of the bottom of the cylinder.
For solution (1) pass 2.0 litres of the gas being examined through a mixture of 0.1 ml of 0.01M *hydrochloric acid* and 50 ml of *carbon dioxide-free water.* For solution (2) use 50 ml of *carbon dioxide-free water.* For solution (3) add 0.2 ml of 0.01M *hydrochloric acid* to 50 ml of *carbon dioxide-free water.* To each solution add 0.1 ml of a 0.02% w/v solution of *methyl red* in *ethanol (70%).*

The intensity of the colour of solution (1) is between those of solutions (2) and (3).

Carbon dioxide Use the apparatus described in the test for Acidity or alkalinity. Pass 1.0 litre through 50 ml of a clear 4.73% w/v solution of *barium hydroxide.* Any turbidity produced in the resulting solution is not more intense than that produced in a reference solution prepared by adding 1 ml of a 0.11% w/v solution of *sodium hydrogen carbonate* in *carbon dioxide-free water* to 50 ml of a 4.73% w/v solution of *barium hydroxide* (300 ppm v/v).

Carbon monoxide Carry out the *limit test for carbon monoxide in medicinal gases*, Appendix IX E, using 5 litres of the gas being examined and 5 litres of *argon* for the blank determination. The difference between the titrations is not more than 0.5 ml (10 ppm v/v).

Halogens and hydrogen sulphide Use the apparatus described in the test for Acidity or alkalinity. Pass 20.0 litres through a mixture of 49 ml of *water* and 1 ml of a 4.25% w/v solution of *silver nitrate* with a flow rate not exceeding 15 litres per hour; the solution does not darken. Any opalescence produced is not more intense than that produced by treating in the same manner a mixture of 1 ml of a 4.25% w/v solution of *silver nitrate*, 40 ml of *chloride standard solution (5 ppm Cl)*, 0.15 ml of 2M *nitric acid* and diluting to 50 ml with *water*, allow to stand protected from light for 5 minutes. Compare 100-mm layers as prescribed in Appendix IV A (10 ppm Cl w/v).

Nitric oxide and nitrogen dioxide Use two of the cylinders described in the test for Acidity or alkalinity connected in series. Examine separately both the liquid and gaseous phases of the gas being examined. To obtain the liquid phase invert the cylinder. The liquid vaporises on leaving the valve.
For solution A dissolve 1 g of *sulphanilic acid* in a mixture of 10 ml of *glacial acetic acid* and 180 ml of *water.* For solution B dissolve 0.2 g of N-(1-naphthyl)ethylene-diamine dihydrochloride in 10 ml of a 50% v/v solution of *glacial acetic acid*, heating gently, and dilute to 200 ml with *water.* Mix 9 volumes of solution A with 1 volume of solution B (reagent A).
In the first cylinder place 15 ml of a solution containing 2.5% w/v of *potassium permanganate* and 1.2% v/v of *sulphuric acid (96%).* Place 20 ml of reagent A in the second cylinder and connect the outlet tube of the first cylinder to the inlet tube of the second cylinder. Pass 2.5 litres of the gas being examined through the reagents at a rate of 15 litres per hour. Prepare a reference solution by adding 0.25 ml of a 0.00616% w/v solution of *sodium nitrite* to 20 ml of reagent A. Allow both the sample solution and the reference solution to stand for 10 minutes. For both the liquid and gaseous phases, any red colour in the sample solution is not more intense than that in the reference solution (2 ppm v/v of NO + NO₂).

Water Carry out Method III for the *determination of water*, Appendix IX C (120 ppm v/v).

Assay Carry out Method II for the *assay of medicinal gases*, Appendix VIII J, using 100 ml. Use a cylinder of the gas being examined from which at least 1% w/w of the contents has been removed.

Storage Nitrous Oxide should be kept under pressure in an approved metal cylinder.

Labelling The metal container should be painted blue and carry a label stating 'Nitrous Oxide'. In addition 'Nitrous Oxide' or the symbol 'N₂O' should be stencilled in paint on the shoulder of the cylinder.

Action and use General anaesthetic; analgesic.

Noradrenaline Acid Tartrate ☆

$C_8H_{11}NO_3,C_4H_6O_6,H_2O$ 337.3   *69815-49-2*

Noradrenaline Acid Tartrate is (*R*)-2-amino-1-(3,4-dihydroxyphenyl)ethanol hydrogen tartrate monohydrate. It contains not less than 98.5 per cent and not more than 101.0 per cent of $C_8H_{11}NO_3,C_4H_6O_6$, calculated with reference to the anhydrous substance.

Characteristics A white or almost white, crystalline powder; odourless.

Solubility Freely soluble in *water*; slightly soluble in *ethanol (96%)*; practically insoluble in *chloroform* and in *ether*.

Identification *Test A may be omitted if tests B, C, D, E and F are carried out. Tests B, D and E may be omitted if tests A, C and F are carried out.*
A. Dissolve 2 g in 20 ml of a 0.5% w/v solution of *sodium metabisulphite* and add 10M *ammonia* until alkaline. Allow the mixture to stand in ice for 1 hour, filter and retain the filtrate. Wash the precipitate with three 2-ml quantities of *water*, followed by 5 ml of *ethanol (96%)* and 5 ml of *ether* and dry the precipitate at a pressure of 1.5 to 2.5 kPa for 3 hours. The *infra-red absorption spectrum* of the residue, Appendix II A, is concordant with the spectrum of noradrenaline base prepared by the same method from a suitable quantity of *noradrenaline acid tartrate EPCRS*.
B. The *light absorption*, Appendix II B, in the range 250 to 350 nm of a 0.005% w/v solution in 0.01M *hydrochloric acid* exhibits a maximum only at 279 nm. The A(1%, 1 cm) at 279 nm is 79 to 85.
C. The *specific optical rotation*, determined in a 2.0% w/v solution of the dried precipitate obtained in test A in 0.5M *hydrochloric acid*, is −44° to −48°, Appendix V F.
D. To 1 ml of a 0.1% w/v solution add 10 ml of *phthalate buffer pH 3.6* and 1 ml of 0.05M *iodine*. Allow to stand for 5 minutes and add 2 ml of 0.1M *sodium thiosulphate*. A faint red colour is produced.
E. To 1 ml of a 0.1% w/v solution add 1 ml of a 1.0% v/v solution of *2,5-diethoxytetrahydrofuran* in *glacial acetic acid*. Heat at 80° for 2 minutes, cool in ice and add 3 ml of a 2.0% w/v solution of *4-dimethylaminobenzaldehyde* in a mixture of 1 volume of *hydrochloric acid* and 19 volumes of *glacial acetic acid*. Mix and allow to stand for 2 minutes. An intense pink colour is produced.
F. 0.2 ml of the filtrate obtained in test A yields *reaction B* characteristic of tartrates, Appendix VI.

Clarity and colour of solution A 2.0% w/v solution is *clear*, Appendix IV A, and not more intensely coloured than *reference solution BY₅*, Appendix IV B, Method I.

Adrenaline Carry out the method for *thin-layer chromatography*, Appendix III A, using *silica gel G* as the coating substance and a mixture of 100 volumes of *acetone*, 100 volumes of *dichloromethane* and 1 volume of *anhydrous formic acid* as the mobile phase. Apply separately to the chromatoplate, as bands 20 mm × 2 mm, 6 µl of each of solutions (1), (2) and (3) and 12 µl of solution (4). Solutions (1), (2) and (3) are solutions in *water* prepared immediately before use containing (1) 2.5% w/v of the substance being examined, (2) 0.125% w/v of *adrenaline acid tartrate EPCRS* and (3) 0.025% w/v of *adrenaline acid tartrate EPCRS*. Solution (4) is a mixture of equal volumes of solutions (1) and (3). Allow to dry and spray the bands with a saturated solution of *sodium hydrogen carbonate*. Allow the plate to dry in air, spray the bands twice with *acetic anhydride*, drying between the two sprayings, and heat the plate at 50° for 90 minutes. After removal of the plate, allow it to dry in air and spray with a freshly prepared mixture of 8 volumes of *methanol*, 2 volumes of *ethylenediamine* and 2 volumes of a 0.5% w/v solution of *potassium hexacyano-ferrate(III)*. Dry the plate at 60° for 10 minutes and examine under *ultra-violet light (254 nm and 365 nm)*. In the chromatogram obtained with solution (1) any band with a higher Rf value than the principal band is not more intense than the corresponding band in the chromatogram obtained with solution (3). The test is not valid unless the chromatogram obtained with solution (4) shows a clearly separated band corresponding to the most intense band in the chromatogram obtained with solution (2) at a higher Rf value than the most intense band.

Phenones Dissolve 40 mg in sufficient 0.01M *hydrochloric acid* to produce 20 ml. The *absorbance* of the resulting solution at 310 nm is not more than 0.20, Appendix II B.

Sulphated ash Not more than 0.1%, Appendix IX A, Method II. Use 0.5 g.

Water 4.5 to 5.8% w/w, Appendix IX C. Use 0.5 g.

Assay Dissolve 0.3 g in *anhydrous glacial acetic acid*, warming if necessary, and carry out Method I for *non-aqueous titration*, Appendix VIII A, using *crystal violet solution* as indicator, until a bluish-green colour is obtained. Each ml of 0.1M *perchloric acid VS* is equivalent to 0.03193 g of $C_8H_{11}NO_3,C_4H_6O_6$.

Storage Noradrenaline Acid Tartrate should be kept in an airtight container or preferably in a sealed tube under vacuum or under an inert gas and protected from light. It darkens in colour on exposure to air and light.

Preparation
Noradrenaline Injection

Action and use Beta-adrenoceptor agonist.

The title of the monograph in the European Pharmacopœia is Noradrenaline Tartrate. In some countries the material described in this monograph may be known as Levarterenol Acid Tartrate.

Norethisterone ☆

$C_{20}H_{26}O_2$ 298.4   68-22-4

Norethisterone is 17β-hydroxy-19-nor-17α-pregn-4-en-20-yn-3-one. It contains not less than 98.0 per cent and not more than 102.0 per cent of $C_{20}H_{26}O_2$, calculated with reference to the dried substance.

Characteristics A white or yellowish-white, crystalline powder. It melts at about 206°, with decomposition.

Solubility Practically insoluble in *water*; slightly soluble in *ethanol (96%)*; soluble in 30 parts of *chloroform*.

Identification *Test A may be omitted if tests B, C, D and E are carried out. Tests C and D may be omitted if tests A, B and E are carried out.*

A. The *infra-red absorption spectrum*, Appendix II A, is concordant with the spectrum of *norethisterone EPCRS*. If the spectra obtained are not concordant dissolve the substances in *chloroform IR*, evaporate to dryness on a water-bath and prepare new spectra of the residues.

B. Complies with the test for *identification of steroids*, Appendix III A, using *impregnating solvent I* and *mobile phase G* and applying separately to the chromatoplate 2 µl of each of two solutions in *chloroform* containing (1) 0.1% w/v of the substance being examined and (2) 0.1% w/v of *norethisterone EPCRS*. The principal spot in the chromatogram obtained with solution (1) is similar in position, colour, fluorescence and size to that in the chromatogram obtained with solution (2).

C. Dissolve 2 mg in 2 ml of *ethanol (96%)*, add 1 ml of *ammoniacal silver nitrate solution* and heat on a water-bath. The solution becomes turbid and a white precipitate is produced which becomes grey on heating. A silver mirror is deposited on the walls of the tube.

D. Dissolve 2 mg in a cooled mixture of 2 ml of *absolute ethanol* and 2 ml of *sulphuric acid* and heat to 70°. The resulting solution appears bluish-violet when examined under transmitted light and red in reflected light. The solution exhibits a bright red fluorescence when examined under ultra-violet light (365 nm).

E. Dissolve 2 mg in 2 ml of *ethanol (96%)* and add 1 ml of a 1% w/v solution of *butylated hydroxytoluene* in *ethanol (96%)* and 2 ml of *1M sodium hydroxide*. Heat at 80° for 30 minutes and cool. A yellowish-pink colour is produced.

Clarity and colour of solution A 2.0% w/v solution in *1,4-dioxan* is clear, Appendix IV A, and not more intensely coloured than *reference solution Y_6*, Appendix IV B, Method II.

Light absorption Measure the *absorbance* of a 0.001% w/v solution in *ethanol (96%)* at the maximum at 240 nm, Appendix II B. The A(1%, 1 cm) at the maximum at 240 nm is 550 to 590.

Specific optical rotation In a 1% w/v solution in *1,4-dioxan*, −33° to −37°, Appendix V F.

Related substances Carry out the method for *thin-layer chromatography*, Appendix III A, using as the coating substance a suitable silica gel containing a fluorescent indicator with an optimal intensity at 254 nm (Merck silica gel 60 F254 is suitable) and a mixture of 90 volumes of *chloroform* and 10 volumes of *acetone* as the mobile phase. Apply separately to the chromatoplate 10 µl as two 5-µl applications of each of the following solutions in the mobile phase. Solutions (1) and (2) contain 0.5% w/v and 0.0025% w/v respectively of the substance being examined. Solution (3) contains 0.025% w/v each of the substance being examined and *ethisterone EPCRS*. After removal of the plate, allow it to dry in air, spray with *ethanolic sulphuric acid (20%)*, heat at 100° to 105° for 5 minutes and examine under *ultra-violet light (365 nm)*. Any *secondary spot* in the chromatogram obtained with solution (1) is not more intense than the spot in the chromatogram obtained with solution (2). The test is not valid unless the chromatogram obtained with solution (3) shows two clearly separated principal spots of equal intensities.

Loss on drying When dried at 105° for 3 hours, loses not more than 0.5% of its weight. Use 1 g.

Assay Dissolve 0.2 g in 40 ml of *tetrahydrofuran*, add 10 ml of a 10% w/v solution of *silver nitrate* and titrate with *0.1M sodium hydroxide VS*, using *bromocresol green solution* as indicator. Repeat the operation without the substance being examined. The difference between the titrations represents the amount of sodium hydroxide required. Each ml of *0.1M sodium hydroxide VS* is equivalent to 0.02984 g of $C_{20}H_{26}O_2$.

Storage Norethisterone should be kept in a well-closed container and protected from light.

Preparation

Norethisterone Tablets

Action and use Progestogen.

Norethisterone Acetate

$C_{22}H_{28}O_3$ 340.5   51-98-9

Norethisterone Acetate is 3-oxo-19-nor-17α-pregn-4-en-20-yn-17β-yl acetate. It contains not less than 97.0 per cent and not more than 102.0 per cent of $C_{22}H_{28}O_3$, calculated with reference to the dried substance.

Characteristics A white or creamy-white, crystalline powder; odourless or almost odourless.

Solubility Practically insoluble in *water*; soluble in 12.5 parts of *ethanol (96%)* and in 4 parts of *acetone*; soluble in *chloroform*; sparingly soluble in *ether*.

Identification A. The *infra-red absorption spectrum*, Appendix II A, is concordant with the *reference spectrum* of norethisterone acetate.

B. Complies with the test for the *identification of steroids*, Appendix III A, using *impregnating solvent II* and *mobile phase D*.

C. Yields the *reaction* characteristic of acetyl groups, Appendix VI.

D. *Melting point*, about 163°, Appendix V A.

Light absorption *Absorbance* of a 0.001% w/v solution in *ethanol (96%)* at the maximum at 240 nm, 0.49 to 0.52, Appendix II B.

Specific optical rotation In a 2% w/v solution in *1,4-dioxan*, −32° to −38°, Appendix V F.

Loss on drying When dried to constant weight at 105°, loses not more than 0.5% of its weight. Use 1 g.

Sulphated ash Not more than 0.1%, Appendix IX A.

Assay Dissolve 0.2 g in 40 ml of *tetrahydrofuran*, add 10 ml of a 10% w/v solution of *silver nitrate* and titrate with 0.1M *sodium hydroxide VS* determining the end-point potentiometrically. Repeat the operation without the substance being examined. The difference between the titrations represents the amount of sodium hydroxide required. Each ml of 0.1M *sodium hydroxide VS* is equivalent to 0.03405 g of $C_{22}H_{28}O_3$.

Storage Norethisterone Acetate should be protected from light.

Action and use Progestogen.

Nortriptyline Hydrochloride

$C_{19}H_{21}N,HCl$ 299.8   *894-71-3*

Nortriptyline Hydrochloride is 3-(10,11-dihydro-5*H*-dibenzo[*a,d*]cyclohept-5-ylidene)-propyl(methyl)amine hydrochloride. It contains not less than 98.0 per cent and not more than 101.0 per cent of $C_{19}H_{21}N,HCl$, calculated with reference to the dried substance.

Characteristics A white or almost white powder; odour, slight and characteristic.

Solubility Soluble in 50 parts of *water* and in 10 parts of *ethanol (96%)*; freely soluble in *chloroform*; practically insoluble in *ether*.

Identification A. Dissolve 0.1 g in 10 ml of *water*, make alkaline with 1M *sodium hydroxide*, extract with 5 ml of *chloroform* and evaporate to dryness using a current of nitrogen. The *infra-red absorption spectrum* of the oily residue, Appendix II A, is concordant with the *reference spectrum* of nortriptyline.

B. The *light absorption*, Appendix II B, in the range 230 to 350 nm of a 0.001% w/v solution in *methanol* exhibits a maximum only at 239 nm. The *absorbance* at 239 nm is about 0.96.

C. Dissolve 50 mg in 3 ml of warm *water*, cool and add 0.05 ml of a 2.5% w/v solution of *quinhydrone* in *methanol*. A red colour is produced slowly (distinction from amitriptyline).

D. Yields *reaction A* characteristic of chlorides, Appendix VI.

E. *Melting point*, about 218°, Appendix V A.

Dibenzosuberone Carry out the method for *thin-layer chromatography*, Appendix III A, using *silica gel G* as the coating substance and a mixture of 70 volumes of *toluene* and 30 volumes of *carbon tetrachloride* as the mobile phase but allowing the solvent front to ascend 12 cm above the line of application. Apply separately to the chromatoplate 5 μl of each of two solutions in *ethanol (96%)* containing (1) 2.0% w/v of the substance being examined and (2) 0.0010% w/v of *dibenzosuberone*. After removal of the plate, allow it to dry in air until the odour of solvent is no longer detectable, spray with *sulphuric acid* containing 4% v/v of *formaldehyde solution* and examine immediately under *ultra-violet light (365 nm)*. Any spot corresponding to dibenzosuberone in the chromatogram obtained with solution (1) is not more intense than the spot in the chromotogram obtained with solution (2).

Loss on drying When dried to constant weight at 105°, loses not more than 0.5% of its weight. Use 1 g.

Sulphated ash Not more than 0.1%, Appendix IX A.

Assay Carry out Method I for *non-aqueous titration*, Appendix VIII A, using 0.5 g and *1-naphtholbenzein solution* as indicator. Each ml of 0.1M *perchloric acid VS* is equivalent to 0.02998 g of $C_{19}H_{21}N,HCl$.

Storage Nortriptyline Hydrochloride should be protected from light.

Preparations
Nortriptyline Capsules
Nortriptyline Tablets

Action and use Antidepressant.

Noscapine ☆

$C_{22}H_{23}NO_7$ 413.4   *128-62-1*

Noscapine is (3*S*)-6,7-dimethoxy-3-[(5*R*)-5,6,7,8-tetrahydro-4-methoxy-6-methyl-1,3-dioxolo[4,5-*g*]isoquinolin-5-yl]phthalide. It contains not less than 98.5 per cent and not more than 100.5 per cent of $C_{22}H_{23}NO_7$, calculated with reference to the dried substance.

Characteristics Colourless crystals or a white, crystalline powder.

Solubility Practically insoluble in *water*; very slightly soluble in boiling *water*; slightly soluble in *ethanol (96%)* and in *ether*; soluble in *acetone* and in *chloroform*. It dissolves in strong acids; on dilution with water, the base may be precipitated.

Identification *Test A may be omitted if tests B, C and D are carried out. Tests B, C and D may be omitted if test A is carried out.*

A. The *infra-red absorption spectrum*, Appendix II A, is concordant with the spectrum of *noscapine EPCRS*.

B. The *light absorption*, Appendix II B, in the range 250 to 350 nm of a 0.005% w/v solution in *methanol* exhibits maxima at 291 nm and 310 nm. The ratio of the *absorbance* at the maximum at 310 nm to that at the maximum at 291 nm is 1.2 to 1.3.

C. Complies with the test for Specific optical rotation.

D. *Melting point*, 174° to 177°, Appendix V A, Method I.

Clarity and colour of solution A 2% w/v solution in *acetone* is *clear*, Appendix IV A, and not more intensely coloured than *reference solution Y₆*, Appendix IV B, Method II.

Specific optical rotation In a solution prepared by dissolving 0.5 g in sufficient 0.1M *hydrochloric acid* to produce 25 ml, +42° to +48°, Appendix V F.

Related substances Carry out the method for *thin-layer chromatography*, Appendix III A, using *silica gel G* as the coating substance and a mixture of 60 volumes of *acetone*, 60 volumes of *toluene*, 9 volumes of *ethanol (96%)* and 3 volumes of 13.5M *ammonia* as the mobile phase. Apply separately to the chromatoplate 10 µl of each of two solutions of the substance being examined in *acetone* containing (1) 2.5% w/v and (2) 0.0125% w/v. After removal of the plate, dry it in a current of air and spray with *dilute potassium iodobismuthate solution*. Any *secondary spot* in the chromatogram obtained with solution (1) is not more intense than the spot in the chromatogram obtained with solution (2).

Loss on drying When dried to constant weight at 100° to 105°, loses not more than 1.0% of its weight. Use 0.5 g.

Sulphated ash Not more than 0.1%, Appendix IX A, Method II. Use 1 g.

Assay Dissolve 0.35 g in 40 ml of *anhydrous glacial acetic acid*, warming gently, and carry out Method I for *non-aqueous titration*, Appendix VIII A, determining the end-point potentiometrically. Each ml of 0.1M *perchloric acid VS* is equivalent to 0.04134 g of $C_{22}H_{23}NO_7$.

Storage Noscapine should be kept in a well-closed container and protected from light.

Preparation

Noscapine Linctus

Action and use Cough suppressant.

Noscapine Hydrochloride ☆

$C_{22}H_{23}NO_7$,HCl,H₂O   467.9   *912-60-7*

Noscapine Hydrochloride is (3S)-6,7-dimeth-oxy-3-[(5R)-5,6,7,8-tetrahydro-4-methoxy-6-methyl-1,3-dioxolo[4,5-g]isoquinolin-5-yl]-phthalide hydrochloride monohydrate. It contains not less than 98.5 per cent and not more than 100.5 per cent of $C_{22}H_{23}NO_7$,HCl, calculated with reference to the dried substance.

Characteristics Colourless crystals or a white, crystalline powder; hygroscopic. It melts at about 200°, with decomposition.

Solubility Freely soluble in *water*, in *ethanol (96%)* and in *chloroform*; practically insoluble in *ether*. Aqueous solutions are faintly acidic; the base may be precipitated when the solutions are allowed to stand.

Identification *Test A may be omitted if tests B, C, D and E are carried out. Tests B, C and D may be omitted if tests A and E are carried out.*

A. Dissolve 40 mg in a mixture of 2 ml of *water* and 3 ml of *ethanol (96%)*, add 1 ml of 2M *ammonia* and heat until solution is complete. Allow to cool, if necessary scratch the walls of the tube with a glass rod, filter and reserve the filtrate for test E. The *infra-red absorption spectrum*, Appendix II A, of the precipitate, after washing with *water* and drying at 100° to 105°, is concordant with the spectrum of *noscapine EPCRS*.

B. The *light absorption*, Appendix II B, in the range 250 to 350 nm of a 0.005% w/v solution in *methanol* containing 0.05% v/v of 2M *ammonia* exhibits maxima at 291 nm and 310 nm. The ratio of the *absorbance* at the maximum at 310 nm to that at the maximum at 291 nm is 1.2 to 1.3.

C. Complies with the test for Specific optical rotation.

D. The *melting point* of the precipitate obtained in test A, after washing with *water* and drying at 100° to 105°, is 174° to 177°, Appendix V A, Method I.

E. The filtrate reserved in test A yields *reaction A* characteristic of chlorides, Appendix VI.

Acidity pH of a 2% w/v solution, not less than 3.0, Appendix V L.

Clarity and colour of solution Dissolve 0.5 g in *water*, add 0.3 ml of 0.1M *hydrochloric acid* and dilute to 25 ml with *water*. The solution is *clear*, Appendix IV A, and not more intensely coloured than *reference solution Y₆* or *BY₆*, Appendix IV B, Method II.

Specific optical rotation In a 2.0% w/v solution in 0.01M *hydrochloric acid*, +38.5° to +44.0°, Appendix V F.

Related substances Carry out the method for *thin-layer chromatography*, Appendix III A, using *silica gel G* as the coating substance and a mixture of 60 volumes of *acetone*, 60 volumes of *toluene*, 9 volumes of *ethanol (96%)* and 3 volumes of 13.5M *ammonia* as the mobile phase. Apply separately to the chromatoplate 10 µl of each of two solutions of the substance being examined in *ethanol (96%)* containing (1) 2.5% w/v and (2) 0.0125% w/v. After removal of the plate, dry it in a current of air and spray with *dilute potassium iodobismuthate solution*. Any *secondary spot* in the chromatogram obtained with solution (1) is not more intense than the spot in the chromatogram obtained with solution (2).

Loss on drying When dried to constant weight at 100° to 105°, loses 3.5 to 6.5% of its weight. Use 0.2 g.

Sulphated ash Not more than 0.1%, Appendix IX A, Method II. Use 1 g.

Assay Dissolve 0.4 g in 10 ml of *anhydrous glacial acetic acid*, with heating, cool, add 6 ml of *mercury(II) acetate solution* and carry out Method I for *non-aqueous titration*, Appendix VIII A, determining the end-point potentiometrically. Each ml of 0.1M *perchloric acid VS* is equivalent to 0.04499 g of $C_{22}H_{23}NO_7$,HCl.

Storage Noscapine Hydrochloride should be kept in a well-closed container and protected from light.

Action and use Cough suppressant.

Nutmeg Oil

Nutmeg Oil is obtained by distillation from the dried kernels of the seeds of *Myristica fragrans* Houtt.

Characteristics A clear, colourless, pale yellow or pale green liquid, visibly free from water; odour, that of nutmeg.

Optical rotation East Indian oil, +10° to +25°; West Indian oil, +25° to +45°, Appendix V F.

Refractive index East Indian oil, 1.475 to 1.488; West Indian oil, 1.472 to 1.477, Appendix V E.

Solubility in ethanol Soluble, at 20°, East Indian oil, in 3 volumes of *ethanol (90%)*; West Indian oil, in 4 volumes of *ethanol (90%)*, Appendix X M.

Weight per ml East Indian oil, 0.885 to 0.915 g; West Indian oil, 0.860 to 0.880 g, Appendix V G.

Residue on evaporation Not more than 3.0% when determined by the method for *residue on evaporation of volatile oils*, Appendix X M. Use 2 g and heat for 4 hours.

Storage Nutmeg Oil should be kept in a well-filled, well-closed container, protected from light and stored at a temperature not exceeding 25°.

Action and use Flavour.

Labelling The label states whether the contents are East Indian oil or West Indian oil.

Nystatin ☆

1400-61-9

Nystatin is an antifungal substance produced by the growth of certain strains of *Streptomyces noursei*. It contains mainly tetraenes, the principal component being nystatin A1. The potency is not less than 4400 Units per mg, calculated with reference to the dried substance.

Characteristics A yellow or slightly brown powder; hygroscopic.

Solubility Very slightly soluble in *water*; practically insoluble in *ethanol (96%)*, in *chloroform* and in *ether*; slightly soluble in *methanol*; freely soluble in *dimethylformamide*.

Identification A. The *light absorption* of the final solution obtained in the test for Light absorption, Appendix II B, exhibits four maxima, at 230, 291, 305 and 319 nm, and a shoulder at 280 nm. The ratios of the *absorbances* at the maxima at 291 nm and 319 nm to the *absorbance* at the maximum at 305 nm are 0.61 to 0.73 and 0.83 to 0.96, respectively. The ratio of the *absorbance* at the maximum at 230 nm to that at the shoulder at 280 nm is 0.83 to 1.25.

B. To 2 mg add 0.1 ml of *hydrochloric acid*. A brown colour is produced.

C. To 2 mg add 0.1 ml of *sulphuric acid*. A brown colour is produced which becomes violet on standing.

Light absorption Dissolve 0.1 g in a mixture of 5.00 ml of *glacial acetic acid* and 50 ml of *methanol*, add sufficient *methanol* to produce 100 ml and dilute 1 ml to 100 ml with *methanol*. The *absorbance* of the resulting solution, Appendix II B, measured within 30 minutes of preparation, at the maximum at 305 nm is not less than 0.60. Use in the reference cell a solution prepared in exactly the same manner but omitting the substance being examined.

Heavy metals 1.0 g complies with *limit test C for heavy metals*, Appendix VII (20 ppm). Use 2 ml of *lead standard solution (10 ppm Pb)* to prepare the standard.

Loss on drying When dried over *phosphorus pentoxide* at 60° at a pressure not exceeding 0.1 kPa for 3 hours, loses not more than 5.0% of its weight. Use 1 g.

Sulphated ash Not more than 3.5%, Appendix IX A, Method II. Use 1 g.

Assay Carry out the following procedure protected from light. Dissolve 75 mg in sufficient *dimethylformamide* to produce 50 ml, dilute 10 ml of the resulting solution to 200 ml with a solution containing 9.56% w/v of *potassium dihydrogen orthophosphate* and 11.5% v/v of 1M *potassium hydroxide* and carry out the *biological assay of antibiotics*, Appendix XIV A. The precision of the assay is such that the fiducial limits of error are not less than 95% and not more than 105% of the estimated potency.

Storage Nystatin should be kept in an airtight container, protected from light and stored at a temperature of 2° to 8°.

Labelling The label states (1) the number of Units per mg; (2) the date after which the material is not intended to be used; (3) the conditions under which it should be stored; (4) whether or not it is intended for oral administration.

Preparations
Nystatin Ointment
Nystatin Oral Suspension
Nystatin Pessaries
Nystatin Tablets

Action and use Antifungal.

Nystatin intended for oral administration complies with the following additional requirement.

Abnormal toxicity Complies with the *test for abnormal toxicity*, Appendix XIV L. Inject intraperitoneally a suspension containing not less than 600 Units in 0.5 ml of a 0.5% w/v solution of *acacia*.

Octaphonium Chloride

PhCH₂·ṄEt₂·CH₂·CH₂·O—⟨benzene ring⟩—CMe₂·CH₂·CMe₂·CH₃   Cl⁻

$C_{27}H_{42}ClNO,H_2O$ 450.1   *15687-40-8*

Octaphonium Chloride is benzyldiethyl{2-[4-(1,1,3,3-tetramethylbutyl)phenoxy]ethyl}-ammonium chloride monohydrate. It contains not less than 98.0 per cent and not more than 100.5 per cent of $C_{27}H_{42}ClNO,H_2O$.

Characteristics A white, crystalline powder; odourless or almost odourless.

Solubility Soluble in 5 parts of *water*; soluble in *ethanol (96%)* and in *chloroform*.

Identification A. The *light absorption*, Appendix II B, in the range 230 to 350 nm of a 0.046% w/v solution in *ethanol (96%)* exhibits four maxima, at 263, 269, 274 and 282 nm. The *absorbance* at 263 nm is about 1.14, at 269 nm, about 1.36, at 274 nm, about 1.34 and at 282 nm, about 1.14.

B. To 5 ml of a 1% w/v solution add 1.5 ml of 2M *nitric acid*. A white precipitate is produced which is soluble in *ethanol (96%)*.

C. To 5 ml of a 1% w/v solution add 1.5 ml of a 5% w/v solution of *mercury(II) chloride*. A white precipitate is produced which is soluble in *ethanol (96%)*.

D. Dissolve 0.25 g in 1 ml of *sulphuric acid*, add 0.1 g of *potassium nitrate*, heat on a water-bath for 5 minutes, cool, dilute to 10 ml with *water*, add 0.5 g of *zinc powder* and heat on a water-bath for 5 minutes. To 2 ml of the clear supernatant liquid add 0.5 ml of *sodium nitrite solution*, cool in ice and add to 3 ml of *2-naphthol solution*. An orange-red colour is produced.

E. Yields *reaction A* characteristic of chlorides, Appendix VI.

Acidity pH of a 1% w/v solution, 5.0 to 6.0, Appendix V L.

Non-quaternised amines Carry out the Assay using a further 25 ml of the original solution and 10 ml of 0.1M *hydrochloric acid* in place of the sodium hydroxide. The difference between the volume of 0.05M *potassium iodate VS* required in this titration and that required in the Assay titration is not more than 0.5 ml for each g of substance taken.

Sulphated ash Not more than 0.1%, Appendix IX A.

Water 3.5 to 4.5%, Appendix IX C. Use 0.5 g.

Assay Dissolve 2 g in sufficient *water* to produce 100 ml. Transfer 25 ml to a separating funnel and add 25 ml of *chloroform*, 10 ml of 0.1M *sodium hydroxide* and 10.0 ml of a freshly prepared 5.0% w/v solution of *potassium iodide*. Shake well, allow to separate and discard the chloroform layer. Wash the aqueous layer with three 10-ml quantities of *chloroform* and discard the washings. Add 40 ml of *hydrochloric acid*, allow to cool and titrate with 0.05M *potassium iodate VS* until the deep brown colour is almost discharged. Add 2 ml of *chloroform* and continue the titration, shaking vigorously, until the chloroform layer no longer changes colour. Carry out a blank titration on a mixture of 10.0 ml of the freshly prepared potassium iodide solution, 20 ml of *water* and 40 ml of *hydrochloric acid*. The difference between the titrations represents the amount of potassium iodate required. Each ml of 0.05M *potassium iodate VS* is equivalent to 0.04501 g of $C_{27}H_{42}ClNO,H_2O$.

Action and use Antiseptic; detergent.

In some countries the material described in this monograph may be known as Octafonium Chloride.

Octyl Gallate

HO
HO—⬡—CO·O(CH₂)₇·CH₃
HO

$C_{15}H_{22}O_5$ 282.3   *1034-01-1*

Octyl Gallate is octyl 3,4,5-trihydroxybenzoate.

Characteristics A white or creamy-white powder; odourless or almost odourless.

Solubility Practically insoluble in *water*; soluble in 2.5 parts of *ethanol (96%)*, in 1 part of *acetone*, in 0.7 part of *methanol*, in 7 parts of *propane-1,2-diol*, in 30 parts of *chloroform*, in 3 parts of *ether* and in 33 parts of *arachis oil*.

Identification A. The *light absorption*, Appendix II B, in the range 230 to 350 nm of a 0.002% w/v solution in *methanol* exhibits a maximum only at 275 nm. The *absorbance* at 275 nm is about 0.75.

B. Carry out the method for *gas chromatography*, Appendix III B, using a solution prepared in the following manner. Boil 0.5 g with 50 ml of 5M *sodium hydroxide* under a reflux condenser for 10 minutes, cool and extract with 50 ml of *ether*.

The chromatographic procedure may be carried out using a glass column (1.5 m × 4 mm) packed with *acid-washed, silanised diatomaceous support* (80 to 100 mesh) coated with 10% w/w of free fatty acid phase (Supelco FFAP is suitable) and maintained at 180°.

The principal peak in the chromatogram has the same retention time as *octan-1-ol*, examined under the same conditions.

C. Dissolve 5 mg in a mixture of 25 ml of *acetone* and 25 ml of *water* and add 0.5 ml of *iron(III) chloride solution*. A purplish-black colour is produced which rapidly becomes bluish-black.

Melting point 100° to 102°, Appendix V A.

Acidity Dissolve 0.4 g in 50 ml of *acetone*, add 50 ml of *carbon dioxide-free water* and titrate with 0.1M *sodium hydroxide VS*, using *bromocresol green solution* as indicator, to the blue colour indicative of pH 5.0. Repeat the operation without the substance being examined. The difference between the titrations does not exceed 0.1 ml.

Chloride Shake 0.50 g with 100 ml of *water* at 60° for 10 minutes, cool and filter. 15 ml of the filtrate complies with the *limit test for chlorides*, Appendix VII (0.07%).

Sulphate Shake 0.25 g with 30 ml of *water* at 60° for 10 minutes, cool and filter. 15 ml of the filtrate complies with the *limit test for sulphates*, Appendix VII (0.12%).

Loss on drying When dried to constant weight at 70°, loses not more than 0.5% of its weight. Use 1 g.

Sulphated ash Not more than 0.1%, Appendix IX A.

Storage Octyl Gallate should be kept in a well-closed container and protected from light. Contact with metals should be avoided.

Action and use Antioxidant.

Oestradiol Benzoate ☆

$C_{25}H_{28}O_3$ 376.5   *50-50-0*

Oestradiol Benzoate is estra-1,3,5(10)-triene-3,17β-diol 3-benzoate. It contains not less than 97.0 per cent and not more than 103.0 per cent of $C_{25}H_{28}O_3$, calculated with reference to the dried substance.

Characteristics Colourless crystals or a white or almost white, crystalline powder.

Solubility Practically insoluble in *water*; slightly soluble in *ethanol (96%)* and in fixed oils; soluble in 50 parts of *acetone*.

Identification *Test A may be omitted if tests B, C and D are carried out. Tests C and D may be omitted if tests A and B are carried out.*

A. The *infra-red absorption spectrum*, Appendix II A, is concordant with the spectrum of *estradiol benzoate*

EPCRS. If the spectra are not concordant, prepare new spectra using 5% w/v solutions in *chloroform IR*.

B. In the test for Related substances, the principal spot in the chromatogram obtained with solution (2) corresponds to that in the chromatogram obtained with solution (4) when examined in daylight and under *ultra-violet light (365 nm)*.

C. To 1 mg add 0.5 ml of a 5% w/v solution of *ammonium molybdate* in *sulphuric acid*; a yellowish-green colour is produced which exhibits an intense green fluorescence when examined under ultra-violet light (365 nm). Add 1 ml of *sulphuric acid* followed by 9 ml of *water*; the solution becomes pink with a yellowish fluorescence.

D. *Melting point*, 191° to 198°, Appendix V A, Method I.

Specific optical rotation In a 1% w/v solution in *1,4-dioxan*, +57° to +63°, Appendix V F.

Related substances Carry out the method for *thin-layer chromatography*, Appendix III A, using *silica gel G* as the coating substance and a mixture of 90 volumes of *toluene* and 10 volumes of *ethanol (96%)* as the mobile phase. Apply separately to the chromatoplate 5 µl of each of the following solutions in a mixture of 9 volumes of *chloroform* and 1 volume of *methanol*. Solutions (1), (2) and (3) contain 2.0% w/v, 0.1% w/v and 0.020% w/v respectively of the substance being examined. Solution (4) contains 0.1% w/v of *estradiol benzoate EPCRS*. After removal of the plate, allow it to dry in air until the odour of the solvent is no longer detectable, heat at 110° for 10 minutes, spray with *ethanolic sulphuric acid (20%)*, heat again at 110° for 10 minutes and examine under *ultra-violet light (365 nm)*. Any *secondary spot* in the chromatogram obtained with solution (1) is not more intense than the spot in the chromatogram obtained with solution (3).

Loss on drying When dried at 100° to 105° for 3 hours, loses not more than 0.5% of its weight. Use 0.5 g.

Sulphated ash Not more than 0.2%, Appendix IX A. Use 0.5 g.

Assay Dissolve 25 mg in sufficient *ethanol (96%)* to produce 250 ml. Dilute 10 ml to 100 ml with *ethanol (96%)* and measure the *absorbance* of the resulting solution at the maximum at 231 nm, Appendix II B. Calculate the content of $C_{25}H_{28}O_3$ taking 500 as the value of A(1%, 1 cm) at the maximum at 231 nm.

Storage Oestradiol Benzoate should be kept in a well-closed container and protected from light.

Preparation
Oestradiol Injection

Action and use Oestrogen.

In some countries the material described in this monograph may be known as Estradiol Benzoate.

Oleic Acid

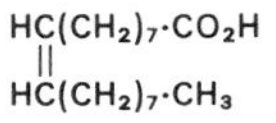

HC(CH₂)₇·CO₂H
‖
HC(CH₂)₇·CH₃

$C_{18}H_{34}O_2$ 282.5   *112-80-1*

Oleic Acid may be obtained by the hydrolysis of fats or fixed oils and separation of the liquid acids by expression or other suitable means. It consists chiefly of $C_{17}H_{33}CO_2H$.

Characteristics A yellowish to pale brown, oily liquid; odour, characteristic.

Solubility Practically insoluble in *water*; very soluble in *ethanol (96%)*, in *chloroform*, in *ether* and in *petroleum spirit (boiling range, 40° to 60°)*.

Acid value 195 to 202, Appendix X B.

Iodine value 85 to 92 (*iodine monochloride method*), Appendix X E.

Weight per ml 0.889 to 0.895 g, Appendix V G.

Mineral acids Shake 5 ml with 5 ml of *water*, allow the liquids to separate and filter through paper moistened with *water*. The filtrate is not acidic to *methyl orange solution*.

Neutral fats and mineral oils Boil 1 ml with 5 ml of 0.5M *sodium carbonate* and 25 ml of *water* in a large flask. The solution, while hot, is clear or at most opalescent.

Congealing point Dry about 10 ml by heating to 110° with frequent stirring, transfer to a test-tube about 20 mm in diameter, cool and when at 15° immerse the tube in a suitable water-bath so that the cooling takes place at the rate of 2° per minute. Stir the sample with a thermometer; it does not become cloudy until the temperature has fallen to 10°. On further cooling it congeals to a white solid or semi-solid mass at about 4°.

Sulphated ash Not more than 0.1% w/w, Appendix IX A.

Storage Oleic Acid should be kept in a well-filled, well-closed container and protected from light. On exposure to air it darkens in colour and the odour becomes more pronounced.

Olive Oil ☆

Olive Oil is the fixed oil obtained by cold expression or other suitable mechanical means from the ripe drupes of *Olea europaea* L.

Characteristics A clear, yellow or greenish-yellow, transparent liquid; odour and taste, characteristic. When cooled it begins to become cloudy at 10° and becomes a soft mass at about 0°.

Solubility Practically insoluble in *ethanol (96%)*; miscible with *chloroform*, with *ether* and with petroleum spirit.

Identification Carry out the test for *identification of fixed oils by thin-layer chromatography*, Appendix X N. The chromatogram obtained from the oil being examined is concordant with the *typical chromatogram* for olive oil. For certain types of olive oil the difference in the sizes of spots E and F is less pronounced than in the figure.

Acid value Not more than 2.0, Appendix X B. Use 5 g dissolved in 50 ml of the prescribed mixture of solvents.

Light absorption The *absorbance* of a 1% w/v solution in *cyclohexane* at the maximum at 270 nm is not more than 0.20, Appendix II B. The ratio of the *absorbance* at 232 nm to that at 270 nm is more than 8.

Peroxide value Not more than 15, Appendix X F.

Relative density 0.910 to 0.916, Appendix V G.

Unsaponifiable matter Not more than 1.5% w/w when determined by the following method. To 5 g of the oil in a 150-ml flask add 50 ml of 2M *ethanolic potassium hydroxide* and heat under a reflux condenser on a water-bath for 1 hour, shaking frequently. Add 50 ml of *water* through the condenser, shake, allow to cool and transfer the contents of the flask to a separating funnel, rinsing the flask with 50 ml of *petroleum spirit (boiling range, 40° to 60°)*

in portions and adding the rinsings to the separating funnel. Shake vigorously for 1 minute, allow to separate and transfer the aqueous layer to a second separating funnel. If an emulsion forms add small quantities of *ethanol (96%)* or of a concentrated solution of *potassium hydroxide*. Extract the aqueous layer with two 50-ml quantities of *petroleum spirit (boiling range, 40° to 60°)* and combine the organic layers in a third separating funnel. Wash with three 50-ml quantities of *ethanol (50%)*, transfer the petroleum spirit layer to a weighed 250-ml flask, rinse the separating funnel with small quantities of *petroleum spirit (boiling range, 40° to 60°)* and add the rinsings to the flask. Evaporate the solvent on a water-bath, dry at 100° to 105° for 15 minutes with the flask in a horizontal position, allow to cool and weigh. Repeat the drying for successive 15-minute periods until the loss in weight between two successive weighings does not exceed 0.1%. Dissolve the residue in 20 ml of *ethanol (96%)* previously neutralised to 0.1 ml of *bromophenol blue solution* and, if necessary, titrate with 0.1M *hydrochloric acid VS*. Calculate the percentage content of unsaponifiable matter from the expression $100(a - 0.032b)/w$ where a is the weight, in g, of the residue, b is the volume, in ml, of 0.1M hydrochloric acid required and w is the weight, in g, of oil taken. The test is not valid if $0.032b$ is greater than 5% of a and must be repeated.

Foreign fixed oils Carry out the test for *foreign oils by gas chromatography*, Appendix X N. The fatty-acid fraction of the oil has the following composition.

Saturated fatty acids of chain length less than C_{16} Not more than 0.1%.

Palmitic acid 7.5 to 20.0%.

Palmitoleic acid (equivalent chain length on polyethylene glycol adipate 16.3) Not more than 3.5%.

Stearic acid 0.5 to 3.5%.

Oleic acid (equivalent chain length on polyethylene glycol adipate 18.3) 56.0 to 85.0%.

Linoleic acid (equivalent chain length on polyethylene glycol adipate 18.9) 3.5 to 20.0%.

Linolenic acid (equivalent chain length on polyethylene glycol adipate 19.7) Not more than 1.5%.

Arachidic acid Not more than 0.5%.

Gadoleic acid (equivalent chain length on polyethylene glycol adipate 20.3) Not more than 0.2%.

Behenic acid Not more than 0.2%.

Erucic acid (equivalent chain length on polyethylene glycol adipate 22.3) Not more than 0.1%.

Sterols *Separation of the sterol fraction* Carry out the method for *thin-layer chromatography*, Appendix III A, using a 0.5-mm layer of *silica gel G* to coat the chromatoplate and a mixture of 85 volumes of *heptane* and 15 volumes of *acetone* as the mobile phase, but allowing the solvent front to ascend 18 cm above the line of application. Use three plates, each plate being divided into two equal parts. To one half of each plate apply separately, as a band 10 mm × 3 mm, 5 µl of solution (4) and, as a band 40 mm × 3 mm, 0.1 ml of solution (1) or solution (2) or solution (3) (chromatograms A). To the other half of each plate apply, as a band 40 mm × 3 mm, 0.1 ml of solution (1) or solution (2) or solution (3) to correspond with the first half of the plate (chromatograms B). Solutions (1), (2) and (3) are solutions in *chloroform* containing 5% w/v of the unsaponifiable matter, prepared as described in the test for Unsaponifiable matter but omitting the final titration, of

(1) the oil being examined, (2) *rapeseed oil* and (3) *sunflower oil*. Solution (4) is a 5% w/v solution of *cholesterol* in *chloroform*. After removal of the plates, dry them in a current of nitrogen, place a sheet of glass over each of the chromatograms B and spray the plates with a 5% w/v solution of *potassium permanganate*. The chromatogram obtained with solution (4) shows a band due to cholesterol and the chromatograms A obtained with solutions (1), (2) and (3) each show a band with a similar Rf value due to sterols. From each of the chromatograms B remove an area of the coating corresponding to the area occupied by the sterol band in the appropriate chromatogram A and place into separate 50-ml flasks. To each flask add 15 ml of hot *chloroform*, shake and filter through a sintered-glass filter (BS porosity No. 3); wash each filter with three 15-ml quantities of *chloroform*, evaporate the filtrate and washings to dryness in a current of nitrogen and determine the weight of the residue.

Determination of the sterols Carry out the following operations protected from humidity and prepare the solutions immediately before use. Carry out the method for *gas chromatography*, Appendix III B, using the following solutions in a freshly prepared mixture of 9 volumes of *anhydrous pyridine*, 3 volumes of *hexamethyldisilazane* and 1 volume of *trimethylchlorosilane*. For solution (1) add 20 µl of the solvent mixture per mg to the sterols separated from the oil being examined, allow to stand in a desiccator over *phosphorus pentoxide* for 30 minutes, centrifuge and use the supernatant liquid. For solution (2) add 20 µl of the solvent mixture per mg to a mixture of 1 part of cholesterol and 9 parts of the sterols separated from rapeseed oil, allow to stand in a desiccator over *phosphorus pentoxide* for 30 minutes, centrifuge and use the supernatant liquid. For solution (3) add 20 µl of the solvent mixture per mg to the sterols separated from sunflower oil, allow to stand in a desiccator over *phosphorus pentoxide* for 30 minutes, centrifuge and use the supernatant liquid.

The chromatographic procedure may be carried out using a glass column (1 to 2 m × 3 to 4 mm) packed with *diatomaceous support* coated with 2 to 4% w/w of methyl silicone gum (SE-30 is suitable), maintaining the column at 275° and the injection port and the detector at 285°.

The chromatogram obtained with solution (2) shows four major peaks corresponding to cholesterol, brassicasterol, campesterol and β-sitosterol at retention times relative to cholesterol of about 1.0, 1.1, 1.3 and 1.6 respectively; other peaks may also be present. The chromatogram obtained with solution (3) shows four major peaks corresponding to campesterol, stigmasterol, β-sitosterol and Δ^7-stigmasterol, at retention times relative to cholesterol of about 1.3, 1.4, 1.6 and 1.8 respectively; other peaks may also be present. In the chromatogram obtained with solution (1) identify any peaks corresponding to brassicasterol, β-sitosterol, cholesterol, Δ^7-stigmasterol, campesterol and stigmasterol and calculate the percentage content of each of the last-named five components in the sterol fraction of the oil being examined using the expression $100A/S$ where A is the area of the peak due to the component being determined and S is the sum of the areas of the peaks corresponding to the six named sterols.

The sterol fraction of the oil contains more than 93% of β-sitosterol, less than 0.5% of cholesterol, less than 0.5% of Δ^7-stigmasterol and less than 4% of campesterol. The content of Δ^7-stigmasterol is less than the content of campesterol. Any other sterols present at relative retention times identical with those of β-sitosterol and Δ⁷-stigmasterol are to be calculated as β-sitosterol and Δ⁷-stigmasterol respectively.

Sesame oil Shake 10 ml for about 1 minute with a mixture of 0.5 ml of a 0.35% v/v solution of *furfuraldehyde* in *acetic anhydride* and 4.5 ml of *acetic anhydride* in a cylinder closed with a ground-glass stopper, filter through paper impregnated with *acetic anhydride* and add 0.2 ml of *sulphuric acid* to the filtrate. No bluish-green colour is produced.

Storage Olive Oil should be kept in a well-filled, well-closed container and protected from light. Olive Oil intended for use in the manufacture of a parenteral dosage form should be kept in a glass container.

Labelling When the addition of antioxidants is authorised, the name and quantity of the added antioxidant are stated on the label.

The label states if the contents are suitable for use in the manufacture of a parenteral dosage form.

Olive Oil intended for use in the manufacture of a parenteral dosage form complies with the requirements stated above with the following modifications and with the additional test for Water.

Acid value Not more than 0.5, Appendix X B.

Peroxide value Not more than 5.0, Appendix X F.

Water Not more than 0.1%, Appendix IX C. Use 10 g dissolved in a mixture of equal volumes of *chloroform* and *anhydrous methanol*.

Opium
Raw Opium

Opium is the latex obtained by incision from the unripe capsules of *Papaver somniferum* L., dried or partly dried by heat or spontaneous evaporation, and worked into somewhat irregularly-shaped masses. It is known in commerce as Indian opium. It contains not less than 9.5 per cent of morphine, calculated as anhydrous morphine, $C_{17}H_{19}NO_3$.

Characteristics Odour, strong and characteristic.

Macroscopical Usually occurs in roughly cubical to irregularly-shaped pieces or soft masses weighing about 900 g and wrapped in plastic material; internally dark brown, smooth and homogeneous.

Microscopical The following structures are usually to be found in the residue left after removing the amorphous latex by exhaustion with *water*: poppy capsule represented by occasional fragments of epidermis composed of small five- to six-sided cells with strongly thickened walls and sometimes with stellate lumina; stomata infrequent, *anomocytic*, 17 μm wide and 25 μm long or sometimes circular. Pollen grains occasional, sub-spherical, with 3 pores, 16 to 40 μm, usually 20 to 30 μm, in diameter.

Assay Triturate 8 g in a mortar with 10 ml of *water* until a perfectly uniform mixture is produced. Add a further 20 ml of *water* and 2 g of *calcium hydroxide* and mix very thoroughly. Transfer the mixture to a tared flask, rinsing the mortar with successive small quantities of *water*

sufficient to produce 90 g. Stopper the flask and allow to stand for 30 minutes, shaking occasionally. Filter and collect 52 ml of the filtrate, representing 5 g of the substance being examined. Transfer to a small conical flask, add 5 ml of *ethanol (90%)* and 25 ml of *ether*, stopper the flask, shake, add 2.0 g of *ammonium chloride*, shake for 5 minutes and allow to stand for 30 minutes, shaking occasionally, making the total time of shaking about 15 minutes. Allow to stand overnight. Decant the ether layer as completely as possible into a funnel fitted with a tightly packed plug of absorbent cotton, rinse the flask and its contents with a further 10 ml of *ether* and again decant through the filter. Wash the filter with 5 ml of *ether*, added slowly and in portions, and pour the aqueous liquid into the filter without attempting to remove all the crystals. When all the liquid has passed through, wash the flask and filter with *morphinated water* until the filtrate is free from chloride. Wash the crystals on the filter back into the flask, add 30 ml of 0.05M *sulphuric acid VS*, boil, cool and titrate the excess of acid with 0.1M *sodium hydroxide VS* using *methyl red solution* as indicator. Each ml of 0.05M *sulphuric acid VS* is equivalent to 0.02853 g of $C_{17}H_{19}NO_3$. To the amount indicated by the titration add 0.052 g to correct for loss of morphine due to its solubility.

Preparations
Prepared Opium
Opium Tincture

Action and use Narcotic analgesic.

When Opium is prescribed, Prepared Opium shall be dispensed.

Prepared Opium
Powdered Opium

Prepared Opium is Opium dried at a moderate temperature, reduced to a *fine* or *moderately fine powder* and adjusted by the addition of powdered Lactose suitably coloured with burnt sugar, or of powdered cocoa husk, to contain 9.5 to 10.5 per cent of morphine, calculated as anhydrous morphine, $C_{17}H_{19}NO_3$.

Characteristics A light brown powder consisting of yellowish-brown or brownish-red particles; odour, characteristic of opium.

Microscopical The residue left after exhaustion with *water* exhibits the structures described under Opium. If powdered cocoa husk, in the form of brown fragments, is present the following additional characteristics are to be seen. Spirally-thickened vessels about 10 to 20 μm wide, in groups of one to six, embedded in spongy parenchyma composed of thin-walled cells about 40 to 60 μm long and wide, with arm-like projections; projections from adjacent cells united to one another to enclose almost circular intercellular spaces. Stone-cells derived from a single sclerenchymatous layer, individual cells thick-walled, about 5 to 10 μm wide and 10 to 30 μm long, rectangular to polyhedral in shape. Mucilage as fragments staining in *ruthenium red solution*.

Assay Carry out the Assay described under Opium. Each ml of 0.05M *sulphuric acid VS* is equivalent to 0.02853 g of $C_{17}H_{19}NO_3$. To the amount indicated by the titration add 0.052 g to correct for loss of morphine due to its solubility.

Storage Prepared Opium should be kept in a well-closed container.

Action and use Narcotic analgesic.

Orange Oil

Orange Oil is obtained by mechanical means from the fresh peel of the sweet orange, *Citrus sinensis* (L.) Osbeck.

Characteristics A yellow to yellowish-brown liquid, visibly free from water; odour, that of orange.

Optical rotation +94° to +99°, Appendix V F. On distillation, the first 10% of the distillate has an optical rotation the same as, or only slightly lower than, the original oil.

Refractive index 1.472 to 1.476, Appendix V E.

Solubility in ethanol Soluble at 20°, in 7 parts of *ethanol (90%)*, Appendix X M. A bright solution is rarely obtained due to the presence of waxy non-volatile substances.

Weight per ml 0.842 to 0.848 g, Appendix V G.

Residue on evaporation 1.0 to 5.0% when determined by the method for *residue on evaporation of volatile oils*, Appendix X M. Use 2 g and heat for 4 hours.

Content of aldehydes Not less than 1.0% w/w, calculated as decanal, $C_{10}H_{20}O$. Carry out the method for the *determination of aldehydes*, Appendix X K, using 10 g, omitting the *toluene* and using a volume, not less than 7 ml, of *hydroxylamine solution in ethanol (60%)* that exceeds by 1 to 2 ml the volume of 0.5M *potassium hydroxide in ethanol (60%) VS* required. Each ml of 0.5M *potassium hydroxide in ethanol (60%) VS* is equivalent to 0.07876 g of $C_{10}H_{20}O$.

Storage Orange Oil should be kept in a well-filled, well-closed container, protected from light and stored at a temperature not exceeding 25°.

Action and use Flavour.

Terpeneless Orange Oil

Terpeneless Orange Oil may be prepared by concentrating Orange Oil under reduced pressure until most of the terpenes have been removed or by solvent partition.

Characteristics A clear, yellow or orange-yellow liquid, visibly free from water; odour and taste, those of orange.

Optical rotation Not more than +60°, Appendix V F.

Refractive index 1.461 to 1.473, Appendix V E.

Solubility in ethanol Soluble, at 20°, in 1 part of *ethanol (90%)*, Appendix X M.

Weight per ml 0.855 to 0.880 g, Appendix V G.

Content of aldehydes Not less than 18% w/w, calculated as decanal, $C_{10}H_{20}O$. Carry out the method for the *determination of aldehydes*, Appendix X K, using 1.5 g, omitting the *toluene* and using a volume, not less than 7 ml, of *hydroxylamine solution in ethanol (60%)* that exceeds by 1 to 2 ml the volume of 0.5M *potassium hydroxide in ethanol (60%) VS* required. Each ml of 0.5M *potassium hydroxide in ethanol (60%) VS* is equivalent to 0.07876 g of $C_{10}H_{20}O$.

Storage Terpeneless Orange Oil should be kept in a well-filled, well-closed container, protected from light and stored at a temperature not exceeding 25°.

Preparation
Compound Orange Spirit

Action and use Flavour.

Dried Bitter-Orange Peel

Dried Bitter-Orange Peel is the dried outer part of the pericarp of the ripe, or nearly ripe, fruit of *Citrus aurantium* L.

Characteristics Odour, aromatic; taste, aromatic and bitter.

Macroscopical In strips or pieces; outer surface dark orange-red and somewhat rough from the presence of numerous minute pits, each corresponding to an oil gland; inner surface with only a small remnant of white, spongy pericarp. Fracture, short.

Microscopical Epidermis of small polyhedral cells. Tissue subjacent to the epidermis parenchymatous, many of the cells containing prismatic crystals of calcium oxalate. Numerous large oil glands and small vascular strands embedded in the parenchyma.

Volatile oil Not less than 2.5% v/w, Appendix XI E. Use 20 g, crushed under *water*, and distil for 3 hours.

Preparations
Orange Peel Infusion
Orange Tincture

Orciprenaline Sulphate

$(C_{11}H_{17}NO_3)_2,H_2SO_4$ 520.6   5874-97-5

Orciprenaline Sulphate is 1-(3,5-dihydroxyphenyl)-2-isopropylaminoethanol sulphate containing variable amounts of water and methanol of crystallisation. It contains not less than 98.0 per cent and not more than 102.0 per cent of $(C_{11}H_{17}NO_3)_2,H_2SO_4$, calculated with reference to the anhydrous, methanol-free substance.

Characteristics A white, crystalline powder; odourless or almost odourless.

Solubility Soluble in 2 parts of *water* and in 1 part of *ethanol (96%)*; practically insoluble in *chloroform* and in *ether*.

Identification A. The *infra-red absorption spectrum*, Appendix II A, is concordant with the *reference spectrum* of orciprenaline sulphate.

B. The *light absorption*, Appendix II B, in the range 240 to 350 nm of a 0.015% w/v solution in 0.01M *hydrochloric acid* exhibits a broad maximum at 278 nm. The *absorbance* over the range 276 to 280 nm is about 1.0.

C. To 1 ml of a 1% w/v solution add 0.2 ml of a saturated solution of *mercury(II) acetate*. A yellow colour is produced.

D. Yields the *reactions* characteristic of sulphates, Appendix VI.

E. *Melting point*, about 205°, Appendix V A.

Acidity pH of a 10% w/v solution, 4.0 to 5.5, Appendix V L.

Phenones *Absorbance* of a 2% w/v solution in 0.01M *hydrochloric acid* at 328 nm, not more than 0.16, Appendix II B.

Heavy metals Dissolve 2.0 g in 10 ml of *water* containing 0.25 ml of 6M *acetic acid* and add 2 ml of *hydrogen sulphide solution*. No darkening occurs.

Iron The residue obtained in the test for Sulphated ash complies with the *limit test for iron*, Appendix VII (20 ppm). Use *iron standard solution (2 ppm Fe)* to prepare the standard.

Methanol Carry out the method for *gas chromatography*, Appendix III B, using three solutions in *water* containing (1) 0.50% v/v of *methanol* and 0.50% v/v of *ethanol (96%)* (internal standard), (2) 10% w/v of the substance being examined and (3) 10% w/v of the substance being examined and 0.50% v/v of the internal standard.

The chromatographic procedure may be carried out using a glass column (1.5 m × 4 mm) packed with porous polymer beads (80 to 100 mesh) (Porapak Q is suitable) and maintained at 140°.

Calculate the percentage w/w of *methanol* taking 0.792 g as its weight per ml at 20°. The sum of the content of methanol and the content of water determined below is not more than 6.0% w/w.

Sulphated ash Not more than 0.1%, Appendix IX A. Use 1.0 g.

Water Not more than 2.0% w/w, Appendix IX C. Use 1.2 g.

Assay Carry out Method I for *non-aqueous titration*, Appendix VIII A, using 0.75 g and *crystal violet solution* as indicator. Each ml of 0.1M *perchloric acid VS* is equivalent to 0.05206 g of $(C_{11}H_{17}NO_3)_2,H_2SO_4$.

Storage Orciprenaline Sulphate should be protected from light.

Preparations
Orciprenaline Injection
Orciprenaline Tablets

Action and use Beta-adrenoceptor agonist.

Orphenadrine Citrate

$C_{18}H_{23}NO,C_6H_8O_7$ 461.5   *4682-36-4*

Orphenadrine Citrate is dimethyl[2-(2-methyl-benzhydryloxy)ethyl]amine dihydrogen citrate. It contains not less than 98.5 per cent and not more than 101.0 per cent of $C_{18}H_{23}NO,C_6H_8O_7$, calculated with reference to the dried substance.

Characteristics A white or almost white, crystalline powder; odourless or almost odourless.

Solubility Soluble in 70 parts of *water*; slightly soluble in *ethanol (96%)*; practically insoluble in *chloroform* and in *ether*.

Identification A. The *light absorption*, Appendix II B, in the range 230 to 350 nm of a 0.06% w/v solution in *ethanol (96%)* exhibits three maxima, at 258, 264 and 271 nm. The *absorbance* at 258 nm is about 0.68, at 264 nm, about 0.72 and at 271 nm, about 0.47.

B. Dissolve 50 mg in 10 ml of *ethanol (50%)*, add 10 ml of *trinitrophenol solution* and allow to stand. The *melting point* of the precipitate, after recrystallisation from *ethanol (96%)*, is about 89° or about 107°, Appendix V A.

C. Dissolve 5 mg in 2 ml of *sulphuric acid*. An orange-red colour is produced.

D. To 1 g add 10 ml of *water* and 2 ml of 5M *sodium hydroxide*, shake with two 10-ml quantities of *chloroform* and discard the chloroform. Heat the aqueous solution to boiling with an excess of *mercury(II) sulphate solution*, filter if necessary and boil the resulting solution with 0.2 ml of *potassium permanganate solution*. The solution is decolorised and a white precipitate is produced.

Melting point 135° to 138°, Appendix V A.

Lead Not more than 10 ppm when determined by the following method. Heat 1.5 g with 7.5 ml of *nitric acid* in a long-necked flask until the first reaction has subsided, add 2.5 ml of *sulphuric acid* and continue heating until the solution is colourless, adding, dropwise, more *nitric acid* if necessary. Cool, add 10 ml of *water*, evaporate to low volume, cool and dilute to 25 ml with *water* (solution A). To 15 ml of the solution add 1 g of *citric acid*. Transfer the solution to a *Nessler cylinder* and make alkaline with 5M *ammonia*. In a second *Nessler cylinder* mix 5 ml of solution A and 1 g of *citric acid*, make alkaline with 5M *ammonia* and add 1 ml of *lead standard solution (10 ppm Pb)*. Treat the contents of each cylinder, respectively, in the following manner. Add 1 ml of *potassium cyanide solution PbT*; the solutions should not be more than faintly opalescent. If the colours of the solutions differ, equalise them by the addition of a few drops of a highly diluted solution of burnt sugar or other non-reactive substance. Dilute to 50 ml with *water*, add 0.1 ml of a filtered 10% w/v solution of *sodium sulphide* and mix thoroughly. Compare the colours of the two solutions by a suitable method, such as by light reflected from a white tile through the Nessler cylinders. The colour of the solution in the first cylinder is less intense than that of the solution in the second cylinder.

Quaternary ammonium salt Carry out the method for *thin-layer chromatography*, Appendix III A, using *silica gel G* as the coating substance and a mixture of 50 volumes of *propan-2-ol*, 30 volumes of *butyl acetate*, 15 volumes of *water* and 5 volumes of 13.5M *ammonia* as the mobile phase. Apply separately to the chromatoplate 5 µl of each of two solutions in *methanol* containing (1) 1.0% w/v of the substance being examined and (2) 0.0050% w/v of *ethyldimethyl[2-(2-methylbenzhydryloxy)ethyl]ammonium chloride BPCRS*. After removal of the plate, allow it to dry in air and spray with *dilute potassium iodobismuthate solution*. Any spot corresponding to ethyldimethyl[2-(2-methylbenzhydryloxy)ethyl]ammonium hydroxide in the chromatogram obtained with solution (1) is not more intense than the spot in the chromatogram obtained with solution (2).

Secondary amine Carry out the method for *thin-layer chromatography*, Appendix III A, using *silica gel GF254* as the coating substance and a mixture of 96 volumes of *butan-1-ol* and 4 volumes of 13.5M *ammonia* as the mobile phase. Apply separately to the chromatoplate 10 µl of each of two solutions in *methanol* containing (1) 4.0% w/v of the substance being examined and (2) 0.020% w/v of *methyl[2-(2-methylbenzhydryloxy)ethyl]amine hydrochloride BPCRS*. After removal of the plate, allow it to dry in air and examine under *ultra-violet light (254 nm)*. Spray the plate with *dilute potassium iodobismuthate solution* and examine again. Using both methods of visualisation any spot corresponding to methyl[2-(2-methylbenzhydryloxy)-ethyl]amine in the chromatogram obtained with solution (1) is not more intense than the spot in the chromatogram obtained with solution (2).

Loss on drying When dried to constant weight at 105°, loses not more than 0.5% of its weight. Use 1 g.

Sulphated ash Not more than 0.1%, Appendix IX A.

Assay Carry out Method I for *non-aqueous titration*, Appendix VIII A, using 1 g and *1-naphtholbenzein solution* as indicator. Each ml of 0.1M *perchloric acid VS* is equivalent to 0.04615 g of $C_{18}H_{23}NO,C_6H_8O_7$.

Storage Orphenadrine Citrate should be kept in a well-closed container and protected from light.

Action and use Skeletal muscle relaxant.

Orphenadrine Hydrochloride

$C_{18}H_{23}NO,HCl$ 305.9   *341-69-5*

Orphenadrine Hydrochloride is dimethyl[2-(2-methylbenzhydryloxy)ethyl]amine hydrochloride. It contains not less than 98.5 per cent and not more than 101.0 per cent of $C_{18}H_{23}NO$, HCl, calculated with reference to the dried substance.

Characteristics A white or almost white, crystalline powder; odourless or almost odourless.

Solubility Soluble in 1 part of *water*, in 1 part of *ethanol (96%)* and in 2 parts of *chloroform*; practically insoluble in *ether*.

Identification A. The *light absorption*, Appendix II B, in the range 230 to 350 nm of a 0.06% w/v solution in

ethanol (96%) exhibits three maxima, at 258, 264 and 271 nm. The *absorbance* at 258 nm is about 1.07, at 264 nm, about 1.13 and at 271 nm, about 0.73.

B. Dissolve 5 mg in 2 ml of *sulphuric acid*. An orange-red colour is produced.

C. Dissolve 50 mg in 10 ml of *ethanol (50%)*, add 10 ml of *trinitrophenol solution* and allow to stand. The *melting point* of the precipitate, after recrystallisation from *ethanol (96%)*, is about 89° or about 107°, Appendix V A.

D. Yields *reaction A* characteristic of chlorides, Appendix VI.

Melting point 159° to 162°, Appendix V A.

Lead Not more than 10 ppm when determined by the following method. Heat 1.5 g with 7.5 ml of *nitric acid* in a long-necked flask until the first reaction has subsided, add 2.5 ml of *sulphuric acid* and continue heating until the solution is colourless, adding, dropwise, more *nitric acid* if necessary. Cool, add 10 ml of *water*, evaporate to low volume, cool and dilute to 25 ml with *water* (solution A). To 15 ml of the solution add 1 g of *citric acid*. Transfer the solution to a *Nessler cylinder* and make alkaline with 5M *ammonia*. In a second *Nessler cylinder* mix 5 ml of solution A and 1 g of *citric acid*, make alkaline with 5M *ammonia* and add 1 ml of *lead standard solution (10 ppm Pb)*. Treat the contents of each cylinder, respectively, in the following manner. Add 1 ml of *potassium cyanide solution PbT*; the solutions should not be more than faintly opalescent. If the colours of the solutions differ, equalise them by the addition of a few drops of a highly diluted solution of burnt sugar or other non-reactive substance. Dilute to 50 ml with *water*, add 0.1 ml of a filtered 10% w/v solution of *sodium sulphide* and mix thoroughly. Compare the colours of the two solutions by a suitable method, such as by light reflected from a white tile through the Nessler cylinders. The colour of the solution in the first cylinder is not more intense than that of the solution in the second cylinder.

Quaternary ammonium salt Carry out the method for *thin-layer chromatography*, Appendix III A, using *silica gel G* as the coating substance and a mixture of 50 volumes of *propan-2-ol*, 30 volumes of *butyl acetate*, 15 volumes of *water* and 5 volumes of 13.5M *ammonia* as the mobile phase. Apply separately to the chromatoplate 5 µl of each of two solutions in *methanol* containing (1) 1.0% w/v of the substance being examined and (2) 0.0050% w/v of *ethyldimethyl[2-(2-methylbenzhydryloxy)ethyl]ammonium chloride BPCRS*. After removal of the plate, allow it to dry in air and spray with *dilute potassium iodobismuthate solution*. Any spot corresponding to ethyldimethyl[2-(2-methylbenzhydryloxy)ethyl]ammonium hydroxide in the chromatogram obtained with solution (1) is not more intense than the spot in the chromatogram obtained with solution (2).

Secondary amine Carry out the method for *thin-layer chromatography*, Appendix III A, using *silica gel GF254* as the coating substance and a mixture of 96 volumes of *butan-1-ol* and 4 volumes of 13.5M *ammonia* as the mobile phase. Apply separately to the chromatoplate 10 µl of each of two solutions in *methanol* containing (1) 4.0% w/v of the substance being examined and (2) 0.020% w/v of *methyl[2-(2-methylbenzhydryloxy)ethyl]amine hydrochloride BPCRS*. After removal of the plate, allow it to dry in air and examine under *ultra-violet light (254 nm)*. Spray the plate with *dilute potassium iodobismuthate solution* and examine again. Using both methods of visualisation any spot corresponding to methyl[2-(2-methylbenzhydryl-oxy)ethyl]amine in the chromatogram obtained with solution (1) is not more intense than the spot in the chromatogram obtained with solution (2).

Loss on drying When dried to constant weight at 105°, loses not more than 0.5% of its weight. Use 1 g.

Sulphated ash Not more than 0.1%, Appendix IX A.

Assay Carry out Method I for *non-aqueous titration*, Appendix VIII A, using 1 g, 20 ml of *mercury(II) acetate solution* and *1-naphtholbenzein solution* as indicator. Each ml of 0.1M *perchloric acid VS* is equivalent to 0.03059 g of $C_{18}H_{23}NO,HCl$.

Storage Orphenadrine Hydrochloride should be kept in a well-closed container and protected from light.

Preparation
Orphenadrine Hydrochloride Tablets

Action and use Used in treatment of Parkinson's disease.

Oxazepam

$C_{15}H_{11}ClN_2O_2$ 286.7   *604-75-1*

Oxazepam is 7-chloro-1,3-dihydro-3-hydroxy-5-phenyl-1,4-benzodiazepin-2-one. It contains not less than 98.5 per cent and not more than 101.0 per cent of $C_{15}H_{11}ClN_2O_2$, calculated with reference to the dried substance.

Characteristics A white or almost white, crystalline powder; odourless or almost odourless.

Solubility Practically insoluble in *water*; slightly soluble in *ethanol (96%)* and in *chloroform*.

Identification A. The *infra-red absorption spectrum*, Appendix II A, is concordant with the *reference spectrum* of oxazepam.
B. The *light absorption*, Appendix II B, in the range 210 to 350 nm of a 0.0008% w/v solution in *ethanol (96%)* exhibits two maxima, at 230 nm and 316 nm. The *absorbance* at 230 nm is about 1.0.

Related substances Carry out the method for *thin-layer chromatography*, Appendix III A, using a silica gel F254 precoated chromatoplate (Merck silica gel 60 F254 plates are suitable) and a mixture of 100 volumes of *chloroform* and 10 volumes of *methanol* as the mobile phase. Apply separately to the plate 20 μl of each of three solutions of the substance being examined in *acetone* containing (1) 0.50% w/v, (2) 0.0010% w/v and (3) 0.00050% w/v. After removal of the plate, allow it to dry in air and examine under *ultra-violet light (254 nm)*. Any *secondary spot* in the chromatogram obtained with solution (1) is not more intense than the spot in the chromatogram obtained with solution (2) and not more than one such spot is more intense than the spot in the chromatogram obtained with solution (3).

Loss on drying When dried to constant weight at 105° at a pressure not exceeding 0.7 kPa, loses not more than 0.5% of its weight. Use 1 g.

Sulphated ash Not more than 0.1%, Appendix IX A.

Assay Dissolve 0.5 g in a mixture of 10 ml of *anhydrous glacial acetic acid* and 90 ml of *acetic anhydride* and carry out Method I for *non-aqueous titration*, Appendix VIII A, determining the end-point potentiometrically. Each ml of 0.1M *perchloric acid VS* is equivalent to 0.02867 g of $C_{15}H_{11}ClN_2O_2$.

Storage Oxazepam should be kept in a well-closed container and protected from light.

Preparations
Oxazepam Capsules
Oxazepam Tablets

Action and use Anxiolytic.

Oxprenolol Hydrochloride

$C_{15}H_{23}NO_3,HCl$ 301.8   *6452-73-9*

Oxprenolol Hydrochloride is 1-(2-allyloxy-phenoxy)-3-isopropylaminopropan-2-ol hydrochloride. It contains not less than 98.5 per cent and not more than 101.0 per cent of $C_{15}H_{23}NO_3,HCl$, calculated with reference to the dried substance.

Characteristics A white to slightly cream, crystalline powder; odourless or almost odourless.

Solubility Soluble in less than 1 part of *water* and in 1.5 parts of *ethanol (96%)*; very slightly soluble in *ether*.

Identification A. Dissolve 0.1 g in 10 ml of *ethyl acetate* with the aid of heat, allow to cool in a stream of water, induce crystallisation by prolonged scratching with a glass rod, filter and dry the residue at 60° at a pressure not exceeding 0.7 kPa. The *infra-red absorption spectrum* of the residue, Appendix II A, is concordant with the *reference spectrum* of oxprenolol hydrochloride.
B. The *light absorption*, Appendix II B, in the range 230 to 350 nm of a 0.016% w/v solution in 0.01M *hydrochloric acid* exhibits a maximum only at 273 nm. The *absorbance* at 273 nm is about 1.2.
C. Dissolve 0.2 g in 10 ml of *water*, make alkaline with 1.25M *sodium hydroxide* and extract with two 5-ml quantities of *ether*. Wash the combined extracts with *water* until the washings are free from alkali, shake with *anhydrous sodium sulphate*, filter and evaporate the filtrate to dryness. The *melting point* of the residue is about 76°, Appendix V A.
D. Yields *reaction A* characteristic of chlorides, Appendix VI.

Acidity pH of a 5.0% w/v solution, 4.0 to 6.0, Appendix V L.

Colour of solution A 20.0% w/v solution is not more intensely coloured than *reference solution Y_5*, Appendix IV B, Method I.

Melting point 106° to 109°, Appendix V A.

Heavy metals 1.0 g complies with *limit test C for heavy metals*, Appendix VII (10 ppm). Use 1 ml of *lead standard solution (10 ppm Pb)* to prepare the standard.

Related substances Carry out the method for *thin-layer chromatography*, Appendix III A, using *silica gel HF254* as the coating substance and a mixture of 90 volumes of *chloroform* and 10 volumes of *methanol* as the mobile phase, but standing a beaker containing 13.5M *ammonia* in the tank and allowing the solvent front to ascend 10 cm above the line of application. Apply separately to the chromatoplate 5 μl of each of three solutions in *water* containing (1) 2.0% w/v of the substance being examined, (2) 0.010% w/v of *1-(3-allyl-2-hydroxyphenoxy)-3-isopropyl-aminopropan-2-ol hydrochloride BPCRS* and (3) 0.010% w/v of *1-(2-hydroxyphenoxy)-3-isopropylamino-propan-2-ol hydrochloride BPCRS*. After removal of the plate, dry it at 40° for 10 minutes, allow to cool and spray with a freshly prepared solution containing 0.5% w/v of *potassium hexacyanoferrate(III)* and 6.0% w/v of *iron(III) chloride hexahydrate*. Any *secondary spots* in the chromatogram obtained with solution (1) are not more intense than the proximate spots in the chromatograms obtained with solutions (2) and (3).

Loss on drying When dried to constant weight at 60° at a pressure not exceeding 0.7 kPa, loses not more than 0.5% of its weight. Use 1 g.

Sulphated ash Not more than 0.1%, Appendix IX A.

Assay Carry out Method I for *non-aqueous titration*, Appendix VIII A, using 0.4 g, 20 ml of *mercury(II) acetate solution* and *1-naphtholbenzein solution* as indicator. Each ml of 0.1M *perchloric acid VS* is equivalent to 0.03018 g of $C_{15}H_{23}NO_3,HCl$.

Preparation
Oxprenolol Tablets

Action and use Beta-adrenoceptor antagonist.

Oxygen ☆

O_2 32.00   *7782-44-7*

Oxygen contains not less than 99.0 per cent v/v of O_2.

Deliver the gas at a steady rate of 4 litres per hour for the following tests unless otherwise specified.

Characteristics A colourless gas; odourless; tasteless.

Solubility At 20° and at a pressure of 101.3 kPa, soluble in about 32 volumes of *water*.

Identification A. Causes a glowing splinter of wood to burst into flame.
B. Shake with *alkaline pyrogallol solution*. The gas being examined is absorbed and the solution becomes dark brown.

Acidity or alkalinity Use a hermetically closed, flat-bottomed, glass cylinder with dimensions such that 50 ml of liquid reaches a height of 12 to 14 cm, fitted with an outlet tube and with an inlet tube with an orifice 1 mm in internal diameter reaching to within 2 mm of the bottom of the cylinder.

For solution (1) pass 2.0 litres of the gas being examined through a mixture of 0.1 ml of 0.01M *hydro-chloric acid* and 50 ml of *carbon dioxide-free water*. For solution (2) use 50 ml of *carbon dioxide-free water*. For solution (3) add 0.2 ml of 0.01M *hydrochloric acid* to 50 ml of *carbon dioxide-free water*. To each solution add 0.1 ml of a 0.02% w/v solution of *methyl red* in *ethanol (70%)*.

The intensity of the colour of solution (1) is between those of solutions (2) and (3).

Carbon dioxide Use the apparatus described in the test for Acidity or alkalinity. Pass 1.0 litre through 50 ml of a clear 4.73% w/v solution of *barium hydroxide*. Any turbidity produced in the resulting solution is not more intense than that produced in a reference solution prepared by adding 1 ml of a 0.11% w/v solution of *sodium hydrogen carbonate* in *carbon dioxide-free water* to 50 ml of a 4.73% w/v solution of *barium hydroxide* (300 ppm v/v).

Carbon monoxide Carry out the *limit test for carbon monoxide in medicinal gases*, Appendix IX E, using 7.5 litres of the gas being examined and 7.5 litres of *argon* for the blank determination. The difference between the titrations is not more than 0.4 ml (5 ppm v/v).

Oxidising substances Use the apparatus described in the test for Acidity or alkalinity. Carry out the procedure protected from light. Pass 5.0 litres of the gas being examined through a mixture of 50 ml of freshly prepared *potassium iodide and starch solution* and 0.2 ml of *glacial acetic acid*. No change is observed when compared with a reference solution prepared at the same time and in the same manner but through which the gas has not been passed.

Assay Carry out Method I for the *assay of medicinal gases*, Appendix VIII J, using a freshly prepared mixture of 21 ml of a 56% w/v solution of *potassium hydroxide* and 130 ml of a 20% w/v solution of *sodium dithionite* as the absorbing solution.

Storage Oxygen should be kept under pressure in an approved metal cylinder. Valves and taps should not be lubricated with oil or grease.

Labelling The shoulder of the metal cylinder should be painted white and the remainder should be painted black. The cylinder should carry a label stating 'Oxygen'. In addition, 'Oxygen' or the symbol 'O₂' should be stencilled in paint on the shoulder of the cylinder.

Oxymetholone

$C_{21}H_{32}O_3$ 332.5   *434-07-1*

Oxymetholone is 17β-hydroxy-2-hydroxy-methylene-17α-methyl-5α-androstan-3-one. It contains not less than 97.0 per cent and not more than 103.0 per cent of $C_{21}H_{32}O_3$, calculated with reference to the dried substance.

Characteristics A white to creamy-white crystalline powder; odourless or almost odourless.

Solubility Practically insoluble in *water*; soluble in 50 parts of *ethanol (96%)* and in 9 parts of *chloroform*; slightly soluble in *ether*.

Identification A. The *infra-red absorption spectrum*, Appendix II A, is concordant with the *reference spectrum* of oxymetholone.

B. The *light absorption*, Appendix II B, in the range 230 to 350 nm of a 0.002% w/v solution in 0.01M *ethanolic sodium hydroxide* exhibits a maximum only at 315 nm. The *absorbance* at 315 nm is about 1.1.

C. The *light absorption*, Appendix II B, in the range 230 to 350 nm of a 0.003% w/v solution in 0.01M *ethanolic hydrochloric acid* exhibits a maximum only at 277 nm. The *absorbance* at 277 nm is about 1.0.

D. Complies with the test for *identification of steroids*, Appendix III A, using *impregnating solvent II* and *mobile phase D*.

Melting point 175° to 180°, Appendix V A.

Specific optical rotation In a 2% w/v solution in *1,4-dioxan*, +34° to +38°, Appendix V F.

Related substances Carry out the method for *thin-layer chromatography*, Appendix III A, using *silica gel G* as the coating substance and a mixture of 98 volumes of *toluene* and 2 volumes of *absolute ethanol* as the mobile phase. Apply separately to the chromatoplate 10 µl of each of two solutions of the substance being examined in a mixture of equal volumes of *ethanol (96%)* and *chloroform* containing (1) 1.0% w/v and (2) 0.0050% w/v. After removal of the plate, allow it to dry in air and spray with *vanillin—ethanolic sulphuric acid reagent*. Any *secondary spot* in the chromatogram obtained with solution (1) is not more intense than the spot in the chromatogram obtained with solution (2).

Loss on drying When dried to constant weight at 105°, loses not more than 0.5% of its weight. Use 1 g.

Sulphated ash Not more than 0.1%, Appendix IX A.

Assay Dissolve 0.1 g in sufficient 0.01M *ethanolic sodium hydroxide* to produce 200 ml, dilute 5 ml to 250 ml with 0.01M *ethanolic sodium hydroxide* and measure the *absorbance* of the resulting solution at the maximum at 315 nm, Appendix II B. Calculate the content of $C_{21}H_{32}O_3$ taking 547 as the value of A(1%, 1 cm) at the maximum at 315 nm.

Storage Oxymetholone should be kept free from contact with ferrous metals and protected from light.

Preparation
Oxymetholone Tablets

Action and use Anabolic steroid.

Oxyphenbutazone ☆

$C_{19}H_{20}N_2O_3,H_2O$ 342.4   *129-20-4*

Oxyphenbutazone is 4-butyl-2-(4-hydroxy-phenyl)-1-phenylpyrazolidine-3,5-dione mono-hydrate. It contains not less than 99.0 per cent and not more than 101.0 per cent of $C_{19}H_{20}N_2O_3$, calculated with reference to the anhydrous substance.

Characteristics A white, crystalline powder.

Solubility Practically insoluble in *water*; soluble in 3 parts of *ethanol (96%)*, in 20 parts of *chloroform* and in 20 parts of *ether*. It dissolves in dilute solutions of alkali hydroxides.

Identification *Test A may be omitted if tests B, C and D are carried out. Tests B and D may be omitted if tests A and C are carried out.*

A. The *infra-red absorption spectrum*, Appendix II A, is concordant with the spectrum of *oxyphenbutazone EPCRS* when examined as 6% w/v solutions in *dichloromethane*.

B. The *light absorption*, Appendix II B, in the range 230 to 350 nm of a 0.001% w/v solution in 0.01M *sodium hydroxide* exhibits a maximum at 254 nm. The A(1%, 1 cm) at 254 nm is 710 to 770.

C. To 2 ml of a 1% w/v solution in *ethanol (96%)* add 2 ml of a 0.1% w/v solution of *dichloroquinonechloroimine* in *ethanol (96%)* and 1 ml of *sodium carbonate solution*. An intense green colour is produced.

D. To 0.1 g add 1 ml of *glacial acetic acid* and 2 ml of *hydrochloric acid* and boil under a reflux condenser for 30 minutes. Cool, add 10 ml of *water* and filter. To the filtrate add 3 ml of a 0.7% w/v solution of *sodium nitrite*; a yellow colour is produced. To 1 ml of the resulting solution add a solution of 10 mg of *2-naphthol* in 5 ml of a 10.6% w/v solution of *anhydrous sodium carbonate*; an orange to orange-red precipitate is produced.

Clarity of solution To 0.50 g add a mixture of 12 ml of 1M *sodium hydroxide* and 8 ml of a 7.5% w/v solution of *glycine*, shake for 1 minute and maintain at 25° for exactly 60 minutes (solution A). The solution is *clear*, Appendix IV A.

Light absorption *Absorbance* of a 4-cm layer of solution A at 420 nm, measured immediately after preparation, not more than 0.40, Appendix II B.

Heavy metals 1.0 g complies with *limit test C for heavy metals*, Appendix VII (20 ppm). Use 2 ml of *lead standard solution (10 ppm Pb)* to prepare the standard.

Related substances Carry out the method for *thin-layer chromatography*, Appendix III A, using *silica gel HF254* as the coating substance and a mixture of 80 volumes of *chloroform* and 20 volumes of *glacial acetic acid* containing 0.02% w/v of *butylated hydroxytoluene* as the mobile phase. To prepare the chromatoplate allow the solvent front to ascend 4 cm, remove the plate and dry it in a current of cold air for 1 minute. Without delay and under a current of nitrogen, apply separately to the plate 5 µl of each of the following solutions prepared immediately before use. For solution (1) dissolve 0.1 g in 5 ml of a solution containing 0.02% w/v of *butylated hydroxytoluene* in *absolute ethanol*. For solution (2) dilute 1 ml of solution (1) to 200 ml with the ethanolic butylated hydroxytoluene solution. Develop immediately, allowing the solvent front to ascend 10 cm above the line of application. After removal of the plate, allow it to dry in a current of cold air for 15 minutes and examine under *ultra-violet light (254 nm)*. Any *secondary spot* in the chromatogram obtained with solution (1) is not more intense than the spot in the chromatogram obtained with solution (2).

Sulphated ash Not more than 0.1%, Appendix IX A, Method II. Use 1 g.

Water 5.0 to 6.0% w/w, Appendix IX C. Use 0.5 g.

Assay Dissolve 0.3 g in 25 ml of *acetone* and titrate with 0.1M *sodium hydroxide VS* using *bromothymol blue solution* as indicator and continuing the titration until the blue colour persists for at least 15 seconds. Repeat the operation without the substance being examined. The difference between the titrations represents the amount of sodium hydroxide required. Each ml of 0.1M *sodium hydroxide VS* is equivalent to 0.03244 g of $C_{19}H_{20}N_2O_3$.

Storage Oxyphenbutazone should be protected from light.

Preparation

Oxyphenbutazone Eye Ointment

Action and use Anti-inflammatory; analgesic.

Oxytetracycline ☆

Oxytetracycline Dihydrate

$C_{22}H_{24}N_2O_9$ 460.5   *79-57-2*

Oxytetracycline is (4S,4aR,5S,5aR,6S,12aS)-4-dimethylamino-1,4,4a,5,5a,6,11,12a-octahydro-3,5,6,10,12,12a-hexahydroxy-6-methyl-1,11-dioxonaphthacene-2-carboxamide, a substance produced by the growth of certain strains of *Streptomyces rimosus* or obtained by any other means. It contains a variable quantity of water. The potency is not less than 930 Units per mg, calculated with reference to the anhydrous substance.

Characteristics A yellow, crystalline powder; odourless.

Solubility Very slightly soluble in *water*. It dissolves in dilute acids and alkalis.

Identification A. Complies with the test for *identification of tetracyclines*, Appendix III A, using the following solutions. Solution (1) contains 0.05% w/v each of the substance being examined, *chlortetracycline hydrochloride EPCRS, demeclocycline hydrochloride EPCRS, doxycycline hyclate EPCRS* and *tetracycline hydrochloride EPCRS*. Solution (2) contains 0.05% w/v each of *chlortetracycline hydrochloride EPCRS, demeclocycline hydrochloride EPCRS, doxycycline hyclate EPCRS* and *tetracycline hydrochloride EPCRS*.

B. A 0.02% w/v solution in *hydrochloric acid* is yellow and exhibits a green fluorescence when examined under ultra-violet light (365 nm).

C. To 2 mg add 5 ml of *sulphuric acid*; a deep red colour is produced. Add the solution to 2.5 ml of *water*; the colour changes to yellow.

D. Dissolve 10 mg in a mixture of 1 ml of 2M *nitric acid* and 5 ml of *water*. Shake and add 1 ml of a 1.7% w/v solution of *silver nitrate*. Any opalescence produced is not more intense than that in a solution prepared in the same manner but omitting the substance being examined.

Acidity or alkalinity pH of a 1% w/v suspension, 4.5 to 7.5, Appendix V L.

Light absorption Dissolve 20 mg in sufficient *0.1M chloride buffer pH 2.0* to produce 100 ml and dilute 10 ml of the resulting solution to 100 ml with the same buffer solution. The A(1%, 1 cm) at 353 nm is 290 to 310, Appendix II B.

Specific optical rotation In a 1% w/v solution in 0.1M *hydrochloric acid*, −203° to −216°, Appendix V F. Allow the solution to stand protected from light for 30 minutes before measurement.

Light-absorbing impurities A. Dissolve 20 mg in sufficient of a mixture of 1 volume of 1M *hydrochloric acid* and 99 volumes of *methanol* to produce 10 ml. The *absorbance* at 430 nm, when measured within 1 hour of preparing the solution, is not more than 0.25, Appendix II B.

B. Dissolve 0.1 g in sufficient of a mixture of 1 volume of 1M *hydrochloric acid* and 99 volumes of *methanol* to produce 10 ml. The *absorbance* at 490 nm, when measured within 1 hour of preparing the solution, is not more than 0.20, Appendix II B.

Heavy metals 0.5 g complies with *limit test C for heavy metals*, Appendix VII (50 ppm). Use 2.5 ml of *lead standard solution (10 ppm Pb)* to prepare the standard.

Sulphated ash Not more than 0.5%, Appendix IX A, Method II. Use 1 g.

Water 4.0 to 8.0% w/w, Appendix IX C. Use 0.25 g.

Assay Carry out the *biological assay of antibiotics*, Appendix XIV A. The precision of the assay is such that the fiducial limits of error are not less than 95% and not more than 105% of the estimated potency.

Storage Oxytetracycline should be kept in a well-closed container and protected from light.

Labelling The label states (1) the date after which the material is not intended to be used; (2) the conditions under which it should be stored.

Preparation

Oxytetracycline Tablets

Action and use Antibacterial.

Oxytetracycline Calcium

$(C_{22}H_{23}N_2O_9)_2Ca$ 958.9   *15251-48-6*

Oxytetracycline Calcium is the calcium salt of (4S,4aR,5S,5aR,6S,12aS)-4-dimethylamino-1,4,4a,5,5a,6,11,12a-octahydro-3,5,6,10,12,12a-hexahydroxy-6-methyl-1,11-dioxonaphthacene-2-carboxamide, a substance produced by the growth of certain strains of *Streptomyces rimosus*, or obtained by any other means. It contains not less than 90.0 per cent and not more than 100.5 per cent of $(C_{22}H_{23}N_2O_9)_2Ca$, calculated with reference to the anhydrous substance.

Characteristics A pale yellow to greenish-fawn, crystalline powder.

Solubility Practically insoluble in *water*; soluble in dilute acids. It dissolves slowly in 5M *ammonia*.

Identification A. Carry out the method for *thin-layer chromatography*, Appendix III A, using a cellulose precoated chromatoplate (Merck cellulose plates are suitable). Spray the plate uniformly with *citro-phosphate buffer pH 4.5* until traces of moisture appear and dry the plate at 50° for 30 minutes. Use a mixture of 60 volumes of *ethyl acetate*, 30 volumes of *acetone* and 6 volumes of *water* as the mobile phase. Apply separately to the plate 1 μl of each of three solutions in 0.01M *methanolic hydrochloric acid* containing (1) 0.05% w/v of the substance being examined and 0.05% w/v of *tetracycline hydrochloride EPCRS*, (2) 0.05% w/v of *tetracycline hydrochloride EPCRS* and (3) 0.05% w/v of *oxytetracycline EPCRS*. As a fourth spot apply 1 μl of a mixture of equal volumes of solution (3) and a solution in 0.01M *methanolic hydrochloric acid* containing 0.05% w/v of the substance being examined. Spray the plate very finely and evenly with a 5% w/v solution of *2,4,6-collidine*, freshly prepared at 5°, until traces of moisture appear. Place the plate in the unlined tank so that it is not in contact with the mobile phase and leave to become impregnated with the vapour of the solvent for 1 hour before development. After removal of the plate, allow it to dry in air, expose to the vapour of 13.5M *ammonia* and examine immediately under *ultra-violet light (365 nm)*; the time of exposure to the ammonia vapour and the choice of intensity of the ultra-violet light should be such as to allow visualisation of the spots corresponding to the reference substances.

Compared with the chromatogram obtained with solution (2), the chromatogram obtained with solution (1) shows an additional spot corresponding in position to the spot in the chromatogram obtained with solution (3). The principal spot in the fourth chromatogram appears as a single compact spot.

B. To 2 mg add 5 ml of *sulphuric acid*; a deep red colour is produced. Add the solution to 2.5 ml of *water*; the colour changes to yellow.

C. Dissolve 2 mg in 10 ml of *hydrochloric acid*; the solution is yellow. When examined under ultra-violet light (365 nm), the solution exhibits a green fluorescence.

D. Yields *reaction B* characteristic of calcium salts, Appendix VI.

Acidity or alkalinity pH of a 2.5% w/v suspension, 6.0 to 7.5, Appendix V L.

Light absorption *Absorbance* of a 0.002% w/v solution in *0.1M chloride buffer pH 2.0* at the maximum at 353 nm, 0.56 to 0.61, Appendix II B.

Specific optical rotation In a 1% w/v solution in 0.1M *hydrochloric acid*, −194° to −210°, Appendix V F. Allow the solution to stand protected from light for 30 minutes before measurement.

Light-absorbing impurities A. Dissolve 0.2 g in 6 ml of 1M *hydrochloric acid* and add sufficient *methanol* to produce 100 ml. The *absorbance* at 430 nm, when measured within 1 hour of preparing the solution, is not more than 0.30, Appendix II B.

B. Dissolve 1 g in 6 ml of 1M *hydrochloric acid* and add sufficient *methanol* to produce 100 ml. The *absorbance* at 490 nm, when measured within 1 hour of preparing the solution, is not more than 0.20, Appendix II B.

Calcium 3.90 to 4.20%, calculated with reference to the anhydrous substance, when determined by the following method. Transfer about 1 g, accurately weighed, to a long-necked digestion flask, cautiously add 10 ml of *nitric acid* and mix. Allow to stand for 5 minutes, add a glass bead and heat on a water-bath for 5 minutes. Remove from the water-bath, cautiously add 5 ml of 9M *perchloric*

acid and heat, adding further 5-ml quantities of the perchloric acid at intervals until the liquid is almost colourless. Add 0.1 ml of *nitric acid* and allow any further reaction to subside. Do not allow the volume of the liquid in the flask to be reduced below 3 ml at any stage in the oxidation. Wash the walls of the flask with 40 ml of *water*, collecting the washings in the flask, and boil for 3 to 4 minutes to expel chlorine. Cool, transfer the contents of the flask to a conical flask with the aid of *water* and dilute to about 200 ml with *water*. Adjust to pH 9 with 5M *sodium hydroxide* and then add 100 ml of *water* followed by 12 ml of 10M *sodium hydroxide* and mix. Add about 15 mg of *calconcarboxylic acid mixture* and titrate with 0.05M *disodium edetate VS* until the colour changes from violet to full blue. Each ml of 0.05M *disodium edetate VS* is equivalent to 0.002004 g of Ca.

Water Not more than 15.0% w/w, Appendix IX C. Use 0.5 g.

Assay Dissolve 0.3 g of *sulphadimidine* (internal standard) in sufficient *methanol* to produce 500 ml (solution A). Carry out the method for *high-performance liquid chromatography*, Appendix III D, using the following solutions. For solution (1) dissolve 50 mg of *oxytetracycline hydrochloride BPCRS* in 10 ml of 0.1M methanolic hydrochloric acid, prepared by diluting 25.0 ml of 1M *hydrochloric acid* to 250 ml with *methanol*, and add 20 ml of solution A and sufficient *methanol (15%)* to produce 100 ml. For solution (2) dissolve 50 mg of the substance being examined in 10 ml of the 0.1M methanolic hydrochloric acid and add 20 ml of *methanol* and sufficient *methanol (15%)* to produce 100 ml. Prepare solution (3) in the same manner as solution (2) but adding 20 ml of solution A in place of the 20 ml of methanol.

The chromatographic procedure may be carried out using (a) a stainless steel column (20 cm × 5 mm) packed with *strong cation exchanger (5 μm)**, (b) as the mobile phase with a flow rate of 0.7 ml per minute, a solution prepared by dissolving 3.4 g of *potassium dihydrogen orthophosphate* and 9.3 g of *disodium edetate* in 650 ml of *water*, adding sufficient *methanol* to produce 1000 ml and adjusting the pH to 5.3 with 0.1M *sodium hydroxide* and (c) a detection wavelength of 263 nm.

Calculate the content of $(C_{22}H_{23}N_2O_9)_2Ca$ from the declared content of $C_{22}H_{24}N_2O_9$ in *oxytetracycline hydrochloride BPCRS*. Each mg of $C_{22}H_{24}N_2O_9$ is equivalent to 1.041 mg of $(C_{22}H_{23}N_2O_9)_2Ca$.

Storage Oxytetracycline Calcium should be kept in a well-closed container, protected from light and stored at a temperature not exceeding 15°.

Labelling The label states (1) the date after which the material is not intended to be used; (2) the conditions under which it should be stored.

Action and use Antibacterial.

*It is recommended that freshly packed columns should be conditioned by eluting with about 10 column volumes of 0.025M *potassium dihydrogen orthophosphate*, followed by the mobile phase for several hours until the peak due to oxytetracycline exhibits satisfactory symmetry.

Oxytetracycline Hydrochloride ☆

C₂₂H₂₄N₂O₉,HCl   496.9   2058-46-0

Oxytetracycline Hydrochloride is the hydrochloride of (4S,4aR,5S,5aR,6S,12aS)-N-4-dimethylamino-1,4,4a,5,5a,6,11,12a-octahydro-3,5,6,10,12,12a-hexahydroxy-6-methyl-1,11-dioxonaphthacene-2-carboxamide, a substance produced by the growth of certain strains of *Streptomyces rimosus* or obtained by any other means. The potency is not less than 860 Units per mg, calculated with reference to the anhydrous substance.

Characteristics A yellow, crystalline powder; odourless; hygroscopic.

Solubility Soluble in 2 parts of *water* and in 45 parts of *ethanol (96%)*. Solutions in *water* become turbid on standing due to the precipitation of oxytetracycline.

Identification A. Complies with the test for *identification of tetracyclines*, Appendix III A, using the following solutions. Solution (1) contains 0.05% w/v each of the substance being examined, *chlortetracycline hydrochloride EPCRS*, *demeclocycline hydrochloride EPCRS*, *doxycycline hyclate EPCRS* and *tetracycline hydrochloride EPCRS*. Solution (2) contains 0.05% w/v each of *chlortetracycline hydrochloride EPCRS*, *demeclocycline hydrochloride EPCRS*, *doxycycline hyclate EPCRS* and *tetracycline hydrochloride EPCRS*.

B. A 0.02% w/v solution in *hydrochloric acid* is yellow and exhibits a greenish-yellow fluorescence when examined under ultra-violet light (365 nm).

C. To 2 mg add 5 ml of *sulphuric acid*; a deep red colour is produced. Add the solution to 2.5 ml of *water*; the colour changes to yellow.

D. Yields *reaction A* characteristic of chlorides, Appendix VI.

Acidity pH of a 1% w/v solution, 2.3 to 2.9, Appendix V L.

Light absorption Dissolve 20 mg in sufficient *0.1M chloride buffer pH 2.0* to produce 100 ml and dilute 10 ml of the resulting solution to 100 ml with the same buffer solution. The A(1%, 1 cm) at 353 nm is 270 to 290, Appendix II B.

Specific optical rotation In a 1% w/v solution in 0.1M *hydrochloric acid*, −188° to −200°, Appendix V F. Allow the solution to stand protected from light for 30 minutes before measurement.

Light-absorbing impurities A. Dissolve 20 mg in sufficient of a mixture of 1 volume of 1M *hydrochloric acid* and 99 volumes of *methanol* to produce 10 ml. The *absorbance* at 430 nm, when measured within 1 hour of preparing the solution, is not more than 0.50, Appendix II B.

B. Dissolve 0.1 g in sufficient of a mixture of 1 volume of 1M *hydrochloric acid* and 99 volumes of *methanol* to produce 10 ml. The *absorbance* at 490 nm, when measured within 1 hour of preparing the solution, is not more than 0.20, Appendix II B.

Heavy metals 0.5 g complies with *limit test C for heavy metals*, Appendix VII (50 ppm). Use 2.5 ml of *lead standard solution (10 ppm Pb)* to prepare the standard.

Sulphated ash Not more than 0.5%, Appendix IX A, Method II. Use 1 g.

Water Not more than 2.0%, Appendix IX C. Use 0.5 g.

Assay Carry out the *biological assay of antibiotics*, Appendix XIV A. The precision of the assay is such that the fiducial limits of error are not less than 95% and not more than 105% of the estimated potency.

Storage Oxytetracycline Hydrochloride should be kept in an airtight container and protected from light. If the material is intended for use in the manufacture of a parenteral dosage form the container should be sterile, tamper-evident and sealed so as to exclude micro-organisms.

Labelling The label on the container states (1) the date after which the material is not intended to be used; (2) the conditions under which it should be stored; (3) whether or not it is intended for use in the manufacture of a parenteral dosage form.

Preparation
Oxytetracycline Capsules

Action and use Antibacterial.

Oxytetracycline Hydrochloride intended for use in the manufacture of a parenteral dosage form complies with the following additional requirements.

Pyrogens Complies with the *test for pyrogens*, Appendix XIV K. Use per kg of the rabbit's weight 1 ml of a solution in *water for injections* containing 5 mg per ml.

Sterility Complies with the *test for sterility*, Appendix XVI A.

Fractionated Palm Kernel Oil

Fractionated Palm Kernel Oil is obtained by expression of the natural oil from the kernels of *Elaeis guineensis* followed by selective solvent fractionation and hydrogenation.

Characteristics A white, solid, brittle fat; odourless or almost odourless.

Solubility Practically insoluble in *water* and in *ethanol (96%)*; miscible with *chloroform*, with *ether* and with *petroleum spirit (boiling range, 40° to 60°)*.

Acid value Not more than 0.2, Appendix X B.

Iodine value Not more than 6.0 (*iodine bromide method*), Appendix X E.

Melting point 31° to 36°, Appendix V A, Method IV.

Refractive index At 50°, 1.445 to 1.447, Appendix V E.

Saponification value 246 to 250, Appendix X G.

Peroxides Dissolve 5 g in 15 ml of *chloroform*, add 20 ml of *glacial acetic acid* and 0.5 ml of a saturated solution of *potassium iodide*, mix well, allow to stand in the dark for exactly 1 minute, add 30 ml of *water* and titrate with 0.01M *sodium thiosulphate VS* using *starch mucilage* as indicator. Not more than 0.5 ml of 0.01M *sodium thiosulphate VS* is required.

Storage Fractionated Palm Kernel Oil should be stored at a temperature not exceeding 25°.

Action and use Suppository basis.

The standards of this monograph encompass several different suppository bases. The selection of a basis for a particular suppository formulation should be appropriate to the product concerned and it may be necessary to apply more restrictive standards for a particular application.

Pancreatin

Pancreatin is a preparation of mammalian pancreas containing enzymes having protease, lipase and amylase activity. It may contain Sodium Chloride. Pancreatin contains in 1 mg not less than 1.4 Units of free protease activity, not less than 20 Units of lipase activity and not less than 24 Units of amylase activity. Pancreatin is prepared in conditions designed to minimise the degree of microbial contamination.

Characteristics A white or buff amorphous powder; free from unpleasant odour.

Solubility Soluble or partly soluble in *water* forming a slightly turbid solution; practically insoluble in *ethanol (96%)* and in *ether.*

Identification A. Triturate 0.5 g with 10 ml of *water* and adjust to pH 8.0 by the addition of 1M *sodium hydroxide* using *cresol red solution* as indicator. Divide the resulting solution into two equal portions. Boil one portion [solution (1)] and leave the other untreated [solution (2)]. To each add a few shreds of *congo red fibrin,* warm to 38° to 40° and maintain at this temperature for 1 hour. Solution (2) is stained red and solution (1) is colourless or not more than slightly pink.

B. Triturate 0.25 g with 10 ml of *water* and adjust to pH 8.0 by the addition of 1M *sodium hydroxide* using *cresol red solution* as indicator. Divide the resulting solution into two equal portions. Boil one portion [solution (1)] and leave the other untreated [solution (2)]. Dissolve 0.1 g of *soluble starch* in 100 ml of boiling *water,* boil for 2 minutes, cool and dilute to 150 ml with *water.* Add solution (1) to half the starch mucilage and solution (2) to the remainder and maintain the mixtures at 38° to 40° for 5 minutes. To 1 ml of each mixture add 10 ml of *iodine solution.* The liquid containing solution (2) retains the colour of the solution of iodine and the liquid containing solution (1) acquires an intense blue colour.

Fat Extract 1 g with *petroleum spirit (boiling range, 40° to 60°)* for 3 hours in an apparatus for the *continuous extraction of drugs,* Appendix XI F, evaporate the extract and dry the residue at 105° for 2 hours. The residue weighs not more than 30 mg.

Loss on drying When dried at 60° at a pressure not exceeding 0.7 kPa for 4 hours, loses not more than 5.0% of its weight. Use 0.5 g.

Microbial contamination 1 g is free from *Escherichia coli;* 10 g is free from salmonellae, Appendix XVI B1.

Assay Carry out the *assay of pancreatin,* Appendix XIV E3.

Storage Pancreatin should be kept in a well-closed container and stored at a temperature not exceeding 15°.

Labelling The label states (1) the minimum number of Units of activity of free protease, lipase and amylase per mg; (2) the name of any added substance; (3) the date after which the material is not intended to be used; (4) the conditions under which it should be stored.

Preparations
Pancreatin Granules
Pancreatin Tablets

Action and use Enzymes used in pancreatic deficiency.

Pancreatic Extract ☆

Pancreatic Extract is prepared from fresh or frozen mammalian pancreases. It contains enzymes having protease, lipase and amylase activity. Pancreatic Extract contains in 1 mg not less than 1.0 Unit of total protease activity, not less than 15 Units of lipase activity and not less than 12 Units of amylase activity. Pancreatic Extract is prepared in conditions designed to minimise the degree of microbial contamination.

Characteristics A slightly brown amorphous powder; odour, faint and characteristic.

Solubility Partly soluble in *water;* practically insoluble in *ethanol (96%)* and in *ether.*

Identification A. Triturate 0.5 g with 10 ml of *water* and adjust to pH 8.0 by the addition of 0.1M *sodium hydroxide* using *cresol red solution* as indicator. Divide the resulting suspension into two equal portions. Boil one portion [suspension (1)] and leave the other untreated [suspension (2)]. To each add a few shreds of *congo red fibrin,* warm to 38° to 40° and maintain at this temperature for 1 hour. Suspension (2) is stained red and suspension (1) is colourless or not more than slightly pink.

B. Triturate 0.25 g with 10 ml of *water* and adjust to pH 8.0 by the addition of 0.1M *sodium hydroxide* using *cresol red solution* as indicator. Divide the resulting solution into two equal portions. Boil one portion [solution (1)] and leave the other untreated [solution (2)]. Dissolve 0.1 mg of *soluble starch* in 100 ml of boiling *water,* boil for 2 minutes, cool and dilute to 150 ml with *water.* Add solution (1) to half the starch mucilage and solution (2) to the remainder and maintain the mixtures at 38° to 40° for 5 minutes. To 1 ml of each mixture add 10 ml of *iodine solution.* The liquid containing solution (2) retains the colour of the solution of iodine and the liquid containing solution (1) acquires an intense blue colour.

Fat Extract 1.0 g with *petroleum spirit (boiling range, 40° to 60°)* for 3 hours, evaporate the extract and dry the residue at 100° to 105° for 2 hours. The residue weighs not more than 50 mg (5.0%).

Loss on drying When dried at 60° at a pressure not exceeding 0.7 kPa for 4 hours, loses not more than 5.0% of its weight. Use 0.5 g.

Microbial contamination* 1 g is free from *Escherichia coli;* 10 g is free from salmonellae, Appendix XVI B1.

Assay Carry out the *assay of pancreatin,* Appendix XIV E3, with the following modifications.

Determine the total protease activity by carrying out the method described for free protease activity but preparing the solution of the substance being examined as follows. Triturate for 5 minutes an amount of the substance being examined containing approximately 100 Units of protease activity with 25 ml of *calcium chloride solution* cooled to 5°. Dilute to 100 ml with the cooled calcium chloride solution. To 10 ml of the resulting suspension add 10 ml of *enterokinase solution,* mix and maintain at 35° for 15 minutes. Cool and dilute with sufficient *borate buffer solution pH 7.5,* cooled to 2° to 8°, so that the estimated total protease activity corresponds to the activity of the Standard Preparation.

Storage Pancreatic Extract should be kept in an airtight container and stored at a temperature not exceeding 15°.

Labelling The label states (1) the minimum number of Units of activity of total protease, lipase and amylase per mg; (2) the name of any added substance; (3) the date after which the material is not intended to be used; (4) the conditions under which it should be stored.

The title of the monograph in the European Pharmacopœia is Pancreas Powder.

*In certain states party to the Convention on the Elaboration of a European Pharmacopœia, Pancreatic Extract may be required to comply with a limit for a total viable aerobic count of 10^4 micro-organisms per gram, determined by plate count, Appendix XVI B2.

Pancuronium Bromide

$C_{35}H_{60}Br_2N_2O_4$ 732.7   15500-66-0

Pancuronium Bromide is 1,1'-(3α,17β-diacetoxy-5α-androstan-2β,16β-ylene)bis(1-methylpiperidinium) dibromide. It contains not less than 98.0 per cent and not more than 102.0 per cent of $C_{35}H_{60}Br_2N_2O_4$, calculated with reference to the dried substance.

Characteristics White or almost white crystals or crystalline powder; odourless; hygroscopic.

Solubility Soluble in 1 part of *water*, in 5 parts of *ethanol (96%)*, in 5 parts of *chloroform*, in 4 parts of *dichloromethane* and in 1 part of *methanol*; practically insoluble in *ether*.

Identification A. The *infra-red absorption spectrum*, Appendix II A, is concordant with the *reference spectrum* of pancuronium bromide.
B. Dissolve 5 mg in 10 ml of *water* and add 10 ml of *1,2-dichloroethane* followed by 1 ml of *methyl orange solution*. Shake, centrifuge, allow the layers to separate and acidify the organic layer with 1M *sulphuric acid*. A red colour is produced.
C. Yields the *reactions* characteristic of bromides, Appendix VI.

Specific optical rotation In a 3% w/v solution, +38° to +42°, Appendix V F.

Related substances Carry out the method for *thin-layer chromatography*, Appendix III A, using a silica gel precoated chromatoplate (Machery Nagel plates are suitable) and as the mobile phase the upper layer obtained by shaking together 60 volumes of *butan-1-ol*, 48 volumes of a 20% w/v solution of *ammonium chloride*, 40 volumes of *pyridine* and 12 volumes of *glacial acetic acid*. Use an unlined tank closed with an ungreased lid and develop the chromatogram immediately after introducing the mobile phase into the tank. Apply separately to the plate 2 µl of each of four solutions in a 0.9% w/v solution of *sodium chloride* containing (1) 0.50% w/v of the substance being examined, (2) 0.010% w/v of *dacuronium bromide BPCRS*, (3) 0.0050% w/v of the substance being examined and (4) 0.50% w/v of *pancuronium bromide BPCRS*. At a fifth point apply 4 µl of a mixture of equal volumes of solutions (2) and (4). Allow the solvent front to ascend to within 1 cm of the top of the plate. After removal of the plate, allow the solvent to evaporate and heat at 120° for 1 hour. Allow to cool to room temperature, spray with *ethanolic sulphuric acid (10%)* and heat at 120° for 1 hour. Any spot corresponding to dacuronium bromide in the chromatogram obtained with solution (1) is not more intense than the spot in the chromatogram obtained with solution (2). Any other *secondary spot* in the chromatogram obtained with solution (1) is not more intense than the spot in the chromatogram obtained with solution (3). The test is not valid unless the chromatogram obtained with the solution prepared by mixing solutions (2) and (4) shows two clearly separated spots.

Loss on drying When dried at 105° for 3 hours, loses not more than 1.0% of its weight in excess of the percentage determined in the test for Water. Use 1 g.

Sulphated ash Not more than 0.1%, Appendix IX A.

Water 5.0 to 8.0% w/w, Appendix IX C. Use 0.3 g.

Assay Carry out Method I for *non-aqueous titration*, Appendix VIII A, using 0.3 g, 20 ml of *mercury(II) acetate solution* and *1-naphtholbenzein solution* as indicator. Each ml of 0.1M *perchloric acid VS* is equivalent to 0.03663 g of $C_{35}H_{60}Br_2N_2O_4$.

Storage Pancuronium Bromide should be kept in a well-closed container and stored at a temperature of 2° to 8°.

Preparation
Pancuronium Injection

Action and use Neuromuscular blocking substance used to produce relaxation during anaesthesia.

Papaverine Hydrochloride ☆

$C_{20}H_{21}NO_4,HCl$ 375.9   61-25-6

Papaverine Hydrochloride is 6,7-dimethoxy-1-(3,4-dimethoxybenzyl)isoquinoline hydrochloride. It contains not less than 99.0 per cent and not more than 101.0 per cent of $C_{20}H_{21}NO_4,HCl$, calculated with reference to the dried substance.

Characteristics White or almost white crystals or a white or almost white, crystalline powder; odourless.

Solubility Soluble in 40 parts of *water*; slightly soluble in *ethanol (96%)*; soluble in *chloroform*; practically insoluble in *ether*.

Identification A. The *light absorption*, Appendix II B, in the range 230 to 270 nm of a 0.0005% w/v solution in

0.01M *hydrochloric acid* exhibits a maximum at 250 nm. The A(1%, 1 cm) at 250 nm is 1590 to 1670. The *light absorption*, in the range 270 to 350 nm of a 0.0025% w/v solution in 0.01M *hydrochloric acid* exhibits two maxima, at 280 to 290 nm and 303 to 313 nm. The A(1%, 1 cm) at these maxima are 140 to 200 and 200 to 250 respectively.
B. To 10 mg add 3 ml of *acetic anhydride*, add cautiously 0.15 ml of *sulphuric acid* and heat on a water-bath for 3 to 4 minutes. A yellow colour with a green fluorescence is produced.
C. To 10 ml of a 2% w/v solution in *carbon dioxide-free water* add dropwise 10M *ammonia* and allow to stand. The *melting point* of the precipitate, after washing with water and drying, is 146° to 149°, Appendix V A, Method I.
D. Yields the *reaction* characteristic of alkaloids, Appendix VI.
E. Yields *reaction A* characteristic of chlorides, Appendix VI.

Acidity pH of a 2% w/v solution, prepared with the aid of gentle heat, 3.0 to 4.0, Appendix V L.

Clarity and colour of solution A 2.0% w/v solution in *carbon dioxide-free water*, prepared with the aid of gentle heat, is *clear*, Appendix IV A, and not more intensely coloured than *reference solution GY₆*, Appendix IV B, Method II.

Readily carbonisable substances To 50 mg add 5 ml of *sulphuric acid (96% w/w)*. Any colour that is produced within 15 minutes is not more intense than that of *reference solution R₄ or Y₄*, Appendix IV B, Method I.

Related substances Carry out the method for *thin-layer chromatography*, Appendix III A, using *silica gel GF254* as the coating substance and a mixture of 70 volumes of *toluene*, 20 volumes of *ethyl acetate* and 10 volumes of *diethylamine* as the mobile phase. Apply separately to the chromatoplate 10 μl of each of the following solutions. For solution (1) dissolve 0.5 g of the substance being examined in sufficient of a mixture of equal volumes of *ethanol (96%)* and *water* to produce 10 ml. For solution (2) dissolve 50 mg of *codeine* in sufficient of a mixture of equal volumes of *ethanol (96%)* and *water* to produce 100 ml. After removal of the plate, warm it until the odour of diethylamine is no longer detectable and examine under *ultra-violet light (254 nm)*. Any *secondary spot* in the chromatogram obtained with solution (1) is not more intense than the spot in the chromatogram obtained with solution (2).

Loss on drying When dried to constant weight at 100° to 105°, loses not more than 1.0% of its weight. Use 1 g.

Sulphated ash Not more than 0.1%, Appendix IX A, Method II. Use the residue obtained in the test for Loss on drying.

Assay Dissolve 0.3 g in 30 ml of *anhydrous glacial acetic acid* and carry out Method I for *non-aqueous titration*, Appendix VIII A, adding 6 ml of *mercury(II) acetate solution* and using 0.05 ml of *crystal violet solution* as indicator. Each ml of 0.1M *perchloric acid VS* is equivalent to 0.03759 g of $C_{20}H_{21}NO_4,HCl$.

Storage Papaverine Hydrochloride should be kept in a well-closed container and protected from light.

Action and use Antispasmodic.

Paracetamol ☆

$C_8H_9NO_2$ 151.2   *103-90-2*

Paracetamol is 4′-hydroxyacetanilide. It contains not less than 99.0 per cent and not more than 101.0 per cent of $C_8H_9NO_2$, calculated with reference to the dried substance.

Characteristics A white, crystalline powder; odourless.

Solubility Soluble in 70 parts of *water* and in 7 parts of *ethanol (96%)*; very slightly soluble in *chloroform* and in *ether*.

Identification *Test A may be omitted if tests B, C, D and E are carried out. Tests B, C and D may be omitted if tests A and E are carried out.*
A. The *infra-red absorption spectrum*, Appendix II A, is concordant with the spectrum of *paracetamol EPCRS*.
B. Dissolve 50 mg in sufficient *methanol* to produce 100 ml. To 1 ml of the solution add 0.5 ml of 0.1M *hydrochloric acid* and dilute to 100 ml with *methanol*. Protect the resulting solution from light and immediately measure the *absorbance* at the maximum at 249 nm, Appendix II B. The A(1%, 1 cm) at 249 nm is about 880.
C. Boil 0.1 g in 1 ml of *hydrochloric acid* for 3 minutes, add 10 ml of *water* and cool; no precipitate is produced. Add 0.05 ml of 0.0167M *potassium dichromate*; a violet colour is produced which does not turn red.
D. Yields the *reaction* characteristic of acetyl groups, Appendix VI, heating over a naked flame.
E. *Melting point*, 168° to 172°, Appendix V A, Method I.

Heavy metals Dissolve 1.0 g in sufficient of a mixture of 85 volumes of *acetone* and 15 volumes of *water* to produce 20 ml. 12 ml of the resulting solution complies with *limit test B for heavy metals*, Appendix VII (20 ppm). Prepare the standard using lead standard solution (1 ppm Pb) obtained by diluting *lead standard solution (100 ppm Pb)* with the acetone—water mixture.

4-Aminophenol Dissolve 0.50 g in sufficient *methanol (50%)* to produce 10 ml. Add 0.2 ml of *sodium nitroprusside—carbonate solution*, mix and allow to stand for 30 minutes. The solution is not more intensely coloured than 10 ml of a solution prepared at the same time and in the same manner using 0.5 g of *4-aminophenol-free paracetamol* and incorporating 0.5 ml of a 0.005% w/v solution of *4-aminophenol* in *methanol (50%)*.

Related substances Carry out the method for *thin-layer chromatography*, Appendix III A, using *silica gel GF254* as the coating substance and a mixture of 65 volumes of *chloroform*, 25 volumes of *acetone* and 10 volumes of *toluene* as the mobile phase, but allowing the solvent front to ascend 14 cm above the line of application in an unsaturated tank. Apply separately to the chromatoplate 200 μl of solution (1) and 40 μl of each of solutions (2), (3) and (4). For solution (1) transfer 1.0 g of the substance being examined, finely powdered, to a ground-glass-stoppered 15-ml centrifuge tube, add 5 ml of *peroxide-free ether*, shake mechanically for 30 minutes, centrifuge at 1000 revolutions per minute for 15 minutes or until a clear supernatant liquid is obtained and decant the supernatant liquid. For solution (2) dilute 1 ml of solution (1) to 10 ml with *ethanol (96%)*. Solution (3) contains 0.005% w/v of *4-chloroacetanilide* in *ethanol (96%)*. For solution (4) dissolve 0.25 g of *4-chloro-acetanilide* and 0.1 g of the substance being examined in sufficient *ethanol (96%)* to produce 100 ml. After removal of the plate, dry it in a current of warm air and examine under *ultra-violet light (254 nm)*. Any spot corresponding to 4-chloroacetanilide in the chromatogram obtained with solution (1) is not more intense than the spot in the chromatogram obtained with solution (3). Any other *secondary spot* in the chromatogram obtained with solution (2) is not more intense than the spot in the chromatogram obtained with solution (3). The test is not valid unless the chromatogram obtained with solution (4) shows two clearly separated principal spots, the spot corresponding to the substance being examined having the lower Rf value.

Loss on drying When dried to constant weight at 100° to 105°, loses not more than 0.5% of its weight. Use 1 g.

Sulphated ash Not more than 0.1%, Appendix IX A, Method II. Use 1 g.

Assay Dissolve 0.3 g in a mixture of 10 ml of *water* and 30 ml of 1M *sulphuric acid*. Boil under a reflux condenser for 1 hour, cool and dilute to 100 ml with *water*. To 20 ml of the solution add 40 ml of *water*, 40 g of *water* in the form of ice, 15 ml of 2M *hydrochloric acid* and 0.1 ml of *ferroin sulphate solution* and titrate with 0.1M *ammonium cerium(IV) sulphate VS* until a yellow colour is produced. Repeat the operation without the substance being examined. The difference between the titrations represents the amount of ammonium cerium(IV) sulphate required. Each ml of 0.1M *ammonium cerium(IV) sulphate VS* is equivalent to 0.007560 g of $C_8H_9NO_2$.

Storage Paracetamol should be kept in a well-closed container and protected from light.

Preparations
Paediatric Paracetamol Oral Solution
Paracetamol Oral Suspension
Paracetamol Tablets

Action and use Analgesic and antipyretic.

Hard Paraffin

Hard Paraffin is a mixture of solid hydrocarbons obtained from petroleum or from shale oil.

Characteristics A colourless or white substance, frequently showing a crystalline structure; odourless or almost odourless, even when freshly cut; slightly greasy to the touch. It burns with a luminous flame. When melted the liquid is free from fluorescence by daylight.

Solubility Practically insoluble in *water* and in *ethanol (96%)*; soluble in *chloroform* and in *ether*.

Acidity or alkalinity Boil 5 g with 10 ml of *ethanol (90%)* previously neutralised to *litmus solution*. The suspension is neutral to *litmus solution*.

Solidifying point 50° to 57°, Appendix V B, with the following modifications. Place in the inner test-tube sufficient of the melted substance to fill the tube to a depth of about 50 mm. Stir the substance gently and steadily, without scraping the wall of the tube, while the tube and its contents are allowed to cool. The temperature

at which the level of the mercury in the thermometer remains stationary for a short time is taken as the solidifying point.

Sulphated ash Not more than 0.1%, Appendix IX A.

Liquid Paraffin ☆

Liquid Paraffin is a purified mixture of liquid saturated hydrocarbons obtained from petroleum.

Characteristics A transparent, colourless, oily liquid, free from fluorescence by daylight; odourless or almost odourless and giving not more than a faint odour when heated.

Solubility Practically insoluble in *water*; sparingly soluble in *ethanol (96%)*; soluble in *chloroform*, in *ether* and in hydrocarbons.

Acidity or alkalinity To 10 ml add 20 ml of boiling *water*, shake vigorously for 1 minute, allow to separate and filter the aqueous layer. To 10 ml of the filtrate add 0.1 ml of *dilute phenolphthalein solution*. The solution is colourless and not more than 0.1 ml of 0.1M *sodium hydroxide* is required to change the colour of the solution to pink.

Relative density 0.827 to 0.890, Appendix V G.

Dynamic viscosity 110 to 230 mPa s when determined at 19.9° to 20.1°, Appendix V H, Method II.

Polycyclic aromatic hydrocarbons Extract 25 ml of *hexane UV* in a 125-ml all-glass separating funnel with an ungreased tap with two 5-ml quantities of *dimethyl sulphoxide UV* and discard the extracts. Add 25.0 ml of the substance being examined, mix, add 5 ml of *dimethyl sulphoxide UV*, shake vigorously for 1 minute and allow to stand until two clear layers are produced. Transfer the lower layer to a second, similar separating funnel, add 2 ml of *hexane UV* and shake vigorously. Allow to separate and measure the *light absorption* of the lower layer (solution A), Appendix II B, in the range 260 to 420 nm using in the reference cell the clear lower layer obtained by shaking 5 ml of *dimethyl sulphoxide UV* with 25 ml of *hexane UV* for 1 minute. Measure the *absorbance* of a 0.00070% w/v solution of *naphthalene* in *2,2,4-trimethyl-pentane UV* at 275 nm using *2,2,4-trimethylpentane UV* in the reference cell. The *absorbance* of solution A at all wavelengths in the range 260 to 420 nm is not more than one third of that of the naphthalene solution at 275 nm.

Readily carbonisable substances Use a test-tube (about 125 mm × 18 mm) fitted with a glass stopper and graduated at 5 ml and 10 ml and which has been washed with *chromic—sulphuric acid mixture*, rinsed with *water* and dried. To 5 ml add 5 ml of a solution of *nitrogen-free sulphuric acid* containing 95.0 to 95.5% w/w of H_2SO_4. Insert the stopper and shake as vigorously as possible in the longitudinal direction of the tube for 5 seconds. Loosen the stopper, immediately place the tube in a water-bath, supporting it so as to prevent contact of the tube with the bottom and side of the bath, and heat for 10 minutes. At the end of the second, fourth, sixth and eighth minutes remove the tube from the bath and shake as vigorously as possible in the longitudinal direction of the tube for 5 seconds. At the end of the tenth minute remove the tube and allow to stand for 10 minutes. The upper layer may be hazy but is unchanged in colour. The lower layer is not more intensely coloured than a mixture prepared by the addition of 1.5 ml of *red primary solution*, 3.0 ml of *yellow primary solution* and 0.5 ml of *blue primary solution* to 2 ml of a solution prepared by mixing 2.5 ml of *hydrochloric acid* with sufficient *water* to produce 100 ml, Appendix IV B, Method I.

Solid paraffins Place a suitable quantity, previously dried by heating at 100° for 2 hours and cooled in a desiccator over *sulphuric acid*, in a glass tube having an internal diameter of approximately 25 mm. Close the tube and immerse in ice. After 4 hours the liquid is sufficiently clear that a black line 0.5 mm in width held vertically behind the tube is easily seen.

Storage Liquid Paraffin should be protected from light.

Preparations

Liquid Paraffin Oral Emulsion

Liquid Paraffin and Magnesium Hydroxide Oral Emulsion

Action and use Faecal softener.

Light Liquid Paraffin ☆

Light Liquid Paraffin is a purified mixture of liquid saturated hydrocarbons obtained from petroleum.

Characteristics A transparent, colourless, oily liquid, free from fluorescence by daylight; odourless or almost odourless and giving not more than a faint odour when heated.

Solubility Practically insoluble in *water*; sparingly soluble in *ethanol (96%)*; soluble in *chloroform*, in *ether* and in hydrocarbons.

Acidity or alkalinity; Polycyclic aromatic hydrocarbons; Readily carbonisable substances; Solid paraffins Complies with the requirements stated under Liquid Paraffin.

Relative density 0.810 to 0.875, Appendix V G.

Dynamic viscosity 25 to 80 mPa s when determined at 19.9° to 20.1°, Appendix V H, Method II.

Storage Light Liquid Paraffin should be protected from light.

White Soft Paraffin

White Petroleum Jelly

White Soft Paraffin is a semi-solid mixture of hydrocarbons obtained from petroleum and bleached.

Characteristics A white, translucent, soft unctuous mass, retaining these characteristics on storage and when melted and allowed to cool without stirring; not more than slightly fluorescent by daylight, even when melted; odourless when rubbed on the skin.

Solubility Practically insoluble in *water* and in *ethanol (96%)*; soluble in *chloroform*, in *ether* and in *petroleum spirit (boiling range, 40° to 60°)*, the solutions sometimes showing a slight opalescence.

Acidity or alkalinity Boil 5 g with 10 ml of *ethanol (96%)* previously neutralised to *litmus solution*. The extract is neutral to *litmus solution*.

Light absorption *Absorbance* of a 0.05% w/v solution in *2,2,4-trimethylpentane UV* at 290 nm, not more than 0.5, Appendix II B.

Melting point 38° to 56°, Appendix V A, Method III.

Foreign organic matter Heat 1 g until fumes appear. No acrid odour is evolved.

Sulphated ash Not more than 0.1%, Appendix IX A.

Storage White Soft Paraffin should be protected from light.

Yellow Soft Paraffin

Yellow Petroleum Jelly

Yellow Soft Paraffin is a semi-solid mixture of hydrocarbons obtained from petroleum.

Characteristics A pale yellow to yellow, translucent, soft unctuous mass, retaining these characteristics on storage and when melted and allowed to cool without stirring; not more than slightly fluorescent by daylight, even when melted; odourless when rubbed on the skin.

Solubility Practically insoluble in *water* and in *ethanol (96%)*; soluble in *chloroform*, in *ether* and in *petroleum spirit (boiling range, 40° to 60°)*, the solutions sometimes showing a slight opalescence.

Acidity or alkalinity Boil 5 g with 10 ml of *ethanol (96%)* previously neutralised to *litmus solution*. The extract is neutral to *litmus solution*.

Light absorption *Absorbance* of a 0.05% w/v solution in *2,2,4-trimethylpentane UV* at 290 nm, not more than 0.75, Appendix II B.

Melting point 38° to 56°, Appendix V A, Method III.

Foreign organic matter Heat 1 g until fumes appear. No acrid odour is evolved.

Sulphated ash Not more than 0.1%, Appendix IX A.

Storage Yellow Soft Paraffin should be protected from light.

Paraldehyde ☆

$C_6H_{12}O_3$ 132.2   *123-63-7*

Paraldehyde is 2,4,6-trimethyl-1,3,5-trioxane, the trimer of acetaldehyde. It may contain a suitable proportion of antioxidant.

Characteristics A clear, colourless or pale yellow liquid; odour, strong and characteristic. At low temperatures it solidifies to produce a crystalline mass.

Solubility Soluble in 9 parts of *water*, but less soluble in boiling *water*; miscible with *ethanol (96%)*, with *chloroform*, with *ether* and with volatile oils.

Identification A. A 10.0% v/v solution in *carbon dioxide-free water* (solution A) is *clear*, Appendix IV A, but becomes turbid on warming.

B. Heat 5 ml with 0.1 ml of 1M *sulphuric acid*. Acetaldehyde, recognisable by its odour, is evolved.

C. To 5 ml of solution A add 5 ml of *ammoniacal silver nitrate solution* in a test-tube and heat on a water-bath. Silver is deposited as a mirror on the side of the tube.

Acidity Titrate 50 ml of solution A with 0.1M *sodium hydroxide VS* using 0.05 ml of *dilute phenolphthalein solution* as indicator. Not more than 1.5 ml of 0.1M *sodium hydroxide VS* is required to change the colour of the solution.

Distillation range Not more than 10% distils below 123° and not less than 95% distils below 126°, Appendix V C.

Freezing point 10° to 13°, Appendix V B.

Refractive index 1.403 to 1.406, Appendix V E.

Relative density 0.991 to 0.996, Appendix V G.

Acetaldehyde Shake 5 ml with a mixture of 5 ml of *ethanol (60%)*, 5 ml of *hydroxylamine solution in ethanol (60%)* and 0.2 ml of *methyl orange solution*. Not more than 0.8 ml of 0.5M *sodium hydroxide VS* is required to change the colour of the solution to a pure yellow.

Peroxides To 50 ml of solution A in a stoppered vessel add 5 ml of 1M *sulphuric acid* and 10 ml of 1M *potassium iodide*, close the vessel and allow to stand protected from light for 15 minutes. Titrate with 0.1M *sodium thiosulphate VS* using 1 ml of *starch solution* as indicator, allow to stand for 5 minutes and, if necessary, complete the titration. Not more than 2.0 ml of 0.1M *sodium thiosulphate VS* is required.

Non-volatile matter Evaporate 5 ml on a water-bath and dry at 105° for 1 hour. The residue weighs not more than 3 mg (0.06% w/v).

Storage Paraldehyde should be kept in a small, well-filled, airtight container, protected from light and stored at a temperature of 8° to 15°. When solidified, the whole of the contents of the container should be liquefied before use.

Labelling The label states the name and proportion of any antioxidant.

Preparation
Paraldehyde Injection

Action and use Anticonvulsant.

Penicillamine

D-Penicillamine

$$HS-\underset{\underset{CH_3}{|}}{\overset{\overset{CH_3}{|}}{C}}-\underset{\underset{NH_2}{|}}{\overset{\overset{H}{|}}{C}}-CO_2H$$

$C_5H_{11}NO_2S$ 149.2   52-67-5

Penicillamine is 3,3-dimethyl-D-cysteine. It contains not less than 95.0 per cent and not more than 100.5 per cent of $C_5H_{11}NO_2S$, calculated with reference to the dried substance.

Characteristics A white or almost white, finely crystalline powder; odour, characteristic.

Solubility Soluble in 9 parts of *water*; slightly soluble in *ethanol (96%)*; practically insoluble in *chloroform* and in *ether*.

Identification A. Dissolve 20 mg in 4 ml of *water* and add 2 ml of *phosphotungstic acid solution*. A deep blue colour is produced on standing for a few minutes.

B. Dissolve 0.5 g in 5 ml of warm *acetone* containing 0.5 ml of *hydrochloric acid*, cool in ice and scratch the inside of the tube with a glass rod; a white precipitate is produced. Filter, wash the precipitate with *acetone* and dry in a current of air. A 1% w/v solution of the precipitate is dextrorotatory.

C. Dissolve 10 mg in 5 ml of *water* and add 0.05 ml of 5M *sodium hydroxide* and 20 mg of *ninhydrin*. An intense blue or violet-blue colour is produced immediately.

Acidity pH of a 1% w/v solution, 4.5 to 5.5, Appendix V L.

Specific optical rotation In a 5% w/v solution in 1M *sodium hydroxide*, −58° to −68°, Appendix V F.

Mercuric salts Not more than 40 ppm when determined by the following method. Disperse 1 g in 10 ml of *water* in a stoppered flask, add 0.2 ml of 9M *perchloric acid* and swirl to dissolve. Add 1 ml of *ammonium pyrrolidine-dithiocarbamate solution*, mix, add 2 ml of *4-methylpentan-2-one*, shake well for 1 minute and add sufficient *water* to produce 25 ml. Determine by *atomic absorption spectrophotometry*, Appendix II D, introducing the methylpentanone layer into the flame, measuring at 254 nm and using *4-methylpentan-2-one* in place of *water*. Use *mercury solution ASp*, suitably diluted with *water*, for the standard solutions, adjusted to contain the same concentrations of 9M *perchloric acid*, *ammonium pyrrolidinedithiocarbamate solution* and *4-methylpentan-2-one* as the solution being examined.

Penicillamine disulphide Carry out the method for *thin-layer chromatography*, Appendix III A, using *silica gel G* as the coating substance and a mixture of 50 volumes of *butyl acetate*, 30 volumes of *butan-1-ol*, 30 volumes of *methanol*, 20 volumes of *water* and 5 volumes of 6M *acetic acid* as the mobile phase. Apply separately to the chromatoplate 5 µl of each of two solutions containing (1) 2.0% w/v of the substance being examined and (2) 0.040% w/v of D-*penicillamine disulphide*. After removal of the plate, allow it to dry in air and spray with a 2% w/v solution of *ninhydrin* in *ethanol (96%)*. Heat at 105° for 5 minutes or until spots begin to appear. Any spot corresponding to penicillamine disulphide in the chromatogram obtained with solution (1) is not more intense than the spot in the chromatogram obtained with solution (2).

Benzylpenicilloic acid and benzylpenicillin Carry out the method described in the test for Penicillamine disulphide using as solution (2) a 0.020% w/v solution of the substance being examined. After removal of the chromatoplate, allow it to dry in air and spray with a mixture of 100 ml of a 1% w/v solution of *soluble starch*, 6 ml of *glacial acetic acid* and 3 ml of *iodine solution*. Any *secondary spot* in the chromatogram obtained with solution (1) is not more intense than the spot in the chromatogram obtained with solution (2).

Loss on drying When dried to constant weight at 60° at a pressure not exceeding 0.7 kPa, loses not more than 0.5% of its weight. Use 1 g.

Sulphated ash Not more than 1.0%, Appendix IX A.

Assay Dissolve 0.1 g in 50 ml of *water*, add 5 ml of 1M *sodium hydroxide* and 0.2 ml of a 0.1% w/v solution of *dithizone* in *ethanol (96%)* and titrate with 0.02M *mercury(II) nitrate VS*. Each ml of 0.02M *mercury(II) nitrate VS* is equivalent to 0.005968 g of $C_5H_{11}NO_2S$.

Preparation
Penicillamine Tablets

Action and use Used in treatment of rheumatoid arthritis and in treatment of lead poisoning.

Pentagastrin

Boc-βAla-Trp-Met-Asp-Phe—NH₂

$C_{37}H_{49}N_7O_9S$ 767.9   5534-95-2

Pentagastrin is a pentapeptide that stimulates gastric secretion of acid. It contains not less than 97.0 per cent and not more than 103.0 per cent of $C_{37}H_{49}N_7O_9S$, calculated with reference to the dried substance.

Characteristics A white or almost white powder.

Solubility Practically insoluble in *water*; slightly soluble in *ethanol (96%)*; soluble in *5M ammonia* and in *dimethylformamide*.

Identification A. The *light absorption*, Appendix II B, in the range 230 to 350 nm of a 0.010% w/v solution in 0.01M *ammonia* exhibits maxima at 280 nm and 288 nm and an inflection at 275 nm.
B. Carry out the method for *thin-layer chromatography*, Appendix III A, using *silica gel G* as the coating substance on each of three chromatoplates and the following solvent systems as the mobile phases: (A) a mixture of 75 volumes of *butan 2-ol* and 25 volumes of a 3% v/v solution of 13.5M *ammonia*, (B) the upper layer produced by shaking together 50 volumes of *water*, 40 volumes of *butan-1-ol* and 10 volumes of *glacial acetic acid* and allowing to separate and (C) a mixture of 50 volumes of *glacial acetic acid*, 25 volumes of *ether* and 25 volumes of *water*. Apply separately to each plate 2 µl of each of two solutions in 0.1M *ammonia* containing (1) 0.5% w/v of the substance being examined and (2) *pentagastrin BPCRS* containing 0.5% w/v of pentagastrin. After removal of the plates, allow them to dry in air, heat at 100° for 2 minutes, spray with a 1.0% w/v solution of *4-dimethylaminobenzaldehyde* in a mixture of 3 volumes of *methanol* and 1 volume of *hydrochloric acid* and heat at 100° until purple spots are produced (about 2 minutes). Examine by transmitted light. On each plate, the principal spot in the chromatogram obtained with solution (1) corresponds to that in the chromatogram obtained with solution (2).

Light absorption Ratio of the *absorbance* of a 0.010% w/v solution in 0.01M *ammonia* at the maximum at 280 nm to that at the maximum at 288 nm, 1.12 to 1.22, Appendix II B.

Specific optical rotation In a 1% w/v solution in *dimethylformamide*, −25.0° to −29.0°, Appendix V F.

Amino acids β-Alanine, 11.0 to 12.2%, aspartic acid, 16.4 to 18.2%, methionine, 18.4 to 20.4% and phenylalanine, 20.4 to 22.6%, when determined by *amino acid analysis*, Appendix III G, using 1 mg. Standardise the apparatus with 1 mg of an equimolar mixture of β-alanine, aspartic acid, methionine and phenylalanine.

Related substances Carry out the method for *thin-layer chromatography*, Appendix III A, using *silica gel G* as the coating substance and a mixture of 100 volumes of *ether*, 20 volumes of *glacial acetic acid* and 10 volumes of *water*

as the mobile phase. Apply separately to the chromato-plate 10 µl of each of two solutions of the substance being examined in a mixture of 24 volumes of *methanol* and 1 volume of 13.5M *ammonia* containing (1) 0.50% w/v and (2) 0.010% w/v. After removal of the plate, allow it to dry in air, heat at 100° for 2 minutes, spray with a 1.0% w/v solution of *4-dimethylaminobenzaldehyde* in a mixture of 3 volumes of *methanol* and 1 volume of *hydrochloric acid* and heat at 100° until purple spots are produced (about 2 minutes). Examine by transmitted light. Any *secondary spot* in the chromatogram obtained with solution (1) is not more intense than the spot in the chromatogram obtained with solution (2).

Loss on drying When dried over *phosphorus pentoxide* at a pressure not exceeding 0.7 kPa for 24 hours, loses not more than 0.5% of its weight. Use 1 g.

Assay Dissolve 5 mg in sufficient 0.01M *ammonia* to produce 100 ml and measure the *absorbance* at the maximum at 280 nm, Appendix II B. Calculate the content of $C_{37}H_{49}N_7O_9S$ taking 70 as the value of A(1%, 1 cm) at the maximum at 280 nm.

Storage Pentagastrin should be protected from light.

Preparation
Pentagastrin Injection

Action and use Peptide stimulating gastric secretion.

Pentamidine Isethionate

$C_{19}H_{24}N_4O_2,2C_2H_6O_4S$ 592.7   140-64-7

Pentamidine Isethionate is 4,4'-(pentamethyl-enedioxy)dibenzamidine bis(2-hydroxyethane-sulphonate). It contains not less than 98.5 per cent and not more than 102.5 per cent of $C_{19}H_{24}N_4O_2,2C_2H_6O_4S$, calculated with reference to the dried substance.

Characteristics White or almost white crystals or powder; odourless or almost odourless; hygroscopic.

Solubility Soluble in 10 parts of *water*; slightly soluble in *ethanol (96%)*; practically insoluble in *chloroform* and in *ether*.

Identification A. The *infra-red absorption spectrum*, Appendix II A, is concordant with the *reference spectrum* of pentamidine isethionate.
B. The *light absorption*, Appendix II B, in the range 230 to 350 nm of a 0.002% w/v solution in 0.01M *hydrochloric acid* exhibits a maximum only at 262 nm. The *absorbance* at 262 nm is about 0.95.
C. To 10 ml of a 0.05% w/v solution add 1 ml of a 0.1% w/v solution of *glyoxal sodium bisulphite* and 1 ml of a solution prepared by dissolving 4 g of *boric acid* in a mixture of 27 ml of 1M *sodium hydroxide* and sufficient *water* to produce 100 ml. Heat on a water-bath for 10 minutes. A magenta colour is produced.

Acidity pH of a 5% w/v solution, 4.5 to 6.5, Appendix V L.

Melting point 188° to 192°, Appendix V A.

Ammonium isethionate To 1 g in a test-tube about 4 cm in diameter add 10 ml of *water* and 20 ml of 1M *sodium* *hydroxide*. Immediately insert a stopper carrying a splash head and an aspirator tube about 0.5 cm in diameter. Connect the splash head to two test-tubes in series, each containing 20 ml of 0.01M *sulphuric acid VS*. Heat the tube containing the substance being examined in a water-bath at 45° to 50° and, maintaining this temperature, draw a current of air, previously passed through 1M *sulphuric acid*, through the liquids in the series of tubes for 3 hours at such a rate that the bubbles are just too rapid to count. Titrate the combined solutions from the two absorption tubes with 0.02M *sodium hydroxide VS* using *methyl red— methylene blue solution* as indicator. Not less than 36.5 ml is required.

Related substances Carry out the method for *thin-layer chromatography*, Appendix III A, using a silica gel F254 precoated chromatoplate (Merck silica gel 60 F254 plates are suitable) activated by heating at 105° for 1 hour and as the mobile phase the upper layer obtained by shaking together 100 volumes of *water*, 80 volumes of *butan-1-ol* and 20 volumes of *glacial acetic acid*. Apply separately to the plate 10 μl of each of two solutions of the substance being examined in *methanol* containing (1) 5.0% w/v and (2) 0.025% w/v. After removal of the plate, allow it to dry in air and examine under *ultra-violet light (254 nm)*. Any *secondary spot* in the chromatogram obtained with solution (1) is not more intense than the spot in the chromatogram obtained with solution (2).

Loss on drying When dried to constant weight at 105°, loses not more than 4.0% of its weight. Use 1 g.

Sulphated ash Not more than 0.1%, Appendix IX A.

Assay Carry out Method I for the *determination of nitrogen*, Appendix VIII H, using 0.4 g and 9 ml of *nitrogen-free sulphuric acid*. Each ml of 0.05M *sulphuric acid VS* is equivalent to 0.01482 g of $C_{19}H_{24}N_4O_2,2C_2H_6O_4S$.

Storage Pentamidine Isethionate should be kept in a well-closed container.

Preparation
Pentamidine Injection

Action and use Anti-protozoal.

Pentazocine

$C_{19}H_{27}NO$ 285.4   *359-83-1*

Pentazocine is $(2R\star,6R\star,11R\star)$-1,2,3,4,5,6-hexahydro-6,11-dimethyl-3-(3-methylbut-2-enyl)-2,6-methano-3-benzazocin-8-ol. It contains not less than 98.0 per cent and not more than 101.0 per cent of $C_{19}H_{27}NO$, calculated with reference to the dried substance.

Characteristics A white or creamy-white powder; odourless or almost odourless.

Solubility Practically insoluble in *water*; soluble in 15 parts of *ethanol (96%)*, in 2 parts of *chloroform* and in 33 parts of *ether*.

Identification A. The *infra-red absorption spectrum*, Appendix II A, is concordant with the *reference spectrum* of pentazocine (form A).
B. To 1 mg in a porcelain crucible add 0.5 ml of a 1% w/v solution of *ammonium molybdate* in *sulphuric acid*. An intense blue colour is produced which changes to bluish-green, green and finally, on standing, yellow.
C. Dissolve 5 mg in 5 ml of *sulphuric acid*, add 0.05 ml of a 9% w/v solution of *iron(III) chloride* and mix; a yellow colour is produced which deepens slightly in intensity on warming. On the addition of 0.05 ml of *nitric acid* the yellow colour is unchanged.

Melting point 150° to 155°, Appendix V A.

Light absorption To 0.1 g add 20 ml of *water* and 1 ml of 1M *hydrochloric acid*, shake to dissolve and add sufficient *water* to produce 100 ml. To 10 ml add 1 ml of 1M *hydrochloric acid* and dilute to 100 ml with *water*. The *absorbance* of the resulting solution at the maximum at 278 nm is 0.67 to 0.71, Appendix II B.

Related substances Carry out the method for *thin-layer chromatography*, Appendix III A, using a silica gel F254 precoated chromatoplate (Merck silica gel 60 F254 plates are suitable) and a mixture of 94 volumes of *chloroform*, 3 volumes of *isopropylamine* and 3 volumes of *methanol* as the mobile phase. Apply separately to the plate 10 μl of each of four solutions of the substance being examined in *chloroform* containing (1) 2.0% w/v, (2) 0.020% w/v, (3) 0.010% w/v and (4) 0.0050% w/v. After removal of the plate, allow it to dry in air and examine under *ultra-violet light (254 nm)*. Heat the plate at 105° for 15 minutes, allow to cool, expose to iodine vapour and re-examine under *ultra-violet light (254 nm)*. In the chromatogram obtained with solution (1) any *secondary spot* is not more intense than the spot in the chromatogram obtained with solution (2), not more than one such spot is more intense than the spot in the chromatogram obtained with solution (3) and not more than four such spots are more intense than the spot in the chromatogram obtained with solution (4).

Loss on drying When dried at 60° at a pressure not exceeding 0.7 kPa for 4 hours, loses not more than 1.0% of its weight. Use 1 g.

Sulphated ash Not more than 0.1%, Appendix IX A.

Assay Carry out Method I for *non-aqueous titration*, Appendix VIII A, using 0.6 g and *crystal violet solution* as indicator. Each ml of 0.1M *perchloric acid VS* is equivalent to 0.02854 g of $C_{19}H_{27}NO$.

Storage Pentazocine should be kept in a well-closed container and protected from light.

Preparation
Pentazocine Injection

Action and use Analgesic.

Pentazocine Hydrochloride

$C_{19}H_{27}NO,HCl$ 321.9   *64024-15-3*

Pentazocine Hydrochloride is $(2R\star,6R\star,11R\star)$-1,2,3,4,5,6-hexahydro-6,11-dimethyl-3-(3-methylbut-2-enyl)-2,6-methano-3-benzazocin-8-ol hydrochloride. It contains not less than 98.0 per cent and not more than 101.0 per cent of C$_{19}$H$_{27}$NO,HCl, calculated with reference to the dried substance.

Characteristics A white or pale cream powder; odourless or almost odourless.

Solubility Soluble in 42 parts of *water*, in 16 parts of *ethanol (96%)* and in 8 parts of *chloroform*; practically insoluble in *ether*.

Identification A. The *infra-red absorption spectrum*, Appendix II A, is concordant with the *reference spectrum* of pentazocine hydrochloride.

B. To 1 mg in a porcelain crucible add 0.5 ml of a 1% w/v solution of *ammonium molybdate* in *sulphuric acid*. An intense blue colour is produced which changes to bluish-green, green and finally, on standing, yellow.

C. Dissolve 5 mg in 5 ml of *sulphuric acid*, add 0.05 ml of a 9% w/v solution of *iron(III) chloride* and mix; a yellow colour is produced which deepens slightly in intensity on warming. On the addition of 0.05 ml of *nitric acid* the yellow colour is unchanged.

D. Yields *reaction A* characteristic of chlorides, Appendix VI.

Acidity pH of a 1% w/v solution, 4.0 to 6.0, Appendix V L.

Light absorption Dissolve 0.1 g in 10 ml of 1M *hydrochloric acid* and add sufficient *water* to produce 100 ml. Dilute 10 ml to 100 ml with *water*. The *absorbance* of the resulting solution at the maximum at 278 nm is 0.59 to 0.63, Appendix II B.

Related substances Carry out the method for *thin-layer chromatography*, Appendix III A, using a silica gel F254 precoated chromatoplate (Merck silica gel 60 F254 plates are suitable) and a mixture of 94 volumes of *chloroform*, 3 volumes of *isopropylamine* and 3 volumes of *methanol* as the mobile phase. Apply separately to the plate 10 μl of each of four solutions of the substance being examined in *chloroform* containing (1) 2.0% w/v, (2) 0.020% w/v, (3) 0.010% w/v and (4) 0.0050% w/v. After removal of the plate, allow it to dry in air and examine under *ultra-violet light (254 nm)*. Heat the plate at 105° for 15 minutes, allow to cool, expose to iodine vapour and re-examine under *ultra-violet light (254 nm)*. In the chromatogram obtained with solution (1) any *secondary spot* is not more intense than the spot in the chromatogram obtained with solution (2), not more than one such spot is more intense than the spot in the chromatogram obtained with solution (3) and not more than four such spots are more intense than the spot in the chromatogram obtained with solution (4).

Loss on drying When dried to constant weight at 100° at a pressure not exceeding 0.7 kPa, loses not more than 1.0% of its weight. Use 1 g.

Sulphated ash Not more than 0.1%, Appendix IX A.

Assay Carry out Method I for *non-aqueous titration*, Appendix VIII A, using 0.5 g and *crystal violet solution* as indicator. Each ml of 0.1M *perchloric acid VS* is equivalent to 0.03219 g of C$_{19}$H$_{27}$NO,HCl.

Storage Pentazocine Hydrochloride should be kept in a well-closed container and protected from light.

Preparation
Pentazocine Tablets

Action and use Analgesic.

Pentobarbitone ☆

C$_{11}$H$_{18}$N$_2$O$_3$ 226.3   76-74-4

Pentobarbitone is 5-ethyl-5-(1-methylbutyl)-barbituric acid. It contains not less than 99.0 per cent and not more than 101.0 per cent of C$_{11}$H$_{18}$N$_2$O$_3$, calculated with reference to the dried substance.

Characteristics Colourless crystals or a white, crystalline powder; odourless.

Solubility Very slightly soluble in *water*; freely soluble in *absolute ethanol*, in *chloroform* and in *ether*. It dissolves in aqueous solutions of alkali hydroxides and carbonates and in aqueous ammonia.

Identification A. Complies with the test for *identification of barbiturates*, Appendix III A.

B. To 10 mg add 10 mg of *vanillin* and 2 ml of *sulphuric acid*, mix and heat for 2 minutes on a water-bath; a brownish-red colour is produced. Cool and add cautiously 5 ml of *absolute ethanol (96%)*; the colour changes to violet and then to blue.

C. Determine the *melting point* of the substance being examined, Appendix V A, Method I. Mix equal quantities of the substance being examined and *pentobarbital EPCRS* and determine the *melting point* of the mixture. The difference between the melting points, which are about 133°, is not more than 2°.

Acidity Boil 1 g for 2 minutes with 50 ml of *water*, cool and filter. To 10 ml of the filtrate add 0.15 ml of *methyl red solution*. The solution is orange-yellow and not more than 0.1 ml of 0.1M *sodium hydroxide VS* is required to change the colour of the solution to a pure yellow.

Clarity and colour of solution Dissolve 1.0 g in a mixture of 4 ml of 2M *sodium hydroxide* and 6 ml of *water*. The solution is *clear*, Appendix IV A, and not more intensely coloured than *reference solution Y$_6$*, Appendix IV B, Method II.

Isomer Dissolve 0.3 g in 5 ml of a 5% w/v solution of *anhydrous sodium carbonate*, heating gently if necessary. Add a solution of 0.3 g of *4-nitrobenzyl chloride* in 10 ml of *ethanol (96%)* and heat under a reflux condenser for 30 minutes. Cool to 25°, filter and wash the precipitate with five 5-ml quantities of *water*. Heat the precipitate with 25 ml of *ethanol (96%)* in a small flask under a reflux condenser until dissolved (about 10 minutes), cool to 25° and, if necessary, scratch the wall of the flask with a glass rod to induce crystallisation. Filter, wash the precipitate with two 5-ml quantities of *water* and dry at 100° to 105° for 30 minutes. The *melting point* of the dried precipitate is 136° to 148°, Appendix V A, Method I.

Related substances Complies with the test for *related substances in barbiturates*, Appendix III A.

Loss on drying When dried to constant weight at 100° to 105°, loses not more than 0.5% of its weight. Use 1 g.

Sulphated ash Not more than 0.1%, Appendix IX A, Method II. Use 1 g.

Assay Dissolve 0.1 g in 5 ml of *pyridine*, add 10 ml of *silver nitrate—pyridine reagent* and titrate with 0.1M *ethanolic sodium hydroxide VS*, using 0.5 ml of *thymolphthalein solution* as indicator, until a pure blue colour is obtained. Repeat the operation without the substance being examined. The difference between the titrations represents the amount of sodium hydroxide required. Each ml of 0.1M *ethanolic sodium hydroxide VS* is equivalent to 0.01131 g of $C_{11}H_{18}N_2O_3$.

Action and use Hypnotic.

The title of the monograph in the European Pharmacopœia is Pentobarbital.

Pentobarbitone Sodium ☆

$C_{11}H_{17}N_2NaO_3$ 248.3   *57-53-0*

Pentobarbitone Sodium is sodium 5-ethyl-5-(1-methylbutyl)barbiturate. It contains not less than 99.0 per cent and not more than 101.5 per cent of $C_{11}H_{17}N_2NaO_3$, calculated with reference to the dried substance.

Characteristics A white, crystalline powder; hygroscopic.

Solubility Very soluble in *water* and in *ethanol (96%)*; practically insoluble in *ether*.

Identification A. To 10 ml of a 10% w/v solution add 5 ml of 2M *acetic acid*. A white, crystalline precipitate is produced which, after washing with *water* and drying at 100° to 105°, complies with the following test.

Carry out the test for Related substances but allow the solvent front to ascend 18 cm above the line of application and use the following solutions. For solution (1) dissolve 25 mg of the precipitate in *ethanol (96%)* and dilute to 25 ml with the same solvent. Solution (2) contains 0.1% w/v of *pentobarbital EPCRS* in *ethanol (96%)*. After removal of the plate, examine immediately under *ultra-violet light (254 nm)*. The principal spot in the chromatogram obtained with solution (1) is similar in position and size to that in the chromatogram obtained with solution (2).

B. To 10 mg add 10 mg of *vanillin* and 2 ml of *sulphuric acid*, mix and heat on a water-bath for 2 minutes; a reddish-brown colour is produced. Cool and add 5 ml of *ethanol (96%)*; the colour changes to violet and then to blue.

C. Determine the *melting points*, Appendix V A, Method I, of the dried precipitate obtained in test A and of a mixture of equal parts of the dried precipitate and *pentobarbital EPCRS*. The difference between the melting points, which are about 131°, is not greater than 2°.

D. Ignite 1 g. The residue yields *reaction A* characteristic of sodium salts, Appendix VI.

Alkalinity pH of a freshly prepared 10% w/v solution, 9.6 to 11.0, Appendix V L.

Heavy metals To 7.5 ml of a 10% w/v solution add 2.5 ml of 2M *acetic acid* and 2.5 ml of *acetate buffer pH 3.5*, filter and dilute the filtrate to 15 ml with *water*. 12 ml of the solution complies with *limit test A for heavy metals*, Appendix VII (20 ppm). In preparing the sample solution replace the buffer solution with *water*. Use *lead standard solution (1 ppm Pb)* to prepare the standard.

Free pentobarbitone Not more than 3.5% when determined by the following method. Dissolve 2 g in 75 ml of *dimethylformamide*, warming gently if necessary, and titrate with 0.1M *sodium methoxide VS*, using 0.25 ml of a 1% w/v solution of *thymol blue* in *dimethylformamide* as indicator, until the colour changes from olive green to blue. Repeat the operation without the substance being examined. The difference between the titrations represents the amount of sodium methoxide required. Each ml of 0.1M *sodium methoxide VS* is equivalent to 0.02263 g of pentobarbitone.

Isomer Dissolve 0.3 g in 5 ml of a 5% w/v solution of *anhydrous sodium carbonate*, heating gently if necessary. Add 10 ml of a 3% w/v solution of *4-nitrobenzyl chloride* in *ethanol (96%)* and heat under a reflux condenser for 30 minutes. Cool to 25°, scratch the walls of the vessel with a glass rod if necessary to induce crystallisation, filter and wash the precipitate with five 5-ml quantities of *water*. Heat the precipitate with 25 ml of *ethanol (96%)* in a small flask under a reflux condenser until dissolved (about 10 minutes), cool to 25° and, if necessary, scratch the wall of the flask with a glass rod to induce crystallisation. Filter, wash the precipitate with two 5-ml quantities of *water* and dry at 100° to 105° for 30 minutes. The *melting point* of the dried precipitate is 136° to 148°, Appendix V A, Method I.

Related substances Carry out the method for *thin-layer chromatography*, Appendix III A, using *silica gel GF254* as the coating substance and the lower layer of a mixture of 80 volumes of *chloroform*, 15 volumes of *ethanol (96%)* and 5 volumes of 13.5M *ammonia* as the mobile phase. Apply separately to the chromatoplate 10 µl of each of two solutions of the substance being examined in *ethanol (96%)* containing (1) 2.0% w/v and (2) 0.010% w/v. After removal of the plate, examine it immediately under *ultra-violet light (254 nm)*. Spray the plate with *diphenyl-carbazone—mercury reagent*, allow to dry in air, spray with *ethanolic potassium hydroxide solution* previously diluted 1 in 5 with *aldehyde-free ethanol (96%)*, heat at 100° to 105° for 5 minutes and examine immediately in daylight. By both methods of visualisation, any *secondary spot* in the chromatogram obtained with solution (1) is not more intense than the spot in the chromatogram obtained with solution (2).

Loss on drying When dried to constant weight at 100° to 105°, loses not more than 3.0% of its weight. Use 1 g.

Assay Dissolve 0.2 g in 15 ml of a 12.75% w/v solution of *silver nitrate* in *pyridine* and titrate with 0.1M *ethanolic sodium hydroxide VS*, using 0.5 ml of *thymolphthalein solution* as indicator, until a pure blue colour is obtained. Repeat the operation without the substance being examined. The difference between the titrations represents the amount of sodium hydroxide required. Each ml of 0.1M *ethanolic sodium hydroxide VS* is equivalent to 0.02483 g of $C_{11}H_{17}N_2NaO_3$.

Storage Pentobarbitone Sodium should be kept in an airtight container.

Preparations
Pentobarbitone Capsules
Pentobarbitone Tablets

Action and use Hypnotic.

The title of the monograph in the European Pharmacopœia is Pentobarbital Sodium.

Peppermint Leaf ☆

Peppermint Leaf consists of the dried leaves of *Mentha × piperita* L.

Characteristics Odour, characteristic and penetrating; taste, aromatic and characteristic.

Macroscopical Leaf, entire or broken, thin, fragile often crumpled, green to brownish-green, and in some varieties with brownish-purple veins; lamina 3 to 9 cm long and 1 to 3 cm wide, oval or lanceolate, apex acuminate, margin sharply dentate, base asymmetrical; venation pinnate, prominent on the lower surface, lateral veins leaving the midrib at an angle of about 45°; lower surface slightly pubescent and with glandular trichomes visible under a hand lens (6×) as bright yellowish points; petiole, grooved, 5 to 10 mm long.

Microscopical Lower epidermal cells, in surface view, isodiametric with sinuous and pitted anticlinal walls, cuticle striated over the veins; stomata *diacytic*, numerous on the lower surface, absent or very rare on the upper surface; covering trichomes, short, conical, unicellular or bicellular, or elongated and uniseriate, three- to eight-celled, with striated cuticle; glandular trichomes of two types (a) unicellular base with small, rounded unicellular head 15 to 25 μm in diameter and (b) unicellular base with large oval head, 55 to 70 μm in diameter, consisting of eight radiating cells; upper epidermal cells with sinuous and pitted anticlinal walls. Leaf dorsiventral with a single layer of palisade cells and four to six layers of spongy mesophyll. Midrib containing collateral bundles with narrow medullary rays and sub-epidermal collenchyma. Calcium oxalate crystals absent.

Identification Carry out the method for *thin-layer chromatography*, Appendix III A, using *silica gel GF254* as the coating substance and a mixture of 95 volumes of *toluene* and 5 volumes of *ethyl acetate* as the mobile phase. Apply separately to the chromatoplate, as bands 20 mm × 3 mm, 20 μl of solution (1) and 10 μl of solution (2). For solution (1) add 2 ml of *dichloromethane* to 0.2 g of the freshly bruised leaves, shake for a few minutes, filter, evaporate the filtrate to dryness at 40° and dissolve the residue in 0.1 ml of *toluene*. For solution (2) dissolve 50 mg of (−)-*menthol*, 20 μl of *cineole*, 10 mg of *thymol* and 10 μl of *menthyl acetate* in sufficient *toluene* to produce 10 ml. After removal of the plate, allow it to dry in air until the odour of the solvent in no longer detectable and examine under *ultra-violet light (254 nm)*. In the chromatogram obtained with solution (1) there are no quenching bands at Rf values slightly lower than that of the faint band due to thymol in the chromatogram obtained with solution (2) (carvone and pulegone). Spray the plate with *anisaldehyde solution* and examine while heating at 100° to 105° for 5 to 10 minutes. The chromatogram obtained with solution (2) shows, in order of increasing Rf value, a deep blue to violet band (menthol), a violet-blue to brown band (cineole), a pink band (thymol) and a bluish-violet band (menthyl acetate). The chromatogram obtained with solution (1) shows an intense band corresponding to menthol, a faint band corresponding to cineole, a bluish-violet band corresponding to menthyl acetate and at a slightly lower Rf value a greenish band (menthone). The chromatogram obtained with solution (1) does not show intense greyish-green or faint bluish-grey bands at Rf values between those of cineole and thymol in the chromatogram obtained with solution (2) (carvone, pulegone, isomenthone). The chromatogram obtained with solution (1) shows an intense reddish-violet band near the solvent front (hydrocarbons) and a brownish-yellow band (menthofuran) at a slightly lower Rf value. Other less intensely coloured bands may also be seen.

Foreign matter Not more than 5% of stem; diameter of the stems, not greater than 1 mm; not more than 2% of foreign elements, Appendix XI D, Test B. Use 10 g.

Not more than 10% of leaf showing brown stains due to *Puccinia menthae*.

Acid-insoluble ash Not more than 1.5%, Appendix XI K, Method II. Use 1 g, in powder.

Water Not more than 11.0%, Appendix IX C, Method II. Use 20 g.

Volatile oil Not less than 1.2% v/w, Appendix XI E, using a 500-ml flask, 200 ml of *water* as the distillation liquid and 0.50 ml of *xylene* in the graduated tube. Use 20 g and distil at a rate of 2 to 4 ml per minute for 2 hours.

Storage Peppermint Leaf should be kept in a well-closed container and protected from light.

Action and use Carminative.

Peppermint Oil ☆

Peppermint Oil is obtained by steam distillation from the aerial parts of the flowering plant of *Mentha × piperita* L. It contains not less than 4.5 per cent w/w and not more than 10.0 per cent w/w of esters, calculated as menthyl acetate, $C_{12}H_{22}O_2$, not less than 44.0 per cent w/w of free alcohols, calculated as menthol, $C_{10}H_{20}O$, and not less than 15.0 per cent w/w and not more than 32.0 per cent w/w of ketones, calculated as menthone, $C_{10}H_{18}O$.

Characteristics A colourless, pale yellow or greenish-yellow liquid; odour, characteristic; taste, characteristic followed by a sensation of cold.

Identification Carry out the method for *thin-layer chromatography*, Appendix III A, using *silica gel GF254* as the coating substance and a mixture of 95 volumes of *toluene* and 5 volumes of *ethyl acetate* as the mobile phase. Apply separately to the chromatoplate, as bands 20 mm × 3 mm, 20 μl of solution (1) and 10 μl of solution (2). Solution (1) contains 1% w/v of the oil in *toluene*. For solution (2) dissolve 50 mg of (−)-*menthol*, 20 μl of *cineole*, 10 mg of *thymol* and 10 μl of *menthyl acetate* in sufficient *toluene* to produce 10 ml. After removal of the plate, allow it to dry in air until the odour of solvent is no longer detectable and examine under *ultra-violet light (254 nm)*. In the chromatogram obtained with solution (1) there are no quenching bands at Rf values slightly lower than that of the faint band due to thymol in the chromatogram obtained with solution (2) (carvone and pulegone). Spray the plate with *anisaldehyde solution* and examine in daylight while heating at 100° to 105° for 5 to 10 minutes. The chromatogram obtained with solution (2) shows, in order of increasing Rf value, an intense blue to violet band (menthol) in the lower third, a violet-blue to brown band (cineole), a pink band (thymol) and a violet-blue band (menthyl acetate). The chromatogram obtained with solution (1) shows an intense band corresponding to menthol, a band corresponding to cineole, a violet-blue band corresponding to menthyl acetate and at a slightly lower Rf value a greenish band (menthone). The chromatogram obtained with solution (1) does not show intense greyish-green or faint bluish-grey bands at Rf values between those of cineole and thymol in the chromatogram obtained with solution (2) (carvone, pulegone, isomenthone). The chromatogram obtained with solution (1) shows an intense reddish-violet band near the solvent front (hydrocarbons) and a brownish-yellow band (menthofuran) at a slightly lower Rf value; other less intensely coloured bands may also be seen.

Acidity To 2 g add 0.25 ml of *dilute phenolphthalein solution*. Not more than 0.1 ml of 0.5M *ethanolic potassium hydroxide VS* is required to change the colour of the solution.

Optical rotation $-16°$ to $-30°$, Appendix V F.

Refractive index 1.460 to 1.467, Appendix V E.

Relative density 0.900 to 0.912, Appendix V G.

Solubility in ethanol Soluble in 4 volumes of *ethanol (70%)*, Appendix X M. The solution may show an opalescence.

Dimethyl sulphide Distil 25 ml, collect the first 1 ml of the distillate and carefully superimpose it on 5 ml of a 6.5% w/v solution of *mercury(II) chloride*. No white film is produced within 1 minute at the interface of the two liquids.

Fixed oils and resinified volatile oils Complies with the test for *fixed oils and resinified volatile oils*, Appendix X M.

Assay *For esters* To 2 g in a borosilicate-glass flask add 2 ml of *ethanol (90%)* and 0.25 ml of *dilute phenolphthalein solution* and neutralise with 0.5M *ethanolic potassium hydroxide*. Add 25 ml of 0.5M *ethanolic potassium hydroxide VS* and a few pieces of porous pot and heat under a reflux condenser on a water-bath for 30 minutes. Add 1 ml of *dilute phenolphthalein solution* and immediately titrate with 0.5M *hydrochloric acid VS*. Repeat the operation without the oil. The difference between the titrations represents the volume of alkali required to saponify the esters. Each ml of 0.5M *ethanolic potassium hydroxide VS* is equivalent to 0.09915 g of esters, calculated as menthyl acetate, $C_{12}H_{22}O_2$.

For free alcohols To 1 g in a dry acetylation flask, of 125- to 150-ml volume, add 3 ml of a mixture of 1 volume of *acetic anhydride* and 3 volumes of *pyridine*. Determine the weight of the acetylation mixture to the nearest mg, keeping the flask well closed while weighing. Boil under a reflux condenser in a water-bath for 3 hours, maintaining the water level 2 to 3 cm above the level of the liquid in the flask throughout. Remove the flask from the bath and add 50 ml of *water* through the condenser, remove the condenser and wash the walls of the flask with 10 ml of *water*. Allow to stand for 15 minutes and titrate with 0.5M *sodium hydroxide VS* using 1 ml of *dilute phenolphthalein solution* as indicator. Repeat the operation without the oil. The difference between the titrations represents the volume of sodium hydroxide required. Each ml of 0.5M *sodium hydroxide VS* is equivalent to 0.07815 g of free alcohols, calculated as menthol, $C_{10}H_{20}O$. If the quantities of acetic anhydride in pyridine used in the two determinations differ by more than 5 mg, adjust the volume of alkali used in the second titration by

multiplying by a/b where a is the weight, in g, of acetic anhydride in pyridine used in the first test and b is the weight, in g, of acetic anhydride in pyridine used in the second test.

For ketones To 2 g add 25 ml of *hydroxylamine solution in ethanol (96%)*, heat on a water-bath for 1 hour, allow to cool, add about 1 mg of *methyl orange* and titrate with 0.5M *ethanolic potassium hydroxide VS* until an orange-yellow colour is obtained. Repeat the heating for further periods of 1 hour until, after cooling, not more than 0.1 ml of 0.5M *ethanolic potassium hydroxide VS* is required to neutralise the solution. Each ml of 0.5M *ethanolic potassium hydroxide VS* is equivalent to 0.0771 g of ketones, calculated as menthone, $C_{10}H_{18}O$.

Storage Peppermint Oil should be kept in a well-filled, airtight container and protected from light and heat.

Preparations
Concentrated Peppermint Emulsion
Peppermint Spirit

Action and use Flavour.

Perphenazine

$C_{21}H_{26}ClN_3OS$ 404.0   *58-39-9*

Perphenazine is 2-{4-[3-(2-chlorophenothiazin-10-yl)propyl]piperazin-1-yl}ethanol. It contains not less than 99.0 per cent and not more than 101.0 per cent of $C_{21}H_{26}ClN_3OS$, calculated with reference to the dried substance.

Characteristics A white or creamy-white powder; odourless or almost odourless.

Solubility Practically insoluble in *water*; soluble in 20 parts of *ethanol (96%)*, in 1 part of *chloroform* and in 80 parts of *ether*. It dissolves readily in 2M *hydrochloric acid*.

Identification A. The *infra-red absorption spectrum*, Appendix II A, is concordant with the *reference spectrum* of perphenazine.

B. The *light absorption*, Appendix II B, in the range 230 to 350 nm of a 0.0014% w/v solution in *absolute ethanol* exhibits a maximum at 258 nm and a less well-defined maximum at 315 nm. The *absorbance* at 258 nm is about 1.3.

C. Dissolve 5 mg in 2 ml of *sulphuric acid* and allow to stand for 5 minutes. A red colour is produced.

Melting point 96° to 100°, Appendix V A.

Related substances Complies with the test for *related substances in phenothiazines*, Appendix III A, using *mobile phase C* and applying separately to the chromatoplate 10 µl of each of two freshly prepared solutions of the substance being examined in *ethanol (96%)* containing (1) 1.0% w/v and (2) 0.0050% w/v.

Loss on drying When dried to constant weight at 65°, loses not more than 0.5% of its weight. Use 1 g.

Sulphated ash Not more than 0.1%, Appendix IX A.

Assay Carry out Method I for *non-aqueous titration*, Appendix VIII A, using 0.5 g and *crystal violet solution* as indicator. Each ml of 0.1M *perchloric acid VS* is equivalent to 0.02020 g of $C_{21}H_{26}ClN_3OS$.

Storage Perphenazine should be protected from light.

Preparations
Perphenazine Injection
Perphenazine Tablets

Action and use Antipsychotic; antiemetic.

Pethidine Hydrochloride ☆

$C_{15}H_{21}NO_2,HCl$ 283.8   *50-13-5*

Pethidine Hydrochloride is ethyl 1-methyl-4-phenylpiperidine-4-carboxylate hydrochloride. It contains not less than 99.0 per cent and not more than 101.0 per cent of $C_{15}H_{21}NO_2,HCl$, calculated with reference to the dried substance.

Characteristics A white, crystalline powder.

Solubility Very soluble in *water*; freely soluble in *ethanol (96%)* and in *chloroform*; practically insoluble in *ether*.

Identification *Test A may be omitted if tests B, C and D are carried out. Tests B and D may be omitted it tests A and C are carried out.*

A. The *infra-red absorption spectrum*, Appendix II A, is concordant with the European Pharmacopœia reference spectrum of pethidine hydrochloride.

B. Dissolve 0.1 g in 10 ml of *absolute ethanol* and add 10 ml of a 1% w/v solution of *2,4,6-trinitrophenol*. A crystalline precipitate is produced which, after washing with *water* and drying at 100° to 105°, has a *melting point* of 186° to 193°, Appendix V A, Method I. Mix a portion of the dried precipitate with an equal quantity of the substance being examined. The *melting point* of the mixture is not less than 20° lower than that of the precipitate.

C. A 1% w/v solution yields *reaction A* characteristic of chlorides, Appendix VI.

D. *Melting point*, 187° to 190°, Appendix V A, Method I.

Acidity or alkalinity To 10 ml of a 2% w/v solution in *carbon dioxide-free water* add 0.2 ml of *methyl red solution* and 0.2 ml of 0.01M *sodium hydroxide VS*; the solution is yellow. Add 0.3 ml of 0.01M *hydrochloric acid VS*; the solution is red.

Clarity and colour of solution A 2.0% w/v solution in *carbon dioxide-free water* is *clear*, Appendix IV A, and *colourless*, Appendix IV B, Method II.

Related substances Carry out the method for *thin-layer chromatography*, Appendix III A, using *kieselguhr G* as the coating substance but allowing the solvent front to ascend 12 cm above the line of application. Impregnate the dry chromatoplate by placing it in a tank containing 9 volumes of *acetone* and 1 volume of *2-phenoxyethanol* so that the plate dips about 5 mm beneath the surface of the liquid, allowing the impregnating solvent to ascend at least 15 cm, removing the plate from the tank and drying

in a current of air. Use immediately, with the flow of the mobile phase in the direction in which impregnation was carried out. Use as the mobile phase the upper layer obtained by shaking together 100 volumes of *petroleum spirit (boiling range, 40° to 60°)*, 8 volumes of *2-phenoxyethanol* and 1 volume of *diethylamine* and allowing to settle.

Apply separately to the plate 5 μl of each of the following solutions. For solution (1) dissolve 0.1 g in 5 ml of *water*, add 0.5 ml of 10M *sodium hydroxide* and 2 ml of *ether* and shake; allow the layers to separate and use the upper layer. For solution (2) dilute 0.5 ml of solution (1) to 50 ml with *ether*. After removal of the plate, allow it to dry in air for 10 minutes, return the plate to the tank and repeat the development. Remove the plate, allow it to dry in air for 10 minutes and spray with a 0.2% w/v solution of *2,7-dichlorofluorescein* in *methanol*. Allow to stand for 5 minutes and spray with *water* until the background is white to pale yellow. Examine in daylight. The chromatograms show red to orange spots. Any *secondary spot* in the chromatogram obtained with solution (1) is not more intense than the spot in the chromatogram obtained with solution (2). Examine without delay under *ultra-violet light (365 nm)*. The chromatograms show spots with intense yellow fluorescence. Any *secondary spot* in the chromatogram obtained with solution (1) is not more intense than the spot in the chromatogram obtained with solution (2).

Loss on drying When dried to constant weight at 100° to 105°, loses not more than 0.5% of its weight. Use 1 g.

Sulphated ash Not more than 0.1%, Appendix IX A, Method II. Use 1 g.

Assay Dissolve 0.2 g in 30 ml of *anhydrous glacial acetic acid*, add 5 ml of *mercury(II)* acetate solution and carry out Method I for *non-aqueous titration*, Appendix VIII A, using *crystal violet solution* as indicator. Each ml of 0.1M *perchloric acid VS* is equivalent to 0.02838 g of $C_{15}H_{21}NO_2,HCl$.

Storage Pethidine Hydrochloride should be kept in an airtight container and protected from light.

Preparations
Pethidine Injection
Pethidine Tablets

Action and use Narcotic analgesic.

Phenazone ☆

$C_{11}H_{12}N_2O$ 188.2   *60-80-0*

Phenazone is 2,3-dimethyl-1-phenyl-3-pyrazolin-5-one. It contains not less than 99.0 per cent and not more than 100.5 per cent of $C_{11}H_{12}N_2O$, calculated with reference to the dried substance.

Characteristics Colourless crystals or a white, crystalline powder.

Solubility Very soluble in *water*, in *ethanol (96%)* and in *chloroform*; sparingly soluble in *ether*.

Identification *Test A may be omitted if tests B, C and D are carried out. Tests B and C may be omitted if tests A and D are carried out.*

A. The *infra-red absorption spectrum*, Appendix II A, is concordant with the spectrum of *phenazone EPCRS*.

B. To 1 ml of a 5.0% w/v solution in *carbon dioxide-free water* (solution A) add 4 ml of *water* and 0.5 ml of a 1.3% w/v solution of *iron(III) chloride hexahydrate*. A red colour is produced which is discharged on the addition of 1M *sulphuric acid*.

C. To 1 ml of solution A add 4 ml of *water*, 0.25 ml of 1M *sulphuric acid* and 1 ml of *sodium nitrite solution*. A green colour is produced.

D. *Melting point*, 109° to 113°, Appendix V A, Method I.

Acidity or alkalinity To 10 ml of solution A add 0.1 ml of *dilute phenolphthalein solution*; the solution is colourless. Add 0.2 ml of 0.01M *sodium hydroxide VS*; the solution is red. Add 0.25 ml of *methyl red solution* and 0.4 ml of 0.01M *hydrochloric acid VS*; the solution is red or yellowish-red.

Clarity and colour of solution Solution A is *clear*, Appendix IV A, and *colourless*, Appendix IV B, Method II.

Heavy metals Solution A complies with *limit test A for heavy metals*, Appendix VII (20 ppm). Use *lead standard solution (1 ppm Pb)* to prepare the standard.

Chloride 10 ml of solution A, diluted to 15 ml, complies with the *limit test for chlorides*, Appendix VII (100 ppm).

Sulphate A 10.0% w/v solution complies with the *limit test for sulphates*, Appendix VII (100 ppm).

Loss on drying When dried over *phosphorus pentoxide* at 60° at a pressure of 1.5 to 2.5 kPa for 6 hours, loses not more than 1.0% of its weight. Use 1 g.

Sulphated ash Not more than 0.1%, Appendix IX A, Method II. Use 1 g.

Assay Dissolve 0.15 g in 20 ml of *water*, add 2 g of *sodium acetate* and 25 ml of 0.05M *iodine VS* and allow to stand protected from light for 30 minutes. Add 25 ml of *ethanol (96%)*, shake until the precipitate is dissolved and titrate the excess of iodine with 0.1M *sodium thiosulphate VS* using 1 ml of *starch solution*, added towards the end of the titration, as indicator. Repeat the operation without the substance being examined. The difference between the titrations represents the amount of iodine required. Each ml of 0.05M *iodine VS* is equivalent to 0.00941 g of $C_{11}H_{12}N_2O$.

Storage Phenazone should be kept in a well-closed container and protected from light.

Phenelzine Sulphate

$CH_2 \cdot CH_2 \cdot NH \cdot NH_2 \quad ,H_2SO_4$

$C_8H_{12}N_2,H_2SO_4$　　234.3　　*156-51-4*

Phenelzine Sulphate is phenethylhydrazine hydrogen sulphate. It contains not less than 98.0 per cent and not more than 100.5 per cent of $C_8H_{12}N_2,H_2SO_4$, calculated with reference to the dried substance.

Characteristics A white powder or pearly platelets; odour, pungent.

Solubility Soluble in 7 parts of *water*; practically insoluble in *ethanol (96%)*, in *chloroform* and in *ether*.

Identification A. The *light absorption*, Appendix II B, in the range 230 to 350 nm of a 0.1% w/v solution in 0.05M *sulphuric acid* exhibits three well-defined maxima, at 252, 258 and 263 nm. The *absorbance* at 252 nm is about 0.62, at 258 nm, about 0.77 and at 263 nm, about 0.58.

B. Dissolve 0.1 g in 5 ml of *water*, make alkaline with 5M *sodium hydroxide* and add 1 ml of *potassium cupri-tartrate solution*. A red precipitate is produced.

C. Yields the *reactions* characteristic of sulphates, Appendix VI.

Melting point 164° to 168°, Appendix V A.

Loss on drying When dried over *phosphorus pentoxide* at a pressure not exceeding 0.7 kPa for 24 hours, loses not more than 1.0% of its weight. Use 1 g.

Sulphated ash Not more than 0.1%, Appendix IX A.

Assay Dissolve 0.25 g in 50 ml of *water*, add 1.5 g of *sodium hydrogen carbonate* and 50 ml of 0.05M *iodine VS*, close the flask and allow to stand for 90 minutes. Add 20 ml of 2M *hydrochloric acid* and titrate with 0.1M *sodium thiosulphate VS* using *starch mucilage*, added towards the end of the titration, as indicator. Repeat the operation without the substance being examined. The difference between the titrations represents the amount of iodine required. Each ml of 0.05M *iodine VS* is equivalent to 0.005857 g of $C_8H_{12}N_2,H_2SO_4$.

Storage Phenelzine Sulphate should be kept in a well-closed container and protected from light.

Preparation
Phenelzine Tablets

Action and use Monoamine oxidase inhibitor.

Phenethicillin Potassium

PhOCHMe·CO·NH— ... CO₂K

$C_{17}H_{19}KN_2O_5S$　　402.5　　*132-93-4*

Phenethicillin Potassium is a mixture of the potassium salts of (6R)-[(2R)-2-phenoxypropionamido]penicillanic acid and (6R)-[(2S)-2-phenoxypropionamido]penicillanic acid. It contains not less than 97.0 per cent and not more than 100.5 per cent of $C_{17}H_{19}KN_2O_5S$, calculated with reference to the anhydrous substance.

Characteristics A white or almost white powder.

Solubility Soluble in 1.5 parts of *water* and in 85 parts of *ethanol (96%)*; slightly soluble in *absolute ethanol* and in *chloroform*; practically insoluble in *ether*.

Identification A. The *infra-red absorption spectrum*, Appendix II A, is concordant with the *reference spectrum* of phenethicillin potassium.

B. Dissolve 10 mg in 10 ml of *water* and add 0.5 ml of *neutral red solution*. Add sufficient 0.01M *sodium hydroxide* to produce a permanent orange colour and then add

1.0 ml of *penicillinase solution*. The colour changes rapidly to red.

C. Heat 0.5 g with 10 ml of 5M *hydrochloric acid* under a reflux condenser for 4 hours, cool, add a mixture of 7 ml of 5M *sodium hydroxide* and 7 ml of *water* and extract with successive 10-ml quantities of *ether* until complete extraction is effected. Wash the combined ether extracts with *water*, filter through *anhydrous sodium sulphate* and evaporate the filtrate to dryness. The *melting point* of the residue, after recrystallisation from *petroleum spirit (boiling range, 40° to 60°)*, is about 116°, Appendix V A.

D. Ignite. The residue yields the *reactions* characteristic of potassium salts, Appendix VI.

Acidity or alkalinity pH of a 10% w/v solution, 5.5 to 7.5, Appendix V L.

Specific optical rotation In a 1% w/v solution in a solution containing 0.2% w/v of *dipotassium hydrogen orthophosphate* and 0.8% w/v of *potassium dihydrogen orthophosphate*, +217° to +244°, Appendix V F.

Iodine-absorbing substances Not more than 3%, calculated with reference to the anhydrous substance, when determined by the following method. Dissolve 0.125 g in sufficient *mixed phosphate buffer pH 7.0* to produce 25 ml. To 10 ml add 10 ml of *mixed phosphate buffer pH 4.0* and 10 ml of 0.01M *iodine VS* and titrate immediately with 0.01M *sodium thiosulphate VS* using *starch mucilage*, added towards the end of the titration, as indicator. Repeat the operation without the substance being examined. The difference between the titrations represents the amount of iodine-absorbing substances present. Each ml of 0.01M *sodium thiosulphate VS* is equivalent to 0.000425 g of iodine-absorbing substances.

Water Not more than 1.5% w/w, Appendix IX C. Use 1.5 g.

Assay Dissolve 0.25 g in sufficient *water* to produce 500 ml and dilute 10 ml to 100 ml with *water*. Place two 2-ml aliquots of the resulting solution in separate stoppered tubes. To one tube add 10 ml of *imidazole—mercury reagent*, mix, stopper the tube and immerse in a water-bath at 60° for exactly 25 minutes, swirling occasionally. Remove from the water-bath and cool rapidly to 20° (solution A). To the second tube add 10 ml of *water* and mix (solution B). Without delay measure the *absorbances* of solutions A and B at the maximum at 325 nm, Appendix II B, using in the reference cell a mixture of 2 ml of *water* and 10 ml of *imidazole—mercury reagent* for solution A and *water* for solution B. Calculate the content of $C_{17}H_{19}KN_2O_5S$ from the difference between the absorbances of solutions A and B, from the difference obtained by repeating the operation using *phenethicillin potassium BPCRS* in place of the substance being examined and from the declared content of $C_{17}H_{19}KN_2O_5S$ in *phenethicillin potassium BPCRS*.

Storage Phenethicillin Potassium should be kept in a well-closed container.

Labelling The label states (1) the date after which the material is not intended to be used; (2) the conditions under which it should be stored.

Preparations
Phenethicillin Capsules
Phenethicillin Oral Solution
Phenethicillin Tablets

Action and use Antibacterial.

Phenindamine Tartrate

$C_{19}H_{19}N,C_4H_6O_6$ 411.5   *569-59-5*

Phenindamine Tartrate is 2,3,4,9-tetrahydro-2-methyl-9-phenyl-1*H*-indeno[2,1-*c*]pyridine hydrogen tartrate. It contains not less than 98.5 per cent and not more than 101.0 per cent of $C_{19}H_{19}N,C_4H_6O_6$, calculated with reference to the dried substance.

Characteristics A white or almost white, voluminous powder; odourless or almost odourless.

Solubility Soluble in 70 parts of *water*; slightly soluble in *ethanol (96%)*; practically insoluble in *chloroform* and in *ether*.

Identification A. The *light absorption*, Appendix II B, in the range 230 to 300 nm of a 0.004% w/v solution exhibits a maximum only at 259 nm. The *absorbance* at 259 nm is about 0.88.

B. Dissolve 25 mg in 5 ml of *sulphuric acid*. An orange-brown colour is produced which is discharged when the solution is carefully diluted with 20 ml of *water*.

C. Dissolve 0.5 g in 15 ml of hot *water*, add a slight excess of 5M *sodium hydroxide*, filter and neutralise the filtrate to *litmus paper* with 2M *hydrochloric acid*. The solution yields *reaction B* characteristic of tartrates, Appendix VI.

D. *Melting point*, 160° to 162°, Appendix V A. When heated to 163° it resolidifies and it melts again at about 168°, with decomposition.

Acidity pH of a 1% w/v solution, 3.4 to 3.9, Appendix V L.

Loss on drying When dried to constant weight at 105°, loses not more than 1.0% of its weight. Use 1 g.

Sulphated ash Not more than 0.1%, Appendix IX A.

Assay Dissolve 0.7 g in 40 ml of warm *water*, cool, add 10 ml of *sodium carbonate solution* and extract with successive quantities of 25, 10 and 10 ml of *chloroform*, washing each extract with the same 15 ml of *water* and filtering into a dry flask. Titrate the combined extracts, which should be clear and free from droplets of water, with 0.05M *perchloric acid VS* using *oracet blue B solution* as indicator. Each ml of 0.05M *perchloric acid VS* is equivalent to 0.02057 g of $C_{19}H_{19}N,C_4H_6O_6$.

Storage Phenindamine Tartrate should be kept in a well-closed container and protected from light.

Preparation
Phenindamine Tablets

Action and use Histamine H_1-receptor antagonist.

Phenindione

$C_{15}H_{10}O_2$ 222.2   *83-12-5*

Phenindione is 2-phenylindane-1,3-dione. It contains not less than 98.0 per cent and not more than 100.5 per cent of $C_{15}H_{10}O_2$, calculated with reference to the dried substance.

Characteristics Soft, white or creamy-white crystals; odourless or almost odourless.

Solubility Very slightly soluble in *water*; slightly soluble in *ethanol (96%)* and in *ether*; freely soluble in *chloroform*. Solutions are yellow to red in colour.

Identification A. The *infra-red absorption spectrum*, Appendix II A, is concordant with the *reference spectrum* of phenindione.
B. Dissolve 0.1 g in 30 ml of *ethanol (96%)* with the aid of heat, cool and add sufficient *ethanol (96%)* to produce 50 ml. Dilute 10 ml to 250 ml with 0.1M *sodium hydroxide* and further dilute 5 ml to 100 ml with 0.1M *sodium hydroxide*. The *absorbance* of the resulting solution at the maximum at 278 nm is about 1.1 and at the maximum at 330 nm is about 0.32, Appendix II B.
C. To 1 g add 50 ml of *ethanol (96%)* and 0.5 ml of *aniline*, heat gently under a reflux condenser for 3 hours, cool in ice and filter. The *melting point* of the residue, after washing with 2 ml of *ethanol (96%)* and recrystallising from *chloroform*, is about 225°, Appendix V A.

Melting point 148° to 151°, Appendix V A.

Related substances Carry out in subdued light the method for *thin-layer chromatography*, Appendix III A, using a silica gel F254 precoated chromatoplate (Merck silica gel 60 F254 plates are suitable) and as the mobile phase a solution containing 0.02% w/v of *butylated hydroxytoluene* in a mixture of 80 volumes of *toluene*, 20 volumes of *ethyl acetate* and 4 volumes of *glacial acetic acid*. Allow the solvent front to ascend 4 cm, remove the plate and dry it in a current of cold air for 1 minute. Without delay apply separately to the plate 10 µl of each of three solutions of the substance being examined in *dichloromethane* containing (1) 1.0% w/v, (2) 0.020% w/v and (3) 0.0050% w/v and develop immediately. After removal of the plate, allow it to dry in a current of warm air and examine under *ultra-violet light (254 nm)*. Any *secondary spot* in the chromatogram obtained with solution (1) is not more intense than the spot in the chromatogram obtained with solution (2) and not more than one such spot is more intense than the spot in the chromatogram obtained with solution (3).

Loss on drying When dried at 105° for 2 hours, loses not more than 1.0% of its weight. Use 1 g.

Sulphated ash Not more than 0.1%, Appendix IX A.

Assay To 0.3 g add 50 ml of *ethanol (96%)* and warm until solution is effected. Cool to room temperature, add 10 ml of a 10% v/v solution of *bromine* in *ethanol (96%)* and allow to stand for 10 minutes, shaking occasionally. Add 1 g of *2-naphthol* and shake until the colour of the bromine is discharged. Remove any vapour of bromine in the flask with a current of air, add 50 ml of *water* and 10 ml of *potassium iodide solution* and titrate the liberated iodine with 0.1M *sodium thiosulphate VS* using *starch mucilage* as indicator. Each ml of 0.1M *sodium thiosulphate VS* is equivalent to 0.01111 g of $C_{15}H_{10}O_2$.

Storage Phenindione should be kept in a well-closed container.

Preparation
Phenindione Tablets

Action and use Anticoagulant.

Pheniramine Maleate

$C_{16}H_{20}N_2,C_4H_4O_4$ 356.5   *132-20-7*

Pheniramine Maleate is dimethyl[3-phenyl-3-(2-pyridyl)propyl]amine hydrogen maleate. It contains not less than 99.0 per cent and not more than 101.0 per cent of $C_{16}H_{20}N_2,C_4H_4O_4$, calculated with reference to the dried substance.

Characteristics A white or almost white, crystalline powder; odourless or almost odourless.

Solubility Soluble in 0.3 part of *water*, in 2.5 parts of *ethanol (96%)* and in 1.5 parts of *chloroform*; very slightly soluble in *ether*.

Identification A. The *infra-red absorption spectrum*, Appendix II A, is concordant with the *reference spectrum* of pheniramine maleate.
B. The *light absorption*, Appendix II B, in the range 230 to 350 nm of a 0.004% w/v solution in 0.1M *hydrochloric acid* exhibits a maximum at 265 nm and an inflection at 262 nm. The *absorbance* at 265 nm is about 0.83.
C. Dissolve 0.5 g in 5 ml of *water*, add 2 ml of 13.5M *ammonia* and extract with three 5-ml quantities of *chloroform*. Evaporate the aqueous extract to dryness, add 0.2 ml of 1M *sulphuric acid* and 5 ml of *water*, extract with four 25-ml quantities of *ether* and evaporate the combined ether extracts to dryness in a current of warm air. To the residue add 50 mg of *resorcinol* and 1 ml of *sulphuric acid*, heat in a water-bath for 2 minutes, shake well, heat in a water-bath for a further 30 minutes and cool in ice. Carefully add 5 ml of *water*; a yellow colour is produced. To 2 ml of the solution add 3 ml of a 50% w/v solution of *ammonium acetate*, previously cooled in ice; a pink colour is produced which persists for at least 10 minutes in the cooled solution.

Acidity pH of a 1% w/v solution, 4.5 to 5.5, Appendix V L.

Melting point 106° to 109°, Appendix V A.

Related substances Carry out the method for *thin-layer chromatography*, Appendix III A, using *silica gel G* as the coating substance and a mixture of 50 volumes of *cyclohexane*, 40 volumes of *chloroform* and 10 volumes of *diethylamine* as the mobile phase. Apply separately to the chromatoplate 10 µl of each of three solutions of the substance being examined in *methanol* containing (1) 2.0% w/v, (2) 0.020% w/v and (3) 0.0040% w/v. After removal of the plate, allow it to dry in air and spray with *dilute potassium iodobismuthate solution*. Any *secondary spot* in the chromatogram obtained with solution (1) is not more intense than the spot in the chromatogram obtained with solution (2) and not more than one such spot is more intense than the spot in the chromatogram obtained with solution (3).

Loss on drying When dried to constant weight at 60° at a pressure not exceeding 0.7 kPa, loses not more than 0.5% of its weight. Use 1 g.

Sulphated ash Not more than 0.1%, Appendix IX A.

Assay Carry out Method I for *non-aqueous titration*, Appendix VIII A, using 0.5 g and *1-naphtholbenzein solution* as indicator. Each ml of 0.1M *perchloric acid VS* is equivalent to 0.01782 g of $C_{16}H_{20}N_2,C_4H_4O_4$.

Storage Pheniramine Maleate should be protected from light.

Action and use Histamine H_1-receptor antagonist.

Phenobarbitone ☆

$C_{12}H_{12}N_2O_3$ 232.2   *50-06-6*

Phenobarbitone is 5-ethyl-5-phenylbarbituric acid. It contains not less than 99.0 per cent and not more than 101.0 per cent of $C_{12}H_{12}N_2O_3$, calculated with reference to the dried substance.

Characteristics Colourless crystals or a white, crystalline powder; odourless.

Solubility Very slightly soluble in *water*; freely soluble in *ethanol (96%)*; sparingly soluble in *chloroform*; soluble in *ether*. It dissolves in aqueous solutions of alkali hydroxides and carbonates and in aqueous ammonia.

Identification *Test A may be omitted if tests B, C and D are carried out. Tests B and D may be omitted if tests A and C are carried out.*
A. The *infra-red absorption spectrum*, Appendix II A, is concordant with the spectrum of *phenobarbital EPCRS*.
B. Complies with the test for *identification of barbiturates*, Appendix III A.
C. Determine the *melting point* of the substance being examined, Appendix V A, Method I. Mix equal quantities of the substance being examined and *phenobarbital EPCRS* and determine the *melting point* of the mixture. The difference between the melting points, which are about 176°, is not greater than 2°.
D. Yields the *reaction* characteristic of non-nitrogen substituted barbiturates, Appendix VI.

Acidity Mix 1 g with 50 ml of *water*, boil for 2 minutes and filter. To 10 ml of the filtrate add 0.15 ml of *methyl red solution*. The solution is orange-yellow and not more than 0.1 ml of 0.1M *sodium hydroxide VS* is required to change the colour of the solution to a pure yellow.

Clarity and colour of solution Dissolve 1.0 g in 4 ml of 2M *sodium hydroxide* and 6 ml of *water*. The solution is *clear*, Appendix IV A, and not more intensely coloured than *reference solution* Y_6, Appendix IV B, Method II.

Related substances Complies with the test for *related substances in barbiturates*, Appendix III A.

Loss on drying When dried to constant weight at 100° to 105°, loses not more than 0.5% of its weight. Use 1 g.

Sulphated ash Not more than 0.1%, Appendix IX A, Method II. Use 1 g.

Assay Dissolve 0.1 g in 5 ml of *pyridine*, add 0.5 ml of *thymolphthalein solution* and 10 ml of *silver nitrate—pyridine reagent* and titrate with 0.1M *ethanolic sodium hydroxide VS* until a pure blue colour is obtained. Repeat the operation without the substance being examined. The difference between the titrations represents the amount of sodium hydroxide required. Each ml of 0.1M *ethanolic sodium hydroxide VS* is equivalent to 0.01161 g of $C_{12}H_{12}N_2O_3$.

Preparations
Phenobarbitone Elixir
Phenobarbitone Tablets

Action and use Sedative; anticonvulsant.

The title of the monograph in the European Pharmacopœia is Phenobarbital.

Phenobarbitone Sodium
Soluble Phenobarbitone

$C_{12}H_{11}N_2NaO_3$ 254.2   *57-30-7*

Phenobarbitone Sodium is sodium 5-ethyl-5-phenylbarbiturate. It contains not less than 98.0 per cent and not more than 100.5 per cent of $C_{12}H_{11}N_2NaO_3$, calculated with reference to the dried substance.

Characteristics A white powder; odourless or almost odourless; hygroscopic.

Solubility Soluble in 3 parts of *water* and in 25 parts of *ethanol (96%)*; practically insoluble in *chloroform* and in *ether*.

Identification A. Heat 0.2 g of the residue obtained in the Assay on a water-bath with 15 ml of *ethanol (25%)* until dissolved, filter while hot and allow to cool. Filter, wash the crystals with a small quantity of *ethanol (25%)*, dry at 105° and heat in a sealed tube at 105° for 1 hour. The *infra-red absorption spectrum* of the residue, Appendix II A, is concordant with the *reference spectrum* of phenobarbitone.
B. Dissolve 50 mg of the dried crystals obtained in test A in 2 ml of a 0.2% w/v solution of *cobalt(II) acetate* in *methanol*, warm, add 50 mg of powdered *sodium tetraborate* and heat to boiling. A bluish-violet colour is produced.
C. A 5% w/v solution is alkaline to *litmus solution*. On acidification with 2M *hydrochloric acid* it yields a white precipitate.
D. Ignite about 0.1 g. The residue, when moistened with *hydrochloric acid* and introduced on a platinum wire into a flame, imparts a yellow colour to the flame.
E. 1 g dissolves completely in 20 ml of *ethanol (90%)* (distinction from barbitone sodium).
F. The *melting point* of the dried crystals obtained in test A is about 175°, Appendix V A.

Alkalinity pH of a 10% w/v solution, not more than 11, Appendix V L.

Neutral and basic substances Dissolve 1 g in a mixture of 2 ml of 5M *sodium hydroxide* and 13 ml of *water* and shake for 1 minute with 25 ml of *ether*. Wash the ethereal layer with three 5-ml quantities of *water*, evaporate the ether and dry the residue at 105° for 1 hour. The residue weighs not more than 3 mg.

Loss on drying When dried to constant weight at 130°, loses not more than 7.0% of its weight. Use 1 g.

Assay Dissolve 0.5 g in 15 ml of *water*, add 5 ml of 2M *hydrochloric acid* and extract with 50 ml of *ether* and then with successive 25-ml quantities of *ether* until complete extraction is effected. Wash the combined extracts with two 5-ml quantities of *water* and wash the combined aqueous extracts with two 10-ml quantities of *ether*. Add the ether to the main ethereal extract, evaporate to low bulk, add 2 ml of *absolute ethanol*, evaporate to dryness and dry the residue to constant weight at 105°. Each g of residue is equivalent to 1.095 g of $C_{12}H_{11}N_2NaO_3$.

Storage Phenobarbitone Sodium should be kept in a well-closed container.

Preparations
Phenobarbitone Injection
Phenobarbitone Sodium Tablets

Action and use Anticonvulsant.

In some countries the material described in this monograph may be known as Phenobarbital Sodium.

Phenol

C₆H₆O   94.11   *108-95-2*

Phenol contains not less than 99.0 per cent and not more than 100.5 per cent of C_6H_6O.

Characteristics Colourless or faintly pink, needle-shaped crystals or crystalline masses; odour, characteristic and not tarry; deliquescent; caustic.

Solubility Soluble in 12 parts of *water*; freely soluble in *ethanol (96%)*, in *chloroform*, in *ether*, in *glycerol* and in fixed and volatile oils.

Identification A. The *infra-red absorption spectrum*, Appendix II A, is concordant with the *reference spectrum* of phenol. Melt a sufficient quantity, prepare a thin film between two potassium bromide plates previously warmed to 60° and record the spectrum immediately. The film must remain liquid during the production of the spectrum.

B. Dissolve 0.5 g in 2 ml of 13.5M *ammonia*; the solution is *clear*, Appendix IV A. Dilute to 100 ml with 13.5M *ammonia* and to 2 ml add 0.05 ml of *sodium hypochlorite solution (3% Cl)* and allow to stand at room temperature; a deep blue colour is produced.

C. Add *bromine water* to a 1% w/v solution. A white precipitate is produced, which, on the continued addition of *bromine water* at first dissolves, then reappears and becomes permanent.

Acidity Mix 5 ml of the solution obtained in the test for Clarity and colour of solution with 5 ml of *water* and add 0.05 ml of *methyl orange solution*. A yellow but no orange or red colour is produced.

Clarity and colour of solution A solution of 1.0 g in 15 ml of *water* at 20° is *clear*, Appendix IV A, and not more intensely coloured than *reference solution R₇*, Appendix IV B, Method II.

Freezing point 40° to 41°, Appendix V B, but with the following modifications. After determining the approximate freezing point and remelting the crystals, insert the inner tube into the jacket with the temperature of the cooling bath 6° to 8° below the expected freezing point. Measure the temperature at intervals of 30 seconds, with continuous and gentle stirring, so that a seed crystal is present as the temperature of the substance being examined falls to that at which crystallisation commences. The freezing point corresponds to the first five consecutive readings during which the temperature remains constant within 0.05°. If super-cooling occurs, the constant temperature may be observed immediately after the temperature rise, provided that the rise does not exceed 1°. If a constant temperature is not obtained over the first five readings after the rise in temperature, take six readings beginning with the point at which the maximum temperature is first attained. Plot the readings against time and draw a straight line to lie evenly between the first and second and between the fifth and sixth of the six points. Extrapolate this line until it intersects the portion of the curve before the temperature rise. Take the point of intersection as the freezing point.

Non-volatile matter When heated on a water-bath and dried at 105°, leaves not more than 0.05% of residue. Use 5 g.

Assay Dissolve 2 g in sufficient *water* to produce 1000 ml. Transfer 25 ml to a 500-ml glass-stoppered flask, add 50 ml of 0.05M *bromine VS* and 5 ml of *hydrochloric acid*, stopper, allow to stand for 30 minutes, swirling occasionally, and allow to stand for a further 15 minutes. Add 5 ml of a 20% w/v solution of *potassium iodide*, taking care to avoid loss of bromine, shake thoroughly and titrate with 0.1M *sodium thiosulphate VS* until only a faint yellow colour remains. Add 0.2 ml of *starch mucilage* and 10 ml of *chloroform* and complete the titration with vigorous shaking. Repeat the operation without the substance being examined. The difference between the titrations represents the amount of bromine required. Each ml of 0.05M *bromine VS* is equivalent to 0.001569 g of C_6H_6O.

Storage Phenol should be kept in a well-closed container, protected from light and stored at a temperature not exceeding 15°.

Preparations
Phenol Glycerin
Oily Phenol Injection
Phenol and Glycerol Injection

Action and use Antiseptic; antimicrobial preservative; antipruritic.

Liquefied Phenol

Phenol	800 g
Purified Water	sufficient to produce 1000 g

Warm the Phenol on a water-bath until it is melted, add the Purified Water and mix thoroughly.

Content of phenol, C_6H_6O 77.0 to 81.5% w/w.

Characteristics A colourless or faintly coloured liquid; odour, characteristic and not tarry; caustic.

Solubility Soluble in 11 parts of *water*; miscible with *ethanol (96%)*, with *ether* and with *glycerol*.

Identification A. To 10 ml of a 1% v/v solution add 0.05 ml of *iron(III) chloride test-solution*. A violet colour is produced.

B. Add *bromine water* to a 1% w/v solution. A white precipitate is produced, which, on the continued addition of *bromine water*, at first dissolves, then reappears and becomes permanent.

C. When heated, the temperature at which distillation occurs gradually rises but does not exceed 183°.

Clarity and colour of solution A solution of 1.0 ml in 14 ml of *water*, at 20°, is *clear*, Appendix IV A, and not more intensely coloured than *reference solution R_7*, Appendix IV B, Method II.

Weight per ml 1.055 to 1.060 g, Appendix V G.

Non-volatile matter When heated on a water-bath and dried at 105°, leaves not more than 0.05% w/v of residue.

Assay Dissolve 2.5 g in sufficient *water* to produce 50 ml, transfer 25 ml to a 500-ml glass-stoppered flask and add 50 ml of 0.05M *bromine VS* and 5 ml of *hydrochloric acid*, stopper, swirl occasionally during 30 minutes and allow to stand for 15 minutes. Add 5 ml of a 20% w/v solution of *potassium iodide* taking care to avoid loss of bromine, shake thoroughly and titrate with 0.1M *sodium thiosulphate VS* until only a faint yellow colour remains. Add 0.1 ml of *starch mucilage* and 10 ml of *chloroform* and complete the titration with vigorous shaking. Repeat the operation without the material being examined. The difference between the titrations represents the amount of bromine required. Each ml of 0.05M *bromine VS* is equivalent to 0.001569 g of C_6H_6O. Using the weight per ml, calculate the percentage w/v of C_6H_6O.

Storage Liquefied Phenol should be kept in a well-closed container and protected from light. Liquefied Phenol may congeal or deposit crystals if stored at a temperature below 4°. It should be completely melted before use.

Action and use Antiseptic; antimicrobial preservative; antipruritic.

Note When Phenol is to be mixed with collodion, fixed oils or paraffins, melted Phenol should be used and not Liquefied Phenol.

Phenolphthalein

$C_{20}H_{14}O_4$ 318.3   77-09-8

Phenolphthalein is 3,3-bis(4-hydroxyphenyl)-phthalide. It contains not less than 98.0 per cent and not more than 102.0 per cent of $C_{20}H_{14}O_4$, calculated with reference to the dried substance.

Characteristics A white or yellowish-white, crystalline or amorphous powder; odourless or almost odourless.

Solubility Practically insoluble in *water*; soluble in *ethanol (96%)* and in *ether*.

Identification Dissolves in dilute solutions of alkali hydroxides and in hot solutions of alkali carbonates forming a red solution which is decolorised by dilute acids.

Melting point 258° to 263°, Appendix V A.

Heavy metals Mix 5.0 g with 200 ml of *water* in a long-necked, round-bottomed flask, add 15 ml of *nitric acid*, bring gently to the boil and continue boiling until the volume of the liquid is reduced to about 20 ml. Allow to cool, add 10 ml of *sulphuric acid* and mix. Heat to boiling and add small, successive quantities of *nitric acid*, cooling before each addition, until a colourless liquid is obtained. Heat until white fumes are evolved and if darkening occurs at this stage continue the treatment with *nitric acid*, finally heating until white fumes are again evolved. Allow the colourless liquid to cool, add 25 ml of a saturated solution of *ammonium oxalate* and boil until the slight froth completely subsides. Cool and dilute to 100 ml with *water*. To 20 ml of the resulting solution add 10 ml of *water* and 2 g of *citric acid*, dissolve, make alkaline with 5M *ammonia* and add 1 ml of *potassium cyanide solution PbT*. Transfer to a separating funnel, add 10 ml of *dithizone solution* and shake vigorously. Allow the liquids to separate and reserve the lower layer. Repeat the extraction with two 5-ml quantities of *dithizone solution*. If, after the third extraction, the chloroform layer is bright red, continue the extraction with further 5-ml quantities of *dithizone solution* until the colour of the chloroform layer no longer changes to bright red. Wash the mixed chloroform solutions by shaking with 10 ml of *water* and then extract with two 10-ml quantities of 2M *hydrochloric acid*. Wash the combined extracts with 10 ml of *chloroform*. 12 ml of the resulting solution complies with *limit test A for heavy metals*, Appendix VII (20 ppm). Use *lead standard solution (1 ppm Pb)* to prepare the standard.

Fluoran 0.50 g dissolves completely in a mixture of 4 ml of 1M *sodium hydroxide* and 50 ml of *water*.

Loss on drying When dried to constant weight at 105°, loses not more than 1.0% of its weight. Use 1 g.

Sulphated ash Not more than 0.1%, Appendix IX A.

Assay Dissolve 0.1 g in 100 ml of *ethanol (96%)*, dilute 5 ml to 50 ml with *ethanol (96%)* and evaporate 5 ml of the resulting solution to dryness on a water-bath. Dissolve the residue in sufficient *glycine buffer pH 11.3* to produce 100 ml, mix and immediately measure the *absorbance* at the maximum at 555 nm, Appendix II B. Calculate the content of $C_{20}H_{14}O_4$ taking 1055 as the value of A(1%, 1 cm) at the maximum at 555 nm.

Action and use Laxative.

Phenolsulphonphthalein ☆

$C_{19}H_{14}O_5S$ 354.4   *143-74-8*

Phenolsulphonphthalein is 4,4'-(3*H*-2,1-benz-oxathiol-3-ylidene)diphenol *S,S*-dioxide. It contains not less than 98.0 per cent and not more than 102.0 per cent of $C_{19}H_{14}O_5S$, calculated with reference to the dried substance.

Characteristics A bright red to dark red, crystalline powder; odourless.

Solubility Very slightly soluble in *water*; slightly soluble in *ethanol (96%)*.

Identification A. Dissolve 10 mg in sufficient of a 1% w/v solution of *sodium carbonate* to produce 200 ml. Dilute 5 ml of the solution to 100 ml with the same solvent. The *light absorption* of the resulting solution, Appendix II B, in the range 400 to 630 nm exhibits a maximum only at 558 nm. The A(1%, 1 cm) at the maximum is 1900 to 2100.

B. Dissolve 10 mg in 1 ml of 2M *sodium hydroxide* and dilute to 10 ml with *water*; the solution is deep red. To 5 ml of the solution add a slight excess of 1M *sulphuric acid*; the solution becomes orange.

C. To 5 ml of the solution used in test B add 1 ml of 0.05M *bromine VS* and 1 ml of 2M *hydrochloric acid*, shake, allow to stand for 15 minutes and make alkaline with 2M *sodium hydroxide*. An intense violet-blue colour is produced.

Related substances Carry out the method for *thin-layer chromatography*, Appendix III A, using *silica gel GF254* as the coating substance and a mixture of 100 volumes of *2-methylbutan-2-ol*, 25 volumes of *glacial acetic acid* and 25 volumes of *water* as the mobile phase. Apply separately to the chromatoplate 10 µl of each of two solutions of the substance being examined in 0.1M *sodium hydroxide* containing (1) 2.0% w/v and (2) 0.010% w/v. After removal of the plate, allow it to dry in air until the odour of solvent is no longer detectable. Expose the plate to ammonia vapour and examine under *ultra-violet light (254 nm)*. Not more than one *secondary spot* is visible in the chromatogram obtained with solution (1) and any such spot is not more intense than the spot in the chromatogram obtained with solution (2).

Insoluble matter To 1 g, finely powdered, add 12 ml of a 4.2% w/v solution of *sodium hydrogen carbonate* and allow to stand for 1 hour, shaking frequently. Add sufficient *water* to produce 100 ml and allow to stand for 15 hours. Centrifuge at 2000 to 3000 *g* for 30 minutes, decant the supernatant liquid and wash the residue with 25 ml of a 1% w/v solution of *sodium hydrogen carbonate* and then with 25 ml of *water* and dry at 100° to 105°. The residue weighs not more than 5 mg (0.5%).

Loss on drying When dried to constant weight at 100° to 105°, loses not more than 1.0% of its weight. Use 1 g.

Sulphated ash Not more than 0.2%, Appendix IX A, Method II. Use 0.5 g.

Assay Dissolve 0.9 g in 15 ml of 1M *sodium hydroxide VS* and dilute to 250 ml with *water*. To 10 ml of the solution add 25 ml of *glacial acetic acid*, 20 ml of 0.0167M *potassium bromate VS*, 5 ml of a 10% w/v solution of *potassium bromide* and 5 ml of *hydrochloric acid*, stopper the flask and allow to stand protected from light for 15 minutes. Add 10 ml of a 10% w/v solution of *potassium iodide* and titrate immediately with 0.1M *sodium thiosulphate VS* using 0.1 ml of *starch solution* as indicator. Each ml of 0.0167M *potassium bromate VS* is equivalent to 0.00443 g of $C_{19}H_{14}O_5S$.

Action and use Diagnostic aid.

The title of the monograph in the European Pharmacopœia is Phenolsulfonphthalein.

Phenoxybenzamine Hydrochloride

$C_{18}H_{22}ClNO,HCl$ 340.3   *63-92-3*

Phenoxybenzamine Hydrochloride is benzyl-(2-chloroethyl)1-methyl-2-phenoxyethylamine hydrochloride. It contains not less than 98.5 per cent and not more than 101.0 per cent of $C_{18}H_{22}ClNO,HCl$, calculated with reference to the dried substance.

Characteristics A white or almost white, crystalline powder; odourless or almost odourless.

Solubility Sparingly soluble in *water*; soluble in 9 parts of *ethanol (96%)* and in 9 parts of *chloroform*.

Identification A. The *infra-red absorption spectrum*, Appendix II A, is concordant with the *reference spectrum* of phenoxybenzamine hydrochloride.

B. Dissolve 0.5 g in 50 ml of *ethanol-free chloroform* and extract with three 20-ml quantities of 0.01M *hydrochloric acid*. Filter the chloroform layer through absorbent cotton and dilute 5 ml of the filtrate to 250 ml with *ethanol-free chloroform*. The *light absorption* of the resulting solution, Appendix II B, in the range 250 to 350 nm exhibits two maxima, at 272 nm and 279 nm. The *absorbance* at 272 nm is about 1.1 and at 279 nm is about 0.90.

C. Yields the *reactions* characteristic of chlorides, Appendix VI.

Melting point 137.5° to 140°, Appendix V A.

Related substances Carry out the method for *thin-layer chromatography*, Appendix III A, using *silica gel G* as the coating substance and a mixture of 80 volumes of *acetone* and 20 volumes of *chloroform* as the mobile phase. Apply separately to the chromatoplate 10 µl of each of two freshly prepared solutions of the substance being examined in *methanol* containing (1) 2.0% w/v and (2) 0.010% w/v. After removal of the plate, allow it to dry in air and spray with *dilute potassium iodobismuthate solution*. Any *secondary spot* in the chromatogram obtained with solution (1) is not more intense than the spot in the chromatogram obtained with solution (2).

Loss on drying When dried over *phosphorus pentoxide* at a pressure not exceeding 0.7 kPa for 24 hours, loses not more than 0.5% of its weight. Use 1 g.

Sulphated ash Not more than 0.1%, Appendix IX A.

Assay Carry out Method I for *non-aqueous titration*, Appendix VIII A, using 0.6 g and *oracet blue B solution* as indicator. Each ml of 0.1M *perchloric acid VS* is equivalent to 0.03403 g of $C_{18}H_{22}ClNO,HCl$.

Preparation
Phenoxybenzamine Capsules

Action and use Alpha-adrenoceptor antagonist.

Phenoxyethanol

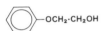

$C_8H_{10}O_2$ 138.2   *122-99-6*

Phenoxyethanol is 2-phenoxyethanol. It contains not less than 99.0 per cent and not more than 100.5 per cent of $C_8H_{10}O_2$.

Characteristics A colourless, slightly viscous liquid; odour, faint and pleasant.

Solubility Soluble in 43 parts of *water*, in 50 parts of *arachis oil* and in 50 parts of *olive oil*; miscible with *ethanol* (96%), with *acetone* and with *glycerol*.

Identification A. The *infra-red absorption spectrum*, Appendix II A, is concordant with the *reference spectrum* of phenoxyethanol.
B. The *light absorption*, Appendix II B, in the range 240 to 350 nm of a 0.01% w/v solution exhibits two maxima, at 269 nm and 275 nm. The *absorbance* at 269 nm is about 0.98 and at 275 nm is about 0.78.
C. Shake 2 ml with a mixture of 4 g of *potassium permanganate*, 5.4 g of *sodium carbonate* and 75 ml of *water* for 30 minutes and filter. Saturate the filtrate with *sodium chloride* and acidify with *hydrochloric acid*. The *melting point* of the precipitate, after recrystallisation from *water* and drying, is about 99°, Appendix V A.

Weight per ml 1.105 to 1.110 g, Appendix V G.

Phenol Dissolve 1 g in 50 ml of *chloroform*, shake with 10 ml of 0.2M *sodium hydroxide* and wash the aqueous layer with two 20-ml quantities of *chloroform*. Dilute the aqueous layer to 100 ml with *water*. The *absorbance* of the resulting solution at the maximum at 287 nm is not more than 0.27, Appendix II B.

Related substances Carry out the method for *gas chromatography*, Appendix III B, using three solutions in *chloroform* containing (1) 0.50% w/v of each of the substance being examined and *methyl laurate* (internal standard), (2) 50% w/v of the substance being examined

and (3) 50% w/v of the substance being examined and 0.50% w/v of the internal standard,

The chromatographic procedure may be carried out using a glass column (1.5 m × 4 mm) packed with *acid-washed, silanised diatomaceous support* (80 to 100 mesh) coated with 3% w/v of phenyl methyl silicone fluid (50% phenyl) (OV-17 is suitable) and maintained at 130°.

In the chromatogram obtained with solution (3) the ratio of the sum of the areas of any *secondary peaks* to the area of the peak due to the internal standard is not greater than the ratio of the area of the peak due to the substance being examined to that of the peak due to the internal standard in the chromatogram obtained with solution (1).

Assay To 2 g add 10 ml of freshly prepared *acetic anhydride-pyridine solution*, heat on a water-bath for 45 minutes, add 10 ml of *water*, heat for a further 2 minutes, cool, add 10 ml of *butan-1-ol*, shake vigorously and titrate the excess of acid with 1M *sodium hydroxide VS* using *phenolphthalein solution* as indicator. Repeat the operation without the substance being examined, cooling before carefully adding the 10 ml of *water*. The difference between the titrations represents the amount of acetic anhydride required by the phenoxyethanol. Each ml of 1M *sodium hydroxide VS* is equivalent to 0.1382 g of $C_8H_{10}O_2$.

Action and use Antimicrobial preservative; also used topically in treatment of bacterial infections.

Phenoxymethylpenicillin ☆

$C_{16}H_{18}N_2O_5S$ 350.4   *87-08-1*

Phenoxymethylpenicillin is (6R)-6-(2-phenoxy-acetamido)penicillanic acid, produced by the growth of certain strains of *Penicillium notatum* or related organisms on a culture medium containing an appropriate precursor, or obtained by any other means. It contains not less than 95.0 per cent and not more than 100.5 per cent of penicillins, calculated as $C_{16}H_{18}N_2O_5S$, with reference to the anhydrous substance.

Characteristics A white, crystalline powder; odourless or with a slight, characteristic odour.

Solubility Very slightly soluble in *water*; soluble in 7 parts of *ethanol* (96%); practically insoluble in fixed oils and in *liquid paraffin*.

Identification *Test A may be omitted if tests B, C and D are carried out. Tests B, C and D may be omitted if test A is carried out.*
A. The *infra-red absorption spectrum*, Appendix II A, is concordant with the spectrum of *phenoxymethylpenicillin EPCRS*.
B. Complies with the test for Acidity.
C. Dissolve 0.1 g in sufficient *0.0067M mixed phosphate buffer pH 7.0* to produce 100 ml. Dilute 10 ml with sufficient *0.0067M mixed phosphate buffer pH 7.0* to produce 100 ml (solution A). To 10 ml of solution A add 0.5 ml of *dilute penicillinase solution* and allow to stand at

30° for 10 minutes (solution B). To 5 ml of solution A and to 5 ml of solution B, in separate test-tubes, add 10 ml of *acetate buffer pH 4.6* and 5 ml of *0.0005M iodine*. Mix the contents of each tube and add, to each, 0.1 ml of *starch solution*. The mixture obtained with solution A is blue. The mixture obtained with solution B remains colourless.

D. Yields the *reaction* characteristic of penicillins and cephalosporins, Appendix VI.

Acidity pH of a 0.5% w/v solution, 2.4 to 4.0, Appendix V L.

Light absorption The *absorbance* of a 0.1% w/v solution in *0.1M sodium hydroxide* at 306 nm is not more than 0.36, Appendix II B. The *absorbance* of a 0.02% w/v solution in *0.1M sodium hydroxide* at the maximum at 274 nm is not less than 0.56.

Specific optical rotation In a 1% w/v solution in *butan-1-ol*, +186° to +200°, Appendix V F.

Phenoxyacetic acid Carry out the method for *thin-layer chromatography*, Appendix III A, using *silica gel G* as the coating substance and a mixture of 80 volumes of *chloroform*, 15 volumes of *anhydrous formic acid* and 5 volumes of *methanol* as the mobile phase. Apply separately to the chromatoplate 10 μl of each of two solutions containing (1) 2.0% w/v of the substance being examined in *methanol* and (2) 0.010% w/v of *phenoxyacetic acid* in *phosphate buffer pH 6.6*. After removal of the plate, dry it in a current of warm air and spray with a 0.15% w/v solution of *potassium permanganate* in *sulphuric acid (5%)*. Any spot corresponding to phenoxyacetic acid in the chromatogram obtained with solution (1) is not more intense than the spot in the chromatogram obtained with solution (2).

Water Not more than 0.5% w/w, Appendix IX C. Use 1 g.

Assay Dissolve 50 mg in 5 ml of *1M sodium hydroxide*, add 5 ml of *water* and allow to stand for 15 minutes. Add 5 ml of *1M nitric acid*, 20 ml of *acetate buffer pH 4.6* and 20 ml of *water*. Titrate at 35° to 40° with *0.02M mercury(II) nitrate VS* determining the end-point potentiometrically using a platinum or mercury indicator electrode and a mercury—mercury(I) sulphate reference electrode; titrate slowly so that the titration takes about 15 minutes and disregard any preliminary inflection on the titration curve. Each ml of *0.02M mercury(II) nitrate VS* is equivalent to 0.007008 g of total penicillins, calculated as $C_{16}H_{18}N_2O_5S$.

To 0.25 g add 25 ml of *water* and 25 ml of *acetate buffer pH 4.6* and shake until solution is complete. Titrate immediately at room temperature with *0.02M mercury(II) nitrate VS*, determining the end-point as above. Each ml of *0.02M mercury(II) nitrate VS* is equivalent to 0.007008 g of degradation products, calculated as $C_{16}H_{18}N_2O_5S$. Subtract the percentage of degradation products from the percentage of total penicillins; the difference is the content of penicillins, calculated as $C_{16}H_{18}N_2O_5S$.

Storage Phenoxymethylpenicillin should be kept in an airtight container.

Labelling The label states (1) the date after which the material is not intended to be used; (2) the conditions under which it should be stored.

Action and use Antibacterial.

Phenoxymethylpenicillin Calcium
Penicillin V Calcium

$(C_{16}H_{17}N_2O_5S)_2Ca,2H_2O$ 774.9   *147-48-8*

Phenoxymethylpenicillin Calcium is calcium (6R)-6-(2-phenoxyacetamido)penicillanate dihydrate. It contains not less than 94.0 per cent and not more than 100.5 per cent of penicillins calculated as $(C_{16}H_{17}N_2O_5S)_2Ca$ with reference to the anhydrous substance.

Characteristics A white, crystalline powder.

Solubility Slowly soluble in 120 parts of *water*; practically insoluble in fixed oils and in *liquid paraffin*.

Identification A. The *infra-red absorption spectrum*, Appendix II A, is concordant with the *reference spectrum* of phenoxymethylpenicillin calcium.

B. Dissolve 10 mg in 10 ml of *water* and add 0.5 ml of *neutral red solution*. Add sufficient *0.01M sodium hydroxide* to produce a permanent orange colour and then add 1.0 ml of *penicillinase solution*. The colour changes rapidly to red.

C. Ignite. The residue yields the *reactions* characteristic of calcium salts, Appendix VI.

Acidity or alkalinity pH of a 0.5% w/v solution, 5.0 to 7.5, Appendix V L.

Light absorption The *absorbance* of a 0.1% w/v solution in *0.1M sodium hydroxide* at 306 nm is not more than 0.33, Appendix II B. The *absorbance* of a 0.02% w/v solution in *0.1M sodium hydroxide* at the maximum at 274 nm is not less than 0.50.

Phenoxyacetic acid Carry out the method for *thin-layer chromatography*, Appendix III A, using *silica gel G* as the coating substance and a mixture of 80 volumes of *chloroform*, 15 volumes of *anhydrous formic acid* and 5 volumes of *methanol* as the mobile phase. Apply separately to the chromatoplate 5 μl of each of two solutions in *methanol* containing (1) 4.0% w/v of the substance being examined and (2) 0.020% w/v of *phenoxyacetic acid*. After removal of the plate, dry it in a current of warm air and spray with a 0.15% w/v solution of *potassium permanganate* in *sulphuric acid (5%)*. Any spot corresponding to phenoxyacetic acid in the chromatogram obtained with solution (1) is not more intense than the spot in the chromatogram obtained with solution (2).

Water 4.2 to 5.1% w/w, Appendix IX C. Use 0.5 g.

Assay Dissolve 0.1 g in sufficient *water* to produce 100 ml. To 10 ml in a stoppered flask add 5 ml of *1M sodium hydroxide* and allow to stand for 20 minutes. Add 20 ml of a freshly prepared buffer solution containing 5.44% w/v of *sodium acetate* and 2.40% w/v of *glacial acetic acid*, 5 ml of *1M hydrochloric acid* and 25 ml of *0.01M iodine VS*, close the flask with a wet stopper and allow to stand for 20 minutes, protected from light. Titrate the excess of iodine with *0.02M sodium thiosulphate VS* using *starch mucilage*, added towards the end of the titration, as indicator. To a further 10 ml of the solution add 20 ml of the buffer solution and 25 ml of *0.01M iodine VS*, allow to stand for 20 minutes and titrate with *0.02M sodium thiosulphate VS* using *starch mucilage*, added towards the end of the titration, as indicator. The difference between the titrations represents the volume of *0.01M iodine VS* equivalent to the penicillins present.

Calculate the content of penicillins as $(C_{16}H_{17}N_2O_5S)_2Ca$ from the difference obtained by carrying out the assay at the same time using *phenoxymethylpenicillin potassium BPCRS* in place of the substance being examined and the declared equivalent content of $(C_{16}H_{17}N_2O_5S)_2Ca$ in *phenoxymethylpenicillin potassium BPCRS*.

Storage Phenoxymethylpenicillin Calcium should be kept in a well-closed container.

Preparation
Phenoxymethylpenicillin Oral Suspension

Action and use Antibacterial.

Phenoxymethylpenicillin Potassium ☆
Penicillin V Potassium

$C_{16}H_{17}KN_2O_5S$ 388.5   *132-98-9*

Phenoxymethylpenicillin Potassium is potassium (6*R*)-6-(2-phenoxyacetamido)-penicillanate, produced by the growth of certain strains of *Penicillium notatum* or related organisms on a culture medium containing an appropriate precursor, or obtained by any other means. It contains not less than 95.0 per cent and not more than 100.5 per cent of penicillins, calculated as $C_{16}H_{17}KN_2O_5S$ with reference to the anhydrous substance.

Characteristics A white, crystalline powder; odourless or with a slight, characteristic odour.

Solubility Soluble in 1.5 parts of *water*; practically insoluble in *chloroform*, in *ether*, in fixed oils and in *liquid paraffin*.

Identification *Test A may be omitted if tests B, C and D are carried out. Tests B and D may be omitted if tests A and C are carried out.*
A. The *infra-red absorption spectrum*, Appendix II A, is concordant with the spectrum of *phenoxymethylpenicillin potassium EPCRS*.
B. Dissolve 0.1 g in sufficient *0.0067M mixed phosphate buffer pH 7.0* to produce 100 ml. Dilute 10 ml with sufficient *0.0067M mixed phosphate buffer pH 7.0* to produce 100 ml (solution A). To 10 ml of solution A add 0.5 ml of *dilute penicillinase solution* and allow to stand at 30° for 10 minutes (solution B). To 5 ml of solution A and to 5 ml of solution B, in separate test-tubes, add 10 ml of *acetate buffer pH 4.6* and 5 ml of 0.0005M *iodine*. Mix the contents of each tube and add, to each, 0.1 ml of *starch solution*. The mixture obtained with solution A is blue. The mixture obtained with solution B remains colourless.
C. Yields *reaction A* characteristic of potassium salts, Appendix VI.
D. Yields the *reaction* characteristic of penicillins and cephalosporins, Appendix VI.

Acidity or alkalinity pH of a 0.5% w/v solution, 5.5 to 7.5, Appendix V L.

Light absorption The *absorbance* of a 0.1% w/v solution in 0.1M *sodium hydroxide* at 306 nm is not more than 0.33, Appendix II B. The *absorbance* of a 0.02% w/v solution in 0.1M *sodium hydroxide* at the maximum at 274 nm is not less than 0.50.

Specific optical rotation In a 1% w/v solution in *carbon dioxide-free water*, +215° to +230°, Appendix V F.

Phenoxyacetic acid Carry out the method for *thin-layer chromatography*, Appendix III A, using *silica gel G* as the coating substance and a mixture of 80 volumes of *chloroform*, 15 volumes of *anhydrous formic acid* and 5 volumes of *methanol* as the mobile phase. Apply separately to the chromatoplate 10 μl of each of two solutions in *phosphate buffer pH 6.6* containing (1) 2.0% w/v of the substance being examined and (2) 0.010% w/v of *phenoxyacetic acid*. After removal of the plate, dry it in a current of warm air and spray with a 0.15% w/v solution of *potassium permanganate* in *sulphuric acid* (5%). Any spot corresponding to phenoxyacetic acid in the chromatogram obtained with solution (1) is not more intense than the spot in the chromatogram obtained with solution (2).

Water Not more than 1.0% w/w, Appendix IX C. Use 1 g.

Assay Dissolve 50 mg in 5 ml of 1M *sodium hydroxide*, add 5 ml of *water* and allow to stand for 15 minutes. Add 5 ml of 1M *nitric acid*, 20 ml of *acetate buffer pH 4.6* and 20 ml of *water*. Titrate at 35° to 40° with 0.02M *mercury(II) nitrate VS* determining the end-point potentiometrically using a platinum or mercury indicator electrode and a mercury—mercury(I) sulphate reference electrode; titrate slowly so that the titration takes about 15 minutes and disregard any preliminary inflection on the titration curve. Each ml of 0.02M *mercury(II) nitrate VS* is equivalent to 0.00777 g of total penicillins, calculated as $C_{16}H_{17}KN_2O_5S$.

To 0.25 g add 25 ml of *water* and 25 ml of *acetate buffer pH 4.6* and shake until solution is complete. Titrate immediately at room temperature with 0.02M *mercury(II) nitrate VS*, determining the end-point as above. Each ml of 0.02M *mercury(II) nitrate VS* is equivalent to 0.00777 g of degradation products, calculated as $C_{16}H_{17}KN_2O_5S$. Subtract the percentage of degradation products from the percentage of total penicillins; the difference is the content of penicillins, calculated as $C_{16}H_{17}KN_2O_5S$.

Storage Phenoxymethylpenicillin Potassium should be kept in an airtight container.

Labelling The label states (1) the date after which the material is not intended to be used; (2) the conditions under which it should be stored.

Preparations
Phenoxymethylpenicillin Capsules
Phenoxymethylpenicillin Oral Solution
Phenoxymethylpenicillin Oral Suspension
Phenoxymethylpenicillin Tablets

Action and use Antibacterial.

Phentolamine Mesylate

$C_{17}H_{19}N_3O,CH_4O_3S$ 377.5   *65-28-1*

Phentolamine Mesylate is 3-[*N*-(2-imidazolin-2-ylmethyl)-*p*-toluidino]phenol methanesulphonate. It contains not less than 99.0 per cent and not more than 100.5 per cent of $C_{17}H_{19}N_3O,CH_4O_3S$, calculated with reference to the dried substance.

Characteristics A white, crystalline powder; odourless or almost odourless; slightly hygroscopic.

Solubility Soluble in 1 part of *water* and in 5 parts of *ethanol (96%)*; slightly soluble in *chloroform*.

Identification A. The *infra-red absorption spectrum*, Appendix II A, is concordant with the *reference spectrum* of phentolamine mesylate.

B. The *light absorption*, Appendix II B, in the range 230 to 350 nm of a 0.004% w/v solution exhibits a maximum only at 278 nm. The *absorbance* at 278 nm is about 0.99.

C. Dissolve 0.5 g in 5 ml of *ethanol (96%)* and 5 ml of 0.1M *hydrochloric acid* and add 2 ml of a 0.5% w/v solution of *ammonium metavanadate*. A light green precipitate is produced.

D. Mix 50 mg with 0.2 g of powdered *sodium hydroxide*, heat to fusion and continue the heating for a few seconds longer. Cool, add 0.5 ml of *water* and a slight excess of 2M *hydrochloric acid* and warm. Sulphur dioxide is evolved, which turns moistened *starch—iodate paper* blue.

E. *Melting point* of the residue obtained in the Assay, about 138°, Appendix V A.

Acidity or alkalinity Dissolve 0.10 g in 10 ml of *carbon dioxide-free water*. The solution is not alkaline to *methyl red solution* and requires not more than 0.05 ml of 0.1M *sodium hydroxide VS* to make it alkaline.

Melting point 177° to 181°, Appendix V A.

Related substances Carry out the method for *thin-layer chromatography*, Appendix III A, using *silica gel G* as the coating substance and a mixture of 85 volumes of *butan-2-one*, 15 volumes of *acetone* and 5 volumes of 13.5M *ammonia* as the mobile phase. Apply separately to the chromatoplate 10 µl of each of two solutions of the substance being examined in *ethanol (96%)* containing (1) 2.0% w/v and (2) 0.010% w/v. After removal of the plate, allow it to dry in air and spray with *dilute potassium iodobismuthate solution*. Any *secondary spot* in the chromatogram obtained with solution (1) is not more intense than the spot in the chromatogram obtained with solution (2).

Loss on drying When dried to constant weight at 105°, loses not more than 0.5% of its weight. Use 1 g.

Sulphated ash Not more than 0.1%, Appendix IX A.

Assay Dissolve 0.1 g in 40 ml of *water*, add 20 ml of a 20% w/v solution of *trichloroacetic acid*, allow to stand for 3 hours, filter, wash the residue with two 5-ml quantities of *water* and dry to constant weight at 105°. Each g of residue is equivalent to 0.8487 g of $C_{17}H_{19}N_3O,CH_4O_3S$.

Storage Phentolamine Mesylate should be kept in a well-closed container and protected from light.

Preparation
Phentolamine Injection

Action and use Alpha-adrenoceptor antagonist.

Phenylbutazone ☆

$C_{19}H_{20}N_2O_2$ 308.4   *50-33-9*

Phenylbutazone is 4-butyl-1,2-diphenyl-pyrazolidine-3,5-dione. It contains not less than 99.0 per cent and not more than 101.0 per cent of $C_{19}H_{20}N_2O_2$, calculated with reference to the dried substance.

Characteristics A white or almost white, crystalline powder; practically odourless.

Solubility Practically insoluble in *water*; sparingly soluble in *ethanol (96%)*; soluble in 1.25 parts of *chloroform* and in 15 parts of *ether*. It dissolves in aqueous solutions of the alkali hydroxides.

Identification *Test A may be omitted if tests B, C and D are carried out. Tests B and C may be omitted if tests A and D are carried out.*

A. The *infra-red absorption spectrum*, Appendix II A, is concordant with the spectrum of *phenylbutazone EPCRS*.

B. Dissolve 30 mg in 25 ml of *methanol*, add 50 ml of 1M *sodium hydroxide* and dilute to 100 ml with *water*. Dilute 5 ml to 250 ml with *water*. The *light absorption* of the resulting solution, Appendix II B, in the range 240 to 350 nm exhibits a maximum at 264 nm. The A(1%, 1 cm) at 264 nm is 650 to 700. Use a solution containing 0.5 ml of *methanol*, 1.0 ml of 1M *sodium hydroxide* and 98.5 ml of *water* in the reference cell.

C. To 0.1 g add 1 ml of *glacial acetic acid* and 2 ml of *hydrochloric acid* and heat under a reflux condenser for 30 minutes. Cool, add 10 ml of *water* and filter. Add to the filtrate 3 ml of 0.1M *sodium nitrite*; a yellow colour is produced. To 1 ml of the solution add a solution containing 10 mg of *2-naphthol* in 5 ml of a 10.6% w/v solution of *anhydrous sodium carbonate*; a reddish-brown to reddish-violet precipitate is produced.

D. *Melting point*, 104° to 107°, Appendix V A, Method I.

Acidity or alkalinity Heat to boiling 1 g with 50 ml of *water*, cool with shaking in a stoppered vessel and filter. To 25 ml of the filtrate add 0.5 ml of *dilute phenolphthalein solution*; the solution is colourless and not more than 0.5 ml of 0.01M *sodium hydroxide VS* is required to change the colour of the solution. Add 0.6 ml of 0.01M *hydrochloric acid VS* and 0.1 ml of *methyl red solution*; the solution is red or orange.

Clarity of solution Dissolve 1.0 g in 20 ml of 2M *sodium hydroxide* with shaking and allow to stand at 25° for 3 hours (solution A). The solution is *clear*, Appendix IV A.

Light absorption *Absorbance* of a 4-cm layer of solution A at 420 nm, not more than 0.20, Appendix II B.

Heavy metals 1.0 g complies with *limit test C for heavy metals*, Appendix VII (20 ppm). Use 2 ml of *lead standard solution (10 ppm Pb)* to prepare the standard.

Related substances Carry out the method for *thin-layer chromatography*, Appendix III A, using *silica gel GF254* as the coating substance and a mixture of 50 volumes of *chloroform*, 40 volumes of *cyclohexane* and 10 volumes of *glacial acetic acid* as the mobile phase but allowing the solvent front to ascend 10 cm above the line of application. Before use spray the chromatoplate evenly with a 2% w/v solution of *sodium metabisulphite* until wet, dry in air for 15 minutes, heat at 120° for 30 minutes and allow to cool. Apply separately to the plate 5 µl of each of the following solutions prepared immediately before use and develop immediately. For solution (1) dissolve 0.2 g in a mixture of equal volumes of *chloroform* and *absolute ethanol* containing 0.02% w/v of *butylated hydroxytoluene* and dilute to 5 ml with the same solvent mixture. For solution (2) dilute 1 ml of solution (1) to 200 ml with the same solvent mixture. After removal of the plate, dry it in a current of warm air for 10 minutes and examine under *ultra-violet light (254 nm)*. Any *secondary spot* in the chromatogram obtained with solution (1) is not more intense than the spot in the chromatogram obtained with solution (2).

Loss on drying When dried over *phosphorus pentoxide* at 80° at a pressure of 1.5 to 2.5 kPa for 4 hours, loses not more than 0.2% of its weight. Use 1 g.

Sulphated ash Not more than 0.1%, Appendix IX A, Method II. Use 1 g.

Assay Dissolve 0.5 g in 25 ml of *acetone* and titrate with 0.1M *sodium hydroxide VS*, using 0.5 ml of *bromothymol blue solution* as indicator, until a blue colour is obtained that persists for 15 seconds. Repeat the operation without the substance being examined. The difference between the titrations represents the amount of sodium hydroxide required. Each ml of 0.1M *sodium hydroxide VS* is equivalent to 0.03084 g of $C_{19}H_{20}N_2O_2$.

Storage Phenylbutazone should be protected from light.

Preparation
Phenylbutazone Tablets

Action and use Anti-inflammatory; analgesic.

Phenylephrine Hydrochloride

$C_9H_{13}NO_2,HCl$ 203.7   *61-76-7*

Phenylephrine Hydrochloride is (*S*)-1-(3-hydroxyphenyl)-2-methylaminoethanol hydrochloride. It contains not less than 98.5 per cent and not more than 101.0 per cent of $C_9H_{13}NO_2,HCl$, calculated with reference to the dried substance.

Characteristics A white or almost white, crystalline powder; odourless or almost odourless.

Solubility Soluble in 2 parts of *water*, in 4 parts of *ethanol (96%)* and in 2 parts of *glycerol*.

Identification A. The *infra-red absorption spectrum*, Appendix II A, is concordant with the *reference spectrum* of phenylephrine hydrochloride.
B. The *light absorption*, Appendix II B, in the range 230 to 350 nm of a 0.01% w/v solution in 0.5M *sulphuric acid* exhibits a maximum only at 273 nm. The *absorbance* at 273 nm is about 0.90.
C. Dissolve 10 mg in 1 ml of *water* and add 0.05 ml of *copper sulphate solution* and 1 ml of 5M *sodium hydroxide*; a

violet colour is produced. Add 1 ml of *ether* and shake; the ether layer remains colourless.
D. Yields the *reactions* characteristic of chlorides, Appendix VI.

Melting point 141° to 144°, Appendix V A.

Specific optical rotation In a 2% w/v solution, −43° to −47°, Appendix V F.

Sulphate Dissolve 0.25 g in 60 ml of *water*. 15 ml of the resulting solution complies with the *limit test for sulphates*, Appendix VII (0.24%).

Phenones *Absorbance* of a 0.2% w/v solution at 310 nm, not more than 0.20, Appendix II B.

Related substances Carry out in subdued light the method for *thin-layer chromatography*, Appendix III A, using a silica gel precoated chromatoplate (Merck silica gel 60 plates are suitable) and a mixture of 80 volumes of *propan-2-ol*, 15 volumes of 13.5M *ammonia* and 5 volumes of *chloroform* as the mobile phase. Apply separately to the plate 10 µl of each of two solutions of the substance being examined in *methanol* containing (1) 2.0% w/v and (2) 0.010% w/v. After removal of the plate, allow it to dry in air and spray with *sodium diazobenzenesulphonate solution*. Any *secondary spot* in the chromatogram obtained with solution (1) is not more intense than the spot in the chromatogram obtained with solution (2).

Loss on drying When dried to constant weight at 105°, loses not more than 1.0% of its weight. Use 1 g.

Sulphated ash Not more than 0.2%, Appendix IX A.

Assay Carry out Method I for *non-aqueous titration*, Appendix VIII A, using 0.5 g, 20 ml of *mercury(II) acetate solution* and *1-naphtholbenzein solution* as indicator. Each ml of 0.1M *perchloric acid VS* is equivalent to 0.02037 g of $C_9H_{13}NO_2,HCl$.

Storage Phenylephrine Hydrochloride should be kept in a well-closed container and protected from light.

Preparation
Phenylephrine Injection

Action and use Sympathomimetic.

Phenylmercuric Borate ☆

Phenylmercuric Borate is a compound consisting of equimolecular proportions of phenylmercury orthoborate and phenylmercury hydroxide ($C_{12}H_{13}BHg_2O_4$) or of the dehydrated form (metaborate, $C_{12}H_{11}BHg_2O_3$) or a mixture of the two compounds. It contains not less than 64.5 per cent and not more than 66.0 per cent of Hg and not less than the equivalent of 9.8 per cent and not more than the equivalent of 10.3 per cent of borates expressed as H_3BO_3, both calculated with reference to the dried substance.

Characteristics Colourless, shiny crystals or a white or slightly yellowish, crystalline powder; odourless or almost odourless.

Solubility Slightly soluble in *water* and in *ethanol (96%)*.

Identification A. Dissolve 0.25 g by sprinkling on the surface of boiling *water*, allow to cool and dilute to 25 ml with *water* (solution A). To 2 ml of solution A add 8 ml of

water and 0.1 ml of *sodium sulphate solution*. A white precipitate is produced which darkens slowly on heating.
B. To 0.1 g add 0.5 ml of *nitric acid*, heat until a dark brown colour is produced and transfer the solution with 20 ml of *water* into a beaker. The odour characteristic of nitrobenzene is produced.
C. Dissolve 20 mg in 2 ml of *methanol*. A clear, colourless solution is produced which when ignited burns with a green-edged flame.

Clarity and colour of solution Solution A is *clear*, Appendix IV A, and *colourless*, Appendix IV B, Method II.

Ionised mercury To 10 ml of solution A add 2 ml of 1M *potassium iodide* and 3 ml of 2M *hydrochloric acid* and filter; the filtrate is colourless. Wash the precipitate with 3 ml of *water* and to the combined filtrate and washings add 2 ml of 2M *sodium hydroxide* and dilute to 20 ml with *water*. 12 ml of the solution complies with *limit test A for heavy metals*, Appendix VII (100 ppm). Use a mixture of 2.5 ml of *lead standard solution (2 ppm Pb)* and 7.5 ml of *water* to prepare the standard.

Loss on drying When dried at 45° for 15 hours, loses not more than 3.5% of its weight. Use 0.5 g.

Assay *For Hg* Dissolve 0.3 g in 100 ml of *water* and add 3 ml of *nitric acid*. Titrate with 0.1M *ammonium thiocyanate VS*, using 2 ml of *ammonium iron(III) sulphate solution* as indicator, until a persistent reddish-yellow colour is obtained. Each ml of 0.1M *ammonium thiocyanate VS* is equivalent to 0.02006 g of Hg.

For borate Dissolve 0.6 g in 25 ml of *water* by heating, dissolve 10 g of D-*sorbitol* in the hot solution and cool. Titrate with 0.1M *sodium hydroxide VS*, using 0.5 ml of *dilute phenolphthalein solution* as indicator, until a persistent pink colour is obtained. Repeat the operation without the substance being examined. The difference between the titrations represents the amount of sodium hydroxide required. Each ml of 0.1M *sodium hydroxide VS* is equivalent to 0.00618 g of H_3BO_3.

Storage Phenylmercuric Borate should be kept in a well-closed container and protected from light.

Action and use Antiseptic; antimicrobial preservative.

Phenylmercuric Nitrate

$C_{12}H_{11}Hg_2NO_4$ 634.4   *55-68-5*

Phenylmercuric Nitrate is basic phenylmercury nitrate. It contains not less than 98.0 per cent and not more than 102.0 per cent of $C_{12}H_{11}Hg_2NO_4$, calculated with reference to the dried substance.

Characteristics White or yellowish-white, lustrous plates or a white, crystalline powder; odourless or almost odourless.

Solubility Very slightly soluble in *water* and in *ethanol (96%)*. It dissolves in *glycerol* and in fixed oils.

Identification A. To 10 ml of a saturated solution add 0.1 ml of *sodium sulphide solution*; a white precipitate is produced. Boil the mixture and allow to stand; the precipitate becomes black.
B. Heat 0.5 g with 0.5 g of *zinc powder*, 0.5 g of *reduced iron* and 5 ml of 5M *sodium hydroxide*. Ammonia is evolved.

C. Heat 50 mg with 7.5 ml of *iodine solution* and remove the excess of iodine with 0.1M *sodium thiosulphate*. A characteristic, aromatic odour is produced.
D. *Melting point*, about 188°, with decomposition, Appendix V A. Regulate the rate of rise of temperature to 5° per minute.

Acidity A 0.02% w/v solution in *carbon dioxide-free water* is neutral to *bromocresol green solution*.

Mercuric salts and heavy metals Heat 0.10 g with 15 ml of *water*, cool, filter and add 0.1 ml of *sodium sulphide solution* to the filtrate. The resulting precipitate shows no immediate colour.

Loss on drying When dried over *phosphorus pentoxide* at a pressure not exceeding 0.7 kPa for 24 hours, loses not more than 1.0% of its weight. Use 1 g.

Assay Boil 0.3 g with 5 ml of an 85% w/v solution of *formic acid*, 15 ml of *water* and 1 g of *zinc powder* under a reflux condenser for 30 minutes. Wash the condenser with 10 ml of *water*. Retaining as much as possible of the precipitate in the flask, filter and wash the precipitate with *water* until the washings are neutral to *litmus paper*. Dissolve any precipitate on the filter in a mixture of 20 ml of *nitric acid* and 10 ml of *water* and return the solution to the flask. Reattach the condenser and boil for 10 minutes. Wash the condenser with 10 ml of *water*. Disconnect the condenser, heat the flask on a water-bath for 3 minutes and add 0.5 g of *urea* and sufficient 0.02M *potassium permanganate* to produce a permanent pink colour. Cool, decolorise with a few drops of *hydrogen peroxide solution (20 vol)* and titrate with 0.1M *ammonium thiocyanate VS* using *ammonium iron(III) sulphate solution* as indicator. Each ml of 0.1M *ammonium thiocyanate VS* is equivalent to 0.01586 g of $C_{12}H_{11}Hg_2NO_4$.

Action and use Antiseptic; antimicrobial preservative.

Phenylpropanolamine Hydrochloride

$C_9H_{13}NO,HCl$ 187.7   *154-41-6*

Phenylpropanolamine Hydrochloride is (1*RS*),(2*SR*)-2-amino-1-phenylpropan-1-ol hydrochloride. It contains not less than 99.0 per cent and not more than 102.0 per cent of $C_9H_{13}NO,HCl$, calculated with reference to the dried substance.

Characteristics A white to creamy-white, crystalline powder; odourless or almost odourless.

Solubility Soluble in 2.5 parts of *water* and in 9 parts of *ethanol (96%)*; practically insoluble in *chloroform* and in *ether*.

Identification A. The *infra-red absorption spectrum*, Appendix II A, is concordant with the *reference spectrum* of phenylpropanolamine hydrochloride.
B. The *light absorption*, Appendix II B, in the range 230 to 350 nm of a 0.1% w/v solution in 0.1M *hydrochloric acid* exhibits three maxima, at 251, 257 and 262 nm. The *absorbance* at 251 nm is about 0.74, at 257 nm, about 0.94 and at 262 nm, about 0.72.

C. Dissolve 0.5 g in 20 ml of *water*, add 10 ml of 1M *sodium hydroxide* and extract with three 25-ml quantities of *ether*, washing each extract with the same 5 ml of *water*. Dry the combined ether extracts by shaking with *anhydrous sodium carbonate*, filter and evaporate the ether. The *melting point* of the residue, after drying at 80° for 2 hours, is about 102°, Appendix V A.

D. Yields the *reactions* characteristic of chlorides, Appendix VI.

Acidity pH of a 3% w/v solution, 4.5 to 6.0, Appendix V L.

Melting point 193° to 196°, Appendix V A.

(1RS,2RS)-Norpseudoephedrine Not more than 1.0% when determined by the following method. Carry out the method for *high-performance liquid chromatography*, Appendix III D, using solutions in the mobile phase containing (1) 0.010% w/v of *(1RS,2RS)-norpseudoephedrine hydrochloride BPCRS*, (2) 1.0% w/v of the substance being examined and (3) 0.10% w/v of the substance being examined and 0.10% w/v of *(1RS,2RS)-norpseudoephedrine hydrochloride BPCRS*.

The chromatographic procedure may be carried out using (a) a stainless steel column (20 cm × 4 mm) packed with *stationary phase C* (5 μm) (Nucleosil C18 is suitable), (b) 0.05M *dioctyl sodium sulphosuccinate* in a mixture of *methanol*, *water* and *glacial acetic acid* (60 volumes of *methanol*, 40 volumes of *water* and 1 volume of *glacial acetic acid* is usually suitable) as the mobile phase with a flow rate of 1 ml per minute and (c) a detection wavelength of 257 nm.

The area of any peak corresponding to *(1RS,2RS)-norpseudoephedrine* in the chromatogram obtained with solution (2) is not greater than that of the area of the peak due to *(1RS,2RS)-norpseudoephedrine* in the chromatogram obtained with solution (1). The test is not valid unless the *resolution factor* between the peaks due to *(1RS,2RS)-norpseudoephedrine* and phenylpropanolamine in the chromatogram obtained with solution (3) is more than 2.0, the *column efficiency* is not less than 15,000 theoretical plates per metre with respect to the peak due to phenylpropanolamine and the retention time of the peak due to phenylpropanolamine is not more than 30 minutes.

Phenones *Absorbance* of a 2% w/v solution in 0.01M *hydrochloric acid* at 283 nm, not more than 0.30, Appendix II B.

Loss on drying When dried to constant weight at 100° to 105°, loses not more than 0.5% of its weight. Use 1 g.

Sulphated ash Not more than 0.1%, Appendix IX A.

Assay Carry out Method I for *non-aqueous titration*, Appendix VIII A, using 0.6 g, 20 ml of *mercury(II) acetate solution* and *1-naphtholbenzein solution* as indicator. Each ml of 0.1M *perchloric acid VS* is equivalent to 0.01877 g of $C_9H_{13}NO,HCl$.

Action and use Sympathomimetic.

Phenytoin

$C_{15}H_{12}N_2O_2$ 252.3   *57-41-0*

Phenytoin is 5,5-diphenylimidazolidine-2,4-dione. It contains not less than 99.0 per cent and not more than 101.0 per cent of $C_{15}H_{12}N_2O_2$, calculated with reference to the dried substance.

Characteristics A white or almost white, crystalline powder; odourless or almost odourless.

Solubility Very slightly soluble in *water*; soluble in 70 parts of *ethanol (96%)*; slightly soluble in *chloroform* and in *ether*.

Identification A. The *infra-red absorption spectrum*, Appendix II A, is concordant with the *reference spectrum* of phenytoin.

B. To 0.1 g add 0.5 ml of 1M *sodium hydroxide*, 10 ml of a 10% w/v solution of *pyridine* and 1 ml of *copper sulphate—pyridine reagent* and allow to stand for 10 minutes. A blue precipitate is produced.

C. *Melting point*, about 295°, with decomposition, Appendix V A.

Clarity and colour of solution A solution of 1.0 g in a mixture of 20 ml of *water* and 5 ml of 1M *sodium hydroxide* is *clear*, Appendix IV A, and not more intensely coloured than *reference solution BY_6*, Appendix IV B, Method I.

Heavy metals Moisten the residue obtained in the test for Sulphated ash with 2 ml of *hydrochloric acid* and evaporate to dryness. Dissolve the residue in *water* and add sufficient *water* to produce 20 ml. 12 ml of the resulting solution complies with *limit test A for heavy metals*, Appendix VII (20 ppm). Use *lead standard solution (1 ppm Pb)* to prepare the standard.

Benzilic acid Dissolve 0.1 g in 5 ml of *sulphuric acid*. Any red colour produced is not more intense than that of a 0.002% w/v solution of *benzilic acid* in *sulphuric acid*.

Benzil and benzophenone Carry out the method for *thin-layer chromatography*, Appendix III A, using *silica gel GF254* as the coating substance and a mixture of 75 volumes of *hexane* and 30 volumes of *1,4-dioxan* as the mobile phase but allowing the solvent front to ascend 12 cm above the line of application. Apply separately to the chromatoplate 5 μl of each of the following solutions. Solution (1) contains 2.0% w/v of the substance being examined in a mixture of 1 volume of *glacial acetic acid* and 9 volumes of *acetone*. Solution (2) contains 0.0040% w/v of *benzophenone* in *ethanol (96%)*. Solution (3) contains 0.0040% w/v of *benzil* in *ethanol (96%)*. After removal of the plate, allow the solvent to evaporate and examine under *ultra-violet light (254 nm)*. In the chromatogram obtained with solution (1) any spots corresponding to benzophenone and benzil are not more intense than the spots in the chromatograms obtained with solutions (2) and (3) respectively.

Loss on drying When dried to constant weight at 105°, loses not more than 0.5% of its weight. Use 1.0 g.

Sulphated ash Not more than 0.1%, Appendix IX A. Use 1.0 g.

Assay Dissolve 0.5 g in 25 ml of *dimethylformamide* and carry out Method II for *non-aqueous titration*, Appendix VIII A, using 0.1M *sodium methoxide VS* as titrant and *quinaldine red solution* as indicator. Each ml of 0.1M *sodium methoxide VS* is equivalent to 0.02523 g of $C_{15}H_{12}N_2O_2$.

Storage Phenytoin should be kept in a well-closed container.

Preparation
Phenytoin Oral Suspension

Action and use Anticonvulsant.

Phenytoin Sodium ☆

$C_{15}H_{11}N_2NaO_2$ 274.3   *630-93-3*

Phenytoin Sodium is the sodium derivative of 5,5-diphenylimidazolidine-2,4-dione. It contains not less than 98.5 per cent and not more than 100.5 per cent of $C_{15}H_{11}N_2NaO_2$, calculated with reference to the anhydrous substance.

Characteristics A white, crystalline powder; slightly hygroscopic.

Solubility Soluble in *water* and in *ethanol (96%)*; practically insoluble in *chloroform* and in *ether*.

Identification *Test A may be omitted if tests B and C are carried out. Test B may be omitted if tests A and C are carried out.*

A. Dissolve 0.1 g in 20 ml of *water*, acidify with 2M *hydrochloric acid* and extract with three 30-ml quantities of *chloroform*. Wash the combined chloroform extracts with *water*, evaporate and dry the residue at 100° to 105°. The *infra-red absorption spectrum* of the residue, Appendix II A, is concordant with the spectrum of the residue obtained by treating 0.1 g of *phenytoin sodium EPCRS* in the same manner.

B. Heat 10 mg with 1 ml of *water* and 0.05 ml of 10M *ammonia* until boiling begins. Add 0.05 ml of a 5% w/v solution of *copper(II) sulphate* in 2M *ammonia* and shake. A pink, crystalline precipitate is produced.

C. Ignite 1 g and cool. Add 2 ml of *water* to the residue and neutralise the solution with *hydrochloric acid*. Filter and dilute the filtrate to 4 ml with *water*. 0.1 ml of the resulting solution yields *reaction B* characteristic of sodium salts, Appendix VI.

Clarity and colour of solution Suspend 1.0 g in 5 ml of *water* and dilute to 20 ml with 0.1M *sodium hydroxide*. The solution is *clear*, Appendix IV A, and not more intensely coloured than *reference solution BY$_6$*, Appendix IV B, Method II.

Heavy metals 2.0 g complies with *limit test C for heavy metals*, Appendix VII (10 ppm). Use 2 ml of *lead standard solution (10 ppm Pb)* to prepare the standard.

Free phenytoin Dissolve 0.3 g in 10 ml of a mixture of equal volumes of *pyridine* and *water* and add 0.5 ml of *dilute phenolphthalein solution* and 3 ml of *silver nitrate—pyridine reagent*. Not more than 1.0 ml of 0.1M *sodium hydroxide* is required to change the colour of the solution to pink.

Related substances Carry out the method for *thin-layer chromatography*, Appendix III A, using as the coating substance a suitable silica gel containing a fluorescent indicator with an optimal intensity at 254 nm (Merck silica gel 60 F254 is suitable) and a mixture of 45 volumes of *chloroform*, 45 volumes of *propan-2-ol* and 10 volumes of 13.5M *ammonia* as the mobile phase. Apply separately to the chromatoplate 10 μl of each of four solutions in *methanol* containing (1) 4% w/v of the substance being examined, (2) 0.04% w/v of the substance being examined, (3) 0.020% w/v of *benzophenone* and (4) 0.020% w/v of *benzil* and allow to dry in a current of cold air for 2 minutes. After removal of the plate, dry it at 80° for 5 minutes and examine under *ultra-violet light (254 nm)*. In the chromatogram obtained with solution (1) any spot corresponding to benzophenone is not more intense than the spot in the chromatogram obtained with solution (3), any spot corresponding to benzil is not more intense than the spot in the chromatogram obtained with solution (4) and any other *secondary spot* is not more intense than the spot in the chromatogram obtained with solution (2).

Water Not more than 3.0% w/w, Appendix IX C. Use 1 g.

Assay Suspend 0.18 g in 2 ml of *water*, add 8 ml of 0.05M *sulphuric acid VS* and heat gently for 1 minute. Add 30 ml of *methanol*, cool and titrate potentiometrically with 0.1M *sodium hydroxide VS*. After the first inflection, add 5 ml of *silver nitrate—pyridine reagent*, mix and complete the titration. Record the volume of 0.1M *sodium hydroxide VS* added between the two inflections. Each ml of 0.1M *sodium hydroxide VS* is equivalent to 0.02743 g of $C_{15}H_{11}N_2NaO_2$.

Storage Phenytoin Sodium should be kept in an airtight container.

Preparations
Phenytoin Capsules
Phenytoin Injection
Phenytoin Tablets

Action and use Anticonvulsant.

Pholcodine ☆

$C_{23}H_{30}N_2O_4,H_2O$ 416.5   *509-67-1*

Pholcodine is (5*R*,6*S*)-4,5-epoxy-9a-methyl-3-(2-morpholinoethoxy)morphin-7-en-6-ol monohydrate. It contains not less than 98.5 per cent and not more than 100.5 per cent of $C_{23}H_{30}N_2O_4$, calculated with reference to the dried substance.

Characteristics Colourless crystals or a white or almost white, crystalline powder.

Solubility Soluble in 50 parts of *water*; freely soluble in *ethanol (96%)* and in *acetone*; very soluble in *chloroform*; slightly soluble in *ether*. It dissolves in dilute mineral acids.

Identification *Test A may be omitted if tests B and C are carried out. Tests B and C may be omitted if test A is carried out.*

A. The *infra-red absorption spectrum*, Appendix II A, is concordant with the European Pharmacopœia reference spectrum of pholcodine.

B. To 10 ml of a 0.1% w/v solution add 75 ml of *water* and 10 ml of 1M *sodium hydroxide* and dilute to 100 ml with *water*. The *light absorption* of the resulting solution, Appendix II B, in the range 230 to 350 nm exhibits a maximum at 284 nm. The A(1%, 1 cm) at 284 nm is 36 to 38.

C. Dissolve 50 mg in 1 ml of *sulphuric acid* and add 0.05 ml of a 10% w/v solution of *ammonium molybdate*; a pale blue colour is produced which changes to deep blue on gentle warming. Add 0.05 ml of 2M *nitric acid*; the colour changes to brownish-red.

Specific optical rotation In a 2% w/v solution in *ethanol (96%)*, −94° to −98°, Appendix V F.

Related substances Carry out the method for *thin-layer chromatography*, Appendix III A, using *silica gel G* as the coating substance and a mixture of 70 volumes of *ethanol (96%)*, 70 volumes of *toluene*, 65 volumes of *acetone* and 5 volumes of 13.5M *ammonia* as the mobile phase. Apply separately to the chromatoplate 10 μl of each of three solutions of the substance being examined in *chloroform* containing (1) 2.5% w/v, (2) 0.025% w/v and (3) 0.0125% w/v. After removal of the plate, dry it in a current of air and spray with *dilute potassium iodobismuthate solution*. In the chromatogram obtained with solution (1) any *secondary spot* is not more intense than the spot in the chromatogram obtained with solution (2) and not more than one such spot of higher Rf value than the principal spot is more intense than the spot in the chromatogram obtained with solution (3).

Morphine Dissolve 0.10 g in 5 ml of 0.1M *hydrochloric acid*, add 2 ml of a 1% w/v solution of *sodium nitrite*, allow to stand for 15 minutes and add 3 ml of 6M *ammonia*. The solution is not more intensely coloured than *reference solution B₄*, Appendix IV B, Method II (about 0.13%).

Loss on drying When dried to constant weight at 100° to 105°, loses 3.9 to 4.5% of its weight. Use 0.5 g.

Sulphated ash Not more than 0.1%, Appendix IX A, Method II. Use 1 g.

Assay Dissolve 0.18 g in 50 ml of *anhydrous glacial acetic acid*, warming gently, and carry out Method I for *non-aqueous titration*, Appendix VIII A, determining the end-point potentiometrically at the second inflection. Each ml of 0.1M *perchloric acid VS* is equivalent to 0.01993 g of $C_{23}H_{30}N_2O_4$.

Storage Pholcodine should be kept in a well-closed container.

Preparations
Pholcodine Linctus
Strong Pholcodine Linctus

Action and use Cough suppressant.

Phosphoric Acid ☆

H_3PO_4 98.0   7664-38-2

Phosphoric Acid contains not less than 84.0 per cent w/w and not more than 90.0 per cent w/w of H_3PO_4.

Characteristics A clear, colourless, syrupy liquid; corrosive. When kept at a low temperature it may solidify,

producing a mass of colourless crystals which do not melt until the temperature reaches 28°. It has a relative density of about 1.7.

Solubility Miscible with *water* and with *ethanol (96%)*.

Identification A. Dilute with *water*. The solution is strongly acidic.

B. Dilute 10.0 g to 150 ml with *water* (solution A). Solution A, when neutralised with 2M *sodium hydroxide*, yields the *reactions* characteristic of phosphates, Appendix VI.

Clarity and colour of solution Solution A is *clear*, Appendix IV A, and *colourless*, Appendix IV B, Method II.

Arsenic 7.5 ml of solution A complies with the *limit test for arsenic*, Appendix VII (2 ppm).

Heavy metals To 2.5 g add 4 ml of 6M *ammonia* and dilute to 25 ml with *water*. 12 ml of the resulting solution complies with *limit test A for heavy metals*, Appendix VII (10 ppm). Use *lead standard solution (1 ppm Pb)* to prepare the standard.

Iron 3 ml of solution A diluted to 10 ml with *water* complies with the *limit test for iron*, Appendix VII (50 ppm).

Chloride 15 ml of solution A complies with the *limit test for chlorides*, Appendix VII (50 ppm).

Sulphate 1.5 g diluted to 15 ml with *distilled water* complies with the *limit test for sulphates*, Appendix VII (100 ppm).

Substances precipitated with ammonia To 10 ml of solution A add 8 ml of 6M *ammonia*. Any opalescence produced is not more intense than that of a mixture of 10 ml of solution A and 8 ml of *water*.

Hypophosphorous acid and phosphorous acid To 5 ml of solution A add 2 ml of a 1.7% w/v solution of *silver nitrate* and heat on a water-bath for 5 minutes. The appearance of the solution does not change.

Assay To 1 g add a solution of 10 g of *sodium chloride* in 30 ml of *water* and titrate with 1M *sodium hydroxide VS* using *dilute phenolphthalein solution* as indicator. Each ml of 1M *sodium hydroxide VS* is equivalent to 0.04900 g of H_3PO_4.

Storage Phosphoric Acid should be kept in a well-closed, glass container.

Preparation
Dilute Phosphoric Acid
The title of the monograph in the European Pharmacopœia is Concentrated Phosphoric Acid.

Dilute Phosphoric Acid ☆

Dilute Phosphoric Acid contains not less than 9.5 and not more than 10.5 per cent w/w of H_3PO_4 and is prepared by mixing 115 g of Phosphoric Acid and 885 g of Purified Water.

Identification A. It is strongly acidic.

B. Dilute 86.0 g to 150 ml with *water* (solution A). The resulting solution, when neutralised with *sodium hydroxide*, yields the *reactions* characteristic of phosphates, Appendix VI.

Clarity and colour of solution Solution A is *clear*, Appendix IV A, and *colourless*, Appendix IV B, Method II.

Arsenic 7.5 ml of solution A complies with the *limit test for arsenic*, Appendix VII (0.2 ppm).

Heavy metals To 20 g add 4 ml of *6M ammonia* and dilute to 25 ml with *water*. 12 ml of the resulting solution complies with *limit test A for heavy metals*, Appendix VII (1 ppm). Use a mixture of 8 ml of *lead standard solution (1 ppm Pb)* and 2 ml of *water* to prepare the standard.

Iron 3 ml of solution A diluted to 10 ml with *water* complies with the *limit test for iron*, Appendix VII (6 ppm).

Chloride 15 ml of solution A complies with the *limit test for chlorides*, Appendix VII (6 ppm).

Sulphate 15 ml of the substance being examined complies with the *limit test for sulphates*, Appendix VII (10 ppm).

Substances precipitated with ammonia To 10 ml of solution A add 8 ml of *6M ammonia*. Any opalescence produced is not more intense than that of a mixture of 10 ml of solution A and 8 ml of *water*.

Hypophosphorous acid and phosphorous acid To 5 ml of solution A add 2 ml of a 1.7% w/v solution of *silver nitrate* and heat on a water-bath for 5 minutes. The appearance of the solution is unchanged.

Assay To 8.6 g add a solution of 10 g of *sodium chloride* in 30 ml of *water* and titrate with *1M sodium hydroxide VS* using *dilute phenolphthalein solution* as indicator. Each ml of *1M sodium hydroxide VS* is equivalent to 0.04900 g of H_3PO_4.

Phthalylsulphathiazole ☆

$C_{17}H_{13}N_3O_5S_2$ 403.4   *85-73-4*

Phthalylsulphathiazole is 4′-(thiazol-2-ylsulphamoyl)phthalanilic acid. It contains not less than 98.5 per cent and not more than 101.5 per cent of $C_{17}H_{13}N_3O_5S_2$, calculated with reference to the dried substance.

Characteristics White or yellowish-white, crystalline powder; odourless.

Solubility Practically insoluble in *water*, in *chloroform* and in *ether*; slightly soluble in *ethanol (96%)* and in *acetone*; freely soluble in *dimethylformamide*.

Identification *Test A may be omitted if tests B, C, D and E are carried out. Tests B and C may be omitted if tests A, D and E are carried out.*

A. The *infra-red absorption spectrum*, Appendix II A, is concordant with the spectrum of *phthalylsulfathiazole EPCRS*.

B. Heat 0.1 g with 0.5 g of *resorcinol* and 0.3 ml of *sulphuric acid* on a water-bath until a homogeneous mixture is obtained, cool, add 5 ml of *2M sodium hydroxide* and dilute 0.1 ml of the brownish-red mixture with 25 ml of *water*. An intense green fluorescence is produced which disappears on acidification.

C. To 0.1 g add 3 ml of *1M sulphuric acid* and 0.5 g of *zinc powder*. Fumes are evolved which turn *lead acetate paper* black.

D. Boil 2 g with 8.5 ml of *2M sodium hydroxide* under a reflux condenser for 30 minutes. Cool, add 17.5 ml of *2M hydrochloric acid*, shake vigorously and filter. Neutralise the filtrate with *2M sodium hydroxide*, filter, wash the precipitate with *water* and recrystallise from *water*. The *melting point* of the crystals, after drying at 100° to 105°, is 200° to 203°, Appendix V A, Method I.

E. 2 ml of a 0.005% w/v solution of the crystals obtained in test D in *0.1M hydrochloric acid* yields the *reaction characteristic of primary aromatic amines*, Appendix VI, producing an orange precipitate.

Acidity Shake 2 g with 20 ml of *water* continuously for 30 minutes. Filter and to 10 ml of the filtrate add 0.1 ml of *dilute phenolphthalein solution*. Not more than 0.2 ml of *0.1M sodium hydroxide VS* is required to change the colour of the solution.

Clarity and colour of solution A 5.0% w/v solution in *1M sodium hydroxide* is *clear*, Appendix IV A, and not more intensely coloured than *reference solution BY_5*, Appendix IV B, Method II.

Heavy metals 1.0 g complies with *limit test C for heavy metals*, Appendix VII (20 ppm). Use 2 ml of *lead standard solution (10 ppm Pb)* to prepare the standard.

Sulphathiazole and related aromatic amines Dissolve 5 mg in a mixture of 25 ml of *ethanol (96%)*, 3.5 ml of *water* and 6 ml of *2M hydrochloric acid* previously cooled to 15°. Cool rapidly in ice, immediately add 1 ml of a 0.25% w/v solution of *sodium nitrite*, allow to stand for 3 minutes, add 2.5 ml of a 4% w/v solution of *sulphamic acid* and allow to stand for 5 minutes. Add 1 ml of a 0.4% w/v solution of *N-(1-naphthyl)ethylenediamine dihydrochloride* and dilute to 50 ml with *water*. The *absorbance* of the resulting solution at 550 nm, Appendix II B, is not more than that of a solution prepared at the same time and in the same manner using a mixture of 25 ml of *ethanol (96%)*, 2.5 ml of *water*, 6 ml of *2M hydrochloric acid* and 1 ml of a solution containing 10 mg of *sulphathiazole* and 0.5 ml of *hydrochloric acid* in 100 ml and beginning at the words 'Cool rapidly in ice . . .'.

Loss on drying When dried to constant weight at 100° to 105°, loses not more than 2.0% of its weight. Use 1 g.

Sulphated ash Not more than 0.1%, Appendix IX A, Method II. Use 1 g.

Assay Dissolve 0.3 g in 40 ml of *dimethylformamide* and titrate with *0.1M sodium hydroxide VS* using 0.2 ml of *thymolphthalein solution* as indicator until a blue colour is obtained. Repeat the operation without the substance being examined. The difference between the titrations represents the amount of sodium hydroxide required. Each ml of *0.1M sodium hydroxide VS* is equivalent to 0.02017 g of $C_{17}H_{13}N_3O_5S_2$.

Storage Phthalylsulphathiazole should be protected from light.

Action and use Antibacterial.

Physostigmine Salicylate ☆

Eserine Salicylate

$C_{15}H_{21}N_3O_2,C_7H_6O_3$ 413.5   *57-64-7*

Physostigmine Salicylate is (3aS,8aR)-1,2,3, 3a,8,8a-hexahydro-1,3a,8-trimethyl-pyrrolo[2,3-b]indol-5-yl methylcarbamate salicylate. It contains not less than 98.5 per cent and not more than 101.0 per cent of $C_{15}H_{21}N_3O_2,C_7H_6O_3$, calculated with reference to the dried substance.

Characteristics Colourless or almost colourless crystals which gradually turn red on exposure to air and light, more rapidly in the presence of moisture; odourless. It melts at about 182° with decomposition.

Solubility Soluble in 90 parts of *water* and in 25 parts of *ethanol (96%)*; soluble in *chloroform*; very slightly soluble in *ether*. Aqueous solutions are unstable.

Identification *Test A may be omitted if tests B, C and D are carried out. Tests C and D may be omitted if tests A and B are carried out.*
A. The *infra-red absorption spectrum*, Appendix II A, is concordant with the spectrum of *physostigmine salicylate EPCRS*.
B. In the test for Related substances, the principal spot in the chromatogram obtained with solution (2) is similar in position, colour and size to that in the chromatogram obtained with solution (3).
C. Heat 10 mg in a porcelain dish with 0.15 ml of 6M *ammonia*; an orange solution is produced. The residue obtained on evaporation is soluble in *ethanol (96%)* producing a blue solution. Add 0.1 ml of *glacial acetic acid*; the colour changes to violet and on dilution with *water* exhibits an intense red fluorescence.
D. A 0.9% w/v solution in *carbon dioxide-free water* yields *reaction A* characteristic of salicylates, Appendix VI.

Acidity Dissolve 0.900 g without heating in 95 ml of *carbon dioxide-free water* prepared from *distilled water* and dilute to 100 ml with the same solvent (solution A). The pH of the solution, examined immediately after preparation, is 5.1 to 5.9, Appendix V L.

Clarity and colour of solution Solution A, examined immediately after preparation, is *clear*, Appendix IV A, and *colourless*, Appendix IV B, Method II.

Specific optical rotation In solution A, −90° to −94°, Appendix V F.

Sulphate Solution A complies with the *limit test for sulphates*, Appendix VII (0.1%).

Eseridine To 5 ml of solution A add a few crystals of *potassium iodate* and 0.05 ml of 2M *hydrochloric acid*, add 2 ml of *chloroform* and shake. The chloroform layer does not turn violet within 1 minute.

Related substances Carry out the method for *thin-layer chromatography*, Appendix III A, using *silica gel G* as the coating substance and a mixture of 100 volumes of *cyclohexane*, 23 volumes of *propan-2-ol* and 2 volumes of 13.5M *ammonia* as the mobile phase. Apply separately to the chromatoplate 20 μl of each of four solutions in *ethanol (96%)* containing (1) 2% w/v of the substance being examined, (2) 0.1% w/v of the substance being examined, (3) 0.1% w/v of *physostigmine salicylate EPCRS* and (4) 0.01% w/v of *physostigmine salicylate EPCRS*. After removal of the plate, dry it in a current of cold air, carry out a second chromatographic development in the same direction, remove the plate again, allow it to dry in air and spray with *freshly prepared acetic potassium iodobismuthate solution* and then with *hydrogen peroxide solution (10 vol)*. Examine the plate within 2 minutes. Any *secondary spot* in the chromatogram obtained with solution (1) is not more intense than the spot in the chromatogram obtained with solution (4).

Loss on drying When dried to constant weight at 100° to 105°, loses not more than 1.0% of its weight. Use 1 g.

Sulphated ash Not more than 0.1%, Appendix IX A, Method II. Use the residue obtained in the test for Loss on drying.

Assay Dissolve 0.35 g in 50 ml of a mixture of equal volumes of *chloroform* and *anhydrous glacial acetic acid* and carry out Method I for *non-aqueous titration*, Appendix VIII A, determining the end-point potentiometrically. Each ml of 0.1M *perchloric acid VS* is equivalent to 0.04135 g of $C_{15}H_{21}N_3O_2,C_7H_6O_3$.

Storage Physostigmine Salicylate should be kept in an airtight container and protected from light. An aqueous solution of Physostigmine Salicylate becomes red on exposure to air and preferably should be freshly prepared; if stored, it should be kept in a sealed container.

Action and use Used in treatment of glaucoma.

Physostigmine Sulphate

Eserine Sulphate

$(C_{15}H_{21}N_3O_2)_2,H_2SO_4$ 648.8   *64-47-1*

Physostigmine Sulphate is (3aS,8aR)-1,2,3, 3a,8,8a-hexahydro-1,3a,8-trimethyl-pyrrolo[2,3-b]indol-5-yl methylcarbamate sulphate. It contains not less than 97.0 per cent and not more than 101.0 per cent of $(C_{15}H_{21}N_3O_2)_2,H_2SO_4$, calculated with reference to the dried substance.

Characteristics A white or almost white, microcrystalline powder; odourless or almost odourless; deliquescent.

Solubility Soluble in less than 1 part of *water* and in less than 1 part of *ethanol (96%)*; slightly soluble in *ether*.

Identification A. Dissolve 0.05 g in 2 ml of *water* and add 1M *sodium hydroxide*, dropwise. A white precipitate is produced which dissolves in excess 1M *sodium hydroxide* to produce a red solution.
B. Warm 5 mg with 0.3 ml of 5M *ammonia*. A yellowish-red solution is produced which on evaporation yields a bluish residue.

C. The residue obtained in test B is soluble in *ethanol (96%)* producing a blue solution which, on addition of 6M *acetic acid*, appears blue by transmitted light and exhibits a red fluorescence which is intensified by dilution with *water*. The residue is also soluble in *sulphuric acid*, producing a green solution which, on the gradual addition of *ethanol (96%)*, changes to red but reverts to green when the ethanol is evaporated.

D. Yields the *reactions* characteristic of sulphates, Appendix VI.

Acidity pH of a 1% w/v solution, 3.5 to 5.5, Appendix V L.

Melting point 143° to 147°, Appendix V A.

Specific optical rotation In a 2% w/v solution, −116° to −120°, Appendix V F.

Loss on drying When dried to constant weight at 105°, loses not more than 1.0% of its weight. Use 1 g.

Sulphated ash Not more than 0.1%, Appendix IX A.

Assay Dissolve 0.17 g in 25 ml of *water*, make alkaline by the addition of 1 g of *sodium hydrogen carbonate* and extract with three 25-ml quantities of *chloroform*, filtering each extract through a dry filter paper. Combine the extracts, add 25 ml of *anhydrous glacial acetic acid* and carry out Method I for *non-aqueous titration*, Appendix VIII A, using 0.02M *perchloric acid VS* and *crystal violet solution* as indicator. Each ml of 0.02M *perchloric acid VS* is equivalent to 0.006488 g of $(C_{15}H_{21}N_3O_2)_2,H_2SO_4$.

Storage Physostigmine Sulphate should be kept in a well-closed container and protected from light. An aqueous solution of Physostigmine Sulphate becomes red on exposure to air and preferably should be freshly prepared; if stored, it should be kept in a sealed container.

Preparation
Physostigmine Eye Drops

Action and use Used in treatment of glaucoma.

Phytomenadione
Vitamin K$_1$

$C_{31}H_{46}O_2$ 450.7   *84-80-0*

Phytomenadione is 2-methyl-3-phytyl-1,4-naphthaquinone. It contains not less than 97.0 per cent and not more than 102.0 per cent of $C_{31}H_{46}O_2$.

Characteristics A clear, deep yellow oil; odourless or almost odourless.

Solubility Practically insoluble in *water*; soluble in 70 parts of *ethanol (96%)*; freely soluble in *chloroform*, in *ether* and in fixed oils.

Identification A. The *light absorption*, Appendix II B, in the range 230 to 350 nm of a 0.002% w/v solution in

2,2,4-trimethylpentane exhibits four maxima, at 243, 249, 261 and 270 nm. The *absorbance* at 243 nm is about 0.80, at 249 nm, about 0.84, at 261 nm, about 0.77 and at 270 nm, about 0.78. The spectrum also exhibits minima at 228, 246, 254 and 266 nm. The ratio of the *absorbance* at the minimum at 254 nm to that at the maximum at 249 nm is 0.70 to 0.75.

B. The *light absorption*, Appendix II B, in the range 230 to 350 nm of a 0.02% w/v solution in *2,2,4-trimethylpentane* exhibits a maximum at 327 nm and a minimum at 285 nm. The *absorbance* at the maximum at 327 nm is about 1.4 and at the minimum at 285 nm is about 0.44.

C. To 0.05 ml add 10 ml of *methanol* and 1 ml of a 20% w/v solution of *potassium hydroxide* in *methanol*; a green colour is produced. Heat gently; the colour changes to purple and, on standing, to reddish-brown.

Refractive index 1.526 to 1.528, Appendix V E.

Related substances Carry out in subdued light the method for *thin-layer chromatography*, Appendix III A, using *silica gel GF254* as the coating substance and a mixture of 80 volumes of *cyclohexane*, 20 volumes of *ether* and 1 volume of *methanol* as the mobile phase. Apply separately to the chromatoplate 10 µl of each of two solutions in *2,2,4-trimethylpentane* containing (1) 0.50% w/v of the substance being examined and (2) 0.0050% w/v of *2-methyl-1,4-naphthoquinone*. After removal of the plate, allow it to dry in air and examine under *ultra-violet light (254 nm)*. Any *secondary spot* in the chromatogram obtained with solution (1) is not more intense than the spot in the chromatogram obtained with solution (2).

Sulphated ash Not more than 0.1%, Appendix IX A.

Assay Carry out the following procedure in subdued light. Dissolve 0.1 g in sufficient *2,2,4-trimethylpentane* to produce 100 ml. Dilute 10 ml to 100 ml with *2,2,4-trimethylpentane*, dilute 10 ml of this solution to 100 ml with the same solvent and measure the *absorbance* of the resulting solution at the maximum at 249 nm, Appendix II B. Calculate the content of $C_{31}H_{46}O_2$ taking 420 as the value of A(1%, 1 cm) at the maximum at 249 nm.

Storage Phytomenadione should be kept in a well-closed container and protected from light.

Preparations
Phytomenadione Injection
Phytomenadione Tablets

Pilocarpine Hydrochloride

$C_{11}H_{16}N_2O_2,HCl$ 244.7   *54-71-7*

Pilocarpine Hydrochloride is (3S,4R)-3-ethyl-dihydro-4-[(1-methyl-1H-imidazol-5-yl)methyl]-furan-2(3H)-one hydrochloride. It contains not less than 99.0 per cent and not more than 101.0 per cent of $C_{11}H_{16}N_2O_2,HCl$, calculated with reference to the dried substance.

Characteristics Colourless crystals or a white, crystalline powder; odourless or almost odourless; hygroscopic.

Solubility Soluble in less than 1 part of *water* and in 3 parts of *ethanol (96%)*; slightly soluble in *chloroform*; practically insoluble in *ether*.

Identification A. Dissolve 10 mg in 5 ml of *water*, add 0.1 ml of 1M *sulphuric acid*, 1 ml of *hydrogen peroxide solution (20 vol)*, 1 ml of *toluene* and 0.05 ml of *potassium chromate solution*, shake well and allow to separate. The toluene layer is bluish-violet and the aqueous layer remains yellow.

B. Yields the *reactions* characteristic of chlorides, Appendix VI.

Acidity pH of a 0.5% w/v solution, 3.8 to 5.2, Appendix V L.

Melting point 200° to 205°, Appendix V A.

Specific optical rotation In a 2% w/v solution, +89.0° to +93.0°, Appendix V F.

Nitrate Dissolve 50 mg in 5 ml of *water* and carefully add the solution to 5 ml of a 0.1% w/v solution of *diphenyl-amine* in *sulphuric acid*, ensuring that the liquids do not mix. No blue colour is produced at the liquid interface.

Foreign alkaloids Carry out the method for *thin-layer chromatography*, Appendix III A, using *silica gel G* as the coating substance and a mixture of 125 volumes of *chloroform*, 100 volumes of *acetone* and 2 volumes of 13.5M *ammonia* as the mobile phase. Apply to the chromatoplate 5 µl of a 5.0% w/v solution of the substance being examined in *water*. After removal of the plate, allow it to dry in air and spray with *dilute potassium iodobismuthate solution*. No *secondary spot* is revealed in the chromatogram.

Loss on drying When dried at 105° for 2 hours, loses not more than 1.0% of its weight. Use 1 g.

Sulphated ash Not more than 0.1%, Appendix IX A.

Assay Carry out Method I for *non-aqueous titration*, Appendix VIII A, using 0.5 g. Each ml of 0.1M *perchloric acid VS* is equivalent to 0.02447 g of $C_{11}H_{16}N_2O_2,HCl$.

Storage Pilocarpine Hydrochloride should be kept in a well-closed container and protected from light.

Preparation
Pilocarpine Eye Drops

Action and use Used in treatment of glaucoma.

Pilocarpine Nitrate ☆

$C_{11}H_{16}N_2O_2,HNO_3$ 271.3   *148-72-1*

Pilocarpine Nitrate is (3*S*,4*R*)-3-ethyldihydro-4-[(1-methyl-1*H*-imidazol-5-yl)methyl]furan-2(3*H*)-one nitrate. It contains not less than 98.5 per cent and not more than 101.0 per cent of $C_{11}H_{16}N_2O_2,HNO_3$, calculated with reference to the dried substance.

Characteristics Colourless crystals or a white, crystalline powder; odourless. It melts at about 174°, with decomposition.

Solubility Soluble in 8 parts of *water*; sparingly soluble in *ethanol (96%)*; practically insoluble in *chloroform* and in *ether*.

Identification *Test A may be omitted if tests B, C, D and E are carried out. Tests B and D may be omitted if tests A, C and E are carried out.*

A. The *infra-red absorption spectrum*, Appendix II A, is concordant with the spectrum of *pilocarpine nitrate EPCRS*.

B. In the test for Related substances, the principal spot in the chromatogram obtained with solution (2) is similar in position, colour and size to the spot in the chromatogram obtained with solution (3).

C. Complies with the test for Specific optical rotation.

D. Dissolve 10 mg in 2 ml of *water*, add 0.05 ml of a 5% w/v solution of *potassium dichromate*, 1 ml of *hydrogen peroxide solution (10 vol)* and 2 ml of *chloroform* and shake. A violet colour is produced in the chloroform layer.

E. Yields *reaction A* characteristic of nitrates, Appendix VI.

Acidity pH of a 5% w/v solution, 3.5 to 4.5, Appendix V L.

Clarity and colour of solution A 5.0% w/v solution in *carbon dioxide-free water* (solution A) is *clear*, Appendix IV A, and not more intensely coloured than *reference solution* Y_6, Appendix IV B, Method II.

Specific optical rotation In solution A, +80° to +83°, Appendix V F.

Iron 10 ml of solution A complies with the *limit test for iron*, Appendix VII (10 ppm). Use 5 ml of *iron standard solution (1 ppm Fe)* and 5 ml of *water* to prepare the standard.

Chloride Solution A complies with the *limit test for chlorides*, Appendix VII (70 ppm).

Related substances Carry out the method for *thin-layer chromatography*, Appendix III A, using *silica gel G* as the coating substance and a mixture of 85 volumes of *chloroform*, 14 volumes of *methanol* and 1 volume of 13.5M *ammonia* as the mobile phase. Apply separately to the chromatoplate 10 µl of each four solutions in *water* containing (1) 3% w/v of the substance being examined, (2) 0.1% w/v of the substance being examined, (3) 0.1% w/v of *pilocarpine nitrate EPCRS* and (4) 0.03% w/v of *pilocarpine nitrate EPCRS*. After removal of the plate, dry it at 100° to 105° for 10 minutes, allow to cool and spray with *acetic potassium iodobismuthate solution*. Any *secondary spot* in the chromatogram obtained with solution (1) is not more intense than the spot in the chromatogram obtained with solution (4).

Loss on drying When dried to constant weight at 100° to 105°, loses not more than 0.5% of its weight. Use 0.1 g.

Sulphated ash Not more than 0.1%, Appendix IX A, Method II. Use 0.5 g.

Assay Dissolve 0.25 g in 30 ml of *anhydrous glacial acetic acid* and carry out Method I for *non-aqueous titration*, Appendix VIII A, determining the end-point potentiometrically. Each ml of 0.1M *perchloric acid VS* is equivalent to 0.02713 g of $C_{11}H_{16}N_2O_2,HNO_3$.

Storage Pilocarpine Nitrate should be kept in a well-closed container and protected from light.

Action and use Used in treatment of glaucoma.

Pindolol

OCH₂·CH·CH₂·NHPrⁱ
|
OH

$C_{14}H_{20}N_2O_2$ 248.3   *13523-86-9*

Pindolol is 1-(indol-4-yloxy)-3-isopropyl-aminopropan-2-ol. It contains not less than 98.5 per cent and not more than 101.0 per cent of $C_{14}H_{20}N_2O_2$, calculated with reference to the dried substance.

Characteristics A white or almost white, crystalline powder; odourless or almost odourless.

Solubility Practically insoluble in *water*; slightly soluble in *absolute ethanol* and in *chloroform*; sparingly soluble in *methanol*.

Identification A. The *infra-red absorption spectrum*, Appendix II A, is concordant with the *reference spectrum* of pindolol.
B. The *light absorption*, Appendix II B, in the range 230 to 350 nm of a 0.004% w/v solution in *methanol* exhibits two maxima, at 264 nm and at 287 nm, and a shoulder at 275 nm. The *absorbance* at 264 nm is about 1.36 and at 287 nm is about 0.78.
C. Dissolve 20 mg in a mixture of 1 volume of *glacial acetic acid* and 99 volumes of *methanol* and dilute to 5 ml with the same solvent mixture. Further dilute 1 ml of this solution to 50 ml with the same solvent mixture. To 2 ml of the resulting solution add 1 ml of *dilute dimethyl-aminobenzaldehyde reagent*. A violet-blue colour is produced.
D. *Melting point*, about 171°, Appendix V A.

Clarity and colour of solution A 5.0% w/v solution in 1M *acetic acid* is *clear*, Appendix IV A, and not more intensely coloured than *reference solution BY₄* or *B₄*, Appendix IV B, Method II.

Related substances Carry out in subdued light the method for *thin-layer chromatography*, Appendix III A, using a silica gel precoated chromatoplate (Merck silica gel 60 plates are suitable) and a mixture of 150 volumes of *dichloromethane*, 47 volumes of *methanol* and 3 volumes of *anhydrous formic acid* as the mobile phase. Apply separately to the plate as bands 5 µl of each of three solutions of the substance being examined in a mixture of 1 volume of *glacial acetic acid* and 99 volumes of *methanol* containing (1) 0.40% w/v, prepared immediately before use and applied to the plate as the last solution, (2) 0.0028% w/v and (3) 0.0012% w/v. After removal of the plate, spray immediately with a 1% w/v solution of *4-dimethylaminobenzaldehyde* in a mixture of equal volumes of *hydrochloric acid* and *ethanol (96%)* and warm at 50° for 20 minutes. Any band with an Rf value of about 0.1 in the chromatogram obtained with solution (1) is not more intense than the band in the chromatogram obtained with solution (2). Any other *secondary band* in the chromatogram obtained with solution (1) is not more intense than the band in the chromatogram obtained with solution (3).

Loss on drying When dried to constant weight at 100° to 105°, loses not more than 0.5% of its weight. Use 1 g.

Sulphated ash Not more than 0.1%, Appendix IX A.

Assay Dissolve 0.2 g in 80 ml of *methanol* and titrate with 0.1M *hydrochloric acid VS* determining the end-point potentiometrically. Each ml of 0.1M *hydrochloric acid VS* is equivalent to 0.02483 g of $C_{14}H_{20}N_2O_2$.

Storage Pindolol should be kept in a well-closed container and protected from light.

Preparation
Pindolol Tablets

Action and use Beta-adrenoceptor antagonist.

Piperazine Adipate ☆

$C_4H_{10}N_2,C_6H_{10}O_4$ 232.3   *142-88-1*

Piperazine Adipate contains not less than 98.0 per cent and not more than 101.0 per cent of $C_4H_{10}N_2,C_6H_{10}O_4$, calculated with reference to the anhydrous substance.

Characteristics A white, crystalline powder. It melts at about 250°, with decomposition.

Solubility Soluble in 18 parts of *water*; practically insoluble in *ethanol (96%)*.

Identification *Test A may be omitted if tests B and C are carried out. Tests B and C may be omitted if test A is carried out.*
A. The *infra-red absorption spectrum*, Appendix II A, is concordant with the spectrum of *piperazine adipate EPCRS*.
B. In the test for Related substances examine the chromatoplate after spraying with the ninhydrin solutions. The principal spot in the chromatogram obtained with solution (2) is similar in position, colour and size to that in the chromatogram obtained with solution (3).
C. To 10 ml of a 5% w/v solution add 5 ml of *hydrochloric acid* and extract with three 10-ml quantities of *ether*. Evaporate the combined ether extracts to dryness. The *melting point* of the residue, after washing with *water* and drying at 100° to 105°, is 150° to 154°, Appendix V A, Method I.

Clarity and colour of solution A 5.0% w/v solution is *clear*, Appendix IV A, and not more intensely coloured than *reference solution B₈*, Appendix IV B, Method II.

Heavy metals A 5.0% w/v solution complies with *limit test A for heavy metals*, Appendix VII (20 ppm). Use *lead standard solution (1 ppm Pb)* to prepare the standard.

Related substances Carry out the method for *thin-layer chromatography*, Appendix III A, using a suitable silica gel as the coating substance (Merck silica gel 60 precoated chromatoplates are suitable) and a freshly prepared mixture of 80 volumes of *acetone* and 20 volumes of 13.5M *ammonia* as the mobile phase. Apply separately to the chromatoplate 5 µl of each of six solutions in a mixture of 3 volumes of 13.5M *ammonia* and 2 volumes of *absolute ethanol* containing (1) 10% w/v of the substance being examined, (2) 1.0% w/v of the substance being examined, (3) 1% w/v of *piperazine adipate EPCRS*, (4) 0.025% w/v of *ethylenediamine*, (5) 0.025% w/v of *triethylenediamine* and (6) 0.025% w/v of *triethylenediamine* and 1.0% w/v of the substance being examined. After removal of the plate, dry it at 105°, spray with a 0.3% w/v solution of *ninhydrin* in a mixture of 3 volumes of *glacial acetic acid* and 100 volumes of *butan-1-ol* and then with a 0.15% w/v solution of *ninhydrin* in *absolute ethanol* and dry at 105° for 10 minutes. Any *secondary spot* in the chromatogram obtained with solution (1) is not more intense than the spot in the chromatogram obtained with solution (4). Spray the plate with 0.1M *iodine VS* and allow to stand for 10 minutes. Any spot corresponding to triethylenediamine in the chromatogram obtained with solution (1) is not more intense than the spot in the chromatogram obtained with solution (5). The test is not valid unless the chromatogram obtained with solution (6) shows a spot due to triethylenediamine clearly separated from the principal spot. Disregard any spot on the line of application.

Sulphated ash Not more than 0.1%, Appendix IX A, Method II. Use 1 g.

Water Not more than 0.5%, Appendix IX C. Use 1 g.

Assay Dissolve 0.1 g in 10 ml of *anhydrous glacial acetic acid* with gentle heating and dilute to 70 ml with the same solvent. Carry out Method I for *non-aqueous titration*, Appendix VIII A, using 0.25 ml of *naphtholbenzein solution* as indicator and titrating until the colour of the solution changes from brownish-yellow to green. Each ml of 0.1M *perchloric acid VS* is equivalent to 0.01161 g of $C_4H_{10}N_2,C_6H_{10}O_4$.

Storage Piperazine Adipate should be kept in a well-closed container.

Action and use Anthelmintic.

Piperazine Citrate ☆

$(C_4H_{10}N_2)_3,2C_6H_8O_7$ 643   *41372-10-5*

Piperazine Citrate contains not less than 98.0 per cent and not more than 101.0 per cent of $(C_4H_{10}N_2)_3,2C_6H_8O_7$, calculated with reference to the anhydrous substance. It contains a variable amount of water.

Characteristics A white, granular powder. After drying at 100° to 105° it melts at about 190°.

Solubility Soluble in 1.5 parts of *water*; practically insoluble in *ethanol (96%)* and in *ether*.

Identification *Test A may be omitted if tests B and C are carried out. Tests B and C may be omitted if test A is carried out.*

A. The *infra-red absorption spectrum*, Appendix II A, is concordant with the spectrum of *piperazine citrate EPCRS*. Dry the substances at 120° for 5 hours, powder, taking care to avoid the uptake of moisture, and immediately record the spectra.

B. In the test for Related substances examine the chromatoplate after spraying with the ninhydrin solutions. The principal spot in the chromatogram obtained with solution (2) is similar in position, colour and size to that in the chromatogram obtained with solution (3).

C. A 10% w/v solution yields the *reactions* characteristic of citrates, Appendix VI.

Clarity and colour of solution A 5.0% w/v solution is *clear*, Appendix IV A, and not more intensely coloured than *reference solution B_8*, Appendix IV B, Method II.

Heavy metals A 5.0% w/v solution complies with *limit test A for heavy metals*, Appendix VII (20 ppm). Use *lead standard solution (1 ppm Pb)* to prepare the standard.

Water 10.0 to 14.0% w/w, Appendix IX C. Use 0.3 g.

Related substances Complies with the test described under Piperazine Adipate, using *piperazine citrate EPCRS* in place of *piperazine adipate EPCRS* to prepare solution (3).

Sulphated ash Not more than 0.1%, Appendix IX A, Method II. Use 1 g.

Assay Dissolve 0.1 g in 10 ml of *anhydrous glacial acetic acid* with gentle heating and dilute to 70 ml with the same solvent. Carry out Method I for *non-aqueous titration*, Appendix VIII A, using 0.25 ml of *naphtholbenzein solution* as indicator and titrating until the colour of the solution changes from brownish-yellow to green. Each ml of 0.1M *perchloric acid VS* is equivalent to 0.01071 g of $(C_4H_{10}N_2)_3,2C_6H_8O_7$.

Storage Piperazine Citrate should be kept in a well-closed container.

Preparation
Piperazine Citrate Elixir

Action and use Anthelmintic.

Piperazine Hydrate ☆

$C_4H_{10}N_2,6H_2O$ 194.2   *142-63-2*

Piperazine Hydrate contains not less than 98.0 per cent and not more than 101.0 per cent of $C_4H_{10}N_2,6H_2O$.

Characteristics Colourless, deliquescent crystals. It melts at about 43°.

Solubility Freely soluble in *water* and in *ethanol (96%)*; very slightly soluble in *ether*.

Identification *Test A may be omitted if tests B and C are carried out. Tests B and C may be omitted if test A is carried out.*

A. The *infra-red absorption spectrum*, Appendix II A, is concordant with the spectrum of *piperazine hydrate EPCRS*. Dry the substances over *phosphorus pentoxide* at a pressure of 1.5 to 2.5 kPa for 48 hours, powder, taking care to avoid the uptake of moisture, and immediately record the spectra.

B. In the test for Related substances examine the chromatoplate after spraying with the ninhydrin solutions. The principal spot in the chromatogram obtained with solution (2) is similar in position, colour and size to that in the chromatogram obtained with solution (3).

C. Dissolve 0.5 g in 5 ml of 2M *sodium hydroxide*, add 0.2 ml of *benzoyl chloride* and mix. Continue to add 0.2-ml quantities of *benzoyl chloride* until precipitation is complete. Filter and wash the precipitate with a total of 10 ml of *water* added in small quantities. Dissolve the precipitate in 2 ml of hot *ethanol (96%)*, pour the solution into 5 ml of *water*, allow to stand for 4 hours and filter. The *melting point* of the crystals, after washing with *water* and drying at 100° to 105°, is 191° to 196°, Appendix V A, Method I.

Alkalinity pH of a 5% w/v solution, 10.5 to 12.0, Appendix V L.

Clarity and colour of solution A 5.0% w/v solution in *carbon dioxide-free water* is *clear*, Appendix IV A, and not more intensely coloured than *reference solution B₈*, Appendix IV B, Method II.

Heavy metals A 5.0% w/v solution in *carbon dioxide-free water* complies with *limit test A for heavy metals*, Appendix VII (20 ppm). Use *lead standard solution (1 ppm Pb)* to prepare the standard.

Related substances Complies with the test described under Piperazine Adipate, using *piperazine hydrate EPCRS* in place of *piperazine adipate EPCRS* to prepare solution (3).

Sulphated ash Not more than 0.1%, Appendix IX A, Method II. Use 1 g.

Assay Dissolve 80 mg in 10 ml of *anhydrous glacial acetic acid* with gentle heating and dilute to 70 ml with the same solvent. Carry out Method I for *non-aqueous titration*, Appendix VIII A, using 0.25 ml of *naphtholbenzein solution* as indicator and titrating until the colour of the solution changes from brownish-yellow to green. Each ml of 0.1M *perchloric acid VS* is equivalent to 0.00971 g of $C_4H_{10}N_2,6H_2O$.

Storage Piperazine Hydrate should be kept in an airtight container and protected from light.

Action and use Anthelmintic.

Piperazine Phosphate

$C_4H_{10}N_2,H_3PO_4,H_2O$ 202.1   *18534-18-4*

Piperazine Phosphate contains not less than 98.5 per cent and not more than 100.5 per cent of $C_4H_{10}N_2,H_3PO_4$, calculated with reference to the anhydrous substance.

Characteristics A white, crystalline powder; odourless or almost odourless.

Solubility Soluble in 60 parts of *water*; practically insoluble in *ethanol (96%)*.

Identification A. Dissolve 0.1 g in 5 ml of *water*, add 0.5 g of *sodium hydrogen carbonate*, 0.5 ml of a 5% w/v solution of *potassium hexacyanoferrate(III)* and 0.1 ml of *mercury*. Shake vigorously for 1 minute and allow to stand for 20 minutes. A reddish colour is produced slowly.
B. Dissolve 0.2 g in 5 ml of 2M *hydrochloric acid*, add with stirring 1 ml of a 50% w/v solution of *sodium nitrite* and cool in ice for 15 minutes, stirring if necessary to induce crystallisation. The *melting point* of the crystals, after washing with 10 ml of ice-cold *water* and drying at 105°, is about 159°, Appendix V A.
C. A solution yields the *reactions* characteristic of phoshates, Appendix VI.

Acidity pH of a 1% w/v solution, 6.0 to 6.5, Appendix V L.

Heavy metals Dissolve 2.0 g in 20 ml of 2M *acetic acid*. 12 ml of the resulting solution complies with *limit test A for heavy metals*, Appendix VII (20 ppm). Use *lead standard solution (2 ppm Pb)* to prepare the standard.

Water 8.0 to 9.5% w/w, Appendix IX C. Use 0.25 g.

Assay Dissolve 0.2 g in a mixture of 3.5 ml of 0.5M *sulphuric acid* and 10 ml of *water*. Add 100 ml of *trinitro-phenol solution*, heat on a water-bath for 15 minutes and allow to stand for 1 hour. Filter through a sintered-glass filter (BS porosity No. 4) and wash the residue with successive 10-ml quantities of a mixture of equal volumes of a saturated solution of *2,4,6-trinitrophenol* and *water* until the washings are free from sulphate. Wash the residue with five 10-ml quantities of *absolute ethanol* and dry to constant weight at 100° to 105°. Each g of residue is equivalent to 0.3382 g of $C_4H_{10}N_2,H_3PO_4$.

Preparation
Piperazine Phosphate Tablets

Action and use Anthelmintic.

Podophyllum Resin
Podophyllin

Podophyllum Resin is the resin obtained from the dried rhizomes and roots of *Podophyllum hexandrum* Royle (*P. emodi* Wall.) or, more rarely, of *Podophyllum peltatum* L.

Characteristics An amorphous powder varying in colour from light brown to greenish-yellow, or brownish-grey masses; odour, characteristic; caustic.

Solubility Partly soluble in hot *water*, from which it is precipitated on cooling, in *chloroform*, in *ether* and in 5M *ammonia*.

Identification Add 0.4 g, finely powdered, to 3 ml of *ethanol (60%)*, then add 0.5 ml of 1M *potassium hydroxide*, shake gently and allow to stand. The resin of *P. hexandrum* produces a stiff jelly; the resin of *P. peltatum* does not gelatinise.

Matter insoluble in ethanol (96%) Shake 1 g, finely powdered, with 20 ml of *ethanol (96%)* for 5 minutes, filter through a sintered-glass crucible (BS porosity No. 2), wash the filter with *ethanol (96%)* and dry at 105°. The residue weighs not more than 25 mg.

Matter insoluble in 5M ammonia Shake 0.5 g, finely powdered, with 30 ml of 5M *ammonia* for 30 minutes at about 20°; filter through a sintered-glass crucible (BS porosity No. 2) and wash the flask and filter with 30 ml of *water*, the time taken for filtering and washing being not more than 10 minutes. Dry the filter and residue to constant weight at 105°. The residue from the resin of *P. hexandrum* weighs not less than 0.18 g and not more than 0.30 g; the residue from the resin of *P. peltatum* weighs not more than 50 mg.

Loss on drying When dried to constant weight at 105°, loses not more than 5.0% of its weight. Use 1 g.

Sulphated ash Not more than 1.0%, Appendix IX A.

Storage Podophyllum Resin should be kept in a well-closed container and protected from light. On exposure to light, or to temperatures above 25°, it becomes darker in colour.

Labelling The label states the botanical source.

Preparation
Compound Podophyllin Paint

Action and use Used in treatment of warts.

Poldine Methylsulphate

$$PH_2CCO \cdot OCH_2 \overset{OH}{\underset{N}{\overset{Me}{\underset{+}{\overset{Me}{\mid}}}}} \quad CH_3 \cdot SO_4^-$$

$C_{22}H_{29}NO_7S$ 451.5   *1545-80-2*

Poldine Methylsulphate is 2-benziloyloxy-methyl-1,1-dimethylpyrrolidinium methyl-sulphate. It contains not less than 98.5 per cent and not more than 100.5 per cent of $C_{22}H_{29}NO_7S$, calculated with reference to the dried substance.

Characteristics A white, crystalline powder; odourless or almost odourless.

Solubility Soluble in 1 part of *water* and in 20 parts of *ethanol (96%)*; slightly soluble in *chloroform*.

Identification A. The *infra-red absorption spectrum*, Appendix II A, is concordant with the *reference spectrum* of poldine methylsulphate.
B. The *light absorption*, Appendix II B, in the range 250 to 350 nm of a 0.1% w/v solution exhibits maxima at 252 nm and 258 nm and inflections at 262, 264 and 268 nm. The *absorbance* at 252 nm is about 0.85 and at 258 nm is about 0.99.
C. Dissolve 2 mg in 10 ml of *water*, add 20 ml of *ammonium cobaltothiocyanate solution* and 5 ml of *chloroform* and shake well. The chloroform layer becomes blue.

Acidity or alkalinity pH of a 1.0% w/v solution, 5.0 to 7.0, Appendix V L.

Melting point 137° to 142°, Appendix V A.

Related substances Carry out the method for *thin-layer chromatography*, Appendix III A, using a silica gel precoated chromatoplate (Merck silica gel 60 plates are suitable) and a mixture of 60 volumes of *chloroform*, 30 volumes of *methanol*, 5 volumes of *formic acid* and 5 volumes of *water* as the mobile phase. Apply separately to the chromatoplate 20 µl of each of two solutions of the substance being examined in a mixture of 5 volumes of *methanol* and 1 volume of *formic acid* containing (1) 1.0% w/v and (2) 0.010% w/v. After removal of the plate, allow it to dry in air, spray with *sulphuric acid (50%)* and heat at 110° for 10 minutes. Any pink *secondary spot* in the chromatogram obtained with solution (1) is not more intense than the spot in the chromatogram obtained with solution (2).

Loss on drying When dried to constant weight at 80°, loses not more than 0.5% of its weight. Use 1 g.

Sulphated ash Not more than 0.1%, Appendix IX A.

Assay Dissolve 0.5 g in 10 ml of *water* in a stoppered flask, add 0.05 ml of *cresol red solution* and, if necessary, sufficient 0.05M *sodium hydroxide* to produce a pale pink colour. Add 20 ml of 0.1M *sodium hydroxide VS*, stopper the flask and allow to stand for 10 minutes at 25°. Titrate with 0.1M *hydrochloric acid VS* using *cresol red solution* as indicator. Repeat the operation without the substance being examined. The difference between the titrations represents the amount of alkali required. Each ml of 0.1M *sodium hydroxide VS* is equivalent to 0.04515 g of $C_{22}H_{29}NO_7S$.

Preparation
Poldine Tablets

Action and use Antispasmodic.

In some countries the material described in this monograph may be known as Poldine Metilsulfate.

Polymyxin B Sulphate ☆

$$RCO-A_2bu-Thr-A_2bu-\overset{\overline{\begin{array}{c}N\gamma\end{array}}}{A_2bu}-A_2bu-DPhe-Leu-A_2bu-A_2bu-Thr \quad +H_2SO_4$$

Polymyxin	R
B_1	$-CH_2 \cdot (CH_2)_5 \cdot CHMe \cdot CH_3$
B_2	$-CH_2 \cdot (CH_2)_4 \cdot CHMe \cdot CH_3$

1405-20-5

Polymyxin B Sulphate is a mixture of the sulphates of polypeptides produced by the growth of certain strains of *Bacillus polymyxa* or obtained by any other means. The potency is not less than 6500 Units per mg, calculated with reference to the dried substance.

Characteristics A white or almost white powder; almost odourless; hygroscopic.

Solubility Soluble in *water*; slightly soluble in *ethanol (96%)*.

Identification A. Carry out the method for *thin-layer chromatography*, Appendix III A, protected from light using *silica gel G* as the coating substance and a mixture of 75 parts of *phenol* and 25 parts of *water* as the mobile phase, but allowing the solvent front to ascend 12 cm above the line of application. Apply separately to the chromatoplate, as 10-mm bands, 5 µl of each of the following solutions. For solution (1) dissolve 5 mg of the substance being examined in a mixture of 0.5 ml of *hydrochloric acid* and 0.5 ml of *water*, heat in a sealed tube at 135° for 5 hours, evaporate to dryness on a water-bath, continue to heat until the odour of hydrogen chloride is no longer detectable and dissolve the residue in 0.5 ml of *water*. Solutions (2) to (5) are solutions in *water* containing (2) 0.2% w/v of *L-leucine*, (3) 0.2% w/v of *L-threonine*, (4) 0.2% w/v of *L-phenylalanine* and (5) 0.2% w/v of *L-serine*. Place the plate in the tank so that it is not in contact with the mobile phase and expose it to the vapour of the mobile phase for at least 12 hours.

After removal of the plate, heat it at 100° to 105° and spray with *ethanolic ninhydrin solution*. Heat the plate at 110° for 5 minutes. The chromatogram obtained with solution (1) shows bands corresponding to those in the chromatograms obtained with solutions (2), (3) and (4) but does not show a band corresponding to that in the chromatogram obtained with solution (5). The chromatogram obtained with solution (1) also shows a band with a very low Rf value (2,4-diaminobutyric acid).
B. Dissolve 2 mg in 5 ml of *water* and add 5 ml of 2.5M *sodium hydroxide*. Shake and add 0.25 ml of a 1% w/v solution of *copper(II) sulphate* dropwise, shaking after each addition. A reddish-violet colour is produced.
C. Yields *reaction A* characteristic of sulphates, Appendix VI.

Acidity or alkalinity pH of a 2% w/v solution, 5.0 to 7.0, Appendix V L.

Specific optical rotation In a 2% w/v solution, −78° to −90°, Appendix V F.

Sulphate 15.5 to 17.5% of SO₄, calculated with reference to the dried substance, when determined by the following method. Dissolve 0.25 g in 100 ml of *water*, adjust the pH to 11 with 13.5M *ammonia* and add 10 ml of 0.1M *barium chloride VS*. Titrate with 0.1M *disodium edetate VS* using 0.5 mg of *metalphthalein* as indicator. When the colour of the solution begins to change add 50 ml of *ethanol (96%)* and continue the titration until the violet-blue colour disappears. Each ml of 0.1M *barium chloride VS* is equivalent to 0.009606 g of SO₄.

Phenylalanine 9 to 12%, calculated with reference to the dried substance, when determined by the following method. Dissolve 0.375 g (*w*) in sufficient 0.1M *hydrochloric acid* to produce 100 ml and measure the *absorbance* of the resulting solution at the maxima at 252, 258 and 264 nm and at 280 and 300 nm, Appendix II B. Calculate the percentage content of phenylalanine from the expression

$$9.4787(A_{258} - 0.5A_{252} + 0.5A_{264} - 1.8A_{280} + 0.8A_{300})/w,$$

where A_{252}, A_{258}, A_{264}, A_{280} and A_{300} are the absorbances at 252, 258, 264, 280 and 300 nm, respectively.

Loss on drying When dried over *phosphorus pentoxide* at 60° at a pressure not exceeding 0.7 kPa for 3 hours, loses not more than 6.0% of its weight. Use 1 g.

Sulphated ash Not more than 0.75%, Appendix IX A, Method II. Use 1 g.

Assay Carry out the *biological assay of antibiotics*, Appendix XIV A. The precision of the assay is such that the fiducial limits of error are not less than 95% and not more than 105% of the estimated potency.

Storage Polymyxin B Sulphate should be kept in an airtight container and protected from light. If it is intended for use in the manufacture of a parenteral dosage form the container should be sterile, tamper-evident and sealed so as to exclude micro-organisms.

Labelling The label states (1) the number of Units per mg; (2) the date after which the material is not intended to be used; (3) the conditions under which it should be stored; (4) whether or not it is intended for use in the manufacture of a parenteral dosage form.

Preparation Polymyxin and Bacitracin Eye Ointment

Action and use Antibacterial.

Polymyxin B Sulphate intended for use in the manufacture of a parenteral dosage form complies with the following additional requirements.

Abnormal toxicity Complies with the *test for abnormal toxicity*, Appendix XIV L. Use 0.1 mg dissolved in 0.5 ml of *saline solution*, the injection occupying not more than 60 seconds. The specified time is 48 hours.

Pyrogens Complies with the *test for pyrogens*, Appendix XIV K. Use per kg of the rabbit's weight 1 ml of *water for injections* containing 1.5 mg per ml.

Sterility Complies with the *test for sterility*, Appendix XVI A.

Polysorbate 20 ☆

Polyoxyethylene 20 Sorbitan Monolaurate

9005-64-5

Polysorbate 20 is a mixture of partial lauric esters of sorbitol and its mono- and dianhydrides copolymerised with approximately 20 moles of ethylene oxide for each mole of sorbitol and its anhydrides. The lauric acid used for the esterification may contain variable amounts of other fatty acids.

Characteristics A clear or slightly opalescent, oily, yellowish or brownish-yellow liquid. It has a relative density of about 1.10.

Solubility Miscible with *water*, with *absolute ethanol*, with *ethyl acetate* and with *methanol*; practically insoluble in fixed oils and in *liquid paraffin*.

Identification A. Dissolve 0.5 g in *water* at about 50° and dilute to 10 ml with the same solvent; the solution produces a prolific foam on shaking. Add 0.5 g of *sodium chloride* and heat to boiling; the resulting cloudiness disappears during cooling to about 50°.
B. Heat 4 g under a reflux condenser on a water-bath for 30 minutes with 40 ml of a 5% w/v solution of *potassium hydroxide*. Allow to cool to about 80°, acidify with 20 ml of 2M *nitric acid* and boil for about 10 minutes under a reflux condenser in order to destroy the emulsion. The fatty acid separates on the surface as an oily liquid. Allow to cool to room temperature and extract with 50 ml of *petroleum spirit (boiling range, 50° to 70°)* avoiding vigorous shaking. Wash the organic phase with three 5-ml quantities of *water* and evaporate the organic phase on a water-bath. The *acid value* of the residue, Appendix X B, is 245 to 300. Use 0.3 g.
C. Dissolve 0.1 g in 5 ml of *chloroform*, add 0.1 g of *potassium thiocyanate* and 0.1 g of *cobalt(II) nitrate* and stir with a glass rod. A blue colour is produced.

Acid value Not more than 2.0, Appendix X B. Use 5 g.

Hydroxyl value 96 to 108, Appendix X D, Method II. Use 2 g.

Iodine value Not more than 5.0 (*iodine bromide method*), Appendix X E.

Saponification value 40 to 50, Appendix X G, Method II. Use 15 ml of 0.5M *ethanolic potassium hydroxide VS* and dilute with 50 ml of *water* before carrying out the titration.

Heavy metals 2.0 g complies with *limit test C for heavy metals*, Appendix VII (10 ppm). Use 2 ml of *lead standard solution (10 ppm)* to prepare the standard.

Reducing substances Dissolve 2 g in 25 ml of hot *water*, add 25 ml of 1M *sulphuric acid* and 0.1 ml of *ferroin sulphate solution* and titrate with 0.01M *ammonium cerium(IV) nitrate VS* until the colour change from red to greenish-blue persists for 30 seconds. Repeat the operation without the substance being examined. The difference between the titrations represents the amount of ammonium cerium(IV) nitrate required. Not more than 2.0 ml of 0.01M *ammonium cerium(IV) nitrate VS* is required.

Sulphated ash Not more than 0.2% when determined by the following method. To 2 g in a silica or platinum crucible add 0.5 ml of *sulphuric acid* and heat on a water-bath for 2 hours. Carefully ignite at a low temperature until thoroughly charred. Add 2 ml of *nitric acid* and 0.25 ml of *sulphuric acid*, cautiously heat until white fumes are evolved and then ignite at 600° until the carbon is entirely burned off. Allow to cool, weigh and repeat the operation for periods of 15 minutes until two successive weighings do not differ by more than 0.5 mg.

Water Not more than 3.0% w/w, Appendix IX C. Use 1 g.

Storage Polysorbate 20 should be kept in an airtight container and protected from light.

Action and use Non-ionic surface-active agent.

Polysorbate 60 ☆
Polyoxyethylene 20 Sorbitan Monostearate

9005-67-8

Polysorbate 60 is a mixture of partial stearic esters of sorbitol and its mono- and dianhydrides copolymerised with approximately 20 moles of ethylene oxide for each mole of sorbitol and its anhydrides. The stearic acid used for the esterification may contain variable amounts of other fatty acids, especially palmitic acid.

Characteristics A yellowish-brown semi-gel becoming a clear liquid above 25°. It has a relative density of about 1.10.

Solubility Miscible with *water*, with *absolute ethanol*, with *ethyl acetate* and with *methanol*; practically insoluble in fixed oils and in *liquid paraffin*.

Identification A. Dissolve 0.5 g in *water* at about 50° and dilute to 10 ml with the same solvent; the solution produces a prolific foam on shaking. Add 0.5 g of *sodium chloride* and heat to boiling; the resulting cloudiness disappears during cooling to about 50°.
B. Heat 4 g under a reflux condenser on a water-bath for 30 minutes with 40 ml of a 5% w/v solution of *potassium hydroxide*. Allow to cool to about 80°, acidify with 20 ml of 2M *nitric acid* and boil for about 10 minutes under a reflux condenser in order to destroy the emulsion. The fatty acid separates on the surface as an oily liquid. Allow to cool to room temperature and extract with 50 ml of *petroleum spirit (boiling range, 50° to 70°)* avoiding vigorous shaking. Wash the organic phase with three 5-ml quantities of *water* and evaporate the organic phase on a water-bath. The *acid value* of the residue, Appendix X B, is 190 to 220. Use 0.5 g.
C. Dissolve 0.1 g in 5 ml of *chloroform*, add 0.1 g of *potassium thiocyanate* and 0.1 g of *cobalt(II) nitrate* and stir with a glass rod. A blue colour is produced.

Acid value Not more than 2.0, Appendix X B. Use 5 g.

Hydroxyl value 81 to 96, Appendix X D, Method II. Use 2 g.

Iodine value Not more than 5.0 *(iodine bromide method)*, Appendix X E.

Saponification value 45 to 55, Appendix X G, Method II. Use 15 ml of 0.5M *ethanolic potassium hydroxide VS* and dilute with 50 ml of *water* before carrying out the titration.

Heavy metals; Reducing substances; Sulphated ash; Water Complies with the tests described under Polysorbate 20.

Storage Polysorbate 60 should be kept in an airtight container and protected from light.

Action and use Non-ionic surface-active agent.

Polysorbate 80 ☆
Polyoxyethylene 20 Sorbitan Mono-oleate

9005-65-6

Polysorbate 80 is a mixture of partial oleic esters of sorbitol and its mono- and dianhydrides copolymerised with approximately 20 moles of ethylene oxide for each mole of sorbitol and its anhydrides.

Characteristics A clear, oily, yellowish or brownish-yellow liquid. It has a relative density of about 1.08 and a viscosity, at 25°, of about 400 mPa s.

Solubility Miscible with *water*, with *absolute ethanol*, with *ethyl acetate* and with *methanol*; practically insoluble in fixed oils and in *liquid paraffin*.

Identification A. Dissolve 0.5 g in *water* at about 50° and dilute to 10 ml with the same solvent; the solution produces a prolific foam on shaking. Add 0.5 g of *sodium chloride* and heat to boiling; the resulting cloudiness disappears during cooling to about 50°.
B. Heat 4 g under a reflux condenser on a water-bath for 30 minutes with 40 ml of a 5% w/v solution of *potassium hydroxide*. Allow to cool to about 80°, acidify with 20 ml of 2M *nitric acid* and boil for about 10 minutes under a reflux condenser in order to destroy the emulsion. Cool to 50° and centrifuge. The fatty acid separates on the surface as an oily liquid. Allow to cool to room temperature and extract with 50 ml of *petroleum spirit (boiling range, 50° to 70°)* avoiding vigorous shaking. Wash the organic phase with three 5-ml quantities of *water* and evaporate the organic phase on a water-bath. Superimpose the residue so obtained on a mixture of 2 ml of *nitric acid* and 3 ml of *water*. Carefully add, in small portions, 0.5 g of *sodium nitrite* and allow to stand at room temperature. The fatty acid layer becomes solid within 4 hours.
C. To 2 ml of a 5% w/v solution add 0.5 ml of *bromine water*. The bromine is decolorised.
D. Dissolve 0.1 g of 5 ml of *chloroform*, add 0.1 g of *potassium thiocyanate* and 0.1 g of *cobalt(II) nitrate* and stir with a glass rod. A blue colour is produced.

Acid value Not more than 2.0, Appendix X B. Use 5 g.

Hydroxyl value 65 to 80, Appendix X D, Method II. Use 2 g.

Iodine value 18 to 24 *(iodine bromide method)*, Appendix X E.

Saponification value 45 to 55, Appendix X G, Method II. Use 15 ml of 0.5M *ethanolic potassium hydroxide VS* and dilute with 50 ml of *water* before carrying out the titration.

Heavy metals; Sulphated ash; Water Complies with the tests described under Polysorbate 20.

Reducing substances Dissolve 2 g in 25 ml of hot *water*, add 25 ml of 1M *sulphuric acid* and 0.1 ml of *ferroin sulphate solution* and titrate with 0.01M *ammonium cerium(IV) nitrate VS* until the colour change from red to greenish-blue persists for 30 seconds. Repeat the operation without the substance being examined. The difference between the titrations represents the amount of ammonium cerium(IV) nitrate required. Not more than 5.0 ml of 0.01M *ammonium cerium(IV) nitrate VS* is required.

Storage Polysorbate 80 should be kept in an airtight container and protected from light.

Action and use Non-ionic surface-active agent.

Polythiazide

$C_{11}H_{13}ClF_3N_3O_4S_3$ 439.9   *346-18-9*

Polythiazide is 6-chloro-3,4-dihydro-2-methyl-3-(2,2,2-trifluoroethylthiomethyl)-1,2,4-benzo-thiadiazine-7-sulphonamide 1,1-dioxide. It contains not less than 97.0 per cent and not more than 102.0 per cent of $C_{11}H_{13}ClF_3N_3O_4S_3$, calculated with reference to the dried substance.

Characteristics A white or almost white, crystalline powder; odour, alliaceous.

Solubility Practically insoluble in *water* and in *chloroform*; soluble in 40 parts of *ethanol (96%)*.

Identification A. The *infra-red absorption spectrum*, Appendix II A, is concordant with the *reference spectrum* of polythiazide.

B. The *light absorption*, Appendix II B, in the range 230 to 350 nm of a 0.002% w/v solution in *methanol* exhibits a maximum at 268 nm and a less well-defined maximum at 317 nm. The *absorbance* at 268 nm is about 1.0.

C. Carry out the method for *thin-layer chromatography*, Appendix III A, using *silica gel GF254* as the coating substance and a mixture of 50 volumes of *toluene*, 30 volumes of *ether* and 20 volumes of *acetone* as the mobile phase. Apply separately to the chromatoplate 20 μl of each of two solutions in *methanol* containing (1) 0.02% w/v of the substance being examined and (2) 0.02% w/v of *polythiazide BPCRS*. After removal of the plate, allow it to dry in air until the odour of solvent is no longer detectable, examine under *ultra-violet light (254 nm)* and then reveal the spots using *Method I*. The principal spot in the chromatogram obtained with solution (1) corresponds in colour and intensity to that in the chromatogram obtained with solution (2).

Related substances Carry out the method for *thin-layer chromatography*, Appendix III A, using *silica gel G* as the coating substance and a mixture of 90 volumes of *chloroform* and 10 volumes of *methanol* as the mobile phase. Apply separately to the chromatoplate 5 μl of solution (1) and quantities of 1, 2, 3, 4 and 5 μl of solution (2). Solutions (1) and (2) are solutions of the substance being examined in *acetone* containing (1) 1.0% w/v and (2) 0.020% w/v. After removal of the plate, allow it to dry in air and reveal the spots using *Method I*. Assess the intensity of each *secondary spot* in the chromatogram obtained with solution (1) by reference to the spots in the chromatograms obtained with the

applications of solution (2). The sum of the intensities so assessed does not exceed 3% and no such spot is more intense than the spot in the chromatogram obtained with 5 μl of solution (2).

Loss on drying When dried to constant weight at 105°, loses not more than 1.0% of its weight. Use 1 g.

Sulphated ash Not more than 0.1%, Appendix IX A.

Assay Dissolve 0.1 g in sufficient *methanol* to produce 250 ml, dilute 5 ml to 200 ml with *methanol* and measure the *absorbance* of the resulting solution at the maximum at 268 nm, Appendix II B. Calculate the content of $C_{11}H_{13}ClF_3N_3O_4S_3$ taking 500 as the value of A(1%, 1 cm) at the maximum at 268 nm.

Preparation
Polythiazide Tablets

Action and use Diuretic.

Potassium Acetate

$C_2H_3O_2K$ 98.14   *127-08-2*

Potassium Acetate contains not less than 99.0 per cent and not more than 101.0 per cent of $C_2H_3O_2K$, calculated with reference to the dried substance.

Characteristics Colourless crystals or a white, crystalline powder; odourless or almost odourless.

Solubility Soluble in 0.5 part of *water* and in 2 parts of *ethanol (96%)*.

Identification Yields the *reactions* characteristic of potassium salts and of acetates, Appendix VI.

Alkalinity pH of a 5% w/v solution, 7.5 to 9.5, Appendix V L.

Aluminium Dissolve 4.0 g in 100 ml of *water* and add 10 ml of *acetate buffer pH 6.0*. The resulting solution complies with the *limit test for aluminium*, Appendix VII (1 ppm).

Arsenic 0.50 g complies with the *limit test for arsenic*, Appendix VII (2 ppm).

Calcium 0.10 g complies with the *limit test for calcium*, Appendix VII (100 ppm).

Heavy metals A 25% w/v solution complies with *limit test A for heavy metals*, Appendix VII (4 ppm). Use *lead standard solution (1 ppm Pb)* to prepare the standard.

Magnesium A 0.10% w/v solution complies with the *limit test for magnesium*, Appendix VII (0.1%).

Sodium Not more than 0.5% when determined by Method II for *atomic emission spectrophotometry*, Appendix II D, using a 1% w/v solution and measuring at 589 nm. Use *sodium solution ASp*, diluted if necessary with *water*, for the standard solution.

Chloride 0.14 g complies with the *limit test for chlorides*, Appendix VII (350 ppm).

Nitrate Dissolve 1.0 g in 10 ml of *water* and add 5 mg of *sodium chloride*, 0.05 ml of *indigo carmine solution* and, with stirring, 10 ml of *nitrogen-free sulphuric acid*. A blue colour is produced which persists for at least 10 minutes.

Sulphate 0.25 g complies with the *limit test for sulphates*, Appendix VII (600 ppm).

Readily oxidisable substances Dissolve 2.0 g in 100 ml of boiling *water*, add 6 ml of 5M *sulphuric acid* and 0.3 ml of 0.02M *potassium permanganate*, mix and boil gently for 5 minutes. The pink colour is not completely discharged.

Loss on drying When dried to constant weight at 105°, loses not more than 5.0% of its weight. Use 1 g.

Assay Carry out Method I for *non-aqueous titration*, Appendix VIII A, using 0.2 g and *crystal violet solution* as indicator. Each ml of 0.1M *perchloric acid VS* is equivalent to 0.009814 g of $C_2H_3O_2K$.

Storage Potassium Acetate should be kept in a well-closed container.

Action and use Used in solutions for haemodialysis and peritoneal dialysis.

Potassium Bromide ☆

KBr   119.0   *7758-02-3*

Potassium Bromide contains not less than 98.0 per cent and not more than 100.5 per cent of KBr, calculated with reference to the dried substance.

Characteristics Colourless crystals or a white, crystalline powder; odourless.

Solubility Freely soluble in *water* and in *glycerol*; slightly soluble in *ethanol (96%)*.

Identification A. A 10.0% w/v solution in *carbon dioxide-free water* (solution A) yields the *reactions* characteristic of potassium salts, Appendix VI.
B. Yields the *reactions* characteristic of bromides, Appendix VI.

Acidity or alkalinity To 10 ml of solution A add 0.1 ml of *bromothymol blue solution*. Not more than 0.5 ml of either 0.01M *hydrochloric acid VS* or 0.01M *sodium hydroxide VS* is required to change the colour of the solution.

Clarity and colour of solution Solution A is *clear*, Appendix IV A, and *colourless*, Appendix IV B, Method II.

Barium To 5 ml of solution A add 5 ml of *distilled water* and 1 ml of 1M *sulphuric acid*. After 15 minutes the solution is not more opalescent than a mixture of 5 ml of solution A and 6 ml of *distilled water*.

Heavy metals 12 ml of solution A complies with *limit test A for heavy metals*, Appendix VII (10 ppm). Use *lead standard solution (1 ppm Pb)* to prepare the standard.

Iron 5 ml of solution A diluted to 10 ml with *water* complies with the *limit test for iron*, Appendix VII (20 ppm).

Magnesium and alkaline-earth metals 10 g complies with the *limit test for magnesium and alkaline-earth metals*, Appendix VII. Not more than 5.0 ml of 0.01M *disodium edetate VS* is required (200 ppm, calculated as Ca).

Bromate To 10 ml of solution A add 1 ml of *starch solution*, 0.1 ml of *potassium iodide solution* and 0.25 ml of 0.5M *sulphuric acid* and allow to stand protected from light. No blue or violet colour is produced after 5 minutes.

Chloride Dissolve 1 g in 20 ml of 2M *nitric acid*, add 5 ml of *hydrogen peroxide solution (100 vol)* and heat on a water-bath until the solution is completely decolorised. Wash down the sides of the flask with *water*, heat on a water-bath for 15 minutes, cool and dilute to 50 ml with *water*. Add 5 ml of 0.1M *silver nitrate VS* and 1 ml of *dibutyl phthalate* and titrate with 0.1M *ammonium thiocyanate VS* using 5 ml of *ammonium iron(III) sulphate solution* as indicator. Not more than 1.7 ml of 0.1M *silver nitrate VS* is used (0.6%).

Iodide To 5 ml of solution A add 0.15 ml of a 10.5% w/v solution of *iron(III) chloride hexahydrate* and shake with 2 ml of *chloroform*. The chloroform layer remains *colourless*, Appendix IV B, Method I.

Sulphate 15 ml of solution A complies with the *limit test for sulphates*, Appendix VII (100 ppm).

Loss on drying When dried at 100° to 105° for 3 hours, loses not more than 1.0% of its weight. Use 1 g.

Assay Dissolve 2 g in sufficient *water* to produce 100 ml. To 10 ml of the solution add 50 ml of *water*, 5 ml of 2M *nitric acid*, 25 ml of 0.1M *silver nitrate VS* and 2 ml of *dibutyl phthalate*. Shake and titrate with 0.1M *ammonium thiocyanate VS* using 2 ml of *ammonium iron(III) sulphate solution* as indicator and shaking vigorously towards the end-point. Correct for the amount of chloride present, as determined in the test for Chloride. Each ml of 0.1M *silver nitrate VS* is equivalent to 0.01190 g of KBr.

Action and use Sedative.

Potassium Chloride ☆

KCl   74.6   *7447-40-7*

Potassium Chloride contains not less than 99.0 per cent and not more than 100.5 per cent of KCl, calculated with reference to the dried substance.

Characteristics Colourless crystals or a white, crystalline powder; odourless.

Solubility Soluble in 3 parts of *water*; practically insoluble in *absolute ethanol*.

Identification A. A 10.0% w/v solution in *carbon dioxide-free water* (solution A) yields the *reactions* characteristic of potassium salts, Appendix VI.
B. Yields the *reactions* characteristic of chlorides, Appendix VI.

Acidity or alkalinity To 50 ml of solution A add 0.1 ml of *bromothymol blue solution*. Not more than 0.5 ml of either 0.01M *hydrochloric acid VS* or 0.01M *sodium hydroxide VS* is required to change the colour of the solution.

Clarity and colour of solution Solution A is *clear*, Appendix IV A, and *colourless*, Appendix IV B, Method II.

Barium To 5 ml of solution A add 5 ml of *distilled water* and 1 ml of 1M *sulphuric acid*. After 15 minutes the solution is not more opalescent than a mixture of 5 ml of solution A and 6 ml of *distilled water*.

Heavy metals 12 ml of solution A complies with *limit test A for heavy metals*, Appendix VII (10 ppm). Use *lead standard solution (1 ppm Pb)* to prepare the standard.

Iron 5 ml of solution A diluted to 10 ml with *water* complies with the *limit test for iron*, Appendix VII (20 ppm).

Magnesium and alkaline-earth metals 10 g complies with the *limit test for magnesium and alkaline-earth metals*, Appendix VII. Not more than 5.0 ml of 0.01M *disodium edetate VS* is required (200 ppm, calculated as Ca).

Bromide Dissolve 1.0 g in sufficient *water* to produce 100 ml. To 0.5 ml of the solution add 9 ml of *water*, 1 ml of *buffered phenol red solution* and 0.05 ml of a freshly prepared 2% w/v solution of *chloramine T*, shake for 15 seconds and add 0.15 ml of 0.1M *sodium thiosulphate VS*. Any violet colour produced is not more intense than that of a solution prepared at the same time and in the same manner using 0.5 ml of a 0.0015% w/v solution of *potassium bromide* and 9 ml of *water* (0.1%).

Iodide Moisten 5.0 g by the dropwise addition of a solution recently prepared by mixing 25 ml of *iodide-free starch solution*, 2 ml of 0.5M *sulphuric acid*, 0.15 ml of *sodium nitrite solution* and 25 ml of *water* and examine the mixture in daylight. No particle shows any trace of blue colour within 5 minutes.

Sulphate 5 ml of solution A diluted to 15 ml with *distilled water* complies with the *limit test for sulphates*, Appendix VII (300 ppm).

Loss on drying When dried at 100° to 105° for 3 hours, loses not more than 1.0% of its weight. Use 1 g.

Assay Dissolve 1.3 g in sufficient *water* to produce 100 ml. To 10 ml add 50 ml of *water*, 5 ml of 2M *nitric acid*, 25 ml of 0.1M *silver nitrate VS* and 2 ml of *dibutyl phthalate*. Shake and titrate with 0.1M *ammonium thiocyanate VS* using 2 ml of *ammonium iron(III) sulphate solution* as indicator, until the solution becomes reddish-yellow. Each ml of 0.1M *silver nitrate VS* is equivalent to 0.00746 g of KCl.

Labelling The label states whether or not the material is suitable for use in the manufacture of a parenteral dosage form or for the preparation of haemodialysis solutions.

Preparations

Oral Rehydration Salts

Potassium Chloride and Glucose Intravenous Infusion

Potassium Chloride and Sodium Chloride Intravenous Infusion

Potassium Chloride, Sodium Chloride and Glucose Intravenous Infusion

Action and use Used in treatment of potassium deficiency.

Potassium Chloride intended for use in the manufacture of a parenteral dosage form or for the preparation of haemodialysis solutions complies with the following additional requirement.

Sodium Not more than 0.1% of Na when determined by *atomic emission spectrophotometry*, Appendix II D, using a 1% w/v solution and measuring at 589 nm. Use *sodium solution ASp*, suitably diluted with *water*, for the standard solution.

Potassium Citrate ☆

$$\begin{array}{l} CH_2 \cdot CO_2K \\ | \\ HOCCO_2K \\ | \\ CH_2 \cdot CO_2K \end{array}$$

$C_6H_5K_3O_7,H_2O$ 324.4   *6100-05-6*

Potassium Citrate is tripotassium 2-hydroxypropane-1,2,3-tricarboxylate monohydrate. It contains not less than 99.0 per cent and not more than 101.0 per cent of $C_6H_5K_3O_7$, calculated with reference to the anhydrous substance.

Characteristics Transparent crystals or a white, granular powder; hygroscopic.

Solubility Very soluble in *water*; practically insoluble in *ethanol (96%)*.

Identification A. 0.5 ml of a 10.0% w/v solution in *carbon dioxide-free water* prepared from *distilled water* (solution A) yields *reaction B* characteristic of potassium salts, Appendix VI.

B. To 1 ml of solution A add 4 ml of *water*. The solution yields *reaction A* characteristic of citrates, Appendix VI.

Acidity or alkalinity To 10 ml of solution A add 0.1 ml of *dilute phenolphthalein solution*. Not more than 0.2 ml of either 0.1M *hydrochloric acid VS* or 0.1M *sodium hydroxide VS* is required to change the colour of the solution.

Clarity and colour of solution Solution A is *clear*, Appendix IV A, and *colourless*, Appendix IV B, Method II.

Heavy metals 12 ml of solution A complies with *limit test A for heavy metals*, Appendix VII (10 ppm). Use *lead standard solution (1 ppm Pb)* to prepare the standard.

Sodium Not more than 0.3% of Na when determined by *atomic emission spectrophotometry*, Appendix II D, Method II, measuring at 589 nm. Prepare the test solution by adding 1 ml of 2M *hydrochloric acid* to 10 ml of solution A and diluting to 100 ml with *distilled water*. Use a solution of *sodium chloride* in *distilled water* containing the equivalent of 0.1% of Na, suitably diluted with *distilled water*, for the standard solution.

Chloride Dilute 10 ml of solution A to 15 ml with *water*. The resulting solution complies with the *limit test for chlorides*, Appendix VII (50 ppm).

Oxalate Dissolve 0.50 g in 4 ml of *water*, add 3 ml of *hydrochloric acid* and 1 g of *granulated zinc* and heat on a water-bath for 1 minute. Allow to stand for 2 minutes, decant into 0.25 ml of a 1% w/v solution of *phenylhydrazine hydrochloride*, heat to boiling, cool rapidly, add an equal volume of *hydrochloric acid* and 0.25 ml of a 5% w/v solution of *potassium hexacyanoferrate(III)*, shake and allow to stand for 30 minutes. Any pink colour produced is not more intense than that produced by treating 4 ml of a 0.005% w/v solution of *oxalic acid* at the same time and in the same manner (300 ppm, calculated as anhydrous oxalic acid).

Sulphate To 10 ml of solution A add 2 ml of 7M *hydrochloric acid* and dilute to 15 ml with *distilled water*. The solution complies with the *limit test for sulphates*, Appendix VII (150 ppm).

Readily carbonisable substances Heat 0.20 g, in powder, with 10 ml of *sulphuric acid (96% w/w)* on a water-bath at

89° to 91° for 60 minutes and cool rapidly. The solution is not more intensely coloured than *reference solution Y₂* or *GY₂*, Appendix IV B, Method II.

Water 4.0 to 7.0% w/w, Appendix IX C. Use 0.5 g. After adding the substance being examined, stir for 15 minutes before titrating.

Assay Dissolve 0.15 g in 20 ml of *anhydrous glacial acetic acid*, heat to about 50°, allow to cool and carry out Method I for *non-aqueous titration*, Appendix VIII A, using 0.25 ml of *1-naphtholbenzein solution* as indicator and titrating until a green colour is obtained. Each ml of 0.1M *perchloric acid VS* is equivalent to 0.01021 g of $C_6H_5K_3O_7$.

Storage Potassium Citrate should be kept in an airtight container.

Preparation
Potassium Citrate Mixture

Action and use Systemic alkalinising substance.

Potassium Hydroxide

Caustic Potash

KOH   56.11   *1310-58-3*

Potassium Hydroxide contains not less than 85.0 per cent of total alkali, calculated as KOH, and not more than 4.0 per cent of K_2CO_3.

Characteristics White sticks, pellets or fused masses; dry, hard, brittle and showing a crystalline fracture; very deliquescent. Strongly alkaline and corrosive. Rapidly absorbs carbon dioxide.

Solubility Completely or almost completely soluble in 1 part of *water*; soluble in 3 parts of *ethanol (96%)*; very soluble in boiling *absolute ethanol*.

Identification A solution is strongly alkaline and when neutralised with 2M *hydrochloric acid* yields the *reactions* characteristic of potassium salts, Appendix VI.

Aluminium, iron and matter insoluble in hydrochloric acid Boil 5 g with 40 ml of 2M *hydrochloric acid*, cool, make alkaline with 5M *ammonia*, boil, filter and wash with a 2.5% w/v solution of *ammonium nitrate*. The insoluble residue, after ignition, weighs not more than 5 mg.

Arsenic 0.25 g dissolved in 25 ml of *water* complies with the *limit test for arsenic*, Appendix VII (4 ppm).

Heavy metals Dissolve 2.0 g in 20 ml of *water*. 12 ml of the resulting solution complies with *limit test A for heavy metals*, Appendix VII (10 ppm). Use *lead standard solution (1 ppm Pb)* to prepare the standard.

Sodium Not more than 1.0% of Na when determined by the following method. Dissolve 1.0 g in 50 ml of *water*, add 5 ml of 5M *sulphuric acid* and dilute to 100 ml with *water*. Dilute 1 ml to 10 ml with *water* and determine by Method II for *atomic emission spectrophotometry*, Appendix II D, measuring at 589 nm. Use *sodium solution ASp*, suitably diluted with *water*, for the standard solution.

Chloride Dissolve 0.50 g in 50 ml of *water*, add 1.6 ml of *nitric acid* and dilute to 100 ml with *water*. 15 ml of the resulting solution complies with the *limit test for chlorides*, Appendix VII (0.07%).

Sulphate Dissolve 0.50 g in 30 ml of *water*, add 4.5 ml of 2M *hydrochloric acid* and dilute to 60 ml with *water*. 15 ml of the resulting solution complies with the *limit test for sulphates*, Appendix VII (0.12%).

Assay Dissolve 2 g in 25 ml of *water*, add 5 ml of *barium chloride solution* and titrate with 1M *hydrochloric acid VS* using *phenolphthalein solution* as indicator. Add *bromophenol blue solution* to the solution in the flask and continue the titration with 1M *hydrochloric acid VS*. Each ml of 1M *hydrochloric acid VS* used in the second titration is equivalent to 0.06911 g of K_2CO_3. Each ml of 1M *hydrochloric acid VS* used in the combined titrations is equivalent to 0.05611 g of total alkali, calculated as KOH.

Storage Potassium Hydroxide should be kept in a well-closed container.

Preparation
Potassium Hydroxide Solution

Potassium Hydroxyquinoline Sulphate

Potassium Hydroxyquinoline Sulphate is an equimolecular mixture of quinolin-8-ol sulphate monohydrate, $(C_9H_7NO)_2,H_2SO_4,H_2O$, and potassium sulphate, K_2SO_4. It contains not less than 50.6 per cent and not more than 52.6 per cent of C_9H_7NO, and not less than 29.5 per cent and not more than 32.5 per cent of K_2SO_4, calculated with reference to the anhydrous substance.

Characteristics A pale yellow, microcrystalline powder; odourless or almost odourless. It partly liquefies between 172° and 184°.

Solubility Freely soluble in *water*; insoluble in *ether*; on extraction with hot *absolute ethanol* a residue of potassium sulphate and a solution of quinolin-8-ol sulphate are obtained.

Identification A. To 5 ml of a 5% w/v solution add dropwise, with shaking, 5M *sodium hydroxide* until a heavy precipitate is produced. Filter, wash with *water* and dry at a pressure not exceeding 0.7 kPa for 3 hours. The *infrared absorption spectrum* of the residue, Appendix II A, is concordant with the *reference spectrum* of quinolin-8-ol.
B. To 5 ml of a 5% w/v solution add 0.5 ml of *iron(III) chloride test-solution*. A dark green colour is produced.
C. Yields *reaction A* characteristic of potassium salts, Appendix VI.
D. Yields *reaction A* characteristic of sulphates, Appendix VI.

Water Not more than 5.0% w/w, Appendix IX C. Use 0.5 g.

Assay *For C_9H_7NO* Dissolve 0.35 g in 50 ml of *water* and 20 ml of *hydrochloric acid*, add 50 ml of 0.05M *bromine VS*, stopper the flask and shake for 15 minutes. Allow to stand for 15 minutes, add 80 ml of *water* and 10 ml of *potassium iodide solution* and titrate with 0.1M *sodium thiosulphate VS* using *starch mucilage*, added towards the end of the titration, as indicator. Repeat the operation without the substance being examined. The difference between the titrations represents the amount of bromine required. Each ml of 0.05M *bromine VS* is equivalent to 0.003629 g of C_9H_7NO.

For K₂SO₄ Prepare a solution of suitable strength with *water*. Carry out the method for *atomic emission spectrophotometry*, Appendix II D, measuring at 766.5 nm and using *potassium solution ASp*, suitably diluted with *water*, for the standard solution. Each g of potassium is equivalent to 2.2284 g of K₂SO₄.

Preparation
Potassium Hydroxyquinoline Sulphate and Benzoyl Peroxide Cream.

Action and use Used in treatment of acne.

Potassium Iodide ☆

KI   166.0   *7681-11-0*

Potassium Iodide contains not less than 99.0 per cent and not more than 100.5 per cent of KI, calculated with reference to the dried substance.

Characteristics Colourless crystals or a white powder; odourless.

Solubility Soluble in 0.7 parts of *water*, in 23 parts of *ethanol (96%)* and in 2 parts of *glycerol*.

Identification A 10.0% w/v solution in *carbon dioxide-free water* (solution A) yields the *reactions* characteristic of potassium salts and of iodides, Appendix VI.

Alkalinity To 12.5 ml of solution A add 0.1 ml of *bromothymol blue solution*. Not more than 0.5 ml of 0.01M *hydrochloric acid VS* is required to change the colour of the solution.

Clarity and colour of solution Solution A is *clear*, Appendix IV A, and *colourless*, Appendix IV B, Method II.

Heavy metals 12 ml of solution A complies with *limit test A for heavy metals*, Appendix VII (10 ppm). Use *lead standard solution (1 ppm Pb)* to prepare the standard.

Iron 5 ml of solution A complies with the *limit test for iron*, Appendix VII (20 ppm).

Iodate To 10 ml of solution A add 0.25 ml of *iodide-free starch solution* and 0.2 ml of 1M *sulphuric acid* and allow to stand protected from light for 2 minutes. No blue colour is produced.

Sulphate 10 ml of solution A diluted to 15 ml with *distilled water* complies with the *limit test for sulphates*, Appendix VII (150 ppm).

Thiosulphate To 10 ml of solution A add 0.1 ml of *starch solution* and 0.1 ml of 0.005M *iodine*. A blue colour is produced.

Loss on drying When dried at 100° to 105° for 3 hours, loses not more than 1.0% of its weight. Use 1 g of the powdered substance.

Assay Dissolve 1.5 g in sufficient *water* to produce 100 ml. To 20 ml of the solution add 40 ml of *hydrochloric acid* and titrate with 0.05M *potassium iodate VS* until the colour changes from red to yellow. Add 5 ml of *chloroform* and continue the titration, shaking vigorously, until the chloroform is decolorised. Each ml of 0.05M *potassium iodate VS* is equivalent to 0.01660 g of KI.

Storage Potassium Iodide should be kept in a well-closed container and protected from light.

Action and use Antithyroid.

Potassium Nitrate

KNO₃   101.1   *7767-79-1*

Potassium Nitrate contains not less than 99.0 per cent and not more than 100.5 per cent of KNO₃.

Characteristics Colourless crystals or a white, crystalline powder.

Solubility Soluble in 3.3 parts of *water*.

Identification Yields the *reactions* characteristic of potassium salts and of nitrates, Appendix VI.

Arsenic Heat 1.0 g in a porcelain dish with 5 ml of *sulphuric acid* and 5 ml of *water* until white fumes are evolved, cool, add 5 ml of *water* and again heat until white fumes are evolved, cool and dilute to 50 ml with *water*. 25 ml of the resulting solution complies with the *limit test for arsenic*, Appendix VII (2 ppm).

Heavy metals Dissolve 1.0 g in 20 ml of *water*. 12 ml of the resulting solution complies with *limit test A for heavy metals*, Appendix VII (20 ppm). Use *lead standard solution (1 ppm Pb)* to prepare the standard.

Sodium Not more than 0.1% of Na when determined by Method II for *atomic emission spectrophotometry*, Appendix II D, using a 1.0% w/v solution and measuring at 589 nm. Use *sodium solution ASp*, suitably diluted with *water*, for the standard solution.

Ammonium compounds Warm 1 g with 10 ml of 5M *sodium hydroxide*. No odour of ammonia is detectable.

Chloride Dissolve 1.0 g in 100 ml of *water*. 15 ml of the resulting solution complies with the *limit test for chlorides*, Appendix VII (330 ppm).

Sulphate Dissolve 0.50 g in 60 ml of *water*. 15 ml of the resulting solution complies with the *limit test for sulphates*, Appendix VII (0.12%).

Assay Dissolve 0.3 g in 300 ml of *water* in an ammonia-distillation apparatus, add 3 g of *Devarda's alloy* and 10 ml of 5M *sodium hydroxide* and distil. Collect the distillate in 50 ml of 0.1M *hydrochloric acid VS* and titrate the excess of acid with 0.1M *sodium hydroxide VS* using *methyl red solution* as indicator. Repeat the operation without the substance being examined. The difference between the titrations represents the acid required to neutralise the ammonia produced from the potassium nitrate. Each ml of 0.1M *hydrochloric acid VS* is equivalent to 0.01011 g of KNO₃.

Potassium Permanganate ☆

KMnO₄   158.0   *7722-64-7*

Potassium Permanganate contains not less than 99.0 per cent and not more than 100.5 per cent of KMnO₄.

Characteristics A dark purple or brownish-black, granular powder or dark purple or almost black crystals, usually having a metallic lustre. It decomposes on contact with certain organic substances.

Solubility Soluble in 16 parts of *water*; freely soluble in boiling *water*.

Identification A. Dissolve 50 mg in 5 ml of *water* and add 1 ml of *absolute ethanol* and 0.3 ml of 2M *sodium hydroxide*;

a green colour is produced. Heat the solution to boiling; a dark brown precipitate is produced.

B. Filter the final mixture obtained in test A. The filtrate yields *reaction B* characteristic of potassium salts, Appendix VI.

Colour of solution Dissolve 0.75 g in 25 ml of *distilled water*, add 3 ml of *ethanol (96%)*, boil for 2 to 3 minutes, cool, dilute to 30 ml with *distilled water* and filter. The filtrate (solution A) is *colourless*, Appendix IV B, Method II.

Chloride 10 ml of solution A diluted to 15 ml with *water* complies with the *limit test for chlorides*, Appendix VII (200 ppm).

Sulphate 12 ml of solution A diluted to 15 ml with *distilled water* complies with the *limit test for sulphates*, Appendix VII (500 ppm).

Water-insoluble matter Dissolve 0.5 g in 50 ml of *water*, heat to boiling, filter through a tared, sintered-glass filter (BS porosity No. 4 is suitable) and wash with *water* until the filtrate is colourless. The residue, after drying to constant weight at 100° to 105°, weighs not more than 5 mg (1.0%).

Assay Dissolve 0.3 g in sufficient *water* to produce 100 ml. To 20 ml add 20 ml of *water*, 1 g of *potassium iodide* and 10 ml of 2M *hydrochloric acid* and titrate the liberated iodine with 0.1M *sodium thiosulphate VS* using *starch solution* as indicator. Each ml of 0.1M *sodium thiosulphate VS* is equivalent to 0.003160 g of $KMnO_4$.

Action and use Antiseptic.

Potassium Sorbate

$C_6H_7KO_2$ 150.2   *590-00-1*

Potassium Sorbate is potassium (*E*,*E*)-hexa-2,4-dienoate. It contains not less than 99.0 per cent and not more than 101.0 per cent of $C_6H_7KO_2$, calculated with reference to the anhydrous substance.

Characteristics White or creamy-white pellets or powder; odour, faint and characteristic.

Solubility Soluble in less than 1 part of *water* and in 70 parts of *ethanol (96%)*; very slightly soluble in *acetone*.

Identification A. The *infra-red absorption spectrum*, Appendix II A, is concordant with the *reference spectrum* of potassium sorbate.

B. The *light absorption*, Appendix II B, in the range 230 to 350 nm of a 0.0005% w/v solution in 0.1M *hydrochloric acid* exhibits a maximum only at 264 nm. The *absorbance* at 264 nm is about 0.89.

C. To a solution containing 10 mg in 2 ml of *water* add *bromine water* dropwise. The bromine solution is decolorised.

D. Ignite. The residue yields the *reactions* characteristic of potassium salts, Appendix VI.

Acidity or alkalinity Dissolve 2 g in 20 ml of *water* and add *phenolphthalein solution*. Not more than 0.5 ml of

either 0.1M *sodium hydroxide VS* or 0.1M *hydrochloric acid VS* is required to neutralise the solution.

Aldehyde Dissolve 1 g in a mixture of 50 ml of *propan-2-ol* and 30 ml of *water*, adjust the solution to pH 4 with 1M *hydrochloric acid* and dilute to 100 ml with *water*. To 10 ml of the solution add 1 ml of *decolorised magenta solution* and allow to stand for 30 minutes. Any colour produced is not more intense than that produced by adding 1 ml of *decolorised magenta solution* to a mixture of 1.5 ml of *acetaldehyde standard solution (100 ppm)*, 4 ml of *propan-2-ol* and 4.5 ml of *water* (0.15%, calculated as C_2H_4O).

Arsenic Mix 0.50 g with 2 ml of *bromine water*, evaporate to dryness on a water-bath, ignite gently, cool, dissolve the residue, disregarding any carbon, in a mixture of 5 ml of *water* and 2 ml of *brominated hydrochloric acid* and remove the excess bromine by the addition of *tin(II) chloride solution AsT*. The solution complies with the *limit test for arsenic*, Appendix VII (2 ppm).

Heavy metals 2.0 g complies with *limit test C for heavy metals*, Appendix VII (120 ppm), but using 4M *hydrochloric acid* in place of 2M *hydrochloric acid* and 4 ml of *lead standard solution (10 ppm Pb)* to prepare the standard.

Water Not more than 1.0% w/w, Appendix IX C. Use 2.5 g.

Assay Carry out Method I for *non-aqueous titration*, Appendix VIII A, using 0.5 g and *crystal violet solution* as indicator. Each ml of 0.1M *perchloric acid VS* is equivalent to 0.01502 g of $C_6H_7KO_2$.

Storage Potassium Sorbate should be kept in a well-closed container, protected from light and stored at a temperature not exceeding 15°.

Action and use Antimicrobial preservative.

Povidone

$(C_6H_9NO)_n$ *9003-39-8*

Povidone is poly(2-oxopyrrolidin-1-ylethylene). It consists of linear polymers of 1-vinyl-pyrrolidin-2-one having a K-value in the range 10 to 95. It contains not less than 11.5 per cent and not more than 12.8 per cent of nitrogen, N, calculated with reference to the anhydrous substance.

Characteristics A fine, white or very slightly cream-coloured powder; odourless or almost odourless.

Solubility Soluble in *water*, in *ethanol (96%)* and in *chloroform*; practically insoluble in *ether*.

Identification A. To 0.5 ml of a 10.0% w/v solution (solution A) add 5 ml of *water*, 10 ml of 1M *hydrochloric acid* and 2 ml of a 10% w/v solution of *potassium dichromate*. An orange-yellow precipitate is produced.

B. To 1 ml of solution A add 0.2 ml of *dimethylamino-benzaldehyde solution* and 0.1 ml of *sulphuric acid*. A pink colour is produced.

C. To 0.1 ml of solution A add 5 ml of *water* and 0.2 ml of *iodine solution*. A deep red colour is produced.

Clarity and colour of solution For Povidone having a nominal K-value of 15 or less, a 7.0% w/v solution is *clear*, Appendix IV A, and not more intensely coloured than *reference solution B_6 or BY_6*, Appendix IV B, Method II.

For Povidone having a nominal K-value of more than 15, solution A is *clear*, Appendix IV A, and not more intensely coloured than *reference solution B_6 or BY_6*, Appendix IV B, Method II.

K-Value For Povidone having a nominal value of 15 or less, 85.0 to 115.0% of the declared value, and for Povidone having a nominal value of more than 15, 90.0 to 108.0% of the declared value, determined by the following method.

If the nominal value is 18 or less, prepare a 5% w/v solution; if the nominal value is more than 18 prepare a 1% w/v solution. Allow to stand for 1 hour and carry out Method II for the *determination of viscosity*, Appendix V H, at 24.8 to 25.2° using a size no. 1 viscometer. Calculate the K-value (K_0) from the expression

$$K_0 = \frac{1.5 \log z - 1}{0.15 + 0.003c} + \frac{\sqrt{300c \log z + (c + 1.5c \log z)^2}}{0.15c + 0.003c^2}$$

where c is the weight, in g, on an anhydrous basis of the substance contained in 100 ml of the solution being examined and z is the viscosity relative to that of *water*.

Aldehydes Not more than 0.2%, calculated as C_2H_4O, when determined by the following method. Boil 10 g in 180 ml of 4.5M *sulphuric acid* under a reflux condenser for 45 minutes, cool, fit a distillation head, distil and collect 100 ml of distillate in a mixture of iced *water* and 20 ml of 1M *hydroxylamine hydrochloride*, previously adjusted to pH 3.1. Titrate with 0.1M *sodium hydroxide VS* to pH 3.1 and carry out a blank titration; not more than 4.6 ml is required.

Heavy metals 12 ml of solution A complies with *limit test A for heavy metals*, Appendix VII (10 ppm). Use *lead standard solution (1 ppm Pb)* to prepare the standard.

Vinylpyrrolidone monomer Dissolve 10 g in 80 ml of *water* and add 1 g of *sodium acetate*. Titrate with 0.05M *iodine VS* until a persistent colour is obtained and add an excess of 3.0 ml of the iodine solution. Allow to stand for 10 minutes and titrate the excess of iodine with 0.1M *sodium thiosulphate VS* using 3 ml of *starch mucilage*, added towards the end of the titration, as indicator. Repeat the operation without the substance being examined. The difference between the titrations represents the amount of iodine required. Not more than 3.6 ml of 0.05M *iodine VS* is required (0.2%).

Sulphated ash Not more than 0.1%, Appendix IX A, Method II. Use 1 g.

Water Not more than 5.0% w/w, Appendix IX C. Use 0.5 g.

Assay Carry out Method III for the *determination of nitrogen*, Appendix VIII H, using 0.3 g and 11 ml of *nitrogen-free sulphuric acid*. To destroy the organic substance repeat the addition of *hydrogen peroxide solution (100 vol)* three to six times until a clear and slightly green solution is produced and continue heating for a further 4 hours.

Storage Povidone should be kept in an airtight container.

Labelling The label states the viscosity in terms of a K-value.

Action and use Pharmaceutical aid.

In some countries the material described in this monograph may be known as Polyvidone.

Prazosin Hydrochloride

$C_{19}H_{21}N_5O_4,HCl$ 419.9   *19237-84-4*

Prazosin Hydrochloride is 2-[4-(2-furoyl)-piperazin-1-yl]-6,7-dimethoxyquinazolin-4-yl-amine hydrochloride. It contains not less than 98.5 per cent and not more than 101.0 per cent of $C_{19}H_{21}N_5O_4,HCl$, calculated with reference to the anhydrous substance.

Characteristics A white or almost white powder; odourless or almost odourless.

Solubility Very slightly soluble in *water*; slightly soluble in *ethanol (96%)* and in *methanol*; practically insoluble in *acetone* and in *chloroform*.

Identification A. Dissolve 50 mg in 20 ml of *ethanol (50%)*, add 2 ml of 1M *potassium hydroxide*, extract with two 25-ml quantities of *dichloromethane*, evaporate the combined extracts and dry the residue at 60° at a pressure not exceeding 2 kPa. The *infra-red absorption spectrum* of the residue, Appendix II A, is concordant with the *reference spectrum* of prazosin.

B. The *light absorption*, Appendix II B, in the range 220 to 400 nm of a 0.0007% w/v solution in 0.01M *methanolic hydrochloric acid* exhibits three maxima, at 247, 330 and 343 nm. The *absorbance* at 247 nm is about 0.95, at 330 nm, about 0.19 and at 343 nm, about 0.18.

C. 2 ml of a solution prepared by dissolving 25 mg in 30 ml of *ethanol (96%)* yields *reaction A* characteristic of chlorides, Appendix VI.

Heavy metals Dissolve the residue obtained in the test for Sulphated ash in sufficient 2M *nitric acid* to produce 50 ml. The resulting solution complies with *limit test A for heavy metals*, Appendix VII (50 ppm). Use *lead standard solution (1 ppm Pb)* to prepare the standard.

Iron Not more than 100 ppm when determined by the following method. To 1.0 g add slowly about 35 drops of *nitric acid*. After fuming has subsided ignite by slowly raising the temperature from 150° to 1000°, maintaining the final temperature for 1 hour. Cool, dissolve the residue in 20 ml of 2M *nitric acid*, evaporate to about 5 ml, dilute to 25 ml with 0.2M *nitric acid* and examine the resulting solution by *atomic absorption spectrophotometry*, Appendix II D, measuring at 248 nm and using *iron solution ASp* to prepare the standard solutions. Reserve about 10 ml of the solution for the test for Nickel.

Nickel Not more than 50 ppm when determined by *atomic absorption spectrophotometry*, Appendix II D, on the final solution prepared in the test for Iron. Measure at 232 nm and use *nickel solution ASp* to prepare the standard solutions.

Related substances Carry out the method for *thin-layer chromatography*, Appendix III A, using a *silica gel GF254* precoated chromatoplate (Analchem plates are suitable) and a mixture of 95 volumes of *ethyl acetate* and 5 volumes of *diethylamine* as the mobile phase. Apply separately to the plate 10 µl of each of seven solutions in a mixture of

10 volumes of *chloroform*, 10 volumes of *methanol* and 1 volume of *diethylamine* containing (1) 1.0% w/v of the substance being examined, (2) 0.0020% w/v of the substance being examined, (3) 0.0020% w/v of *2-chloro-6,7-dimethoxyquinazolin-4-ylamine BPCRS*, (4) 0.0020% w/v of *1-(2-furoyl)piperazine BPCRS*, (5) 0.0020% w/v of *1,4-di(2-furoyl)piperazine BPCRS*, (6) 0.0020% w/v of *6,7-dimethoxy-2-piperazin-1-ylquinazolin-4-ylamine BPCRS* and (7) 0.0020% w/v of *2,2'-piperazin-1,4-diyl-bis(6,7-dimethoxyquinazolin-4-ylamine) BPCRS*. After removal of the plate, allow it to dry in air and examine under *ultra-violet light (254 nm)*. In the chromatogram obtained with solution (1) any spots corresponding to 2-chloro-6,7-dimethoxyquinazolin-4-ylamine, 1-(2-furoyl)piperazine, 1,4-di(2-furoyl)piperazine, 6,7-dimethoxy-2-piperazin-1-ylquinazolin-4-ylamine and 2,2'-piperazin-1,4-diyl-bis(6,7-dimethoxyquinazolin-4-ylamine) are not more intense than the corresponding spots in the chromatogram obtained with solutions (3), (4), (5), (6) and (7) and any other *secondary spot* is not more intense than the spot in the chromatogram obtained with solution (2).

Sulphated ash Not more than 0.2%, Appendix IX A. Use 1.0 g.

Water Not more than 0.5% w/w, Appendix IX C. Use 2 g dissolved in a mixture of equal volumes of *chloroform* and *methanol*.

Assay Dissolve 0.35 g in 50 ml of *anhydrous glacial acetic acid* and carry out Method I for *non-aqueous titration*, Appendix VIII A, using 7 ml of *mercury(II) acetate solution* and determining the end-point potentiometrically. Each ml of 0.1M *perchloric acid VS* is equivalent to 0.04199 g of $C_{19}H_{21}N_5O_4,HCl$.

Storage Prazosin Hydrochloride should be kept in a well-closed container and protected from light.

Preparation
Prazosin Tablets

Action and use Antihypertensive.

Prednisolone ☆

$C_{21}H_{28}O_5$ 360.4   *50-24-8*

Prednisolone is 11β,17α,21-trihydroxypregna-1,4-diene-3,20-dione. It contains not less than 96.0 per cent and not more than 104.0 per cent of $C_{21}H_{28}O_5$, calculated with reference to the dried substance.

Characteristics A white or almost white, crystalline powder; hygroscopic. It melts at about 230°, with decomposition.

Solubility Very slightly soluble in *water*; soluble in 27 parts of *absolute ethanol*; soluble in *methanol*; sparingly soluble in *acetone*; slightly soluble in *chloroform*.

Identification *Tests A and B may be omitted if tests C and D are carried out. Tests C and D may be omitted if tests A and B are carried out.*

A. The *infra-red absorption spectrum*, Appendix II A, is concordant with the spectrum of *prednisolone EPCRS*. If the spectra are not concordant, dissolve each substance in the minimum volume of *acetone*, evaporate to dryness on a water-bath and prepare new spectra of the residues.

B. Carry out the method for *thin-layer chromatography*, Appendix III A, using *silica gel GF254* as the coating substance, a mixture of 77 volumes of *dichloromethane*, 15 volumes of *ether*, 8 volumes of *methanol* and 1.2 volumes of *water* as the first mobile phase and a mixture of 80 volumes of *ether*, 15 volumes of *toluene* and 5 volumes of *butan-1-ol* saturated with *water* as the second mobile phase. Apply separately to the chromatoplate 2 μl of each of two solutions in a mixture of 9 volumes of *chloroform* and 1 volume of *methanol* containing (1) 0.25% w/v of the substance being examined and (2) 0.25% w/v of *prednisolone EPCRS* and develop the chromatogram successively with each mobile phase. After removal of the plate, allow it to dry in air and examine under *ultra-violet light (254 nm)*. The principal spot in the chromatogram obtained with solution (1) corresponds to that in the chromatogram obtained with solution (2). Spray with *ethanolic sulphuric acid (20%)*, heat at 120° for 10 minutes or until spots are produced, allow to cool and examine the chromatograms in daylight and under *ultra-violet light (365 nm)*. The principal spot in the chromatogram obtained with solution (1) is similar in colour in daylight, fluorescence under ultra-violet light (365 nm), position and size to that in the chromatogram obtained with solution (2).

C. Carry out the method for *thin-layer chromatography*, Appendix III A, using the coating substance prescribed in the test for Related substances, a mixture of 77 volumes of *dichloromethane*, 15 volumes of *ether*, 8 volumes of *methanol* and 1.2 volumes of *water* as the first mobile phase and a mixture of 80 volumes of *ether*, 15 volumes of *toluene* and 5 volumes of *butan-1-ol* saturated with *water* as the second mobile phase. Apply separately to the chromatoplate 5 μl of each of solutions (1) and (3) and 50 μl of each of solutions (2) and (4), applying the latter two in small quantities in order to obtain small spots. For solution (1) dissolve 25 mg of the substance being examined in sufficient *methanol* to produce 5 ml (solution A). Dilute 2 ml of this solution to 10 ml with *chloroform*. For solution (2) transfer 0.4 ml of solution A to a stoppered glass tube (100 mm × 20 mm) and evaporate the solvent under a stream of nitrogen with gentle heating. Add 2 ml of a 15% v/v solution of *glacial acetic acid* and 50 mg of *sodium bismuthate*, stopper the tube and shake the suspension for 1 hour protected from light. Add 2 ml of a 15% v/v solution of *glacial acetic acid* and filter into a 50-ml separating funnel, washing the filter with two 5-ml quantities of *water*. Shake the clear filtrate with 10 ml of *dichloromethane*, wash the organic layer with 5 ml of 1M *sodium hydroxide* and two 5-ml quantities of *water* and dry over *anhydrous sodium sulphate*. For solution (3) dissolve 25 mg of *prednisolone EPCRS* in *methanol* and dilute to 5 ml with the same solvent (solution B); dilute 2 ml of this solution to 10 ml with *chloroform*. Prepare solution (4) in the same manner as solution (2) but using 0.4 ml of solution B in place of solution A. Develop the chromatogram successively with each mobile phase.

After removal of the plate, allow it to dry in air and examine under *ultra-violet light (254 nm)*. The principal spots in the chromatograms obtained with solutions (1) and (2) correspond to those in the chromatograms obtained with solutions (3) and (4) respectively. Spray with *ethanolic sulphuric acid (20%)* and heat at 120° for 10 minutes or until spots are produced and allow to cool. Examine the chromatograms in daylight and in *ultra-violet light (365 nm)*. The principal spot in each of the chromatograms obtained with solutions (1) and (2) is similar in colour in daylight, fluorescence in ultra-violet light (365 nm), position and size to the principal spot in the chromatograms obtained with solutions (3) and (4) respectively. The principal spots in the chromatograms obtained with solutions (2) and (4) have Rf values distinctly higher than those of the principal spots in the chromatograms obtained with solutions (1) and (2) respectively.

D. Add 2 mg to 2 ml of *sulphuric acid* and shake to dissolve; within 5 minutes an intense red colour is produced with a reddish-brown fluorescence when examined in ultra-violet light (365 nm). Add the solution to 10 ml of *water* and mix; the colour is discharged and there is a yellow fluorescence in ultra-violet light.

Light absorption Dissolve 10 mg in sufficient *ethanol (96%)* to produce 100 ml and dilute 10 ml to 100 ml with the same solvent. The A(1%, 1 cm) of the resulting solution at the maximum at 240 nm is 400 to 430, Appendix II B.

Specific optical rotation In a 1% w/v solution in *1,4-dioxan*, +96° to +120°, Appendix V F.

Related substances Carry out the method for *thin-layer chromatography*, Appendix III A, using as the coating substance a suitable silica gel containing a fluorescent indicator with an optimal intensity at 254 nm (Merck silica gel 60 F254 is suitable) and a mixture of 77 volumes of *dichloromethane*, 15 volumes of *ether*, 8 volumes of *methanol* and 1.2 volumes of *water* as the mobile phase. Apply separately to the chromatoplate 5 μl of each of the following solutions in a mixture of 9 volumes of *chloroform* and 1 volume of *methanol*. Solutions (1), (2) and (3) contain 1.0%, 0.020% and 0.010% w/v respectively of the substance being examined. Solution (4) contains 0.10% w/v each of the substance being examined and *hydrocortisone EPCRS*. After removal of the plate, allow it to dry in air and examine under *ultra-violet light (254 nm)*. Any *secondary spot* in the chromatogram obtained with solution (1) is not more intense than the spot in the chromatogram obtained with solution (2) and not more than one such spot is more intense than the spot in the chromatogram obtained with solution (3). The test is not valid unless the chromatogram obtained with solution (4) shows two clearly separated principal spots.

Loss on drying When dried at 100° to 105° for 3 hours, loses not more than 1.0% of its weight. Use 0.5 g.

Assay Carry out the *tetrazolium assay of steroids*, Appendix VIII P, and calculate the content of $C_{21}H_{28}O_5$ from the *absorbance* obtained by repeating the operation using *prednisolone EPCRS* in place of the substance being examined.

Storage Prednisolone should be kept in a well-closed container and protected from light.

Preparation
Prednisolone Tablets
Action and use Corticosteroid.

Prednisolone Sodium Phosphate

$C_{21}H_{27}Na_2O_8P$ 484.4   *125-02-0*

Prednisolone Sodium Phosphate is disodium 11β,17α-dihydroxy-3,20-dioxopregna-1,4-dien-21-yl orthophosphate. It contains not less than 96.0 per cent and not more than 103.0 per cent of $C_{21}H_{27}Na_2O_8P$, calculated with reference to the anhydrous substance.

Characteristics A white or almost white powder; odourless or almost odourless; hygroscopic.

Solubility Soluble in 3 parts of *water*; slightly soluble in *absolute ethanol*; practically insoluble in *chloroform*.

Identification *Test A may be omitted if tests B, C and D are carried out. Tests B and C may be omitted if tests A and D are carried out.*

A. Dissolve 50 mg in 1 ml of *deuterium oxide* containing 0.1% w/v of *sodium 3-trimethylsilylpropanesulphonate*. The *nuclear magnetic resonance spectrum*, Appendix II C, is concordant with the spectrum of a similar solution of *prednisolone sodium phosphate BPCRS*.

B. Carry out the method for *thin-layer chromatography*, Appendix III A, using *silica gel G* as the coating substance and a freshly prepared mixture of 60 volumes of *butan-1-ol*, 20 volumes of *acetic anhydride* and 20 volumes of *water* as the mobile phase. Apply separately to the chromatoplate 2 μl of each of the following solutions in *methanol*. Solution (1) contains 0.25% w/v of the substance being examined. Solution (2) contains 0.25% w/v of *prednisolone sodium phosphate BPCRS*. Solution (3) is a mixture of equal volumes of solutions (1) and (2). Solution (4) is a mixture of equal volumes of solution (1) and a 0.25% w/v solution of *betamethasone sodium phosphate BPCRS* in *methanol*. After removal of the plate, allow it to dry in air, spray with *ethanolic sulphuric acid (20%)*, heat at 120° for 10 minutes, allow to cool and examine under *ultra-violet light (365 nm)*. The principal spot in the chromatogram obtained with solution (1) corresponds to that in the chromatogram obtained with solution (2). The principal spot in the chromatogram obtained with solution (3) appears as a single compact spot and the chromatogram obtained with solution (4) shows two principal spots with almost identical Rf values.

C. Dissolve 2 mg in 2 ml of *sulphuric acid* and allow to stand for 2 minutes. A dark red colour is produced (distinction from betamethasone sodium phosphate, dexamethasone sodium phosphate and hydrocortisone sodium phosphate).

D. Heat gently 40 mg with 2 ml of *sulphuric acid* until white fumes are evolved, add *nitric acid* dropwise until oxidation is complete and cool. Add 2 ml of *water*, heat until white fumes are again evolved, cool, add 10 ml of *water* and neutralise to *litmus paper* with 5M *ammonia*. The solution yields *reaction A* characteristic of sodium salts and *reaction B* characteristic of phosphates, Appendix VI.

Alkalinity pH of a 0.5% w/v solution, 7.5 to 9.0, Appendix V F.

Specific optical rotation In a 1% w/v solution, +94° to +100°, Appendix V F.

Inorganic phosphate Dissolve 25.0 mg in 10 ml of *water*, add 4 ml of 1M *sulphuric acid*, 1 ml of a 10% w/v solution of *ammonium molybdate* and 2 ml of *methylaminophenol—sulphite reagent* and allow to stand for 15 minutes. Add sufficient *water* to produce 25 ml and allow to stand for a further 15 minutes. The *absorbance* of a 4-cm layer of the resulting solution, Appendix II B, at 730 nm is not more than the absorbance of a 4-cm layer of a solution prepared by treating 10 ml of a 0.0036% w/v solution of *potassium dihydrogen orthophosphate* in the same manner, beginning at the words 'add 4 ml . . .'.

Free prednisolone and other derivatives Carry out Method A for *related foreign steroids*, Appendix III A, applying 1 μl of each of three solutions in *methanol* containing (1) 1.0% w/v of the substance being examined, (2) 0.020% of *prednisolone 21-acetate* and (3) 0.020% w/v of *prednisolone*. Any *secondary spot* corresponding to prednisolone in the chromatogram obtained with solution (1) is not more intense than the spot in the chromatogram obtained with solution (3). Any other *secondary spot* is not more intense than the spot in the chromatogram obtained with solution (2). The principal spot in the chromatogram obtained with solution (1) remains on the line of application.

Water Not more than 8.0% w/w, Appendix IX C. Use 0.5 g.

Assay Dissolve 0.15 g in sufficient *water* to produce 200 ml. Dilute 5 ml to 250 ml with *water* and measure the *absorbance* of the resulting solution at the maximum at 247 nm, Appendix II B. Calculate the content of $C_{21}H_{27}Na_2O_8P$ taking 312 as the value of A(1%, 1 cm) at the maximum at 247 nm.

Storage Prednisolone Sodium Phosphate should be kept in a well-closed container and protected from light.

Preparation
Prednisolone Sodium Phosphate Injection

Action and use Corticosteroid.

Prednisone ☆

$C_{21}H_{26}O_5$ 358.4   *53-03-2*

Prednisone is 17α,21-dihydroxypregna-1,4-diene-3,11,20-trione. It contains not less than 96.0 per cent and not more than 104.0 per cent of $C_{21}H_{26}O_5$, calculated with reference to the dried substance.

Characteristics A white or almost white, crystalline powder. It melts at about 230° with decomposition.

Solubility Practically insoluble in *water*; slightly soluble in *ethanol (96%)* and in *chloroform*.

Identification *Tests A and B may be omitted if tests C and D are carried out. Tests C and D may be omitted if tests A and B are carried out.*

A. The *infra-red absorption spectrum*, Appendix II A, is concordant with the spectrum of *prednisone EPCRS*. If the spectra are not concordant, dissolve each substance in the minimum volume of *acetone*, evaporate to dryness on a water-bath and prepare new spectra of the residues.

B. Examine the chromatograms obtained in the test for Related substances under *ultra-violet light (254 nm)*. The principal spot in the chromatogram obtained with solution (2) corresponds to the principal spot in the chromatogram obtained with solution (5). Spray the plate with *ethanolic sulphuric acid (20%)* and heat at 120° for 10 minutes or until the spots are produced. Allow to cool and examine in daylight and under *ultra-violet light (365 nm)*. The principal spot in the chromatogram obtained with solution (2) is similar in colour in daylight, fluorescence in ultra-violet light (365 nm), position and size to the principal spot in the chromatogram obtained with solution (5).

C. Carry out the method for *thin-layer chromatography*, Appendix III A, using the coating substance and mobile phase prescribed in the test for Related substances. Apply separately to the chromatoplate 5 μl of each of solutions (1) and (3) and 50 μl of each of solutions (2) and (4), applying the latter two in small quantities in order to obtain compact spots. For solution (1) dissolve 25 mg of the substance being examined in *methanol* and dilute to 5 ml with the same solvent (solution A). Dilute 2 ml of this solution to 10 ml with *chloroform*. For solution (2) transfer 0.4 ml of solution A to a stoppered glass tube (100 mm × 20 mm) and evaporate the solvent with gentle heating under a stream of nitrogen. Add 2 ml of a 15% v/v solution of *glacial acetic acid* and 50 mg of *sodium bismuthate*, stopper the tube and shake the suspension for 1 hour, protected from light. Add 2 ml of a 15% v/v solution of *glacial acetic acid* and filter into a 50-ml separating funnel, washing the filtrate with two 5-ml quantities of *water*. Shake the clear filtrate with 10 ml of *dichloromethane*, wash the organic layer with 5 ml of 1M *sodium hydroxide* and two 5-ml quantities of *water* and dry over *anhydrous sodium sulphate*. For solution (3) dissolve 25 mg of *prednisone EPCRS* in *methanol* and dilute to 5 ml with the same solvent (solution B). Dilute 2 ml of the solution to 10 ml with *chloroform*. For solution (4) proceed as for solution (2) but using 0.4 ml of solution B in place of solution A.

After removal of the plate, allow it to dry in air and examine under *ultra-violet light (254 nm)*. The principal spots in the chromatograms obtained with solutions (1) and (2) correspond to those in the chromatograms obtained with solutions (3) and (4) respectively. Spray with *ethanolic sulphuric acid (20%)* and heat at 120° for 10 minutes or until the spots are produced. Examine the chromatograms in daylight and in *ultra-violet light (365 nm)*. The principal spot in each of the chromatograms obtained with solutions (1) and (2) is similar in colour in daylight, fluorescence in ultra-violet light (365 nm), position and size to the principal spot in each of the chromatograms obtained with solutions (3) and (4) respectively. The principal spots in the chromatograms obtained with solutions (2) and (4) have Rf values distinctly higher than those of the principal spots in the chromatograms obtained with solutions (1) and (3).
D. Add 2 mg to 2 ml of *sulphuric acid* and shake to dissolve; a yellow colour is produced within 5 minutes which exhibits a blue fluorescence in ultra-violet light (365 nm). Add the solution to 10 ml of *water* and mix; the yellow colour fades but the blue fluorescence in ultra-violet light remains.

Light absorption Dissolve 10 mg in sufficient *ethanol (96%)* to produce 100 ml and dilute 10 ml to 100 ml with the same solvent. The A(1%, 1 cm) of the resulting solution at the maximum at 240 nm is 405 to 435, Appendix II B.

Specific optical rotation In a 1% w/v solution in *1,4-dioxan*, +167° to +175°, Appendix V F.

Related substances Carry out the method for *thin-layer chromatography*, Appendix III A, using as the coating substance a suitable silica gel containing a fluorescent indicator with an optimal intensity at 254 nm (Merck silica gel 60 F254 is suitable) and a mixture of 77 volumes of *dichloromethane*, 15 volumes of *ether*, 8 volumes of *methanol* and 1.2 volumes of *water* as the mobile phase. Apply separately to the chromatoplate 5 µl of each of the following solutions in a mixture of 9 volumes of *chloroform* and 1 volume of *methanol*. Solutions (1), (2), (3) and (4) contain 1.0% w/v, 0.10% w/v, 0.020% w/v and 0.010 w/v respectively of the substance being examined. Solution (5) contains 0.10% w/v of *prednisone EPCRS*. Solution (6) contains 0.10% w/v each of the substance being examined and *betamethasone EPCRS*. After removal of the plate, allow it to dry in air and examine under *ultra-violet light (254 nm)*. Any *secondary spot* in the chromatogram obtained with solution (1) is not more intense than the spot in the chromatogram obtained with solution (3) and not more than one such spot is more intense than the spot in the chromatogram obtained with solution (4). The test is not valid unless the chromatogram obtained with solution (6) shows two clearly separated principal spots.

Loss on drying When dried at 100° to 105° for 3 hours, loses not more than 1.0% of its weight. Use 0.5 g.

Assay Carry out the *tetrazolium assay of steroids*, Appendix VIII P, and calculate the content of $C_{21}H_{26}O_5$ from the *absorbance* obtained by repeating the operation using *prednisone EPCRS* in place of the substance being examined.

Storage Prednisone should be kept in a well-closed container and protected from light.

Preparation
Prednisone Tablets

Action and use Corticosteroid.

Prenylamine Lactate

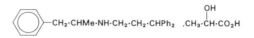

$C_{24}H_{27}N,C_3H_6O_3$ 419.6   *69-43-2*

Prenylamine Lactate is 2-benzhydrylethyl-(α-methylphenethyl)amine lactate. It contains not less than 98.5 per cent and not more than 101.0 per cent of $C_{24}H_{27}N,C_3H_6O_3$, calculated with reference to the dried substance.

Characteristics A white, crystalline powder; odourless or almost odourless.

Solubility Very slightly soluble in *water* and in *ether*; soluble in 5 parts of *ethanol (96%)* and in 2 parts of *chloroform*.

Identification A. The *infra-red absorption spectrum*, Appendix II A, is concordant with the *reference spectrum* of prenylamine lactate.
B. The *light absorption*, Appendix II B, in the range 230 to 350 nm of a 0.05% w/v solution in *methanol* exhibits three maxima, at 253, 258 and 268 nm. The *absorbance* at 253 nm is about 0.62, at 258 nm, about 0.74 and at 268 nm, about 0.45.
C. Dissolve 25 mg in 0.1 ml of *methanol* and add 1 ml of *sulphuric acid*. Heat for 2 minutes at 85°, allow to cool and add a few mg of *4-hydroxybiphenyl*. A violet-red colour is produced.

Melting point 137° to 140°, Appendix V A.

Related substances Carry out the method for *thin-layer chromatography*, Appendix III A, using *silica gel G* as the coating substance and a mixture of 92 volumes of *ethanol (96%)*, 7 volumes of *water* and 1 volume of 13.5M *ammonia* as the mobile phase. Apply separately to the chromatoplate 10 µl of each of two solutions of the substance being examined in *chloroform* containing (1) 5.0% w/v and (2) 0.010% w/v. After removal of the plate, allow it to dry in air and expose to iodine vapour for 10 minutes. Any brown *secondary spot* in the chromatogram obtained with solution (1) is not more intense than the spot in the chromatogram obtained with solution (2). Disregard any blue spot due to lactate.

Loss on drying When dried at 60° at a pressure not exceeding 0.7 kPa for 3 hours, loses not more than 1.0% of its weight. Use 1 g.

Sulphated ash Not more than 0.1%, Appendix IX A.

Assay Carry out Method I for *non-aqueous titration*, Appendix VIII A, using 0.5 g and *1-naphtholbenzein solution* as indicator. Each ml of 0.1M *perchloric acid VS* is equivalent to 0.04196 g of $C_{24}H_{27}N,C_3H_6O_3$.

Storage Prenylamine Lactate should be kept in a well-closed container and protected from light.

Preparation
Prenylamine Tablets

Action and use Vasodilator.

Prilocaine Hydrochloride

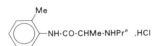

C₁₃H₂₀N₂O,HCl   256.8   *1786-81-8*

Prilocaine Hydrochloride is 2-propylamino-propiono-*o*-toluidide hydrochloride. It contains not less than 99.0 per cent and not more than 101.0 per cent of $C_{13}H_{20}N_2O,HCl$, calculated with reference to the dried substance.

Characteristics A white, crystalline powder; odourless or almost odourless.

Solubility Soluble in 5 parts of *water* and in 6 parts of *ethanol (96%)*; practically insoluble in *ether*.

Identification A. The *infra-red absorption spectrum*, Appendix II A, is concordant with the *reference spectrum* of prilocaine hydrochloride.
B. Dissolve 0.25 g in 10 ml of *water* and make the solution alkaline with 5M *sodium hydroxide*; an oily liquid is produced. Dissolve the oily liquid in 1 ml of *ethanol (96%)*, add 0.5 ml of a 10% w/v solution of *cobalt(II) chloride* and shake for 2 minutes; a bluish-green precipitate is produced.
C. Yields *reaction A* characteristic of chlorides, Appendix VI.

Acidity or alkalinity Dissolve 0.2 g in 10 ml of *carbon dioxide-free water* and titrate with 0.02M *sodium hydroxide VS* or 0.02M *hydrochloric acid VS* using *bromocresol green solution* as indicator. Not more than 0.20 ml of either 0.02M *sodium hydroxide VS* or 0.02M *hydrochloric acid VS* is required to change the colour of the solution.

Melting point 167° to 169°, Appendix V A.

Copper To 0.50 g in 10 ml of *water* add 0.25 ml of 0.05M *disodium edetate* and allow to stand for 2 minutes. Add 0.2 g of *citric acid*, 1 ml of 5M *ammonia* and 1 ml of *sodium diethyldithiocarbamate solution* to the solution and extract with 10 ml of *carbon tetrachloride* for 2 minutes. The colour of the extract is not more intense than that of the extract obtained when 10 ml of a mixture of 3 volumes of *copper standard solution (10 ppm Cu)* and 197 volumes of *water* is treated in the same manner (10 ppm).

Iron Ignite 1.0 g with 1 g of *anhydrous sodium carbonate*, cool, dissolve the residue in sufficient of a mixture of 1 volume of 2M *hydrochloric acid* and 2 volumes of *water* to produce 10 ml. The resulting solution complies with the *limit test for iron*, Appendix VII (10 ppm).

Related substances Carry out the method for *thin-layer chromatography*, Appendix III A, using a silica gel F254 precoated chromatoplate (Merck silica gel 60 F254 plates are suitable), an unlined chromatographic tank and, as the mobile phase, the upper layer (which may be slightly opalescent) obtained by shaking a mixture of 80 volumes of *toluene*, 25 volumes of *ethyl acetate* and 3 volumes of 13.5M *ammonia*. Apply separately to the plate 20 μl of each of three solutions of the substance being examined in *ethanol (96%)* containing (1) 10% w/v, (2) 0.020% w/v and (3) 0.010% w/v. After removal of the plate, allow it to dry in air and examine under *ultra-violet light (254 nm)*. Expose the plate to iodine vapour for at least 2 hours. Any *secondary spot* in the chromatogram obtained with solution (1) is not more intense than the spot in the chromatogram obtained with solution (2) and not more than one such spot is more intense than the spot in the chromatogram obtained with solution (3).

Loss on drying When dried to constant weight at 105°, loses not more than 0.5% of its weight. Use 1 g.

Sulphated ash Not more than 0.1%, Appendix IX A.

Assay Carry out Method I for *non-aqueous titration*, Appendix VIII A, using 0.25 g, 7 ml of *mercury(II) acetate solution* and *1-naphtholbenzein solution* as indicator. Each ml of 0.1M *perchloric acid VS* is equivalent to 0.02568 g of $C_{13}H_{20}N_2O,HCl$.

Storage Prilocaine Hydrochloride should be kept in a well-closed container.

Action and use Local anaesthetic.

Primaquine Phosphate

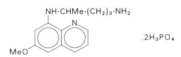

C₁₅H₂₁N₃O,2H₃PO₄   455.3   *63-45-6*

Primaquine Phosphate is 4-amino-1-methyl-butyl(6-methoxy-8-quinolyl)amine diortho-phosphate. It contains not less than 97.5 per cent and not more than 100.5 per cent of $C_{15}H_{21}N_3O,2H_3PO_4$, calculated with reference to the dried substance.

Characteristics An orange-red, crystalline powder; odourless or almost odourless.

Solubility Soluble in 16 parts of *water*; practically insoluble in *chloroform* and in *ether*.

Identification A. Dissolve 0.1 g in 10 ml of *water*, add 2 ml of 2M *sodium hydroxide* and extract with two 20-ml quantities of *chloroform*, reserving the aqueous layer for test C. Wash the chloroform extracts with *water*, dry with *anhydrous sodium sulphate*, evaporate to dryness and dissolve the residue in 2 ml of *chloroform IR*. The *infra-red absorption spectrum* of the resulting solution, Appendix II A, is concordant with the *reference spectrum* of primaquine.
B. The *light absorption*, Appendix II B, in the range 250 to 300 nm of a 0.003% w/v solution in 0.01M *hydrochloric acid* exhibits two maxima, at 265 nm and 282 nm. The *absorbance* at 265 nm is about 0.99 and at 282 nm is about 0.98.
C. The aqueous layer obtained in test A, after neutralisation with 2M *nitric acid*, yields the *reactions* characteristic of phosphates, Appendix VI.

Acidity pH of a 1% w/v solution, 2.5 to 3.5, Appendix V L.

Loss on drying When dried to constant weight at 105°, loses not more than 0.5% of its weight. Use 1 g.

Assay Dissolve 0.2 g in 40 ml of *anhydrous glacial acetic acid* with gentle heating and carry out Method I for *non-aqueous titration*, Appendix VIII A, determining the end-point potentiometrically. Each ml of 0.1M *perchloric acid VS* is equivalent to 0.02277 g of $C_{15}H_{21}N_3O,2H_3PO_4$.

Storage Primaquine Phosphate should be protected from light.

Preparation
Primaquine Tablets

Action and use Antimalarial.

Primidone

$C_{12}H_{14}N_2O_2$ 218.3   125-33-7

Primidone is 5-ethylperhydro-5-phenyl-pyrimidine-4,6-dione. It contains not less than 99.0 per cent and not more than 100.5 per cent of $C_{12}H_{14}N_2O_2$, calculated with reference to the dried substance.

Characteristics A white, crystalline powder; odourless or almost odourless.

Solubility Very slightly soluble in *water*; slightly soluble in *ethanol (96%)*; practically insoluble in most other organic solvents.

Identification A. The *infra-red absorption spectrum*, Appendix II A, is concordant with the *reference spectrum* of primidone.
B. Dissolve 0.1 g in 5 ml of *chromotropic acid solution* and heat in a water-bath for 30 minutes. A pinkish-blue colour is produced.
C. *Melting point*, about 280°, Appendix V A.

Heavy metals To 2.0 g of the substance being examined in a Kjeldahl flask add 20 ml of a mixture of 4 volumes of *nitric acid* and 1 volume of *perchloric acid* and heat carefully until any initial reaction has subsided. Cool, carefully add 4 ml of *sulphuric acid* and heat until the nitric acid volatilises and a vigorous reaction occurs to complete the oxidation. Remove the source of heat and add 5 ml of a mixture of 4 volumes of *nitric acid* and 1 volume of *perchloric acid*. Allow the reaction to subside and continue heating until the residual sulphuric acid begins to fume. Allow to cool and dilute carefully with 20 ml of *water*. Transfer the solution to a beaker and evaporate to dryness. To the cooled residue add 2 ml of *hydrochloric acid* and slowly evaporate to dryness on a water-bath. Add to the residue 10 ml of 1M *hydrochloric acid*, digest for 10 minutes on the water-bath and cool. Neutralise the solution with 13.5M *ammonia* and adjust the acidity to pH 3 to 4 by the careful addition of *glacial acetic acid*. Dilute to about 35 ml with *water*, add 10 ml of *hydrogen sulphide solution*, dilute to 50 ml with *water*, mix and allow to stand for 10 minutes. The resulting solution is not more intensely coloured than a standard prepared in the same manner but using 2 ml of *lead standard solution (10 ppm Pb)* in place of the substance being examined (10 ppm).

2-Ethyl-2-phenylmalondiamide Dissolve 25 mg of *octadecan-1-ol* (internal standard) in sufficient *pyridine* to produce 50 ml (solution A). Carry out the method for *gas chromatography*, Appendix III B, using the following solutions. For solution (1) add 2 ml of solution A and 1 ml of N,O-*bis(trimethylsilyl)acetamide* to 2 ml of a

0.050% w/v solution of *2-ethyl-2-phenylmalondiamide* in *pyridine*, mix, allow to stand at 100° for 5 minutes, cool and dilute to 10 ml with *pyridine*. Prepare solution (2) in the same manner as solution (3) but use 0.1 g of the substance being examined in 4 ml of *pyridine* and omit the addition of solution A. For solution (3) mix 0.1 g of the substance being examined with 2 ml of *pyridine*, add 2 ml of solution A and 1 ml of N,O-*bis-(trimethylsilyl)acetamide*, allow to stand at 100° for 5 minutes, cool and dilute to 10 ml with *pyridine*.

The chromatographic procedure may be carried out using a glass column (1.5 m × 4 mm) packed with *acid-washed, silanised diatomaceous support* (100 to 120 mesh) coated with 3% w/w of phenyl methyl silicone fluid (50% phenyl) (OV-17 is suitable) and maintained at 170°.

In the chromatogram obtained with solution (3) the ratio of the area of the peak derived from 2-ethyl-2-phenylmalondiamide to the area of the peak derived from the internal standard is not greater than the corresponding ratio in the chromatogram obtained with solution (1).

Loss on drying When dried to constant weight at 130°, loses not more than 0.5% of its weight. Use 1 g.

Sulphated ash Not more than 0.1%, Appendix IX A.

Assay Carry out Method I for the *determination of nitrogen*, Appendix VIII H, using 0.2 g and 8 ml of *nitrogen-free sulphuric acid*. Each ml of 0.05M *sulphuric acid VS* is equivalent to 0.01091 g of $C_{12}H_{14}N_2O_2$.

Preparations
Primidone Oral Suspension
Primidone Tablets

Action and use Anticonvulsant.

Probenecid ☆

$C_{13}H_{19}NO_4S$ 285.4   57-66-9

Probenecid is 4-(dipropylsulphamoyl)benzoic acid. It contains not less than 99.0 per cent and not more than 101.0 per cent of $C_{13}H_{19}NO_4S$, calculated with reference to the dried substance.

Characteristics A white or almost white, crystalline powder; odourless.

Solubility Practically insoluble in *water*; sparingly soluble in *ethanol (96%)* and in *chloroform*; soluble in *acetone*; slightly soluble in *ether*.

Identification *Test A may be omitted if tests B, C and D are carried out. Tests B and C may be omitted if tests A and D are carried out.*
A. The *infra-red absorption spectrum*, Appendix II A, is concordant with the spectrum of *probenecid EPCRS*.
B. The *light absorption*, Appendix II B, in the range 220 to 350 nm of a 0.001% w/v solution in a mixture of 1 volume of 0.1M *hydrochloric acid* and 9 volumes of *ethanol (96%)* exhibits two maxima, at 223 nm and 248 nm. The A(1%, 1 cm) at the maximum at 248 nm is 310 to 350.
C. Dissolve 0.2 g in the minimum volume of 2M *ammonia* (about 0.6 ml) and add 3 ml of a 1.7% w/v solution of

silver nitrate. A white precipitate is produced which dissolves in an excess of aqueous ammonia.

D. *Melting point*, 197° to 202°, Appendix V A, Method I.

Acidity Heat 2 g with 100 ml of *water* on a water-bath for 30 minutes, cool, restore to the original volume with *water*, filter and titrate 50 ml of the filtrate with 0.1M *sodium hydroxide VS* using *dilute phenolphthalein solution* as indicator. Not more than 0.5 ml of 0.1M *sodium hydroxide VS* is required to change the colour of the solution.

Clarity and colour of solution A 10.0% w/v solution in 1M *sodium hydroxide* is *clear*, Appendix IV A, and not more intensely coloured than *reference solution* Y_6, Appendix IV B, Method II.

Heavy metals 1.0 g complies with *limit test C for heavy metals*, Appendix VII (20 ppm). Use 2 ml of *lead standard solution (10 ppm Pb)* to prepare the standard.

Related substances Carry out the method for *thin-layer chromatography*, Appendix III A, using *silica gel GF254* as the coating substance and a mixture of 55 volumes of *toluene*, 20 volumes of *di-isopropyl ether*, 15 volumes of *chloroform* and 10 volumes of *glacial acetic acid* as the mobile phase. Apply separately to the chromatoplate 20 μl of each of two solutions of the substance being examined in *acetone* containing (1) 1.0% w/v and (2) 0.0050% w/v. After removal of the plate, allow it to dry in air and examine under *ultra-violet light (254 nm)*. Any *secondary spot* in the chromatogram obtained with solution (1) is not more intense than the spot in the chromatogram obtained with solution (2).

Loss on drying When dried to constant weight at 100° to 105°, loses not more than 0.5% of its weight. Use 1 g.

Sulphated ash Not more than 0.1%, Appendix IX A, Method II. Use 1 g.

Assay Dissolve 0.25 g in 50 ml of *ethanol (96%)*, shaking and heating gently if necessary, and titrate with 0.1M *sodium hydroxide VS* determining the end-point potentiometrically. Each ml of 0.1M *sodium hydroxide VS* is equivalent to 0.02854 g of $C_{13}H_{19}NO_4S$.

Preparation
Probenecid Tablets

Action and use Used in treatment of gout and to delay renal excretion of penicillins and cephalosporins.

Procainamide Hydrochloride

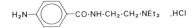

$C_{13}H_{21}N_3O,HCl$ 271.8   *614-39-1*

Procainamide Hydrochloride is 4-amino-*N*-(2-diethylaminoethyl)benzamide hydrochloride. It contains not less than 98.0 per cent and not more than 101.0 per cent of $C_{13}H_{21}N_3O,HCl$, calculated with reference to the dried substance.

Characteristics A white to yellowish-white, crystalline powder; odourless or almost odourless; hygroscopic.

Solubility Soluble in 0.25 part of *water* and in 2 parts of *ethanol (96%)*; slightly soluble in *chloroform*; practically insoluble in *ether*.

Identification A. The *infra-red absorption spectrum*, Appendix II A, is concordant with the *reference spectrum* of procainamide hydrochloride.

B. The *light absorption*, Appendix II B, in the range 230 to 350 nm of a 0.002% w/v solution in 0.02M *sodium hydroxide* exhibits a maximum only at 275 nm. The *absorbance* at 275 nm is about 1.2.

C. Dissolve 1 g in 10 ml of *water*, add 10 ml of 5M *sodium hydroxide* and extract with 10 ml of *chloroform*. Add 10 ml of *toluene* to the extract, dry over *anhydrous sodium sulphate* and filter. Mix the filtrate with 5 ml of dry *pyridine*, add 1 ml of *benzoyl chloride* dropwise, heat on a water-bath for 30 minutes and pour into 100 ml of 2.5M *sodium hydroxide*. Extract with 10 ml of *ether*, wash the extract with 20 ml of *water*, dilute with 30 ml of *ether* and allow to crystallise. The *melting point* of the crystals, after recrystallisation from *ethanol (45%)*, is about 186°, Appendix V A.

D. Yields the *reactions* characteristic of chlorides, Appendix VI.

Acidity pH of a 10% w/v solution, 5.0 to 6.5, Appendix V L.

Melting point 165° to 169°, Appendix V A.

Heavy metals A 10.0% w/v solution complies with *limit test A for heavy metals*, Appendix VII (10 ppm). Use *lead standard solution (1 ppm Pb)* to prepare the standard.

Related substances Carry out the method for *thin-layer chromatography*, Appendix III A, using *silica gel G* as the coating substance and a mixture of 70 volumes of *chloroform*, 30 volumes of *methanol* and 0.7 volume of 13.5M *ammonia* as the mobile phase. Apply separately to the chromatoplate 10 μl of each of two solutions of the substance being examined in *methanol* containing (1) 2.0% w/v and (2) 0.010% w/v and then at each point of application 10 μl of a 20% v/v solution of 13.5M *ammonia* in *methanol*. After removal of the plate, allow it to dry in air and spray with *ethanolic dimethylaminobenzaldehyde solution*. Any *secondary spot* in the chromatogram obtained with solution (1) is not more intense than the spot in the chromatogram obtained with solution (2).

Loss on drying When dried to constant weight at 105°, loses not more than 1.0% of its weight. Use 1 g.

Sulphated ash Not more than 0.1%, Appendix IX A.

Assay Dissolve 0.5 g in 75 ml of *water*, add 10 ml of *hydrochloric acid* and titrate with 0.1M *sodium nitrite VS*, using 1 ml of *ferrocyphen solution* as indicator, until a violet colour is produced that is stable for not less than 3 minutes. Repeat the operation without the substance being examined. The difference between the titrations represents the amount of sodium nitrite required. Each ml of 0.1M *sodium nitrite VS* is equivalent to 0.02718 g of $C_{13}H_{21}N_3O,HCl$.

Storage Procainamide Hydrochloride should be kept in a well-closed container.

Preparations
Procainamide Injection
Procainamide Tablets

Action and use Anti-arrhythmic.

Procaine Hydrochloride ☆

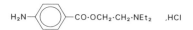

C₁₃H₂₀N₂O₂,HCl   272.8   51-5-8

Procaine Hydrochloride is 2-diethylaminoethyl 4-aminobenzoate hydrochloride. It contains not less than 99.0 per cent and not more than 101.0 per cent of $C_{13}H_{20}N_2O_2,HCl$, calculated with reference to the dried substance.

Characteristics Colourless crystals or a white, crystalline powder; odourless.

Solubility Soluble in 1 part of *water* and in 25 parts of *ethanol (96%)*; slightly soluble in *chloroform*; practically insoluble in *ether*.

Identification *Test A may be omitted if tests B, C, D, E and F are carried out. Tests B, C and D may be omitted if tests A, E and F are carried out.*
A. The *infra-red absorption spectrum*, Appendix II A, is concordant with the spectrum of *procaine hydrochloride EPCRS*.
B. To 5 mg add 0.5 ml of *fuming nitric acid*, evaporate to dryness on a water-bath, cool, dissolve the residue in 5 ml of *acetone* and add 1 ml of 0.1M *ethanolic potassium hydroxide*. A reddish-brown colour is produced.
C. To 0.2 ml of a 5% w/v solution in *carbon dioxide-free water* add 2 ml of *water* and 0.5 ml of 1M *sulphuric acid*, shake and add 1 ml of a 0.1% w/v solution of *potassium permanganate*. The colour is immediately discharged.
D. 2 ml of a 0.05% w/v solution in *carbon dioxide-free water* yields the *reaction* characteristic of primary aromatic amines, Appendix VI.
E. Yields *reaction A* characteristic of chlorides, Appendix VI.
F. *Melting point*, 154° to 158°, Appendix V A, Method I.

Acidity Dissolve 2.5 g in sufficient *water* to produce 50 ml and dilute 4 ml to 10 ml with the same solvent. The pH of the resulting solution is 5.0 to 6.5, Appendix V L.

Clarity and colour of solution A 5.0% w/v solution in *carbon dioxide-free water* is *clear*, Appendix IV A, and *colourless*, Appendix IV B, Method II.

Heavy metals Complies with *limit test E for heavy metals*, Appendix VII, preparing the solution by dissolving 1.0 g in sufficient *water* to produce 25 ml and using 10 ml of the filtrate. Use 2 ml of *lead standard solution (1 ppm Pb)* to prepare the standard (5 ppm).

Related substances Carry out the method for *thin-layer chromatography*, Appendix III A, using *silica gel GF254* as the coating substance and a mixture of 80 volumes of *dibutyl ether*, 16 volumes of n-*hexane* and 4 volumes of *glacial acetic acid* as the mobile phase but allowing the solvent front to ascend 10 cm above the line of application. Apply separately to the chromatoplate 5 μl of each of two solutions in *water* containing (1) 10.0% w/v of the substance being examined and (2) 0.0050% w/v of *4-aminobenzoic acid*. After removal of the plate, dry it at 100° to 105° for 10 minutes and examine under *ultra-violet light (254 nm)*. Any *secondary spot* in the chromatogram obtained with solution (1) is not more intense than the spot in the chromatogram obtained with solution (2). The principal spot remains on the line of application.

Loss on drying When dried to constant weight at 100° to 105°, loses not more than 0.5% of its weight. Use 1 g.

Sulphated ash Not more than 0.1%, Appendix IX A, Method II. Use 1 g.

Assay Dissolve 0.4 g in 50 ml of 2M *hydrochloric acid*, add 3 g of *potassium bromide*, cool, if necessary, in ice and carry out the method for *amperometric titration*, Appendix VIII B. Each ml of 0.1M *sodium nitrite VS* is equivalent to 0.02728 g of $C_{13}H_{20}N_2O_2,HCl$.

Storage Procaine Hydrochloride should be protected from light.

Action and use Local anaesthetic.

Procaine Penicillin ☆

C₁₃H₂₀N₂O₂,C₁₆H₁₈N₂O₄S,H₂O   588.7   6130-64-9

Procaine Penicillin is 2-diethylaminoethyl 4-aminobenzoate (6R)-6-(2-phenylacetamido)-penicillanate monohydrate. It contains not less than 96.0 per cent and not more than 102.0 per cent of penicillins, calculated as $C_{13}H_{20}N_2O_2,C_{16}H_{18}N_2O_4S$, and not less than 39.0 per cent and not more than 42.0 per cent of procaine, $C_{13}H_{20}N_2O_2$, both calculated with reference to the anhydrous substance.

Characteristics A white, crystalline powder.

Solubility Slightly soluble in *water*; freely soluble in *ethanol (96%)*.

Identification *Test A may be omitted if tests B, C and D are carried out. Tests B, C and D may be omitted if test A is carried out.*
A. The *infra-red absorption spectrum*, Appendix II A, is concordant with the spectrum of *procaine benzylpenicillin EPCRS*.
B. Prepare a 0.01% w/v solution of the substance being examined in *0.0067M mixed phosphate buffer pH 7.0* (solution A). To 10 ml of solution A add 0.5 ml of a solution prepared by diluting 1 ml of *penicillinase solution* to 10 ml with *water* and allow to stand at 30° for 10 minutes (solution B). To 5 ml of solution A and to 5 ml of solution B, in separate test-tubes, add 10 ml of *acetate buffer pH 4.6* and 5 ml of 0.0005M *iodine*. Mix the contents of each tube and add, to each, 0.1 ml of *starch solution*. The mixture obtained with solution A is blue; the mixture obtained with solution B remains colourless.
C. Yields the *reaction* characteristic of penicillins and cephalosporins, Appendix VI.
D. Yields the *reaction* characteristic of primary aromatic amines, Appendix VI, producing a bright, orange-red precipitate.

Acidity or alkalinity pH of a 0.33% w/v solution, 5.0 to 7.5, Appendix V L.

Specific optical rotation Dissolve 0.25 g in sufficient of a mixture of 3 volumes of *acetone* and 2 volumes of *water* to produce 25 ml. The *specific optical rotation* in the resulting solution is +165° to +180°, Appendix V F.

Water 3.0 to 4.2% w/w, Appendix IX C. Use 0.5 g.

Assay *For penicillins* Dissolve 70 mg in 1 ml of *methanol*, add 5 ml of *water* and 5 ml of 1M *sodium hydroxide* and allow to stand for 15 minutes. Add 5 ml of 1M *nitric acid*,

20 ml of *acetate buffer pH 4.6* and 20 ml of *water*. Titrate at 35° to 40° with 0.02M *mercury(II) nitrate VS*. Determine the end-point potentiometrically using a platinum or mercury indicator electrode and a mercury—mercury(I) sulphate reference electrode; titrate slowly so that the titration takes about 15 minutes and disregard any preliminary inflection on the titration curve. Each ml of 0.02M *mercury(II) nitrate VS* is equivalent to 0.01141 g of total penicillins, calculated as $C_{13}H_{20}N_2O_2,C_{16}H_{18}N_2O_4S$.

Dissolve 0.25 g in 25 ml of *methanol* and add 25 ml of *acetate buffer pH 4.6*. Titrate immediately at room temperature with 0.02M *mercury(II) nitrate VS* determining the end-point as above. Each ml of 0.02M *mercury(II) nitrate VS* is equivalent to 0.01141 g of degradation products, calculated as $C_{13}H_{20}N_2O_2,C_{16}H_{18}N_2O_4S$. Subtract the percentage of degradation products found from the percentage of total penicillins found; the difference is the content of penicillins, calculated as $C_{13}H_{20}N_2O_2$, $C_{16}H_{18}N_2O_4S$.

For procaine Dissolve 0.1 g in sufficient *methanol* to produce 100 ml, dilute 5 ml to 250 ml with *water* and measure the *absorbance* of the resulting solution at the maximum at 290 nm, Appendix II B. Calculate the content of $C_{13}H_{20}N_2O_2$ taking 777 as the value of A(1%, 1 cm) at the maximum at 290 nm.

Storage Procaine Penicillin should be kept in an airtight container, protected from moisture and stored at a temperature not exceeding 30°. If the material is intended for use in the manufacture of a parenteral dosage form, the container should be sterile, tamper-evident and sealed so as to exclude micro-organisms.

Labelling The label states (1) the date after which the material is not intended to be used; (2) the conditions under which it should be stored; (3) whether or not it is intended for use in the manufacture of a parenteral dosage form.

Preparations
Procaine Penicillin Injection
Fortified Procaine Penicillin Injection

Action and use Antibacterial.

300 mg is approximately equivalent to 200 mg of benzylpenicillin.

Procaine Penicillin intended for use in the manufacture of a parenteral dosage form complies with the following additional requirements.

Pyrogens Complies with the *test for pyrogens*, Appendix XIV K. Use per kg of the rabbit's weight 0.5 ml of a solution in *sodium chloride injection* containing 5 mg per ml.

Sterility Complies with the *test for sterility*, Appendix XVI A.

The title of the monograph in the European Pharmacopœia is Procaine Benzylpenicillin.

Prochlorperazine Maleate ☆

$C_{20}H_{24}ClN_3S,2C_4H_4O_4$ 606.1   *84-02-6*

Prochlorperazine Maleate is 2-chloro-10-[3-(4-methylpiperazin-1-yl)propyl]phenothiazine di(hydrogen maleate). It contains not less than 98.0 per cent and not more than 101.0 per cent of $C_{20}H_{24}ClN_3S,2C_4H_4O_4$, calculated with reference to the dried substance.

Characteristics A white or pale yellow, crystalline powder; almost odourless.

Solubility Very slightly soluble in *water* and in *ethanol* (96%); practically insoluble in *chloroform* and in *ether*.

Identification *Test A may be omitted if tests B, C and D are carried out. Test B may be omitted if tests A, C and D are carried out.*

A. The *infra-red absorption spectrum*, Appendix II A, is concordant with the spectrum of *prochlorperazine maleate EPCRS*.

B. Carry out the following procedure protected from light. The *light absorption*, Appendix II B, in the range 280 to 350 nm of a 0.010% w/v solution in 0.1M *hydrochloric acid*, examined immediately after preparation, exhibits a maximum at 305 nm. Dilute 10 ml of the solution to 100 ml with the same solvent and examine immediately. The *light absorption* in the range 230 to 280 nm exhibits a maximum at 255 nm. The A(1%, 1 cm) at the maximum at 255 nm is 525 to 575.

C. Carry out the test for *identification of phenothiazines*, Appendix III A, but applying 4 μl of each of the following solutions. Solution (1) contains 0.1% w/v of the substance being examined in a mixture of equal volumes of *methanol* and *chloroform*. Solution (2) contains 0.1% w/v of *prochlorperazine maleate EPCRS* in the same solvent mixture.

D. Suspend 0.2 g in a mixture of 3 ml of *water* and 2 ml of 5M *sodium hydroxide* and shake with three 5-ml quantities of *ether*. To 0.1 ml of the aqueous layer add a solution of 10 mg of *resorcinol* in 3 ml of *sulphuric acid* and heat in a water-bath for 15 minutes; no colour is produced. To the remainder of the aqueous layer add 2 ml of *bromine solution*, heat in a water-bath for 15 minutes, then heat to boiling and cool. To 0.1 ml of the solution add a solution of 10 mg of *resorcinol* in 3 ml of *sulphuric acid* and heat in a water-bath for 15 minutes; a blue colour is produced.

Acidity pH of a saturated solution, 3.0 to 4.0, Appendix V L.

Related substances Complies with the test for *related substances in phenothiazines*, Appendix III A, using *mobile phase A*.

Loss on drying When dried to constant weight at 100° to 105°, loses not more than 1.0% of its weight. Use 1 g.

Sulphated ash Not more than 0.1%, Appendix IX A. Use 1 g.

Assay Dissolve 0.2 g in 50 ml of *anhydrous glacial acetic acid* and carry out Method I for *non-aqueous titration*,

Appendix VIII A, determining the end-point potentiometrically. Each ml of 0.1M *perchloric acid VS* is equivalent to 0.03031 g of $C_{20}H_{24}ClN_3S,2C_4H_4O_4$.

Storage Prochlorperazine Maleate should be kept in a well-closed container and protected from light.

Preparation
Prochlorperazine Tablets

Action and use Antipsychotic; antiemetic.

Prochlorperazine Mesylate

$C_{20}H_{24}ClN_3S,2CH_4SO_3$ 556.2   *5132-55-8*

Prochlorperazine Mesylate is 2-chloro-10-[3-(4-methylpiperazin-1-yl)propyl]phenothiazine di(methanesulphonate). It contains not less than 98.0 per cent and not more than 101.0 per cent of $C_{20}H_{24}ClN_3S,2CH_4SO_3$, calculated with reference to the dried substance.

Characteristics A white or almost white powder; odourless or almost odourless.

Solubility Soluble in less than 0.5 part of *water* and in 40 parts of *ethanol (96%)*; slightly soluble in *chloroform*; practically insoluble in *ether*.

Identification A. The *infra-red absorption spectrum*, Appendix II A, is concordant with the *reference spectrum* of prochlorperazine mesylate.
B. The *light absorption*, Appendix II B, in the range 230 to 350 nm of a 0.0014% w/v solution in *absolute ethanol* containing 0.01% v/v of 13.5M *ammonia* exhibits a maximum at 258 nm and a less well-defined maximum at 313 nm. The *absorbance* at 258 nm is about 0.88.
C. Dissolve 5 mg in 2 ml of *sulphuric acid* and allow to stand for 5 minutes. A red colour is produced.
D. Mix 50 mg with 0.2 g of powdered *sodium hydroxide*, heat to fusion and continue the heating for a few seconds longer. Cool, add 0.5 ml of *water* and a slight excess of 2M *hydrochloric acid* and warm. Sulphur dioxide is evolved which turns moistened *starch—iodate paper* blue.

Acidity pH of a 2% w/v solution, 2.0 to 3.0, Appendix V L.

Related substances Complies with the test for *related substances in phenothiazines*, Appendix III A, using *mobile phase A* and dissolving the substance being examined in *methanol* containing 0.5% v/v of 13.5M *ammonia*.

Loss on drying When dried to constant weight at 100° at a pressure not exceeding 0.7 kPa, loses not more than 1.0% of its weight. Use 1 g.

Sulphated ash Not more than 0.1%, Appendix IX A.

Assay Dissolve 0.8 g in 10 ml of *water*, add 5 ml of 1M *sodium hydroxide* and extract by shaking with successive quantities of 50, 25, 25 and 25 ml of *ether*. Wash the combined ether extracts with 5 ml of *water*, shake the washings with 5 ml of *ether*, add the ether to the combined ether extracts and evaporate the ether. Add 2 ml of *absolute ethanol* to the residue, evaporate to dryness and carry out Method I for *non-aqueous titration*, Appendix VIII A, using *1-naphtholbenzein solution* as indicator. Each ml of 0.1M *perchloric acid VS* is equivalent to 0.02831 g of $C_{20}H_{24}ClN_3S,2CH_4SO_3$.

Storage Prochlorperazine Mesylate should be protected from light.

Preparation
Prochlorperazine Injecton

Action and use Antipsychotic; antiemetic.

Procyclidine Hydrochloride

$C_{19}H_{29}NO,HCl$ 323.9   *1508-76-5*

Procyclidine Hydrochloride is 1-cyclohexyl-1-phenyl-3-pyrrolidin-1-ylpropan-1-ol hydrochloride. It contains not less than 99.0 per cent and not more than 101.0 per cent of $C_{19}H_{29}NO,HCl$, calculated with reference to the dried substance.

Characteristics A white, crystalline powder; odourless or almost odourless.

Solubility Soluble in 40 parts of *water* and in 15 parts of *ethanol (96%)*; practically insoluble in *acetone* and in *ether*.

Identification A. The *infra-red absorption spectrum*, Appendix II A, is concordant with the *reference spectrum* of procyclidine hydrochloride.
B. Dissolve 0.25 g in 10 ml of *water*, make alkaline with 5M *ammonia* and extract with three 10-ml quantities of *ether*. Dry the combined extracts over *anhydrous sodium sulphate*, filter, remove the ether and scratch the residue with a glass rod to induce solidification. The *melting point* of the residue is about 85°, Appendix V A.
C. Yields the *reactions* characteristic of chlorides, Appendix VI.

Acidity pH of a 1% w/v solution, 4.5 to 6.5, Appendix V L.

Related substances A. Carry out the method for *thin-layer chromatography*, Appendix III A, using *silica gel GF254* as the coating substance and a mixture of 100 volumes of *ether* and 1 volume of 13.5M *ammonia* as the mobile phase. Apply separately to the chromatoplate 5 µl of each of three solutions in *chloroform* containing (1) 2.0% w/v of the substance being examined, (2) 0.0040% w/v of *1-phenyl-3-pyrrolidinopropan-1-one hydrochloride BPCRS* and (3) 0.010% w/v of the substance being examined. After removal of the plate, dry it at 105° for 15 minutes and examine under *ultra-violet light (254 nm)*. Any spot corresponding to 1-phenyl-3-pyrrolidinopropan-1-one in the chromatogram obtained with solution (1) is not more intense than the spot in the chromatogram obtained with solution (2). Spray the plate with *dilute potassium iodobismuthate solution*. Any *secondary spot* in the chromatogram obtained with solution (1) is not more intense than the spot in the chromatogram obtained with solution (3).
B. Carry out the method for *gas chromatography*, Appendix III B, using the following solutions. For solution (1) add 5 ml of 1.25M *sodium hydroxide* to 20 ml of a 0.015% w/v solution of the substance being examined and mix. Extract with two 20-ml quantities of *ether*, add to the combined extracts 5 ml of a 0.06% w/v solution of *triphenylethylene* (internal standard) in *ether*, shake with *anhydrous sodium sulphate* and filter; evaporate the filtrate and dissolve the residue in 1 ml of *ether*. Prepare solution

(2) in the same manner as solution (1) but using 20 ml of a 0.50% w/v solution of the substance being examined and omitting the addition of the internal standard solution. Prepare solution (3) in the same manner as solution (1) but using 20 ml of a 0.50% w/v solution of the substance being examined.

The chromatographic procedure may be carried out using a glass column (1.5 m × 4 mm) packed with *acid-washed, silanised diatomaceous support* (HP Chromosorb W is suitable) (80 to 100 mesh), coated with 10% w/w of modified polyethylene glycol 20M (SP-1000 is suitable) and 2% w/w of *potassium hydroxide* and maintained at 240°, and using on-column injection.

The ratio of the sum of the areas of the *secondary peaks* to the area of the peak due to the internal standard in the chromatogram obtained with solution (3) is not more than the ratio of the area of the principal peak to the area of the internal standard peak in the chromatogram obtained with solution (1).

Loss on drying When dried to constant weight at 105°, loses not more than 0.5% of its weight. Use 1 g.

Sulphated ash Not more than 0.1%, Appendix IX A.

Assay Carry out Method I for *non-aqueous titration*, Appendix VIII A, using 0.7 g and *crystal violet solution* as indicator. Each ml of 0.1M *perchloric acid VS* is equivalent to 0.03239 g of $C_{19}H_{29}NO,HCl$.

Preparation
Procyclidine Tablets

Action and use Used in treatment of Parkinson's disease.

Progesterone ☆

$C_{21}H_{30}O_2$ 314.5   *57-83-0*

Progesterone is pregn-4-ene-3,20-dione. It contains not less than 97.0 per cent and not more than 103.0 per cent of $C_{21}H_{30}O_2$, calculated with reference to the dried substance.

Characteristics Colourless crystals or a white or slightly yellowish-white, crystalline powder.

Solubility Practically insoluble in *water*; soluble in 8 parts of *ethanol (96%)* and in less than 1 part of *chloroform*; sparingly soluble in *acetone*, in *1,4-dioxan*, in *ether* and in fixed oils.

Identification A. The *infra-red absorption spectrum*, Appendix II A, is concordant with the spectrum of *progesterone EPCRS*. If the spectra obtained are not concordant, prepare new spectra using 5% w/v solutions in *chloroform IR*.

B. Carry out the method for *thin-layer chromatography*, Appendix III A, using as the coating substance a suitable silica gel containing a fluorescent indicator with an optimal intensity at 254 nm (Merck silica gel 60 F254 is suitable) and a mixture of 66 volumes of *chloroform* and 33 volumes of *ethyl acetate* as the mobile phase. Apply separately to the chromatoplate 5 µl of each of two solutions in a mixture of 9 volumes of *chloroform* and 1 volume of *methanol* containing (1) 0.1% w/v of the substance being examined and (2) 0.1% w/v of *progesterone EPCRS*. After removal of the plate, allow it to dry in air and examine under *ultra-violet light (254 nm)*. The principal spot in the chromatogram obtained with solution (1) is similar in position and size to the spot in the chromatogram obtained with solution (2). Spray the plate with *ethanolic sulphuric acid (20%)*, heat at 120° for 15 minutes, allow to cool and examine in daylight and under *ultra-violet light (365 nm)*. The principal spot in the chromatogram obtained with solution (1) is similar in position, colour in daylight, fluorescence in ultra-violet light and size to the spot in the chromatogram obtained with solution (2).

C. *Melting point*, 128° to 132°, Appendix V A, Method I.

Specific optical rotation In a 1% w/v solution in *absolute ethanol*, +186° to +194°, Appendix V F.

Related substances Carry out the method for *thin-layer chromatography*, Appendix III A, using *silica gel G* as the coating substance and a mixture of 66 volumes of *chloroform* and 33 volumes of *ethyl acetate* as the mobile phase. Apply separately to the chromatoplate 5 µl of each of two solutions of the substance being examined in a mixture of 9 volumes of *chloroform* and 1 volume of *methanol* containing (1) 1.0% w/v and (2) 0.010% w/v. After removal of the plate, allow it to dry in air, spray with a saturated solution of *potassium dichromate* in *sulphuric acid (70%)*, heat at 130° for 30 minutes and allow to cool. Any *secondary spot* in the chromatogram obtained with solution (1) is not more intense than the spot in the chromatogram obtained with solution (2).

Loss on drying When dried at 100° to 105° for 2 hours, loses not more than 0.5% of its weight. Use 0.5 g.

Assay Dissolve 25 mg in sufficient *ethanol (96%)* to produce 250 ml, dilute 5 ml to 50 ml with the same solvent and measure the *absorbance* of the resulting solution at the maximum at 241 nm, Appendix II B. Calculate the content of $C_{21}H_{30}O_2$ taking 535 as the value of A(1%, 1 cm) at the maximum at 241 nm.

Storage Progesterone should be kept in a well-closed container and protected from light.

Preparation
Progesterone Injection

Action and use Progestogen.

Proguanil Hydrochloride

$C_{11}H_{16}ClN_5,HCl$ 290.2   *637-32-1*

Proguanil Hydrochloride is 1-(4-chlorophenyl)-5-isopropylbiguanide hydrochloride. It contains not less than 99.0 per cent and not more than 101.0 per cent of $C_{11}H_{16}ClN_5,HCl$, calculated with reference to the dried substance.

Characteristics A white, crystalline powder; odourless or almost odourless.

Solubility Slightly soluble in *water*, more soluble in hot *water*; soluble in 40 parts of *ethanol (96%)*; practically insoluble in *chloroform* and in *ether*.

Identification A. The *infra-red absorption spectrum*, Appendix II A, is concordant with the *reference spectrum* of proguanil hydrochloride.

B. The *light absorption*, Appendix II B, in the range 220 to 350 nm of a 0.001% w/v solution in *methanol* exhibits a maximum at 258 nm and a shoulder at 233 nm. The *absorbance* at 258 nm is about 0.82.

C. To 15 ml of a saturated solution add 2 ml of 5M *sodium hydroxide* and extract with 20 ml of *ether*. Wash the ether extract with *water* and evaporate to dryness at 105°. The *melting point* of the residue is about 131°, Appendix V A.

D. Yields the *reactions* characteristic of chlorides, Appendix VI.

Acidity or alkalinity To 35 ml of *water* maintained at 60° to 65° add 0.2 ml of *methyl red—methylene blue solution*, neutralise with 0.01M *sodium hydroxide VS* or 0.01M *hydrochloric acid VS*, add 0.4 g of the substance being examined and stir until dissolved. The resulting solution is not acidic and requires for neutralisation not more than 0.2 ml of 0.01M *hydrochloric acid VS*.

4-Chloroaniline Dissolve 0.10 g in 1 ml of 2M *hydrochloric acid*, add sufficient *water* to produce 20 ml, cool to 5°, add 1 ml of 0.05M *sodium nitrite*, allow to stand at 5° for 5 minutes, add 2 ml of a 5% w/v solution of *ammonium sulphamate* and allow to stand for 10 minutes. Add 2 ml of a 0.1% w/v solution of N-*(1-naphthyl)ethylenediamine dihydrochloride*, dilute to 50 ml with *water* and allow to stand for 30 minutes. Any magenta colour produced is not more intense than that produced by treating in the same manner and at the same time 20 ml of a 0.000125% w/v solution of *4-chloroaniline*.

Related substances Carry out the method for *high-performance liquid chromatography*, Appendix III D, using solutions of the substance being examined in the mobile phase containing (1) 0.00010% w/v and (2) 0.010% w/v.

The chromatographic procedure may be carried out using (a) a stainless steel column (10 cm × 5 mm) packed with *stationary phase C* (5 μm) (Nucleosil C18 is suitable), (b) 0.01M *sodium hexanesulphonate* in a mixture of 120 volumes of *methanol*, 80 volumes of *water* and 1 volume of *glacial acetic acid* as the mobile phase with a flow rate of 1 ml per minute and (c) a detection wavelength of 254 nm.

The sum of the areas of the *secondary peaks* in the chromatogram obtained with solution (2) is not greater than the area of the principal peak in the chromatogram obtained with solution (1).

Loss on drying When dried to constant weight at 105°, loses not more than 0.5% of its weight. Use 1 g.

Sulphated ash Not more than 0.1%, Appendix IX A.

Assay Carry out Method I for *non-aqueous titration*, Appendix VIII A, using 0.3 g and determining the end-point potentiometrically. Each ml of 0.1M *perchloric acid VS* is equivalent to 0.01451 g of $C_{11}H_{16}ClN_5,HCl$.

Storage Proguanil Hydrochloride should be protected from light.

Preparation
Proguanil Tablets

Action and use Antimalarial.

Promazine Hydrochloride

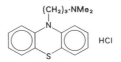

$C_{17}H_{20}N_2S,HCl$ 320.9   *53-60-1*

Promazine Hydrochloride is dimethyl(3-phenothiazin-10-ylpropyl)amine hydrochloride. It contains not less than 99.0 per cent and not more than 101.0 per cent of $C_{17}H_{20}N_2S,HCl$, calculated with reference to the dried substance.

Characteristics A white or almost white, crystalline powder; odourless or almost odourless; slightly hygroscopic.

Solubility Soluble in 1 part of *water*, in 2 parts of *ethanol (96%)* and in 2 parts of *chloroform*.

Identification A. The *infra-red absorption spectrum*, Appendix II A, is concordant with the *reference spectrum* of promazine hydrochloride.

B. The *light absorption*, Appendix II B, in the range 230 to 350 nm of a 0.001% w/v solution in 0.01M *hydrochloric acid* exhibits a maximum at 252 nm and a less well-defined maximum at 302 nm. The *absorbance* at 252 nm is about 0.93.

C. Dissolve 5 mg in 2 ml of *sulphuric acid* and allow to stand for 5 minutes. An orange colour is produced.

D. Yields *reaction A* characteristic of chlorides, Appendix VI.

Acidity pH of a 5% w/v solution, 4.2 to 5.4, Appendix V L.

Melting point 177° to 181°, Appendix V A.

Related substances Complies with the test for *related substances in phenothiazines*, Appendix III A, using *mobile phase A* and as solutions (1) and (2) solutions of the substance being examined in *methanol* containing (1) 1.0% w/v and (2) 0.0050% w/v.

Loss on drying When dried to constant weight at 105°, loses not more than 0.5% of its weight. Use 1 g.

Sulphated ash Not more than 0.1%, Appendix IX A.

Assay Dissolve 0.6 g in 100 ml of *acetone* and carry out Method I for *non-aqueous titration*, Appendix VIII A, using 3 ml of a saturated solution of *methyl orange* in *acetone* as indicator. Each ml of 0.1M *perchloric acid VS* is equivalent to 0.03209 g of $C_{17}H_{20}N_2S,HCl$.

Storage Promazine Hydrochloride should be kept in a well-closed container and protected from light.

Preparations
Promazine Injection
Promazine Tablets

Action and use Antipsychotic.

Promethazine Hydrochloride ☆

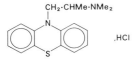

$C_{17}H_{20}N_2S,HCl$ 320.9   *58-33-3*

Promethazine Hydrochloride is dimethyl-[1-methyl-2-(phenothiazin-10-yl)ethyl]amine hydrochloride. It contains not less than 98.5 per cent and not more than 101.0 per cent of $C_{17}H_{20}N_2S,HCl$, calculated with reference to the dried substance.

Characteristics A white or faintly yellowish, crystalline powder. It melts at about 222°, with decomposition.

Solubility Soluble in 0.6 part of *water*, in 9 parts of *ethanol (96%)* and in 2 parts of *chloroform*; practically insoluble in *ether*.

Identification *Test A may be omitted if tests B, C and D are carried out. Test C may be omitted if tests A, B and D are carried out.*
A. The *infra-red absorption spectrum*, Appendix II A, is concordant with the spectrum of *promethazine hydrochloride EPCRS*.
B. Complies with the test for *identification of phenothiazines*, Appendix III A.
C. Dissolve 0.25 g in 25 ml of *water*, add slowly, with stirring, 25 ml of a 1% w/v solution of *2,4,6-trinitrophenol* and allow the mixture to stand for 10 minutes. The *melting point* of the precipitate, after washing with a small quantity of *water*, recrystallising from *ethanol (96%)* and drying, is about 160°, with decomposition, Appendix V A, Method I.
D. 5 ml of 1% w/v solution yields *reaction B* characteristic of chlorides, Appendix VI.

Acidity pH of a freshly prepared 10% w/v solution, 4.0 to 5.0, Appendix V L.

Related substances Carry out the test for *related substances in phenothiazines*, Appendix III A, using *mobile phase B* and applying separately to the chromatoplate 10 μl of each of three freshly prepared solutions in a mixture of 95 volumes of *methanol* and 5 volumes of *diethylamine* containing (1) 2.0% w/v of the substance being examined, (2) 0.020% w/v of *isopromethazine hydrochloride EPCRS* and (3) 0.010% w/v of *promethazine hydrochloride EPCRS*. Any spot corresponding to isopromethazine in the chromatogram obtained with solution (1) is not more intense than the spot in the chromatogram obtained with solution (2). Any other *secondary spot* in the chromatogram obtained with solution (1) is not more intense than the spot in the chromatogram obtained with solution (3).

Loss on drying When dried to constant weight at 100° to 105°, loses not more than 0.5% of its weight. Use 1 g.

Sulphated ash Not more than 0.1%, Appendix IX A, Method II. Use 1 g.

Assay Dissolve 0.25 g in a mixture of 5 ml of 0.01M *hydrochloric acid* and 50 ml of *ethanol (96%)* and titrate with 0.1M *sodium hydroxide VS* determining the end-point potentiometrically. Calculate the volume added between the two inflections. Each ml of 0.1M *sodium hydroxide VS* is equivalent to 0.03209 g of $C_{17}H_{20}N_2S,HCl$.

Storage Promethazine Hydrochloride should be kept in a well-closed container and protected from light.
Preparations
Promethazine Oral Solution
Promethazine Injection
Promethazine Hydrochloride Tablets
Action and use Histamine H_1-receptor antagonist; antiemetic.

Promethazine Theoclate

$C_{17}H_{20}N_2S,C_7H_7ClN_4O_2$ 499.0   *17693-51-5*

Promethazine Theoclate is the dimethyl[1-methyl-2-(phenothiazin-10-yl)ethyl]amine salt of 8-chlorotheophylline. It contains not less than 98.0 per cent and not more than 101.0 per cent of $C_{17}H_{20}N_2S,C_7H_7ClN_4O_2$, calculated with reference to the dried substance.

Characteristics A white or almost white powder; odourless or almost odourless.

Solubility Very slightly soluble in *water*; soluble in 70 parts of *ethanol (96%)* and in 2.5 parts of *chloroform*; practically insoluble in *ether*.

Identification A. Shake 0.15 g with 2.5 ml of *water*, add 1 ml of 5M *ammonia* and extract with 30 ml of *ether*. Wash the ether extract with 10 ml of *water*, dry with *anhydrous sodium sulphate* and evaporate the ether to dryness. Dissolve the residue in 1 ml of *chloroform IR*. The *infra-red absorption spectrum* of the resulting solution, Appendix II A, is concordant with the *reference spectrum* of promethazine.
B. The *light absorption*, Appendix II B, in the range 230 to 350 nm of a 0.0014% w/v solution in *absolute ethanol* containing 0.01% v/v of 13.5M *ammonia* exhibits a maximum at 255 nm. The *absorbance* at 255 nm is about 1.1.
C. Dissolve 5 mg in 2 ml of *sulphuric acid* and allow to stand for 5 minutes. A red colour is produced.
D. Shake 0.4 g with 10 ml of *water*, add 4 ml of 5M *ammonia*, shake with two 30-ml quantities of *ether* and add 4 ml of *hydrochloric acid* to the aqueous solution. Filter the white precipitate, wash with *water* and dry at 105°. Dissolve 10 mg of the residue in 1 ml of *hydrochloric acid*, add 0.1 g of *potassium chlorate* and evaporate to dryness. A reddish residue remains which becomes purple on exposure to the vapour of 5M *ammonia*.
E. Fuse 50 mg of the residue obtained in test D with 0.5 g of *anhydrous sodium carbonate*, boil the residue with 5 ml of *water*, acidify to *litmus paper* with *nitric acid* and filter. The filtrate yields *reaction A* characteristic of chlorides, Appendix VI.

Chloride Shake 0.3 g with 30 ml of *water* for 2 minutes and filter. 15 ml of the filtrate complies with the *limit test for chlorides*, Appendix VII, but using 2 ml of *nitric acid* in place of 1 ml of 2M *nitric acid* (350 ppm).

Related substances Carry out the test for *related substances in phenothiazines*, Appendix III A, using *mobile phase B* and applying separately to the chromatoplate 10 µl of each of three freshly prepared solutions in a mixture of 95 volumes of *methanol* and 5 volumes of *diethylamine* containing (1) 2.0% w/v of the substance being examined, (2) 0.020% w/v of *isopromethazine hydrochloride EPCRS* and (3) 0.010% w/v of the substance being examined. Any spot in the chromatogram obtained with solution (1) corresponding to isopromethazine is not more intense than the spot in the chromatogram obtained with solution (2). Any other *secondary spot* in the chromatogram obtained with solution (1) is not more intense than the spot in the chromatogram obtained with solution (3).

Loss on drying When dried to constant weight at 105°, loses not more than 0.5% of its weight. Use 1 g.

Sulphated ash Not more than 0.1%, Appendix IX A.

Assay Dissolve 1 g in 200 ml of *acetone* and carry out Method I for *non-aqueous titration*, Appendix VIII A, using 3 ml of a saturated solution of *methyl orange in acetone* as indicator. Each ml of 0.1M *perchloric acid VS* is equivalent to 0.04990 g of $C_{17}H_{20}N_2S,C_7H_7ClN_4O_2$.

Storage Promethazine Theoclate should be kept in a well-closed container and protected from light.

Preparation

Promethazine Theoclate Tablets

Action and use Histamine H_1-receptor antagonist; antiemetic.

In some countries the material described in this monograph may be known as Promethazine Teoclate.

Propanidid

Et₂N·CO·CH₂O— (MeO) —CH₂·CO₂Prⁿ

$C_{18}H_{27}NO_5$ 337.4   *1421-14-3*

Propanidid is propyl 4-diethylcarbamoyl-methoxy-3-methoxyphenylacetate. It contains not less than 98.0 per cent and not more than 101.0 per cent of $C_{18}H_{27}NO_5$.

Characteristics A pale greenish-yellow, viscous liquid; odour, slight.

Solubility Very slightly soluble in *water*; miscible with *ethanol (96%)*, with *chloroform* and with *ether*.

Identification A. The *infra-red absorption spectrum*, Appendix II A, is concordant with the *reference spectrum* of propanidid.
B. The *light absorption*, Appendix II B, in the range 230 to 350 nm of a 0.01% w/v solution in *ethanol (96%)* exhibits a maximum only at 280 nm. The *absorbance* at 280 nm is about 0.82.
C. Boil 0.05 ml with a solution of 0.2 g of *hydroxylamine hydrochloride* in 4 ml of 1M *sodium hydroxide* for 30 seconds, cool, acidify with 5 ml of 0.5M *sulphuric acid* and add 0.05 ml of a 1% w/v solution of *iron(III) chloride*. An intense red colour is produced.

Acidity Dissolve 0.5 g in 20 ml of *methanol* previously neutralised to *phenolphthalein solution* and titrate with

0.02M *sodium hydroxide VS*. Not more than 1.7 ml is required to change the colour of the solution.

Refractive index 1.515 to 1.518, Appendix V E.

Related substances Carry out the method for *thin-layer chromatography*, Appendix III A, using *silica gel G* as the coating substance and a mixture of 60 volumes of *di-isopropyl ether*, 30 volumes of *ethyl acetate* and 10 volumes of *glacial acetic acid* as the mobile phase. Apply separately to the chromatoplate 10 µl of each of two solutions of the substance being examined in *methanol* containing (1) 2.0% w/v and (2) 0.010% w/v. After removal of the plate, allow it to dry in air and heat at 135° for 30 minutes. Cool, spray lightly with a mixture of equal volumes of a 0.5% w/v solution of *potassium permanganate* and a 14% v/v solution of *sulphuric acid* and allow to stand for 15 minutes. Any *secondary spot* in the chromatogram obtained with solution (1) is not larger than the spot in the chromatogram obtained with solution (2).

Free amine Dissolve 5 g in 50 ml of *glacial acetic acid* and carry out Method I for *non-aqueous titration*, Appendix VIII A, determining the end-point potentiometrically. Not more than 2.0 ml of 0.1M *perchloric acid VS* is required.

Sulphated ash Not more than 0.1%, Appendix IX A.

Assay Boil 1 g with 50 ml of 0.1M *ethanolic potassium hydroxide VS* under a reflux condenser for 3 hours, cool, add 10 ml of *water* and titrate the excess of alkali with 0.1M *hydrochloric acid VS* using *phenolphthalein solution* as indicator. Repeat the operation without the substance being examined. The difference between the titrations represents the amount of alkali required. Each ml of 0.1M *ethanolic potassium hydroxide VS* is equivalent to 0.03374 g of $C_{18}H_{27}NO_5$.

Action and use Short-acting intravenous anaesthetic.

Propantheline Bromide

CO·OCH₂·CH₂·ṄPr^i₂
Me
Br⁻

$C_{23}H_{30}BrNO_3$ 448.4   *50-34-0*

Propantheline Bromide is di-isopropylmethyl-[2-(xanthen-9-ylcarbonyloxy)ethyl]ammonium bromide. It contains not less than 98.0 per cent and not more than 102.0 per cent of $C_{23}H_{30}BrNO_3$, calculated with reference to the dried substance.

Characteristics A white or yellowish-white powder; odourless or almost odourless; slightly hygroscopic.

Solubility Very soluble in *water*, in *ethanol (96%)* and in *chloroform*; practically insoluble in *ether*.

Identification *Test A may be omitted if tests B, C, D, E and F are carried out. Tests B, C and D may be omitted if tests A, E and F are carried out.*
A. The *infra-red absorption spectrum*, Appendix II A, is concordant with the *reference spectrum* of propantheline bromide.
B. The *light absorption*, Appendix II B, in the range 240 to 350 nm of a 0.008% w/v solution in *methanol* exhibits two

maxima, at 246 nm and 282 nm. The A(1%, 1 cm) at 246 nm is about 120 and at 282 nm is about 60.

C. Dissolve 0.2 g in 15 ml of *water*, add 1 ml of 10M *sodium hydroxide*, boil for 2 minutes, cool slightly, add 7.5 ml of 2M *hydrochloric acid*, cool and filter. The *melting point* of the residue, after washing with *water*, recrystallising from *ethanol (50%)* and drying at 100° to 105° for 1 hour, is about 215°, Appendix V A.

D. To 10 mg of the crystals obtained in test C add 5 ml of *sulphuric acid*. A bright yellow solution is produced which fluoresces strongly in ultra-violet light (365 nm).

E. Dissolve 50 mg in 0.1 ml of *water* in a 25-ml flask, add 1 ml of a saturated solution of *potassium permanganate* and assemble a micro-distillation apparatus fitted to a reflux condenser and with the outlet tube immersed in 1 ml of *water* in a test tube which is maintained at 0° in ice. Distil fairly vigorously and continue heating for 1 minute after a dry residue has been obtained in the flask. Add to the distillate 0.5 ml of a 20% v/v solution of *morpholine* and 0.5 ml of a freshly prepared 5% w/v solution of *sodium nitroprusside*, maintaining the test tube at 0° in ice. Mix, allow to stand for 5 minutes at 0° and then for 3 minutes at room temperature; no blue colour is produced in the solution or in a blank solution prepared by treating in the same manner a volume of *water* equal to the volume of the distillate. Add to the test solution 1 g of *ammonium sulphate*, mix and allow to stand for 15 minutes at room temperature; a stable, intense pink colour is produced. The blank solution, treated in the same manner, exhibits a brownish-yellow colour.

F. Yields the *reactions* characteristic of bromides, Appendix VI.

Clarity of solution A 3.0% w/v solution is *clear*, Appendix IV A.

Related substances Carry out the method for *thin-layer chromatography*, Appendix III A, using *silica gel GF254* as the coating substance and a mixture of 140 volumes of *1,2-dichloroethane*, 60 volumes of *methanol*, 2.5 volumes of *anhydrous formic acid* and 2.5 volumes of *water* as the mobile phase but allowing the solvent front to ascend 10 cm above the line of application. Apply separately to the chromatoplate 10 µl of each of two solutions of the substance being examined in *chloroform* containing (1) 1.0% w/v and (2) 0.0050% w/v. After removal of the plate, allow it to dry in air and examine under *ultra-violet light (254 nm)*. Any *secondary spot* in the chromatogram obtained with solution (1) is not more intense than the spot in the chromatogram obtained with solution (2).

Loss on drying When dried to constant weight at 100° to 105°, loses not more than 1.0% of its weight. Use 1 g.

Sulphated ash Not more than 0.1%, Appendix IX A, Method II. Use 1 g.

Assay Carry out Method I for *non-aqueous titration*, Appendix VIII A, using 0.4 g, adding 7 ml of *mercury(II) acetate solution* and using *crystal violet solution* as indicator. Each ml of 0.1M *perchloric acid VS* is equivalent to 0.04484 g of $C_{23}H_{30}BrNO_3$.

Storage Propantheline Bromide should be kept in a well-closed container.

Preparation
Propantheline Tablets

Action and use Antispasmodic.

Propranolol Hydrochloride

$$OCH_2 \cdot CH \cdot CH_2 \cdot NHPr' \quad .HCl$$

$C_{16}H_{21}NO_2,HCl$　　295.8　　*318-98-9*

Propranolol Hydrochloride is 1-isopropylamino-3-(1-naphthyloxy)propan-2-ol hydrochloride. It contains not less than 99.0 per cent and not more than 101.0 per cent of $C_{16}H_{21}NO_2,HCl$, calculated with reference to the dried substance.

Characteristics A white or almost white powder; odourless or almost odourless.

Solubility Soluble in 20 parts of *water* and in 20 parts of *ethanol (96%)*; slightly soluble in *chloroform*.

Identification A. Dissolve 0.1 g in 10 ml of *water*, make alkaline with 1M *sodium hydroxide* and extract with 10 ml of *chloroform*. Wash the extract with 5 ml of *water*, dry over *anhydrous sodium sulphate*, evaporate to dryness and dry the residue at 50° for 1 hour at a pressure of 2 kPa. The *infra-red absorption spectrum* of the residue, Appendix II A, is concordant with the *reference spectrum* of propranolol.

B. The *light absorption*, Appendix II B, in the range 230 to 350 nm of a 0.004% w/v solution in *methanol* exhibits three maxima, at 290, 306 and 319 nm. The *absorbance* at 290 nm is about 0.84, at 306 nm, about 0.50 and at 319 nm, about 0.30.

C. Dissolve 0.2 g in 6 ml of *water*, heating gently if necessary, make alkaline with 5M *sodium hydroxide* and extract with two 5-ml quantities of *ether*. Wash the combined extracts with *water* until the washings are free from alkali, dry with *anhydrous sodium sulphate*, filter and evaporate to dryness. The *melting point* of the residue, after drying at 50° at a pressure of 2 kPa for 1 hour, is about 94°, Appendix V A.

D. Yields *reaction A* characteristic of chlorides, Appendix VI.

Acidity pH of a 1% w/v solution, 5.0 to 6.0, Appendix V L.

Related substances Carry out the method for *thin-layer chromatography*, Appendix III A, using *silica gel G* as the coating substance and a mixture of 90 volumes of *toluene* and 10 volumes of *methanol* as the mobile phase. Apply separately to the chromatoplate 10 µl of each of two solutions of the substance being examined in *methanol* containing (1) 10.0% w/v and (2) 0.020% w/v. After removal of the plate, allow it to dry in air, spray with a mixture of 0.5 ml of *anisaldehyde*, 10 ml of *glacial acetic acid*, 85 ml of *methanol* and 5 ml of *sulphuric acid* and heat at 105° for 15 minutes. Any *secondary spot* in the chromatogram obtained with solution (1) is not more intense than the spot in the chromatogram obtained with solution (2).

Loss on drying When dried to constant weight at 105°, loses not more than 0.5% of its weight. Use 1 g.

Sulphated ash Not more than 0.1%, Appendix IX A.

Assay Carry out Method I for *non-aqueous titration*, Appendix VIII A, using 0.7 g and *1-naphtholbenzein* *solution* as indicator. Each ml of 0.1M *perchloric acid VS* is equivalent to 0.02958 g of $C_{16}H_{21}NO_2,HCl$.

Preparations

Propranolol Injection

Propranolol Tablets

Action and use Beta-adrenoceptor antagonist.

Propyl Gallate

$C_{10}H_{12}O_5$ 212.2   *121-79-9*

Propyl Gallate is propyl 3,4,5-trihydroxy-benzoate.

Characteristics A white to creamy-white crystalline powder; odourless or almost odourless.

Solubility Very slightly soluble in *water*; soluble in 3 parts of *ethanol (96%)* and in 3 parts of *ether*; very slightly soluble in *arachis oil*.

Identification A. The *light absorption*, Appendix II B, in the range 230 to 350 nm of a 0.002% w/v solution in *methanol* exhibits a maximum only at 275 nm. The *absorbance* at 275 nm is about 0.98.

B. Carry out the method for *gas chromatography*, Appendix III B, using a solution prepared in the following manner. Boil 0.5 g with 50 ml of 5M *sodium hydroxide* under a reflux condenser for 10 minutes and distil 5 ml.

The chromatographic procedure may be carried out using a glass column (1.5 m × 4 mm) packed with *acid-washed, silanised diatomaceous support* coated with 10% w/w of free fatty acid phase (Supelco FFAP is suitable) and maintained at 80°.

The principal peak in the chromatogram has the same retention time as that of *propan-1-ol*, examined under the same conditions.

C. Dissolve 5 mg in 50 ml of *water* and add 0.05 ml of *iron(III) chloride solution*. A bluish-black colour is produced.

Melting point 148° to 151°, Appendix V A.

Chloride Shake 1.0 g with 100 ml of *water* for 5 minutes and filter. 15 ml of the filtrate complies with the *limit test for chlorides*, Appendix VII (330 ppm).

Sulphate Shake 0.8 g with 100 ml of *water* for 5 minutes and filter. 15 ml of the filtrate complies with the *limit test for sulphates*, Appendix VII (0.12%).

Loss on drying When dried to constant weight at 105°, loses not more than 1.0% of its weight. Use 1 g.

Sulphated ash Not more than 0.1%, Appendix IX A.

Storage Propyl Gallate should be kept in a well-closed container and protected from light. Contact with metals should be avoided.

Action and use Antioxidant.

Propyl Hydroxybenzoate ☆

Propylparaben

$C_{10}H_{12}O_3$ 180.2   *94-13-3*

Propyl Hydroxybenzoate is propyl 4-hydroxy-benzoate. It contains not less than 99.0 per cent and not more than 101.0 per cent of $C_{10}H_{12}O_3$, calculated with reference to the dried substance.

Characteristics A white, crystalline powder.

Solubility Very slightly soluble in *water*; freely soluble in *ethanol (96%)*, in *methanol* and in *ether*.

Identification A. The *light absorption*, Appendix II B, in the range 230 to 280 nm of a 0.0005% w/v solution in *ethanol (96%)* exhibits a maximum only at 258 nm.

B. Dissolve 0.1 g in 2 ml of *ethanol (96%)*, boil and add 0.5 ml of *mercury—nitric acid solution*. A precipitate is produced and the supernatant liquid becomes red.

C. *Melting point*, 95° to 98°, Appendix V A, Method I.

Acidity Dissolve 0.2 g in 5 ml of *ethanol (96%)*, add 5 ml of *carbon dioxide-free water* and 0.1 ml of *bromocresol green solution*. Not more than 0.1 ml of 0.1M *sodium hydroxide VS* is required to change the colour of the solution.

Clarity and colour of solution Dissolve 1.0 g in 10 ml of *ethanol (96%)*. The solution is *clear*, Appendix IV A, and not more intensely coloured than *reference solution BY₆*, Appendix IV B, Method II.

Loss on drying When dried over *phosphorus pentoxide* at 80° at a pressure of 1.5 to 2.5 kPa for 2 hours, loses not more than 0.5% of its weight. Use 1 g.

Sulphated ash Not more than 0.1%, Appendix IX A, Method II. Use 1 g.

Assay To 80 mg add 25 ml of 2M *sodium hydroxide* and boil gently under a reflux condenser for 30 minutes. Cool, add 25 ml of 0.0333M *potassium bromate VS*, 5 ml of a 12.5% w/v solution of *potassium bromide* and 40 ml of *glacial acetic acid*, cool in ice, add 10 ml of *hydrochloric acid*, immediately stopper the flask and allow to stand for 15 minutes. Add 15 ml of 1M *potassium iodide*, mix and titrate the liberated iodine with 0.1M *sodium thiosulphate VS* using 2 ml of *starch solution*, added towards the end of the titration, as indicator. Repeat the operation without the substance being examined. The difference between the titrations represents the amount of potassium bromate required. The volume of 0.0333M *potassium bromate VS* is equivalent to half of the volume of 0.1M *sodium thiosulphate VS* required for the titration. Each ml of 0.0333M *potassium bromate VS* is equivalent to 0.006007 g of $C_{10}H_{12}O_3$.

Action and use Antimicrobial preservative.

The title of the monograph in the European Pharmacopœia is Propyl Parahydroxybenzoate.

Propylene Glycol ☆

OH
|
CH₃·CH·CH₂OH

$C_3H_8O_2$ 76.10   *57-55-6*

Propylene Glycol is propane-1,2-diol.

Characteristics A clear, colourless, viscous liquid; hygroscopic.

Solubility Miscible with *water*, with *ethanol (96%)* and with *chloroform*.

Identification A. Dissolve 0.5 ml in 5 ml of *pyridine* and add 2 g of finely ground *4-nitrobenzoyl chloride*. Boil for 1 minute and pour into 15 ml of *water* with shaking. Filter, wash the precipitate with 20 ml of a saturated solution of *sodium hydrogen carbonate* and then with *water* and dry. Recrystallise from boiling *ethanol (80%)*, filtering while hot. The *melting point* of the crystals, after drying at 100° to 105°, is 123° to 128°, Appendix V A, Method I.
B. *Boiling point*, 184° to 189°, Appendix V D.
C. Complies with the test for Refractive index.
D. Complies with the test for Relative density.

Acidity Mix 10 ml with 40 ml of *water* and add 0.1 ml of *bromothymol blue solution*. The solution is greenish-yellow and not more than 0.05 ml of 0.1M *sodium hydroxide VS* is required to change the colour to blue.

Clarity and colour *Clear*, Appendix IV A, and *colourless*, Appendix IV B, Method II.

Refractive index 1.431 to 1.433, Appendix V E.

Relative density 1.035 to 1.040, Appendix V G.

Heavy metals Mix 3.0 ml with 12 ml of *water*. 12 ml of the resulting solution complies with *limit test A for heavy metals*, Appendix VII (5 ppm). Use *lead standard solution (1 ppm Pb)* to prepare the standard.

Oxidising substances To 10 ml add 5 ml of *water*, 2 ml of 1M *potassium iodide* and 2 ml of 1M *sulphuric acid* and allow to stand in a stoppered vessel protected from light for 15 minutes. Titrate the liberated iodine with 0.05M *sodium thiosulphate VS* using 1 ml of *starch solution* as indicator. Not more than 0.2 ml of 0.05M *sodium thiosulphate VS* is required.

Reducing substances Mix 1 ml with 1 ml of 6M *ammonia* and heat in a water-bath at 60° for 5 minutes. Remove from the water-bath; the solution is not yellow. Immediately add 0.15 ml of 0.1M *silver nitrate*; the solution does not change its appearance within 5 minutes.

Sulphated ash Heat 50 g until it ignites and allow to burn. Cool, moisten the residue with *sulphuric acid* and ignite; repeat the operations. The residue weighs not more than 5 mg (0.01%).

Water Not more than 0.2%, Appendix IX C. Use 5 g.

Storage Propylene Glycol should be kept in an airtight container.

Propyliodone

O=⟨ring⟩N—CH₂·CO₂Prⁿ

$C_{10}H_{11}I_2NO_3$ 447.0   *587-61-1*

Propyliodone is propyl 3,5-di-iodo-4-oxo-pyridin-1-ylacetate. It contains not less than 99.0 per cent and not more than 101.0 per cent of $C_{10}H_{11}I_2NO_3$, calculated with reference to the dried substance.

Characteristics A white or almost white, crystalline powder; odourless or almost odourless.

Solubility Practically insoluble in *water*; slightly soluble in *ethanol (96%)* and in *chloroform*; very slightly soluble in *ether*.

Identification A. The *light absorption*, Appendix II B, in the range 230 to 350 nm of a 0.002% w/v solution in *absolute ethanol* exhibits two maxima, at 239 nm and 281 nm. The *absorbance* at 239 nm is about 0.64 and at 281 nm, about 0.52.
B. Boil 1 g with 10 ml of 1M *sodium hydroxide* under a reflux condenser for 30 minutes, add 10 ml of *water* and acidify to *litmus paper* with *hydrochloric acid*. The *melting point* of the precipitate, after washing with *water* and drying, is about 245°, Appendix V A.
C. Heat 50 mg with *sulphuric acid*. Violet vapours of iodine are evolved.

Acidity Dissolve 1 g in 40 ml of hot *propan-1-ol* previously neutralised to *phenolphthalein solution*, cool and allow to stand in ice for 15 minutes, shaking frequently. Filter, wash the residue with the neutralised propan-1-ol and titrate the combined filtrate and washings with 0.05M *sodium hydroxide VS*, using *phenolphthalein solution* as indicator, until the pink colour persists for 15 seconds. Not more than 0.15 ml of 0.05M *sodium hydroxide VS* is required.

Melting point 187° to 190°, Appendix V A.

Inorganic iodide Shake 2.4 g with 30 ml of *water* for 15 minutes and filter. To 10 ml of the filtrate add 1 ml of 2M *nitric acid*, 1 ml of a 0.2% w/v solution of *sodium nitrite* and 1 ml of *chloroform*, shake and centrifuge. Any purple colour in the chloroform layer is not more intense than that obtained when a mixture of 2 ml of *iodide standard solution (20 ppm I)* and 8 ml of *water* is treated in the same manner.

Loss on drying When dried to constant weight at 105°, loses not more than 0.5% of its weight. Use 1 g.

Sulphated ash Not more than 0.1%, Appendix IX A.

Assay Carry out the method for *oxygen-flask combustion for iodine*, Appendix VIII C, using 15 mg. Each ml of 0.02M *sodium thiosulphate VS* is equivalent to 0.7450 mg of $C_{10}H_{11}I_2NO_3$.

Storage Propyliodone should be protected from light.

Preparations
Propyliodone Suspension
Propyliodone Oily Suspension

Action and use Radio-opaque substance used in investigation of fistulae and sinuses and in bronchography.

Propylthiouracil ☆

C₇H₁₀N₂OS   170.2   51-52-5

Propylthiouracil is 2,3-dihydro-6-propyl-2-thioxopyrimidin-4(1*H*)-one. It contains not less than 98.0 per cent and not more than 100.5 per cent of C₇H₁₀N₂OS, calculated with reference to the dried substance.

Characteristics White or practically white crystals or crystalline powder.

Solubility Very slightly soluble in *water* and in *ether*; sparingly soluble in *ethanol (96%)*. It dissolves in aqueous solutions of alkali hydroxides.

Identification *Test A may be omitted if tests B, C and D are carried out. Tests B and C may be omitted if tests A and D are carried out.*

A. The *infra-red absorption spectrum*, Appendix II A, is concordant with the spectrum of *propylthiouracil EPCRS*. Examine as dispersions of 1 mg in 0.3 g of *potassium bromide IR*.

B. Examine the chromatograms obtained in the test for Thiourea and related substances under ultra-violet light (254 nm) before exposure of the plate to iodine vapour. The principal spot in the chromatogram obtained with solution (2) is similar in position and size to that in the chromatogram obtained with solution (3).

C. To 20 mg add 8 ml of *bromine water* and shake for a few minutes. Boil until the mixture is decolorised, allow to cool and filter. Add 2 ml of a 6.1% w/v solution of *barium chloride*; a white precipitate is produced. Add 5 ml of 2M *sodium hydroxide*; the precipitate does not become violet.

D. *Melting point*, 217° to 221°, Appendix V A, Method I.

Heavy metals Dissolve 1.0 g in the minimum quantity of 6M *ammonia* and dilute to 20 ml with *water*. 12 ml of the resulting solution complies with *limit test A for heavy metals*, Appendix VII (20 ppm). Use *lead standard solution (1 ppm Pb)* to prepare the standard.

Thiourea and related substances Carry out the method for *thin-layer chromatography*, Appendix III A, using *silica gel GF254* as the coating substance and a mixture of 100 volumes of *chloroform*, 12 volumes of *propan-2-ol* and 0.2 volumes of *glacial acetic acid* as the mobile phase. Apply separately to the chromatoplate 10 μl of each of five solutions in *methanol* containing (1) 1.0% w/v of the substance being examined, (2) 0.10% w/v of the substance being examined, (3) 0.10% w/v of *propylthiouracil EPCRS*, (4) 0.00050% w/v of *thiourea* and (5) 0.010% w/v of the substance being examined. After removal of the plate, allow it to dry in air and examine under *ultra-violet light (254 nm)*. Expose the plate to iodine vapour for 10 minutes. Any spot corresponding to thiourea in the chromatogram obtained with solution (1) is not more intense than the spot in the chromatogram obtained with solution (4) and any other *secondary spot* is not more intense than the spot in the chromatogram obtained with solution (5).

Loss on drying When dried to constant weight at 100° to 105°, loses not more than 0.5% of its weight. Use 1 g.

Sulphated ash Not more than 0.1%, Appendix IX A, Method II. Use 1 g.

Assay To 0.3 g add 30 ml of *water* and 30 ml (n₁ ml) of 0.1M *sodium hydroxide VS*, boil and shake until solution is complete. Add 50 ml of 0.1M *silver nitrate* with stirring, boil gently for 5 minutes, cool and titrate with 0.1M *sodium hydroxide VS* determining the end-point potentiometrically (n₂ ml). Record the total volume (n₁ + n₂ ml) of 0.1M *sodium hydroxide VS* added. Each ml of 0.1M *sodium hydroxide VS* is equivalent to 0.008511 g of C₇H₁₀N₂OS.

Storage Propylthiouracil should be kept in a well-closed container and protected from light.

Preparation
Propylthiouracil Tablets

Action and use Antithyroid.

Protamine Sulphate

Protamine Sulphate is a mixture of the sulphates of basic peptides prepared from sperm or mature testes of fish, usually species of Salmonidae and Clupeidae. It binds with heparin in solution, inhibiting its anticoagulant activity; in the conditions described under the Assay this binding produces a precipitate. One milligram of Protamine Sulphate precipitates not less than 100 Units of *heparin sodium EPBRP★* calculated with reference to the dried substance. It is prepared in conditions designed to minimise microbial contamination.

Characteristics A white or almost white powder; hygroscopic.

Solubility Sparingly soluble in *water*; practically insoluble in *ethanol (96%)*, in *chloroform* and in *ether*.

Identification A. Produces a precipitate under the conditions of the Assay.

B. *Specific optical rotation*, in a 1% w/v solution in 0.1M *hydrochloric acid*, −65° to −85°, Appendix V F.

C. Dissolve 0.20 g in *water* and dilute to 10 ml with the same solvent (solution A). To 0.5 ml of solution A add 4.5 ml of *water*, 1.0 ml of a 10% w/v solution of *sodium hydroxide* and 1.0 ml of a 0.02% w/v solution of *1-naphthol* and mix. Cool to 5° and add 0.5 ml of *alkaline sodium hypobromite solution*. An intense red colour is produced.

D. Heat 2 ml of solution A in a water-bath at 60° and add 0.1 ml of *mercury(II) sulphate solution*; no precipitate is produced. Cool the mixture in ice; a precipitate is produced.

E. Yields *reaction A* characteristic of sulphates, Appendix VI.

Clarity and colour of solution To 2.5 ml of solution A add 7.5 ml of *water*. The resulting solution is not more opalescent than *reference suspension II*, Appendix IV A, and not more intensely coloured than *reference solution BY₆* or *Y₆*, Appendix IV B, Method II.

Light absorption Dilute 2.5 ml of solution A to 5.0 ml with *water*. The *absorbance* of the resulting solution at 260 to 280 nm is not more than 0.5, Appendix II B.

Heavy metals 1.0 g complies with *limit test D for heavy metals*, Appendix VII (20 ppm). Use 2 ml of *lead standard solution (10 ppm Pb)* to prepare the standard.

Iron Dissolve 1.0 g in *water* with the aid of heat and dilute to 10 ml with the same solvent. The resulting solution complies with the *limit test for iron*, Appendix VII (10 ppm).

Mercury Not more than 10 ppm of Hg when determined by the following method. Add 20 ml of a mixture of equal volumes of *nitric acid* and *sulphuric acid* to 2 g in a 250-ml flask fitted with a ground-glass stopper, boil under a reflux condenser for 1 hour, cool and carefully dilute with *water*. Boil until nitrous fumes are no longer evolved. Cool, carefully dilute the solution to 200 ml with *water*, mix and filter. Transfer 50 ml of the filtrate to a separating funnel. Shake with successive small quantities of *chloroform* until the chloroform layer remains colourless. To the aqueous layer add 25 ml of 1M *sulphuric acid*, 115 ml of *water* and 10 ml of a 20% w/v solution of *hydroxylamine hydrochloride*. Titrate with *dithizone solution VS*; after each addition, shake the mixture 20 times and towards the end of the titration allow to separate and discard the chloroform layer. Titrate until a bluish-green colour is produced. Calculate the content of mercury using the equivalent of mercury in µg per ml of titrant determined in the standardisation of the dithizone solution.

Nitrogen 21.0 to 26.0%, calculated with reference to the dried substance, when determined by Method IV, Appendix VIII H. Use 10 mg and heat for 3 to 4 hours.

Sulphate 16 to 24% when determined by the following method. Dissolve 0.15 g in 15 ml of *water* in a beaker, add 5 ml of 2M *hydrochloric acid* and heat to boiling. Slowly add to the boiling solution 10 ml of *barium chloride solution*. Cover and heat on a water-bath for 1 hour. Filter and wash the precipitate several times with small quantities of hot *water*. Dry and ignite the residue to constant weight at 600°. Each g of the residue is equivalent to 0.4117 g of sulphate, SO_4.

Loss on drying When dried at 100° to 105° for 3 hours, loses not more than 5.0% of its weight. Use 1 g.

Assay Carry out the *assay of protamine sulphate*, Appendix XIV D4.

Storage Protamine Sulphate should be kept in an airtight container.

If the material is intended for use in the manufacture of a parenteral dosage form, the container should be sterile, tamper-evident and sealed so as to exclude micro-organisms.

Labelling The label states (1) the date after which the material is not intended to be used; (2) the conditions under which it should be stored; (3) whether or not it is intended for use in the manufacture of a parenteral dosage form.

Preparation
Protamine Sulphate Injection

Protamine Sulphate intended for use in the manufacture of a parenteral dosage form complies with the following additional requirements.

Abnormal toxicity Complies with the *test for abnormal toxicity*, Appendix XIV L. Use 0.5 mg dissolved in 0.5 ml of *water for injections*.

Pyrogens Complies with the *test for pyrogens*, Appendix XIV K. Use per kg of the rabbit's weight 1 ml of a solution containing 10 mg per ml.

*This requirement refers to batch no. 1 of *heparin sodium EPBRP* since the potency of protamine sulphate determined by the Assay depends on the potency and average molecular weight of the heparin used.

Prothionamide

$C_9H_{12}N_2S$ 180.3   *14222-60-7*

Prothionamide is 2-propylpyridine-4-carbo-thioamide. It contains not less than 99.0 per cent and not more than 101.0 per cent of $C_9H_{12}N_2S$, calculated with reference to the dried substance.

Characteristics Yellow crystals or crystalline powder; odourless or almost odourless.

Solubility Practically insoluble in *water*; soluble in 30 parts of *ethanol (96%)* and in 16 parts of *methanol*; slightly soluble in *chloroform* and in *ether*.

Identification A. The *infra-red absorption spectrum*, Appendix II A, is concordant with the *reference spectrum* of prothionamide.
B. The *light absorption*, Appendix II B, in the range 230 to 350 nm of a 0.002% w/v solution in *ethanol (96%)* exhibits a maximum only at 291 nm. The *absorbance* at 291 nm is about 0.78.
C. Heat 0.1 g with 5 ml of 1M *hydrochloric acid*. A gas is evolved which turns *lead acetate paper* black.

Acidity Dissolve 2 g in 20 ml of warm *methanol*, add 20 ml of *water*, cool, shake until crystallisation occurs and titrate with 0.1M *sodium hydroxide VS* using *cresol red solution* as indicator. Not more than 0.2 ml is required to change the colour of the solution.

Melting point 140° to 143°, Appendix V A.

Heavy metals Dissolve the residue obtained in the test for Sulphated ash in 1 ml of 2M *hydrochloric acid* and dilute to 20 ml with *water*. 12 ml of the resulting solution complies with *limit test A for heavy metals*, Appendix VII (20 ppm). Use *lead standard solution (1 ppm Pb)* to prepare the standard.

Related substances Carry out in subdued light the method for *thin-layer chromatography*, Appendix III A, using *silica gel GF254* as the coating substance and a mixture of 90 volumes of *chloroform* and 10 volumes of *methanol* as the mobile phase. Apply separately to the chromatoplate 5 µl of each of two solutions of the substance being examined in *methanol* containing (1) 5.0% w/v and (2) 0.025% w/v. After removal of the plate, allow it to dry in air and examine under *ultra-violet light (254 nm)*. Any *secondary spot* in the chromatogram obtained with solution (1) is not more intense than the spot in the chromatogram obtained with solution (2).

Loss on drying When dried to constant weight at 105°, loses not more than 0.5% of its weight. Use 1 g.

Sulphated ash Not more than 0.1%, Appendix IX A, Method II. Use 1.0 g.

Assay Carry out Method I for *non-aqueous titration*, Appendix VIII A, using 0.45 g and *crystal violet solution* as indicator. Each ml of 0.1M *perchloric acid VS* is equivalent to 0.01803 g of $C_9H_{12}N_2S$.

Storage Prothionamide should be protected from light.

Preparation

Prothionamide Tablets

Action and use Antituberculous.

In some countries the material described in this monograph may be known as Protionamide.

Protriptyline Hydrochloride

$C_{19}H_{21}N,HCl$ 299.8   *1225-55-4*

Protriptyline Hydrochloride is 3-(5*H*-dibenzo-[*a,d*]cyclohept-5-yl)propyl(methyl)amine hydrochloride. It contains not less than 99.0 per cent and not more than 101.0 per cent of $C_{19}H_{21}N,HCl$, calculated with reference to the dried substance.

Characteristics A white to yellowish-white powder; odourless or almost odourless.

Solubility Soluble in 2 parts of *water*, in 4.5 parts of *ethanol (96%)* and in 3 parts of *chloroform*; practically insoluble in *ether*.

Identification A. Dissolve 0.1 g in 10 ml of *water*, make alkaline with 1M *sodium hydroxide*, extract with 5 ml of *chloroform*, dry with *anhydrous sodium sulphate* and evaporate the solvent using a current of nitrogen. The *infra-red absorption spectrum* of the oily residue, Appendix II A, is concordant with the *reference spectrum* of protriptyline.

B. The *light absorption*, Appendix II B, in the range 230 to 350 nm of a 0.002% w/v solution in a mixture of 1 volume of 1M *hydrochloric acid* and 9 volumes of *methanol* exhibits a maximum only at 292 nm. The *absorbance* at 292 nm is about 0.93.

C. Dissolve 50 mg in 3 ml of *water* and add 0.05 ml of a 2.5% w/v solution of *quinhydrone* in *methanol*. A red colour is produced slowly.

D. Yields *reaction A* characteristic of chlorides, Appendix VI.

E. *Melting point*, about 168°, Appendix V A.

Acidity pH of a 1% w/v solution, 5.0 to 6.5, Appendix V L.

Loss on drying When dried to constant weight at 60° at a pressure not exceeding 0.7 kPa, loses not more than 0.5% of its weight. Use 1 g.

Sulphated ash Not more than 0.1%, Appendix IX A.

Assay Carry out Method I for *non-aqueous titration*, Appendix VIII A, using 0.7 g and *crystal violet solution* as indicator. Each ml of 0.1M *perchloric acid VS* is equivalent to 0.02998 g of $C_{19}H_{21}N,HCl$.

Storage Protriptyline Hydrochloride should be kept in a well-closed container.

Preparation

Protriptyline Tablets

Action and use Antidepressant.

Proxymetacaine Hydrochloride

$C_{16}H_{26}N_2O_3,HCl$ 330.9   *5875-06-9*

Proxymetacaine Hydrochloride is 2-diethyl-aminoethyl 3-amino-4-propoxybenzoate hydrochloride. It contains not less than 98.0 per cent and not more than 102.0 per cent of $C_{16}H_{26}N_2O_3,HCl$, calculated with reference to the dried substance.

Characteristics A white or almost white, crystalline powder; odourless or almost odourless.

Solubility Soluble in *water* and in *chloroform*; very soluble in *absolute ethanol*; practically insoluble in *ether*.

Identification A. The *infra-red absorption spectrum*, Appendix II A, is concordant with the *reference spectrum* of proxymetacaine hydrochloride.

B. The *light absorption*, Appendix II B, in the range 220 to 350 nm, of a 0.0020% w/v solution exhibits three maxima, at 231, 268 and 310 nm. The *absorbance* at 268 nm is about 0.58 and at 310 nm is about 0.32.

C. A 5% w/v solution yields the *reaction* characteristic of primary aromatic amines and the *reactions* characteristic of chlorides, Appendix VI.

Acidity pH of a 1% w/v solution, 5.7 to 6.4, Appendix V L.

Related substances A. Carry out the method for *thin-layer chromatography*, Appendix III A, using *silica gel GF254* as the coating substance and a mixture of 75 volumes of *toluene*, 30 volumes of *ethyl acetate* and 5 volumes of *diethylamine* as the mobile phase. Apply separately to the chromatoplate 10 µl of each of three solutions of the substance being examined in *methanol* containing (1) 2.0% w/v, (2) 0.020% w/v and (3) 0.010% w/v. After removal of the plate, heat it at 105° for 10 minutes, allow to cool and examine under *ultra-violet light (254 nm)*. Any *secondary spot* in the chromatogram obtained with solution (1) is not more intense than the spot in the chromatogram obtained with solution (2) and not more than one such spot is more intense than the spot in the chromatogram obtained with solution (3). Disregard any spot remaining on the line of application.

B. Carry out the method for *thin-layer chromatography*, Appendix III A, using *silica gel GF254* as the coating substance and a mixture of 80 volumes of *1,4-dioxan*, 20 volumes of *cyclohexane* and 4 volumes of *glacial acetic acid* as the mobile phase. Apply separately to the chromatoplate 10 µl of each of two solutions in *methanol* containing (1) 2.0% w/v of the substance being examined and (2) 0.0050% w/v of *3-amino-4-propoxybenzoic acid BPCRS*. After removal of the plate, allow it to dry in air and examine under *ultra-violet light (254 nm)*. Any *secondary spot* in the chromatogram obtained with solution (1) is not more intense than the spot in the chromatogram obtained with solution (2). The principal spot remains on the line of application.

Loss on drying When dried at 105° for 3 hours, loses not more than 0.5% of its weight. Use 1 g.

Sulphated ash Not more than 0.15%, Appendix IX A.

Assay Carry out Method I for *non-aqueous titration*, Appendix VIII A, using 0.25 g, 20 ml of *mercury(II) acetate solution* and *1-naphtholbenzein solution* as indicator. Each ml of 0.1M *perchloric acid VS* is equivalent to 0.01654 g of $C_{16}H_{26}N_2O_3,HCl$.

Storage Proxymetacaine Hydrochloride should be kept in a well-closed container and protected from light.

Preparation
Proxymetacaine Eye Drops

Action and use Local anaesthetic.

Proxyphylline ☆

$C_{10}H_{14}N_4O_3$ 238.2   *603-00-9*

Proxyphylline is 1,3-dimethyl-7-(2-hydroxy-propyl)purine-2,6(3H,1H)-dione. It contains not less than 98.5 per cent and not more than 101.0 per cent of $C_{10}H_{14}N_4O_3$, calculated with reference to the dried substance.

Characteristics A white, crystalline powder.

Solubility Very soluble in water; soluble in *ethanol (96%)*; freely soluble in *chloroform*; slightly soluble in *ether*.

Identification *Test A may be omitted if tests B, C and D are carried out. Tests C and D may be omitted if tests A and B are carried out.*
A. The *infra-red absorption spectrum*, Appendix II A, is concordant with the spectrum of *proxyphylline EPCRS*. Examine as dispersions of 0.5 to 1 mg in 0.3 g of *potassium bromide*.
B. Dissolve 1 g in 5 ml of *acetic anhydride* and boil under a reflux condenser for 15 minutes. Allow to cool, add 100 ml of a mixture of 4 volumes of *petroleum spirit (boiling range, 50° to 70°)* and 1 volume of *ether* and cool in ice for not less than 20 minutes with occasional shaking. Filter, wash the precipitate with the same solvent mixture and recrystallise from *ethanol (96%)*. The *melting point* of the crystals, after drying over *phosphorus pentoxide* at a pressure of 1.5 to 2.5 kPa, is 87° to 92°, Appendix V A, Method I.
C. Yields the *reaction* characteristic of xanthines, Appendix VI.
D. *Melting point*, 134° to 136°, Appendix V A, Method I.

Acidity or alkalinity To 10 ml of a 5.0% w/v solution in *carbon dioxide-free water* (solution A) add 0.25 ml of

bromothymol blue solution. The solution is yellow or green and not more than 0.4 ml of 0.01M *sodium hydroxide VS* is required to change the colour to blue.

Clarity and colour of solution Solution A is *clear*, Appendix IV A, and *colourless*, Appendix IV B, Method II.

Heavy metals 12 ml of solution A complies with *limit test A for heavy metals*, Appendix VII (20 ppm). Use *lead standard solution (1 ppm Pb)* to prepare the standard.

Chloride Dilute 2.5 ml of solution A to 15 ml with *water*. The solution complies with the *limit test for chlorides*, Appendix VII (400 ppm).

Related substances Carry out the method for *thin-layer chromatography*, Appendix III A, using *silica gel HF254* as the coating substance and a mixture of 90 volumes of *chloroform*, 10 volumes of *absolute ethanol* and 1 volume of 13.5M *ammonia* as the mobile phase. Apply separately to the chromatoplate 10 µl of each of the following freshly prepared solutions. For solution (1) dissolve 0.3 g of the substance being examined in sufficient *methanol (60%)* to produce 10 ml. For solution (2) dilute 1 volume of solution (1) to 100 volumes with *methanol*. For solution (3) dilute 1 volume of solution (1) to 500 volumes with *methanol*. For solution (4) dissolve 10 mg of *theophylline* in *methanol*, add 0.3 ml of solution (1) and dilute to 10 ml with *methanol*. After removal of the plate, allow it to dry in air and examine under *ultra-violet light (254 nm)*. Any *secondary spot* in the chromatogram obtained with solution (1) is not more intense than the spot in the chromatogram obtained with solution (2) and not more than one such spot is more intense than the spot in the chromatogram obtained with solution (3). The test is not valid unless the chromatogram obtained with solution (4) shows two clearly separated principal spots.

Loss on drying When dried to constant weight at 100° to 105°, loses not more than 0.5% of its weight. Use 1 g.

Sulphated ash Not more than 0.1%, Appendix IX A, Method II. Use 1 g.

Assay Dissolve 0.2 g in 3 ml of *anhydrous formic acid*, add 50 ml of *acetic anhydride* and carry out Method I for *non-aqueous titration*, Appendix VIII A, determining the end-point potentiometrically. Each ml of 0.1M *perchloric acid VS* is equivalent to 0.02382 g of $C_{10}H_{14}N_4O_3$.

Storage Proxyphylline should be kept in a well-closed container and protected from light.

Action and use Xanthine bronchodilator.

Pseudoephedrine Hydrochloride

$C_{10}H_{15}NO,HCl$ 201.7   *345-78-8*

Pseudoephedrine Hydrochloride is (1S,2R)-2-methylamino-1-phenylpropan-1-ol hydrochloride. It contains not less than 99.0 per cent and not more than 101.0 per cent of $C_{10}H_{15}NO$, HCl, calculated with reference to the dried substance.

Characteristics A white, crystalline powder; odourless or almost odourless.

Solubility Soluble in 1.6 parts of *water*, in 4 parts of *ethanol (96%)* and in 60 parts of *chloroform*.

Identification A. The *infra-red absorption spectrum*, Appendix II A, is concordant with the *reference spectrum* of pseudoephedrine hydrochloride.

B. The *light absorption*, Appendix II B, in the range 230 to 350 nm of a 0.05% w/v solution exhibits three maxima, at 251, 257 and 263 nm. The *absorbance* at 251 nm is about 0.75, at 257 nm, about 0.98 and at 263 nm, about 0.78.

C. A 5% w/v solution yields *reaction A* characteristic of chlorides, Appendix VI.

Acidity or alkalinity Dissolve 0.2 g in 10 ml of freshly boiled and cooled *water* and titrate with 0.02M *sodium hydroxide VS* or 0.02M *hydrochloric acid VS* using *methyl red solution* as indicator. Not more than 0.1 ml of 0.02M *sodium hydroxide VS* or 0.02M *hydrochloric acid VS* is required to change the colour of the solution.

Clarity and colour of solution A 5.0% w/v solution is not more than very faintly opalescent and is colourless.

Melting point 183° to 186°, Appendix V A.

Specific optical rotation In a 5% w/v solution, using a 2-dm tube, +61.0° to +62.5°, Appendix V F.

Related substances Carry out the method for *thin-layer chromatography*, Appendix III A, using a silica gel precoated chromatoplate (Merck silica gel 60 plates are suitable) and a mixture of 40 volumes of *butyl acetate*, 20 volumes of *acetone*, 20 volumes of *butan-1-ol*, 10 volumes of 5M *ammonia* and 10 volumes of *methanol* as the mobile phase. Apply separately to the plate 10 µl of each of two solutions of the substance being examined in *ethanol (96%)* containing (1) 10% w/v and (2) 0.10% w/v. After removal of the plate, allow it to dry in a current of warm air, spray with a solution containing 0.3 g of *ninhydrin* in a mixture of 100 ml of *butan-1-ol* and 3 ml of *glacial acetic acid* and heat at 120° for 20 minutes. Any *secondary spot* in the chromatogram obtained with solution (1) is not more intense than the spot in the chromatogram obtained with solution (2). Disregard any yellow spot near the line of application.

Loss on drying When dried to constant weight at 105°, loses not more than 0.5% of its weight. Use 1 g.

Sulphated ash Not more than 0.1%, Appendix IX A.

Assay Carry out Method I for *non-aqueous titration*, Appendix VIII A, using 0.5 g and *1-naphtholbenzein solution* as indicator. Each ml of 0.1M *perchloric acid VS* is equivalent to 0.02017 g of $C_{10}H_{15}NO,HCl$.

Action and use Sympathomimetic.

Pyrazinamide

$C_5H_5N_3O$ 123.1   *98-96-4*

Pyrazinamide is pyrazine-2-carboxamide. It contains not less than 99.0 per cent and not more than 100.5 per cent of $C_5H_5N_3O$, calculated with reference to the anhydrous substance.

Characteristics A white or almost white, crystalline powder; odourless or almost odourless.

Solubility Soluble in 70 parts of *water* and in 70 parts of *chloroform*; slightly soluble in *ethanol (96%)*; very slightly soluble in *ether*.

Identification A. Dissolve a sufficient quantity in the minimum volume of *ethanol (96%)* and evaporate to dryness. The *infra-red absorption spectrum* of the residue, Appendix II A, is concordant with the *reference spectrum* of pyrazinamide.

B. The *light absorption*, Appendix II B, in the range 230 to 350 nm of a 0.002% w/v solution exhibits two maxima, at 268 nm and 310 nm. The *absorbance* at 268 nm is about 1.3 and at 310 nm, about 0.11.

C. Boil 20 mg with 5 ml of 5M *sodium hydroxide*. Ammonia, recognisable by its odour, is evolved.

Melting point 188° to 191°, Appendix V A.

Heavy metals Ignite gently 2.0 g until thoroughly charred, cool, add 2 ml of *nitric acid* and 0.25 ml of *sulphuric acid*, heat cautiously until white fumes are evolved and ignite until the residue is free of carbon. Cool, add 2 ml of *hydrochloric acid* evaporate to dryness on a water-bath and dissolve the residue in 20 ml of *water*. 12 ml of the resulting solution complies with *limit test A for heavy metals*, Appendix VII (20 ppm). Use *lead standard solution (2 ppm Pb)* to prepare the standard.

Related substances Carry out the method for *thin-layer chromatography*, Appendix III A, using *silica gel GF254* as the coating substance and a mixture of 60 volumes of *butan-1-ol*, 20 volumes of *glacial acetic acid* and 20 volumes of *water* as the mobile phase but allowing the solvent front to ascend 10 cm above the line of application. Apply separately to the chromatoplate 20 µl of each of two solutions of the substance being examined in a mixture of 9 volumes of *chloroform* and 1 volume of *methanol* containing (1) 1.0% w/v and (2) 0.0020% w/v. After removal of the plate, allow it to dry in air and examine immediately under *ultra-violet light (254 nm)*. Any *secondary spot* in the chromatogram obtained with solution (1) is not more intense than the spot in the chromatogram obtained with solution (2).

Sulphated ash Not more than 0.1%, Appendix IX A.

Water Not more than 0.5% w/w, Appendix IX C. Use 5 g.

Assay Gently boil 0.3 g with 200 ml of *water* and 75 ml of 5M *sodium hydroxide* for 20 minutes in an ammonia-distillation apparatus, collecting any distillate in 50 ml of 0.05M *sulphuric acid VS*. Boil vigorously to complete the distillation of the ammonia and titrate the excess of acid with 0.1M *sodium hydroxide VS* using *methyl red solution* as indicator. Repeat the operation without the substance being examined. The difference between the titrations represents the amount of acid required to neutralise the ammonia formed. Each ml of 0.05M *sulphuric acid VS* is equivalent to 0.01231 g of $C_5H_5N_3O$.

Storage Pyrazinamide should be kept in a well-closed container.

Preparation
Pyrazinamide Tablets

Action and use Antituberculous.

Pyridostigmine Bromide

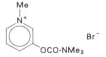

C₉H₁₃BrN₂O₂   261.1   *101-26-8*

Pyridostigmine Bromide is 3-dimethyl-carbamoyloxy-1-methylpyridinium bromide. It contains not less than 98.5 per cent and not more than 101.0 per cent of $C_9H_{13}BrN_2O_2$, calculated with reference to the dried substance.

Characteristics A white or almost white, crystalline powder; odour, agreeable, characteristic; deliquescent.

Solubility Soluble in less than 1 part of *water*, in less than 1 part of *ethanol (96%)* and in 1 part of *chloroform*; practically insoluble in *ether*.

Identification A. The *infra-red absorption spectrum*, Appendix II A, is concordant with the *reference spectrum* of pyridostigmine bromide.
B. The *light absorption*, Appendix II B, in the range 230 to 350 nm of a 0.005% w/v solution exhibits a maximum only at 270 nm. The *absorbance* at 270 nm is about 0.92.
C. Yields the *reactions* characteristic of bromides, Appendix VI.

Acidity Dissolve 0.2 g in 20 ml of *carbon dioxide-free water*. Not more than 0.2 ml of 0.02M *sodium hydroxide VS* (carbonate-free) is required to bring the pH to 7.0.

Melting point 153° to 156°, Appendix V A.

Light absorption Dissolve 50 mg in a mixture of 2 ml of *phosphate buffer pH 7.0* and 8 ml of *water*. The *absorbance* of the resulting solution at 320 nm is not more than 1.0, Appendix II B.

Related substances Carry out the method for *thin-layer chromatography*, Appendix III A, using *silica gel G* as the coating substance and a mixture of 67 volumes of *water*, 30 volumes of *methanol* and 3 volumes of *diethylamine* as the mobile phase. Apply separately to the chromatoplate 10 μl of each of two solutions of the substance being examined in *water* containing (1) 2.0% w/v and (2) 0.010% w/v. After removal of the plate, dry it in a current of warm air, spray with *diazotised nitroaniline solution* and then with 0.1M *sodium hydroxide*. Dry the plate in a current of warm air and spray with *dilute potassium iodobismuthate solution*. Any *secondary spot* in the chromatogram obtained with solution (1) is not more intense than the spot in the chromatogram obtained with solution (2).

Loss on drying When dried to constant weight at 105°, loses not more than 2.0% of its weight. Use 1 g.

Sulphated ash Not more than 0.1%, Appendix IX A.

Assay Carry out Method I for *non-aqueous titration*, Appendix VIII A, using 0.85 g, adding 20 ml of *mercury(II) acetate solution* and using *quinaldine red solution* as indicator. Each ml of 0.1M *perchloric acid VS* is equivalent to 0.02611 g of C₉H₁₃BrN₂O₂.

Storage Pyridostigmine Bromide should be kept in a well-closed container and protected from light.

Preparations
Pyridostigmine Injection
Pyridostigmine Tablets
Action and use Anticholinesterase.

Pyridoxine Hydrochloride ☆
Vitamin B₆

C₈H₁₁NO₃,HCl   205.6   *58-56-0*

Pyridoxine Hydrochloride is 5-hydroxy-6-methylpyridine-3,4-dimethanol hydrochloride. It contains not less than 99.0 per cent and not more than 101.0 per cent of $C_8H_{11}NO_3,HCl$, calculated with reference to the dried substance.

Characteristics A white or almost white, crystalline powder; odourless or almost odourless. It melts at about 205°, with decomposition.

Solubility Soluble in 5 parts of *water* and in 100 parts of *ethanol (96%)*; practically insoluble in *chloroform* and in *ether*.

Identification *Test A may be omitted if tests B, C and D are carried out. Tests B and C may be omitted if tests A and D are carried out.*
A. The *infra-red absorption spectrum*, Appendix II A, is concordant with the spectrum of *pyridoxine hydrochloride EPCRS*.
B. The *light absorption*, Appendix II B, in the range 250 to 350 nm of a 0.001% w/v solution in 0.1M *hydrochloric acid* exhibits a maximum at 288 to 296 nm. The A(1%, 1 cm) at the maximum is 425 to 445. The *light absorption* in the range 220 to 350 nm of a solution prepared by diluting 1 ml of a 0.1% w/v solution in 0.1M *hydrochloric acid* to 100 ml with *0.025M standard phosphate buffer* exhibits two maxima, at 248 to 256 nm and at 320 to 327 nm. The A(1%, 1 cm) at 248 to 256 nm is 175 to 195 and at 320 to 327 nm is 345 to 365.
C. In the test for Related substances the principal spot in the chromatogram obtained with solution (2) is similar in colour, size and position to that in the chromatogram obtained with solution (4).
D. A 5% w/v solution yields *reaction A* characteristic of chlorides, Appendix VI.

Acidity pH of a 5% w/v solution, 2.4 to 3.0, Appendix V L.

Clarity and colour of solution A 5.0% w/v solution is *clear*, Appendix IV A, and not more intensely coloured than *reference solution Y₇*, Appendix IV B, Method II.

Heavy metals 12 ml of a 5.0% w/v solution complies with *limit test A for heavy metals*, Appendix VII (20 ppm). Use *lead standard solution (1 ppm Pb)* to prepare the standard.

Related substances Carry out the method for *thin-layer chromatography*, Appendix III A, using *silica gel G* as the coating substance and a mixture of 65 volumes of *acetone*, 13 volumes of *carbon tetrachloride*, 13 volumes of *tetrahydrofuran* and 9 volumes of 13.5M *ammonia* as the mobile phase, but carrying out the chromatography in an unlined tank. Apply separately to the chromatoplate 2 µl of each of four solutions in *water* containing (1) 10% w/v of the substance being examined, (2) 1.0% w/v of the substance being examined, (3) 0.025% w/v of the substance being examined and (4) 1.0% w/v of *pyridoxine hydrochloride EPCRS*. After removal of the plate, allow it to dry in air and spray with a 5% w/v solution of *sodium carbonate* in a mixture of 70 volumes of *water* and 30 volumes of *ethanol (96%)*. Dry it in a current of air, spray with a 0.1% w/v solution of *dichloroquinonechloroimine* in *ethanol (96%)* and examine immediately. Any *secondary spot* in the chromatogram obtained with solution (1) is not more intense than the spot in the chromatogram obtained with solution (3). Disregard any spots remaining on the line of application.

Loss on drying When dried to constant weight at 100° to 105°, loses not more than 0.5% of its weight. Use 1 g.

Sulphated ash Not more than 0.1%, Appendix IX A, Method II. Use 1 g.

Assay Dissolve 0.15 g in a mixture of 5 ml of *anhydrous glacial acetic acid* and 6 ml of *mercury(II) acetate solution*. Carry out Method I for *non-aqueous titration*, Appendix VIII A, using 0.05 ml of *crystal violet solution* as indicator, until a green colour is produced. Each ml of 0.1M *perchloric acid VS* is equivalent to 0.02056 g of $C_8H_{11}NO_3,HCl$.

Storage Pyridoxine Hydrochloride should be protected from light.

Preparation
Pyridoxine Tablets

Action and use Used in treatment of sideroblastic anaemias.

Pyrimethamine ☆

$C_{12}H_{13}ClN_4$ 248.7   *58-14-0*

Pyrimethamine is 5-(4-chlorophenyl)-6-ethylpyrimidine-2,4-diyldiamine. It contains not less than 99.0 per cent and not more than 101.0 per cent of $C_{12}H_{13}ClN_4$, calculated with reference to the dried substance.

Characteristics Colourless crystals or an almost white, crystalline powder; odourless.

Solubility Practically insoluble in *water*; slightly soluble in *ethanol (96%)* and in *chloroform*; very slightly soluble in *ether*.

Identification *Test A may be omitted if tests B, C and D are carried out. Tests B, C and D may be omitted if test A is carried out.*
A. The *infra-red absorption spectrum*, Appendix II A, is concordant with the spectrum of *pyrimethamine EPCRS*.
B. Dissolve 0.14 g in sufficient *absolute ethanol* to produce 100 ml, dilute 10 ml of the solution to 100 ml with 0.1M *hydrochloric acid* and dilute 10 ml of this solution to

100 ml with the same solvent. The *light absorption* of the resulting solution, Appendix II B, in the range 250 to 300 nm exhibits a maximum at 272 nm and a minimum at 261 nm. The A(1%, 1 cm) at 272 nm is 310 to 330.
C. In the test for Related substances, the principal spot in the chromatogram obtained with solution (2) is similar in position and size to that in the chromatogram obtained with solution (3).
D. *Melting point*, 239° to 243°, Appendix V A, Method I.

Acidity or alkalinity Shake 1.0 g with 50 ml of *water* for 2 minutes and filter (solution A). To 10 ml add 0.05 ml of *phenolphthalein solution*; the solution is colourless and not more than 0.2 ml of 0.01M *sodium hydroxide VS* is required to change the colour to pink. Add 0.4 ml of 0.01M *hydrochloric acid VS* and 0.05 ml of *methyl red solution*; the solution is red or orange.

Clarity and colour of solution Dissolve 0.25 g in sufficient of a mixture of 3 volumes of *dichloromethane* and 1 volume of *methanol* to produce 10 ml. The resulting solution, examined immediately, is *clear*, Appendix IV A, and not more intensely coloured than *reference solution BY_6*, Appendix IV B, Method II.

Sulphate Solution A complies with the *limit test for sulphates*, Appendix VII (80 ppm). Use a mixture of 2.5 ml of *sulphate standard solution (10 ppm SO₄)* and 12.5 ml of *water* to prepare the standard.

Related substances Carry out the method for *thin-layer chromatography*, Appendix III A, using *silica gel GF254* as the coating substance and a mixture of 76 volumes of *toluene*, 12 volumes of *glacial acetic acid*, 8 volumes of *propan-1-ol* and 4 volumes of *chloroform* as the mobile phase, but allowing the solvent front to ascend 10 cm above the line of application. Apply separately to the chromatoplate 20 µl of each of four freshly prepared solutions in a mixture of 9 volumes of *chloroform* and 1 volume of *methanol* containing (1) 1.0% w/v of the substance being examined, (2) 0.1% w/v of the substance being examined, (3) 0.1% w/v of *pyrimethamine EPCRS* and (4) 0.0025% w/v of the substance being examined. After removal of the plate, allow it to dry in air and examine under *ultra-violet light (254 nm)*. Any *secondary spot* in the chromatogram obtained with solution (1) is not more intense than the spot in the chromatogram obtained with solution (4).

Loss on drying When dried for 4 hours at 100° to 105°, loses not more than 0.5% of its weight. Use 0.5 g.

Sulphated ash Not more than 0.1%, Appendix IX A, Method II. Use 1 g.

Assay Dissolve 0.2 g in 25 ml of *anhydrous glacial acetic acid*, heating gently, cool and carry out Method I for *non-aqueous titration*, Appendix VIII A, determining the end-point potentiometrically. Each ml of 0.1M *perchloric acid VS* is equivalent to 0.02487 g of $C_{12}H_{13}ClN_4$.

Storage Pyrimethamine should be protected from light.

Preparation
Pyrimethamine Tablets

Action and use Antimalarial.

Pyroxylin
Cellulose Nitrate

Pyroxylin is a nitrated cellulose obtained by the action of a mixture of nitric and sulphuric acids on wood pulp or cotton linters that have been freed from fatty matter. It must be damped with not less than 25 per cent by weight of Isopropyl Alcohol or of Industrial Methylated Spirit.

CAUTION Compliance is required with the provisions of relevant legislation relating to the storage of, use of and containers used for Pyroxylin.

In the following tests, particular care should be exercised when drying pyroxylin. The material so obtained is explosive and sensitive to ignition by impact or friction and it should be handled as carefully as possible.

Characteristics White or almost white, cuboid granules or fibrous material, the latter resembling absorbent cotton but harsher to the touch and more powdery. Both the granules and the fibrous material appear moist and smell strongly of the damping fluid. Highly flammable.

Solubility Soluble in *glacial acetic acid* and in *acetone*.

Identification Add *water* to a solution in *acetone*. A white, viscid mass is readily precipitated.

Clarity and colour of solution Dissolves at 20° in a mixture of 1 volume of *ethanol (90%)* and 3 volumes of *ether* to produce an almost clear and colourless to pale straw-coloured solution.

Kinematic viscosity 1160 to 2900 mm^2 s^{-1}, Appendix V H, Method III, when determined in a solution prepared in the following manner. To 20 g, previously dried to constant weight by heating on a water-bath at 80° and allowing to cool in a desiccator over silica gel, add 200 ml of a mixture of 19 volumes of *acetone* and 1 volume of *water*. Shake vigorously to prevent the formation of aggregates of partly-solvated pyroxylin and rotate suitably to obtain a homogeneous solution. The viscosity of the solution should be measured within 48 hours.

Nitrogen 11.7 to 12.2%, calculated with reference to the material dried to constant weight by heating on a water-bath at 80° and allowing to cool in a desiccator over silica gel, when determined by the following method. Transfer 0.4 g of the dried substance to a 750-ml round-bottomed flask using 60 ml of *water*, add 20 ml of *hydrogen peroxide solution (20 vol)* and then add slowly, with shaking, 50 ml of a 30% w/w solution of *potassium hydroxide* and 5 ml of *ethanol (96%)*. Agitate slowly for 3 hours or until the substance being examined has dissolved. Add 3 g of *Devarda's alloy* and immediately connect the flask to the spray trap of an ammonia-distillation apparatus, the receiver of which contains 50 ml of 0.1M *hydrochloric acid VS* and 0.15 ml of *methyl red solution*. Allow the reaction to proceed until no further evolution of gas occurs and then heat the contents of the flask to boiling and distil carefully until 30 ml remains in the round-bottomed flask. Rinse the delivery tube into the receiver with *water* and titrate the combined distillate and rinsings with 0.1M *sodium hydroxide VS*. Repeat the operation without the substance being examined. The difference between the titrations represents the amount of acid required to neutralise the ammonia formed. Each ml of 0.1M *hydrochloric acid VS* is equivalent to 0.001401 g of nitrogen.

Storage Pyroxylin should be kept in a well-closed container, loosely packed, protected from light and stored at a temperature not exceeding 15°, remote from fire. The container should be suitably designed to disrupt should the internal pressure reach or exceed 1400 kPa. The amount of damping fluid must not be allowed to fall below 25% w/w; should this happen, the material should be either rewetted or used immediately for the preparation of Collodion.

Preparation
Flexible Collodion

Quillaia
Quillaia Bark

Quillaia is the dried inner part of the bark of *Quillaja saponaria* Molina and of other species of *Quillaja*.

Characteristics Odourless or almost odourless; dust strongly sternutatory.

Macroscopical Pieces flat, up to about 1 metre long, 10 to 20 cm broad and 3 to 10 mm, usually 6 mm, thick. Outer surface brownish-white or pale reddish-brown, longitudinally striated or coarsely reticulated, with occasional blackish-brown patches of adherent outer bark; inner surface yellowish-white, smooth and very hard; fracture splintery and laminated, the broken surface showing numerous large prisms of calcium oxalate as glistening points. Smoothed transversely cut surface appearing chequered, with delicate radial lines representing medullary rays and tangential lines formed by alternating tangential bands of fibrous and non-fibrous phloem.

Microscopical Outer bark, when present, consisting of reddish-brown cork cells alternating with bands of brown parenchyma containing numerous groups of phloem fibres and large prisms of calcium oxalate. Inner bark consisting of alternating bands of tortuous fibres, irregularly enlarged at intervals, about 500 to 1000 μm long and 20 to 50 μm wide and of sieve tissue mixed with parenchyma. Medullary rays mostly three to four, but sometimes up to six cells wide, with occasional pitted, subrectangular sclereids adjacent to the bundles of phloem fibres. Starch granules 5 to 20 μm, usually about 10 μm, in diameter and prisms of calcium oxalate usually 50 to 170 μm long and up to 30 μm wide present in the parenchymatous cells.

Extractive soluble in ethanol (45%) Not less than 22.0%, Appendix XI B.

Acid-insoluble ash Not more than 1.0%, Appendix XI K.

Foreign matter Not more than 2.0%, Appendix XI D.

Preparation
Quillaia Liquid Extract

Action and use Emulsifying agent.

Powdered Quillaia

Powdered Quillaia is Quillaia in powder.

Characteristics Pale buff with a pink tinge. Diagnostic structures: bundles of phloem fibres with unevenly thickened walls; occasional sclereids; calcium oxalate prisms, often in fragments; starch granules and cork cells in small amounts. When shaken with water a copious, persistent froth is produced.

Extractive soluble in ethanol (45%) Not less than 22.0%, Appendix XI B.

Acid-insoluble ash Not more than 1.0%, Appendix XI K.

Preparation
Quillaia Liquid Extract

Action and use Emulsifying agent.

Quinalbarbitone Sodium ☆

Secobarbitone Sodium

$C_{12}H_{17}N_2NaO_3$ 260.3   *309-43-3*

Quinalbarbitone Sodium is sodium 5-allyl-5-(1-methylbutyl)barbiturate. It contains not less than 98.5 per cent and not more than 102.0 per cent of $C_{12}H_{17}N_2NaO_3$, calculated with reference to the dried substance.

Characteristics A white powder; odourless; hygroscopic.

Solubility Soluble in 3 parts of *water*, leaving a small insoluble residue, and in 5 parts of *ethanol (96%)*; practically insoluble in *chloroform* and in *ether*.

Identification *Test A may be omitted if tests B, C, D and E are carried out. Tests B and D may be omitted if tests A, C and E are carried out.*

A. To 10 ml of a 10% w/v solution in *ethanol (50%)* add 90 ml of *water* and 5 ml of 2M *acetic acid*, stir vigorously, add 200 ml of *water* and boil until the precipitate dissolves and no oily particles remain on the surface of the liquid. Allow to cool until a haziness begins to appear in the solution, induce crystallisation if necessary and allow the solution to stand for at least 12 hours. Wash the crystals with three 10-ml quantities of *water* and dry the residue at 80°. The *infra-red absorption spectrum* of the residue, Appendix II A, is concordant with the spectrum obtained using the residue similarly prepared from 0.1 g of *secobarbital sodium EPCRS*.

B. Complies with the test for *identification of barbiturates*, Appendix III A.

C. Determine the *melting point*, Appendix V A, Method I, of the residue obtained in test A. Mix equal parts of the residue with the residue obtained from *secobarbital sodium EPCRS* and determine the melting point of the mixture. The difference between the melting points, which are about 96°, is not greater than 2°.

D. Yields the *reaction* characteristic of non-nitrogen substituted barbiturates, Appendix VI.

E. Yields *reaction A* characteristic of sodium salts, Appendix VI.

Alkalinity pH of a 10% w/v solution, not more than 11, Appendix V L.

Clarity and colour of solution A freshly prepared 10.0% w/v solution in *ethanol (50%)* is *clear*, Appendix IV A, and not more intensely coloured than *reference solution* Y_7, Appendix IV B, Method II.

Related substances Complies with the test for *related substances in barbiturates*, Appendix III A.

Loss on drying When dried to constant weight at 100° to 105°, loses not more than 3.0% of its weight. Use 0.5 g.

Assay Dissolve 0.25 g in 5 ml of *absolute ethanol*, add 10 ml of *silver nitrate—pyridine reagent* and titrate with 0.1M *ethanolic sodium hydroxide VS*, using 0.5 ml of *thymolphthalein solution* as indicator, until a pure blue colour is obtained. Repeat the operation without the substance being examined. The difference between the titrations represents the amount of sodium hydroxide required. Each ml of 0.1M *ethanolic sodium hydroxide VS* is equivalent to 0.02603 g of $C_{12}H_{17}N_2NaO_3$.

Storage Quinalbarbitone Sodium should be kept in an airtight container.

Action and use Hypnotic.

The title of the monograph in the European Pharmacopœia is Secobarbital Sodium.

Quinidine Bisulphate

$C_{20}H_{24}N_2O_2,H_2SO_4$ 422.5   *747-45-5*

Quinidine Bisulphate is (8*R*,9*S*)-6'-methoxy-cinchonan-9-ol hydrogen sulphate. It contains not less than 98.5 per cent and not more than 101.5 per cent of alkaloid hydrogen sulphates, calculated as $C_{20}H_{24}N_2O_2,H_2SO_4$ with reference to the anhydrous substance.

Characteristics Colourless crystals; odourless or almost odourless.

Solubility Soluble in 8 parts of *water* and in 3 parts of *ethanol (96%)*; practically insoluble in *ether*.

Identification A. To 5 ml of a 0.5% w/v solution add 0.1M *sodium hydroxide* dropwise until the solution becomes turbid and then add 0.05 ml of 0.05M *sulphuric acid* to produce a clear solution (solution A). To 2 ml of solution A add 0.15 ml of *bromine water* and 1 ml of 5M *ammonia*. An emerald-green colour is produced.

B. To 2 ml of solution A add 1 ml of *silver nitrate solution*. A white precipitate is produced.

C. Yields the *reactions* characteristic of sulphates, Appendix VI.

Acidity pH of a 1% w/v solution, 2.6 to 3.6, Appendix V L.

Specific optical rotation In a 2% w/v solution in 0.1M *hydrochloric acid*, +246° to +258°, Appendix V F, determined using a 2-dm layer.

Dihydroquinidine bisulphate Not more than 15.0%, calculated with reference to the anhydrous substance, when determined by the following method. Dissolve 0.2 g in 20 ml of *water* and add 0.5 g of *potassium bromide* and 15 ml of 2M *hydrochloric acid*. Titrate slowly with 0.0167M *potassium bromate VS*, using *methyl red solution* as indicator, until a yellow colour is produced. Add a solution of 0.5 g of *potassium iodide* in 200 ml of *water* and stopper the flask immediately. Allow to stand in the dark for 5 minutes and titrate with 0.1M *sodium thiosulphate VS* using *starch solution*, added towards the end of the titration, as indicator. Repeat the operation without the substance being examined. Each ml of 0.0167M *potassium bromate VS* is equivalent to 0.02113 g of $C_{20}H_{24}N_2O_2$, H_2SO_4. Calculate the content of dihydroquinidine bisulphate by subtracting the result from the assay result.

Other cinchona alkaloids Carry out the method for *thin-layer chromatography*, Appendix III A, using *silica gel G* as the coating substance and a mixture of 60 volumes of *toluene*, 36 volumes of *ether* and 15 volumes of *diethylamine* as the mobile phase. Apply separately to the chromato-plate 4 μl of each of four solutions in *methanol* containing (1) 1.0% w/v of the substance being examined, (2) 0.025% w/v of *quinine*, (3) 0.025% w/v of *cinchonine* and (4) 1.0% w/v of *quinidine sulphate* and 0.025% w/v of *cinchonine*. After removal of the plate, allow it to dry in air for 15 minutes and repeat the development. Dry the plate at 105° for 30 minutes, allow to cool and spray with *iodoplatinate reagent*. Any *secondary spot* in the chromatogram obtained with solution (1) is not more intense than the spots in the chromatograms obtained with solutions (2) and (3). The test is not valid unless the chromatogram obtained with solution (4) shows two clearly separated principal spots.

Sulphated ash Not more than 0.1%, Appendix IX A.

Water Not more than 5.0% w/w, Appendix IX C. Use 1 g.

Titratable cation 75.3 to 79.6%, calculated with reference to the anhydrous substance, when determined by the following method. To the combined aqueous solutions reserved in the Assay add 0.1 ml of *phenolphthalein solution* and titrate with 0.1M *hydrochloric acid VS*. Each ml of 0.1M *sodium hydroxide VS* is equivalent to 0.01632 g of $[C_{20}H_{26}N_2O_2]^{2+}$.

Assay Dissolve 0.45 g in 15 ml of *water*, add 25 ml of 0.1M *sodium hydroxide VS* and extract with three 25-ml quantities of *chloroform*. Wash the combined chloroform extracts with 20 ml of *water*, combine the aqueous solutions and reserve for the test for Titratable cation. Dry the chloroform extracts with *anhydrous sodium sulphate*, evaporate to dryness at a pressure of 2 kPa and dissolve the residue in 50 ml of *anhydrous glacial acetic acid*. Carry out Method I for *non-aqueous titration*, Appendix VIII A, using *crystal violet solution* as indicator. Each ml of 0.1M *perchloric acid VS* is equivalent to 0.02113 g of $C_{20}H_{24}N_2O_2$,H_2SO_4.

Storage Quinidine Bisulphate should be kept in a well-closed container and protected from light.

Action and use Anti-arrhythmic.

Quinidine Sulphate ☆

$(C_{20}H_{24}N_2O_2)_2,H_2SO_4,2H_2O$ 783.0   6591-63-5

Quinidine Sulphate is (8*R*,9*S*)-6'-methoxy-cinchonan-9-ol sulphate dihydrate. It contains not less than 99.0 per cent and not more than 101.0 per cent of alkaloid monosulphates, calculated as $(C_{20}H_{24}N_2O_2)_2,H_2SO_4$ with reference to the dried substance.

Characteristics A white or almost white, crystalline powder or silky, colourless needles; odourless.

Solubility Slightly soluble in *water*; soluble in boiling *water*, in *ethanol (96%)* and in *chloroform*; practically insoluble in *acetone* and in *ether*.

Identification A. In the test for Other cinchona alkaloids the principal spot in the chromatogram obtained with solution (1) corresponds in position, colour and size to that in the chromatogram obtained with solution (5).
B. Dissolve 5 mg in 5 ml of *water*, add 0.2 ml of *bromine water* and 1 ml of 2M *ammonia*. An emerald-green colour is produced.
C. Dissolve 0.1 g in 3 ml of 1M *sulphuric acid* and dilute to 100 ml with *water*. An intense blue fluorescence is produced which disappears almost completely on the addition of 1 ml of *hydrochloric acid*.
D. Dissolve 50 mg in 5 ml of hot *water*, cool, add 1 ml of *silver nitrate solution* and stir with a glass rod. After a few minutes a white precipitate is produced which is soluble in 2M *nitric acid*.
E. Yields *reaction A* characteristic of sulphates, Appendix VI.

Acidity pH of a 1% w/v solution, 6.0 to 6.8, Appendix V L.

Clarity and colour of solution A 2.00% w/v solution in 0.1M *hydrochloric acid* is *clear*, Appendix IV A, and not more intensely coloured than *reference solution GY_6*, Appendix IV B, Method II.

Specific optical rotation In a 2% w/v solution in 0.1M *hydrochloric acid*, +275° to +290°, Appendix V F.

Dihydroquinidine sulphate Not more than 15.0%, calculated with reference to the dried substance, when determined by the following method. Dissolve 0.2 g in 20 ml of *water* and add 0.5 g of *potassium bromide* and 15 ml of 2M *hydrochloric acid*. Titrate slowly with 0.0167M *potassium bromate VS*, using *methyl red solution* as indicator, until a yellow colour is produced. Add a solution of 0.5 g of *potassium iodide* in 200 ml of *water* and stopper the flask immediately. Allow to stand in the dark for 5 minutes and titrate with 0.1M *sodium thiosulphate VS* using 5 ml of *starch solution*, added towards the end of the titration, as indicator. Repeat the operation without the substance being examined. Each ml of 0.0167M *potassium bromate VS* is equivalent to 0.01867 g of $(C_{20}H_{24}N_2O_2)_2$, H_2SO_4. Calculate the content of dihydroquinidine sulphate by subtracting the result from the assay result.

Other cinchona alkaloids Carry out the method for *thin-layer chromatography*, Appendix III A, using *silica gel G* as the coating substance and a mixture of 60 volumes of *toluene*, 36 volumes of *ether* and 15 volumes of *diethylamine* as the mobile phase. Apply separately to the chromato-plate 4 µl of each of five solutions in *methanol* containing (1) 1.0% w/v of the substance being examined, (2) 0.025% w/v of *quinine*, (3) 0.025% w/v of *cinchonine*, (4) 1.0% w/v of *quinidine sulphate EPCRS* and 0.025% w/v of *cinchonine* and (5) 1.0% w/v of *quinidine sulphate EPCRS*. After removal of the plate, allow it to dry in a current of air for 15 minutes and repeat the development. Dry the plate at 105° for 30 minutes, allow to cool and spray with *iodoplatinate reagent*. Any *secondary spot* in the chromato-gram obtained with solution (1) is not more intense than the spots in the chromatograms obtained with solutions (2) and (3). Disregard any spot in the chromato-gram obtained with solution (1) corresponding to the spot with an Rf value slightly lower than that of the principal spot in the chromatogram obtained with solution (5). The test is not valid unless the chromatogram obtained with solution (4) shows two clearly separated spots.

Loss on drying When dried to constant weight at 130°, loses 3.0 to 5.0% of its weight. Use 1 g.

Sulphated ash Not more than 0.1%, Appendix IX A, Method II. Use 1 g.

Assay Dissolve 0.3 g in a mixture of 10 ml of *chloroform* and 20 ml of *acetic anhydride* and carry out Method I for *non-aqueous titration*, Appendix VIII A, determining the end-point potentiometrically. Each ml of 0.1M *perchloric acid VS* is equivalent to 0.02490 g of $(C_{20}H_{24}N_2O_2)_2,H_2SO_4$.

Storage Quinidine Sulphate should be kept in a well-closed container and protected from light.

Preparation

Quinidine Sulphate Tablets

Action and use Anti-arrhythmic.

Quinine Bisulphate

$C_{20}H_{24}N_2O_2,H_2SO_4,7H_2O$ 548.6   *549-56-4*

Quinine Bisulphate is (8*S*,9*R*)-6′-methoxy-cinchonan-9-ol hydrogen sulphate heptahydrate. It contains not less than 98.5 per cent and not more than 101.5 per cent of alkaloid hydrogen sulphates, calculated as $C_{20}H_{24}N_2O_2,H_2SO_4$ with reference to the anhydrous substance.

Characteristics Colourless crystals or a white, crystalline powder; odourless or almost odourless; efflorescent in dry air.

Solubility Soluble in 8 parts of *water* and in 50 parts of *ethanol* (96%).

Identification A. To 5 ml of a 0.5% w/v solution add 0.1M *sodium hydroxide* dropwise until the solution becomes turbid and then add 0.05 ml of 0.05M *sulphuric acid* to produce a clear solution (solution A). To 2 ml of solution A add 0.15 ml of *bromine water* and 1 ml of 5M *ammonia*. An emerald-green colour is produced.

B. To 2 ml of solution A add *silver nitrate solution*. No white precipitate is produced.

C. A solution has a blue fluorescence.

D. Yields the *reactions* characteristic of sulphates, Appendix VI.

Acidity pH of a 1% w/v solution, 2.8 to 3.4, Appendix V L.

Specific optical rotation In a 3% w/v solution in 0.1M *hydrochloric acid*, −208° to −216°, Appendix V F.

Dihydroquinine bisulphate Not more than 10.0%, calculated with reference to the anhydrous substance, when determined by the following method. Dissolve 0.2 g in 20 ml of *water* and add 0.5 g of *potassium bromide* and 15 ml of 2M *hydrochloric acid*. Titrate slowly with 0.0167M *potassium bromate VS*, using *methyl red solution* as indicator, until a yellow colour is produced. Add a solution of 0.5 g of *potassium iodide* in 200 ml of *water* and stopper the flask immediately. Allow to stand in the dark for 5 minutes and titrate with 0.1M *sodium thiosulphate VS* using *starch solution*, added towards the end of the titration, as indicator. Repeat the operation without the substance being examined. Each ml of 0.0167M *potassium bromate VS* is equivalent to 0.02113 g of $C_{20}H_{24}N_2O_2$, H_2SO_4. Calculate the content of dihydroquinine bisulphate by subtracting the result from the assay result.

Other cinchona alkaloids Carry out the method for *thin-layer chromatography*, Appendix III A, using *silica gel G* as the coating substance and a mixture of 60 volumes of *toluene*, 36 volumes of *ether* and 15 volumes of *diethylamine* as the mobile phase. Apply separately to the chromato-plate 4 µl of each of three solutions in *methanol* containing (1) 1.0% w/v of the substance being examined, (2) 0.025% w/v of *cinchonidine* and (3) 1.0% w/v of *quinine sulphate* and 0.025% w/v of *cinchonidine*. After removal of the plate, allow it to dry in air for 15 minutes and repeat the development. Dry the plate at 105° for 30 minutes, allow it to cool and spray with *iodoplatinate reagent*. Any *secondary spot* in the chromatogram obtained with solution (1) is not more intense than the spot in the chromatogram obtained with solution (2). The test is not valid unless the chromatogram obtained with solution (3) shows two clearly separated spots.

Sulphated ash Not more than 0.1%, Appendix IX A.

Water 19.0 to 25.0% w/w, Appendix IX C. Use 0.2 g.

Titratable cation 75.3 to 79.6%, calculated with reference to the anhydrous substance, when determined by the following method. Add to the combined aqueous solutions reserved in the Assay 0.1 ml of *phenolphthalein solution* and titrate with 0.1M *hydrochloric acid VS*. Each ml of 0.1M *sodium hydroxide VS* is equivalent to 0.01632 g of $[C_{20}H_{26}N_2O_2]^{2+}$.

Assay Dissolve 0.45 g in 15 ml of *water*. Add 25 ml of 0.1M *sodium hydroxide VS* and extract with three 25-ml quantities of *chloroform*. Wash the combined chloroform extracts with 20 ml of *water*, combine the aqueous solutions and reserve for the test for Titratable cation. Dry the chloroform extracts with *anhydrous sodium sulphate*, evaporate to dryness at a pressure of 2 kPa and dissolve the residue in 50 ml of *anhydrous glacial acetic acid*. Carry out Method I for *non-aqueous titration*, Appendix VIII A, using *crystal violet solution* as indicator. Each ml of 0.1M *perchloric acid VS* is equivalent to 0.02113 g of $C_{20}H_{24}N_2O_2,H_2SO_4$.

Storage Quinine Bisulphate should be kept in a well-closed container and protected from light.

Preparation

Quinine Bisulphate Tablets

Action and use Antimalarial.

Quinine Dihydrochloride

$C_{20}H_{24}N_2O_2,2HCl$ 397.3   60-93-5

Quinine Dihydrochloride is (8S,9R)-6'-methoxycinchonan-9-ol dihydrochloride. It contains not less than 99.0 per cent and not more than 101.0 per cent of alkaloid dihydrochlorides, calculated as $C_{20}H_{24}N_2O_2,2HCl$, with reference to the dried substance.

Characteristics A white or almost white powder; odourless or almost odourless.

Solubility Soluble in 0.5 part of *water* and in 14 parts of *ethanol (96%)*.

Identification A. To 5 ml of a 0.5% w/v solution add 0.1M *sodium hydroxide* dropwise until the solution becomes turbid and then add 0.05 ml of 0.05M *sulphuric acid* to produce a clear solution (solution A). To 2 ml of solution A add 0.15 ml of *bromine water* and 1 ml of 5M *ammonia*. An emerald-green colour is produced.
B. To 2 ml of solution A and 1 ml of *silver nitrate solution*. No white precipitate is produced.
C. To a 0.5% w/v solution add an equal volume of 1M *sulphuric acid*. An intense blue fluorescence is produced.
D. Yields *reaction A* characteristic of chlorides, Appendix VI.

Acidity pH of a 3% w/v solution, 2.0 to 3.0, Appendix V L.

Specific optical rotation In a 3% w/v solution in 0.1M *hydrochloric acid*, −223° to −229°, Appendix V F.

Barium To 15 ml of a 2.0% w/v solution add 1 ml of 1M *sulphuric acid*. The solution remains clear for at least 15 minutes.

Sulphate 0.125 g complies with the *limit test for sulphates*, Appendix VII (0.12%).

Dihydroquinine dihydrochloride Not more than 10.0%, calculated with reference to the dried substance, when determined by the following method. Dissolve 0.2 g in 20 ml of *water* and add 0.5 g of *potassium bromide* and 15 ml of 2M *hydrochloric acid*. Titrate slowly with 0.0167M *potassium bromate VS*, using *methyl red solution* as indicator, until a yellow colour is produced. Add a solution of 0.5 g of *potassium iodide* in 200 ml of *water* and stopper the flask immediately. Allow to stand in the dark for 5 minutes and titrate with 0.1M *sodium thiosulphate VS* using *starch solution*, added towards the end of the titration, as indicator. Repeat the operation without the substance being examined. Each ml of 0.0167M *potassium bromate VS* is equivalent to 0.01987 g of $C_{20}H_{24}N_2O_2$, 2HCl. Calculate the content of dihydroquinine dihydrochloride by subtracting the result from the assay result.

Other cinchona alkaloids Carry out the method for *thin-layer chromatography*, Appendix III A, using *silica gel G* as the coating substance and a mixture of 60 volumes of *toluene*, 36 volumes of *ether* and 15 volumes of *diethylamine* as the mobile phase. Apply separately to the chromatoplate 4 µl of each of three solutions in *methanol* containing (1) 1.0% w/v of the substance being examined, (2) 0.025% w/v of *cinchonidine* and (3) 1.0% w/v of *quinine sulphate* and 0.025% w/v of *cinchonidine*. After removal of the plate, allow it to dry in air for 15 minutes and repeat the development. Dry the plate at 105° for 30 minutes, allow it to cool and spray with *iodoplatinate reagent*. Any *secondary spot* in the chromatogram obtained with solution (1) is not more intense than the spot in the chromatogram obtained with solution (2). The test is not valid unless the chromatogram obtained with solution (3) shows two clearly separated spots.

Loss on drying When dried to constant weight at 105°, loses not more than 3.0% of its weight. Use 1 g.

Sulphated ash Not more than 0.1%, Appendix IX A.

Titratable cation 79.7 to 84.2%, calculated with reference to the dried substance, when determined by the following method. Dissolve 0.4 g in 10 ml of *water*, add 40 ml of *methanol* and titrate with 0.1M *sodium hydroxide VS* using *phenolphthalein solution* as indicator. Each ml of 0.1M *sodium hydroxide VS* is equivalent to 0.01632 g of $[C_{20}H_{26}N_2O_2]^{2+}$.

Assay Dissolve 0.3 g in a mixture of 50 ml of *anhydrous glacial acetic acid* and 20 ml of *acetic anhydride*, add 10 ml of *mercury(II) acetate solution* and carry out Method I for *non-aqueous titration*, Appendix VIII A, using *crystal violet solution* as indicator. Each ml of 0.1M *perchloric acid VS* is equivalent to 0.01987 g of $C_{20}H_{24}N_2O_2,2HCl$.

Storage Quinine Dihydrochloride should be kept in a well-closed container and protected from light.

Action and use Antimalarial.

Quinine Hydrochloride ☆

$C_{20}H_{24}N_2O_2,HCl,2H_2O$ 396.9   6119-47-7

Quinine Hydrochloride is (8S,9R)-6'-methoxy-cinchonan-9-ol hydrochloride dihydrate. It contains not less than 99.0 per cent and not more than 101.0 per cent of alkaloid hydrochlorides, calculated as $C_{20}H_{24}N_2O_2,HCl$, with reference to the dried substance.

Characteristics Fine, colourless, silky needles often grouped in clusters.

Solubility Soluble in 23 parts of *water*; freely soluble in *ethanol (96%)* and in *chloroform*; very slightly soluble in *ether*. The solution in *chloroform* may not be clear owing to the formation of droplets of water.

Identification A. In the test for Other cinchona alkaloids, the principal spot in the chromatogram obtained with solution (1) corresponds in position, colour and size to that in the chromatogram obtained with solution (4).
B. Dissolve 10 mg in sufficient *water* to produce 10 ml and to 5 ml of the solution add 0.2 ml of *bromine water* and then 1 ml of 2M *ammonia*. An emerald-green colour is produced.
C. Dissolve 0.1 g in 3 ml of 1M *sulphuric acid* and dilute to 100 ml with *water*. An intense blue fluorescence is

produced which disappears almost completely on the addition of 1 ml of *hydrochloric acid*.

D. Yields the *reactions* characteristic of chlorides, Appendix VI.

Acidity pH of a 1% w/v solution, 6.0 to 6.8, Appendix V L.

Clarity and colour of solution A 2.0% w/v solution in *carbon dioxide-free water* is *clear*, Appendix IV A, and not more intensely coloured than *reference solution* Y_6, Appendix IV B, Method II.

Specific optical rotation In a 2% solution in 0.1M *hydrochloric acid*, $-245°$ to $-258°$, Appendix V F.

Barium To 15 ml of a 2.0% w/v solution in *carbon dioxide-free water* add 1 ml of 1M *sulphuric acid* and allow to stand for at least 15 minutes. The solution is not more opalescent than a mixture of 15 ml of the 2.0% w/v solution and 1 ml of *water*.

Sulphate A 2.0% w/v solution in *carbon dioxide-free water* complies with the *limit test for sulphates*, Appendix VII (500 ppm).

Dihydroquinine monohydrochloride Not more than 10.0%, calculated with reference to the dried substance, when determined by the following method. Dissolve 0.2 g in 20 ml of *water* and add 0.5 g of *potassium bromide* and 15 ml of 2M *hydrochloric acid*. Titrate slowly with 0.0167M *potassium bromate VS*, using *methyl red solution* as indicator, until a yellow colour is produced. Add a solution of 0.5 g of *potassium iodide* in 200 ml of *water* and stopper the flask immediately. Allow to stand in the dark for 5 minutes and titrate with 0.1M *sodium thiosulphate VS* using 5 ml of *starch solution*, added towards the end of the titration, as indicator. Repeat the operation without the substance being examined. Each ml of 0.0167M *potassium bromate VS* is equivalent to 0.01804 g of $C_{20}H_{24}N_2O_2,HCl$. Calculate the content of dihydroquinine monohydrochloride by subtracting the result from the assay result.

Other cinchona alkaloids Carry out the method for *thin-layer chromatography*, Appendix III A, using *silica gel G* as the coating substance and a mixture of 60 volumes of *toluene*, 36 volumes of *ether* and 15 volumes of *diethylamine* as the mobile phase. Apply separately to the chromato-plate 4 μl of each of four solutions in *methanol* containing (1) 1.0% w/v of the substance being examined, (2) 0.025% w/v of *cinchonidine*, (3) 1.0% w/v of *quinine sulphate EPCRS* and 0.025% w/v of *cinchonidine* and (4) 1.0% w/v of *quinine sulphate EPCRS*. After removal of the plate, allow it to dry in a current of air for 15 minutes and repeat the development. Dry the plate at 105° for 30 minutes, allow it to cool and spray with *iodoplatinate reagent*. Any *secondary spot* in the chromatogram obtained with solution (1) is not more intense than the spot in the chromatogram obtained with solution (2). Disregard any spot in the chromatogram obtained with solution (1) corresponding to the spot with an Rf value slightly lower than that of the principal spot in the chromatogram obtained with solution (4). The test is not valid unless the chromatogram obtained with solution (3) shows two clearly separated spots.

Loss on drying When dried to constant weight at 100° to 105°, loses 6.0 to 10.0% of its weight. Use 1 g.

Sulphated ash Not more than 0.1%, Appendix IX A, Method II. Use 1 g.

Assay Dissolve 0.3 g in a mixture of 50 ml of *anhydrous glacial acetic acid* and 20 ml of *acetic anhydride*, add 5 ml of *mercury(II) acetate solution* and carry out Method I for *non-aqueous titration*, Appendix VIII A, determining the end-point potentiometrically. Each ml of 0.1M *perchloric acid VS* is equivalent to 0.01804 g of $C_{20}H_{24}N_2O_2,HCl$.

Storage Quinine Hydrochloride should be kept in a well-closed container and protected from light.

Action and use Antimalarial.

Quinine Sulphate ☆

$(C_{20}H_{24}N_2O_2)_2,H_2SO_4,2H_2O$ 783.0   *6119-70-6*

Quinine Sulphate is (8*S*,9*R*)-6'-methoxy-cinchonan-9-ol sulphate dihydrate. It contains not less than 99.0 per cent and not more than 101.0 per cent of alkaloid monosulphates, calculated as $(C_{20}H_{24}N_2O_2)_2,H_2SO_4$ with reference to the dried substance.

Characteristics A white or almost white, crystalline powder or fine colourless needles; odourless.

Solubility Slightly soluble in *water*; sparingly soluble in boiling *water* and in *ethanol* (96%); very slightly soluble in *chloroform*; practically insoluble in *ether*.

Identification A. In the test for Other cinchona alkaloids, the principal spot in the chromatogram obtained with solution (1) corresponds in position, colour and size to the principal spot in the chromatogram obtained with solution (4).

B. Dissolve 5 mg in 5 ml of *water* and add 0.2 ml of *bromine water* and 1 ml of 2M *ammonia*. An emerald-green colour is produced.

C. Dissolve 0.1 g in 3 ml of 1M *sulphuric acid* and dilute to 100 ml with *water*. An intense blue fluorescence is produced which disappears almost completely on the addition of 1 ml of *hydrochloric acid*.

D. Dissolve 45 mg in 5 ml of 2M *hydrochloric acid*. The resulting solution yields *reaction a* characteristic of sulphates, Appendix VI.

Acidity pH of a 1% w/v suspension, 5.7 to 6.6, Appendix V L.

Clarity and colour of solution A 2.0% w/v solution in 0.1M *hydrochloric acid* is *clear*, Appendix IV A, and not more intensely coloured than *reference solution* GY_6, Appendix IV B, Method II.

Specific optical rotation In a 2% solution in 0.1M *hydrochloric acid*, $-237°$ to $-245°$, Appendix V F.

Dihydroquinine sulphate Not more than 10.0%, calculated with reference to the dried substance, when determined by the following method. Dissolve 0.2 g in 20 ml of *water* and add 0.5 g of *potassium bromide* and 15 ml of 2M *hydrochloric acid*. Titrate slowly with 0.0167M *potassium bromate VS*, using *methyl red solution* as indicator, until a yellow colour is produced. Add a solution of 0.5 g of *potassium iodide* in 200 ml of *water* and stopper the flask immediately. Allow to stand in the dark for 5 minutes and titrate with 0.1M *sodium thiosulphate VS* using 5 ml of *starch solution*, added towards the end of the titration, as indicator. Repeat the operation without the substance being examined. Each ml of 0.0167M *potassium bromate VS* is equivalent to 0.01867 g of $(C_{20}H_{24}N_2O_2)_2$, H_2SO_4. Calculate the content of dihydroquinine sulphate by subtracting the result from the assay result.

Other cinchona alkaloids Carry out the method for *thin-layer chromatography*, Appendix III A, using *silica gel G* as the coating substance and a mixture of 60 volumes of *toluene*, 36 volumes of *ether* and 15 volumes of *diethylamine* as the mobile phase. Apply separately to the chromato-plate 4 µl of each of four solutions in *methanol* containing (1) 1.0% w/v of the substance being examined, (2) 0.025% w/v of *cinchonidine*, (3) 1.0% w/v of *quinine sulphate EPCRS* and 0.025% w/v of *cinchonidine* and (4) 1.0% w/v of *quinine sulphate EPCRS*. After removal of the plate, allow it to dry in a current of air for 15 minutes and repeat the development. Dry the plate at 105° for 30 minutes, allow to cool and spray with *iodoplatinate reagent*. Any *secondary spot* in the chromatogram obtained with solution (1) is not more intense than the spot in the chromatogram obtained with solution (2). Disregard any spot in the chromatogram obtained with solution (1) corresponding to the spot with an Rf value slightly lower than that of the principal spot in the chromatogram obtained with solution (4) The test is not valid unless the chromatogram obtained with solution (3) shows two clearly separated spots.

Loss on drying When dried to constant weight at 105°, loses 3.0 to 5.0% of its weight. Use 1 g.

Sulphated ash Not more than 0.1%, Appendix IX A, Method II. Use 1 g.

Assay Dissolve 0.3 g in a mixture of 10 ml of *chloroform* and 20 ml of *acetic anhydride* and carry out Method I for *non-aqueous titration*, Appendix VIII A, determining the end-point potentiometrically. Each ml of 0.1M *perchloric acid VS* is equivalent to 0.02490 g of $(C_{20}H_{24}N_2O_2)_2$,H_2SO_4.

Storage Quinine Sulphate should be kept in a well-closed container and protected from light.

Preparation
Quinine Sulphate Tablets

Action and use Antimalarial.

Reserpine ☆

$C_{33}H_{40}N_2O_9$ 609   *50-55-5*

Reserpine is methyl 11,17α-dimethoxy-18β-(3,4,5-trimethoxybenzoyloxy)-3β,20α-yohim-bane-16β-carboxylate. It contains not less than 99.0 per cent and not more than 101.0 per cent of total alkaloids and not less than 98.0 per cent and not more than 102.0 per cent of $C_{33}H_{40}N_2O_9$, both calculated with reference to the dried substance.

Characteristics Small, white to slightly yellow crystals or crystalline powder, which darken slowly on exposure to light.

Solubility Practically insoluble in *water* and in *ether*; very slightly soluble in *ethanol (96%)*; soluble in 6 parts of *chloroform*.

Identification *Test A may be omitted if tests B, C, D and E are carried out. Tests B, C, D and E may be omitted if test A is carried out.*
A. The *infra-red absorption spectrum*, Appendix II A, is concordant with the spectrum of *reserpine EPCRS*.
B. Dilute 1 ml of a 0.2% w/v solution in *chloroform* to 100 ml with *ethanol (96%)*. The *light absorption* of the resulting solution, Appendix II B, examined immediately after preparation in the range 230 to 350 nm exhibits a maximum at 268 nm. The A(1%, 1 cm) at the maximum is 265 to 285. Over the range 288 to 295 nm the spectrum exhibits a slight minimum and then a shoulder or a slight maximum. Over this range the A(1%, 1 cm) is about 170.
C. To 1 mg add 0.1 ml of a 0.1% w/v solution of *sodium molybdate* in *sulphuric acid*. A yellow colour is produced which changes to blue within 2 minutes.
D. To 1 mg add 0.2 ml of a freshly prepared 1% w/v solution of *vanillin* in *hydrochloric acid*. A rose-pink colour is produced within 2 minutes.
E. Mix 0.5 mg with 5 mg of *4-dimethylaminobenzaldehyde* and 0.2 ml of *glacial acetic acid* and add 0.2 ml of *sulphuric acid*; a green colour is produced. Add 1 ml of *glacial acetic acid*; the colour changes to red.

Specific optical rotation In a solution prepared immediately before use by dissolving 0.25 g in sufficient *chloroform* to produce 25 ml, −116° to −128°, Appendix V F.

Oxidation products *Absorbance* of a 0.02% w/v solution in *glacial acetic acid* at 388 nm, measured immediately after preparation, not more than 0.10, Appendix II B.

Loss on drying When dried over *phosphorus pentoxide* at 60° at a pressure not exceeding 0.7 kPa for 3 hours, loses not more than 0.5% of its weight. Use 0.5 g.

Sulphated ash Not more than 0.1%, Appendix IX A, Method II. Use 0.5 g.

Assay *For total alkaloids* Dissolve 0.5 g in a mixture of 40 ml of *anhydrous glacial acetic acid* and 6 ml of *acetic* *anhydride* and carry out Method I for *non-aqueous titration*, Appendix VIII A, determining the end-point potentiometrically. Each ml of 0.1M *perchloric acid VS* is equivalent to 0.06090 g of total alkaloids.

For C₃₃H₄₀N₂O₉ Carry out the following procedure protected from light. Moisten 25 mg with 2 ml of *ethanol (96%)*, add 2 ml of 0.25M *sulphuric acid* and 10 ml of *ethanol (96%)* and warm gently to dissolve. Cool, dilute to 100 ml with *ethanol (96%)* and dilute 5 ml to 50 ml with the same solvent (solution A). Transfer 10 ml to a boiling tube, add 2 ml of 0.25M *sulphuric acid* and 2 ml of a freshly prepared 0.3% w/v solution of *sodium nitrite*, mix and heat in a water-bath at 55° for 35 minutes. Cool, add 1 ml of a freshly prepared 5% w/v solution of *sulphamic acid* and dilute to 25 ml with *ethanol (96%)*. Measure the *absorbance* of the resulting solution at the maximum at 388 nm, Appendix II B, using in the reference cell a solution prepared by treating a further 10 ml of solution A in the same manner and at the same time but omitting the sodium nitrite solution. Calculate the content of $C_{33}H_{40}N_2O_9$ from the *absorbance* obtained by repeating the operation using *reserpine EPCRS* in place of the substance being examined.

Storage Reserpine should be kept in a well-closed container and protected from light.

Action and use Antihypertensive.

Resorcinol ☆

OH

OH

$C_6H_6O_2$ 110.1   *108-46-3*

Resorcinol is benzene-1,3-diol. It contains not less than 98.5 per cent and not more than 101.0 per cent of $C_6H_6O_2$, calculated with reference to the dried substance.

Characteristics Colourless or slightly pinkish-grey crystals or crystalline powder; odour, characteristic. Turns red on exposure to light and air.

Solubility Soluble in less than 1 part of *water* and in 1 part of *ethanol (96%)*; slightly soluble in *chloroform*; freely soluble in *ether*.

Identification A. Dissolve 0.1 g in 1 ml of *water*, add 1 ml of 10M *sodium hydroxide* and 0.1 ml of *chloroform* and heat; an intense deep red colour is produced. Add a slight excess of *hydrochloric acid*; a pale yellow colour is produced.
B. Thoroughly mix 10 mg with 10 mg of *potassium hydrogen phthalate*, both finely powdered. Heat over a naked flame until an orange-yellow colour is produced, cool, add 2 ml of 1M *sodium hydroxide* and 10 ml of *water* and shake to dissolve. An intense green fluorescence is produced.
C. *Melting point*, 109° to 112°, Appendix V A, Method I.

Acidity or alkalinity To 10 ml of a 10.0% w/v solution in *carbon dioxide-free water* (solution A) add 0.05 ml of *ethanolic bromophenol blue solution*. Not more than 0.05 ml of either 0.1M *hydrochloric acid VS* or 0.1M *sodium hydroxide VS* is required to change the colour of the solution.

Clarity and colour of solution Solution A is *clear*, Appendix IV A, and not more intensely coloured than *reference solution B₅* or *R₅*, Appendix IV B, Method II, and remains so when heated on a water-bath for 5 minutes.

Catechol Mix 2 ml of solution A with 1 ml of *neutral ammonium molybdate solution*. Any yellow colour produced is not more intense than that produced by mixing 2 ml of a 0.01% w/v solution of *catechol* with 1 ml of *neutral ammonium molybdate solution*.

Related substances Carry out the method for *thin-layer chromatography*, Appendix III A, using *silica gel G* as the coating substance and a mixture of 60 volumes of *hexane* and 40 volumes of *ethyl acetate* as the mobile phase. Apply separately to the chromatoplate 2 μl of each of two solutions of the substance being examined in *methanol* containing (1) 5.0% w/v and (2) 0.025% w/v. After removal of the plate, allow it to dry in air for 15 minutes and expose it to iodine vapour. Any *secondary spot* in the chromatogram obtained with solution (1) is not more intense than the spot in the chromatogram obtained with solution (2).

Loss on drying When dried over *anhydrous silica gel* for 4 hours, loses not more than 1.0% of its weight. Use 1 g, in powder.

Sulphated ash Not more than 0.1%, Appendix IX A, Method II. Use 1 g.

Assay Dissolve 0.5 g in sufficient *water* to produce 250 ml. To 25 ml of the solution add 1 g of *potassium bromide*, 50 ml of 0.0167M *potassium bromate VS*, 15 ml of *chloroform* and 15 ml of 7M *hydrochloric acid*. Stopper the flask, shake and allow to stand for 15 minutes protected from light, shaking occasionally. Add 10 ml of a 10% w/v solution of *potassium iodide*, shake thoroughly, allow to stand for 5 minutes and titrate with 0.1M *sodium thiosulphate VS* using 1 ml of *starch solution* as indicator. Each ml of 0.0167M *potassium bromate VS* is equivalent to 0.001835 g of $C_6H_6O_2$.

Storage Resorcinol should be kept in a well-closed container and protected from light.

Action and use Keratolytic.

Rhatany Root ☆
Krameria

Rhatany Root consists of the dried root of *Krameria triandra* Ruiz and Pavon, known in commerce as Peruvian rhatany. It contains not less than 10.0 per cent of tannins.

Characteristics Odourless.

Macroscopical Dark reddish-brown. Thick, knotty crown, bearing nearly straight or somewhat tortuous roots; bark, rugged and scaly in the older pieces, smooth with sharp transverse fissures in the younger pieces, separating readily from the wood. Fracture, fibrous in the bark, splintery in the wood. The smoothed, transversely-cut surface shows a dark brownish-red bark occupying about one-third of the radius; dense, pale, reddish-brown and finely porous wood with numerous fine medullary rays; central heart wood often darker.

Microscopical Bark: cork layer, 1 to 1.5 mm thick, comprising thin-walled cells with dark brownish-red contents; phloem with groups of sieve tissue, arranged radially, alternating with numerous groups of yellow, non-lignified fibres, individual fibres 12 to 30 μm wide, 400 to 1100 μm long, tortuous and with a lumen of varying width. Fibre groups accompanied by files of cells containing calcium oxalate prisms, 2 to 30 μm wide and up to 100 μm long, or crystal sand. Parenchyma containing reddish-brown colouring matter and simple or compound starch granules, mostly round, individual granules 4 to 30 μm in diameter. Numerous medullary rays, uniseriate near the cambium, multiseriate in the outer parts, containing starch. Xylem indistinctly radiate; vessels solitary or in groups of two to five, 20 to 60 μm in diameter, with bordered pits; fibre-tracheids, about 20 μm wide and 200 to 600 μm long surrounding the vessels; intermediary parenchyma in tangential bands one cell wide connecting two medullary rays or extending along a wider arc; cells about 8 to 12 μm wide and 80 to 150 μm long; small amounts of diffuse, lignified parenchyma; numerous uniseriate medullary rays.

Identification A. Macerate 0.1 g, in powder, with 10 ml of *water* for 1 hour and filter. Add 2 ml of a 10% w/v solution of *ammonium iron(II) sulphate* to the filtrate; the liquid becomes cloudy and dark grey. Allow to stand; the supernatant liquid is greyish-green.

B. To 0.5 g, in powder, add 5 ml of *ethanol (96%)*, allow to stand for 2 hours, shaking frequently, and filter. Dilute 1 ml of the brownish-red filtrate to 100 ml with *ethanol (96%)*. Add 0.1 ml of a 10% w/v solution of *iron(III) chloride hexahydrate* in *ethanol (96%)*. A green colour is produced.

Foreign matter Not more than 2%, Appendix IX D, Test B. Not more than 5.0% of the substance being examined consists of crown or root exceeding 25 mm in diameter. Root without bark should be present only in small quantities.

Sulphated ash Not more than 6.0%, Appendix IX A, Method II. Use 1 g, in powder.

Assay To 0.75 g, in *No. 180 powder*, add 150 ml of *water*, boil for 30 minutes in a water-bath, cool in water, dilute to 250 ml with *water*, allow the solids to settle and filter through a 12-cm diameter filter paper, discarding the first 50 ml of the filtrate.

Total polyphenols Dilute 5 ml of the filtrate to 25 ml with *water*, mix 5 ml of this solution with 1 ml of *phosphotungstic acid solution* and dilute to 50 ml with a 15% w/v solution of *sodium carbonate*. Determine the *absorbance* of the resulting solution at 715 nm, Appendix II B, 2 minutes after the addition of the last reagent (A_1).

Polyphenols not precipitated with hide powder To 10 ml of the filtrate add 0.1 g of *hide powder EPCRS*, shake well for 60 minutes and filter. Dilute 5 ml to 25 ml with *water* and complete the procedure described under Total polyphenols, beginning at the words 'mix 5 ml . . .' (A_2). Dissolve 50 mg of *pyrogallol* in *water* and dilute to 100 ml with *water*. Dilute 5 ml to 100 ml with *water* and complete the procedure described under Total polyphenols beginning at the words 'mix 5 ml . . .' (A_3).

Calculate the percentage of tannins in the substance being examined from the expression $13.12(A_1 - A_2)/wA_3$, where w is the weight, in g, of substance taken.

Storage Rhatany Root should be kept in a well-closed container and protected from light

Action and use Astringent.

Powdered Rhatany Root

Powdered Rhatany Root is Rhatany Root in powder. It contains not less than 10.0 per cent of tannins.

Characteristics Reddish-brown. Diagnostic structures: cork cells with dark brown contents; fragments of yellow, tortuous, non-lignified fibres, 12 to 30 μm in diameter, with thick walls without apparent channels and with a variable lumen; phloem parenchyma cells in files containing prisms of calcium oxalate, 2 to 30 μm wide and up to 100 μm long, or crystal sand; fragments of grey xylem fibres with thick walls, very pronounced regularly-occurring channels and a large lumen; vessel fragments with bordered pits, fragments of fibre-tracheids; simple or compound starch granules, 4 to 30 μm in diameter with a stellate hilum, some occurring in the cells of the medullary rays and the xylem parenchyma. The reddish-brown colouring matter turns brownish-green when treated with a 1.3% w/v solution of *iron(III) chloride hexahydrate*.

Identification Complies with the requirements stated under Rhatany Root.

Sulphated ash Not more than 6.0%, Appendix IX A, Method II. Use 1 g.

Assay Carry out the Assay described under Rhatany Root.

Storage Powdered Rhatany Root should be kept in a well-closed container and protected from light.

Action and use Astringent.

Rhubarb ☆

Rhubarb consists of the dried underground parts of *Rheum palmatum* L. or *Rheum officinale* Baillon, or hybrids of these two species, or mixtures of these, separated from the stem, rootlets and most of the bark, frequently divided. It contains not less than 2.5 per cent of hydroxyanthracene derivatives, calculated as rhein, $C_{15}H_8O_6$.

Characteristics Odour, characteristic.

Macroscopical Variable appearance, which may include discoid pieces, up to 10 cm in diameter and 1 to 5 cm in thickness, cylindrical pieces, oval to round or plano-convex pieces. Surface has a pinkish tinge with a reticulum of darker lines. Fracture, granular. Transverse section of rhizome shows narrow outer zone containing a white reticulum with radiating dark lines; a ring of star spot formations of anomalous vascular bundles is usually visible inside this zone. The root shows a more radiate structure.

Microscopical Transverse section shows a ground tissue of thin-walled rounded or occasionally polygonal parenchyma with abundant simple or two- to four-compound starch granules, 2 to 35 μm in size, usually 10 to 20 μm, with star-shaped hilum; some larger cells contain calcium oxalate cluster crystals, up to 100 μm or more in diameter. Phloem, sieve tubes frequently obliterated. Xylem vessels unlignified, reticulately thickened, up to 175 μm wide, in groups of two to five. Medullary rays, one to four cells wide, usually two or three, containing yellowish-orange to brownish-red amorphous masses, which turn red when treated with a 10% w/v solution of *potassium hydroxide*. Star spots each with distinct reddish-brown medullary rays and a circular cambium separating the central white phloem from peripheral xylem, visible on the inside of the peripheral radiate zone. Sclereids and fibres absent.

Identification A. Carry out the method for *thin-layer chromatography*, Appendix III A, using *silica gel G* as the coating substance and a mixture of 75 volumes of *petroleum spirit (boiling range, 60° to 80°)*, 25 volumes of *ethyl acetate* and 1 volume of *anhydrous formic acid* as the mobile phase, but allowing the solvent front to ascend 10 cm above the line of application. Apply separately to the chromatoplate 20 μl of each of the following solutions as bands 20 mm long and not more than 3 mm wide. For solution (1) heat 50 mg of the substance being examined, in *No. 180 powder*, with 30 ml of *water* and 1 ml of *hydrochloric acid* for 15 minutes on a water-bath, allow to cool, extract the liquid with 25 ml of *ether*, dry the ether solution over *anhydrous sodium sulphate*, filter, evaporate the filtrate to dryness and dissolve the residue in 0.5 ml of *ether*. For solution (2) dissolve 5 mg of *emodin* in 5 ml of *ether*. After removal of the plate, allow it to dry in air and examine under *ultra-violet light (365 nm)*. The chromatogram obtained with solution (1) shows orange fluorescent bands at Rf values of about 0.15 due to aloe-emodin, at about 0.25 due to rhein, at about 0.40 due to emodin, at about Rf 0.50 due to physcion and at about 0.55 due to chrysophanol. The band due to emodin corresponds to the band obtained in the chromatogram obtained with solution (2). Place the plate in a chamber containing ammonia vapour. The bands previously observed become red.

B. To 50 mg, in powder, add 25 ml of 2M *hydrochloric acid*, heat on a water-bath for 15 minutes, allow to cool, shake with 20 ml of *ether*, separate the ether layer and shake it with 10 ml of 6M *ammonia*. A red colour is produced in the aqueous layer.

Rheum rhaponticum Carry out the method for *thin-layer chromatography*, Appendix III A, using *silica gel G* as the coating substance and a mixture of 80 volumes of *chloroform* and 20 volumes of *methanol* as the mobile phase, but allowing the solvent front to ascend 12 cm above the line of application. Apply separately to the chromatoplate 20 μl of each of the following solutions as bands 20 mm long and not more than 3 mm wide. For solution (1) heat 0.2 g of the substance being examined, in *No. 180 powder*, with 2 ml of *methanol* under a reflux condenser for 5 minutes, cool, filter and use the filtrate. For solution (2) dissolve 10 mg of *rhaponticin* in 10 ml of *methanol*. After removal of the plate, allow it to dry in air and spray with *phosphomolybdic acid solution*. The chromatogram obtained with solution (1) does not show a blue band near the line of application corresponding to that shown in the chromatogram obtained with solution (2).

Foreign matter Not more than 1%, Appendix XI D, Test B.

Acid-insoluble ash Not more than 1.0%, Appendix XI K, Method II.

Assay Mix 0.1 g, in *No. 180 powder*, with 30 ml of *water* and weigh. Heat under a reflux condenser in a water-bath for 15 minutes, allow to cool, add 50 mg of *sodium hydrogen carbonate*, weigh and restore to the original weight with *water*. Centrifuge, transfer 10 ml of the liquid to a 100-ml round-bottomed flask with a ground-glass neck, add 20 ml of a 10.5% w/v solution of *iron(III) chloride hexahydrate*, mix, heat under a reflux condenser in a water-bath for 20 minutes, add 1 ml of *hydrochloric acid* and continue heating for 20 minutes, shaking frequently. Cool, transfer to a separating funnel and extract with two 25-ml quantities of *ether* previously used to rinse the flask. Combine the ether extracts, wash with two 15-ml quantities of *water*, filter the ether extracts through absorbent cotton and dilute to 100 ml with *ether*. Evaporate 10 ml carefully to dryness, dissolve the residue in 10 ml of a 0.5% w/v solution of *magnesium acetate* in *methanol* and measure the *absorbance* of the resulting solution at 515 nm, Appendix II B, using *methanol* in the reference cell. Calculate the content of $C_{15}H_8O_6$ taking 440 as the value of A(1%, 1 cm) at 515 nm.

Storage Rhubarb should be kept in a well-closed container and protected from light and moisture.

Preparations
Ammoniated Rhubarb and Soda Mixture
Compound Rhubarb Tincture

Action and use Laxative.

Powdered Rhubarb

Powdered Rhubarb is Rhubarb in powder. It contains not less than 2.5 per cent of hydroxy-anthracene derivatives, calculated as rhein, $C_{15}H_8O_6$.

Characteristics Orange or yellowish-brown. Diagnostic structures: calcium oxalate cluster crystals, up to 100 μm or more in diameter, or their fragments; unlignified, reticulately thickened vessels, 20 to 175 μm, mainly 60 to 100 μm, in width; starch granules present; sclereids and fibres absent.

Identification; *Rheum rhaponticum* Complies with the requirements stated under Rhubarb.

Acid-insoluble ash Not more than 1.0%, Appendix XI K.

Assay Carry out the Assay described under Rhubarb. Calculate the content of $C_{15}H_8O_6$ taking 440 as the value of A(1%, 1 cm) at 515 nm.

Storage Powdered Rhubarb should be kept in a well-closed container and protected from light and moisture.

Action and use Laxative.

Riboflavine ☆

$$CH_2OH$$
$$HOCH$$
$$HOCH$$
$$HOCH$$
$$CH_2$$

(structure of riboflavine showing benzopteridine ring system with Me, Me substituents and N, N, O, NH, N, O)

$C_{17}H_{20}N_4O_6$ 376.4   83-88-5

Riboflavine is 3,10-dihydro-7,8-dimethyl-10-[(2S,3S,4R)-2,3,4,5-tetrahydroxypentyl]benzopteridine-2,4-dione. It contains not less than 98.0 per cent and not more than 101.0 per cent of $C_{17}H_{20}N_4O_6$, calculated with reference to the dried substance.

Characteristics A yellow to orange-yellow, crystalline powder; odour, slight.

Solubility Very slightly soluble in *water*; more soluble in *saline solution* than in *water*; practically insoluble in *ethanol (96%)*, in *acetone*, in *chloroform* and in *ether*.

Identification *Test A may be omitted if tests B and C are carried out. Tests B and C may be omitted if test A is carried out.*
A. The *infra-red absorption spectrum*, Appendix II A, is concordant with the spectrum of *riboflavine EPCRS*.
B. Complies with the test for Specific optical rotation.
C. Dissolve 1 mg in 100 ml of *water*. The solution is pale greenish-yellow by transmitted light and by reflected light exhibits an intense yellowish-green fluorescence which disappears on the addition of mineral acids or alkalis.

Acidity or alkalinity To 0.5 g add 25 ml of *carbon dioxide-free water*, boil for 2 minutes, cool and filter. To 10 ml of the filtrate add 0.05 ml of *dilute phenolphthalein solution* and 0.4 ml of 0.01M *sodium hydroxide*; the solution is orange. Add 0.5 ml of 0.01M *hydrochloric acid*; the solution is yellow. Add 0.15 ml of *methyl red solution*; the solution is orange.

Light absorption Dilute a suitable quantity of the final solution obtained in the Assay with an equal volume of *water*. The resulting solution exhibits maxima at 223, 267, 373 and 444 nm. The ratio of the *absorbance* at 373 nm to that at 267 nm is 0.31 to 0.33 and the ratio of the *absorbance* at 444 nm to that at 267 nm is 0.36 to 0.39, Appendix II B.

Specific optical rotation In a 0.5% w/v solution in 0.05M *sodium hydroxide*, $-115°$ to $-135°$, Appendix V F. Measure the angle of rotation within 30 minutes of preparing the solution.

Lumiflavine Shake 25 mg with 10 ml of *ethanol-free chloroform* for 5 minutes and filter. The filtrate is not more intensely coloured than *reference solution BY₆*, Appendix IV B, Method I.

Loss on drying When dried to constant weight at 100° to 105°, loses not more than 1.5% of its weight. Use 1 g.

Sulphated ash Not more than 0.1%, Appendix IX A, Method II. Use the residue obtained in the test for Loss on drying.

Assay Carry out the following procedure in subdued light. Suspend 65 mg in 5 ml of *water*, ensuring that it is completely wetted, and dissolve in 5 ml of 2M *sodium hydroxide*. Immediately add 100 ml of *water* and 2.5 ml of *glacial acetic acid* and dilute to 500 ml with *water*. To 20 ml of this solution add 3.5 ml of a 1.4% w/v solution of *sodium acetate* and dilute to 200 ml with *water*. Measure the *absorbance* of the resulting solution at the maximum at 444 nm, Appendix II B. Calculate the content of $C_{17}H_{20}N_4O_6$ taking 328 as the value of A(1%, 1 cm) at the maximum at 444 nm.

Storage Riboflavine should be kept in an airtight container and protected from light. Solutions, especially in the presence of alkali, deteriorate on exposure to light.

Action and use Component of vitamin B.

In some countries the material described in this monograph may be known as Riboflavin.

Riboflavine Sodium Phosphate
Riboflavine Phosphate (Sodium Salt)

$C_{17}H_{20}N_4NaO_9P,2H_2O$ 514.4   130-40-5

Riboflavine Sodium Phosphate is the dihydrate of the sodium salt of riboflavin-5′-phosphate. It contains the equivalent of not less than 75.0 per cent and not more than 79.0 per cent of $C_{17}H_{20}N_4O_6$, calculated with reference to the dried substance.

Characteristics A yellow to orange-yellow, crystalline powder; odourless or almost odourless; hygroscopic.

Solubility Soluble in 20 parts of *water*; very slightly soluble in *ethanol (96%)*; practically insoluble in *chloroform* and in *ether*.

Identification A. The *light absorption*, Appendix II B, in the range 230 to 350 nm of a 0.001% w/v solution in *phosphate buffer pH 7.0* exhibits a maximum only at 266 nm. The *absorbance* at 266 nm is about 0.61.
B. To 1 ml of a 0.01% w/v solution add 1 ml of 1M *sodium hydroxide*, expose to ultra-violet radiation for 5 minutes, add sufficient 6M *acetic acid* to make the solution acidic to *litmus paper* and shake the mixture with 2 ml of *chloroform*. The chloroform layer exhibits a yellow fluorescence.
C. Dissolve, with the aid of heat, 0.1 g in 1 ml of 5M *hydrochloric acid*, add 10 ml of *ethanol (96%)*, cool in ice, induce crystallisation and filter through a sintered-glass filter (BS porosity No. 4). The *melting point* of the residue, after washing with *ether* and drying, is about 200°, Appendix V A.
D. To 0.5 g add 10 ml of *nitric acid*, evaporate the mixture to dryness on a water-bath, ignite the residue until the carbon is removed, dissolve the final residue in 5 ml of *water* and filter. The filtrate yields the *reactions* characteristic of sodium salts and of phosphates, Appendix VI.

Acidity pH of a 2% w/v solution, 4.0 to 6.3, Appendix V L.

Specific optical rotation In a 1.5% w/v solution in 5M *hydrochloric acid*, $+38°$ to $+42°$, Appendix V F.

Heavy metals To 2.0 g in a silica crucible cautiously add 2 ml of *nitric acid* dropwise followed by 0.25 ml of *sulphuric acid*. Heat cautiously until white fumes are evolved and ignite. Extract the cooled residue with two 2-ml quantities of *hydrochloric acid* and evaporate the extracts to dryness. Dissolve the residue in sufficient 0.1M *acetic acid* to produce 20 ml and carry out *limit test C for heavy metals*, Appendix VII, beginning at the words 'To 12 ml of the resulting solution . . .' (10 ppm). Use 2 ml of *lead standard solution (10 ppm Pb)* to prepare the standard.

Free phosphate Dissolve 0.10 g in sufficient *water* to produce 100 ml. Dilute 5 ml with 5 ml of *water* and add 5 ml of *buffered copper sulphate solution pH 4*, 2 ml of a 3% w/v solution of *ammonium molybdate*, 1 ml of a freshly prepared solution containing 2% w/v of *4-methylamino-phenol sulphate* and 5% w/v of *sodium metabisulphite* and 1 ml of a 3% v/v solution of *perchloric acid*. Add sufficient *water* to produce 25 ml, mix and measure the *absorbance* of the resulting solution at 860 nm, Appendix II B, within 15 minutes of its preparation, using in the reference cell a solution prepared in the same manner but without the substance being examined. The *absorbance* is not greater than that produced by repeating the operation using a solution prepared in the same manner using 7.5 ml of *phosphate standard solution (10 ppm)* and beginning at the words 'add 5 ml of *buffered copper sulphate solution pH 4* . . .' (1.5%).

Lumiflavine To 35 mg add 10 ml of *ethanol-free chloroform*, shake for 5 minutes and filter. The filtrate is not more intensely coloured than a solution prepared by diluting 3 ml of 0.0167M *potassium dichromate VS* to 1000 ml with *water*.

Loss on drying When dried over *phosphorus pentoxide* at 100° at a pressure not exceeding 0.7 kPa for 5 hours, loses not more than 8.0% of its weight. Use 1 g.

Assay Carry out the following procedure in subdued light. Dissolve 0.1 g in 150 ml of *water*, add 2 ml of *glacial acetic acid* and dilute to 1000 ml with *water*. To 10 ml add 3.5 ml of 0.1M *sodium acetate*, dilute to 50 ml with *water* and measure the *absorbance* of the resulting solution at the maximum at 444 nm, Appendix II B. Calculate the content of $C_{17}H_{20}N_4O_6$ taking 323 as the value of A(1%, 1 cm) at the maximum at 444 nm.

Storage Riboflavine Sodium Phosphate should be kept in a well-closed container and protected from light.

Action and use Component of vitamin B.

Rifampicin ☆

$C_{43}H_{58}N_4O_{12}$ 823   *13292-46-1*

Rifampicin is (12*Z*,14*E*,24*E*)-(2*S*,16*S*,17*S*,18*R*, 19*R*,20*R*,21*S*,22*R*,23*S*)-1,2-dihydro-5,6,9,17,19-pentahydroxy-23-methoxy-2,4,12,16,18,20,22-heptamethyl-8-(4-methylpiperazin-1-ylimino-methyl)-1,11-dioxo-2,7-(epoxypentadeca-1,11,13-trienimino)naphtho[2,1-*b*]furan-21-yl acetate. It contains not less than 97.0 per cent and not more than 102.0 per cent of $C_{43}H_{58}N_4O_{12}$, calculated with reference to the dried substance.

Characteristics A brick-red to reddish-brown crystalline powder; practically odourless.

Solubility Slightly soluble in *water*, in *ethanol (96%)*, in *acetone* and in *ether*; soluble in *methanol*; freely soluble in *chloroform*.

Identification A. The *infra-red absorption spectrum*, Appendix II A, is concordant with the spectrum of *rifampicin EPCRS*. Examine the substances as dispersions in *liquid paraffin*.
B. The *light absorption*, Appendix II B, in the range 220 to 500 nm of the final solution obtained in the Assay, exhibits four maxima, at 237, 254, 334 and 475 nm. The ratio of the *absorbance* at the maximum at 334 nm to that at 475 nm is about 1.75.
C. Suspend 25 mg in 25 ml of *water*, shake for 5 minutes and filter. To 5 ml of the filtrate add 1 ml of a 10% w/v solution of *ammonium persulphate* in *phosphate buffer pH 7.4* and shake for a few minutes. The colour changes from orange-yellow to violet-red without the formation of a precipitate.

Acidity pH of a 1% w/v suspension, 4.5 to 6.5, Appendix V L.

Heavy metals 1.0 g complies with *limit test C for heavy metals*, Appendix VII (20 ppm). Use 2 ml of *lead standard solution (10 ppm Pb)* to prepare the standard.

Related substances Carry out the method for *thin-layer chromatography*, Appendix III A, using *silica gel G* as the coating substance, preparing the suspension using *citro-phosphate buffer pH 6.0*, checking the pH and adjusting if necessary. Use a mixture of 85 volumes of *chloroform* and 15 volumes of *methanol* as the mobile phase and allow the solvent front to ascend 12 cm above the line of application. Apply separately to the chromatoplate 20 μl of each of four freshly prepared solutions in *chloroform* containing (1) 2.0% w/v of the substance being examined, (2) 0.010% w/v of *3-formylrifamycin SV EPCRS*, (3) 0.030% w/v of *rifampicin quinone EPCRS* and (4) 0.020% w/v of the substance being examined. After removal of the plate, allow it to dry in air. Any spots corresponding to 3-formylrifamycin SV and rifampicin quinone in the chromatogram obtained with solution (1) are not more intense than the spots in the chromatograms obtained with solutions (2) and (3) respectively and any other *secondary spot* is not more intense than the spot in the chromatogram obtained with solution (4).

Loss on drying When dried at 80° at a pressure not exceeding 0.7 kPa for 4 hours, loses not more than 1.0% of its weight. Use 1 g.

Sulphated ash Not more than 0.1%, Appendix IX A, Method II. Use 2 g.

Assay Dissolve 0.1 g in sufficient *methanol* to produce 100 ml, dilute 2 ml to 100 ml with *phosphate buffer pH 7.4* and measure the *absorbance* of the resulting solution at the maximum at 475 nm, Appendix II B, using the phosphate buffer in the reference cell. Calculate the content of $C_{43}H_{58}N_4O_{12}$ taking 187 as the value of A(1%, 1 cm) at the maximum at 475 nm.

Storage Rifampicin should be kept in an airtight container in an atmosphere of nitrogen, protected from light and stored at a temperature not exceeding 15°.

Labelling The label states (1) the date after which the material is not intended to be used; (2) the conditions under which it should be stored.

Preparations

Rifampicin Capsules

Rifampicin Oral Suspension

Action and use Antituberculous.

Rifamycin Sodium ☆

C_{37}H_{46}NNaO_{12}   720   *14897-39-3*

Rifamycin Sodium is sodium (12*Z*,14*E*,24*E*)-(2*S*,16*S*,17*S*,18*R*,19*R*,20*R*,21*S*,22*R*,23*S*)-21-acetoxy-1,2-dihydro-6,9,17,19-tetrahydroxy-23-methoxy-2,4,12,16,18,20,22-heptamethyl-1,11-dioxo-2,7-(epoxypentadeca-1,11,13-trienimino)-naphtho[2,1-*b*]furan-5-olate, the monosodium salt of rifamycin SV, a substance obtained by chemical transformation of rifamycin B, which is produced during growth of certain strains of *Streptomyces mediterranei*. Rifamycin SV may also be obtained directly from certain *Streptomyces mediterranei* mutants. The potency is not less than 900 Units per mg, calculated with reference to the anhydrous substance.

Characteristics A fine or slightly granular, red powder.

Solubility Soluble in *water*; freely soluble in *absolute ethanol* and in *methanol*; practically insoluble in *chloroform* and in *ether*.

Identification A. Dilute 1 ml of a 0.1% w/v solution in *methanol* to 50 ml with *phosphate buffer pH 7.0*. The *light absorption*, Appendix II B, in the range 250 to 460 nm exhibits two maxima, at 314 nm and 445 nm. The ratio of the *absorbance* at 314 nm to that at 445 nm is 1.55 to 1.65.

B. To 1 ml of a 0.5% w/v solution add 1 ml of a 10% w/v solution of *ammonium persulphate* in *phosphate buffer pH 7.0*; a flocculent brownish-yellow precipitate is produced. After about 2 minutes add 0.5 ml of 1M *sodium carbonate*; the precipitate dissolves completely and the solution becomes violet-red.

C. Yields *reaction A* characteristic of sodium salts, Appendix VI.

Acidity or alkalinity pH of a 5% w/v solution, 6.5 to 7.5, Appendix V L.

Light absorption Dissolve 20 mg in 5 ml of *methanol* and dilute to 100 ml with freshly prepared *phosphate buffer pH 7.0* to which has been added 0.1% w/v of *L-ascorbic acid* immediately before use. Dilute 5 ml of this solution to 50 ml with the phosphate buffer—ascorbic acid solution, allow to stand for 30 minutes and measure the *absorbance*

at the maximum at 445 nm, Appendix II B. The A(1%, 1 cm) is 190 to 210.

Heavy metals 2.0 g complies with *limit test C for heavy metals*, Appendix VII (10 ppm). Use 2 ml of *lead standard solution (10 ppm Pb)* to prepare the standard.

Rifamycin B Carry out the method for *thin-layer chromatography*, Appendix III A, using a chromatoplate prepared in the following manner. Shake thoroughly 27 g of *silanised silica gel HF254* with 60 ml of a mixture of 1 volume of *methanol* and 2 volumes of *water*. Use the slurry to coat the plate, dry it in air for 3 hours and then in a desiccator over *self-indicating silica gel* and use not sooner than 24 hours after preparation. Use as the mobile phase a mixture of 60 volumes of *phosphate buffer pH 7.0* and 40 volumes of *acetone* to which has been added sufficient *L-ascorbic acid* to give a final concentration of 0.1% w/v and allow the solvent front to ascend 10 cm above the line of application. Apply separately to the chromatoplate 5 µl of each of two solutions in *acetone* containing (1) 1.0% w/v of the substance being examined and (2) 0.020% w/v of *rifamycin B EPCRS*. After removal of the plate, allow it to dry in air, protected from light. The chromatogram obtained with solution (1) shows a reddish-yellow spot at an Rf value of about 0.2 and the chromatogram obtained with solution (2) shows a yellow spot at an Rf value of about 0.5. Any yellow spot with an Rf value of 0.5 corresponding to rifamycin B in the chromatogram obtained with solution (1) is not more intense than the spot in the chromatogram obtained with solution (2).

Water 12.0 to 17.0% w/w, Appendix IX C. Use 0.2 g.

Assay Carry out the *biological assay of antibiotics*, Appendix XIV A. The precision of the assay is such that the fiducial limits of error are not less than 95% and not more than 105% of the estimated potency.

Storage Rifamycin Sodium should be kept in an airtight container and protected from light. If the material is intended for use in the manufacture of a parenteral dosage form, the container should be sterile, tamper-evident and sealed so as to exclude micro-organisms.

Labelling The label states (1) the number of Units per mg; (2) the date after which the material is not intended to be used; (3) the conditions under which it should be stored; (4) whether or not it is intended for use in the manufacture of a parenteral dosage form.

Action and use Antibacterial.

Rifamycin sodium intended for use in the manufacture of a parenteral dosage form complies with the following additional requirements.

Abnormal toxicity Complies with the *test for abnormal toxicity*, Appendix XIV L. Use 0.5 ml of a solution in *water for injections* containing 8 mg per ml of the substance being examined.

Depressor substances Complies with the *test for depressor substances*, Appendix XIV M. Use per kg of the cat's weight 0.1 ml of a solution containing 30 mg per ml of the substance being examined.

Pyrogens Complies with the *test for pyrogens*, Appendix XIV K. Use per kg of the rabbit's weight 1 ml of a solution containing 10 mg per ml of the substance being examined.

Sterility Complies with the *test for sterility*, Appendix XVI A.

Saccharin

C₇H₅NO₃S   183.2   *81-07-2*

Saccharin is 1,2-benzisothiazolin-3-one 1,1-dioxide. It contains not less than 99.0 per cent and not more than 100.5 per cent of C₇H₅NO₃S, calculated with reference to the dried substance.

Characteristics White crystals or a white, crystalline powder; odourless or almost odourless.

Solubility Slightly soluble in *water*; soluble in about 25 parts of boiling *water*, in 30 parts of *ethanol (96%)* and in 12 parts of *acetone*; slightly soluble in *chloroform* and in *ether*. It dissolves in 5M *ammonia*, in solutions of alkali hydroxides and, with evolution of carbon dioxide, in solutions of alkali bicarbonates.

Identification A. Mix 20 mg with 40 mg of *resorcinol*, add 0.5 ml of *sulphuric acid* and heat over a small flame until a dark green colour is produced; allow to cool and add 10 ml of *water* and an excess of 5M *sodium hydroxide*. A fluorescent green liquid is produced.
B. Dissolve 0.1 g in 5 ml of a 10% w/v solution of *sodium hydroxide*, evaporate to dryness and gently fuse the residue over a small flame until ammonia is no longer evolved. Allow to cool, dissolve in 20 ml of *water*, make the solution just acidic to *litmus paper*, filter and add 0.05 ml of *iron(III) chloride test-solution*. A violet colour is produced.
C. A saturated solution is acidic to *litmus paper*.

Melting point 226° to 230°, Appendix V A.

Arsenic Mix 0.50 g with 0.3 g of *anhydrous sodium carbonate*, add 1 ml of *bromine water* and mix thoroughly. Evaporate to dryness on a water-bath, gently ignite and add to the cooled residue a mixture of 2.0 ml of *brominated hydrochloric acid* and 0.5 ml of *bromine water*. Add 4 ml of *water* and boil gently, occasionally adding sufficient *bromine water* to maintain a slight excess. Filter and remove the excess of bromine with a sufficient quantity of *tin(II) chloride solution AsT*. The resulting solution complies with the *limit test for arsenic*, Appendix VII (2 ppm).

Heavy metals To 2.0 g in a silica crucible add 4 ml of a 25% w/v solution of *magnesium sulphate* in *sulphuric acid (6%)*. Mix, heat cautiously to ignition over a flame or in an oven at a temperature not exceeding 800° until a white residue is obtained. Allow to cool, moisten the residue with 0.2 ml of *sulphuric acid (6%)*, evaporate and repeat the ignition ensuring that the total period of ignition does not exceed 2 hours. Dissolve the residue using two 5-ml quantities of 2M *hydrochloric acid*, transferring the solution to a 20-ml graduated flask and filtering if necessary. Wash the crucible and filter with *water* and make the combined solution and washings alkaline with 13.5M *ammonia*. Cool, acidify with 6M *acetic acid* and add a further 1.5 ml. Dilute with *water* to 20 ml and filter if necessary. 12 ml of the resulting solution complies with *limit test A for heavy metals*, Appendix VII (10 ppm). Use *lead standard solution (1 ppm Pb)* to prepare the standard.

Related substances Carry out the method for *thin-layer chromatography*, Appendix III A, using *silica gel G* as the coating substance and a mixture of 100 volumes of *chloroform*, 50 volumes of *methanol* and 11.5 volumes of 13.5M *ammonia* as the mobile phase. Apply separately to the chromatoplate 5 µl of each of the following four solutions. For solution (1) dissolve 2.0 g of the substance being examined in 10 ml of a 10% w/v solution of *sodium hydrogen carbonate* and mix well with 12.5 g of white diatomaceous filter-aid (Celite 545 filtration grade is suitable). Transfer to a chromatographic tube (250 mm × 25 mm) fitted with a fritted glass disc and stopcock at the bottom. Pack the contents of the tube by tapping on a padded surface and then by tamping firmly from the top. Elute with *dichloromethane* so that 50 ml of eluate is obtained in about 30 minutes. Evaporate the eluate to dryness and dissolve the residue in 4.0 ml of *acetone*. Solution (2) contains 0.010% w/v of *toluene-2-sulphonamide BPCRS* in *acetone*. Solution (3) contains 0.50% w/v of the substance being examined in *methanol*. Solution (4) contains 0.0050% w/v of *4-sulphamoylbenzoic acid* in *acetone*.

After removal of the plate, dry it in a current of warm air, heat at 105° for 5 minutes and spray the hot plate with *sodium hypochlorite solution* diluted with *water* to contain 0.5% w/v of available chlorine. Dry in a current of cold air until a sprayed area of the plate below the line of application gives at most a faint blue colour with 0.05 ml of a 0.5% w/v solution of *potassium iodide* in *starch mucilage* containing 1% v/v of *glacial acetic acid*; avoid prolonged exposure to cold air. Spray the plate with the same mixture. Any spot corresponding to toluene-2-sulphonamide in the chromatogram obtained with solution (1) is not more intense than the spot in the chromatogram obtained with solution (2) and any spot corresponding to 4-sulphamoylbenzoic acid in the chromatogram obtained with solution (3) is not more intense than the spot in the chromatogram obtained with solution (4).

Readily carbonisable substances Dissolve 0.20 g in 5 ml of *sulphuric acid* and maintain at about 50° for 10 minutes. The solution is not more intensely coloured than *reference solution BY₆*, Appendix IV B, Method II.

Loss on drying When dried to constant weight at 105°, loses not more than 1.0% of its weight. Use 1 g.

Sulphated ash Not more than 0.2%, Appendix IX A.

Assay Dissolve 0.5 g in 75 ml of hot *water*, cool quickly and titrate with 0.1M *sodium hydroxide VS* using *phenolphthalein solution* as indicator. Each ml of 0.1M *sodium hydroxide VS* is equivalent to 0.01832 g of C₇H₅NO₃S.

Action and use Sweetening agent.

Saccharin Sodium
Soluble Saccharin

C₇H₄NNaO₃S   205.2   *6155-57-3*

Saccharin Sodium is the sodium salt of 1,2-benzisothiazolin-3-one 1,1-dioxide. It contains not less than 99.0 per cent and not more than 101.0 per cent of C₇H₄NNaO₃S, calculated with reference to the anhydrous substance.

Characteristics White crystals or a white, crystalline powder; odourless or almost odourless; efflorescent.

Solubility Soluble in 1.5 parts of *water* and in 50 parts of *ethanol (96%)*.

Identification A. Mix 20 mg with 40 mg of *resorcinol*, add 0.5 ml of *sulphuric acid* and heat over a small flame until a dark green colour is produced; allow to cool and add 10 ml of *water* and an excess of 5M *sodium hydroxide*. A fluorescent green liquid is produced.
B. Dissolve 0.1 g in 5 ml of a 10% w/v solution of *sodium hydroxide*, evaporate to dryness and gently fuse the residue over a small flame until ammonia is no longer evolved. Allow to cool, dissolve in 20 ml of *water*, make the solution just acidic to *litmus paper*, filter and add 0.05 ml of *iron(III) chloride test-solution*. A violet colour is produced.
C. The residue on ignition yields the *reactions* characteristic of sodium salts and of sulphates, Appendix VI.

Free acid or alkali To a solution of 1 g in *carbon dioxide-free water* add 5 ml of 0.005M *sulphuric acid VS*, boil, cool and titrate with 0.01M *sodium hydroxide VS* using *phenolphthalein solution* as indicator. 4.5 to 5.5 ml of 0.01M *sodium hydroxide VS* is required to change the colour of the solution.

Melting point of isolated saccharin Dissolve 1 g in 10 ml of *water* and add 1 ml of *hydrochloric acid*. A crystalline precipitate is produced which, when washed and dried, has a *melting point* not lower than 226°, Appendix V A.

Arsenic Mix 0.50 g with 0.3 g of *anhydrous sodium carbonate*, add 1 ml of *bromine water* and mix thoroughly. Evaporate to dryness on a water-bath, gently ignite and add to the cooled residue a mixture of 2 ml of *brominated hydrochloric acid* and 0.5 ml of *bromine water*. Add 4 ml of *water* and boil gently, occasionally adding sufficient *bromine water* to maintain a slight excess. Filter and remove the excess of bromine with a sufficient quantity of *tin(II) chloride solution AsT*. The resulting solution complies with the *limit test for arsenic*, Appendix VII (2 ppm).

Heavy metals A 10.0% w/v solution complies with *limit test A for heavy metals*, Appendix VII (10 ppm). Use *lead standard solution (1 ppm Pb)* to prepare the standard.

Related substances Complies with the test described under Saccharin, using for solution (1) 2.6 g of the substance being examined and for solution (2) a 0.0050% w/v solution of *toluene-2-sulphonamide BPCRS* in *acetone*.

Water 3.0 to 15.0% w/w, Appendix IX C. Use 1 g.

Assay Carry out Method I for *non-aqueous titration*, Appendix VIII A, using 0.3 g and *crystal violet solution* as indicator. Each ml of 0.1M *perchloric acid VS* is equivalent to 0.02052 g of $C_7H_4NNaO_3S$.

Storage Saccharin Sodium should be kept in a well-closed container.

Action and use Sweetening agent.

Salbutamol ☆

HO— (ring) —CH·CH₂·NHBuᵗ with OH above CH and HOCH₂ on ring

$C_{13}H_{21}NO_3$ 239.3   *18559-94-9*

Salbutamol is 1-(4-hydroxy-3-hydroxymethyl-phenyl)-2-(*tert*-butylamino)ethanol. It contains not less than 98.0 per cent and not more than 101.0 per cent of $C_{13}H_{21}NO_3$, calculated with reference to the dried substance.

Characteristics A white or almost white, crystalline powder. It melts at about 155°, with decomposition.

Solubility Soluble in 70 parts of *water* and in 25 parts of *ethanol (96%)*; slightly soluble in *ether*.

Identification *Test A may be omitted if tests B, C and D are carried out. Tests B and D may be omitted if tests A and C are carried out.*
A. The *infra-red absorption spectrum*, Appendix II A, is concordant with the spectrum of *salbutamol EPCRS*.
B. The *light absorption*, Appendix II B, in the range 230 to 350 nm of a 0.008% w/v solution in 0.1M *hydrochloric acid* exhibits a maximum only at 276 nm. The A(1%, 1 cm) at 276 nm is 66 to 75.
C. In the test for Related substances, the principal spot in the chromatogram obtained with solution (2) is similar in position, colour and size to the spot in the chromatogram obtained with solution (3).
D. Dissolve 10 mg in 50 ml of a 2% w/v solution of *sodium tetraborate*, add 1 ml of a 3% w/v solution of *4-aminophenazone*, 10 ml of a 2% w/v solution of *potassium hexacyanoferrate(III)* and 10 ml of *chloroform*, shake and allow to separate. An orange-red colour is produced in the chloroform layer.

Clarity and colour of solution A 2.0% w/v solution in *methanol* is *clear*, Appendix IV A, and not more intensely coloured than *reference solution BY₅*, Appendix IV B, Method II.

Related substances Carry out the method for *thin-layer chromatography*, Appendix III A, using *silica gel G* as the coating substance and a mixture of 50 volumes of *ethyl acetate*, 30 volumes of *propan-2-ol*, 16 volumes of *water* and 4 volumes of 13.5M *ammonia* as the mobile phase. Apply separately to the chromatoplate 5 μl of each of three solutions in *methanol* containing (1) 2.0% w/v of the substance being examined, (2) 0.010% w/v of the substance being examined and (3) 0.010% w/v of *salbutamol EPCRS*. After removal of the plate, allow it to dry in air until the odour of the solvent is no longer detectable, place it for a few minutes in an atmosphere saturated with *diethylamine* and spray with *diazotised sulphanilic acid solution*. Any *secondary spot* in the chromatogram obtained with solution (1) is not more intense than the spot in the chromatogram obtained with solution (3).

Loss on drying When dried to constant weight at 100° to 105°, loses not more than 0.5% of its weight. Use 1 g.

Sulphated ash Not more than 0.1%, Appendix IX A. Method II. Use 1 g.

Assay Carry out Method I for *non-aqueous titration*, Appendix VIII A, using 0.2 g dissolved in 30 ml of *anhydrous glacial acetic acid* and determining the end-point potentiometrically. Each ml of 0.1M *perchloric acid VS* is equivalent to 0.02393 g of $C_{13}H_{21}NO_3$.

Storage Salbutamol should be kept in a well-closed container and protected from light.

Action and use Beta-adrenoceptor agonist.

Salbutamol Sulphate

$(C_{13}H_{21}NO_3)_2,H_2SO_4$ 576.7   *51022-70-9*

Salbutamol Sulphate is 1-(4-hydroxy-3-hydroxymethylphenyl)-2-(*tert*-butylamino)-ethanol sulphate. It contains not less than 98.0 per cent and not more than 101.0 per cent of $(C_{13}H_{21}NO_3)_2,H_2SO_4$, calculated with reference to the dried substance.

Characteristics A white or almost white powder; odourless or almost odourless.

Solubility Soluble in 4 parts of *water*; slightly soluble in *ethanol (96%)*, in *chloroform* and in *ether*.

Identification A. The *infra-red absorption spectrum*, Appendix II A, is concordant with the *reference spectrum* of salbutamol sulphate.

B. The *light absorption*, Appendix II B, in the range 230 to 350 nm of a 0.008% w/v solution in 0.1M *hydrochloric acid* exhibits a maximum only at 276 nm. The *absorbance* at 276 nm is about 0.46.

C. Dissolve 10 mg in 50 ml of a 2% w/v solution of *sodium tetraborate*, add 1 ml of a 3% w/v solution of *4-aminophenazone*, 10 ml of a 2% w/v solution of *potassium hexacyanoferrate(III)* and 10 ml of *chloroform*, shake and allow to separate. An orange-red colour is produced in the chloroform layer.

D. To 2 ml of a 1% w/v solution add 0.1 ml of *iron(III) chloride test-solution*. A violet colour is produced which on addition of 1 ml of *sodium hydrogen carbonate solution* changes to orange. The solution may become opalescent.

E. Yields the *reactions* characteristic of sulphates, Appendix VI.

Boron Not more than 50 ppm when determined by the following method. To 50 mg add 5 ml of a 3% w/v solution of an equimolar mixture of *anhydrous sodium carbonate* and *potassium carbonate*, evaporate to dryness on a water-bath and dry at 120°. Ignite the residue rapidly until the organic matter has been destroyed, allow to cool and add 0.5 ml of *water* and 3 ml of a freshly prepared 0.125% w/v solution of *curcumin* in *glacial acetic acid*. Warm gently to effect solution, allow to cool and add 3 ml of a mixture prepared by adding slowly 5 ml of *sulphuric acid*, with stirring, to 5 ml of *glacial acetic acid*. Mix and allow to stand for 30 minutes. Add sufficient *ethanol (96%)* to produce 100 ml, filter and measure the *absorbance* of the filtrate at the maximum at 555 nm, Appendix II B. Calculate the content of boron from a reference curve prepared from the *absorbances* obtained by treating suitable aliquots of a solution of *boric acid* in the same manner.

Related substances Carry out the method for *thin-layer chromatography*, Appendix III A, using *silica gel G* as the coating substance and a mixture of 50 volumes of *ethyl acetate*, 30 volumes of *propan-2-ol*, 16 volumes of *water*

and 4 volumes of 13.5M *ammonia* as the mobile phase. Apply separately to the chromatoplate 10 µl of each of two solutions in *water* containing (1) 2.0% w/v of the substance being examined and (2) 0.010% w/v of *1-(4-hydroxy-3-methylphenyl)-2-(tert-butylamino)ethanol BPCRS*. After removal of the plate, allow it to dry in air until the odour of the solvent is no longer detectable, place it in an atmosphere saturated with *diethylamine* for a few minutes and spray with *diazotised nitroaniline solution*. Any *secondary spot* in the chromatogram obtained with solution (1) is not more intense than the spot in the chromatogram obtained with solution (2).

Loss on drying When dried to constant weight at 100° at a pressure not exceeding 0.7 kPa, loses not more than 0.5% of its weight. Use 1 g.

Sulphated ash Not more than 0.1%, Appendix IX A.

Assay Carry out Method I for *non-aqueous titration*, Appendix VIII A, using 0.9 g and *oracet blue B solution* as indicator. Each ml of 0.1M *perchloric acid VS* is equivalent to 0.05767 g of $(C_{13}H_{21}NO_3)_2,H_2SO_4$.

Storage Salbutamol Sulphate should be kept in a well-closed container and protected from light.

Preparations
Salbutamol Injection
Salbutamol Tablets

Action and use Beta-adrenoceptor agonist.

Salcatonin ☆

Cys-Ser-Asn-Leu-Ser-Thr-Cys-Val-Leu-Gly-Lys-Leu-Ser-
Gln-Glu-Leu-His-Lys-Leu-Gln-Thr-Tyr-Pro-Arg-Thr-Asn-
Thr-Gly-Ser-Gly-Thr-Pro—NH$_2$

47931-85-1

Salcatonin is a synthetic polypeptide having the structure determined for salmon calcitonin I that lowers the calcium concentration in plasma of mammals by diminishing the rate of bone resorption. It contains not less than 4000 Units per mg, calculated with reference to the peptide content.

Characteristics A white or almost white, light powder.

Solubility Freely soluble in *water*.

Identification A. Causes a hypocalcaemic response when injected as directed under the Assay.

B. Carry out the method for *thin-layer chromatography*, Appendix III A, using *microcrystalline cellulose* as the coating substance and a mixture of 30 volumes of *butan-1-ol*, 24 volumes of *water*, 20 volumes of *pyridine* and 6 volumes of *glacial acetic acid* as the mobile phase. Apply separately to the chromatoplate 1 µl of each of two freshly prepared solutions in 0.1M *acetic acid* containing (1) 0.25% w/v of the substance being examined and (2) 0.25% w/v of *calcitonin (salmon) EPCRS*. After removal of the plate, allow it to dry in air for 1 hour, heat at 110° for 10 minutes and spray the hot plate with a solution prepared immediately before use by diluting *sodium hypochlorite solution* with *water* to contain 0.5% w/v of available chlorine. Dry in a current of cold air until a sprayed area of the plate below the line of application gives at most a very faint blue colour with 0.05 ml of *potassium iodide and starch solution*; avoid prolonged exposure to the cold air. Spray the plate with *potassium iodide and starch solution*. The principal spot in the chromatogram obtained with solution (1) corresponds to that in the chromatogram obtained with solution (2).

C. It contains the amino acids in the proportions specified in the test for Amino acids. It does not contain alanine, methionine, phenylalanine or tryptophan.

Light absorption The *light absorption*, Appendix II B, in the range 250 to 280 nm of a 0.1% w/v solution in 0.01M *hydrochloric acid* exhibits a maximum at 275 nm. The *absorbance* at 275 nm is 0.40 to 0.55, calculated with reference to the peptide content. The ratio of the absorbance at 275 nm to that at 254 nm is not less than 1.6.

Acetic acid Not more than 15% w/w when determined by the method for *gas chromatography*, Appendix III B, using three solutions in *water* containing (1) 0.1% v/v of *glacial acetic acid* and 0.1% v/v of *1,4-dioxan* (internal standard), (2) 1.0% w/v of the substance being examined and (3) 1.0% w/v of the substance being examined and 0.1% v/v of the internal standard.

The chromatographic procedure may be carried out using a glass column (2 m × 2 mm) packed with porous polymer beads (100 to 120 mesh) (Porapak Q is suitable) and maintained at 150°.

Chloride Dissolve 0.7 mg in 15 ml of *water*. The resulting solution complies with the *limit test for chlorides*, Appendix VII (7%).

Related substances A. Carry out the method for *thin-layer chromatography*, Appendix III A, using *microcrystalline cellulose* as the coating substance and a mixture of 42 volumes of *butan-1-ol*, 30 volumes of *water*, 24 volumes of *pyridine* and 4 volumes of *glacial acetic acid* as the mobile phase. Apply separately to the chromatoplate, as bands about 1 cm wide, 10 µl of each of two solutions of the substance being examined in 0.1M *acetic acid* containing (1) 0.20% w/v and (2) 0.010% w/v. After removal of the plate, allow it to dry in air for 1 hour, heat at 110° for 10 minutes and then spray the hot plate with a solution prepared immediately before use by diluting *sodium hypochlorite solution* with *water* to contain 0.5% w/v of available chlorine. Dry in a current of cold air until a sprayed area of the plate below the line of application gives at most a very faint blue colour with 0.05 ml of *potassium iodide and starch solution*; avoid prolonged exposure to the cold air. Spray the plate with *potassium iodide and starch solution*. Any *secondary band* in the chromatogram obtained with solution (1) is not more intense than the band in the chromatogram obtained with solution (2).

B. Carry out the method for *cellulose acetate electrophoresis*, Appendix III F, using an electrolyte solution containing 60% v/v of a mixture of 225 volumes of *water*, 25 volumes of *pyridine* and 1 volume of *glacial acetic acid* and 40% v/v of *formamide*, applying a voltage of 17 volts per cm and allowing electrophoresis to proceed for 1 hour at 5°. Solution (1) is a 1.0% w/v solution of the substance being examined and solution (2) is a 1.0% w/v solution of *calcitonin (salmon) EPCRS*. Any *secondary spot* in the electrophoretogram obtained with solution (1) is not more intense than the corresponding spot in the electrophoretogram obtained with solution (2).

Amino acids Carry out the method for *amino acid analysis*, Appendix III G, using 1.0 mg and a quantity of DL-*norleucine* (internal standard) corresponding to about half the expected number of moles of salcatonin. Heat for 24 hours. Express the content of each amino acid in moles. Calculate the relative proportions of the amino acids taking as equivalent to 1 the sum, divided by 20, of the number of moles of aspartic acid, glutamic acid, proline, glycine, valine, leucine, histidine, arginine and lysine; the values fall within the following limits: aspartic acid, 1.8 to 2.2; glutamic acid, 2.7 to 3.3; proline, 1.7 to 2.3; glycine, 2.7 to 3.3; valine, 0.9 to 1.1; leucine, 4.5 to 5.3; histidine, 0.9 to 1.1; arginine, 0.9 to 1.1; lysine, 1.8 to 2.2; serine, 3.2 to 4.2; threonine, 4.2 to 5.2; tyrosine, 0.7 to 1.1; half-cystine, 1.4 to 2.1.

Peptide Not less than 80.0% when determined in the following manner. Calculate the average number of moles per residue from the sum, divided by 20, of the number of moles of aspartic acid, glutamic acid, proline, glycine, valine, leucine, histidine, arginine and lysine obtained in the test for Amino acids and calculate the percentage peptide content from the expression $343190VA/V_1W$ where W is the weight, in grams, of the substance being examined taken for hydrolysis, A is the average number of moles per residue, V is the final volume of hydrolysate and V_1 is the volume applied to the analyser. The determination is not valid unless the number of moles of norleucine recovered in the test for Amino acids, when corrected for the volume of hydrolysate applied, is within 5% of the amount taken for hydrolysis.

Water Not more than 10% w/w when determined by the method for *gas chromatography*, Appendix III B, using throughout dry glassware which may be siliconised and the following solutions. For solution (1) dilute 50 µl of *anhydrous methanol* (internal standard) with sufficient *anhydrous propan-2-ol* to produce 100 ml. For solution (2) dissolve 2 mg of the substance being examined in 0.5 ml of *anhydrous propan-2-ol*. For solution (3) dissolve 2 mg of the substance being examined in 0.5 ml of solution (1). For solution (4) add 10 µl of *water* to 50 ml of solution (1).

The chromatographic procedure may be carried out using a stainless steel column (1 m × 2 mm) packed with porous polymer beads (60 to 80 mesh) (Chromosorb 102 is suitable) maintained at 114°, helium as the carrier gas and a thermal conductivity detector maintained at 150°.

From the chromatograms obtained and taking into account any water detectable in solution (1), calculate the percentage w/w of water taking 0.9972 g as its weight per ml at 20°.

Total acetic acid and water Not more than 20% w/w when determined by adding together the percentages of acetic acid and water found by the methods described above.

Assay Carry out the *biological assay of salcatonin*, Appendix XIV C2. The estimated potency is not less than 80% and not more than 125% of the stated potency. The fiducial limits of error are not less than 64% and not more than 156% of the stated potency.

Storage Salcatonin should be kept in a well-closed container, protected from light and stored at a temperature of 2° to 8°. Under these conditions it may be expected to retain its potency for not less than 2 years.

Labelling The label states (1) the number of Units in the container; (2) the number of Units per mg; (3) the date after which the material is not intended to be used; (4) the conditions under which the material should be stored.

Preparation
Salcatonin Injection

Action and use Hypocalcaemic hormone.

The title of the monograph in the European Pharmacopœia is Calcitonin (Salmon).

Salicylic Acid ☆

CO₂H
OH

$C_7H_6O_3$ 138.1   *69-72-7*

Salicylic Acid is 2-hydroxybenzoic acid. It contains not less than 99.0 per cent and not more than 100.5 per cent of $C_7H_6O_3$, calculated with reference to the dried substance.

Characteristics White or colourless, acicular crystals or a white, crystalline powder.

Solubility Slightly soluble in *water*; freely soluble in *ethanol (96%)* and in *ether*; sparingly soluble in *chloroform*.

Identification *Test A may be omitted if tests B and C are carried out. Test B may be omitted if tests A and C are carried out.*
A. The *infra-red absorption spectrum*, Appendix II A, is concordant with the spectrum of *salicylic acid EPCRS*.
B. Dissolve 30 mg in 5 ml of 0.05M *sodium hydroxide*, neutralise if necessary and dilute to 20 ml with *water*. 1 ml of the solution yields *reaction A* characteristic of salicylates, Appendix VI.
C. *Melting point*, 158° to 161°, Appendix V A, Method I.

Clarity and colour of solution Dissolve 1.0 g in 10 ml of *ethanol (96%)*. The resulting solution is *clear*, Appendix IV A, and *colourless*, Appendix IV B, Method II.

Heavy metals Dissolve 2.0 g in 15 ml of *ethanol (96%)* and add 5 ml of *water*. 12 ml of the resulting solution complies with *limit test B for heavy metals*, Appendix VII (20 ppm). Use *lead standard solution (100 ppm Pb)*, diluted with a mixture of 3 volumes of *ethanol (96%)* and 1 volume of *water* to contain 2 µg of Pb per ml, to prepare the standard.

Chloride Dissolve 2.5 g in 50 ml of boiling *distilled water*, cool and filter. Reserve 15 ml of the filtrate for the test for Sulphate. Dilute 10 ml of the remaining filtrate to 15 ml with *water*. The resulting solution complies with the *limit test for chlorides*, Appendix VII (100 ppm).

Sulphate 15 ml of the filtrate reserved in the test for Chloride complies with the *limit test for sulphates*, Appendix VII (200 ppm).

Loss on drying When dried to constant weight in a desiccator, loses not more than 0.5% of its weight. Use 1 g.

Sulphated ash Not more than 0.1%, Appendix IX A, Method II. Use 2 g.

Assay Dissolve 0.12 g in 30 ml of *ethanol (96%)*, add 20 ml of *water* and titrate with 0.1M *sodium hydroxide VS*, using *phenol red solution* as indicator, until a reddish-violet colour is obtained. Each ml of 0.1M *sodium hydroxide VS* is equivalent to 0.01381 g of $C_7H_6O_3$.

Storage Salicylic Acid should be kept in a well-closed container and protected from light.

Preparations
Salicylic Acid Collodion
Salicylic Acid Lotion
Salicylic Acid Ointment
Coal Tar and Salicylic Acid Ointment
Zinc and Salicylic Acid Paste

Action and use Keratolytic.

Salsalate

CO₂H   OH
OCO

$C_{14}H_{10}O_5$ 258.2   *552-94-3*

Salsalate is *o*-(2-hydroxybenzoyl)salicylic acid. It contains not less than 99.0 per cent and not more than 101.0 per cent of $C_{14}H_{10}O_5$, calculated with reference to the dried substance.

Characteristics A white or almost white powder; odourless or almost odourless.

Solubility Very slightly soluble in *water*; soluble in 6 parts of *ethanol (96%)*, in 8 parts of *chloroform* and in 12 parts of *ether*.

Identification A. The *infra-red absorption spectrum*, Appendix II A, is concordant with the *reference spectrum* of salsalate.
B. Heat 0.2 g to boiling for 3 minutes with 4 ml of 2M *sodium hydroxide*, cool and add 5 ml of 1M *sulphuric acid*. The *melting point* of the precipitate, after washing with *water* and drying at 100° to 105°, is about 158°, Appendix V A.
C. *Melting point*, about 145°, Appendix V A.

Clarity and colour of solution A 10.0% w/v solution in *ethanol (96%)* is *clear*, Appendix IV A, and not more intensely coloured than *reference solution Y₅*, Appendix IV B, Method II.

Heavy metals Dissolve 0.75 g in 9 ml of *acetone* and add 6 ml of *water*. The solution complies with *limit test B for heavy metals*, Appendix VII (15 ppm). Use 10 ml of *lead standard solution (1 ppm Pb)* to prepare the standard.

Chloride Shake 1.5 g with 6 ml of *ethanol (96%)*, dilute with *water* to 50 ml, shake and filter. Reserve 15 ml of the filtrate for the test for Sulphate. 15 ml of the filtrate complies with the *limit test for chlorides*, Appendix VII (110 ppm).

Sulphate 10 ml of the filtrate reserved in the test for chloride, diluted to 15 ml, complies with the *limit test for sulphates*, Appendix VII (500 ppm).

Salicylic acid Not more than 0.5% when determined by the following method. Dissolve 1 g in 20 ml of *chloroform* and extract with four 20-ml quantities of *iron(III) nitrate solution*. Combine and filter the extracts and dilute to 100 ml with *iron(III) nitrate solution*. Measure the *absorbance* of the resulting solution at the maximum at 530 nm, Appendix II B, using *iron(III) nitrate solution* in the reference cell and calculate the content of salicylic acid from the *absorbance* of a solution prepared in the same manner but using 20 ml of a 0.025% w/v solution of *salicylic acid* in *chloroform* in place of the solution being examined.

Related substances Carry out the method for *thin-layer chromatography*, Appendix III A, using *silica gel GF254* as the coating substance and a mixture of 98 volumes of *butan-2-one* and 2 volumes of *glacial acetic acid* as the mobile phase. Apply separately to the chromatoplate 5 μl of each of three solutions in *ethanol (96%)* containing (1) 5.0% w/v of the substance being examined, (2) 0.010% w/v of the substance being examined and (3) 0.05% w/v of *salicylic acid*. After removal of the plate, allow it to dry in a current of air until the odour of acetic acid is no longer detectable. Examine under *ultra-violet light (254 nm)* and spray with a 1% w/v solution of *iron(III) nitrate* in 0.01M *acetic acid*. Under both methods of visualisation any *secondary spot* in the chromatogram obtained with solution (1), other than any spot corresponding to salicylic acid, is not more intense than the spot in the chromatogram obtained with solution (2).

Loss on drying When dried at 60° at a pressure not exceeding 0.7 kPa for 3 hours, loses not more than 0.5% of its weight. Use 1 g.

Sulphated ash Not more than 0.1%, Appendix IX A.

Assay Dissolve 0.5 g in 25 ml of *ethanol (96%)* previously neutralised to *bromothymol blue solution*, add 25 ml of *water* and titrate with 0.1M *sodium hydroxide VS* using *bromothymol blue solution* as indicator. Each ml of 0.1M *sodium hydroxide VS* is equivalent to 0.02582 g of $C_{14}H_{10}O_5$.

Storage Salsalate should be kept in a well-closed container.

Preparation

Salsalate Capsules

Action and use Anti-inflammatory; analgesic.

Selenium Sulphide

SeS₂   143.1   7488-56-4

Selenium Sulphide contains not less than 52.0 per cent and not more than 55.0 per cent of Se.

Characteristics A bright orange to reddish-brown powder; odour, faint, of hydrogen sulphide.

Identification A. Gently boil 50 mg with 5 ml of *nitric acid* for 30 minutes, dilute to 50 ml with *water* and filter. To 5 ml of the filtrate add 10 ml of *water* and 5 g of *urea*, boil, cool and add 2 ml of *potassium iodide solution*. A yellow to orange colour is produced which darkens rapidly on standing.
B. Allow the coloured solution obtained in test A to stand for 10 minutes and filter through *kieselguhr*. The filtrate yields the *reactions* characteristic of sulphates, Appendix VI.

Soluble selenium compounds To 10 g add 100 ml of *water*, mix well, allow to stand for 1 hour with frequent shaking and filter. To 10 ml of the filtrate add 2 ml of 2.5M *formic acid*, dilute to 50 ml with *water*, adjust the pH to 2.0 to 3.0 with 2.5M *formic acid*, add 2 ml of a 0.5% w/v solution of *3,3'-diaminobenzidine tetrahydro-*

chloride in *water*, allow to stand for 45 minutes and adjust the pH to 6.0 to 7.0 with 5M *ammonia*. Shake the solution for 1 minute with 10 ml of *toluene* and allow to separate. The *absorbance* of the toluene solution, Appendix II B, at the maximum at 420 nm is not greater than that of a solution prepared by treating 5 ml of *selenium standard solution (1 ppm Se)* in the same manner (5 ppm, calculated as Se).

Assay To 0.1 g add 25 ml of *fuming nitric acid*, heat on a water-bath for 1 hour, cool and dilute to 100 ml with *water*. To 25 ml of the solution add 10 ml of *potassium iodide solution* and 10 ml of *chloroform* and titrate immediately with 0.02M *sodium thiosulphate VS* until the aqueous layer is a pale straw colour. Stopper the flask, shake vigorously for 30 seconds, add 0.1 ml of *starch mucilage* and continue the titration to the complete absence of blue colour in the aqueous layer. Each ml of 0.02M *sodium thiosulphate VS* is equivalent to 0.0003948 g of Se.

Preparation

Selenium Sulphide Scalp Application

Action and use Used in treatment of dandruff and seborrhoeic dermatitis of the scalp.

Senega Root ☆

Senega

Senega Root consists of the dried root and root crown of *Polygala senega* L. or of certain closely-related species of *Polygala* or a mixture of these.

Characteristics Odour, faint, sweet, slightly rancid or reminiscent of methyl salicylate.

Macroscopical Root crown: greyish-brown, two to five times as wide as the root, forming an irregular head up to 3 cm in diameter consisting of numerous remains of stems and tightly-packed brownish-red buds. Tap root: brown to yellow, from 1 to 8 mm in diameter at the crown, gradually tapering to the tip, up to 10 cm or more in length; occasionally branched, usually tortuous without secondary roots, except that Japanese species and varieties have numerous fibrous rootlets about 4 to 10 cm long; surface transversely and longitudinally striated, often showing a more or less distinct decurrent, elongated, spiral keel. Fracture short, showing yellowish cortex of variable thickness, surrounding a paler central woody area somewhat circular or irregular in shape, according to species.

Microscopical Transverse section of root: cork formed from several layers of thin-walled cells, phelloderm of slightly collenchymatous cells containing droplets of oil; phloem and xylem arrangement usually normal, especially near the crown, but where a keel is present this is formed by increased development of phloem; other anomalous secondary development sometimes occurs resulting in the formation of one or two large wedge-shaped rays in the phloem and xylem composed of parenchymatous cells containing droplets of oil; xylem usually central, consisting of vessels up to 60 μm in diameter, associated with numerous thin-walled tracheids and a few small, lignified, parenchymatous cells.

Identification Carry out the method for *thin-layer chromatography*, Appendix III A, using *silica gel G* as the coating substance and the upper phase of a mixture of 50 volumes of *butan-1-ol*, 40 volumes of *water* and 10 volumes of *glacial acetic acid* as the mobile phase, but allowing the solvent front to ascend 12 cm above the line of application. Apply separately to the chromatoplate 10 μl of solution (1) and 10 μl and 40 μl of solution (2) as bands 20 mm long and not more than 3 mm wide. For solution (1) heat 1 g, in *No. 300 powder*, with 10 ml of *ethanol (70%)* under a reflux condenser for 15 minutes, filter and cool. For solution (2) dissolve 10 mg of *aescin* in sufficient *ethanol (70%)* to produce 10 ml. After removal of the plate, dry it at 100° to 105°, spray with about 10 ml of *anisaldehyde solution* (for a plate 200 mm × 200 mm in size) and heat again at 100° to 105° until the bands due to saponosides turn red. In the chromatogram obtained with solution (1) three to five red bands appear in the lower and middle part of the chromatogram; in the chromatograms obtained with solution (2) greyish-violet bands, due to aescin, appear at the same Rf values. Spray the plate with about 10 ml of a solution containing 2 g of *phosphomolybdic acid* in 10 ml of *ethanol (96%)* (for a plate 200 mm × 200 mm in size) and heat at 100° to 105° until the bands due to saponosides become blue. The size and intensity of the bands in the chromatogram obtained with solution (1) are intermediate between those in the chromatograms obtained with solution (2).

Foreign matter Not more than 2%, Appendix XI D, Test B.

Acid-insoluble ash Not more than 3.0%, Appendix XI K, Method II.

Sulphated ash Not more than 8.0%, Appendix IX A, Method II. Use 1 g, in powder.

Storage Senega Root should be kept in a well-closed container and protected from light.

Action and use Expectorant.

Powdered Senega Root

Powdered Senega Root is Senega Root in powder.

Characteristics Light brown; odour, irritant and sternutatory. Diagnostic structures: longitudinal fragments of lignified tissue made up of pitted tracheids and somewhat larger vessels with numerous bordered pits and with reticulate thickening; yellowish parenchyma and collenchymatous cells containing droplets of oil; occasional fragments of cork and of epidermal tissue with stomata and unicellular trichomes (from the bud scales); starch, crystals and stone cells absent. When shaken with *water*, the powder produces copious frothing.

Identification; Acid-insoluble ash; Sulphated ash Complies with the requirements stated under Senega Root.

Storage Powdered Senega Root should be kept in a well-closed container and protected from light.

Action and use Expectorant.

Alexandrian Senna Fruit ☆

Alexandrian Senna Fruit is the dried fruit of *Cassia senna* L. (*C. acutifolia* Delile). It contains not less than 3.4 per cent of hydroxyanthracene glycosides, calculated as sennoside B.

Characteristics Odour, slight.

Macroscopical Flattened reniform pods, green to greenish-brown at the edges, dark brown in the central area, about 40 to 50 mm long and at least 20 mm wide; stylar point at one end, short stalk at the other; containing six or seven flattened obovate seeds, green to pale brown, with a continuous network of prominent ridges on the testa.

Microscopical Epicarp with strongly cuticularised isodiametrical cells, occasional *anomocytic* or *paracytic* stomata and very few conical, unicellular and warty trichomes; hypodermis with collenchymatous cells; mesocarp with parenchymatous tissue, a layer of prisms of calcium oxalate and containing vascular bundles incompletely surrounded by fibres with a crystal sheath of calcium oxalate prisms; endocarp consisting of thick-walled and interlacing fibres. Seeds, subepidermal layer of palisade cells with thick outer walls; endosperm composed of polyhedral cells with mucilaginous walls.

Identification A. Carry out test A for Identification described under Senna Leaf. The chromatogram obtained with solution (1) shows two reddish-brown bands, due to sennoside B (Rf value 0.1 to 0.2) and sennoside A (Rf value 0.2 to 0.3), with Rf values similar to those in the chromatogram obtained with solution (2). The chromatograms obtained with both solutions also show two reddish-brown bands due to sennoside D (Rf value 0.3 to 0.4) and sennoside C (Rf value 0.4 to 0.5) and between them a red band due to rhein-8-glucoside may be visible.

B. Complies with test B for Identification described under Senna Leaf.

Foreign matter Not more than 1%, Appendix XI D, Test B.

Acid-insoluble ash Not more than 2.0%, Appendix XI K, Method II.

Assay Carry out the Assay described under Senna Leaf. Calculate the percentage content of hydroxyanthracene glycosides expressed as sennoside B taking 240 as the value of A(1%, 1 cm) at the maximum at 515 nm.

Storage Alexandrian Senna Fruit should be protected from light and moisture.

Preparations
Senna Liquid Extract
Senna Tablets

Action and use Stimulant laxative.

The title of the monograph in the European Pharmacopœia is Alexandrian Senna Pods.

Powdered Alexandrian Senna Fruit

Powdered Alexandrian Senna Fruit is Alexandrian Senna Fruit in powder. It contains not less than 3.4 per cent of hydroxyanthracene glycosides, calculated as sennoside B.

Characteristics Brown. Diagnostic structures: epicarp with polygonal cells and a small number of conical warty trichomes and occasional *anomocytic* or *paracytic* stomata; fibres in two crossed layers accompanied by a crystal sheath of calcium oxalate prisms; characteristic palisade cells in the seeds and stratified cells in the endosperm; clusters and prisms of calcium oxalate.

Identification A. Carry out test A for Identification described under Senna Leaf. The chromatogram obtained with solution (1) shows two reddish-brown bands, due to sennoside B (Rf value 0.1 to 0.2) and sennoside A (Rf value 0.2 to 0.3), with Rf values similar to those in the chromatogram obtained with solution (2). The chromatograms obtained with both solutions also show two reddish-brown bands due to sennoside D (Rf value 0.3 to 0.4) and sennoside C (Rf value 0.4 to 0.5) and between them a red band due to rhein-8-glucoside may be visible.

B. Complies with test B for Identification described under Senna Leaf.

Acid-insoluble ash Not more than 2.0%, Appendix XI K.

Assay Carry out the Assay described under Senna Leaf. Calculate the percentage content of hydroxyanthracene glycosides expressed as sennoside B taking 240 as the A(1%, 1 cm) at the maximum at 515 nm.

Storage Powdered Alexandrian Senna Fruit should be protected from light and moisture.

Action and use Stimulant laxative.

Tinnevelly Senna Fruit ☆

Tinnevelly Senna Fruit is the dried fruit of *Cassia angustifolia* Vahl. It contains not less than 2.2 per cent of hydroxyanthracene glycosides, caculated as sennoside B.

Characteristics Odour, slight.

Macroscopical Flattened reniform pods, yellowish-brown to brown at the edges, dark brown in the central area, about 35 to 60 mm long and 14 to 18 mm wide; stylar point at one end, short stalk at the other; containing five to eight flattened, obovate seeds, green to pale brown, with incomplete wavy transverse ridges on the testa.

Microscopical Epicarp with strongly cuticularised isodiametrical cells, occasional *anomocytic* or *paracytic* stomata and very few conical, unicellular and warty trichomes; hypodermis with collenchymatous cells; mesocarp with parenchymatous tissue, a layer of prisms of calcium oxalate and containing vascular bundles incompletely surrounded by fibres with a crystal sheath of calcium oxalate prisms; endocarp consisting of thick-walled and interlacing fibres. Seeds: subepidermal layer of palisade cells with thick outer walls; endosperm composed of polyhedral cells with mucilaginous walls.

Identification A. Carry out test A for Identification described under Senna Leaf. The chromatogram obtained with solution (1) shows two reddish-brown bands due to sennoside B (Rf value 0.1 to 0.2) and sennoside A (Rf value 0.2 to 0.3), with Rf values similar to those in the chromatogram obtained with solution (2). The chromatograms obtained with both solutions also show two reddish-brown bands due to sennoside D (Rf value 0.3 to 0.4) and sennoside C (Rf value 0.4 to 0.5) and between them a red band due to rhein-8-glucoside may be visible.

B. Complies with test B for Identification described under Senna Leaf.

Foreign matter Not more than 1%, Appendix XI D, Test B.

Acid-insoluble ash Not more than 2.0%, Appendix XI K, Method II.

Assay Carry out the Assay described under Senna Leaf. Calculate the percentage content of hydroxyanthracene glycosides expressed as sennoside B taking 240 as the value of A(1%, 1 cm) at the maximum at 515 nm.

Storage Tinnevelly Senna Fruit should be protected from light and moisture.

Preparations
Senna Liquid Extract
Senna Tablets

Action and use Stimulant laxative.

The title of the monograph in the European Pharmacopœia is Tinnevelly Senna Pods.

Powdered Tinnevelly Senna Fruit

Powdered Tinnevelly Senna Fruit is Tinnevelly Senna Fruit in powder. It contains not less than 2.2 per cent of hydroxyanthracene glycosides, calculated as sennoside B.

Characteristics Brown. Diagnostic structures: epicarp with polygonal cells and a small number of conical warty trichomes and occasional *anomocytic* or *paracytic* stomata; fibres in two crossed layers, accompanied by a crystal sheath of calcium oxalate prisms; characteristic palisade cells in the seeds and stratified cells in the endosperm; clusters and prisms of calcium oxalate.

Identification A. Carry out test A for Identification described under Senna Leaf. The chromatogram obtained with solution (1) shows two reddish-brown bands due to sennoside B (Rf value 0.1 to 0.2) and sennoside A (Rf value 0.2 to 0.3), with Rf values similar to those in the chromatogram obtained with solution (2). The chromatograms obtained with both solutions also show two reddish-brown bands due to sennoside D (Rf value 0.3 to 0.4) and and sennoside C (Rf value 0.4 to 0.5) and between them a red band due to rhein-8-glucoside may be visible.

B. Complies with test B for Identification described under Senna Leaf.

Acid-insoluble ash Not more than 2%, Appendix XI K.

Assay Carry out the Assay described under Senna Leaf. Calculate the percentage content of hydroxyanthracene glycosides expressed as sennoside B taking 240 as the value of A(1%, 1 cm) at the maximum at 515 nm.

Storage Powdered Tinnevelly Senna Fruit should be protected from light and moisture.

Action and use Stimulant laxative.

Senna Leaf ☆

Senna Leaf consists of the dried leaflets of Alexandrian or Khartoum senna, *Cassia senna* L. (*C. acutifolia* Delile), or Tinnevelly senna, *C. angustifolia* Vahl, or a mixture of both species. It contains not less than 2.5 per cent of hydroxyanthracene glycosides, calculated as sennoside B.

Characteristics Odour, slight and characteristic.

Macroscopical Alexandrian senna leaf. Greyish-green to brownish-green, thin fragile leaflets, lanceolate, mucronate, asymmetrical at the base, 15 to 40 mm long and 5 to 15 mm wide, the maximum width being at a point slightly below the centre. Lamina slightly undulant, both surfaces covered with fine, short trichomes. Pinnate venation, visible mainly on the lower surface with lateral veins leaving the midrib at about 60° and anastomosing to form a ridge near the margin.

Tinnevelly senna leaf. Yellowish-green to brownish-green leaflets, elongated and lanceolate, slightly asymmetrical at the base, 20 to 50 mm long and 7 to 20 mm wide at the centre. The two surfaces are smooth with a very small number of short trichomes and frequently marked with transverse or oblique lines.

Microscopical Leaf presents an isobilateral structure; epidermal cells tabular with straight anticlinal walls and frequently containing mucilage staining pink with *ruthenium red solution*. Trichomes, unicellular, up to 250 µm long with thick warty walls usually curved near the base and pointing in the direction of the limb; the base surrounded by radial epidermal cells. *paracytic* stomata; palisade parenchyma is interrupted above the midrib where it is replaced by collenchyma. Vascular bundles incompletely surrounded by fibres with a crystal sheath containing calcium oxalate prisms. Occasional cluster crystals of calcium oxalate in the mesophyll.

Identification A. Carry out the method for *thin-layer chromatography*, Appendix III A, using *silica gel G* as the coating substance and a mixture of 40 volumes of *ethyl acetate*, 40 volumes of *propan-1-ol* and 30 volumes of *water* as the mobile phase, but allowing the solvent front to ascend 10 cm above the line of application. Apply separately to the chromatoplate, as bands 20 mm long and not more than 2 mm wide, 10 µl of each of the following solutions. For solution (1) heat to boiling 0.5 g, in *No. 180 powder*, with 5 ml of a mixture of equal volumes of *ethanol (96%)* and *water*, centrifuge and use the supernatant liquid. For solution (2) dissolve 10 mg of *senna extract EPCRS* in 1 ml of a mixture of equal volumes of *ethanol (96%)* and *water*. (A slight residue remains.) After removal of the plate, allow the solvent to evaporate, spray with a 20% v/v solution of *nitric acid*, heat at 120° for 10 minutes, allow to cool and spray with a 5% w/v solution of *potassium hydroxide* in *ethanol (50%)* until the bands appear. The chromatogram obtained with solution (1) shows two reddish-brown bands due to sennoside B (Rf value 0.1 to 0.2) and sennoside A (Rf value 0.2 to 0.3) with Rf values similar to those in the chromatogram obtained with solution (2). The chromatograms obtained with both solutions show two reddish-brown bands due to sennoside D (Rf value 0.3 to 0.4) and sennoside C (Rf value 0.4 to 0.5) and between them a red band due to rhein-8-glucoside may be visible. B. To 25 mg, in *No. 180 powder*, add 50 ml of *water* and 2 ml of *hydrochloric acid*, heat in a water-bath for 15 minutes, allow to cool and shake with 40 ml of *ether*. Dry the ether layer over *anhydrous sodium sulphate*, evaporate 5 ml to dryness, cool and add 5 ml of 6M *ammonia* to the residue; a yellow or orange colour is produced. Heat on a water-bath for 2 minutes; a reddish-violet colour is produced.

Cassia auriculata Mount 50 leaf fragments in an 80% w/v solution of *sulphuric acid*; no carmine red colour appears. Shake 0.2 g, in powder, with 3 ml of *ethanol (96%)* for 3 minutes, filter, add 0.2 g of *decolorising charcoal*, shake and filter. Add an equal volume of a 33% w/v solution of *sulphuric acid* to the filtrate. No red colour is produced either in the cold or after heating for 1 minute on a water-bath.

Foreign matter Not more than 3% of foreign organs and not more than 1% of foreign elements, Appendix XI D, Test B.

Stomatal index Alexandrian senna, 10 to 15, usually 12.5; Tinnevelly senna, 14 to 20, usually 17.5, Appendix XI H.

Acid-insoluble ash Not more than 2.5%, Appendix XI K, Method II.

Assay To 0.15 g, in *No. 180 powder*, add 30 ml of *water*, mix, weigh, heat under a reflux condenser in a water-bath for 15 minutes, allow to cool, weigh and restore to the original weight with *water*. Centrifuge, transfer 20 ml of the supernatant liquid to a 150-ml separating funnel, add 0.1 ml of 2M *hydrochloric acid*, shake with three 15-ml quantities of *chloroform*, allow the layers to separate, discard the chloroform layer, add 0.1 g of *sodium hydrogen carbonate* and shake for 3 minutes. Centrifuge the aqueous layer and transfer 10 ml of the supernatant liquid to a 100-ml round-bottomed flask fitted with a ground-glass neck. Add 20 ml of a 10.5% w/v solution of *iron(III) chloride hexahydrate*, mix, heat under a reflux condenser in a water-bath for 20 minutes, add 1 ml of *hydrochloric acid* and continue heating for 20 minutes, shaking frequently, until the precipitate is dissolved. Cool, transfer the mixture to a separating funnel and shake with three 25-ml quantities of *ether* previously used to rinse the flask; combine the ether extracts and wash with two 15-ml quantities of *water*. Dilute the ether extracts to 100 ml with *ether*, evaporate 10 ml carefully to dryness and dissolve the residue in 10 ml of a 0.5% w/v solution of *magnesium acetate* in *methanol*. Measure the *absorbance* of the resulting solution at 515 nm, Appendix II B, using *methanol* in the reference cell. Calculate the percentage content of hydroxyanthracene glycosides expressed as sennoside B taking 240 as the value of A(1%, 1 cm) at the maximum at 515 nm.

Storage Senna Leaf should be protected from light and moisture.

Action and use Stimulant laxative.

Powdered Senna Leaf

Powdered Senna Leaf is Senna Leaf in powder. It contains not less than 2.5 per cent of hydroxyanthracene glycosides, calculated as sennoside B.

Characteristics Light green to greenish-yellow. Diagnostic structures: polygonal epidermal cells showing *paracytic* stomata. Unicellular trichomes, conical in shape, with warty walls, isolated or attached to fragments of epidermis. Fragments of fibro-vascular bundles with a cryatal sheath containing calcium oxalate prisms. Cluster crystals isolated or in fragments of parenchyma.

Identification Complies with the requirements stated under Senna Leaf.

Cassia auriculata Shake 0.2 g with 3 ml of *ethanol (96%)* for 3 minutes, filter, add 0.2 g of *decolorising charcoal*, shake and filter. Add an equal volume of a 33% w/v solution of *sulphuric acid* to the filtrate. No red colour is produced either in the cold or after heating for 1 minute on a water-bath.

Acid-insoluble ash Not more than 2.5%, Appendix XI K.

Assay Carry out the Assay described under Senna Leaf. Calculate the percentage content of hydroxyanthracene glycosides expressed as sennoside B taking 240 as the value of A(1%, 1 cm) at the maximum at 515 nm.

Storage Powdered Senna Leaf should be protected from light and moisture.

Action and use Stimulant laxative.

Sesame Oil ☆

Sesame Oil is the fixed oil obtained from the ripe seeds of *Sesamum indicum* L. by expression or extraction and subsequent refining.

Characteristics A clear, light yellow liquid; almost odourless. It solidifies to a buttery mass at about $-4°$.

Solubility Practically insoluble in *ethanol (96%)*; miscible with *chloroform*, with *ether* and with petroleum spirit.

Identification A. Carry out the test for *identification of fixed oils by thin-layer chromatography*, Appendix X N. The chromatogram obtained from the oil is concordant with the *typical chromatogram* for sesame oil.
B. Shake 10 ml with a mixture of 4.5 ml of *acetic anhydride* and 0.5 ml of a 0.35% v/v solution of *furfuraldehyde* in *acetic anhydride* in a cylinder fitted with a ground-glass stopper, filter through a filter paper impregnated with *acetic anhydride* and add to the filtrate 0.2 ml of *sulphuric acid*. A bluish-green colour is produced.

Acid value Not more than 0.6, Appendix X B.

Peroxide value Not more than 5.0, Appendix X F.

Refractive index 1.472 to 1.476, Appendix V E.

Relative density 0.915 to 0.923, Appendix V G.

Unsaponifiable matter Not more than 1.8% w/w, Appendix X H, Method II.

Alkaline impurities Complies with the test for *alkaline impurities*, Appendix X N.

Foreign fixed oils Carry out the test for *foreign oils by gas chromatography*, Appendix X N. The fatty-acid fraction of the oil has the following composition.
Saturated fatty acids of chain length less than C_{16} Not more than 0.5%.
Palmitic acid 7.0 to 12.0%.
Stearic acid 3.5 to 6.0%.
Oleic acid 35.0 to 50.0%.
Linoleic acid (equivalent chain length on polyethylene glycol adipate 18.9) 35.0 to 50.0%.
Linolenic acid (equivalent chain length on polyethylene glycol adipate 19.7) Not more than 1.0%.
Arachidic acid Not more than 1.0%.
Gadoleic acid (equivalent chain length on polyethylene glycol adipate 20.3) Not more than 0.5%.
Behenic acid Not more than 0.5%.

Erucic acid (equivalent chain length on polyethylene glycol adipate 22.3) Not more than 0.1%.

Storage Sesame Oil should be kept in a well-filled, well-closed container and protected from light. Sesame Oil intended for use in the manufacture of a parenteral dosage form should be stored in a glass container.

Labelling When the addition of antioxidants is authorised, the name and quantity of the added antioxidant are stated on the label.

The label states if the contents of the container are suitable for parenteral administration.

Sesame oil intended for use in the manufacture of a parenteral dosage form complies with the requirements stated above with the following modification and with the additional test for water.

Acid value Not more than 0.3, Appendix X B.

Water Not more than 0.05%, Appendix IX C. Use 5 g.

Colloidal Anhydrous Silica ☆

SiO_2 60.1   *7631-86-9*

Colloidal Anhydrous Silica contains not less than 99.0 per cent and not more than 100.5 per cent of SiO_2, determined on the substance ignited at 900°.

Characteristics A light, fine, white amorphous powder; odourless. It has a particle size of about 15 μm.

Solubility Practically insoluble in *water* and in mineral acids with the exception of *hydrofluoric acid*. It dissolves in hot solutions of alkali hydroxides. When 1 g is shaken vigorously with 20 ml of *carbon tetrachloride* for 3 minutes a transparent gel is produced.

Identification 20 mg yields the *reaction* characteristic of silicates, Appendix VI.

Acidity Shake 1 g with 30 ml of *carbon dioxide-free water*. The pH of the resulting suspension is 3.5 to 5.5, Appendix V L.

Heavy metals Suspend 2.5 g in sufficient *water* to produce a semi-fluid slurry and dry at 140°. When the dried substance is white, break up the mass using a glass rod, add 25 ml of *1M hydrochloric acid*, boil gently for 5 minutes, stirring frequently, centrifuge for 20 minutes and filter the supernatant liquid through a membrane filter. To the residue in the centrifuge tube add 3 ml of *2M hydrochloric acid* and 9 ml of *water*, boil, centrifuge for 20 minutes and filter the supernatant liquid through the same membrane filter. Wash the residue with small quantities of *water*, combine the filtrates and washings and dilute to 50 ml with *water*. To 20 ml of the solution add 50 mg of *L-ascorbic acid* and 1 ml of *13.5M ammonia*, neutralise with *2M ammonia* and dilute to 25 ml with *water*. 12 ml of the resulting solution complies with *limit test A for heavy metals*, Appendix VII (25 ppm). Use *lead standard solution (1 ppm Pb)* to prepare the standard.

Chloride To 1.0 g add a mixture of 20 ml of *2M nitric acid* and 30 ml of *water*, heat on a water-bath for 15 minutes, shaking frequently, dilute to 50 ml with *water*, filter if necessary and cool. 10 ml of the filtrate diluted to 15 ml with *water* complies with the *limit test for chlorides*, Appendix VII (250 ppm).

Loss on ignition When ignited at 900° in a platinum crucible for 2 hours, loses not more than 5.0% of its weight. Use 0.2 g and allow to cool in a desiccator before weighing.

Assay To the residue obtained in the test for Loss on ignition add 0.2 ml of *sulphuric acid* and sufficient *ethanol (96%)* to moisten the residue completely, add 6 ml of *hydrofluoric acid* and evaporate to dryness on a hot-plate at 95° to 105°, avoiding loss from spitting. Wash the sides of the dish with 6 ml of *hydrofluoric acid*, evaporate to dryness, ignite at 900°, allow to cool in a desiccator and weigh. The difference between the weight of the final residue and that of the residue obtained in the test for Loss on ignition represents the amount of SiO_2 in the amount of substance taken for the test for Loss on ignition.

Action and use Pharmaceutical aid.

Silver Nitrate ☆

AgNO₃   169.9   7761-88-8

Silver Nitrate contains not less than 99.0 per cent and not more than 100.5 per cent of $AgNO_3$.

Characteristics Colourless, transparent crystals or a white, crystalline powder; odourless.

Solubility Soluble in 0.5 part of *water* and in 27 parts of *ethanol (96%)*.

Identification Yields the *reactions* characteristic of silver salts and *reaction A* characteristic of nitrates, Appendix VI.

Acidity or alkalinity To 2 ml of a 4.0% w/v solution (solution A) add 0.1 ml of *bromocresol green solution*; the solution is blue. To 2 ml of solution A add 0.1 ml of *phenol red solution*; the solution is yellow.

Clarity and colour of solution Solution A is *clear*, Appendix IV A, and *colourless*, Appendix IV B, Method II.

Aluminium, bismuth, copper and lead Dissolve 1.0 g in a mixture of 4 ml of 13.5M *ammonia* and 6 ml of *water*. The resulting solution is *clear*, Appendix IV A, and *colourless*, Appendix IV B, Method II.

Foreign salts To 30 ml of solution A add 7.5 ml of 2M *hydrochloric acid*, shake vigorously, heat for 5 minutes on a water-bath, filter and evaporate 20 ml of the filtrate to dryness on a water-bath. The residue, when dried at 100° to 105°, weighs not more than 2 mg (0.3%).

Assay Dissolve 0.3 g in 50 ml of *water*, add 2 ml of 2M *nitric acid* and 2 ml of *ammonium iron(III) sulphate solution* and titrate with 0.1M *ammonium thiocyanate VS* until a reddish-yellow colour is produced. Each ml of 0.1M *ammonium thiocyanate VS* is equivalent to 0.01699 g of $AgNO_3$.

Storage Silver Nitrate should be kept in a well-closed, non-metallic container and protected from light.

Soft Soap

Soft Soap is soap made by the interaction of potassium hydroxide or sodium hydroxide with a suitable vegetable oil or oils or with fatty acids derived therefrom. It yields not less than 44.0 per cent of fatty acids. It may be coloured with chlorophyll or not more than 0.015 per cent of a suitable green soap dye.

Characteristics A yellowish-white to green or brown, unctuous substance.

Solubility Soluble in *water* and in *ethanol (96%)*.

Chlorides and other ethanol-insoluble substances Dissolve 5 g in 100 ml of hot *ethanol (96%)* previously neutralised to *phenolphthalein solution*, filter through a dried and tared filter, wash the residue thoroughly with hot neutralised *ethanol (96%)* and dry to constant weight at 105°. The residue weighs not more than 0.15 g.

Free fatty acid or alkali hydroxide Boil 250 ml of *ethanol (96%)* to remove carbon dioxide, add 0.5 ml of *phenolphthalein solution*, allow to cool to 70° and neutralise, if necessary, with 0.1M *sodium hydroxide VS* or 0.05M *sulphuric acid VS*. To 100 ml of the neutral ethanol add 10 g of the substance being examined and dissolve it as quickly as possible by heating under a reflux condenser. Cool to 70° and, if the solution is not pink, titrate at 70° with 0.1M *sodium hydroxide VS*; not more than 0.2 ml is required. If the solution is pink, add in a thin stream 5 ml of hot *barium chloride solution* previously neutralised to *phenolphthalein solution*, mix thoroughly and titrate with 0.1M *hydrochloric acid VS* until the pink colour disappears; not more than 1.0 ml is required.

Total free alkali To 100 ml of neutral ethanol prepared as described in the test for Free fatty acid or alkali hydroxide add 10 g of the substance being examined and dissolve it as quickly as possible by heating under a reflux condenser. Add immediately 3 ml of 0.5M *sulphuric acid VS* and boil under a reflux condenser on a water-bath for at least 10 minutes. If the solution is not pink, cool to 70° and titrate with 1M *sodium hydroxide VS* until a pink colour is produced. The volume of 0.5M *sulphuric acid VS* neutralised by the substance being examined is not more than 1.0 ml.

Unsaponifiable matter and unsaponified neutral fat Dissolve 5 g in 80 ml of a mixture of 50 ml of *ethanol (96%)* and 100 ml of *water*, without heating more than is necessary, and transfer to a separating funnel, washing the vessel with the remaining 70 ml of the mixture. Extract with 100 ml of *ether* while still slightly warm, run off the ethanolic soap layer into a second separating funnel and extract with 50 ml of *ether*. Repeat the extraction with 50 ml of *ether* and pour the three ether extracts into a separating funnel containing 20 ml of *water*. Rotate the separating funnel without violent shaking and, after allowing the liquids to separate, run off the water. Repeat the washing with *water* in the same manner until the separated washings are not more than faintly turbid when acidified. Wash the ether solution twice by shaking vigorously with 20 ml of 0.5M *potassium hydroxide*, each washing with alkali being immediately followed by washing with 20 ml of *water*, shaking vigorously each time. Acidify the last alkali washing after separation and, if the liquid becomes turbid, repeat the washing with 0.5M *potassium hydroxide* and *water* until the alkali washing remains clear on acidification. Finally wash with successive 20-ml quantities of *water* until the washings do not give a pink colour with *phenolphthalein solution*. Transfer the ether solution to a tared flask and remove the ether. When nearly all the ether has evaporated, add 3 ml of *acetone*. With the aid of a gentle current of air remove the solvent completely from the flask, which is preferably almost entirely immersed in boiling water, held obliquely and rotated. Repeat the last operation until the weight of the residue is constant. The residue weighs not more than 40 mg.

Characteristics of the fatty acids obtained in the Assay

Acid value Not greater than 205, Appendix X B, when determined on 2 to 3 g of the fatty acids, using 0.5M *potassium hydroxide VS* and substituting 0.02805 for 0.00561 in the formula.

Iodine value Not less than 83 (*iodine monochloride method*), Appendix X E.

Solidifying point Not above 31°, Appendix V B, with the following modifications. Where the determination is made at 15° to 20° the 1000-ml beaker and cooling liquid need not be used. Where the room temperature falls outside this range the 1000-ml beaker should contain water maintained at 15° to 20° and the level of this water should not be below the level of the sample in the inner tube.

Transfer about 15 ml of the melted fatty acids to the inner test-tube. Before the temperature of the fatty acids drops to a point 10° above their expected solidifying point, begin agitation in a vertical manner at a rate of 100 complete up and down motions per minute, the stirrer moving through a vertical distance of about 38 mm. Continue stirring in this manner until the temperature has remained constant for 30 seconds or has begun to rise within 30 seconds of ceasing to fall. Discontinue stirring immediately and lift the stirrer out of the sample. Observe the rise in temperature; the highest temperature reached after cessation of stirring is the solidifying point of the fatty acids. When reading the thermometer avoid all undue vibration as this will cause the temperature to drop before reaching the maximum.

Resin Mix 0.5 ml of the melted fatty acids in a test-tube with 2 ml of *acetic anhydride*, warm, shake until clear and cool to 15.5°. Transfer one drop of this solution to a white porcelain tile, place one drop of a cold mixture of equal volumes of *sulphuric acid* and *water* adjacent to it and gently bring the drops together with a glass rod. No transient violet colour is produced.

Assay Dissolve 30 g in 100 ml of *water*, transfer to a separating funnel, acidify with 1M *sulphuric acid* and extract with successive quantities of 50, 40 and 30 ml of *ether*. Mix the ether solutions in a separating funnel and wash with *water* until the washings are free from mineral acid. Transfer the ether solution to a tared flask, remove the ether and dry the residue of fatty acids to constant weight at 80°.

Preparation
Soap Spirit

Soda Lime

8006-28-8

Soda Lime is a mixture of sodium hydroxide, or sodium hydroxide and potassium hydroxide, with calcium hydroxide.

Characteristics White or greyish-white granules, or it may be coloured with an indicator to show when its absorptive capacity is exhausted. It absorbs about 20% of its weight of carbon dioxide.

Solubility Partially soluble in *water*; almost completely soluble in 1M *acetic acid*.

Identification A. When moistened with *hydrochloric acid* and introduced on a platinum wire into a flame, imparts a yellow colour to the flame.
B. A solution in 1M *acetic acid* yields *reaction C* characteristic of calcium salts, Appendix VI.
C. A suspension in *water* is strongly alkaline to *litmus paper*.

Hardness of granules Shake 200 g on a sieve No. 2000 for 3 minutes using a mechanical sieve shaker that reproduces in a uniform manner the circular and tapping motion given to sieves in manual use and has a frequency of oscillation of 282 to 288 cycles per minute. Place 50 g of the retained material in a hardness pan 20 cm in diameter having a concave brass bottom, 7.9 mm thick at the circumference, 3.2 mm thick at the centre and with an inside spherical radius of curvature of 109 cm. Add 15 steel balls, 7.9 mm in diameter, and shake on the mechanical sieve shaker for 30 minutes. Remove the steel balls, transfer the contents of the pan to a sieve No. 2000 and again shake on the mechanical sieve shaker for 3 minutes. The material retained by the sieve weighs not less than 37.5 g.

Size of granules Shake 500 g on a perforated plate of nominal pore size 6.70 mm; not more than 5 g is retained. Then shake on a sieve No. 4750; not more than 50 g is retained. Shake the unretained material on a sieve No. 1400; not more than 20 g passes through. Shake the unretained material on a sieve No. 600; not more than 7.5 g passes through.

Loss on drying When dried to constant weight at 105°, loses 14.0 to 21.0% of its weight. Use 1 g.

Moisture absorption Place 10 g in an open glass dish about 50 mm in diameter and 30 mm high in a desiccator over *sulphuric acid (14%)* and allow it to remain for 24 hours. The increase in weight is not more than 7.5%.

Carbon dioxide absorption Carry out the method for the determination of *absorption of carbon dioxide by soda lime*, Appendix IX D. The *activity* is not less than 120 minutes.

Storage Soda Lime should be kept in a well-closed container.

Action and use Used to absorb carbon dioxide.

Sodium Acetate ☆

$C_2H_3NaO_2,3H_2O$ 136.1   *6131-90-4*

Sodium Acetate* contains not less than 99.0 per cent and not more than 101.0 per cent of $C_2H_3NaO_2$, calculated with reference to the dried substance.

Characteristics Colourless crystals.

Solubility Soluble in 0.8 part of *water* and in 19 parts of *ethanol (96%)*.

Identification Yields *reactions A* and *B* characteristic of sodium salts and *reactions A* and *B* characteristic of acetates, Appendix VI.

Clarity and colour of solution A 10.0% w/v solution in *carbon dioxide-free water* prepared from *distilled water* (solution A) is *clear*, Appendix IV A, and *colourless*, Appendix IV B, Method II.

Alkalinity pH of a 5% w/v solution, 7.5 to 9.0, Appendix V L.

Arsenic 0.5 g complies with the *limit test for arsenic*, Appendix VII (2 ppm).

Calcium and magnesium Mix 200 ml of *water* with 10 ml of *ammonia buffer pH 10.0*, 0.1 ml of *mordant black 11 mixture* and 2 ml of *0.05M zinc chloride*. Add dropwise *0.02M disodium edetate VS* until the colour changes from violet-red to green. To this solution add 10 g of the substance being examined, shake to dissolve and titrate with *0.02M disodium edetate VS* until the green colour is restored. Not more than 0.65 ml of *0.02M disodium edetate VS* is required (50 ppm, calculated as Ca).

Heavy metals 12 ml of solution A complies with *limit test A for heavy metals*, Appendix VII (10 ppm). Use *lead standard solution (1 ppm Pb)* to prepare the standard.

Iron 10 ml of solution A complies with the *limit test for iron*, Appendix VII (10 ppm).

Chloride 2.5 ml of solution A diluted to 15 ml with *water* complies with the *limit test for chlorides*, Appendix VII (200 ppm).

Sulphate 7.5 ml of solution A diluted to 15 ml with *distilled water* complies with the *limit test for sulphates*, Appendix VII (200 ppm).

Reducing substances Dissolve 1.0 g in 100 ml of boiling *water*, add 5 ml of *1M sulphuric acid* and 0.5 ml of *0.002M potassium permanganate*, mix and boil gently for 5 minutes. The pink colour is not completely discharged.

Loss on drying 39.9 to 40.5% when determined by drying 1 g at 130°. Place the substance being examined in the oven while the latter is still cold.

Assay Dissolve 0.25 g in 50 ml of *anhydrous glacial acetic acid*, add 5 ml of *acetic anhydride* and allow to stand for 30 minutes. Carry out Method I for *non-aqueous titration*, Appendix VIII A, using *0.1M perchloric acid VS* and 0.3 ml of *1-naphtholbenzein solution* as indicator. Each ml of *0.1M perchloric acid VS* is equivalent to 0.00820 g of $C_2H_3NaO_2$.

Storage Sodium Acetate should be kept in an airtight container.

*The material described in this monograph is not necessarily suitable for the preparation of dialysis solutions.

Sodium Acid Citrate
Disodium Hydrogen Citrate

$C_6H_6Na_2O_7,1\frac{1}{2}H_2O$ 263.1   *144-33-2*

Sodium Acid Citrate contains not less than 98.0 per cent and not more than 104.0 per cent of $C_6H_6Na_2O_7,1\frac{1}{2}H_2O$.

Characteristics A white powder; odourless or almost odourless.

Solubility Soluble in less than 2 parts of *water*; practically insoluble in *ethanol (96%)*.

Identification Yields the *reactions* characteristic of sodium salts and of citrates, Appendix VI.

Acidity pH of a 3% w/v solution, 4.9 to 5.2, Appendix V L.

Arsenic 0.50 g dissolved in 25 ml of *water* complies with the *limit test for arsenic*, Appendix VII (2 ppm).

Heavy metals Dissolve 1.0 g in 20 ml of *water*. 12 ml of the resulting solution complies with *limit test A for heavy metals*, Appendix VII (20 ppm). Use *lead standard solution (1 ppm Pb)* to prepare the standard.

Chloride Dissolve 1.0 g in 100 ml of *water*. 15 ml of the resulting solution complies with the *limit test for chlorides*, Appendix VII (330 ppm).

Oxalate Dissolve 1.0 g in 4 ml of *water*, add 3 ml of *hydrochloric acid* and 1 g of *granulated zinc* and heat on a water-bath for 1 minute. Allow to stand for 2 minutes, decant the liquid into a test-tube containing 0.25 ml of a 1% w/v solution of *phenylhydrazine hydrochloride* and heat to boiling. Cool rapidly, transfer to a graduated measuring cylinder, add an equal volume of *hydrochloric acid* and 0.25 ml of a 5% w/v solution of *potassium hexacyanoferrate(III)*, shake and allow to stand for 30 minutes. Any red colour produced is not more intense than that produced by treating in the same manner 4 ml of a 0.005% solution of *oxalic acid* (150 ppm).

Sulphate Dissolve 0.50 g in 57 ml of *water* and add 3 ml of *2M hydrochloric acid*. 15 ml of the resulting solution complies with the *limit test for sulphates*, Appendix VII (0.12%).

Readily carbonisable substances Heat 1.0 g, in powder, with 10 ml of *sulphuric acid* for 30 minutes in a water-bath protected from light. Not more than a pale brown colour is produced.

Assay Heat 2 g until carbonised, cool and boil the residue with 50 ml each of *water* and *0.5M hydrochloric acid VS*. Filter, wash the filter with *water* and titrate the excess of acid in the filtrate and washings with *0.5M sodium hydroxide VS* using *methyl orange solution* as indicator. Each ml of *0.5M hydrochloric acid VS* is equivalent to 0.06578 g of $C_6H_6Na_2O_7,1\frac{1}{2}H_2O$.

Action and use Anticoagulant.

Sodium Acid Phosphate ☆

$NaH_2PO_4,2H_2O$ 156.0   *13472-35-0*

Sodium Acid Phosphate contains not less than 98.0 per cent and not more than 100.5 per cent of NaH_2PO_4, calculated with reference to the dried substance.

Characteristics Colourless crystals or a white, crystalline powder; odourless.

Solubility Soluble in 1 part of *water*; very slightly soluble in *ethanol (96%)*.

Identification A. A 10.0% w/v solution in *carbon dioxide-free water* prepared from *distilled water* (solution A) produces an orange colour with 0.1 ml of *methyl red solution* and a green or blue colour with 0.1 ml of *bromocresol green solution*.

B. Solution A neutralised with a 10% w/v solution of *potassium hydroxide* yields *reaction a* characteristic of sodium, Appendix VI.

C. Solution A yields the *reactions* characteristic of phosphates, Appendix VI.

Acidity pH of a mixture of 5 ml of solution A and 5 ml of *carbon dioxide-free water*, 4.2 to 4.5, Appendix V L.

Clarity and colour of solution Solution A is *clear*, Appendix IV A, and *colourless*, Appendix IV B, Method II.

Arsenic 0.50 g complies with the *limit test for arsenic*, Appendix VII (2 ppm).

Heavy metals 12 ml of solution A complies with *limit test A for heavy metals*, Appendix VII (10 ppm). Use *lead standard solution (1 ppm Pb)* to prepare the standard.

Iron 1.0 g complies with the *limit test for iron*, Appendix VII (10 ppm).

Chloride Dilute 2.5 ml of solution A to 15 ml with *water*. The resulting solution complies with the *limit test for chlorides*, Appendix VII (200 ppm).

Sulphate Dilute 5 ml of solution A to 15 ml with *distilled water*. The resulting solution complies with the *limit test for sulphates*, Appendix VII (300 ppm).

Reducing substances To 5 ml of solution A add 0.25 ml of 0.02M *potassium permanganate* and 5 ml of 1M *sulphuric acid* and heat on a water-bath for 5 minutes. The solution retains a faint red colour.

Loss on drying When dried to constant weight at 130°, loses 21.5 to 24.0% of its weight. Use 0.5 g.

Assay Dissolve 2.5 g in 40 ml of *water* and titrate with carbonate-free 1M *sodium hydroxide VS* determining the end-point potentiometrically. Each ml of 1M *sodium hydroxide VS* is equivalent to 0.1200 g of NaH_2PO_4.

Storage Sodium Acid Phosphate should be kept in a well-closed container.

Preparation
Phosphates Enema

The title of the monograph in the European Pharmacopœia is Sodium Dihydrogen Phosphate Dihydrate.

Sodium Aurothiomalate

39377-38-3

Sodium Aurothiomalate consists mainly of the disodium salt of (aurothio)succinic acid. It contains not less than 44.5 per cent and not more than 46.0 per cent of Au and not less than 10.8 per cent and not more than 11.5 per cent of Na, both calculated with reference to the dried substance.

Characteristics A fine, pale yellow powder; odour, slight; hygroscopic.

Solubility Very soluble in *water*.

Identification A. Ignite 0.1 g and dissolve a portion of the residue by warming with 2 ml of a mixture of 3 volumes of *hydrochloric acid* and 1 volume of *nitric acid* and dilute to 20 ml with *water* (solution A). To 0.2 ml add 20 ml of

water, boil, pour the boiling solution into 5 ml of *tin(II) chloride solution* and mix. A purple colour is produced.

B. To 2 ml of solution A add 2 ml of *hydrogen peroxide solution (20 vol)* and 1 ml of 5M *sodium hydroxide*. A precipitate is produced which appears brownish-black by reflected light and bluish-green by transmitted light.

C. Solution A yields a black precipitate with *hydrogen sulphide* which is insoluble in 2M *hydrochloric acid* but soluble in *ammonium polysulphide solution*.

D. Extract a portion of the residue obtained in test A with 10 ml of 2M *hydrochloric acid*. The solution, after neutralisation if necessary, yields the *reactions* characteristic of sodium salts and of sulphates, Appendix VI.

Acidity or alkalinity pH of a 10% w/v solution, 6.0 to 7.0, Appendix V L.

Stability Dissolve 1.0 g in 10 ml of *water*, filter, seal in an ampoule, heat at 100° for 1 hour, cool and add sufficient *water* to produce 100 ml. The solution remains bright and is not more intensely coloured than a 0.01% w/v solution of *potassium hexacyanoferrate(III)*.

Loss on drying When dried over *phosphorus pentoxide* at a pressure not exceeding 0.7 kPa for 24 hours, loses not more than 2.0% of its weight. Use 1 g.

Assay *For Au* Heat 0.2 g with 10 ml of *sulphuric acid* and continue to boil gently until a clear pale yellow liquid is produced. Cool, add about 1 ml of *nitric acid* dropwise and boil again for 1 hour. Cool, dilute with 70 ml of *water*, boil for 5 minutes, filter, wash the residue of gold with hot *water*, dry and ignite for 3 hours at a temperature not lower than 600°.

For Na Evaporate to dryness the filtrate and washings obtained in the Assay for Au, moisten with *sulphuric acid* and ignite for 3 hours at 600°. Each g of residue is equivalent to 0.3237 g of Na.

Storage Sodium Aurothiomalate should be kept in a well-closed container and protected from light.

Preparation
Sodium Aurothiomalate Injection

Action and use Used in treatment of rheumatoid arthritis.

Sodium Benzoate ☆

CO₂Na

$C_7H_5NaO_2$ 144.1   *532-32-1*

Sodium Benzoate contains not less than 99.0 per cent and not more than 100.5 per cent of $C_7H_5NaO_2$, calculated with reference to the dried substance.

Characteristics A white, crystalline or granular powder or flakes; slightly hygroscopic.

Solubility Soluble in 2 parts of *water* and in 90 parts of *ethanol (96%)*.

Identification Yields *reactions A* and *B* characteristic of sodium salts and *reactions B* and *C* characteristic of benzoates, Appendix VI.

Acidity or alkalinity To 20 ml of a 5% w/v solution in *carbon dioxide-free water* add 0.2 ml of *dilute* *phenolphthalein solution.* Not more than 0.2 ml of 0.1M *hydrochloric acid VS* or 0.2 ml of 0.1M *sodium hydroxide VS* is required to change the colour of the solution.

Clarity and colour of solution A 10.0% w/v solution in *carbon dioxide-free water* is *clear*, Appendix IV A, and not more intensely coloured than *reference solution Y6*, Appendix IV B, Method II.

Heavy metals 2.0 g complies with *limit test C for heavy metals*, Appendix VII (10 ppm). Use 2 ml of *lead standard solution (10 ppm Pb)* to prepare the standard.

Halogenated compounds *Ionic chloride* In three 25-ml graduated flasks prepare the following solutions. For solution (1) add 5 ml of *water* to 20 ml of a 10% w/v solution of the substance being examined in *carbon dioxide-free water* and dilute to 50 ml with *ethanol (96%)*; to 4.0 ml of the resulting solution add 3 ml of 2M *sodium hydroxide* and 3 ml of *ethanol (96%)*. For solution (2) add 2 ml of *water* and 5 ml of *ethanol (96%)* to 3 ml of 2M *sodium hydroxide*. For solution (3) add 6 ml of *water* to 4.0 ml of *chloride standard solution (8 ppm Cl)*. In a fourth 25-ml graduated flask place 10 ml of *water*. Label the flasks A, B, C and D respectively. Prepare a solution of 30 g of *ammonium iron(III) sulphate* in 40 ml of *nitric acid*, dilute to 100 ml with *water*, filter if necessary and store protected from light. To each of the flasks A, B, C and D add 5 ml of the iron(III) solution, mix and add dropwise with swirling 2 ml of 2M *nitric acid* and 5 ml of a recently prepared 0.3% w/v solution of *mercury(II) thiocyanate* in *absolute ethanol*. Shake, dilute the contents of each flask to 25 ml with *water* and allow to stand in a water-bath at 20° for 15 minutes. Measure the *absorbance* of a 2-cm layer of solution A at 460 nm using solution B in the reference cell and that of solution C using solution D in the reference cell, Appendix II B. The absorbance of solution A is not more than that of solution C (200 ppm).

Total chlorine For solution (1) add 5 ml of *water* to 20 ml of a 10% w/v solution of the substance being examined in *carbon dioxide-free water* and dilute to 50 ml with *ethanol (96%)*. To 10 ml of the resulting solution add 7.5 ml of 2M *sodium hydroxide* and 0.125 g of *Raney nickel catalyst* and heat on a water-bath for 10 minutes. Allow to cool, filter and wash with three 2-ml quantities of *ethanol (96%)*. Dilute the filtrate and washings to 25 ml with *water*. Prepare solution (2) in the same manner but using a mixture of 5 ml of *water* and 5 ml of *ethanol (96%)* in place of the solution of the substance being examined and beginning at the words 'add 7.5 ml of 2M *sodium hydroxide* . . .'. Solution (3) is a mixture of 6 ml of *chloride standard solution (8 ppm Cl)* and 4 ml of *water*.

To four 25-ml graduated flasks labelled A, B, C and D transfer 10 ml of solution (1), solution (2), solution (3) and *water* respectively. To each flask add 5 ml of the iron(III) solution prepared in the test for ionic chloride, mix and add dropwise with swirling 2 ml of *nitric acid* and 5 ml of a recently prepared 0.3% w/v solution of *mercury(II) thiocyanate* in *absolute ethanol*. Shake, dilute the contents of each flask to 25 ml with *water* and allow to stand in a water-bath at 20° for 15 minutes. Measure the *absorbance* of a 2-cm layer of solution A at 460 nm using solution B in the reference cell and that of solution C using solution D in the reference cell, Appendix II B. The absorbance of solution A is not more than that of solution C (300 ppm).

Loss on drying When dried to constant weight at 100° to 105°, loses not more than 2.0% of its weight. Use 1 g.

Assay Dissolve 0.25 g in 20 ml of *anhydrous glacial acetic acid*, warming to 50° if necessary, cool and carry out Method I for *non-aqueous titration*, Appendix VIII A, using 0.05 ml of *1-naphtholbenzein solution* as indicator. Each ml of 0.1M *perchloric acid VS* is equivalent to 0.01441 g of $C_7H_5NaO_2$.

Storage Sodium Benzoate should be kept in a well-closed container.

Sodium Bicarbonate ☆

NaHCO₃   84.0   *144-55-8*

Sodium Bicarbonate contains not less than 99.0 per cent and not more than 101.0 per cent of NaHCO₃.

Characteristics A white, crystalline powder; odourless. It changes progressively into sodium carbonate when heated in the dry state or in solution.

Solubility Soluble in 11 parts of *water*; practically insoluble in *ethanol (96%)*.

Identification A. To 5 ml of a 5.0% w/v solution in *carbon dioxide-free water* (solution A) add 0.1 ml of *dilute phenolphthalein solution.* A pale pink colour is produced. On heating a gas is evolved and the solution becomes red.
B. Yields *reactions A* and *B* characteristic of sodium salts and *reaction A* characteristic of bicarbonates, Appendix VI.

Clarity and colour of solution Solution A is *clear*, Appendix IV A, and *colourless*, Appendix IV B, Method II.

Ammonium 10 ml of solution A diluted to 15 ml with *water* complies with the *limit test for ammonium*, Appendix VII (20 ppm). Use a mixture of 5 ml of *water* and 10 ml of *ammonium standard solution (1 ppm NH4)* to prepare the standard.

Arsenic 0.50 g complies with the *limit test for arsenic*, Appendix VII (2 ppm).

Calcium Suspend 1.0 g in 10 ml of *water*, neutralise with *hydrochloric acid* and dilute to 15 ml with *water*. The resulting solution complies with the *limit test for calcium*, Appendix VII (100 ppm).

Heavy metals Dissolve 2.0 g in a mixture of 18 ml of *water* and 2 ml of *hydrochloric acid*. 12 ml of the resulting solution complies with *limit test A for heavy metals*, Appendix VII (10 ppm). Use *lead standard solution (1 ppm Pb)* to prepare the standard.

Iron Dissolve 0.50 g in 5 ml of 2M *hydrochloric acid* and dilute to 10 ml with *water*. The resulting solution complies with the *limit test for iron*, Appendix VII (20 ppm).

Carbonate pH of solution A, when freshly prepared, not more than 8.6, Appendix V L.

Chloride To 7 ml of solution A add 2 ml of *nitric acid* and dilute to 15 ml with *water*. The resulting solution complies with the *limit test for chlorides*, Appendix VII (150 ppm).

Sulphate Suspend 1.0 g in 10 ml of *water*, neutralise with *hydrochloric acid* and dilute to 15 ml with *water*. The resulting solution complies with the *limit test for sulphates*, Appendix VII (150 ppm).

Assay Dissolve 1.5 g in 50 ml of *carbon dioxide-free water* and titrate with 1M *hydrochloric acid VS* using 0.2 ml of *methyl orange solution* as indicator. Each ml of 1M *hydrochloric acid VS* is equivalent to 0.0840 g of NaHCO₃.

Preparations
Sodium Bicarbonate Ear Drops
Sodium Bicarbonate Intravenous Infusion
Compound Sodium Bicarbonate Tablets

Action and use Antacid; used in treatment of electrolyte deficiency.

The title of the monograph in the European Pharmacopœia is Sodium Hydrogen Carbonate.

Sodium Butyl Hydroxybenzoate

Sodium Butylparaben

NaO—⟨benzene ring⟩—CO₂Buⁿ

C₁₁H₁₃NaO₃   216.2   *36457-20-2*

Sodium Butyl Hydroxybenzoate is the sodium salt of butyl 4-hydroxybenzoate. It contains not less than 99.0 per cent and not more than 102.0 per cent of C₁₁H₁₃NaO₃, calculated with reference to the anhydrous substance.

Characteristics A white powder; odourless or almost odourless; hygroscopic.

Solubility Soluble in 1 part of *water* and in 10 parts of *ethanol (96%)*.

Identification A. Dissolve 0.5 g in *water* and acidify to *litmus paper* with *hydrochloric acid*. A white precipitate is produced. Wash the precipitate with *water* and dry; reserve a sufficient quantity for tests C and D. The *infrared absorption spectrum* of the precipitate, Appendix II A, is concordant with the *reference spectrum* of butyl hydroxybenzoate.

B. The *light absorption*, Appendix II B, in the range 230 to 350 nm of a 0.001% w/v solution in *ethanol (96%)* exhibits a maximum only at 259 nm. The *absorbance* at 259 nm is about 0.75.

C. Dissolve 0.1 g of the precipitate obtained in test A in 2 ml of *ethanol (96%)*, boil and add 0.5 ml of *mercury—nitric acid solution*. A precipitate is produced slowly and the supernatant liquid becomes red.

D. *Melting point* of the precipitate obtained in test A, about 69°, Appendix V A.

E. The residue on ignition yields the *reactions* characteristic of sodium salts, Appendix VI.

Alkalinity pH of a 0.1% w/v solution, 9.5 to 10.5, Appendix V L.

Clarity of solution Dissolve 1.0 g in 10 ml of *water*. The solution is *clear*, Appendix IV A.

Chloride Dissolve 1.0 g in 100 ml of *water*, add 1 ml of *nitric acid* and filter. 15 ml of the filtrate complies with the *limit test for chlorides*, Appendix VII (330 ppm).

Sulphate Dissolve 0.50 g in 40 ml of *water*, add 3.5 ml of 2M *hydrochloric acid*, dilute to 60 ml with *water* and filter. 15 ml of the filtrate complies with the *limit test for sulphates*, Appendix VII (0.12%).

Related substances Carry out the method for *thin-layer chromatography*, Appendix III A, using a chromatoplate precoated with silica gel F254 the surface of which has been modified with chemically-bonded octadecylsilyl groups (Whatman KC18F plates are suitable) and a mixture of 70 volumes of *methanol*, 30 volumes of *water* and 1 volume of *glacial acetic acid* as the mobile phase. Apply separately to the plate 2 μl of each of two solutions of the substance being examined, prepared by dissolving in *water* and then adding an equal volume of *acetone*, containing (1) 1.0% w/v and (2) 0.040% w/v. After removal of the plate, allow it to dry in air and examine under *ultra-violet light (254 nm)*. Any *secondary spot* in the chromatogram obtained with solution (1) is not more intense than the spot in the chromatogram obtained with solution (2).

Water Not more than 5.0% w/w, Appendix IX C. Use 1 g.

Assay Gently boil 0.1 g under a reflux condenser with 25 ml of 1.25M *sodium hydroxide* for 30 minutes. Allow to cool, add 25 ml of 0.0333M *potassium bromate VS*, 5 ml of a 12.5% w/v solution of *potassium bromide* and 10 ml of *hydrochloric acid* and immediately stopper the flask. Shake for 15 minutes and allow to stand for 15 minutes. Add 25 ml of *potassium iodide solution* and shake vigorously. Titrate the liberated iodine with 0.1M *sodium thiosulphate VS* using *starch mucilage*, added towards the end of the titration, as indicator. The volume of 0.0333M *potassium bromate VS* used is equivalent to half of the volume of 0.1M *sodium thiosulphate VS* required for the titration. Each ml of 0.0333M *potassium bromate VS* is equivalent to 0.007207 g of C₁₁H₁₃NaO₃.

Storage Sodium Butyl Hydroxybenzoate should be kept in a well-closed container.

Action and use Antimicrobial preservative.

Sodium Calciumedetate ☆

NaO₂CCH₂⟩N—CH₂—CH₂—N⟨CH₂·CO₂Na with Ca chelate

C₁₀H₁₂CaN₂Na₂O₈,xH₂O   374.3 (*anhydrous*)
62-33-9 (anhydrous)

Sodium Calciumedetate is the calcium chelate of disodium ethylenediaminetetra-acetate. It contains not less than 98.0 per cent and not more than 102.0 per cent of C₁₀H₁₂CaN₂Na₂O₈, calculated with reference to the anhydrous substance. It contains a variable amount of water of crystallisation.

Characteristics A white or almost white powder; odourless; hygroscopic.

Solubility Soluble in 2 parts of *water*; practically insoluble in *ethanol (96%)*, in *chloroform* and in *ether*.

Identification A. The *infra-red absorption spectrum*, Appendix II A, is concordant with the spectrum of *sodium calcium edetate EPCRS*.

B. Dissolve 0.5 g in 10 ml of *water*, make alkaline to *litmus paper* with 2M *ammonia* and add 3 ml of a 4% w/v solution of *ammonium oxalate*. Not more than a trace of precipitate is produced.

C. Dissolve 2 g in 10 ml of *water*, add 2 ml of a 10% w/v solution of *lead(II) nitrate*, shake and add 3 ml of *potassium iodide solution*; no yellow precipitate is produced. Make alkaline to *litmus paper* with 2M *ammonia* and add 3 ml of a 4% w/v solution of *ammonium oxalate*; a white precipitate is produced.

D. Ignite. The residue yields *reactions A and B* characteristic of sodium salts and *reactions A and B* characteristic of calcium salts, Appendix VI.

Acidity or alkalinity pH of a 20% w/v solution, 6.5 to 8.0, Appendix V L.

Clarity and colour of solution A 5.0% w/v solution is *clear*, Appendix IV A, and *colourless*, Appendix IV B, Method II.

Heavy metals 1.0 g complies with *limit test D for heavy metals*, Appendix VII (20 ppm). Use 2 ml of *lead standard solution (10 ppm Pb)* to prepare the standard.

Iron Dissolve 0.50 g in 40 ml of *water*. 10 ml of the resulting solution complies with the *limit test for iron*, Appendix VII (80 ppm). Add 0.25 g of *calcium chloride* to both solutions before the addition of *mercaptoacetic acid*.

Chloride Dissolve 1.0 g in 20 ml of *water*, add 30 ml of 2M *nitric acid*, allow to stand for 30 minutes, filter and dilute 2.5 ml of the filtrate to 15 ml with *water*. The resulting solution complies with the *limit test for chlorides*, Appendix VII (0.1%).

Disodium edetate Dissolve 5.0 g in 250 ml of *water*, add 10 ml of *ammonia buffer pH 10.0* and 50 mg of *mordant black 11 mixture* and titrate with 0.1M *magnesium chloride VS*. Not more than 1.5 ml of 0.1M *magnesium chloride VS* is required to change the colour of the solution to violet (1.0%).

Water 5.0 to 13.0%, Appendix IX C, Method I B. Use 0.1 g.

Assay Dissolve 0.5 g in 300 ml of *water*, add 2 g of *hexamine* and 2 ml of 2M *hydrochloric acid* and titrate with 0.1M *lead(II) nitrate VS* using 50 mg of *xylenol orange mixture* as indicator. Each ml of 0.1M *lead(II) nitrate VS* is equivalent to 0.03743 g of $C_{10}H_{12}CaN_2Na_2O_8$.

Storage Sodium Calciumedetate should be kept in a well-closed container.

Preparation

Sodium Calciumedetate Injection

Action and use Chelating substance used in treatment of lead poisoning.

The title of the monograph in the European Pharmacopœia is Sodium Calcium Edetate.

Sodium Carbonate Decahydrate ☆

$Na_2CO_3,10H_2O$ 286.1   *497-19-8*

Sodium Carbonate Decahydrate contains not less than 36.7 per cent and not more than 40.0 per cent of Na_2CO_3.

Characteristics Colourless, transparent crystals or a white, crystalline powder; odourless; efflorescent.

Solubility Soluble in 2 parts of *water*; practically insoluble in *ethanol (96%)*.

Identification A. A 10% w/v solution yields *reaction A* characteristic of sodium salts and *reaction A* characteristic of carbonates, Appendix VI.

B. A 10% w/v solution is strongly alkaline.

Clarity and colour of solution A 40% w/v solution is *clear*, Appendix IV A, and not more intensely coloured than *reference solution Y_6*, Appendix IV B, Method II.

Arsenic Dissolve 5.0 g in a mixture of 25 ml of *water* and 5 ml of *hydrochloric acid*, heat the solution to boiling, cool, neutralise with 2M *sodium hydroxide* and dilute to 50 ml with *water* (solution A). 5 ml of solution A complies with the *limit test for arsenic*, Appendix VII (2 ppm).

Heavy metals 12 ml of solution A complies with *limit test A for heavy metals*, Appendix VII (20 ppm). Use *lead standard solution (2 ppm Pb)* to prepare the standard.

Iron 5 ml of solution A diluted to 10 ml with *water* complies with the *limit test for iron*, Appendix VII (20 ppm).

Alkali hydroxide and bicarbonate Dissolve 1.0 g in 20 ml of *water*, add 20 ml of 0.25M *barium chloride* and filter. To 10 ml of the filtrate add 0.1 ml of *dilute phenolphthalein solution*; the solution does not become red. Heat the remainder of the filtrate to boiling for 2 minutes; the solution remains clear.

Chloride Dissolve 1.0 g in a mixture of 5 ml of *water* and 4 ml of 2M *nitric acid* and dilute to 15 ml with *water*. The resulting solution complies with the *limit test for chlorides*, Appendix VII (50 ppm).

Sulphate 15 ml of solution A complies with the *limit test for sulphates*, Appendix VII (100 ppm).

Assay Dissolve 2 g in 25 ml of *water* and titrate with 1M *hydrochloric acid VS* using 0.2 ml of *methyl orange solution* as indicator. Each ml of 1M *hydrochloric acid VS* is equivalent to 0.05299 g of Na_2CO_3.

Storage Sodium Carbonate Decahydrate should be kept in an airtight container.

Sodium Carbonate Monohydrate ☆

Na_2CO_3,H_2O 124.0   *5698-11-6*

Sodium Carbonate Monohydrate contains not less than 83.0 per cent and not more than 87.5 per cent of Na_2CO_3.

Characteristics Colourless crystals or a white, crystalline powder; odourless.

Solubility Soluble in 3 parts of *water*; practically insoluble in *ethanol (96%)*.

Identification A. A 10% w/v solution yields *reaction A* characteristic of sodium salts and *reaction A* characteristic of carbonates, Appendix VI.

B. A 10% w/v solution is strongly alkaline.

Clarity and colour of solution A 20% w/v solution is *clear*, Appendix IV A, and not more intensely coloured than *reference solution Y_6*, Appendix IV B, Method II.

Arsenic Dissolve 2.0 g in a mixture of 25 ml of *water* and 5 ml of *hydrochloric acid*, heat to boiling, cool, neutralise with 2M *sodium hydroxide* and dilute to 50 ml with *water* (solution A). 5 ml of solution A complies with the *limit test for arsenic*, Appendix VII (5 ppm).

Heavy metals 12 ml of solution A complies with *limit test A for heavy metals*, Appendix VII (50 ppm). Use *lead standard solution (2 ppm Pb)* to prepare the standard.

Iron 5 ml of solution A diluted to 10 ml with *water* complies with the *limit test for iron*, Appendix VII (50 ppm).

Alkali hydroxide and bicarbonate Dissolve 0.40 g in 20 ml of *water*, add 20 ml of 0.25M *barium chloride* and filter. To 10 ml of the filtrate add 0.1 ml of *dilute phenolphthalein solution*; the solution does not become red. Heat the remainder of the filtrate to boiling for 2 minutes; the solution remains clear.

Chloride Dissolve 0.40 g in a mixture of 5 ml of *water* and 4 ml of 2M *nitric acid* and dilute to 15 ml with *water*. The resulting solution complies with the *limit test for chlorides*, Appendix VII (125 ppm).

Sulphate 15 ml of solution A complies with the *limit test for sulphates*, Appendix VII (250 ppm).

Assay Dissolve 1 g in 25 ml of *water* and titrate with 1M *hydrochloric acid VS* using 0.2 ml of *methyl orange solution* as indicator. Each ml of 1M *hydrochloric acid VS* is equivalent to 0.05299 g of Na_2CO_3.

Storage Sodium Carbonate Monohydrate should be kept in an airtight container.

Sodium Chloride ☆

NaCl   58.44   *7647-14-5*

Sodium Chloride contains not less than 99.0 per cent and not more than 100.5 per cent of NaCl, calculated with reference to the dried substance.

Characteristics Colourless crystals or a white crystalline powder; odourless.

Solubility Soluble in 3 parts of *water*; slightly soluble in *absolute ethanol*; soluble in 10 parts of *glycerol*.

Identification Yields *reactions A* and *B* characteristic of sodium salts and the *reactions* characteristic of chlorides, Appendix VI.

Acidity or alkalinity To 20 ml of a 20.0% w/v solution in *carbon dioxide-free water* prepared from *distilled water* (solution A) add 0.1 ml of *bromothymol blue solution*. Not more than 0.5 ml of 0.01M *hydrochloric acid VS* or 0.5 ml of 0.01M *sodium hydroxide VS* is required to change the colour of the solution.

Clarity and colour of solution Solution A is *clear*, Appendix IV A, and *colourless*, Appendix IV B, Method II.

Arsenic 5 ml of solution A complies with the *limit test for arsenic*, Appendix VII (1 ppm).

Barium To 2.5 ml of solution A add 7.5 ml of *distilled water* and 1 ml of 1M *sulphuric acid*. After not less than 15 minutes the solution is not more opalescent than a mixture of 2.5 ml of solution A and 8.5 ml of *distilled water*.

Heavy metals Dilute 10 ml of solution A to 20 ml with *water*. 12 ml of the resulting solution complies with *limit test A for heavy metals*, Appendix VII (10 ppm). Use *lead standard solution (1 ppm Pb)* to prepare the standard.

Iron 2.5 ml of solution A diluted to 10 ml with *water* complies with the *limit test for iron*, Appendix VII (20 ppm).

Magnesium and alkaline-earth metals 10.0 g complies with the *limit test for magnesium and alkaline-earth metals*, Appendix VII. Not more than 2.5 ml of 0.01M *disodium edetate VS* is required (100 ppm, calculated as Ca).

Bromide To 10 ml of a 1.0% w/v solution add 1 ml of *buffered phenol red solution* and 0.05 ml of a freshly prepared 2% w/v solution of *chloramine T*, shake for 15 seconds and add 0.15 ml of 0.1M *sodium thiosulphate VS*. Any violet colour produced is not more intense than that of a standard prepared at the same time and in the same manner using 0.5 ml of a 0.0015% w/v solution of *potassium bromide* and 9.5 ml of *water* (50 ppm).

Ferrocyanide Dissolve 2.0 g in 6 ml of *water* and add 0.5 ml of a mixture of 5 ml of a 1% w/v solution of *ammonium iron(III) sulphate* in a 0.25% w/v solution of *sulphuric acid* and 95 ml of a 1% w/v solution of *iron(II) sulphate*. No blue colour is produced within 10 minutes.

Iodide Moisten 5.0 g by the dropwise addition of a solution recently prepared by mixing 25 ml of *iodide-free starch solution*, 2 ml of 0.5M *sulphuric acid*, 0.15 ml of *sodium nitrite solution* and 25 ml of *water*. Examine the mixture in daylight. No particle shows any trace of blue colour within 5 minutes.

Phosphate Dilute 2 ml of solution A to 100 ml with *water*. The resulting solution complies with the *limit test for phosphates*, Appendix VII (25 ppm).

Sulphate 3 ml of solution A diluted to 15 ml with *distilled water* complies with the *limit test for sulphates*, Appendix VII (250 ppm).

Loss on drying When dried at 100° to 105° for 3 hours, loses not more than 1.0% of its weight. Use 1 g.

Assay Dissolve 1 g in sufficient *water* to produce 100 ml. To 10 ml of the solution add 50 ml of *water*, 5 ml of 2M *nitric acid*, 25 ml of 0.1M *silver nitrate VS* and 2 ml of *dibutyl phthalate*, shake and titrate with 0.1M *ammonium thiocyanate VS* using 2 ml of a 10% w/v solution of *ammonium iron(III) sulphate* as indicator and shaking vigorously towards the end-point. Each ml of 0.1M *silver nitrate VS* is equivalent to 0.005844 g of NaCl.

Labelling The label states whether or not the contents of the container are suitable for use in the manufacture of a parenteral dosage form or for the preparation of haemodialysis solutions.

Preparations
Sodium Chloride Eye Lotion
Sodium Chloride Intravenous Infusion
Sodium Chloride Solution
Sodium Chloride Tablets
Compound Sodium Chloride Mouthwash
Oral Rehydration Salts
Potassium Chloride and Sodium Chloride Intravenous Infusion
Potassium Chloride, Sodium Chloride and Glucose Intravenous Infusion
Sodium Chloride and Glucose Intravenous Infusion

Action and use Used in treatment of electrolyte deficiency.

Sodium Chloride intended for use in the manufacture of a parenteral dosage form or for the preparation of haemodialysis solutions complies with the following additional requirement.

Potassium Not more than 500 ppm when determined by *atomic emission spectrophotometry*, Appendix II D, using a 1.0% w/v solution and measuring at 768 nm. Use *potassium solution ASp*, suitably diluted with *water*, for the standard solutions.

Sodium Citrate ☆
Trisodium Citrate

CH₂·CO₂Na
|
HOCCO₂Na
|
CH₂·CO₂Na

$C_6H_5Na_3O_7,2H_2O$ 294.1   *6132-04-2*

Sodium Citrate* is trisodium 2-hydroxy-propane-1,2,3-tricarboxylate dihydrate. It contains not less than 99.0 per cent and not more than 101.0 per cent of $C_6H_5Na_3O_7$, calculated with reference to the anhydrous substance.

Characteristics White, granular crystals or a white, crystalline powder. Slightly deliquescent in moist air.

Solubility Soluble in less than 2 parts of *water*; practically insoluble in *ethanol (96%)*.

Identification A. 1 ml of a 10.0% w/v solution in *carbon dioxide-free water* (solution A) yields *reaction A* characteristic of sodium salts, Appendix VI.
B. 1 ml of solution A yields *reaction A* characteristic of citrates, Appendix VI.

Acidity or alkalinity To 10 ml of solution A add 0.1 ml of *dilute phenolphthalein solution*. Not more than 0.2 ml of either 0.1M *hydrochloric acid VS* or 0.1M *sodium hydroxide VS* is required to change the colour of the solution.

Clarity and colour of solution Solution A is *clear*, Appendix IV A, and *colourless*, Appendix IV B, Method II.

Heavy metals 12 ml of solution A complies with *limit test A for heavy metals*, Appendix VII (10 ppm). Use *lead standard solution (1 ppm Pb)* to prepare the standard.

Chloride 10 ml of solution A diluted to 15 ml with *water* complies with the *limit test for chlorides*, Appendix VII (50 ppm).

Oxalate Dissolve 0.50 g in 4 ml of *water*, add 3 ml of *hydrochloric acid* and 1 g of *granulated zinc* and heat on a water-bath for 1 minute. Allow to stand for 2 minutes, decant the liquid into a test-tube containing 0.25 ml of a 1% w/v solution of *phenylhydrazine hydrochloride* and heat to boiling. Cool rapidly, transfer to a graduated cylinder and add an equal volume of *hydrochloric acid* and 0.25 ml of a 5% w/v solution of *potassium hexacyanoferrate(III)*. Shake and allow to stand for 30 minutes. Any colour produced is not more intense than that produced by treating at the same time and in the same manner 4 ml of a 0.005% w/v solution of *oxalic acid* (300 ppm).

Sulphate To 10 ml of solution A add 2 ml of 7M *hydrochloric acid* and dilute to 15 ml with *distilled water*. The resulting solution complies with the *limit test for sulphates*, Appendix VII (150 ppm).

Readily carbonisable substances Heat 0.20 g, in powder, with 10 ml of *sulphuric acid (96% w/w)* in a water-bath at 89° to 91° for 1 hour. The resulting solution is not more intensely coloured than *reference solution Y_2* or *GY_2*, Appendix IV B, Method II.

Water 11.0 to 13.0% w/w, Appendix IX C. Use 0.3 g. After adding the substance being examined, stir for 15 minutes before titrating.

Assay Dissolve 0.15 g in 20 ml of *anhydrous glacial acetic acid*, warming to about 50°. Allow to cool and carry out Method I for *non-aqueous titration*, Appendix VIII A, using 0.25 ml of *1-naphtholbenzein solution* as indicator. Each ml of 0.1M *perchloric acid VS* is equivalent to 0.008602 g of $C_6H_5Na_3O_7$.

Storage Sodium Citrate should be kept in an airtight container.

Solutions of Sodium Citrate that have been sterilised may, on keeping, cause the separation of small solid particles from a glass container. A solution containing such particles must not be used.

Preparation
Sodium Citrate Tablets

Action and use Systemic alkalinising substance.

*In certain states party to the Convention on the Elaboration of a European Pharmacopœia, Sodium Citrate intended for use in large-volume preparations for parenteral use may be required to comply with the *test for pyrogens*, Appendix XIV K, injecting per kg of the rabbit's weight 10 ml of a freshly prepared solution in Water for Injections containing 10 mg per ml of the substance being examined and 7.5 mg per ml of *pyrogen-free calcium chloride*.

Sodium Cromoglycate

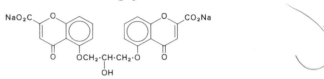

$C_{23}H_{14}Na_2O_{11}$ 512.3   *15826-37-6*

Sodium Cromoglycate is disodium 4,4'-dioxo-5,5'-(2-hydroxytrimethylenedioxy)di(chromene-2-carboxylate). It contains not less than 98.0 per cent and not more than 101.0 per cent of $C_{23}H_{14}Na_2O_{11}$, calculated with reference to the dried substance.

Characteristics A white, crystalline powder; hygroscopic.

Solubility Soluble in 20 parts of *water*; practically insoluble in *ethanol (96%)* and in *chloroform*.

Identification A. The *infra-red absorption spectrum*, Appendix II A, is concordant with the *reference spectrum* of sodium cromoglycate.
B. The *light absorption*, Appendix II B, in the range 230 to 350 nm of a 0.002% w/v solution in *phosphate buffer pH 7.4* exhibits two maxima, at 238 nm and 326 nm. The *absorbance* at 238 nm is about 1.2 and at 326 nm is about 0.32.
C. To 0.1 g add 2 ml of *water* and 2 ml of 1.25M *sodium hydroxide* and boil for 1 minute; a yellow colour is produced. To the hydrolysed solution add 0.5 ml of *diazobenzenesulphonic acid solution*; a blood red colour is produced.
D. Yields the *reactions* characteristic of sodium salts, Appendix VI.

Acidity or alkalinity Dissolve 1 g in 25 ml of freshly boiled and cooled *water*. Not more than 0.25 ml of 0.1M *sodium hydroxide VS* or 0.1M *hydrochloric acid VS* is required to make the solution neutral to *bromothymol blue solution*.

Lead Not more than 10 ppm when determined by the following method. Dissolve 2.5 g in 20 ml of warm *water*.

Cool, add 2 ml of a 10% w/v solution of *citric acid* and 5M *ammonia* until the precipitate dissolves and the solution is alkaline. Add 1 ml of *potassium cyanide solution PbT* and extract with successive 5-ml quantities of a mixture of 1 volume of *dithizone solution* and 10 volumes of *chloroform* until the chloroform layer remains green. Wash the mixed chloroform extracts by shaking with 10 ml of *water* and then extract with two 10-ml quantities of 2M *hydrochloric acid*. Wash the mixed acid solutions with 10 ml of *chloroform* and discard the chloroform. Transfer the solution to a *Nessler cylinder* and make alkaline with 5M *ammonia*. In a second *Nessler cylinder* mix 2 ml of 6M *acetic acid* with 20 ml of 2M *hydrochloric acid*, make alkaline with 5M *ammonia* and add 2.5 ml of *lead standard solution (10 ppm Pb)*. Treat the contents of each cylinder as follows. Add 1 ml of *potassium cyanide solution PbT*; the solutions should not now be more than faintly opalescent. If the colours of the solutions differ, equalise them by the addition of a few drops of a highly diluted solution of burnt sugar or other non-reactive substance. Dilute to 50 ml with *water*, add 0.1 ml of a solution prepared by dissolving 10 g of *sodium sulphide* in sufficient *water* to produce 100 ml and filtering and mix thoroughly. Compare the colours of the two solutions by a suitable method, such as by light reflected from a white tile through the Nessler cylinders; the colour of the solution in the first cylinder is not more intense than that of the solution in the second cylinder.

Oxalate Dissolve 0.10 g in 20 ml of *water*, add 5.0 ml of *iron salicylate solution* and sufficient *water* to produce 50 ml and measure the *absorbance* of a 2-cm layer of the resulting solution at 480 nm, Appendix II B. The *absorbance* is not less than that obtained by repeating the operation using 0.35 mg of *oxalic acid* in place of the substance being examined.

Related substances Carry out the method for *thin-layer chromatography*, Appendix III A, using *silica gel GF254* as the coating substance but omitting the heating and allowing the chromatoplate to stand overnight at room temperature. Use a mixture of 45 volumes of *chloroform*, 45 volumes of *methanol* and 10 volumes of *glacial acetic acid* as the mobile phase. Apply separately to the plate 10 µl of each of two solutions of the substance being examined in a mixture of 1 volume of *acetone*, 4 volumes of *tetrahydrofuran* (that has been freed from stabiliser by passage through a column of suitable alumina) and 6 volumes of *water* containing (1) 2.0% w/v and (2) 0.010% w/v. After removal of the plate, allow it to dry in air and examine under *ultra-violet light (254 nm)*. Any *secondary spot* in the chromatogram obtained with solution (1) with an Rf value higher than that of the principal spot is not more intense than the spot in the chromatogram obtained with solution (2).

Loss on drying When dried to constant weight at 100° at a pressure not exceeding 0.7 kPa, loses not more than 10.0% of its weight. Use 1 g.

Assay Prepare a 0.1M solution of perchloric acid by adding 2.25 ml of *perchloric acid* to 25 ml of *propan-2-ol* and adding sufficient *1,4-dioxan* to produce 250 ml. Standardise the solution by the following method. Dissolve 0.14 g of *potassium hydrogen phthalate* in a mixture of 25 ml of *propane-1,2-diol* and 5 ml of *propan-2-ol* with the aid of heat, cool and add 30 ml of *1,4-dioxan*. Titrate the solution with the perchloric acid solution using a mixture of equal volumes of a 0.2% w/v solution of

methyl orange in *ethanol (96%)* and a 0.2% w/v solution of *xylene cyanol FF* in *ethanol (96%)* as indicator until the colour changes from green to bluish-grey.

Dissolve 0.18 g of the substance being examined in a mixture of 25 ml of *propane-1,2-diol* and 5 ml of *propan-2-ol* with the aid of heat. Cool, add 30 ml of *1,4-dioxan* and titrate with the standardised perchloric acid solution using the same indicator. Each ml of the 0.1M solution of perchloric acid is equivalent to 0.02562 g of $C_{23}H_{14}Na_2O_{11}$.

Storage Sodium Cromoglycate should be kept in a well-closed container.

Preparation

Sodium Cromoglycate Insufflation

Action and use Prophylaxis of allergic conditions.

Sodium Diatrizoate

$C_{11}H_8I_3N_2NaO_4$ 635.9   *537-31-5*

Sodium Diatrizoate is sodium 3,5-diacetamido-2,4,6-tri-iodobenzoate. It contains not less than 98.0 per cent and not more than 101.0 per cent of $C_{11}H_8I_3N_2NaO_4$, calculated with reference to the anhydrous substance.

Characteristics A white powder; odourless or almost odourless.

Solubility Soluble in 2 parts of *water*; slightly soluble in *ethanol (96%)*; practically insoluble in *acetone* and in *ether*.

Identification A. The *infra-red absorption spectrum*, Appendix II A, is concordant with the *reference spectrum* of sodium diatrizoate.

B. Heat 50 mg. Violet vapours of iodine are evolved.

C. To 20 mg add 5 ml of 1M *sodium hydroxide* and boil gently under a reflux condenser for 10 minutes. Cool, add 5 ml of 2M *hydrochloric acid* and cool in ice for 5 minutes. Add 4 ml of a 1% w/v solution of *sodium nitrite*, cool in ice for 5 minutes, add 0.3 g of *sulphamic acid*, swirl gently until effervescence ceases and add 2 ml of a 0.4% w/v solution of N-*(1-naphthyl)ethylenediamine dihydrochloride*. An orange-red colour is produced.

D. Heat 0.5 g with 1 ml of *sulphuric acid* on a water-bath until a pale violet solution is produced, add 2 ml of *ethanol (96%)* and heat again. Ethyl acetate, recognisable by its odour, is produced.

E. Yields the *reactions* characteristic of sodium salts, Appendix VI.

Alkalinity pH of a 50% w/v solution, 7.5 to 9.5, Appendix V L.

Free amine To 1.0 g in a 50-ml glass-stoppered graduated flask add 5 ml of *water*, 10 ml of 0.1M *sodium hydroxide* and 25 ml of *dimethyl sulphoxide*. Stopper the flask, mix the contents by gently swirling and cool in ice, protected from light. After 5 minutes, slowly add 2 ml of *hydrochloric acid*, mix and allow to stand for 5 minutes. Add 2 ml of a 2% w/v solution of *sodium nitrite*, mix and allow to stand for 5 minutes. Add 1 ml of an 8% w/v solution of *sulphamic acid*, mix and allow to stand for 5 minutes. Add 2 ml of a 0.1% w/v solution of N-*(1-naphthyl)ethylene-1,2-diamine dihydrochloride* in a 70% v/v solution of *propane-1,2-diol* and mix. Remove the flask from the ice and allow to stand in water at 22° to 25° for 10 minutes, with occasional gentle shaking. Add sufficient *dimethyl sulphoxide* to produce 50 ml and mix. Within 5 minutes of diluting to 50 ml measure the *absorbance* of the resulting solution at the maximum at 470 nm, Appendix II B, using in the reference cell a solution prepared by treating 5 ml of *water* in the same manner. The absorbance is not more than 0.40.

Inorganic iodide Dissolve 0.80 g in 10 ml of *water*, add sufficient 2M *nitric acid* dropwise to ensure complete precipitation of the iodinated acid and add 3 ml in excess. Filter, wash the precipitate with 5 ml of *water*, add to the filtrate 1 ml of *hydrogen peroxide solution (100 vol)* and 1 ml of *chloroform* and shake. Any purple colour in the chloroform is not more intense than that obtained by adding 2 ml of *iodide standard solution (20 ppm I)* to a mixture of 3 ml of *nitric acid* and sufficient *water* to equal the volume of the test solution, adding 1 ml of *hydrogen peroxide solution (100 vol)* and 1 ml of *chloroform* and shaking (50 ppm).

Water 4.0 to 7.0% w/w, Appendix IX C. Use 0.4 g.

Assay Mix 0.4 g with 12 ml of 5M *sodium hydroxide* and 20 ml of *water*, add 1 g of *zinc powder* and boil under a reflux condenser for 30 minutes. Cool, rinse the condenser with 30 ml of *water*, filter through absorbent cotton and wash the flask and filter with two 20-ml quantities of *water*. To the combined filtrate and washings add 80 ml of *hydrochloric acid*, cool and titrate with 0.05M *potassium iodate VS* until the dark brown solution becomes light brown. Add 5 ml of *chloroform* and continue the titration, shaking well after each addition, until the chloroform becomes colourless. Each ml of 0.05M *potassium iodate VS* is equivalent to 0.02120 g of $C_{11}H_8I_3N_2NaO_4$.

Storage Sodium Diatrizoate should be protected from light.

Preparation
Sodium Diatrizoate Injection

Action and use Radio-opaque substance used in urography.

In some countries the material described in this monograph may be known as Sodium Amidotrizoate.

Sodium Fluoride ☆

NaF   41.99   *7681-49-4*

Sodium Fluoride contains not less than 98.5 per cent and not more than 100.5 per cent of NaF, calculated with reference to the dried substance.

Characteristics A white powder or colourless crystals.

Solubility Soluble in 25 parts of *water*; practically insoluble in *ethanol (96%)*.

Identification A. Dissolve 2.5 g in sufficient *carbon dioxide-free water* without heating to produce 100 ml (solution A). To 2 ml of solution A add 0.5 ml of 0.5M *calcium chloride*. A gelatinous white precipitate is produced which dissolves on adding 5 ml of 0.4M *iron(III) chloride*.

B. Add 4 mg to a mixture of 0.1 ml of *alizarin red S solution* and 0.1 ml of *zirconyl nitrate solution*. The red colour changes to yellow.

C. Yields *reaction A* characteristic of sodium salts, Appendix VI.

Acidity or alkalinity Dissolve 2.5 g of *potassium nitrate* in 40 ml of solution A, dilute to 50 ml with *carbon dioxide-free water*, cool to 0° and add 0.2 ml of *dilute phenolphthalein solution*. If the solution is colourless, not more than 1.0 ml of 0.1M *sodium hydroxide VS* is required to produce a red colour that persists for not less than 15 seconds. If the solution is red, not more than 0.25 ml of 0.1M *hydrochloric acid VS* is required to change the colour of the solution. Reserve the neutralised solution for the test for Fluorosilicate.

Clarity and colour of solution Solution A is *clear*, Appendix IV A, and *colourless*, Appendix IV B, Method II.

Chloride 10 ml of solution A diluted to 15 ml with *water* complies with the *limit test for chlorides*, Appendix VII (200 ppm).

Fluorosilicate Heat to boiling the solution reserved in the test for Acidity or alkalinity and titrate while hot with 0.05M *sodium hydroxide VS* until a permanent pink colour is produced. Not more than 1.5 ml of 0.05M *sodium hydroxide VS* is required.

Sulphate Dissolve 0.25 g in 10 ml of a saturated solution of *boric acid* in *distilled water* and add 5 ml of *distilled water* and 0.6 ml of 7M *hydrochloric acid*. The solution complies with the *limit test for sulphates*, Appendix VII (200 ppm). Prepare the standard by mixing together 0.6 ml of 7M *hydrochloric acid*, 5 ml of *sulphate standard solution (10 ppm SO₄)* and 10 ml of a saturated solution of *boric acid* in *distilled water*.

Loss on drying When dried at 130° for 3 hours, loses not more than 0.5% of its weight. Use 1 g.

Assay To 80 mg add a mixture of 5 ml of *acetic anhydride* and 20 ml of *anhydrous glacial acetic acid* and heat to dissolve. Cool, add 20 ml of *1,4-dioxan* and carry out Method I for *non-aqueous titration*, Appendix VIII A, using 0.1 ml of *crystal violet solution* as indicator. Repeat the operation without the substance being examined. Each ml of 0.1M *perchloric acid VS* is equivalent to 0.004199 g of NaF.

Storage Sodium Fluoride should be kept in a well-closed container.

Action and use Used in prevention of dental caries.

Sodium Fusidate

C$_{31}$H$_{47}$NaO$_6$ 538.7   751-94-0

Sodium Fusidate is sodium (17Z)-16β-acetoxy-3α,11α-dihydroxyfusida-17(20),24-dien-21-oate, an antimicrobial substance produced by the growth of certain strains of *Fusidium coccineum* (K. Tubaki). It contains not less than 97.5 per cent and not more than 100.5 per cent of C$_{31}$H$_{47}$NaO$_6$, calculated with reference to the anhydrous substance.

Characteristics A white or almost white, crystalline powder; slightly hygroscopic.

Solubility Soluble in 1 part of *water* and in 1 part of *ethanol (96%)*; practically insoluble in *acetone* and in *ether*; slightly soluble in *chloroform*.

Identification A. Dissolve 0.1 g in 5 ml of *water*, add 5 ml of *chloroform* and 0.1 ml of a 10% w/w solution of *orthophosphoric acid*, shake vigorously for 1 minute, allow to separate and filter the lower layer through absorbent cotton covered with *anhydrous sodium sulphate*. Repeat the extraction with two 5-ml quantities of *chloroform*, evaporate the combined extracts at a pressure of 2 kPa, dry the residue over *phosphorus pentoxide* at a pressure not exceeding 0.7 kPa for 2 hours and dissolve in 1 ml of *chloroform IR*. The *infra-red absorption spectrum* of the resulting solution, Appendix II A, is concordant with the *reference spectrum* of fusidic acid.

B. Carry out the method described under Related substances, applying separately to the chromatoplate 5 µl of each of two solutions in *ethanol (96%)* containing (1) 0.20% w/v of the substance being examined and (2) 0.24% w/v of *diethanolamine fusidate BPCRS*. The principal spot in the chromatogram obtained with solution (1) corresponds to that in the chromatogram obtained with solution (2).

C. Ignite. The residue yields the *reactions* characteristic of sodium salts, Appendix VI.

Alkalinity pH of a 1.25% w/v solution, 7.5 to 9.0, Appendix V L.

Colour of solution A 15% w/v solution in *carbon dioxide-free water* is not more intensely coloured than *reference solution B$_6$*, Appendix IV B, Method I.

Specific optical rotation Dissolve 1.5 g in 25 ml of *water*, add 0.1 ml of 5M *ammonia* and dilute to 50 ml with *water*. The *specific optical rotation* in the resulting solution is +5° to +8°, Appendix V F.

Related substances Carry out the method for *thin-layer chromatography*, Appendix III A, using *silica gel G* as the coating substance and a mixture of 80 volumes of *chloroform*, 10 volumes of *glacial acetic acid*, 10 volumes of *cyclohexane* and 2.5 volumes of *methanol* as the mobile phase. Apply separately to the chromatoplate 5 µl of each of three solutions in *absolute ethanol* containing (1) 2.0% w/v of the substance being examined, (2) 0.040% w/v of *diethanolamine fusidate BPCRS* and (3) 0.040% w/v of *3-ketofusidic acid BPCRS*. After removal of the plate, dry it at 110° for 10 minutes, spray with *ethanolic sulphuric acid (10%)*, dry at 110° for 10 minutes and examine under *ultra-violet light (365 nm)*. Any red *secondary spot* in the chromatogram obtained with solution (1) is not more intense than the principal spot in the chromatogram obtained with solution (2). Any yellow spot in the chromatogram obtained with solution (1) is not more intense than the principal spot in the chromatogram obtained with solution (3).

Water Not more than 1.5% w/w, Appendix IX C. Use 2.5 g.

Assay Dissolve 0.5 g in a mixture of 15 ml of *water* and 20 ml of *ethanol (96%)*. Titrate with 0.1M *hydrochloric acid VS* to pH 4.1, stirring continuously and determining the end-point potentiometrically. Each ml of 0.1M *hydrochloric acid VS* is equivalent to 0.05387 g of C$_{31}$H$_{47}$NaO$_6$.

Storage Sodium Fusidate should be kept in a well-closed container and protected from light.

Preparations
Sodium Fusidate Capsules
Sodium Fusidate Ointment
Sodium Fusidate Gauze Dressing
Action and use Antibacterial.

Sodium Hydroxide
Caustic Soda

NaOH   40.00   1370-73-2

Sodium Hydroxide contains not less than 97.5 per cent of total alkali, calculated as NaOH, and not more than 2.5 per cent of Na$_2$CO$_3$.

Characteristics White sticks, pellets, spherical particles, fused masses or scales; dry, hard, brittle and showing a crystalline fracture; very deliquescent. Strongly alkaline and corrosive. Rapidly absorbs carbon dioxide.

Solubility Completely or almost completely soluble in 1 part of *water*; very soluble in *ethanol (96%)*.

Identification A solution is strongly alkaline and when neutralised with 2M *hydrochloric acid* yields the *reactions* characteristic of sodium salts, Appendix VI.

Aluminium, iron and matter insoluble in hydrochloric acid Boil 5.0 g with 70 ml of 2M *hydrochloric acid*, cool, make alkaline with 5M *ammonia*, boil, filter and wash with a 2.5% w/v solution of *ammonium nitrate*. The insoluble residue, after ignition, weighs not more than 5 mg.

Arsenic 0.25 g dissolved in 25 ml of *water* complies with the *limit test for arsenic*, Appendix VII (4 ppm).

Heavy metals Dissolve 2.0 g in 20 ml of *water*. 12 ml of the resulting solution complies with *limit test A for heavy metals*, Appendix VII (10 ppm). Use *lead standard solution (1 ppm Pb)* to prepare the standard.

Chloride Dissolve 0.50 g in 50 ml of *water*, add 1.8 ml of *nitric acid* and dilute to 100 ml with *water*. 15 ml of the resulting solution complies with the *limit test for chlorides*, Appendix VII (0.07%).

Sulphate Dissolve 0.50 g in 30 ml of *water*, add 6.2 ml of 2M *hydrochloric acid* and dilute to 55 ml with *water*. 15 ml of the resulting solution complies with the *limit test for sulphates*, Appendix VII (0.12%).

Assay Dissolve 2 g in 25 ml of *water*, add 5 ml of *barium chloride solution* and titrate with 1M *hydrochloric acid VS* using *phenolphthalein solution* as indicator. To the solution in the flask add *bromophenol blue solution* and continue the titration with 1M *hydrochloric acid VS*. Each ml of 1M *hydrochloric acid VS* used in the second titration is equivalent to 0.05299 g of Na_2CO_3. Each ml of 1M *hydrochloric acid VS* used in the combined titrations is equivalent to 0.04000 g of total alkali, calculated as NaOH.

Storage Sodium Hydroxide should be kept in a well-closed container.

Sodium Iodide ☆

NaI   149.9   *7681-82-5*

Sodium Iodide contains not less than 99.0 per cent and not more than 100.5 per cent of NaI, calculated with reference to the dried substance.

Characteristics Colourless crystals or a white crystalline powder; odourless; hygroscopic.

Solubility Soluble in 0.6 part of *water* and in 2 parts of *ethanol (96%)*.

Identification Yields *reactions A* and *B* characteristic of sodium salts and the *reactions* characteristic of iodides, Appendix VI.

Alkalinity To 12.5 ml of a 10.0% w/v solution in *carbon dioxide-free water* (solution A) add 0.1 ml of *bromothymol blue solution*. Not more than 0.7 ml of 0.01M *hydrochloric acid VS* is required to change the colour of the solution.

Clarity and colour of solution Solution A is *clear*, Appendix IV A, and *colourless*, Appendix IV B, Method II.

Heavy metals 12 ml of solution A complies with *limit test A for heavy metals*, Appendix VII (10 ppm). Use *lead standard solution (1 ppm Pb)* to prepare the standard.

Iron 5 ml of solution A diluted to 10 ml with *water* complies with the *limit test for iron*, Appendix VII (20 ppm).

Iodate To 10 ml of solution A add 0.25 ml of *iodide-free starch solution* and 0.2 ml of 1M *sulphuric acid* and allow to stand protected from light for 2 minutes. No blue colour is produced.

Sulphate 10 ml of solution A diluted to 15 ml with *distilled water* complies with the *limit test for sulphates*, Appendix VII (150 ppm).

Thiosulphate To 10 ml of solution A add 0.1 ml of *starch solution*. Not more than 0.1 ml of 0.005M *iodine VS* is required to produce a blue colour.

Loss on drying When dried at 100° to 105° for 3 hours, loses not more than 3.0% of its weight. Use 1 g.

Assay Dissolve 1.3 g in sufficient *water* to produce 100 ml. To 20 ml of the solution add 40 ml of *hydrochloric acid* and titrate with 0.05M *potassium iodate VS* until the colour changes to yellow. Add 5 ml of *chloroform* and

continue the titration, shaking vigorously, until the chloroform layer is decolorised. Each ml of 0.05M *potassium iodate VS* is equivalent to 0.01499 g of NaI.

Storage Sodium Iodide should be kept in a well-closed container and protected from light.

Sodium Lauryl Sulphate ☆

131-21-3

Sodium Lauryl Sulphate is a mixture of sodium alkyl sulphates consisting chiefly of sodium dodecyl sulphate, $CH_3 \cdot (CH_2)_{12} \cdot OSO_3Na$. It contains not less than 85.0 per cent of sodium alkyl sulphates, calculated as $C_{12}H_{25}NaO_4S$.

Characteristics A white or pale yellow powder or crystals; odour, slight but characteristic.

Solubility Freely soluble in *water*, forming an opalescent solution; partly soluble in *ethanol (96%)*.

Identification A. A 1% w/v solution, when shaken, produces copious foam.
B. Mix 0.1 ml of a 1% w/v solution with 0.1 ml of a 0.1% w/v solution of *methylene blue* and 2 ml of 1M *sulphuric acid*, add 2 ml of *chloroform* and shake. The chloroform layer is intensely blue.
C. Mix 10 mg with 10 ml of *ethanol (96%)* and heat to boiling on a water-bath, shaking frequently. Filter immediately and evaporate the ethanol. Dissolve the residue in 8 ml of *water*, add 3 ml of 2M *hydrochloric acid*, evaporate the solution to half its volume and cool. Filter and to the filtrate add 1 ml of 0.25M *barium chloride*. A white crystalline precipitate is produced.
D. Yields *reaction B* characteristic of sodium salts, Appendix VI.

Alkalinity Dissolve 1 g in 100 ml of *carbon dioxide-free water* and add 0.1 ml of *phenol red solution*. Not more than 0.5 ml of 0.1M *hydrochloric acid VS* is required to change the colour of the solution.

Non-esterified alcohols Dissolve 10 g in 100 ml of *water*, add 100 ml of *ethanol (96%)* and extract the solution with three 50-ml quantities of n-*pentane*, adding *sodium chloride*, if necessary, to promote separation of the two layers. Wash the combined organic layers with three 50-ml quantities of *water*. Dry the organic solution over *anhydrous sodium sulphate*, filter and evaporate on a water-bath until the odour of pentane is no longer detectable. Heat the residue at 105° for 15 minutes and cool. The residue weighs not more than 0.4 g.

Sodium chloride and sodium sulphate When determined by the following methods, the sum of the values found is not more than 8.0% w/w.

For NaCl Dissolve 5 g in 50 ml of *water*, add 2M *nitric acid* dropwise until the solution is neutral to *litmus paper*, add 2 ml of a 5% w/v solution of *potassium chromate* and titrate with 0.1M *silver nitrate VS*. Each ml of 0.1M *silver nitrate VS* is equivalent to 0.005844 g of NaCl.

For Na_2SO_4 Dissolve 0.1 g in 40 ml of a mixture of 8 volumes of *propan-2-ol* and 2 volumes of *water*. Adjust the pH to between 2.5 and 4.0 by the addition of 1M *perchloric acid*. Titrate with 0.025M *barium perchlorate VS*, using 0.1 ml of a 0.2% w/v solution of *naphtharson* and 0.1 ml of a 0.0125% w/v solution of *methylene blue* as indicator, until the yellowish-green colour changes to yellowish-pink. Each ml of 0.025M *barium perchlorate VS* is equivalent to 0.003551 g of Na_2SO_4.

Assay Dissolve 1.2 g in sufficient *water* to produce 1000 ml, warming if necessary. To 20 ml add 15 ml of *chloroform* and 10 ml of *dimidium bromide—sulphan blue solution* and titrate with 0.004M *benzethonium chloride VS*, shaking vigorously and allowing the layers to separate after each addition, until the pink colour of the chloroform layer is completely discharged and a greyish-blue colour is produced. Each ml of 0.004M *benzethonium chloride VS* is equivalent to 0.001154 g of sodium alkyl sulphates, calculated as $C_{12}H_{25}NaO_4S$.

Storage Sodium Lauryl Sulphate should be kept in a well-closed container.

Action and use Anionic emulsifying agent.

Sodium Metabisulphite

Sodium Pyrosulphite

$Na_2S_2O_5$ 190.1   *7681-57-4*

Sodium Metabisulphite may be prepared by saturating a solution of sodium hydroxide with sulphur dioxide and allowing crystallisation to occur. It contains not less than 95.0 per cent and not more than 100.5 per cent of $Na_2S_2O_5$.

Characteristics Colourless, prismatic crystals or a white or creamy-white powder; odour, sulphurous.

Solubility Soluble in 2 parts of *water*; slightly soluble in *ethanol (96%)*.

Identification A. Yields the *reactions* characteristic of sodium salts, Appendix VI.
B. A solution decolorises *iodine solution* and the resulting solution yields the *reactions* characteristic of sulphates, Appendix VI.

Acidity A solution is acidic to *phenol red solution*.

Arsenic Mix 0.50 g in a porcelain dish with 5 ml of *water*, 0.25 g of *potassium chlorate* and 3 ml of *hydrochloric acid*, heat to remove chlorine and dilute to 50 ml with *water*. 25 ml of the resulting solution complies with the *limit test for arsenic*, Appendix VII (4 ppm).

Heavy metals Dissolve 1.0 g in 20 ml of *water*. 12 ml of the resulting solution complies with *limit test A for heavy metals*, Appendix VII (40 ppm). Use *lead standard solution (2 ppm Pb)* to prepare the standard.

Thiosulphate Dissolve 1.0 g in 10 ml of 2M *hydrochloric acid* and heat on a water-bath for 10 minutes. Not more than a faint opalescence is produced.

Assay Add 0.2 g to 50 ml of 0.05M *iodine VS*, swirl to dissolve, add 1 ml of *hydrochloric acid* and titrate the excess of iodine with 0.1M *sodium thiosulphate VS*. Each ml of 0.05M *iodine VS* is equivalent to 0.004753 g of $Na_2S_2O_5$.

Storage Sodium Metabisulphite should be kept in a well-closed container. On exposure to air and moisture it is slowly oxidised to sulphate with disintegration of the crystals.

Action and use Antioxidant.

Sodium Methyl Hydroxybenzoate

Sodium Methylparaben

$C_8H_7NaO_3$ 174.1   *5026-62-0*

Sodium Methyl Hydroxybenzoate is the sodium salt of methyl 4-hydroxybenzoate. It contains not less than 99.0 per cent and not more than 102.0 per cent of $C_8H_7NaO_3$, calculated with reference to the anhydrous substance.

Characteristics A white, crystalline powder; odourless or almost odourless; hygroscopic.

Solubility Soluble in 2 parts of *water* and in 50 parts of *ethanol (96%)*; practically insoluble in fixed oils.

Identification A. Dissolve 0.5 g in 5 ml of *water* and acidify to *litmus paper* with *hydrochloric acid*. A white precipitate is produced. Wash the precipitate with *water* and dry; reserve a sufficient quantity for tests B, C and D. The *infra-red absorption spectrum* of the precipitate, Appendix II A, is concordant with the *reference spectrum* of methyl hydroxybenzoate.
B. Boil 10 mg of the precipitate obtained in test A with 10 ml of *water*, cool and add 0.05 ml of *iron(III) chloride test-solution*. A reddish-violet colour is produced.
C. Dissolve 0.1 g of the precipitate obtained in test A in 2 ml of *ethanol (96%)*, boil and add 0.5 ml of *mercury—nitric acid solution*. A precipitate is produced and the supernatant liquid becomes red.
D. The *melting point* of the precipitate obtained in test A is about 126°, Appendix V A.
E. Ignite. The residue yields the *reactions* characteristic of sodium salts, Appendix VI.

Alkalinity pH of a 0.1% w/v solution, 9.5 to 10.5, Appendix V L.

Clarity of solution Dissolve 1.0 g in 10 ml of *water*. The solution is *clear*, Appendix IV A.

Chloride Dissolve 1.0 g in 100 ml of *water*, add 1 ml of *nitric acid* and filter. 15 ml of the filtrate complies with the *limit test for chlorides*, Appendix VII (330 ppm).

Sulphate Dissolve 0.50 g in 40 ml of *water*, add 3.5 ml of 2M *hydrochloric acid*, dilute to 60 ml with *water* and filter. 15 ml of the filtrate complies with the *limit test for sulphates*, Appendix VII (0.12%).

Related substances Carry out the method for *thin-layer chromatography*, Appendix III A, using a chromatoplate precoated with silica gel F254 the surface of which has been modified with chemically-bonded octadecylsilyl groups (Whatman KC18F plates are suitable) and a mixture of 70 volumes of *methanol*, 30 volumes of *water* and 1 volume of *glacial acetic acid* as the mobile phase. Apply separately to the plate 2 µl of each of two solutions of the substance being examined, prepared by dissolving in *water* and then adding an equal volume of *acetone*, containing (1) 1.0% w/v and (2) 0.040% w/v. After removal of the plate, allow it to dry in air and examine under *ultra-violet light (254 nm)*. Any *secondary spot* in the chromatogram obtained with solution (1) is not more intense than the spot in the chromatogram obtained with solution (2).

Water Not more than 5.0% w/w, Appendix IX C. Use 1 g.

Assay Gently boil 0.1 g under a reflux condenser with 25 ml of 1.25M *sodium hydroxide* for 30 minutes. Allow to cool, add 25 ml of 0.0333M *potassium bromate VS*, 5 ml of a 12.5% w/v solution of *potassium bromide* and 10 ml of *hydrochloric acid* and immediately stopper the flask. Shake for 15 minutes and allow to stand for 15 minutes. Add 25 ml of *potassium iodide solution* and shake vigorously. Titrate the liberated iodine with 0.1M *sodium thiosulphate VS* using *starch mucilage*, added towards the end of the titration, as indicator. The volume of 0.0333M *potassium bromate VS* used is equivalent to half of the volume of 0.1M *sodium thiosulphate VS* required for the titration. Each ml of 0.0333M *potassium bromate VS* is equivalent to 0.005804 g of $C_8H_7NaO_3$.

Storage Sodium Methyl Hydroxybenzoate should be kept in a well-closed container.

Action and use Antimicrobial preservative.

Sodium Nitroprusside

$Na_2Fe(CN)_5NO,2H_2O$ 298.0   *13755-38-9*

Sodium Nitroprusside is sodium pentacyano-nitrosylferrate(III) dihydrate. It contains not less than 99.0 per cent and not more than 100.5 per cent of $Na_2Fe(CN)_5NO$, calculated with reference to the anhydrous substance.

Characteristics Reddish-brown crystals or powder; odourless or almost odourless.

Solubility Freely soluble in *water*; slightly soluble in *ethanol (96%)*; very slightly soluble in *chloroform*.

Identification A. The *light absorption*, Appendix II B, in the range 350 to 600 nm of a 1.6% w/v solution exhibits a maximum only at 395 nm. The *absorbance* at 395 nm is about 1.1.
B. Dissolve 20 mg in 2 ml of *water* and add 0.1 ml of *sodium sulphide solution*. A deep purple colour is produced.
C. Yields the *reactions* characteristic of sodium salts, Appendix VI.

Insoluble substances Dissolve 10 g in 50 ml of *water*. Heat the solution on a water-bath for 30 minutes, filter and wash the insoluble matter with *water*. The residue, after drying at 105°, weighs not more than 1 mg.

Chloride Dissolve 1.0 g in 60 ml of *water*. 15 ml of the resulting solution complies with the *limit test for chlorides*, Appendix VII (200 ppm).

Ferricyanide Dissolve 0.50 g in 20 ml of a buffer solution prepared by adjusting the pH of a 10% w/v solution of *ammonium acetate* to 4.62 with 6M *acetic acid* and divide into two equal portions, A and B. To portion B add 1 ml of *ferricyanide standard solution (50 ppm)*, then add to both portions 1 ml of a 0.5% w/v solution of *ammonium iron(II) sulphate* and dilute to 50 ml with *water*. Allow to stand for 1 hour and measure the *absorbance* of each solution at the maximum at 720 nm, Appendix II B. The absorbance of the solution obtained from portion A, using in the reference cell a solution prepared by dissolving 0.25 g of the substance being examined in 10 ml of the buffer and diluting to 50 ml with *water*, is not more than the absorbance of the solution obtained from portion B, using the solution obtained from portion A in the reference cell (0.02%).

Ferrocyanide Dissolve 2.0 g in 40 ml of *water* and divide into two equal portions, A and B. To portion B add 2 ml of *ferrocyanide standard solution (100 ppm)*, then add to

both portions 0.2 ml of *iron(III) chloride test-solution* and dilute to 50 ml with *water*. Allow to stand for 5 minutes and measure the *absorbance* of each solution at the maximum at 695 nm, Appendix II B. The absorbance of the solution obtained from portion A, using a 2% w/v solution of the substance being examined in the reference cell, is not more than the absorbance of the solution obtained from portion B, using the solution obtained from portion A in the reference cell (0.02%).

Sulphate 2.5 g complies with the *limit test for sulphates*, Appendix VII (60 ppm).

Water 9.0 to 15.0% w/w, Appendix IX C, Method I B. Use 1 g.

Assay Dissolve 0.35 g in 100 ml of *water* and add 0.1 ml of 1M *sulphuric acid* and 20 ml of *ethanol (96%)*. Titrate potentiometrically with 0.1M *silver nitrate VS* using a silver—mercury(I) sulphate electrode system. Each ml of 0.1M *silver nitrate VS* is equivalent to 0.01310 g of $Na_2Fe(CN)_5NO$.

Storage Sodium Nitroprusside should be kept in a well-closed container and protected from light.

Preparation
Sodium Nitroprusside Intravenous Infusion.

Action and use Vasodilator.

Sodium Perborate

$NaBO_2,H_2O_2,3H_2O$ 153.9   *7632-04-4*

Sodium Perborate contains not less than 96.0 per cent and not more than 103.0 per cent of $NaBO_2,H_2O_2,3H_2O$.

Characteristics Colourless, prismatic crystals or a white powder, stable in the crystalline form; odourless or almost odourless.

Solubility Soluble in 40 parts of *water*, with some decomposition.

Identification A. Mix 1 ml of a saturated solution with 1 ml of 1M *sulphuric acid* and 0.2 ml of *potassium dichromate solution*, shake with 2 ml of *ether* and allow to stand. A blue colour is produced in the ether layer.
B. The mixture obtained on treating with *sulphuric acid* and *methanol* burns with a greenish flame when ignited.
C. Yields the *reactions* characteristic of sodium salts, Appendix VI.
D. An aqueous solution is alkaline to *litmus solution*.

Arsenic Heat 0.38 g in a porcelain dish with 2 ml of *sulphuric acid* and 2 ml of *water* until white fumes are evolved, cool, add 2 ml of *water* and heat again until white fumes are evolved. Cool, add 50 ml of *water* and 5 ml of *stannated hydrochloric acid* and dilute to 75 ml with *water*. 25 ml of the resulting solution complies with the *limit test for arsenic*, Appendix VII (8 ppm).

Heavy metals Dissolve 2.0 g by heating with 10 ml of 2M *hydrochloric acid*, evaporate to dryness, with stirring, and dissolve the residue in 20 ml of hot *water*. 12 ml of the resulting solution complies with *limit test A for heavy metals*, Appendix VII (10 ppm). Use *lead standard solution (1 ppm Pb)* to prepare the standard.

Iron 6 ml of the solution obtained in the test for Heavy metals diluted to 10 ml with *water* complies with the *limit test for iron*, Appendix VII (80 ppm).

Chloride 0.15 g complies with the *limit test for chlorides*, Appendix VII (330 ppm).

Sulphate 15 ml of a solution prepared by dissolving 0.13 g in 150 ml of *water* complies with the *limit test for sulphates*, Appendix VII (1.2%).

Assay Dissolve 0.3 g in 50 ml of *water*, add 10 ml of 1M *sulphuric acid* and titrate with 0.02M *potassium permanganate VS*. Each ml of 0.02M *potassium permanganate VS* is equivalent to 0.007693 g of $NaBO_2,H_2O_2,3H_2O$.

Storage Sodium Perborate should be kept in an airtight container.

Action and use Antiseptic.

Sodium Phosphate ☆
Disodium Hydrogen Phosphate

$Na_2HPO_4,12H_2O$ 358.1   *7782-85-6*

Sodium Phosphate contains not less than 98.0 per cent and not more than 101.0 per cent of Na_2HPO_4, calculated with reference to the anhydrous substance.

Characteristics Colourless, transparent crystals; strongly efflorescent.

Solubility Very soluble in *water*; practically insoluble in *ethanol (96%)*.

Identification A 10.0% w/v solution in *distilled water* (solution A) yields *reactions A and B* characteristic of sodium salts and the *reactions* characteristic of phosphates, Appendix VI.

Clarity and colour of solution Solution A is *clear*, Appendix IV A, and *colourless*, Appendix IV B, Method II.

Arsenic 5 ml of solution A complies with the *limit test for arsenic*, Appendix VII (2 ppm).

Heavy metals 12 ml of solution A complies with *limit test A for heavy metals*, Appendix VII (10 ppm). Use *lead standard solution (1 ppm Pb)* to prepare the standard.

Iron 5 ml of solution A diluted to 10 ml with *water* complies with the *limit test for iron*, Appendix VII (20 ppm).

Chloride To 2.5 ml of solution A add 10 ml of 2M *nitric acid* and dilute to 15 ml with *water*. The resulting solution complies with the *limit test for chlorides*, Appendix VII (200 ppm).

Sulphate To 3 ml of solution A add 2 ml of 2M *hydrochloric acid* and dilute to 15 ml with *distilled water*. The resulting solution complies with the *limit test for sulphates*, Appendix VII (500 ppm).

Monosodium phosphate The value of the expression $(n_2 - 25)/(25 - n_1)$, where n_1 and n_2 are the titres of 1M *sodium hydroxide VS* obtained in the Assay, does not exceed 0.025.

Reducing substances To 5 ml of solution A add 5 ml of 1M *sulphuric acid* and 0.25 ml of 0.02M *potassium permanganate* and heat on a water-bath for 5 minutes. The red colour is not completely discharged.

Water 57.0 to 61.0%, Appendix IX C, Method I B. Use 0.1 g.

Assay Dissolve 4 g (*w* g) in 25 ml of *water*, add 25 ml of 1M *hydrochloric acid VS* and titrate potentiometrically with 1M *sodium hydroxide VS* until the first inflection of the pH curve is reached (n_1 ml). Continue the titration until the second inflection of the curve is reached; the total volume of sodium hydroxide required is n_2 ml. Determine the percentage content of Na_2HPO_4 from the expression $1420(25 - n_1)/w(100 - d)$, where *d* is the percentage water content.

Storage Sodium Phosphate should be kept in a well-closed container.

Preparation
Phosphates Enema
The title of the monograph in the European Pharmacopœia is Disodium Phosphate Dodecahydrate.

Sodium Propyl Hydroxybenzoate
Sodium Propylparaben

$C_{10}H_{11}NaO_3$ 202.2   *35285-69-9*

Sodium Propyl Hydroxybenzoate is the sodium salt of propyl 4-hydroxybenzoate. It contains not less than 99.0 per cent and not more than 102.0 per cent of $C_{10}H_{11}NaO_3$, calculated with reference to the anhydrous substance.

Characteristics A white, crystalline powder; odourless or almost odourless; hygroscopic.

Solubility Soluble in 1 part of *water*, in 50 parts of *ethanol (96%)* and in 2 parts of *ethanol (50%)*; practically insoluble in fixed oils.

Identification A. Dissolve 0.5 g in 5 ml of *water* and acidify to *litmus paper* with *hydrochloric acid*. A white precipitate is produced. Wash the precipitate with *water* and dry; reserve a portion of the precipitate for test D. The *infra-red absorption spectrum* of the precipitate, Appendix II A, is concordant with the *reference spectrum* of propyl hydroxybenzoate.
B. Boil 10 mg with 10 ml of *water*, cool and add 0.05 ml of *iron(III) chloride test-solution*. A reddish-violet colour is produced.
C. Dissolve 0.1 g in 2 ml of *ethanol (96%)*, boil and add 0.5 ml of *mercury—nitric acid solution*. A precipitate is produced and the supernatant liquid becomes red.
D. *Melting point* of the precipitate obtained in test A, about 95°, Appendix V A.
E. Ignite. The residue yields the *reactions* characteristic of sodium salts, Appendix VI.

Alkalinity pH of a 0.1% w/v solution, 9.5 to 10.5, Appendix V L.

Clarity of solution Dissolve 1.0 g in 10 ml of *water*; the solution is *clear*, Appendix IV A.

Chloride Dissolve 1.0 g in 100 ml of *water*, add 1 ml of *nitric acid* and filter. 15 ml of the filtrate complies with the *limit test for chlorides*, Appendix VII (330 ppm).

Sulphate Dissolve 0.50 g in 40 ml of *water*, add 3.5 ml of 2M *hydrochloric acid*, dilute to 60 ml with *water* and filter. 15 ml of the filtrate complies with the *limit test for sulphates*, Appendix VII (0.12%).

Related substances Carry out the method for *thin-layer chromatography*, Appendix III A, using a chromatoplate precoated with silica gel F254 the surface of which has been modified with chemically-bonded octadecylsilyl groups (Whatman KC18F plates are suitable) and a mixture of 70 volumes of *methanol*, 30 volumes of *water* and 1 volume of *glacial acetic acid* as the mobile phase. Apply separately to the plate 2 μl of each of two solutions of the substance being examined, prepared by dissolving in *water* and then adding an equal volume of *acetone*, containing (1) 1.0% w/v and (2) 0.040% w/v. After removal of the plate, allow it to dry in air and examine under *ultra-violet light (254 nm)*. Any *secondary spot* in the chromatogram obtained with solution (1) is not more intense than the spot in the chromatogram obtained with solution (2).

Water Not more than 5.0% w/w, Appendix IX C. Use 1 g.

Assay Gently boil 0.1 g under a reflux condenser with 25 ml of 1.25M *sodium hydroxide* for 30 minutes. Allow to cool, add 25 ml of 0.0333M *potassium bromate VS*, 5 ml of a 12.5% w/v solution of *potassium bromide* and 10 ml of *hydrochloric acid* and immediately stopper the flask. Shake for 15 minutes and allow to stand for 15 minutes. Add 25 ml of *potassium iodide solution* and shake vigorously. Titrate the liberated iodine with 0.1M *sodium thiosulphate VS* using *starch mucilage*, added towards the end of the titration, as indicator. The volume of 0.0333M *potassium bromate VS* used is equivalent to half of the volume of 0.1M *sodium thiosulphate VS* required for the titration. Each ml of 0.0333M *potassium bromate VS* is equivalent to 0.006740 g of $C_{10}H_{11}NaO_3$.

Storage Sodium Propyl Hydroxybenzoate should be kept in a well-closed container.

Action and use Antimicrobial preservative.

Sodium Salicylate ☆

$C_7H_5NaO_3$ 160.1   *54-21-7*

Sodium Salicylate is sodium 2-hydroxy-benzoate. It contains not less than 99.0 per cent and not more than 101.0 per cent of $C_7H_5NaO_3$, calculated with reference to the dried substance.

Characteristics Colourless, small crystals or shiny flakes or a white, crystalline powder.

Solubility Soluble in 1 part of *water* (concentrated solutions are liable to deposit crystals of the hexahydrate); soluble in 11 parts of *ethanol (96%)*; practically insoluble in *ether*.

Identification *Test A may be omitted if tests B and C are carried out. Test C may be omitted if tests A and B are carried out.*
A. The *infra-red absorption spectrum*, Appendix II A, is concordant with the spectrum of *sodium salicylate EPCRS*.
B. A 10.0% w/v solution in *carbon dioxide-free water* prepared from *distilled water* (solution A) yields *reaction B* characteristic of sodium salts, Appendix VI.
C. Yields the *reactions* characteristic of salicylates, Appendix VI.

Acidity To 20 ml of solution A add 0.1 ml of *phenol red solution*. The solution is yellow and not more than 2.0 ml of 0.01M *sodium hydroxide VS* is required to change the colour to reddish-violet.

Clarity and colour of solution Solution A is *clear*, Appendix IV A, and not more intensely coloured than *reference solution BY₆*, Appendix IV B, Method II.

Heavy metals Dissolve 1.5 g in 5 ml of water and add 10 ml of *ethanol (96%)*. 12 ml of the solution complies with *limit test B for heavy metals*, Appendix VII (20 ppm). Prepare the standard using 10 ml of a standard lead solution (2 ppm Pb) prepared by diluting *lead standard solution (100 ppm Pb)* with a mixture of 5 volumes of *water* and 10 volumes of *ethanol (96%)*.

Chloride To 5 ml of solution A add 5 ml of *water* and 10 ml of 2M *nitric acid* and filter. 10 ml of the filtrate diluted to 15 ml with *water* complies with the *limit test for chlorides*, Appendix VII (200 ppm).

Sulphate 2.5 ml of solution A diluted to 15 ml with *distilled water* complies with the *limit test for sulphates*, Appendix VII (600 ppm).

Loss on drying When dried to constant weight at 100° to 105°, loses not more than 0.5% of its weight. Use 1 g.

Assay Dissolve 0.13 g in 30 ml of *anhydrous glacial acetic acid* and carry out Method I for *non-aqueous titration*, Appendix VIII A, determining the end-point potentiometrically. Each ml of 0.1M *perchloric acid VS* is equivalent to 0.01601 g of $C_7H_5NaO_3$.

Storage Sodium Salicylate should be kept in an airtight container and protected from light.

Preparations
Sodium Salicylate Mixture
Strong Sodium Salicylate Mixture

Action and use Anti-inflammatory; analgesic.

Sodium Starch Glycollate
Sodium Carboxymethyl Starch

Sodium Starch Glycollate is the sodium salt of a poly-α-glucopyranose in which some of the hydroxyl groups are in the form of the carboxy-methyl ether. It contains not less than 2.8 per cent and not more than 4.5 per cent of sodium, Na, calculated with reference to the washed and dried material.

Characteristics A very fine, white or off-white, free-flowing powder; odourless or almost odourless.

Solubility Practically insoluble in *water*; insoluble in most organic solvents.

Identification A. The *infra-red absorption spectrum*, Appendix II A, after suitable expansion of the transmit-tance scale, is concordant with the *reference spectrum* of sodium starch glycollate.
B. To 5 ml of a 2% w/v dispersion add 0.05 ml of 0.005M *iodine*. A dark blue colour is produced.
C. The solution used in the test for Heavy metals yields the *reactions* characteristic of sodium salts, Appendix VI.

Acidity or alkalinity pH of a 2% w/v dispersion in *carbon dioxide-free water*, 5.5 to 7.5, Appendix V L.

Heavy metals To 2.5 g in a silica or platinum crucible add 2 ml of *sulphuric acid (50%)* and heat on a water-bath and then cautiously over a flame to about 600°. Continue heating until all black particles have disappeared, allow to cool, add 0.1 ml of 1M *sulphuric acid*, heat to ignition as before and again allow to cool. Add 0.1 ml of 2M *ammonium carbonate*, evaporate to dryness and cautiously ignite. To the residue add 5 ml of *hydrochloric acid*, evaporate to dryness on a water-bath and dissolve the residue in 50 ml of *water*. 12 ml of the resulting solution complies with *limit test A for heavy metals*, Appendix VII (20 ppm). Use *lead standard solution (1 ppm Pb)* to prepare the standard.

Iron 10 ml of the solution obtained in the test for Heavy metals complies with the *limit test for iron*, Appendix VII (20 ppm).

Sodium chloride Not more than 10.0% when determined by the following method. To 1.0 g add 20 ml of 0.1M *silver nitrate VS* and 30 ml of *nitric acid* and boil carefully for 30 minutes. Cool and add a sufficient volume of a saturated solution of *potassium permanganate* to change the colour of the solution to red. Discharge the colour by the dropwise addition of *hydrogen peroxide solution (10 vol)*, add 3 ml of *dibutyl phthalate* and titrate with 0.1M *ammonium thiocyanate VS* using *ammonium iron(III) sulphate solution* as indicator, shaking vigorously after each addition of titrant. Each ml of 0.1M *silver nitrate VS* is equivalent to 0.005844 g of NaCl.

Sodium glycollate Not more than 2.0% when determined by the following method. To 0.2 g add 5 ml of *glacial acetic acid*, mix well and add 5 ml of *water*, stirring occasionally until solution is complete. Slowly add 50 ml of *acetone* with stirring and then add 1 g of *sodium chloride*. Filter, wash the residue with *acetone* and dilute the filtrate to 100 ml with *acetone*. Transfer 2 ml of this solution to an open flask, heat on a water-bath for exactly 20 minutes, cool, add 5 ml of *naphthalenediol reagent* and mix thoroughly. Add a further 15 ml of the same reagent, mix, cover the flask with aluminium foil and heat on a water-bath for 20 minutes. Cool and dilute to 25 ml with *sulphuric acid*. The *absorbance* of the resulting solution at the maximum at 540 nm, Appendix II B, using *water* in the reference cell, is not more than that of a solution prepared in the following manner. To 5 ml of a 0.062% w/v solution of *glycollic acid*, previously dried at a pressure not exceeding 2 kPa for 16 hours, add 5 ml of *glacial acetic acid*, dilute to 100 ml with *acetone* and complete the procedure described above, beginning at the words 'Transfer 2 ml . . .'.

Loss on drying When dried to constant weight at 105°, loses not more than 10.0% of its weight. Use 1 g.

Assay To 4 g add 350 ml of a mixture of 4 volumes of *ethanol (96%)* and 1 volume of *water*, add 0.25 ml of *phenolphthalein solution* and mix. Add 1M *sodium hydroxide* dropwise until the colour of the suspension becomes faintly pink, shake for 30 minutes and decant through a glass crucible. Repeat this extraction three times, or until a test for chloride ions is negative. Transfer the bulk of the residue to the crucible, wash the residue with *ethanol (96%)* and dry at 110° to constant weight. To 0.5 g of the dried substance add 80 ml of *glacial acetic acid*, heat under a reflux condenser for 2 hours, cool and titrate with 0.1M *perchloric acid VS* determining the end-point potentiometrically. Each ml of 0.1M *perchloric acid VS* is equivalent to 0.002300 g of Na.

Action and use Pharmaceutical aid.

Sodium Stibogluconate

16037-91-5

Sodium Stibogluconate is a pentavalent antimony compound. It contains not less than 30.0 per cent and not more than 34.0 per cent of pentavalent antimony, calculated with reference to the dried and methanol-free substance.

Characteristics A colourless, mostly amorphous powder; odourless or almost odourless.

Solubility Very soluble in *water*; practically insoluble in *ethanol (96%)* and in *ether*.

Identification A. A solution is dextrorotatory.
B. Pass *hydrogen sulphide* into a 5% w/v solution for several minutes. An orange precipitate is produced.
C. When heated, it chars without melting, emitting an odour of burnt sugar and leaving a residue which yields the *reactions* characteristic of antimony compounds and of sodium salts, Appendix VI.

Stability and acidity of solution Heat a solution containing the equivalent of 10% w/v of pentavalent antimony in an autoclave at 115.5° and at a pressure of 170 kPa for 30 minutes. The resulting solution is colourless or almost colourless and has a pH of 5.0 to 5.6, Appendix V L.

Trivalent antimony Dissolve 2 g in 30 ml of *water*, add 15 ml of *hydrochloric acid* and titrate with 0.00833M *potassium bromate VS* using *methyl orange solution* as indicator. Not more than 1.3 ml of 0.00833M *potassium bromate VS* is required.

Chloride Dissolve 2.5 g in 50 ml of *water* and add 2 ml of 2M *nitric acid* and 75 ml of *acetate buffer pH 5.0*. Titrate with 0.1M *silver nitrate VS* determining the end-point potentiometrically. Not more than 3.0 ml of 0.1M *silver nitrate VS* is required.

Methanol Not more than 2.0% w/w when determined by the following method. Carry out the method for *gas chromatography*, Appendix III B, using the following solutions. For solution (1) add 1 ml of a 1.0% v/v solution of *methanol* to 5 ml of a 0.2% v/v solution of *absolute ethanol* (internal standard). For solution (2) add 5 ml of *water* to 0.5 g of the substance being examined and mix in an ultrasonic bath until solution is complete. For solution (3) add 5 ml of a 0.2% v/v solution of the internal standard to 0.5 g of the substance being examined and mix in an ultrasonic bath until solution is complete.

The chromatographic procedure may be carried out using a glass column (1.5 m × 4 mm) packed with porous polymer beads (80 to 100 mesh) (Porapak Q and Chromosorb 101 are suitable) and maintained at 130°.

Calculate the percentage w/w of methanol taking 0.792 g as its weight per ml at 20°.

Undue toxicity Dissolve a suitable quantity in *water for injections* to give a solution containing the equivalent of 28 mg of pentavalent antimony per ml. Inject intravenously 0.3 ml of this solution into each of 10 mice that have been deprived of food for not less than 17 hours. After injection allow the mice access to food and water. None of the mice dies within 24 hours. If one of the mice dies within 24 hours repeat the test. None of the second group of mice dies within 24 hours.

Loss on drying When dried to constant weight at 130° at a pressure not exceeding 0.7 kPa, loses not more than 15.0% of its weight. Use 1 g.

Assay Dissolve 0.16 g in 30 ml of *hydrochloric acid*, add 70 ml of *orthophosphoric acid* and stir carefully until completely mixed. Titrate with 0.05M *ammonium iron(II) sulphate VS* prepared with *sulphuric acid (1%)* and determine the end-point potentiometrically using a platinum electrode and a silver—silver chloride reference electrode. Each ml of 0.05M *ammonium iron(II) sulphate VS* is equivalent to 0.003044 g of pentavalent antimony.

Storage Sodium Stibogluconate should be kept in a well-closed container.

Preparation

Sodium Stibogluconate Injection

Action and use Antiprotozoal.

Anhydrous Sodium Sulphate ☆

Na_2SO_4 142.0   *7681-38-1*

Anhydrous Sodium Sulphate contains not less than 99.0 per cent and not more than 100.5 per cent of Na_2SO_4, calculated with reference to the dried substance.

Characteristics A white powder; odourless; hygroscopic.

Solubility Freely soluble in *water*.

Identification Yields *reactions A* and *B* characteristic of sodium salts and the *reactions* characteristic of sulphates, Appendix VI.

Acidity or alkalinity To 10 ml of a 2.2% w/v solution in *distilled water* (solution A) add 0.1 ml of *bromothymol blue solution*. Not more than 0.5 ml of either 0.01M *hydrochloric acid VS* or 0.01M *sodium hydroxide VS* is required to change the colour of the solution.

Clarity and colour of solution Solution A is *clear*, Appendix IV A, and *colourless*, Appendix IV B, Method II.

Arsenic 10 ml of solution A complies with the *limit test for arsenic*, Appendix VII (5 ppm).

Calcium 10 ml of solution A diluted to 15 ml with *distilled water* complies with the *limit test for calcium*, Appendix VII (450 ppm).

Heavy metals 12 ml of solution A complies with *limit test A for heavy metals*, Appendix VII (45 ppm). Use *lead standard solution (1 ppm Pb)* to prepare the standard.

Iron 5 ml of solution A diluted to 10 ml with *water* complies with the *limit test for iron*, Appendix VII (90 ppm).

Magnesium To 10 ml of solution A add 1 ml of *glycerol*, 0.15 ml of *titan yellow solution*, 0.25 ml of a 2.5% w/v solution of *ammonium oxalate* and 5 ml of 2M *sodium hydroxide* and shake. Any pink colour produced is not more intense than that produced by treating in the same manner a mixture of 5 ml of *magnesium standard solution (10 ppm Mg)* and 5 ml of *water* (200 ppm).

Chloride 5 ml of solution A diluted to 15 ml with *water* complies with the *limit test for chlorides*, Appendix VII (450 ppm).

Loss on drying When dried to constant weight at 130°, loses not more than 5.0% of its weight. Use 1 g.

Assay Dissolve 1.3 g in 50 ml of *water* and pass through a column (200 mm × 20 mm) packed with *strongly acidic ion-exchange resin* at a flow rate of about 4 ml per minute. Elute with *water* (about 300 ml) until 50 ml requires not more than 0.05 ml of 0.1M *sodium hydroxide VS* for neutralisation. Titrate the eluate with 1M *sodium hydroxide VS* using *methyl orange solution* as indicator. Each ml of 1M *sodium hydroxide VS* is equivalent to 0.0710 g of Na_2SO_4.

Storage Anhydrous Sodium Sulphate should be kept in a well-closed container.

Sodium Sulphate ☆

Glauber's Salt

$Na_2SO_4,10H_2O$ 322.2   *7727-73-3*

Sodium Sulphate contains not less than 99.0 per cent and not more than 100.5 per cent of Na_2SO_4, calculated with reference to the dried substance.

Characteristics Colourless, transparent crystals or a white, crystalline powder. It partially dissolves in its own water of crystallisation at about 33°.

Solubility Soluble in 2.5 parts of *water*; practically insoluble in *ethanol (96%)*.

Identification Yields *reactions A* and *B* characteristic of sodium salts and the *reactions* characteristic of sulphates, Appendix VI.

Acidity or alkalinity To 10 ml of a 5.0% w/v solution in *distilled water* (solution A) add 0.1 ml of *bromothymol blue solution*. Not more than 0.5 ml of either 0.01M *hydrochloric acid VS* or 0.01M *sodium hydroxide VS* is required to change the colour of the solution.

Clarity and colour of solution Solution A is *clear*, Appendix IV A, and *colourless*, Appendix IV B, Method II.

Arsenic 10 ml of solution A complies with the *limit test for arsenic*, Appendix VII (2 ppm).

Calcium 10 ml of solution A diluted to 15 ml with *distilled water* complies with the *limit test for calcium*, Appendix VII (200 ppm).

Heavy metals 12 ml of solution A complies with *limit test A for heavy metals*, Appendix VII (20 ppm). Use *lead standard solution (1 ppm Pb)* to prepare the standard.

Iron 5 ml of solution A diluted to 10 ml with *water* complies with the *limit test for iron*, Appendix VII (40 ppm).

Magnesium To 10 ml of solution A add 1 ml of *glycerol*, 0.15 ml of *titan yellow solution*, 0.25 ml of a 4% w/v solution of *ammonium oxalate* and 5 ml of 2M *sodium hydroxide* and shake. Any pink colour produced is not more intense than that produced by treating in the same manner a mixture of 5 ml of *magnesium standard solution (10 ppm Mg)* and 5 ml of *water* (100 ppm).

Chloride 5 ml of solution A diluted to 15 ml with *water* complies with the *limit test for chlorides*, Appendix VII (200 ppm).

Loss on drying When dried at 30° for 1 hour and then at 130° to constant weight, loses 52.0% to 57.0% of its weight. Use 1 g.

Assay Dissolve 3 g in 50 ml of *water* and pass through a column (200 mm × 20 mm) packed with *strongly acidic ion-exchange resin* with a flow rate of about 4 ml per minute. Wash with *water* (about 300 ml) until 50 ml requires not more than 0.05 ml of 0.1M *sodium hydroxide VS* for neutralisation. Titrate the eluate with 1M *sodium hydroxide VS* using *methyl orange solution* as indicator. Each ml of 1M *sodium hydroxide VS* is equivalent to 0.0710 g of Na_2SO_4.

Storage Sodium Sulphate should be kept in a well-closed container.

Action and use Laxative.

The title of the monograph in the European Pharmacopœia is Sodium Sulphate Decahydrate.

Anhydrous Sodium Sulphite

Na_2SO_3 126.04   *7757-83-7*

Anhydrous Sodium Sulphite contains not less than 95.0 per cent and not more than 100.5 per cent of Na_2SO_3.

Characteristics A white, crystalline powder; odourless or almost odourless.

Solubility Soluble in *water*; practically insoluble in *ethanol* (96%).

Identification A. Add a 5% w/v solution to *potassium permanganate solution* previously acidified to *litmus paper* with 1M *sulphuric acid*. The reagent is decolorised.

B. To 5 ml of a 5% w/v solution add 2 ml of a 10% w/v solution of *lead(II) acetate*; a white precipitate is produced. Add 20 ml of 2M *nitric acid*; the precipitate dissolves. Boil the resulting solution for 5 minutes; a white precipitate is produced.

C. Yields the *reactions* characteristic of sodium salts, Appendix VI.

Arsenic Mix 2.0 g in a porcelain dish with 5 ml of *water*, 0.6 g of *potassium chlorate* and 8 ml of *hydrochloric acid*, allow to stand for 1 hour, heat to remove chlorine and dilute to 60 ml with *water*. 15 ml of the resulting solution complies with the *limit test for arsenic*, Appendix VII (2 ppm).

Copper Dissolve 10.0 g in 35 ml of *water*, add 1 ml of a 20% w/v solution of *citric acid* and 1 ml of a freshly prepared and filtered 0.5% w/v solution of *acacia* in cold *water*. Adjust the pH of the solution to 9.0 with 5M *ammonia*, dilute to 50 ml with *water*, add 2 ml of *sodium diethyldithiocarbamate solution*, mix and allow to stand for 2 minutes. Any colour obtained is not more intense than that produced by treating 5 ml of *copper standard solution (10 ppm Cu)* in the same manner (5 ppm).

Iron Dissolve 2.0 g in 12 ml of *water*, add 8 ml of *hydrochloric acid* and evaporate to dryness. Dissolve the residue in a mixture of 1 ml of *hydrochloric acid* and 2 ml of *water* and dilute to 50 ml with *water*. 10 ml of the resulting solution complies with the *limit test for iron*, Appendix VII (25 ppm).

Lead Prepare two solutions as follows. For solution (1) dissolve 0.70 g in 10 ml of 6M *acetic acid*. For solution (2) dissolve 0.20 g in 10 ml of 6M *acetic acid* and add 5 ml of *lead standard solution (1 ppm Pb)*. Make solutions (1) and (2) alkaline with 5M *ammonia* and to each add 1 ml of

potassium cyanide solution PbT. The solutions should be not more than faintly opalescent. If the colours of the solutions differ, equalise by adding about 0.2 ml of a highly diluted solution of burnt sugar or other non-reactive substance. Dilute each solution to 50 ml with *water*, add 0.1 ml of a 10% w/v solution of *sodium sulphide* to each and mix thoroughly. The colour produced in solution (1) is not more intense than that produced in solution (2) when viewed against a white background (10 ppm).

Thiosulphate Dissolve 1.0 g in 10 ml of *water*, add 3 ml of *hydrochloric acid* and heat on a water-bath for 10 minutes. The solution remains clear.

Assay Dissolve 0.25 g in 50 ml of 0.05M *iodine VS*, add 1 ml of *hydrochloric acid* and titrate the excess of iodine with 0.1M *sodium thiosulphate VS* using *starch mucilage* as indicator. Each ml of 0.05M *iodine VS* is equivalent to 0.006302 g of Na_2SO_3.

Storage Anhydrous Sodium Sulphite should be kept in a well-closed container.

Action and use Antioxidant.

Sodium Tetradecyl Sulphate Concentrate

$$CH_3 \quad\quad OSO_3Na \quad\quad CH_2 \cdot CH_3$$
$$CH_3 \cdot CH \cdot CH_2 \cdot CH \cdot CH_2 \cdot CH_2 \cdot CH \cdot CH_2 \cdot CH_2 \cdot CH_2 \cdot CH_3$$

$C_{14}H_{29}NaO_4S$ 316.4   *139-88-8*

Sodium Tetradecyl Sulphate Concentrate is an aqueous gel containing sodium 4-ethyl-1-iso-butyloctyl sulphate. It contains not less than 46.0 per cent w/w and not more than 52.0 per cent w/w of $C_{14}H_{29}NaO_4S$.

Characteristics A clear, colourless gel.

Identification A. Carry out the method for *gas chromatography*, Appendix III B, using the following solutions. For solution (1) boil 0.2 g under a reflux condenser with 20 ml of 2M *hydrochloric acid* for 15 minutes, allow to cool, add 20 ml of *ethanol* (96%) and extract the mixture with two 10-ml quantities of n-*pentane*. Wash the combined pentane extracts with 20 ml of *water* and dry over *anhydrous sodium sulphate*. Solution (2) contains 0.35% w/v of *decan-1-ol* and 0.7% w/v of *dodecan-1-ol* in n-*pentane*.

The chromatographic procedure may be carried out using a glass column (1.5 m × 4 mm) packed with *acid-washed, silanised diatomaceous support* (80 to 100 mesh) coated with 3% w/w of polyethylene glycol (Carbowax 20M is suitable) and maintained at 120°.

The retention time of the principal peak obtained with solution (1) is less than the retention time of the peak due to dodecan-1-ol and more than the retention time of the peak due to decan-1-ol in the chromatogram obtained with solution (2).

B. Mix 0.1 ml of a 2% w/v solution with 0.1 ml of a 0.1% w/v solution of *methylene blue* and 2 ml of 1M *sulphuric acid*, add 2 ml of *chloroform* and shake. The chloroform layer is intensely blue.

C. Mix 20 mg with 10 ml of *ethanol* (96%) and heat to boiling on a water-bath, shaking frequently. Filter immediately and evaporate the ethanol. Dissolve the residue in 8 ml of *water*, add 3 ml of 2M *hydrochloric acid*, evaporate the solution to half its volume and cool. Filter to remove the congealed fatty alcohols and add 1 ml of 0.25M *barium chloride* to the filtrate. A white, crystalline precipitate is produced.

D. Yields *reaction B* characteristic of sodium salts, Appendix VI.

Alkalinity Dissolve 1 g in 100 ml of *water* and add 0.1 ml of *methyl red solution*. If the solution is yellow, not more than 0.5 ml of 0.1M *hydrochloric acid VS* is required to change the colour of the solution.

Non-esterified alcohols Dissolve 10 g in 100 ml of *ethanol (96%)* and extract the solution with three 50-ml quantities of n-*pentane*, adding *sodium chloride* if necessary to promote separation of the two layers. Wash the combined pentane extracts with three 50-ml quantities of *water* and discard the washings. Dry the washed pentane extracts over *anhydrous sodium sulphate*, filter and evaporate on a water-bath until the odour of pentane is no longer detectable. Heat the residue at 105° for 15 minutes and cool. The residue weighs not more than 10 mg.

Chloride Dissolve 33 mg in sufficient *water* to produce 100 ml. 15 ml of the resulting solution complies with the *limit test for chlorides*, Appendix VII (1.0%).

Sulphate Dissolve 1.0 g in sufficient *water* to produce 100 ml. 15 ml of the resulting solution complies with the *limit test for sulphates*, Appendix VII (0.1%).

Sulphated ash 11.5 to 14.5%, Appendix IX A.

Assay Dissolve 2.4 g in sufficient *water* to produce 1000 ml. To 20 ml add 15 ml of *chloroform* and 10 ml of *dimidium bromide—sulphan blue solution* and titrate with 0.004M *benzethonium chloride VS*, shaking vigorously and allowing the layers to separate after each addition, until the pink colour of the chloroform layer is completely discharged and a greyish-blue colour is produced. Each ml of 0.004M *benzethonium chloride VS* is equivalent to 0.001266 g of $C_{14}H_{29}NaO_4S$.

Storage Sodium Tetradecyl Sulphate Concentrate should be kept in a well-closed container, protected from light and stored at a temperature not exceeding 15°.

Preparation

Sodium Tetradecyl Sulphate Injection

Action and use Sclerosant.

Sodium Thiosulphate ☆

Sodium Hyposulphite

$Na_2S_2O_3,5H_2O$ 248.2   *10102-17-7*

Sodium Thiosulphate contains not less than 99.0 per cent and not more than 101.0 per cent of $Na_2S_2O_3,5H_2O$.

Characteristics Colourless, transparent crystals; efflorescent in dry air. It dissolves in its water of crystallisation at about 49°.

Solubility Soluble in 0.5 part of *water*; practically insoluble in *ethanol (96%)*.

Identification A. Decolorises *iodine solution*.

B. To 0.5 ml of a 10.0% w/v solution in *carbon dioxide-free water* prepared from *distilled water* (solution A) add 0.5 ml

of *water* and 2 ml of 0.1M *silver nitrate*. A white precipitate is produced which quickly becomes yellowish, then black.

C. Dilute 2.5 ml of solution A to 5 ml with *water* and add 1 ml of *hydrochloric acid*. A gas is evolved which turns *starch—iodate paper* blue and a precipitate of sulphur is produced.

D. 1 ml of solution A yields *reaction A* characteristic of sodium salts, Appendix VI.

Acidity or alkalinity pH of solution A, 6.0 to 8.4, Appendix V L.

Clarity and colour of solution Solution A is *clear*, Appendix IV A, and *colourless*, Appendix IV B, Method II.

Heavy metals To 10 ml of solution A add 0.05 ml of *sodium sulphide solution* and allow to stand for 2 minutes. Any brown colour produced is not more intense than that produced by treating 10 ml of *lead standard solution (1 ppm Pb)* in the same manner (10 ppm).

Chloride To 5 ml of solution A add 15 ml of 2M *nitric acid*, boil gently for 3 to 4 minutes, cool, filter and dilute the filtrate to 25 ml with *water*. 12.5 ml of the resulting solution, diluted to 15 ml with *water*, complies with the *limit test for chlorides*, Appendix VII (200 ppm).

Sulphate and sulphite Dilute 2.5 ml of solution A to 10 ml with *distilled water*. To 3 ml of this solution add 2 ml of *iodine solution* and gradually add more *iodine solution* dropwise until a very faint persistent yellow colour is produced. The resulting solution, diluted to 15 ml with *distilled water*, complies with the *limit test for sulphates*, Appendix VII (0.2%).

Sulphide To 10 ml of solution A add 0.05 ml of a freshly prepared 5% w/v solution of *sodium nitroprusside*. The solution does not become violet.

Assay Dissolve 0.5 g in 20 ml of *water* and titrate with 0.05M *iodine VS* using 1 ml of *starch solution*, added towards the end of the titration, as indicator. Each ml of 0.05M *iodine VS* is equivalent to 0.02482 g of $Na_2S_2O_3,5H_2O$.

Storage Sodium Thiosulphate should be kept in an airtight container.

Action and use Used in treatment of cyanide poisoning.

Sodium Valproate

$CH_3 \cdot CH_2 \cdot CH_2 \cdot CH \cdot CO_2Na$
$CH_3 \cdot CH_2 \cdot CH_2$

$C_8H_{15}NaO_2$ 166.2   *1069-66-5*

Sodium Valproate is sodium 2-propylpentan-oate. It contains not less than 98.0 per cent and not more than 101.0 per cent of $C_8H_{15}NaO_2$, calculated with reference to the dried substance.

Characteristics A white or almost white, crystalline powder; odourless or almost odourless; deliquescent.

Solubility Soluble in 5 parts of *water* and in 5 parts of *ethanol (96%)*.

Identification A. Dissolve 0.5 g in 5 ml of *water*, add 5 ml of *chloroform* and 1 ml of 2M *hydrochloric acid*, shake vigorously for 1 minute, allow to separate, dry the lower layer with *anhydrous sodium sulphate*, filter and evaporate to dryness. The *infra-red absorption spectrum* of a thin film of the residue, Appendix II A, is concordant with the *reference spectrum* of valproic acid.

B. Dissolve 0.5 g in 5 ml of *water* and add 1 ml of a 10% w/v solution of *cobalt(II) nitrate*. A purple precipitate is produced which is soluble in *carbon tetrachloride*.

C. Yields *reactions B* and *C* characteristic of sodium salts, Appendix VI.

Acidity or alkalinity Dissolve 2 g in 20 ml of *carbon dioxide-free water* and add 0.1 ml of *phenolphthalein solution*. Not more than 1.5 ml of either 0.1M *sodium hydroxide VS* or 0.1M *hydrochloric acid VS* is required to neutralise the solution.

Clarity and colour of solution A 20% w/v solution is not more opalescent than *reference suspension II*, Appendix IV A, and is *colourless*, Appendix IV B, Method I.

Arsenic 0.5 g complies with the *limit test for arsenic*, Appendix VII (2 ppm).

Heavy metals Dissolve 1.0 g in 10 ml of *water*, add 5 ml of 2M *hydrochloric acid*, mix and extract with 30 ml of *ether*. Adjust the pH of the aqueous phase to 7.0 by the dropwise addition of 5M *ammonia* and dilute to 20 ml with *water*. The resulting solution complies with *limit test A for heavy metals*, Appendix VII (20 ppm). Use *lead standard solution (1 ppm Pb)* to prepare the standard.

Iron 0.2 g complies with the *limit test for iron*, Appendix VII (50 ppm).

Chloride Dissolve 0.3 g in 15 ml of *water*, add 2 ml of 2M *nitric acid*, mix and extract with 30 ml of *ether*. Using the aqueous phase carry out the *limit test for chlorides*, Appendix VII, beginning at the words 'immediately add 1 ml of 0.1M *silver nitrate . . .*' (170 ppm).

Sulphate Dissolve 1.5 g in 20 ml of *water*, add 2 ml of 5M *acetic acid*, mix and extract with 40 ml of *ether*. Dilute the aqueous phase to 30 ml with *water* and carry out the *limit test for sulphates*, Appendix VII (200 ppm).

Related substances Carry out the method for *gas chromatography*, Appendix III B, using the following solutions. Solution (1) contains 0.020% w/v of *octanoic acid* (internal standard) in *dichloromethane*. For solution (2) dissolve 0.50 g of the substance being examined in 10 ml of *water*, acidify with 2M *sulphuric acid* and shake with three 20-ml quantities of *dichloromethane*. Wash the combined dichloromethane extracts with 10 ml of *water*, shake with *anhydrous sodium sulphate*, filter and evaporate the filtrate to a volume of about 10 ml at a temperature not exceeding 30° using a rotary evaporator. For solution (3) dissolve 0.50 g of the substance being examined in 10 ml of a 0.020% w/v solution of the internal standard in 0.1M *sodium hydroxide* and continue as described for solution (2), beginning at the words 'acidify with 2M *sulphuric acid . . .*'.

The chromatographic procedure may be carried out using a glass column (1.5 m × 4 mm) packed with *acid-washed, silanised diatomaceous support* (80 to 100 mesh) coated with 15% w/w of *free fatty acid phase* (Supelco FFAP 2-1063 is suitable) and 1% w/w of *orthophosphoric acid* and maintained at 170°.

In the chromatogram obtained with solution (3) the sum of the areas of the *secondary peaks* is not greater than the area of the peak due to the internal standard.

Loss on drying When dried at 105° for 4 hours, loses not more than 2.0% of its weight. Use 1 g.

Assay Carry out Method I for *non-aqueous titration*, Appendix VIII A, using 0.25 g and *oracet blue B* as indicator. Each ml of 0.1M *perchloric acid VS* is equivalent to 0.01662 g of $C_8H_{15}NaO_2$.

Storage Sodium Valproate should be kept in a well-closed container.

Preparations

Sodium Valproate Oral Solution

Sodium Valproate Tablets

Action and use Anticonvulsant.

Sorbic Acid

$C_6H_8O_2$ 112.1   *22500-92-1*

Sorbic Acid is (E,E)-hexa-2,4-dienoic acid. It contains not less than 99.0 per cent and not more than 100.5 per cent of $C_6H_8O_2$, calculated with reference to the anhydrous substance.

Characteristics A white or creamy-white powder; odour, faint and characteristic.

Solubility Slightly soluble in *water* and in fats and fatty oils; soluble in 10 parts of *ethanol (96%)* and in 20 parts of *ether*.

Identification A. The *infra-red absorption spectrum*, Appendix II A, is concordant with the *reference spectrum* of sorbic acid.

B. The *light absorption*, Appendix II B, in the range 230 to 350 nm of a 0.0005% w/v solution in 0.1M *hydrochloric acid* exhibits a maximum only at 264 nm. The *absorbance* at 264 nm is about 1.19.

C. To a saturated solution in *water* add *bromine water* dropwise. The bromine solution is decolorised.

Melting point 133° to 137°, Appendix V A.

Arsenic Mix 0.5 g with 0.3 g of *anhydrous sodium carbonate*, add 1 ml of *bromine water*, mix thoroughly and evaporate to dryness on a water-bath. Gently ignite the residue in a porcelain dish, cool, add 5 ml of *water* and 2 ml of *brominated hydrochloric acid* and remove the excess bromine with *tin(II) chloride solution AsT*. The solution complies with the *limit test for arsenic*, Appendix VII (2 ppm).

Heavy metals 2.0 g complies with *limit test C for heavy metals*, Appendix VII (10 ppm). Use 2 ml of *lead standard solution (10 ppm Pb)* to prepare the standard.

Aldehyde Dissolve 1.0 g in a mixture of 50 ml of *propan-2-ol* and 30 ml of *water*, adjust the solution to pH 4 with 1M *hydrochloric acid* and dilute to 100 ml with *water*. To 10 ml of the solution add 1 ml of *decolorised magenta solution* and allow to stand for 30 minutes. The colour produced is not more intense than that produced by adding 1 ml of *decolorised magenta solution* to a mixture of 1.5 ml of *acetaldehyde standard solution*, 4 ml of *propan-2-ol* and 4.5 ml of *water* (0.15% calculated as C_2H_4O).

Sulphated ash Not more than 0.2%, Appendix IX A.

Water Not more than 0.5%, Appendix IX C. Use 5 g.

Assay Dissolve 1.5 g in 25 ml of *ethanol (96%)* previously neutralised to *phenolphthalein solution* and titrate with 1M *sodium hydroxide VS* using *phenolphthalein solution* as indicator. Each ml of 1M *sodium hydroxide VS* is equivalent to 0.1121 g of $C_6H_8O_2$.

Storage Sorbic Acid should be kept in a well-closed container, protected from light and stored at a temperature not exceeding 15°.

Action and use Antimicrobial preservative.

Sorbitan Monolaurate

1338-39-2

Sorbitan Monolaurate is a mixture of the partial esters of sorbitol and its mono- and di-anhydrides with lauric acid.

Characteristics An amber, viscous liquid; odour, characteristic of fatty acids. It has a weight per ml, at 20°, of about 1.0 g and a viscosity, at 25°, of about 4.5 pascal seconds.

Solubility Practically insoluble but dispersible in *water*; miscible with *ethanol (96%)*; slightly soluble in cottonseed oil.

Identification A. To 5 ml of a 5% w/v dispersion in *water* add 5 ml of 1M *sodium hydroxide*, boil, cool and acidify with 2M *hydrochloric acid*. The solution is strongly opalescent.
B. Heat 4 g under a reflux condenser on a water-bath for 30 minutes with 40 ml of a 5% w/v solution of *potassium hydroxide*. Allow to cool to about 80°, acidify with 20 ml of 2M *nitric acid* and boil for about 10 minutes under a reflux condenser in order to destroy the emulsion. The fatty acid separates on the surface as an oily liquid. Allow to cool to room temperature and extract with 50 ml of *petroleum spirit (boiling range, 40° to 60°)*, avoiding vigorous shaking. Wash the organic phase with three 5-ml quantities of *water* and evaporate the organic phase on a water-bath. The *acid value* of the residue, Appendix X B, is 250 to 300, using 0.3 g and 50 ml of the prescribed solvent.

Acid value 4.0 to 7.0, Appendix X B.

Hydroxyl value 330 to 358, Appendix X D, Method II. Use 1 g.

Saponification value 158 to 170, Appendix X G.

Arsenic Heat gently 3.3 g with 2 ml of *nitric acid* and 0.5 ml of *sulphuric acid* in a long-necked flask until the reaction has subsided. Cool and add carefully in small portions 15 ml of *nitric acid* and 6 ml of *sulphuric acid* taking care to avoid excessive foaming and continue heating, adding further small portions of *nitric acid*, if necessary, until white fumes are evolved and the solution becomes colourless or nearly colourless. Cool, add carefully 10 ml of *water*, evaporate until white fumes are evolved and repeat the addition of *water* and evaporation until all the nitric acid has been removed. Cool and dilute to 100 ml. 10 ml of the resulting solution complies with the *limit test for arsenic*, Appendix VII (3 ppm).

Heavy metals Moisten the residue obtained in the test for Sulphated ash with 0.05 ml of 7M *hydrochloric acid*, add 10 ml of hot *water* and allow to stand for 2 minutes. Add 6M *ammonia* dropwise until the solution is just alkaline and adjust the pH with 2M *acetic acid* to between 3.0 and 4.0. Filter if necessary, wash the dish and the filter with small quantities of *water* and dilute the combined filtrate and washings to 20 ml with *water*. 12 ml of this solution complies with *limit test A for heavy metals*, Appendix VII (10 ppm). Use *lead standard solution (1 ppm Pb)* to prepare the standard.

Sulphated ash Not more than 0.25% when determined by the following method. To 2.0 g in a suitable crucible add sufficient *sulphuric acid* to wet the sample and carefully ignite at a low temperature until thoroughly charred. The crucible may be loosely covered with a lid during the charring. Add 2 ml of *nitric acid* and 0.25 ml of *sulphuric acid*, cautiously heat until white fumes are evolved and then ignite at 500° to 600° until the carbon is entirely burned off. Allow the dish to cool, add 0.2 ml of 1M *sulphuric acid*, heat and ignite as before and allow to cool. Add 0.2 ml of a 16% w/v solution of *ammonium carbonate*. Evaporate and ignite carefully, allow to cool, weigh, ignite again for 5 minutes and repeat the operation until two successive weighings do not differ by more than 0.5 mg.

Action and use Pharmaceutical aid.

In some countries the material described in this monograph may be known as Sorbitan Laurate.

Sorbitan Mono-oleate

1338-43-8

Sorbitan Mono-oleate is a mixture of the partial esters of sorbitol and its mono- and di-anhydrides with oleic acid.

Characteristics An amber, viscous liquid; odour, characteristic of fatty acids. It has a weight per ml, at 20°, of about 1.0 g and a viscosity, at 25°, of about 1 pascal second.

Solubility Practically insoluble but dispersible in *water*; miscible with *ethanol (96%)*.

Identification A. To 5 ml of a 5% w/v dispersion in *water* add 5 ml of 1M *sodium hydroxide*, boil, cool and acidify with 2M *hydrochloric acid*. The solution is strongly opalescent.
B. To a 5% w/v dispersion in *water* add *bromine water* dropwise. The bromine solution is decolorised.

Acid value 5.0 to 8.0, Appendix X B.

Hydroxyl value 193 to 209, Appendix X D, Method II. Use 2 g.

Saponification value 149 to 160, Appendix X G.

Arsenic; Heavy metals; Sulphated ash Complies with the tests described under Sorbitan Monolaurate.

Action and use Pharmaceutical aid.

In some countries the material described in this monograph may be known as Sorbitan Oleate.

Sorbitan Monostearate

HO   OH

CH·CH₂·OCO·C₁₇H₃₅

O

OH

1338-41-6

Sorbitan Monostearate is a mixture of the partial esters of sorbitol and its mono- and di-anhydrides with stearic acid.

Characteristics A pale yellow solid; odour, faint and oily. It has a setting point of about 50°.

Solubility Practically insoluble but dispersible in *water*; slightly soluble in *ethanol (96%)*.

Identification A. To 5 ml of a 5% w/v dispersion in *water* add 5 ml of 1M *sodium hydroxide*, boil, cool and acidify with 2M *hydrochloric acid*. The solution is strongly opalescent.

B. Dissolve 0.5 g in *water* at about 50° and dilute to 10 ml with the same solvent; a copious foam is produced on shaking. Add 0.5 g of *sodium chloride* and heat to boiling; the resulting cloudiness disappears during cooling to about 50°.

C. Heat 4 g under a reflux condenser on a water-bath for 30 minutes with 40 ml of a 5% w/v solution of *potassium hydroxide*. Allow to cool to about 80°, acidify with 20 ml of 2M *nitric acid* and boil for about 10 minutes under a reflux condenser in order to destroy the emulsion; the fatty acid separates on the surface as an oily liquid. Allow to cool to room temperature and extract with 50 ml of *petroleum spirit (boiling range, 40° to 60°)* avoiding vigorous shaking. Wash the organic phase with three 5-ml quantities of *water* and evaporate the organic phase on a water-bath. The *acid value* of the residue, Appendix X B, is about 205, using 0.5 g and 50 ml of the prescribed solvent.

Acid value 5.0 to 10.0, Appendix X B.

Hydroxyl value 235 to 260, Appendix X D, Method II. Use 1.0 g.

Saponification value 147 to 157, Appendix X G.

Arsenic; Heavy metals; Sulphated ash Complies with the tests described under Sorbitan Monolaurate.

Action and use Pharmaceutical aid.

In some countries the material described in this monograph may be known as Sorbitan Stearate.

Sorbitol ☆

CH₂OH

HCOH

HOCH

HCOH

HCOH

CH₂OH

C₆H₁₄O₆   182.2   *30-70-4*

Sorbitol* contains not less than 98.0 per cent and not more than 101.0 per cent of D-glucitol, calculated with reference to the anhydrous substance.

Characteristics A white, crystalline powder; odourless.

Solubility Soluble in 0.5 part of *water* and in 25 parts of *ethanol (96%)*; practically insoluble in *chloroform* and in *ether*.

Identification A. Carry out the method for *thin-layer chromatography*, Appendix III A, using *silica gel G* as the coating substance and a mixture of 70 volumes of *propan-1-ol*, 20 volumes of *ethyl acetate* and 10 volumes of *water* as the mobile phase but allowing the solvent front to ascend 17 cm above the line of application. Apply separately to the chromatoplate 2 μl of each of two solutions in *water* containing (1) 0.25% w/v of the substance being examined and (2) 0.25% w/v of *sorbitol EPCRS*. After removal of the plate, allow it to dry in air and spray with a 0.2% w/v solution of *sodium metaperiodate*. Allow to dry in air for 15 minutes and spray with a 2% w/v solution of *4,4'-methylenebis-N,N-dimethylaniline* in a mixture of 80 volumes of *acetone* and 20 volumes of *glacial acetic acid*. The principal spot in the chromatogram obtained with solution (1) corresponds in position, colour and size to that in the chromatogram obtained with solution (2).

B. To 3 ml of a freshly prepared 10% w/v solution of *catechol* add 6 ml of *sulphuric acid* while cooling in ice. To 3 ml of the mixture add 0.3 ml of a 10.0% w/v solution in *carbon dioxide-free water* prepared from *distilled water* (solution A), mix and heat gently over an open flame for 30 seconds. A pink colour is produced.

C. Dissolve 0.5 g in a mixture of 5 ml of *acetic anhydride* and 0.5 ml of *pyridine* with the aid of heat and allow to stand for 10 minutes. Pour the mixture into 25 ml of *water*, allow to stand in ice for 2 hours and filter. The *melting point* of the residue, after recrystallisation from a small volume of *ethanol (96%)* and drying over *phosphorus pentoxide* at a pressure of 1.5 to 2.5 kPa, is about 100°, Appendix V A, Method I.

Acidity or alkalinity To 10 ml of solution A add 10 ml of *carbon dioxide-free water*. To 10 ml of the resulting solution add 0.1 ml of *dilute phenolphthalein solution*; not more than 0.2 ml of 0.01M *sodium hydroxide VS* is required to change the colour of the solution to pink. To a further 10 ml of the solution add 0.1 ml of *methyl red solution*; not more than 0.3 ml of 0.01M *hydrochloric acid VS* is required to change the colour of the solution to red.

Clarity and colour of solution Solution A is *clear*, Appendix IV A, and *colourless*, Appendix IV B, Method II.

Specific optical rotation Dissolve a mixture of 5 g of the substance being examined and 6.4 g of *sodium tetraborate* in 40 ml of *water*, allow to stand for 1 hour, shaking occasionally, dilute to 50 ml with *water* and filter if necessary. The *specific optical rotation* in the resulting solution is +4.0° to +7.0°, Appendix V F.

Lead Complies with *limit test A for lead in sugars*, Appendix VII (0.5 ppm).

Nickel Complies with the *limit test for nickel in polyols*, Appendix VII (1 ppm).

Chloride 10 ml of solution A diluted to 15 ml with *water* complies with the *limit test for chlorides*, Appendix VII (50 ppm).

Sulphate 15 ml of solution A complies with the *limit test for sulphates*, Appendix VII (100 ppm).

Reducing sugars Dissolve 5 g in 3 ml of *water* with the aid of gentle heat, cool, add 20 ml of *sodium cupri-citrate solution* and a few glass beads, heat in such a manner that the solution boils in 4 minutes and continue boiling for a further 3 minutes. Cool rapidly and add 100 ml of a 2.4% v/v solution of *glacial acetic acid* followed by 20 ml of 0.025M *iodine VS*. Add, shaking continuously, 25 ml of a 6.0% v/v solution of *hydrochloric acid* and, when any precipitate has redissolved, titrate the excess of iodine with 0.05M *sodium thiosulphate VS* using 1 ml of *starch solution*, added towards the end of the titration, as indicator. Not less than 12.8 ml of 0.05M *sodium thiosulphate VS* is required.

Sulphated ash Not more than 0.1%, Appendix IX A, Method II. Use 2 g.

Water Not more than 1.5% w/w, Appendix IX C. Use 1 g.

Assay Dissolve 0.4 g in sufficient *water* to produce 100 ml. Transfer 10 ml to a stoppered flask, add 20 ml of a 2.14% w/v solution of *sodium metaperiodate* and 2 ml of 1M *sulphuric acid* and heat on a water-bath for exactly 15 minutes. Cool, add 3 g of *sodium hydrogen carbonate* in small quantities and 25 ml of 0.1M *sodium arsenite VS*, mix, add 5 ml of a 20% w/v solution of *potassium iodide*, allow to stand for 15 minutes and titrate with 0.05M *iodine VS* until the first trace of yellow colour appears. Repeat the operation without the substance being examined. The difference between the titrations represents the amount of iodine required. Each ml of 0.05M *iodine VS* is equivalent to 0.001822 g of $C_6H_{14}O_6$.

Storage Sorbitol should be kept in a well-closed container.

Preparation

Sorbitol Intravenous Infusion

Action and use For parenteral nutrition.

*In certain states party to the Convention on the Elaboration of a European Pharmacopœia, Sorbitol intended for use in large-volume preparations for parenteral use may be required to comply with the *test for pyrogens*, Appendix XIV K, injecting per kg of the rabbit's weight 10 ml of a solution containing 50 mg per ml.

Sorbitol Solution (70 per cent) (Crystallising) ☆

Sorbitol Solution (70 per cent)

Sorbitol Solution (70 per cent) (Crystallising) is an aqueous solution containing not less than 68.0 per cent and not more than 72.0 per cent w/w of hexitols expressed as D-glucitol.

Characteristics A clear, colourless, viscous liquid; odourless.

Solubility Miscible with *water*, with *glycerol (85%)* and with *propane-1,2-diol*; soluble in *ethanol (96%)*.

Identification A. Carry out the method for *thin-layer chromatography*, Appendix III A, using *silica gel G* as the coating substance and a mixture of 70 volumes of *propan-1-ol*, 20 volumes of *ethyl acetate* and 10 volumes of *water* as the mobile phase but allowing the solvent front to ascend 17 cm above the line of application. Apply separately to the chromatoplate 2 µl of each of two solutions in *water* containing (1) 0.35% w/v of the solution being examined and (2) 0.25% w/v of *sorbitol EPCRS*. After removal of the plate, allow it to dry in air and spray with a 0.2% w/v solution of *sodium metaperiodate*; allow to

dry in air for 15 minutes and spray with a 2% w/v solution of *4,4'-methylenebis-N,N-dimethylaniline* in a mixture of 80 volumes of *acetone* and 20 volumes of *glacial acetic acid*. The principal spot in the chromatogram obtained with solution (1) corresponds in position, colour and size to that in the chromatogram obtained with solution (2).

B. To 3 ml of a freshly prepared 10% w/v solution of *catechol* add 6 ml of *sulphuric acid* while cooling in ice. To 3 ml of the mixture add 0.3 ml of a solution prepared by diluting 7.0 g of the solution being examined to 50 ml with *carbon dioxide-free water* prepared from *distilled water* (solution A), mix and heat gently over an open flame for 30 seconds. A pink colour is produced.

C. Dry 1 g over *phosphorus pentoxide* at 80° at a pressure of 1.5 to 2.5 kPa. Dissolve 0.5 g of the residue in a mixture of 5 ml of *acetic anhydride* and 0.5 ml of *pyridine* with the aid of heat and allow to stand for 10 minutes. Pour the mixture into 25 ml of *water*, allow to stand in ice for 2 hours and filter. The *melting point* of the residue, after recrystallisation from a small volume of *ethanol (96%)* and drying over *phosphorus pentoxide* at a pressure of 1.5 to 2.5 kPa, is about 100°, Appendix V A, Method I.

D. Dilute 7 g with 40 ml of *water*, add 6.4 g of *sodium tetraborate*, allow to stand for 1 hour, shaking occasionally, and dilute to 50 ml with *water*. The *optical rotation* of the resulting solution, Appendix V F, is 0° to +1.5°.

Acidity or alkalinity To 10 ml of solution A add 10 ml of *carbon dioxide-free water*. To 10 ml of the resulting solution add 0.1 ml of *dilute phenolphthalein solution*; not more than 0.2 ml of 0.01M *sodium hydroxide VS* is required to change the colour of the solution to pink. To a further 10 ml of the solution add 0.1 ml of *methyl red solution*; not more than 0.3 ml of 0.01M *hydrochloric acid VS* is required to change the colour of the solution to red.

Clarity and colour of solution Solution A is *clear*, Appendix IV A, and *colourless*, Appendix IV B, Method II.

Refractive index 1.457 to 1.462, Appendix V E.

Relative density Not less than 1.290, Appendix V G.

Lead Complies with *limit test A for lead in sugars*, Appendix VII (0.5 ppm).

Nickel Complies with the *limit test for nickel in polyols*, Appendix VII (1 ppm).

Chloride 7.5 ml of solution A diluted to 15 ml with *water* complies with the *limit test for chlorides*, Appendix VII (50 ppm).

Sulphate 1.5 g diluted to 15 ml with *distilled water* complies with the *limit test for sulphates*, Appendix VII (100 ppm).

Reducing sugars To 5 g add 3 ml of *water*, 20 ml of *sodium cupri-citrate solution* and a few glass beads, heat in such a manner that the solution boils in 4 minutes and continue boiling for a further 3 minutes. Cool rapidly and add 100 ml of a 2.4% v/v solution of *glacial acetic acid* followed by 20 ml of 0.025M *iodine VS*. Add, shaking continuously, 25 ml of a 6.0% v/v solution of *hydrochloric acid* and, when any precipitate has redissolved, titrate the excess of iodine with 0.05M *sodium thiosulphate VS* using 1 ml of *starch solution*, added towards the end of the titration, as indicator. Not less than 12.8 ml of 0.05M *sodium thiosulphate VS* is required.

Sulphated ash Not more than 0.1%, Appendix IX A, Method II. Use 2 g.

Assay Dilute 0.6 g with sufficient *water* to produce 100 ml. Transfer 10 ml to a stoppered flask, add 20 ml of a 2.14% w/v solution of *sodium metaperiodate* and 2 ml of 1M *sulphuric acid* and heat on a water-bath for exactly 15 minutes. Cool, add, in small quantities, 3 g of *sodium hydrogen carbonate* and 25 ml of 0.1M *sodium arsenite VS*, mix, add 5 ml of a 20% w/v solution of *potassium iodide*, allow to stand for 15 minutes and titrate with 0.05M *iodine VS* until the first trace of yellow colour appears. Repeat the operation without the solution being examined. The difference between the titrations represents the amount of iodine required. Each ml of 0.05M *iodine VS* is equivalent to 0.001822 g of $C_6H_{14}O_6$.

Storage Sorbitol Solution (70 per cent) (Crystallising) should be kept in a well-closed container.

Action and use Pharmaceutical aid.

The title of the monograph in the European Pharmacopœia is Sorbitol 70 Per Cent (Crystallising).

Sorbitol Solution (70 per cent) (Non-crystallising) ☆

Sorbitol Solution (70 per cent) (Non-crystallising) is an aqueous solution of hydrogenated, partly hydrolysed starch. It contains not less than 68.0 per cent and not more than 72.0 per cent w/w of solid matter and not less than 62.0 per cent w/w of polyols expressed as D-glucitol.

Characteristics A clear, colourless, viscous liquid; odourless.

Solubility Miscible with *water*, with *glycerol (85%)* and with *propane-1,2-diol*.

Identification A. Complies with test A for Identification described under Sorbitol Solution (70 per cent) (Crystallising).
B. To 3 ml of a freshly prepared 10% w/v solution of *catechol* add 6 ml of *sulphuric acid* while cooling in ice. To 3 ml of the mixture add 0.3 ml of a solution prepared by diluting 7.0 g of the solution being examined to 50 ml with *carbon dioxide-free water* prepared from *distilled water* (solution A), mix and heat gently over an open flame for 30 seconds. A pink colour is produced which becomes deep brownish-red.
C. Dilute 7 g with 40 ml of *water*, add 6.4 g of *sodium tetraborate*, allow to stand for 1 hour, shaking occasionally and dilute to 50 ml with *water*. The *optical rotation* of the resulting solution, Appendix V F, is +1.5° to +3.5°.

Acidity or alkalinity; Clarity and colour of solution; Relative density; Lead; Nickel; Chloride; Sulphate; Reducing sugars; Sulphated ash Complies with the requirements stated under Sorbitol Solution (70 per cent) (Crystallising).

Refractive index 1.455 to 1.465, Appendix V E.

Reducing sugars after hydrolysis To 6 g add 35 ml of *water*, 40 ml of 1M *hydrochloric acid* and a few glass beads and boil under a reflux condenser for 4 hours. Cool, neutralise to *bromothymol blue* with 2M *sodium hydroxide*, cool and dilute to 100 ml with *water*. To 3 ml of the solution add 5 ml of *water*, 20 ml of *sodium cupri-citrate solution* and a few glass beads and carry out the test for

Reducing sugars described under Sorbitol Solution (70 per cent) (Crystallising), beginning at the words 'heat in such a manner . . .'. Not less than 8.0 ml and not more than 14.8 ml of 0.05M *sodium thiosulphate VS* is required.

Assay *For solid matter* Dry 1 g to constant weight over *phosphorus pentoxide* at 80° at a pressure of 1.5 to 2.5 kPa and weigh the residue.

For polyols Carry out the Assay described under Sorbitol Solution (70 per cent) (Crystallising).

Storage Sorbitol Solution (70 per cent) (Non-crystallising) should be kept in a well-closed container.

Action and use Pharmaceutical aid.

The title of the monograph in the European Pharmacopœia is Sorbitol 70 Per Cent (Non-crystallising).

Soya Oil
Soyabean Oil

Soya Oil is the fixed oil obtained from the seeds of *Glycine max* (L.) Merr., refined, deodorised and clarified by filtration at about 0°. It may contain a suitable antioxidant.

Characteristics A pale yellow oil; odourless or almost odourless; taste, bland.

Solubility Almost insoluble in *ethanol (96%)*; miscible with *chloroform*, with *ether* and with *petroleum spirit (boiling range, 40° to 60°)*.

Acid value Not more than 0.6, Appendix X B.

Refractive index 1.466 to 1.470, Appendix V E.

Weight per ml 0.916 to 0.922 g, Appendix V G.

Unsaponifiable matter Not more than 1.5%, Appendix X H.

Stearin Remains bright when maintained at 0° for 16 hours.

Foreign fixed oils Carry out the test for *foreign oils by gas chromatography*, Appendix X N. The fatty-acid fraction of the oil has the following composition.
Palmitic acid 7.0 to 14.0%.
Stearic acid 1.4 to 5.5%.
Oleic acid (equivalent chain length on polyethylene glycol adipate 18.3) 19.0 to 30.0%.
Linoleic acid (equivalent chain length on polyethylene glycol adipate 18.9) 44.0 to 62.0%.
Linolenic acid (equivalent chain length on polyethylene glycol adipate 19.7) 4.0 to 11.0%.

Storage Soya Oil should be kept in a well-filled, well-closed container, protected from light and stored at a temperature not exceeding 25°.

Spearmint Oil

Spearmint Oil is obtained by distillation from fresh flowering plants of *Mentha spicata* L. and *Mentha × cardiaca* (Gray) Bak.

Characteristics A clear, colourless, pale yellow or greenish-yellow liquid when recently distilled, but becoming darker and viscous on keeping; visibly free from water; odour, that of spearmint.

Optical rotation −45° to −60°, Appendix V F.

Refractive index 1.484 to 1.491, Appendix V E.

Solubility in ethanol Soluble, at 20°, in 1 part of *ethanol (80%)*, Appendix X M; the solution may become cloudy when diluted.

Weight per ml 0.917 to 0.934 g, Appendix V G.

Content of carvone Not less than 55.0% w/w, Appendix X L.

Storage Spearmint Oil should be kept in a well-filled, well-closed container, protected from light and stored at a temperature not exceeding 25°.

Action and use Flavour.

Spectinomycin Hydrochloride

$C_{14}H_{24}N_2O_7,2HCl,5H_2O$ 495.4   *22189-32-8*

Spectinomycin Hydrochloride is the penta-hydrate of the dihydrochloride of (2*R*,4a*R*, 5a*R*,6*S*,7*S*,8*R*,9*S*,9a*R*,10a*S*)-perhydro-4a,7,9-trihydroxy-2-methyl-6,8-bis(methylamino)-pyrano[2,3-*b*][1,4]benzodioxin-4-one, an antimicrobial substance produced by *Streptomyces spectabilis* or by any other means. The potency is not less than 780 Units per mg, calculated with reference to the anhydrous substance.

Characteristics A white or almost white, crystalline powder.

Solubility Soluble in 10 parts of *water*; practically insoluble in *ethanol (96%)*, in *chloroform* and in *ether*.

Identification A. The *infra-red absorption spectrum*, Appendix II A, is concordant with the *reference spectrum* of spectinomycin hydrochloride.
B. A 1% w/v solution yields *reaction A* characteristic of chlorides, Appendix VI.

Acidity pH of a 10% w/v solution, 3.8 to 5.6, Appendix V L.

Specific optical rotation In a 10% w/v solution, +15° to +21°, Appendix V F.

Related substances Carry out the method for *thin-layer chromatography*, Appendix III A, using *silica gel G* as the coating substance and a mixture of 50 volumes of *propan-1-ol*, 40 volumes of *water*, 5 volumes of *glacial acetic acid* and 5 volumes of *pyridine* as the mobile phase but allowing the solvent front to ascend 12 cm above the line of application. Apply separately to the chromatoplate 10 μl of each of two solutions of the substance being examined in *water* containing (1) 2.0% w/v and (2) 0.020% w/v. After removal of the plate, allow it to dry in air, spray with a 5% w/v solution of *potassium permanganate* and allow to stand for 2 to 3 minutes. Any *secondary spot* in the chromatogram obtained with solution (1) is not more intense than the spot in the chromatogram obtained with solution (2).

Sulphated ash Not more than 1.0%, Appendix IX A.

Water 16.0 to 20.0% w/w, Appendix IX C. Use 0.2 g.

Assay Carry out the *biological assay of antibiotics*, Appendix XIV A. The precision of the assay is such that the fiducial limits of error are not less than 95% and not more than 105% of the estimated potency.

Storage Spectinomycin Hydrochloride should be kept in a well-closed container and stored at a temperature not exceeding 30°. If it is intended for use in the manufacture of a parenteral dosage form, the container should be sterile and sealed so as to exclude micro-organisms.

Labelling The label states (1) the date after which the material is not intended to be used; (2) the conditions under which it should be stored; (3) whether or not it is intended for use in the manufacture of a parenteral dosage form.

Preparation
Spectinomycin Injection

Action and use Antibacterial.

Spectinomycin Hydrochloride intended for use in the manufacture of a parenteral dosage form complies with the following additional requirements.

Pyrogens Complies with the *test for pyrogens*, Appendix XIV K. Use per kg of the rabbit's weight 1 ml of a solution in *sodium chloride injection* containing 75 mg per ml.

Sterility When intended for use in the manufacture of a parenteral dosage form without further sterilisation, complies with the *test for sterility*, Appendix XVI A.

Spironolactone

$C_{24}H_{32}O_4S$ 416.6   *52-01-7*

Spironolactone is 7α-acetylthio-3-oxo-17α-pregn-4-ene-21,17β-carbolactone. It contains not less than 96.0 per cent and not more than 102.0 per cent of $C_{24}H_{32}O_4S$, calculated with reference to the dried substance.

Characteristics A white to cream powder; odourless or with a slight odour of thioacetic acid.

Solubility Practically insoluble in *water*; soluble in 80 parts of *ethanol (96%)*, in 3 parts of *chloroform* and in 100 parts of *ether*.

Identification A. The *infra-red absorption spectrum*, Appendix II A, is concordant with the *reference spectrum* of spironolactone.
B. Complies with the test for *identification of steroids*, Appendix III A, using *impregnating solvent II* and *mobile phase D*.
C. Shake 10 mg with 2 ml of *sulphuric acid (50%)*; an orange solution with an intense yellowish-green fluorescence is produced. Heat the solution gently; the colour becomes deep red and fumes of hydrogen sulphide

are evolved that turn *lead acetate paper* black. Pour the solution into *water*; a greenish-yellow, opalescent solution is produced.

D. *Melting point*, about 205°, Appendix V A.

Specific optical rotation In a 1% w/v solution in *chloroform*, −33.0° to −37.0°, Appendix V F.

Chromium Mix 0.20 g with 1 g of *potassium carbonate* and 0.3 g of *potassium nitrate* in a platinum crucible, heat gently until fused and ignite at 600° to 650° until the carbon is removed. Cool, dissolve the residue as completely as possible in 10 ml of *water* with the aid of gentle heat, filter and add sufficient *water* to produce 20 ml. To 10 ml add 0.5 g of *urea* and just acidify with *sulphuric acid (14%)*. When effervescence ceases, add a further 1 ml of *sulphuric acid (14%)*, dilute to 20 ml with *water* and add 0.5 ml of *diphenylcarbazide solution*. Any colour produced is not more intense than that produced by adding 1 ml of *sulphuric acid (14%)* to 0.50 ml of a freshly prepared 0.00283% w/v solution of *potassium dichromate*, diluting to 20 ml with *water* and adding 0.5 ml of *diphenylcarbazide solution*.

Mercapto compounds Shake 2 g with 20 ml of *water*, filter and titrate 10 ml of the filtrate with 0.005M *iodine VS* using *starch mucilage* as indicator. Not more than 0.1 ml of 0.005M *iodine VS* is required.

Related substances Carry out the method for *thin-layer chromatography*, Appendix III A, using a silica gel precoated chromatoplate (Merck silica gel 60 plates are suitable) and *butyl acetate* as the mobile phase. Apply separately to the chromatoplate 5 μl of each of two solutions of the substance being examined in *chloroform* containing (1) 2.0% w/v and (2) 0.020% w/v. After removal of the plate, allow the solvent to evaporate at room temperature, return the plate to the tank and again allow the solvent front to ascend 15 cm above the line of application. Remove the plate, allow the solvent to evaporate at room temperature, spray with *methanolic sulphuric acid (10%)* and heat at 105° for 10 minutes. Any *secondary spot* in the chromatogram obtained with solution (1) is not more intense than the spot in the chromatogram obtained with solution (2).

Loss on drying When dried to constant weight at 105°, loses not more than 0.5% of its weight. Use 1 g.

Sulphated ash Not more than 0.1%, Appendix IX A.

Assay Dissolve 10 mg in sufficient *methanol* to produce 100 ml, dilute 10 ml to 100 ml with *methanol* and measure the *absorbance* of the resulting solution at the maximum at 238 nm, Appendix II B. Calculate the content of $C_{24}H_{32}O_4S$ taking 470 as the value of A(1%, 1 cm) at the maximum at 238 nm.

Storage Spironolactone should be protected from light.

Preparation
Spironolactone Tablets

Action and use Diuretic.

Squill

Squill consists of the bulb of *Drimia maritima* (L.) Stearn, collected soon after the plant has flowered, divested of its dry, outer, membranous coats, cut into transverse slices and dried. It is known in commerce as white squill.

Characteristics Odourless or almost odourless.

Macroscopical Transverse slices, about 5 to 8 mm thick, occurring as straight or curved triangular pieces about 5 to 50 mm long and 3 to 8 mm wide at mid-point, tapering towards each end, yellowish-white, texture horny, somewhat translucent, breaking with an almost glassy fracture when quite dry, but readily absorbing moisture when exposed to the air and becoming tough and flexible; transversely cut surface showing a single row of prominent, vascular bundles near the concave edge and numerous smaller bundles scattered throughout the mesophyll.

Microscopical Epidermis: cells polygonal and axially elongated, one to two times longer than wide, cuticle thick, stratified; stomata very rare, *anomocytic*, and nearly circular in outline, about 50 to 60 μm in diameter; mesophyll of colourless, thin-walled parenchyma containing very occasional starch granules, many cells containing bundles of acicular crystals of calcium oxalate embedded in mucilage, crystals up to about 1 mm long and about 1 to 15 μm wide; other cells containing sinistrin; vascular bundles collateral, scattered throughout the mesophyll; xylem vessels with spiral and annular wall thickening; trichomes absent.

Identification The mucilage contained in the cells of the mesophyll is stained red with *alkaline corallin solution* but produces no red colour with *ruthenium red solution* and no purple colour with 0.01M *iodine*.

Acid-insoluble ash Not more than 1.5%, Appendix XI K, Method I.

Extractive soluble in ethanol (60%) Not less than 68.0%, Appendix XI B. Use material that has been dried for 1 hour at 105° and powdered.

Storage Squill should be stored in a dry place at a temperature not exceeding 25°.

Preparations
Squill Liquid Extract
Squill Oxymel

Powdered Squill

Powdered Squill is Squill in powder.

Characteristics White or yellowish-white; very hygroscopic. Diagnostic structures: abundant, acicular crystals of calcium oxalate, the larger ones frequently broken, some embedded in mucilage which is stained red with *alkaline corallin solution* but produces no colour with 0.01M *iodine*; lignified vessels with spiral and annular thickening; fragments of epidermis with very infrequent stomata.

Identification; Acid-insoluble ash; Extractive soluble in ethanol (60%) Complies with the requirements stated under Squill.

Storage Powdered Squill should be kept in a desiccated atmosphere and stored at a temperature not exceeding 25°.

Action and use Expectorant.

Indian Squill

Indian Squill consists of the bulb of *Drimia indica* (Roxb.) J P Jessop, collected soon after the plant has flowered, divested of dry, outer membranous coats and usually cut longitudinally into slices and dried.

Characteristics Odourless or almost odourless.

Macroscopical Curved or irregularly shaped strips, about 10 to 50 mm long, 3 to 10 mm wide and 1 to 3 mm thick, frequently tapering towards the ends, occasionally grouped three or four together and attached to a portion of the axis; ridged in the direction of their length and varying in colour from pale yellowish-brown to buff; brittle when dry, but tough and flexible when exposed to air.

Microscopical Epidermis: cells tetrahedral to hexahedral, thin-walled, three to five times longer than wide, having a thick, striated cuticle; stomata rare, *anomocytic*, circular in outline, 40 to 42 μm in diameter; mesophyll of thin-walled polygonal cells containing mucilage, some cells also containing bundles of acicular crystals of calcium oxalate, 20 to 900 μm in length; vascular bundles collateral, scattered throughout the mesophyll; xylem vessels with spiral and annular wall thickening; trichomes and starch absent.

Identification The mucilage contained in the cells of the mesophyll is stained red with *alkaline corallin solution* and reddish-purple with 0.01M *iodine*.

Ash Not more than 6.0%, Appendix XI J.

Storage Indian Squill should be stored in a dry place at a temperature not exceeding 25°.

Preparation
Squill Oxymel

Action and use Expectorant.

Powdered Indian Squill

Powdered Indian Squill is Indian Squill in powder.

Characteristics Buff coloured; very hygroscopic. Diagnostic structures: numerous acicular crystals of calcium oxalate, the larger ones frequently broken; abundant cells containing mucilage, some with embedded calcium oxalate crystals; the mucilage is stained red with *alkaline corallin solution* and reddish-purple with 0.01M *iodine*; lignified vessels with spiral and annular thickening; fragments of epidermis with very infrequent stomata.

Identification The mucilage contained in the cells of the mesophyll is stained red with *alkaline corallin solution* and reddish-purple with 0.01M *iodine*.

Ash Not more than 6.0%, Appendix XI J.

Storage Powdered Indian Squill should be kept in a desiccated atmosphere and stored at a temperature not exceeding 25°.

Action and use Expectorant.

Stanozolol

$C_{21}H_{32}N_2O$ 328.5   *10418-03-8*

Stanozolol is 17α-methyl-2'*H*-5α-androst-2-eno[3,2-*c*]pyrazol-17β-ol. It contains not less than 98.0 per cent and not more than 101.0 per cent of $C_{21}H_{32}N_2O$, calculated with reference to the dried substance.

Characteristics A white or almost white, crystalline powder.

Solubility Practically insoluble in *water*; sparingly soluble in *ethanol (96%)* and in *chloroform*; soluble in *dimethylformamide*.

Identification A. Dissolve 20 mg in the minimum volume of *chloroform* and evaporate to dryness in a stream of nitrogen at room temperature. The *infra-red absorption spectrum* of the residue, Appendix II A, is concordant with the *reference spectrum* of stanozolol.

B. The *light absorption*, Appendix II B, in the range 220 to 350 nm of a 0.004% w/v solution in a mixture of equal volumes of 0.2M *hydrochloric acid* and *methanol* exhibits a maximum only at 230 nm. The *absorbance* at 230 nm is about 0.80.

C. To 2 mg add 3 ml of *dimethylaminobenzaldehyde reagent*. A yellow colour develops which exhibits a green fluorescence when viewed under ultra-violet light (365 nm).

D. *Melting point*, about 236°, Appendix V A.

Specific optical rotation In a 1% w/v solution in *chloroform*, +34° to +40°, Appendix V F.

Related substances Carry out the method for *thin-layer chromatography*, Appendix III A, using *silica gel H* as the coating substance and a mixture of 90 volumes of *chloroform* and 10 volumes of *methanol* as the mobile phase. Apply separately to the chromatoplate 5 μl of each of two solutions of the substance being examined in a mixture of 1 volume of *methanol* and 4 volumes of *chloroform* containing (1) 2.0% w/v and (2) 0.010% w/v. After removal of the plate, allow it to dry in air, spray with *ethanolic sulphuric acid (20%)*, heat at 105° for 15 minutes and examine under *ultra-violet light (365 nm)*. Any *secondary spot* in the chromatogram obtained with solution (1) is not more intense than the spot in the chromatogram obtained with solution (2).

Loss on drying When dried to constant weight at 100° at a pressure not exceeding 0.7 kPa, loses not more than 1.0% of its weight. Use 1 g.

Assay Dissolve 0.7 g in 50 ml of *anhydrous glacial acetic acid* and carry out Method I for *non-aqueous titration*, Appendix VIII A, determining the end-point potentiometrically. Each ml of 0.1M *perchloric acid VS* is equivalent to 0.03285 g of $C_{21}H_{32}N_2O$.

Storage Stanozolol should be kept in a well-closed container and protected from light.

Preparation
Stanozolol Tablets

Action and use Anabolic steroid.

Starches ☆

Starches are obtained from the caryopsis of maize, *Zea mays* L., of rice, *Oryza sativa* L., or of wheat, *Triticum aestivum* L., or from the tuber of the potato, *Solanum tuberosum* L.

Characteristics Very fine, white powders which creak when pressed between the fingers. Maize starch may be slightly yellowish.

The presence of granules showing cracks or edge irregularities is exceptional in starches other than Wheat Starch; Wheat Starch may contain granules with cracks on the edges.

Solubility Practically insoluble in cold *water* and in *ethanol* (96%).

Identification A. Heat to boiling a suspension of 1 g in 50 ml of *water* for 1 minute and cool. Starches other than Potato Starch give a thin, cloudy mucilage; Potato Starch gives a thicker, more transparent mucilage.
B. Mix 0.05 ml of 0.005M *iodine* with 1 ml of the mucilage obtained in test A. A dark blue colour is produced which disappears on heating and reappears on cooling.

Acidity Add 10 g of the starch to 100 ml of *ethanol (70%)* previously neutralised to 0.5 ml of *dilute phenolphthalein solution*, shake for 1 hour, filter and titrate 50 ml of the filtrate with 0.1M *sodium hydroxide VS*. Not more than 2.0 ml of 0.1M *sodium hydroxide VS* is required to change the colour of the solution.

Foreign matter Not more than traces of cell debris are present.

Microbial contamination* 1.0 g is free from *Escherichia coli*, Appendix XVI B1.

Storage Starches should be kept in airtight containers.

Labelling The label states the type of starch.

Action and use Pharmaceutical aid.

MAIZE STARCH

Maize Starch is obtained from the caryopsis of *Zea mays* L. It complies with the requirements for Starches and with the following additional requirements.

Characteristics *Microscopical* Angular, polyhedral granules, 2 to 23 μm in size, or rounded granules, 25 to 32 μm in diameter. Central hilum consisting of a distinct cavity or two- to five-rayed cleft; no concentric striations. Viewed under polarised light a distinct black cross is seen, intersecting at the hilum.

Loss on drying When dried to constant weight at 100° to 105°, loses not more than 15.0% of its weight. Use 1 g.

Sulphated ash Not more than 0.6%, Appendix IX A, Method II. Use 1 g.

POTATO STARCH

Potato Starch is obtained from the tuber of *Solanum tuberosum* L. It complies with the requirements for Starches and with the following additional requirements.

Characteristics *Microscopical* Single granules either irregular, ovoid or pear-shaped, 30 to 100 μm in size, or rounded, 10 to 35 μm in size; compound granules rare, consisting of groups of two to four elements. Eccentric hilum, with clearly visible concentric striations. Viewed under polarised light a distinct black cross is seen, intersecting at the hilum.

Iron Shake 1.5 g with 15 ml of 2M *hydrochloric acid* and filter. The filtrate complies with the *limit test for iron*, Appendix VII (10 ppm).

Loss on drying When dried to constant weight at 100° to 105°, loses not more than 20.0% of its weight. Use 1 g.

Sulphated ash Not more than 0.6%, Appendix IX A, Method II. Use 1 g.

RICE STARCH

Rice Starch is obtained from the caryopsis of *Oryza sativa* L. It complies with the requirements for Starches and with the following additional requirements.

Characteristics *Microscopical* Polyhedral granules 2 to 5 μm in size, either isolated or aggregated in ovoid masses 10 to 20 μm in size. Central hilum poorly visible; no concentric striations. Viewed under polarised light a distinct black cross is seen, intersecting at the hilum.

Loss on drying When dried to constant weight at 100° to 105°, loses not more than 15.0% of its weight. Use 1 g.

Sulphated ash Not more than 1.0%, Appendix IX A, Method II. Use 1 g.

WHEAT STARCH

Wheat Starch is obtained from the caryopsis of *Triticum aestivum* L. (*T. vulgare* Vill.). It complies with the requirements for Starches and with the following additional requirements.

Characteristics *Microscopical* Large discoid or, more rarely, reniform granules, 10 to 45 μm in size; profile, elliptical and fusiform, slit along the main axis. Small rounded or polyhedral granules, 2 to 10 μm in size. Granules of intermediate size very rarely occur. Hilum and striations discernible only with difficulty. Viewed under polarised light a distinct black cross is seen, intersecting at the hilum.

Loss on drying When dried to constant weight at 100° to 105°, loses not more than 15.0% of its weight. Use 1 g.

Sulphated ash Not more than 0.6%, Appendix IX A, Method II. Use 1 g.

In tropical and subtropical countries where starch obtained from the sources described under Starches is not available, Tapioca Starch obtained from the rhizomes of *Manihot utilissima* Pohl may be used, provided that it complies with the requirements for Starches and with the following additional requirements.

TAPIOCA STARCH

Characteristics *Microscopical* Principally simple granules, subspherical, muller-shaped or rounded polyhedral; smaller granules 5 to 10 μm, larger granules 20 to 35 μm in diameter; hilum, central, punctate, linear or triradiate; striations, faint, concentric; compound granules, few, of two to three unequal components.

Loss on drying When dried to constant weight at 100° to 105°, loses not more than 15.0% of its weight. Use 1 g.

Sulphated ash Not more than 0.6%, Appendix IX A, Method II. Use 1 g.

*In certain states party to the Convention on the Elaboration of a European Pharmacopœia, Starches may be required to comply with a limit for a total viable aerobic count of 10^3 bacteria and 10^2 fungi per gram, determined by plate count, Appendix XVI B2.

Sterculia

Sterculia Gum; Karaya Gum

Sterculia is the gum obtained from *Sterculia urens* Roxb. and other species of *Sterculia*.

Characteristics Odour, that of acetic acid.

Macroscopical Irregular or vermiform pieces, about 5 to 20 mm thick; greyish-white with a brown or pink tinge; surface striated.

Microscopical When powdered and mounted in *ethanol (96%)* it appears as small, transparent, angular particles of various sizes and shapes; the particles lose their sharp edges when water is added and each gradually swells until a large, indefinite, almost structureless mass results; when mounted in *ruthenium red solution* the particles are stained red; no starch particles are visible when mounted in a 0.25% w/v solution of *iodine*.

Solubility Sparingly soluble in *water*, but swells into a homogeneous, adhesive, gelatinous mass. Practically insoluble in *ethanol (96%)*.

Identification A. Add 1 g to 80 ml of *water* and allow to stand for 24 hours, shaking occasionally. A tacky and viscous granular mucilage is produced.
B. Boil 4 ml of the mucilage obtained in test A with 0.5 ml of *hydrochloric acid*, add 1 ml of 5M *sodium hydroxide*, filter, add 3 ml of *potassium cupri-tartrate solution* to the filtrate and heat. A red precipitate is produced.
C. Warm 0.5 g with 2 ml of 5M *sodium hydroxide*. A brown colour is produced.

Acid-insoluble ash Not more than 1.0%, Appendix XI K.

Ash Not more than 7.0%, Appendix XI J.

Volatile acid Not less than 14.0%, calculated as acetic acid, $C_2H_4O_2$, when determined by the following method. To 1 g contained in a 700-ml long-necked flask add 100 ml of *water* and 5 ml of *orthophosphoric acid*, allow to stand for several hours, or until the gum is completely swollen, and boil gently under a reflux condenser for 2 hours. Steam-distil until 800 ml of distillate is obtained and the acid residue measures about 20 ml and titrate the distillate with 0.1M *sodium hydroxide VS* using *phenol-phthalein solution* as indicator. Repeat the operation without the gum. The difference between the titrations represents the amount of alkali required to neutralise the volatile acid. Each ml of 0.1M *sodium hydroxide VS* is equivalent to 0.006005 g of volatile acid, calculated as $C_2H_4O_2$.

Microbial contamination 1.0 g is free from *Escherichia coli*, Appendix XVI B1.

Storage Sterculia should be stored in a dry place at a temperature not exceeding 25°.

Action and use Pharmaceutical aid.

Powdered Sterculia

Powdered Sterculia is Sterculia in powder.

Characteristics White or buff with a distinct odour of acetic acid; transparent, angular, microscopic fragments which, when treated with water, swell and finally disappear.

Identification; Acid-insoluble ash; Ash Complies with the requirements stated under Sterculia.

Volatile acid Not less than 10.0%, calculated as acetic acid, $C_2H_4O_2$, when determined by the method described under Sterculia.

Microbial contamination 1.0 g is free from *Escherichia coli*, Appendix XVI B1.

Storage Powdered Sterculia should be kept in a well-closed container and stored at a temperature not exceeding 25°.

Action and use Pharmaceutical aid.

Stilboestrol ☆

Diethylstilboestrol

$C_{18}H_{20}O_2$ 268.4   56-53-1

Stilboestrol is (E)-αβ-diethylstilbene-4,4′-diol. It contains not less than 97.0 per cent and not more than 101.0 per cent of $C_{18}H_{20}O_2$, calculated with reference to the dried substance.

Characteristics A white or almost white, crystalline powder. It melts at about 172°.

Solubility Practically insoluble in *water*; soluble in 5 parts of *ethanol (96%)*, in 40 parts of *arachis oil* and in 3 parts of *ether*; slightly soluble in *chloroform*. It dissolves in aqueous solutions of alkali hydroxides.

Identification *Test A may be omitted if tests B, C and D are carried out. Tests B and C may be omitted if tests A and D are carried out.*
A. The *infra-red absorption spectrum*, Appendix II A, is concordant with the spectrum of *diethylstilbestrol EPCRS*.
B. The *light absorption*, Appendix II B, in the range 230 to 450 nm of the irradiated solution prepared as directed in the Assay exhibits two maxima, at 292 nm and 418 nm.
C. In the test for Mono- and di-methyl ethers the principal spot in the chromatogram obtained with solution (2) is similar in position, colour and size to that in the chromatogram obtained with solution (3).
D. Dissolve 0.5 mg in 0.2 ml of *glacial acetic acid*, add 1 ml of *orthophosphoric acid* and heat on a water-bath for 3 minutes. A deep yellow colour is produced.

4,4′-Dihydroxystilbene and related ethers *Absorbance* of a 1% w/v solution in *absolute ethanol* at 325 nm, Appendix II B, not more than 0.50.

Mono- and di-methyl ethers Carry out the method for *thin-layer chromatography*, Appendix III A, using *silica gel G* as the coating substance and a mixture of 90 volumes of *toluene* and 10 volumes of *diethylamine* as the mobile phase. Apply separately to the chromatoplate 1 μl of each of the following solutions in *ethanol (96%)*. Solutions (1) and (2) contain 10% and 0.50% w/v respectively of the substance being examined. Solution (3) contains 0.50% w/v of *diethylstilbestrol EPCRS*. Solutions (4) and (5) contain 0.050% w/v of *diethylstilbestrol monomethyl ether EPCRS* and *diethylstilbestrol dimethyl ether EPCRS* respectively. Solution (6) contains

0.25% w/v each of *dienestrol EPCRS* and *diethylstilbestrol EPCRS*. After removal of the plate, allow it to dry in air, spray with *ethanolic sulphuric acid (20%)* and heat at 120° for 10 minutes. Any *secondary spots* in the chromatogram obtained with solution (1) corresponding to the mono- and di-methyl ethers of stilboestrol are not more intense than the spots in the chromatograms obtained with solutions (4) and (5) respectively. Stilboestrol produces one or sometimes two spots. The test is not valid unless the chromatogram obtained with solution (6) shows two clearly separated principal spots.

Loss on drying When dried to constant weight at 100° to 105°, loses not more than 0.5% of its weight. Use 1 g.

Sulphated ash Not more than 0.1%, Appendix IX A, Method II. Use 1.0 g.

Assay Dissolve 20 mg in sufficient *absolute ethanol* to produce 100 ml and dilute 10 ml to 100 ml with the same solvent. To 25 ml of the resulting solution add 25 ml of a solution prepared by dissolving 1 g of *dipotassium hydrogen orthophosphate* in 55 ml of *water*, transfer a portion of the mixture to a 1-cm closed quartz cell, place the cell about 5 cm from a low-pressure, short-wave 2- to 20-watt mercury lamp and irradiate for 5 minutes. Measure the *absorbance* of the irradiated solution at the maximum at 418 nm, Appendix II B, using *water* in the reference cell. Continue the irradiation for successive periods of 3 to 15 minutes, depending on the power of the lamp, and repeat the measurement of the absorbances until the maximum absorbance (about 0.7) is obtained. If necessary adjust the geometry of the irradiation apparatus to obtain a maximum reproducible absorbance at 418 nm. Calculate the content of $C_{18}H_{20}O_2$ from the *absorbance* obtained by repeating the operation using *diethylstilbestrol EPCRS* in place of the substance being examined.

Storage Stilboestrol should be kept in a well-closed container and protected from light.

Preparations
Stilboestrol Pessaries
Stilboestrol Tablets

Action and use Oestrogen.

The title of the monograph in the European Pharmacopœia is Diethylstilbestrol.

Stramonium Leaf ☆

Stramonium Leaf consists of the dried leaf or the dried leaf, flowering tops and occasionally fruits of *Datura stramonium* L. and its varieties. It contains not less than 0.25 per cent of total alkaloids, calculated as hyoscyamine with reference to the material dried at 100° to 105°. The alkaloids consist mainly of those of the hyoscyamine—atropine group together with hyoscine.

Characteristics Odour, unpleasant.

Macroscopical Leaves: dark brownish-green to greyish-green on the upper surface, paler on the lower surface, often much twisted and shrunken during drying, thin and brittle; lamina 8 to 25 cm long and 7 to 15 cm wide; ovate or triangular-ovate, dentately lobed with an acuminate apex and often unequal at the base. Young leaves pubescent on veins; older leaves nearly glabrous. Pinnate venation, secondary veins leaving the midrib at about 45° and running directly into the apices of the lobes. Veins conspicuous, concave on the upper surface, convex on the lower. Stems: green or purplish-green, slender, curved and twisted, wrinkled longitudinally and sometimes wrinkled transversely, branched dichasially, with a single flower or an immature fruit in the fork. Flowers: borne erect upon short pedicels; calyx, gamosepalous, with five lobes; each sepal has an acute longitudinal fold; corolla, plicate, trumpet-shaped; brownish-white or purplish. Immature fruits capsular, usually covered with numerous short, stiff emergences; seeds brown to black, with minutely pitted testa.

Microscopical Leaf: epidermal cells with more or less sinuous anticlinal walls and smooth cuticle; covering and glandular trichomes present, being more numerous on young leaves; covering trichomes uniseriate and conical, composed of three to five cells with warty walls; glandular trichomes short and clavate, with two to seven cells in the head. Stomata *anisocytic*, more frequent on the lower epidermis. Mesophyll dorsiventral, with single palisade layer under which is a crystal layer with each cell containing cluster crystals of calcium oxalate, 10 to 30 µm long, or occasional prisms or microsphenoidal crystals; no crystals present in cells adjoining the veins. Midrib contains an arc of several bicollateral vascular bundles and collenchyma between the upper and lower parts of the epidermis. Fragments of stem: epidermis with uniseriate covering trichomes up to 800 µm long, with warty walls, intraxylary phloem and xylem with wide reticulately-thickened vessels; parenchymatous cells of pith contain calcium oxalate crystals similar to those in the leaf. Corolla: inner epidermis with uniseriate covering trichomes about 40 µm long on the lower part. Many cells of the mesophyll of the calyx and corolla contain cluster crystals, or occasionally prisms, of calcium oxalate.

Identification A. Shake 1 g, in powder, with 10 ml of 0.05M *sulphuric acid* for 2 minutes, filter, add 1 ml of 13.5M *ammonia* and 5 ml of *water* to the filtrate, extract cautiously with 15 ml of *chloroform* to avoid the formation of an emulsion, dry the chloroform layer over *anhydrous sodium sulphate* and filter. Evaporate the chloroform in a porcelain dish, add 0.5 ml of *fuming nitric acid* and evaporate to dryness on a water-bath. Add 10 ml of *acetone* and, dropwise, a 3% w/v solution of *potassium hydroxide* in *ethanol (96%)*. A deep violet colour is produced.

B. Carry out the method for *thin-layer chromatography*, Appendix III A, using *silica gel G* as the coating substance and a mixture of 90 volumes of *acetone*, 7 volumes of *water* and 3 volumes of 13.5M *ammonia* as the mobile phase, but allowing the solvent front to ascend 10 cm above the line of application. Apply separately to a chromatoplate, 200 mm × 200 mm in size, as bands 20 mm × 3 mm, 1 cm apart, 10 µl and 20 µl of each of the following solutions. For solution (1) add 15 ml of 0.05M *sulphuric acid* to 0.4 g of the leaf, in *No. 180 powder*, shake for 15 minutes, filter and wash the filter with 0.05M *sulphuric acid* until 20 ml of filtrate is obtained; add 1 ml of 13.5M *ammonia* to the filtrate, extract with two 10-ml quantities of *peroxide-free ether*, separate the ether layer, by centrifugation if necessary, dry the combined ether extracts over *anhydrous sodium sulphate*, filter, evaporate to dryness on a water-bath and dissolve the residue in 0.5 ml of *methanol*. For solution (2) dissolve 50 mg of *hyoscyamine sulphate* in 9 ml of *methanol* (solution A) and dissolve 15 mg of *hyoscine hydrobromide* in 10 ml of *methanol* (solution B); mix 3.8 ml of solution A with 4.2 ml of solution B and dilute to 10 ml with *methanol*.

After removal of the plate, dry it at 100° to 105° for 15 minutes, allow to cool and spray with 10 ml of *modified potassium iodobismuthate solution* until the bands become visible as orange or brown on a yellow background. The bands in the chromatograms obtained with solution (1) are similar in colour and Rf values to those obtained in the chromatograms obtained with solution (2) (hyoscyamine in the lower third; hyoscine in the upper third) and are at least equal in size. Faint secondary bands may appear, particularly in the middle of the chromatogram obtained with 20 µl of solution (1) or near the line of application in the chromatogram obtained with 10 µl of solution (1). Spray the plate with a freshly prepared 10% w/v solution of *sodium nitrite* until transparent and examine after 15 minutes. The colour due to hyoscyamine in the chromatograms changes from brown to reddish-brown but not to greyish-blue (atropine); any secondary bands are no longer visible.

Foreign matter Not more than 3% of stem with a diameter exceeding 5 mm, Appendix XI D, Test B.

Acid-insoluble ash Not more than 4.0%, Appendix XI K, Method II.

Assay Reduce 50 g, selected from a well-mixed sample, to *No. 180 powder* and determine the moisture content of 2 g by drying to constant weight at 100° to 105°. Moisten 10 g with a mixture of 5 ml of 10M *ammonia*, 10 ml of *ethanol* (96%) and 30 ml of *peroxide-free ether* and mix thoroughly. Transfer the mixture to a small percolator with the aid of the extracting mixture if necessary, allow to macerate for 4 hours and then percolate with a mixture of 1 volume of *chloroform* and 3 volumes of *peroxide-free ether* until *complete extraction* of the alkaloids is effected. Concentrate the percolate to about 50 ml by distillation on a water-bath and transfer to a separating funnel with the aid of *peroxide-free ether*. Add a quantity of *peroxide-free ether* at least 2.1 times the volume of the percolate to produce a liquid considerably less dense than water. Extract the solution with not less than three 20-ml quantities of 0.25M *sulphuric acid*, separating the layers by centrifugation if necessary, and transfer each acid extract to a second separating funnel. Make the combined extracts alkaline with 10M *ammonia* and extract with three 30-ml quantities of *chloroform*. Combine the chloroform extracts, add 4 g of *anhydrous sodium sulphate* and allow to stand for 30 minutes, shaking occasionally. Decant the chloroform and wash the sodium sulphate with three 10-ml quantities of *chloroform*. Evaporate the combined chloroform extracts and washings to dryness on a water-bath and heat the residue at 100° to 105° for 15 minutes. Dissolve the residue in several ml of *chloroform*, add 20 ml of 0.01M *sulphuric acid VS*, remove the chloroform by evaporation on a water-bath and titrate the excess acid with 0.02M *sodium hydroxide VS* using *methyl red solution* as indicator. Each ml of 0.01M *sulphuric acid VS* is equivalent to 0.005788 g of total alkaloids, calculated as hyoscyamine.

Storage Stramonium Leaf should be kept in a airtight container and protected from light.

Preparation

Prepared Stramonium

Action and use Antispasmodic.

Powdered Stramonium Leaf

Powdered Stramonium Leaf is Stramonium Leaf in powder. It contains not less than 0.25 per cent of total alkaloids, calculated as hyoscyamine with reference to the material dried at 100° to 105°. The alkaloids consist mainly of those of the hyoscyamine—atropine group together with hyoscine.

Characteristics Green to greyish-green; odour that of the unground drug. Diagnostic structures: fragments of leaf lamina showing slightly sinuous-walled epidermal cells and numerous *anisocytic* stomata; conical, warty-walled covering trichomes, expanded at the base, frequently fragmented; fewer clavate, glandular trichomes; fragments of the crystal layer of the mesophyll with each cell, except those adjacent to the veins, containing one or more cluster crystals of calcium oxalate; occasional fibres and reticulately-thickened vessels from the stem; subspherical pollen grains, 60 to 80 µm in diameter; numerous isolated cluster crystals of calcium oxalate, 10 to 30 µm long, and occasional prisms and microsphenoidal crystals.

Identification Complies with the tests for Identification described under Stramonium Leaf.

Acid-insoluble ash Not more than 4.0%, Appendix XI K.

Assay Carry out the Assay described under Stramonium Leaf.

Storage Powdered Stramonium Leaf should be kept in an airtight container and protected from light.

Action and use Antispasmodic.

Prepared Stramonium ☆

Prepared Stramonium is Stramonium Leaf in *No. 180 powder* adjusted, if necessary, by the addition of Lactose or of stramonium leaf powder of lower alkaloidal content to contain 0.23 to 0.27 per cent of total alkaloids, calculated as hyoscyamine with reference to the material dried at 100° to 105°.

Characteristics Grey to greenish-grey powder. Diagnostic structures as described under Stramonium Leaf; additionally, when mounted in *glycerol (85%)*, crystals of lactose may be seen.

Identification Complies with the tests for Identification described under Stramonium Leaf.

Acid-insoluble ash Not more than 4.0%, Appendix XI K, Method II.

Loss on drying When dried to constant weight at 100° to 105°, loses not more than 5.0% of its weight. Use 1 g.

Assay Carry out the Assay described under Stramonium Leaf.

Storage Prepared Stramonium should be kept in an airtight container and protected from light.

Streptokinase ☆

Streptokinase is a preparation of a protein obtained from culture filtrates of certain strains of *Streptococcus haemolyticus* group C. It has the property of combining with human plasminogen to form plasminogen activator and is purified to contain not less than 600 Units of streptokinase activity per µg of nitrogen before addition of any stabiliser or carrier. It usually contains a buffer and may be stabilised by the addition of suitable substances such as Albumin Solution.

Characteristics A white powder or a white friable solid; hygroscopic.

Solubility Freely soluble in *water*.

Identification A. Place 0.5 ml of citrated human, canine or rabbit plasma in a haemolysis tube maintained in a water-bath at 37°. Add 0.1 ml of a solution of the substance being examined containing 10,000 Units of streptokinase activity per ml in *citro-phosphate buffer pH 7.2* and 0.1 ml of a solution of *thrombin* containing 20 Units per ml in *citro-phosphate buffer pH 7.2* and shake immediately; a clot forms and lyses within 30 minutes. Repeat the procedure using citrated bovine plasma; lysis does not occur within 1 hour.

B. Dissolve 0.6 g of agar in 50.0 ml of *mixed barbitone buffer pH 8.6*, heating until a clear solution is obtained. Place glass plates (50 mm × 50 mm) that are free from traces of grease on a level surface. Apply to each plate 4 ml of the agar solution and allow to cool until set. Bore a hole 6 mm in diameter in the centre of the agar and an appropriate number of holes (not exceeding six) at distances of 11 mm from the central hole removing the residual agar by means of a cannula connected to a vacuum pump. Place a quantity of 80 µl of goat or rabbit antistreptokinase serum containing 10,000 units of antistreptokinase activity per ml in the central hole and 80 µl of a solution of the substance being examined containing 125,000 Units of streptokinase activity per ml in each of the surrounding holes. Place the plates in a humidified tank for 24 hours.

Only one precipitation arc is produced which is well defined and localised between the application point of the serum and each hole containing the solution of the substance being examined.

Acidity or alkalinity pH of a solution containing 5,000 Units per ml, 6.8 to 7.5, Appendix V L.

Streptodornase Introduce 0.5 ml of a 0.1% w/v solution of *sodium deoxyribonucleate* in *imidazole buffer pH 6.5* into each of eight centrifuge tubes. To each of the first two tubes add 0.25 ml of *imidazole buffer pH 6.5* and 0.25 ml of a solution of the substance being examined in *imidazole buffer pH 6.5* containing 150,000 Units of streptokinase activity per ml (solution A) followed immediately by 3.0 ml of 0.25M *perchloric acid*. Mix the contents of each tube, centrifuge for 5 minutes at 3000 *g* and measure the *absorbance* of each of the supernatant liquids at 260 nm, Appendix II B, using a mixture of 1.0 ml of *imidazole buffer pH 6.5* and 3.0 ml of 0.25M *perchloric acid* in the reference cell. Let the sum of the two absorbances be A_1. To each of the remaining six tubes add, respectively, 0.25, 0.25, 0.125, 0.125, 0 and 0 ml of *imidazole buffer pH 6.5*, followed by 0.25 ml of solution A and finally 0, 0, 0.125, 0.125, 0.25 and 0.25 ml respectively of a solution of the Standard Preparation of streptokinase—streptodornase containing 20 Units of streptodornase activity per ml in *imidazole buffer pH 6.5*. Mix the contents of each tube, incubate at 37° for 15 minutes and add to each tube 3.0 ml of 0.25M *perchloric acid*. Mix the contents of each tube, centrifuge and measure the *absorbance* of each of the supernatant liquids at 260 nm, Appendix II B, using the mixture specified above in the reference cell. Let the sum of the absorbances of the liquids in the third and fourth tubes be A_2, that of the liquids in the fifth and sixth tubes be A_3 and that of the liquids in the seventh and eighth tubes be A_4. $(A_2 - A_1)$ is less than $0.5 (A_3 + A_4) - A_2$.

Streptolysin Dissolve a quantity of the substance being examined equivalent to 500,000 Units of streptokinase activity in 0.5 ml of a mixture of 9 volumes of *saline solution* and 1 volume of *citro-phosphate buffer pH 7.2* in a haemolysis tube. Add 0.4 ml of a 2.3% w/v solution of *sodium thioglycollate* and incubate in a water-bath at 37° for 10 minutes. Add 0.1 ml of a solution of a reference preparation of human antistreptolysin O containing 5 Units per ml and incubate at 37° for 5 minutes. Add 1 ml of *rabbit erythrocyte suspension*, continue the incubation for 30 minutes and centrifuge at about 1000 *g*. The *absorbance* of the supernatant liquid at 550 nm, Appendix II B, is not more than 1.5 times the *absorbance* obtained by repeating the above procedure using 0.5 ml of the mixture of saline solution and citro-phosphate buffer pH 7.2 in place of the solution containing the substance being examined.

Loss on drying When dried over *phosphorus pentoxide* at a pressure not exceeding 2.7 Pa for 24 hours, loses not more than 4.0% of its weight.

Assay Carry out the *biological assay of streptokinase*, Appendix XIV E4. The estimated potency is not less than 90% and not more than 111% of the stated potency. The fiducial limits of error are not less than 80% and not more than 125% of the stated potency.

Storage Streptokinase should be kept in a sealed container and protected from light. Under these conditions it may be expected to retain its potency for 3 years. If the contents are intended for use in the manufacture of a parenteral dosage form, the container should be sterile.

Labelling The label states (1) the number of Units of streptokinase activity in the container; (2) the number of Units of streptokinase activity per mg calculated with reference to the dried preparation; (3) the name and quantity of any added substances; (4) the date after which the material is not intended to be used; (5) the conditions under which it should be stored; (6) whether or not it is intended for use in the manufacture of a parenteral dosage form.

Preparation
Streptokinase Injection

Action and use Fibrinolytic enzyme.

Streptokinase intended for use in the manufacture of a parenteral dosage form complies with the following additional requirements.

Abnormal toxicity Complies with the *test for abnormal toxicity*, Appendix XIV L. Use a solution containing 50,000 Units in 0.5 ml of *water for injections*. The injection should occupy 15 to 20 seconds.

Pyrogens Complies with the *test for pyrogens*, Appendix XIV K. Use 20,000 Units per kg of the rabbit's weight dissolved in not more than 1 ml of *water for injections*.

Sterility Complies with the *test for sterility*, Appendix XVI A.

Streptomycin Sulphate ☆

$(C_{21}H_{39}N_7O_{12})_2,3H_2SO_4$ 1457   *3810-74-0*

Streptomycin Sulphate is the sulphate of *O*-2-deoxy-2-methylamino-α-L-glucopyranosyl-(1→2)-*O*-5-deoxy-3-*C*-formyl-α-L-lyxofuranosyl-(1→4)-*N*^{1},*N*^{3}-diamidino-D-streptamine, a substance produced by the growth of certain strains of *Streptomyces griseus* or obtained by any other means. It may contain added stabilisers. The potency is not less than 720 Units per mg, calculated with reference to the dried substance.

Characteristics A white or almost white powder; hygroscopic; odourless or almost odourless.

Solubility Very soluble in *water*; practically insoluble in *ethanol (96%)*, in *chloroform* and in *ether*.

Identification A. Carry out the method for *thin-layer chromatography*, Appendix III A, using a 7% w/v solution of *potassium dihydrogen orthophosphate* as the mobile phase and a chromatoplate prepared in the following manner. Mix 0.3 g of *carbomer* (Carbopol 934 is suitable) with 240 ml of *water*, allow to stand with moderate stirring for 1 hour, adjust to pH 7 by the gradual addition with constant shaking of 2M *sodium hydroxide* and add 30 g of *silica gel H*. Spread a uniform layer of the resulting suspension 0.75 mm thick. Heat the plate at 110° for 1 hour, allow to cool and use immediately. Apply separately to the plate 10 μl of each of three solutions in *water* containing (1) 0.10% w/v of the substance being examined, (2) 0.10% w/v of *streptomycin sulphate EPCRS* and (3) 0.10% w/v of *streptomycin sulphate EPCRS*, 0.10% w/v of *neomycin sulphate EPCRS* and 0.10% w/v of *kanamycin monosulphate EPCRS*. Allow the solvent front to ascend 12 cm above the line of application. After removal of the plate, dry it in a current of warm air, spray with a mixture of equal volumes of a 0.2% w/v solution of

naphthalene-1,3-diol in *ethanol (96%)* and *sulphuric acid (46%)* and heat at 150° for 5 to 10 minutes. The principal spot in the chromatogram obtained with solution (1) is similar in position, colour and size to that in the chromatogram obtained with solution (2). The test is not valid unless the chromatogram obtained with solution (3) shows three clearly separated principal spots.

B. Dissolve 5 to 10 mg in 4 ml of *water* and add 1 ml of 1M *sodium hydroxide*. Heat in a water-bath for 4 minutes. Add a slight excess of 2M *hydrochloric acid* and 0.1 ml of a 10% w/v solution of *iron(III) chloride hexahydrate*. A violet colour is produced.

C. Dissolve 0.1 g in 2 ml of *water* and add 1 ml of *dilute 1-naphthol solution* and 2 ml of a mixture of equal volumes of *dilute sodium hypochlorite solution* and *water*. A red colour is produced.

D. Dissolve 10 mg in 5 ml of *water* and add 1 ml of 1M *hydrochloric acid*. Heat in a water-bath for 2 minutes. Add 2 ml of a 0.5% w/v solution of *1-naphthol* in 1M *sodium hydroxide* and heat in a water-bath for 1 minute. A faint yellow colour is produced.

E. Yields *reaction A* characteristic of sulphates, Appendix VI.

Acidity or alkalinity pH of a 25% w/v solution, 4.5 to 7.0, Appendix V L.

Clarity and colour of solution A 25.0% w/v solution in *carbon dioxide-free water* is not more intensely coloured than degree 3 of the appropriate range of *reference solutions*, Appendix IV B, Method II. The solution, after standing protected from light at a temperature of about 20° for 24 hours, is not more opalescent than *reference suspension II*, Appendix IV A.

Sulphate 18.0 to 21.5%, calculated with reference to the dried substance, when determined by the following method. Dissolve 0.25 g in 100 ml of *water*, adjust the pH to 11 with 13.5M *ammonia* and add 10 ml of 0.1M *barium chloride VS* and 0.5 mg of *metalphthalein*. Titrate the excess of barium chloride with 0.1M *disodium edetate VS*, adding 50 ml of *ethanol (96%)* when the colour of the solution begins to change and continuing the titration until the violet-blue colour disappears. Each ml of 0.1M *barium chloride VS* is equivalent to 0.009606 g of sulphate, SO_4^{2-}.

Colorimetric test Dissolve 0.100 g in sufficient *water* to produce 100 ml. To 5 ml add 5 ml of 0.2M *sodium hydroxide* and heat in a water-bath for exactly 10 minutes. Cool in ice for exactly 5 minutes, add 3 ml of a 1.5% w/v solution of *ammonium iron(III) sulphate* in 0.25M *sulphuric acid* and sufficient *water* to produce 25 ml and mix. Exactly 20 minutes after the addition of the ammonium iron(III) sulphate, measure the *absorbance* of a 2-cm layer at the maximum at 525 nm, Appendix II B, using in the reference cell a solution prepared in the same manner but omitting the substance being examined. The absorbance is not less than 90.0% of that obtained by carrying out the procedure at the same time and in the same manner using *streptomycin sulphate EPCRS* in place of the substance being examined, each absorbance being calculated with reference to the dried material.

Streptomycin B Carry out the method for *thin-layer chromatography*, Appendix III A, using *silica gel G* as the coating substance and a mixture of 50 volumes of *toluene*, 25 volumes of *glacial acetic acid* and 25 volumes of *methanol* as the mobile phase but allowing the solvent front to ascend 13 to 15 cm above the line of application.

Apply separately to the chromatoplate 10 µl of each of the following solutions. For solution (1) dissolve 0.20 g of the substance being examined in 5 ml of a freshly prepared mixture of 3 volumes of *sulphuric acid* and 97 volumes of *methanol*, heat under a reflux condenser for 1 hour, cool, wash down the condenser with *methanol* and add sufficient *methanol* to produce 20 ml. For solution (2) dissolve 36 mg of D-*mannose* in 5 ml of a freshly prepared mixture of 3 volumes of *sulphuric acid* and 97 volumes of *methanol*, heat under a reflux condenser for 1 hour, cool, wash down the condenser with *methanol* and add sufficient *methanol* to produce 50 ml. Dilute 5 ml of the resulting solution to 50 ml with *methanol*; this solution contains the equivalent of 0.03% w/v of streptomycin B (1 mg of D-mannose is equivalent to 4.13 mg of streptomycin B). After removal of the plate, allow it to dry in air and spray with a freshly prepared mixture of equal volumes of a 0.2% w/v solution of *naphthalene-1,3-diol* in *ethanol (96%)* and a 20% v/v solution of *sulphuric acid* and heat at 110° for 5 minutes. The spot in the chromatogram obtained with solution (2) is more intense than any corresponding spot in the chromatogram obtained with solution (1).

Loss on drying When dried over *phosphorus pentoxide* at 60° at a pressure not exceeding 0.1 kPa for 24 hours, loses not more than 7.0% of its weight. Use 1 g.

Methanol Carry out the method for *gas chromatography*, Appendix III B, using two solutions in *water* containing (1) 0.0120% w/v of *methanol* and (2) 4.00% w/v of the substance being examined.

The chromatographic procedure may be carried out using a glass column (1.5 to 2.0 m × 2 to 4 mm) packed with porous polymer heads (80 to 100 mesh) (Porapak Q is suitable) and maintained at a constant temperature of 120° to 140° with the inlet port and the detector at a temperature at least 50° higher than that of the column and using 30 to 40 ml per minute as the flow rate of the carrier gas.

The area of any peak corresponding to methanol in the chromatogram obtained with solution (2) is not greater than that of the peak in the chromatogram obtained with solution (1) (0.3%).

Sulphated ash Not more than 1.0%, Appendix IX A, Method II. Use 1 g.

Assay Carry out the *biological assay of antibiotics*, Appendix XIV A. The precision of the assay is such that the fiducial limits of error are not less than 95% and not more than 105% of the estimated potency.

Storage Streptomycin Sulphate should be kept in an airtight container and protected from moisture. If it is intended for use in the manufacture of a parenteral dosage form, the container should be sterile, tamper-evident and sealed so as to exclude micro-organisms.

Labelling The label states (1) the equivalent weight of streptomycin base in the container; (2) the name and quantity of any added stabiliser; (3) the date after which the material is not intended to be used; (4) the conditions under which it should be stored; (5) whether or not it is intended for use in the manufacture of a parenteral dosage form.

Preparation
Streptomycin Injection

Action and use Antituberculous.

When streptomycin is prescribed or demanded, Streptomycin Sulphate shall be dispensed or supplied. The quantity of streptomycin prescribed or demanded shall be interpreted as referring to streptomycin base and the corresponding amount of Streptomycin Sulphate shall be dispensed or supplied.

Streptomycin Sulphate intended for use in the manufacture of a parenteral dosage form is free from depressor substances and complies with the following additional requirements.

Abnormal toxicity Complies with the *test for abnormal toxicity*, Appendix XIV L. Use 1 mg dissolved in 0.5 ml of *water for injections*.

Pyrogens Complies with the *test for pyrogens*, Appendix XIV K. Use per kg of the rabbit's weight 2.0 ml of a solution in *water for injections* containing 6 mg per ml.

Sterility Complies with the *test for sterility*, Appendix XVI A.

Succinylsulphathiazole ☆

$$HO_2CCO \cdot CH_2 \cdot CH_2 \cdot CO \cdot NH \text{---} \langle \bigcirc \rangle \text{---} SO_2 \cdot NH \text{---} \langle \text{thiazole} \rangle$$

C$_{13}$H$_{13}$N$_3$O$_5$S$_2$,H$_2$O   373.4   *116-43-8*

Succinylsulphathiazole is 4-(*N*-thiazol-2-yl-sulphamoyl)succinanilic acid. It contains not less than 99.0 per cent and not more than 101.0 per cent of C$_{13}$H$_{13}$N$_3$O$_5$S$_2$, calculated with reference to the dried substance.

Characteristics A white or yellowish-white, crystalline powder; odourless.

Solubility Very slightly soluble in *water*; slightly soluble in *ethanol (96%)*; practically insoluble in *ether*. It dissolves in aqueous solutions of alkali hydroxides and carbonates.

Identification *Test A may be omitted if tests B, C, D and E are carried out. Tests C, D and E may be omitted if tests A and B are carried out.*
A. The *infra-red absorption spectrum*, Appendix II A, is concordant with the spectrum of *succinylsulfathiazole EPCRS*. If the spectra obtained are not concordant, recrystallise the substances from hot *water*, dry the crystals carefully between two sheets of filter paper and prepare new spectra.
B. In a borosilicate glass tube mix 0.1 g with 0.5 g of *hydroquinone* and 1 ml of *sulphuric acid* and heat in a bath of glycerol at 135° for 10 minutes. Cool in ice and add, with shaking, 15 ml of *water*. Add 5 ml of *toluene*, shake for 10 seconds and allow to stand for 2 minutes. An intense pink colour is produced in the toluene layer.
C. Heat 0.1 g in a test-tube over a small flame. Fumes are evolved which turn *lead acetate paper* black.
D. Boil 2 g for 10 minutes with 10 ml of *water* and 10 ml of 10M *sodium hydroxide*. Cool and adjust to pH 3.0 with 7M *hydrochloric acid*. Cool, adjust to pH 7 with *sodium hydrogen carbonate solution* and filter. The *melting point* of the precipitate, after washing with *water* and drying at 105°, is 196° to 204°, Appendix V A, Method I.
E. 2 ml of a 0.005% w/v solution of the precipitate obtained in test D in 0.1M *hydrochloric acid* yields the

reaction characteristic of primary aromatic amines, Appendix VI, producing an orange precipitate.

Acidity Shake 2 g with 20 ml of *water* continuously for 30 minutes. Filter and to 10 ml of the filtrate add 0.1 ml of *dilute phenolphthalein solution*. Not more than 2 ml of 0.1M *sodium hydroxide VS* is required to change the colour of the solution.

Clarity and colour of solution A 5.0% w/v solution in a mixture of 5 volumes of 2M *sodium hydroxide* and 15 volumes of *water* is *clear*, Appendix IV A, and not more intensely coloured than *reference solution* Y_4 or BY_4, Appendix IV B, Method II.

Heavy metals 1.0 g complies with *limit test D for heavy metals*, Appendix VII (20 ppm). Use 2 ml of *lead standard solution (10 ppm Pb)* to prepare the standard.

Sulphathiazole and related aromatic amines Dissolve 20 mg in a mixture of 25 ml of *ethanol (96%)*, 3.5 ml of *water* and 6 ml of 2M *hydrochloric acid* previously cooled to 15°. Cool rapidly in ice, immediately add 1 ml of a 0.25% w/v solution of *sodium nitrite*, allow to stand for 3 minutes, add 2.5 ml of a 4% w/v solution of *sulphamic acid* and allow to stand for 5 minutes. Add 1 ml of a 0.4% w/v solution of *N-(1-naphthyl)ethylene-1,2-diamine dihydrochloride* and dilute to 50 ml with *water*. The *absorbance* of the resulting solution at 550 nm, Appendix II B, is not more than that of a solution prepared at the same time and in the same manner using a mixture of 25 ml of *ethanol (96%)*, 2 ml of *water*, 6 ml of 2M *hydrochloric acid* and 1.5 ml of a solution containing 10 mg of *sulphathiazole* and 0.5 ml of *hydrochloric acid* in 100 ml and beginning at the words 'Cool rapidly in ice . . .'.

Loss on drying When dried to constant weight at 100° to 105°, loses 4.0 to 5.5% of its weight. Use 1 g.

Sulphated ash Not more than 0.1%, Appendix IX A, Method II. Use 1 g.

Assay Dissolve 0.3 g in 100 ml of a mixture of 1 volume of *hydrochloric acid* and 2 volumes of *water*, boil for 1 hour under a reflux condenser and carry out the method for *amperometric titration*, Appendix VIII B. Each ml of 0.1M *sodium nitrite VS* is equivalent to 0.03554 g of $C_{13}H_{13}N_3O_5S_2$.

Storage Succinylsulphathiazole should be protected from light.

Action and use Antibacterial.

Sucrose ☆
Refined Sugar

$C_{12}H_{22}O_{11}$ 342.3   *57-30-1*

Sucrose is β-D–fructofuranosyl-α-D-glucopyranoside.

Characteristics Lustrous, dry, colourless crystals or a white, crystalline powder; odourless; taste, sweet.

Solubility Soluble in 0.5 part of *water*; slightly soluble in *ethanol (96%)*; freely soluble in *ethanol (70%)*.

Identification A. Carry out the method for *thin-layer chromatography*, Appendix III A, using *silica gel G* as the coating substance and a mixture of 50 volumes of *1,2-dichloroethane*, 25 volumes of *anhydrous glacial acetic acid*, 15 volumes of *methanol* and 10 volumes of *water*, measured accurately, as the mobile phase. Apply separately to the chromatoplate 2 μl of each of three solutions in *methanol (60%)* containing (1) 0.05% w/v of the substance being examined, (2) 0.05% w/v of *sucrose EPCRS* and (3) 0.05% w/v each of *fructose EPCRS*, *glucose EPCRS*, *lactose EPCRS* and *sucrose EPCRS*. Thoroughly dry the points of application before developing the chromatogram. After removal of the plate, dry it in a current of warm air and repeat the development after renewing the mobile phase. After removal of the plate, dry it in a current of warm air, spray with a 0.5% w/v solution of *thymol* in *ethanolic sulphuric acid (5%)* and heat at 130° for 10 minutes. The principal spot in the chromatogram obtained with solution (1) is similar in position, colour and size to that in the chromatogram obtained with solution (2). The test is not valid unless the chromatogram obtained with solution (3) shows four clearly separated principal spots.

B. Dilute 1 ml of a 50% w/v solution to 100 ml with *water*. To 5 ml of the solution add 2 ml of 2M *sodium hydroxide* and 0.15 ml of 0.5M *copper(II) sulphate*; the solution is clear and blue and remains so on boiling. To the hot solution add 4 ml of 2M *hydrochloric acid*, heat to boiling and add 4 ml of 2M *sodium hydroxide*; an orange precipitate is produced immediately.

Acidity or alkalinity To 10 ml of a 50.0% w/v solution in *carbon dioxide-free water* prepared from *distilled water* (solution A) add 0.3 ml of *dilute phenolphthalein solution*. The solution is colourless and not more than 0.3 ml of 0.01M *sodium hydroxide VS* is required to change the colour of the solution to pink.

Clarity, colour and odour of solution Solution A is *clear*, Appendix IV A, not more intensely coloured than *reference solution* Y_6, Appendix IV B, Method II, and odourless.

Specific optical rotation In a 20% w/v solution, +66.2° to +66.8°, Appendix V F.

Barium To 10 ml of solution A add 1 ml of 1M *sulphuric acid*. When examined immediately and after 1 hour any opalescence is not more intense than that of a mixture of 1 ml of *distilled water* and 10 ml of solution A.

Lead Complies with *limit test A for lead in sugars*, Appendix VII (0.5 ppm).

Sulphite Dissolve 5.0 g in *water*, add 2 ml of 0.1M *sodium hydroxide* and dilute to 50 ml with *water*. To 10 ml of the solution add 1 ml of a 31% w/v solution of *hydrochloric acid*, 2 ml of *faded magenta solution* and 2 ml of a 0.5% v/v solution of *formaldehyde*. Allow to stand for 30 minutes and measure the *absorbance* at the maximum at 583 nm, Appendix II B. The absorbance is not more than that of a standard prepared in the following manner. To 3 ml of a 0.0076% w/v solution of *sodium metabisulphite* add 4 ml of 0.1M *sodium hydroxide* and dilute to 100 ml with *water*. Treat 10 ml of the resulting solution in the same manner as the test solution beginning at the words 'add 1 ml of a 31% w/v solution . . .'. Use in the reference cell a solution prepared in the same manner using 10 ml of *water* (15 ppm of SO_2).

Dextrins To 2 ml of solution A add 8 ml of *water*, 0.05 ml of 2M *hydrochloric acid* and 0.05 ml of 0.05M *iodine*. The solution remains yellow.

Glucose and invert sugar To 10 ml of solution A add 1 ml of 1M *sodium hydroxide* and 1 ml of a 0.1% w/v solution of *methylene blue*, mix and place in a water-bath for 2 minutes. Remove from the water-bath and examine immediately. The blue colour does not disappear completely. Disregard any blue colour at the air—solution interface.

Foreign colouring matter A. Filter 100 ml of solution A through a glass-fibre filter 2.4 cm in diameter. The filter is not coloured blue. (The filter complies with the following requirements: mean basic weight, 52 g m^{-2}; thickness, 0.25 mm; mean pore size, 1.0 μm.)
B. To 100 ml of solution A in a ground-glass-stoppered tube add 1 ml of *dilute hypophosphorous acid* and allow to stand for 1 hour. No unpleasant odour is detectable.
C. Examine solution A under ultra-violet light (365 nm). Any fluorescence is not more intense than that of a solution containing 0.4 ppm of *quinine sulphate* in 0.005M *sulphuric acid*.

Sulphated ash Not more than 0.02% when determined in the following manner. Dissolve 5 g in 5 ml of *water*, add 2 ml of *sulphuric acid*, evaporate to dryness and ignite to constant weight.

Storage Sucrose should be kept in a well-closed container.

Preparation
Syrup

Sulfadoxine

C$_{12}$H$_{14}$N$_4$O$_4$S   310.3   *2447-57-6*

Sulfadoxine is N^1-(5,6-dimethoxypyrimidin-4-yl)sulphanilamide. It contains not less than 99.0 per cent and not more than 101.0 per cent of C$_{12}$H$_{14}$N$_4$O$_4$S, calculated with reference to the dried substance.

Characteristics A white or creamy-white, crystalline powder; odourless or almost odourless.

Solubility Very slightly soluble in *water*; slightly soluble in *ethanol (96%)* and in *methanol*; practically insoluble in *ether*.

Identification A. The *infra-red absorption spectrum*, Appendix II A, is concordant with the *reference spectrum* of sulfadoxine.
B. The *light absorption*, Appendix II B, in the range 230 to 350 nm of a 0.0006% w/v solution in 0.1M *sodium hydroxide* exhibits a maximum only at 272 nm. The *absorbance* at 272 nm is about 0.45.
C. Yields the *reaction* characteristic of primary aromatic amines, Appendix VI, producing an orange-red precipitate.

Acidity Heat 1 g with 50 ml of *carbon dioxide-free water* at about 70° for 5 minutes, cool quickly to 20° and filter. 25 ml of the filtrate requires not more than 0.25 ml of 0.1M *sodium hydroxide VS* for titration to pH 7.0, Appendix V L.

Clarity and colour of solution A 5.0% w/v solution in 3M *hydrochloric acid* is *clear*, Appendix IV A, and not more intensely coloured than *reference solution BY$_5$*, Appendix IV B, Method I.

Melting point 197° to 200°, Appendix V A.

Heavy metals 1.0 g complies with *limit test C for heavy metals*, Appendix VII (20 ppm). Use 2 ml of *lead standard solution (10 ppm Pb)* to prepare the standard.

Related substances Complies with test B for *related substances in sulphonamides*, Appendix III A, using as solution (2) a 0.0025% w/v solution of *sulphanilamide*.

Loss on drying When dried to constant weight at 100° to 105°, loses not more than 0.5% of its weight. Use 1 g.

Sulphated ash Not more than 0.1%, Appendix IX A.

Assay Dissolve 0.5 g in a mixture of 75 ml of *water* and 10 ml of *hydrochloric acid* and carry out the method for *amperometric titration*, Appendix VIII B. Each ml of 0.1M *sodium nitrite VS* is equivalent to 0.03103 g of C$_{12}$H$_{14}$N$_4$O$_4$S.

Storage Sulfadoxine should be protected from light.

Action and use Antimalarial.

Sulindac

C$_{20}$H$_{17}$FO$_3$S   356.4   *38194-50-2*

Sulindac is (*Z*)-5-fluoro-2-methyl-1-(4-methyl-sulphinylbenzylidene)indene-3-acetic acid. It contains not less than 99.0 per cent and not more than 101.0 per cent of C$_{20}$H$_{17}$FO$_3$S, calculated with reference to the dried substance.

Characteristics A yellow, crystalline powder; odourless or almost odourless.

Solubility Very slightly soluble in *water* and in *ether*; sparingly soluble in *ethanol (96%)*; soluble in *chloroform*.

Identification A. The *infra-red absorption spectrum*, Appendix II A, is concordant with the *reference spectrum* of sulindac.
B. The *light absorption*, Appendix II B, in the range 230 to 350 nm of a 0.002% w/v solution in 0.1M *methanolic hydrochloric acid* exhibits two maxima, at 284 nm and 327 nm, and a less well-defined maximum at 258 nm. The *absorbance* at 284 nm is about 0.84 and at 327 nm is about 0.74.

Heavy metals 2.0 g complies with *limit test D for heavy metals*, Appendix VII (10 ppm). Use 2 ml of *lead standard solution (10 ppm Pb)* to prepare the standard.

Related substances Carry out the method for *high-performance liquid chromatography*, Appendix III D, using two solutions of the substance being examined in the mobile phase containing (1) 0.0020% w/v and (2) 0.20% w/v.

The chromatographic procedure may be carried out using (a) a stainless steel column (30 cm × 3.9 mm) packed with *stationary phase a* (10 μm) (μPorasil is suitable), (b) a mixture of 400 volumes of *ethanol-free chloroform*, 100 volumes of *ethyl acetate*, 4 volumes of *ethanol (96%)* and 1 volume of *glacial acetic acid* as the mobile phase with a flow rate of 2 ml per minute and (c) a detection wavelength of 280 nm.

In the chromatogram obtained with solution (2) the sum of the areas of the *secondary peaks* is not greater than the area of the peak obtained with solution (1).

Loss on drying When dried to constant weight at 100° at a pressure not exceeding 0.7 kPa, loses not more than 0.5% of its weight. Use 1 g.

Sulphated ash Not more than 0.1%, Appendix IX A.

Assay Dissolve 0.7 g in 80 ml of *methanol* and titrate with 0.1M *sodium hydroxide VS* determining the end-point potentiometrically. Each ml of 0.1M *sodium hydroxide VS* is equivalent to 0.03564 g of $C_{20}H_{17}FO_3S$.

Storage Sulindac should be kept in a well-closed container and protected from light.

Preparation
Sulindac Tablets

Action and use Anti-inflammatory; analgesic.

Sulphacetamide Sodium ☆
Soluble Sulphacetamide

H_2N—⟨⟩—$SO_2 \cdot NCO \cdot CH_3$ (with Na)

$C_8H_9N_2NaO_3S,H_2O$ 254.2   6209-17-2

Sulphacetamide Sodium is the monohydrate of the sodium salt of N^1-acetylsulphanilamide. It contains not less than 99.0 per cent and not more than 101.0 per cent of $C_8H_9N_2NaO_3S$, calculated with reference to the anhydrous substance.

Characteristics A white or yellowish-white, crystalline powder; odourless.

Solubility Soluble in 1.5 parts of *water*; slightly soluble in *ethanol (96%)*; practically insoluble in *chloroform* and in *ether*.

Identification *Test A may be omitted if tests B, C, D, E and F are carried out. Tests B, C, D and E may be omitted if tests A and F are carried out.*
A. The *infra-red absorption spectrum*, Appendix II A, is concordant with the spectrum of *sulfacetamide sodium EPCRS*.
B. The *light absorption*, Appendix II B, in the range 230 to 350 nm of a 0.001% w/v solution in *citro-phosphate buffer pH 7.0* exhibits a maximum only at 255 nm. The A(1%, 1 cm) at 255 nm is 660 to 720.
C. Dissolve 1 g in 10 ml of *water*, add 6 ml of 2M *acetic acid* and filter. Wash the precipitate with cold *water* and dry at 100° to 105° for 4 hours. The *melting point* of the precipitate is 181° to 185°, Appendix V A, Method I.
D. Dissolve 0.1 g of the precipitate obtained in test C in 5 ml of *ethanol (96%)*, add 0.2 ml of *sulphuric acid* and heat. Ethyl acetate, recognisable by its odour, is produced.
E. Dissolve 0.1 g of the precipitate obtained in test C in 1 ml of *water* with the aid of heat. The solution yields the

reaction characteristic of primary aromatic amines, Appendix VI, producing an orange-red precipitate.
F. A 5% w/v solution yields the *reactions* characteristic of sodium salts, Appendix VI.

Alkalinity pH of a 5% w/v solution, 8.0 to 9.5, Appendix V L.

Clarity and colour of solution A 5.0% w/v solution in *carbon dioxide-free water* is *clear*, Appendix IV A, and not more intensely coloured than *reference solution GY₄*, Appendix IV B, Method II.

Heavy metals Dissolve 2.5 g in sufficient *distilled water* to produce 25 ml, add 25 ml of 2M *acetic acid*, shake for 30 minutes and filter (solution A). 12 ml of the solution complies with *limit test A for heavy metals*, Appendix VII (20 ppm). Use *lead standard solution (1 ppm Pb)* to prepare the standard.

Sulphate 15 ml of solution A complies with the *limit test for sulphates*, Appendix VII (200 ppm).

Related substances Carry out the method for *thin-layer chromatography*, Appendix III A, using *silica gel HF254* as the coating substance and a mixture of 50 volumes of *butan-1-ol*, 25 volumes of *absolute ethanol*, 25 volumes of *water* and 10 volumes of 13.5M *ammonia* as the mobile phase. Apply separately to the chromatoplate 5 µl of each of four solutions in *water* containing (1) 10.0% w/v of the substance being examined, (2) 0.050% w/v of *sulphanilamide*, (3) 0.025% w/v of *sulphanilamide* and (4) 0.050% w/v of *sulphanilamide* in solution (1). After removal of the plate, allow it to dry in air and spray with a 2% w/v solution, prepared without heating, of *4-dimethylaminobenzaldehyde* in a 55% v/v solution of *hydrochloric acid*. Any *secondary spot* in the chromatogram obtained with solution (1) is not more intense than the spot in the chromatogram obtained with solution (2) and not more than one such spot is more intense than the spot in the chromatogram obtained with solution (3). The test is not valid unless the chromatogram obtained with solution (4) shows two clearly separated principal spots.

Water 6.0 to 8.0% w/w, Appendix IX C. Use 0.2 g.

Assay Dissolve 0.5 g in a mixture of 50 ml of *water* and 20 ml of 2M *hydrochloric acid* and add 3 g of *potassium bromide*. Cool the solution in ice and carry out the method for *amperometric titration*, Appendix VIII B. Each ml of 0.1M *sodium nitrite VS* is equivalent to 0.02362 g of $C_8H_9N_2NaO_3S$.

Storage Sulphacetamide Sodium should be protected from light.

Preparations
Sulphacetamide Eye Drops
Sulphacetamide Eye Ointment

Action and use Antibacterial.

Sulphadiazine ☆

C₁₀H₁₀N₄O₂S   250.3   68-35-9

Sulphadiazine is N^1-(pyrimidin-2-yl)sulph-anilamide. It contains not less than 99.0 per cent and not more than 101.0 per cent of $C_{10}H_{10}N_4O_2S$, calculated with reference to the dried substance.

Characteristics White, yellowish-white or pinkish-white crystals or crystalline powder. It melts at about 255°, with decomposition.

Solubility Practically insoluble in *water* and in *chloroform*; very slightly soluble in *ethanol (96%)*; slightly soluble in *acetone*. It dissolves in aqueous solutions of alkali hydroxides and in dilute mineral acids.

Identification *Test A may be omitted if tests B, C and D are carried out. Tests C and D may be omitted if tests A and B are carried out.*
A. The *infra-red absorption spectrum*, Appendix II A, is concordant with the spectrum of *sulfadiazine EPCRS*.
B. In the test for Related substances, the principal spot in the chromatogram obtained with solution (2) corresponds in position and size to the principal spot in the chromatogram obtained with solution (4).
C. Heat 3 g in a test-tube inclined at an angle of 45° with the lower part immersed in a silicone oil-bath at about 270°. It decomposes and a white or yellowish-white sublimate is produced. The *melting point* of the sublimate, after recrystallisation from *toluene* and drying at 100°, is 123° to 127°, Appendix V A, Method I.
D. Dissolve 5 mg in 10 ml of 1M *hydrochloric acid* and dilute 1 ml of this solution to 10 ml with *water*. The solution, without further acidification, yields the *reaction* characteristic of primary aromatic amines, Appendix VI.

Acidity Heat 1.25 g of the finely powdered substance at 70° with 25 ml of *carbon dioxide-free water* for 5 minutes. Cool for about 15 minutes in ice and filter. To 20 ml of the filtrate add 0.1 ml of *bromothymol blue solution*. Not more than 0.2 ml of 0.1M *sodium hydroxide VS* is required to change the colour of the solution.

Colour of solution Dissolve 0.8 g in 10 ml of 1M *sodium hydroxide*. The solution is not more intensely coloured than *reference solution Y₅, BY₅* or *GY₅*, Appendix IV B, Method II.

Heavy metals 1.0 g complies with *limit test D for heavy metals*, Appendix VII (20 ppm). Use 2 ml of *lead standard solution (10 ppm Pb)* to prepare the standard.

Related substances Complies with test C for *related substances in sulphonamides*, Appendix III A.

Loss on drying When dried to constant weight at 100° to 105°, loses not more than 0.5% of its weight. Use 1 g.

Sulphated ash Not more than 0.1%, Appendix IX A, Method II. Use 1 g.

Assay Dissolve 0.2 g in a mixture of 20 ml of 2M *hydrochloric acid* and 50 ml of *water*. Add 3 g of *potassium bromide*, cool in ice and carry out the method for *amperometric titration*, Appendix VIII B. Each ml of 0.1M *sodium nitrite VS* is equivalent to 0.02503 g of $C_{10}H_{10}N_4O_2S$.

Storage Sulphadiazine should be kept in a well-closed container and protected from light.

Preparation
Sulphadiazine Injection

Action and use Antibacterial.

Sulphadimethoxine

C₁₂H₁₄N₄O₄S   310.3   122-11-2

Sulphadimethoxine is N^1-(2,6-dimethoxy-pyrimidin-4-yl)sulphanilamide. It contains not less than 99.0 per cent and not more than 101.0 per cent of $C_{12}H_{14}N_4O_4S$, calculated with reference to the dried substance.

Characteristics A white or creamy-white, crystalline powder; odourless or almost odourless.

Solubility Very slightly soluble in *water*; slightly soluble in *ethanol (96%)*. It dissolves in dilute mineral acids and in aqueous solutions of alkali hydroxides and carbonates.

Identification A. The *infra-red absorption spectrum*, Appendix II A, is concordant with the *reference spectrum* of sulphadimethoxine.
B. Yields the *reaction* characteristic of primary aromatic amines, Appendix VI, producing an orange-red precipitate.

Acidity Heat 1 g with 50 ml of *carbon dioxide-free water* at about 70° for 5 minutes, cool quickly to 20° and filter. 25 ml of the filtrate requires not more than 0.1 ml of 0.1M *sodium hydroxide VS* for titration to pH 7.0, Appendix V L.

Clarity and colour of solution A 5.0% w/v solution in 2M *hydrochloric acid* is *clear*, Appendix IV A, and not more intensely coloured than *reference solution BY₅*, Appendix IV B, Method I.

Melting point 198° to 204°, Appendix V A.

Heavy metals 1.0 g complies with *limit test C for heavy metals*, Appendix VII (20 ppm). Use 2 ml of *lead standard solution (10 ppm Pb)* to prepare the standard.

Related substances Complies with test B for *related substances in sulphonamides*, Appendix III A.

Loss on drying When dried to constant weight at 100° to 105°, loses not more than 0.5% of its weight. Use 1 g.

Sulphated ash Not more than 0.1%, Appendix IX A.

Assay Dissolve 0.5 g in a mixture of 75 ml of *water* and 10 ml of *hydrochloric acid* and carry out the method for *amperometric titration*, Appendix VIII B. Each ml of 0.1M *sodium nitrite VS* is equivalent to 0.03103 g of $C_{12}H_{14}N_4O_4S$.

Storage Sulphadimethoxine should be protected from light.

Preparation
Sulphadimethoxine Tablets

Action and use Antibacterial.

Sulphadimidine ☆

H₂N—⟨benzene ring⟩—SO₂·NH—⟨pyrimidine ring with Me, N, N, Me⟩

$C_{12}H_{14}N_4O_2S$ 278.3   *57-68-1*

Sulphadimidine is N^1-(4,6-dimethylpyrimidin-2-yl)sulphanilamide. It contains not less than 99.0 per cent and not more than 101.0 per cent of $C_{12}H_{14}N_4O_2S$, calculated with reference to the dried substance.

Characteristics White or almost white crystals or powder. It melts at about 197°, with decomposition.

Solubility Very slightly soluble in *water*; slightly soluble in *ethanol (96%)*; practically insoluble in *ether*. It dissolves in dilute mineral acids and in aqueous solutions of alkali hydroxides and carbonates.

Identification *Test A may be omitted if tests B, C and D are carried out. Tests C and D may be omitted if tests A and B are carried out.*
A. The *infra-red absorption spectrum*, Appendix II A, is concordant with the spectrum of *sulfadimidine EPCRS*.
B. In the test for Related substances, the principal spot in the chromatogram obtained with solution (2) corresponds in position and size to the principal spot in the chromatogram obtained with solution (4).
C. Heat 3 g in a test-tube inclined at an angle of 45° with the lower part immersed in a silicone oil-bath at about 270°. It decomposes and a white or yellowish-white sublimate is produced. The *melting point* of the sublimate, after recrystallisation from *toluene* and drying at 100°, is 150° to 154°, Appendix V A, Method I.
D. Dissolve 5 mg in 10 ml of 1M *hydrochloric acid* and dilute 1 ml of this solution to 10 ml with *water*. The solution, without further acidification, yields the *reaction characteristic of primary aromatic amines*, Appendix VI.

Acidity Heat 1.25 g of the finely powdered substance at about 70° for 5 minutes with 25 ml of *carbon dioxide-free water*. Cool in ice for about 15 minutes and filter. To 20 ml of the filtrate add 0.1 ml of *bromothymol blue solution*. Not more than 0.2 ml of 0.1M *sodium hydroxide VS* is required to change the colour of the solution.

Colour of solution A 5.0% w/v solution in 1M *sodium hydroxide* is not more intensely coloured than *reference solution* Y_5, BY_5 or GY_5, Appendix IV B, Method II.

Heavy metals 1.0 g complies with *limit test D for heavy metals*, Appendix VII (20 ppm). Use 2 ml of *lead standard solution (10 ppm Pb)* to prepare the standard.

Related substances Complies with test C for *related substances in sulphonamides*, Appendix III A.

Loss on drying When dried to constant weight at 100° to 105°, loses not more than 0.5% of its weight. Use 1 g.

Sulphated ash Not more than 0.1%, Appendix IX A, Method II. Use 1 g.

Assay Dissolve 0.25 g in 20 ml of 2M *hydrochloric acid* and 50 ml of *water*, add 3 g of *potassium bromide*, cool in ice and carry out the method for *amperometric titration*, Appendix VIII B. Each ml of 0.1M *sodium nitrite VS* is equivalent to 0.02783 g of $C_{12}H_{14}N_4O_2S$.

Storage Sulphadimidine should be kept in a well-closed container and protected from light.

Preparations
Paediatric Sulphadimidine Oral Suspension
Sulphadimidine Injection
Sulphadimidine Tablets

Action and use Antibacterial.

Sulphadimidine Sodium

$C_{12}H_{13}N_4NaO_2S$ 300.3   *1981-58-4*

Sulphadimidine Sodium is the sodium salt of N^1-(4,6-dimethylpyrimidin-2-yl)sulphanilamide. It contains not less than 98.0 per cent and not more than 101.0 per cent of $C_{12}H_{13}N_4NaO_2S$, calculated with reference to the dried substance.

Characteristics White or creamy-white crystals or powder; odourless or almost odourless; hygroscopic.

Solubility Soluble in 2.5 parts of *water* and in 60 parts of *ethanol (96%)*.

Identification A. Dissolve 0.1 g in 10 ml of *water*, acidify with 1M *hydrochloric acid*, filter, wash the precipitate with *water* and dry the residue at 105°. The *infra-red absorption spectrum* of the residue, Appendix II A, is concordant with the *reference spectrum* of sulphadimidine.
B. Acidify a solution with 6M *acetic acid*. A precipitate is produced which, after washing with cold *water* and drying at 105°, yields the *reaction* characteristic of primary aromatic amines, Appendix VI, producing a bright orange-red precipitate.
C. *Melting point* of the washed and dried precipitate obtained in test B, about 198°, Appendix V A.
D. Incinerate 0.5 g. The residue, when moistened with *hydrochloric acid* and introduced on a platinum wire into a flame, imparts a yellow colour to the flame.

Alkalinity pH of a 10% w/v solution, 10.0 to 11.0, Appendix V L.

Clarity and colour of solution A 33.3% w/v solution is *clear*, Appendix IV A, and not more intensely coloured than *reference solution* Y_4, Appendix IV B, Method I.

Related substances Complies with test A for *related substances in sulphonamides*, Appendix III A. Prepare solution (1) by dissolving the substance being examined in 1 volume of 13.5M *ammonia* and then diluting with 9 volumes of *ethanol (96%)* to produce a 1.0% w/v solution.

Loss on drying When dried to constant weight at 105°, loses not more than 2.0% of its weight. Use 1 g.

Assay Dissolve 0.5 g in a mixture of 75 ml of *water* and 10 ml of *hydrochloric acid* and carry out the method for *amperometric titration*, Appendix VIII B. Each ml of 0.1M *sodium nitrite VS* is equivalent to 0.03003 g of $C_{12}H_{13}N_4NaO_2S$.

Storage Sulphadimidine Sodium should be protected from light.

Preparation
Sulphadimidine Injection

Action and use Antibacterial.

Sulphafurazole

Sulfisoxazole

$C_{11}H_{13}N_3O_3S$ 267.3   *127-69-5*

Sulphafurazole is N^1-(3,4-dimethylisoxazol-5-yl)sulphanilamide. It contains not less than 99.0 per cent and not more than 101.0 per cent of $C_{11}H_{13}N_3O_3S$, calculated with reference to the dried substance.

Characteristics A white or yellowish-white, crystalline powder; odourless or almost odourless.

Solubility Practically insoluble in *water*; soluble in 50 parts of *ethanol (96%)*; slightly soluble in *chloroform* and in *ether*; soluble in 30 parts of *sodium hydrogen carbonate solution*.

Identification A. The *infra-red absorption spectrum*, Appendix II A, is concordant with the *reference spectrum* of sulphafurazole.
B. Yields the *reaction* characteristic of primary aromatic amines, Appendix VI, producing an orange-red precipitate.

Acidity Heat 1 g at 70° for 5 minutes with 50 ml of *carbon dioxide-free water*, cool quickly to 20° and filter. 25 ml of the filtrate requires not more than 0.25 ml of 0.1M *sodium hydroxide VS* for titration to pH 7.0, Appendix V L.

Melting point 195° to 198°, Appendix V A.

Clarity and colour of solution A 5.0% w/v solution in 3M *hydrochloric acid* is *clear*, Appendix IV A, and not more intensely coloured than *reference solution Y_5*, Appendix IV B, Method I.

Heavy metals 1.0 g complies with *limit test C for heavy metals*, Appendix VII (20 ppm). Use 2 ml of *lead standard solution (10 ppm Pb)* to prepare the standard.

Related substances Complies with test A for *related substances in sulphonamides*, Appendix III A, but using for solution (1) 0.10% w/v of the substance being examined and for solution (2) 0.00050% w/v of *sulphanilamide* in the prescribed solvent mixture.

Loss on drying When dried to constant weight at 105°, loses not more than 0.5% of its weight. Use 1 g.

Sulphated ash Not more than 0.1%, Appendix IX A.

Assay Dissolve 0.5 g in 50 ml of *acetone* and carry out Method II for *non-aqueous titration*, Appendix VIII A, using 0.1M *tetrabutylammonium hydroxide VS* as titrant and a 0.3% w/v solution of *thymol blue* in *methanol* as indicator. Each ml of 0.1M *tetrabutylammonium hydroxide VS* is equivalent to 0.02673 g of $C_{11}H_{13}N_3O_3S$.

Storage Sulphafurazole should be protected from light.

Preparation
Sulphafurazole Tablets

Action and use Antibacterial.

Sulphamethizole

$C_9H_{10}N_4O_2S_2$ 270.3   *144-82-1*

Sulphamethizole is N^1-(5-methyl-1,3,4-thia-diazol-2-yl)sulphanilamide. It contains not less than 99.0 per cent and not more than 101.0 per cent of $C_9H_{10}N_4O_2S_2$, calculated with reference to the dried substance.

Characteristics Colourless crystals or a white or creamy-white, crystalline powder; odourless or almost odourless.

Solubility Slightly soluble in *water*, in *chloroform* and in *ether*; soluble in 60 parts of boiling *water*, in 25 parts of *ethanol (96%)* and in 15 parts of *acetone*. It dissolves in aqueous solutions of the alkali hydroxides and in dilute mineral acids.

Identification A. The *infra-red absorption spectrum*, Appendix II A, is concordant with the *reference spectrum* of sulphamethizole.
B. Yields the *reaction* characteristic of primary aromatic amines, Appendix VI, producing an orange-red precipitate which darkens on standing.

Acidity Heat 1 g with 50 ml of *carbon dioxide-free water* at about 70° for 5 minutes, cool quickly to 20° and filter. 25 ml of the filtrate requires not more than 0.5 ml of 0.1M *sodium hydroxide VS* for titration to pH 7.0, Appendix V L.

Melting point 208° to 211°, Appendix V A.

Clarity and colour of solution A 5.0% w/v solution in 2M *hydrochloric acid* is *clear*, Appendix IV A, and not more intensely coloured than *reference solution Y_5*, Appendix IV B, Method I.

Heavy metals 1.0 g complies with *limit test C for heavy metals*, Appendix VII (20 ppm). Use 2 ml of *lead standard solution (10 ppm Pb)* to prepare the standard.

Related substances Complies with test A for *related substances in sulphonamides*, Appendix III A.

Loss on drying When dried to constant weight at 105°, loses not more than 0.5% of its weight. Use 1 g.

Sulphated ash Not more than 0.1%, Appendix IX A.

Assay Dissolve 0.5 g in a mixture of 75 ml of *water* and 10 ml of *hydrochloric acid* and carry out the method for *amperometric titration*, Appendix VIII B. Each ml of 0.1M *sodium nitrite VS* is equivalent to 0.02703 g of $C_9H_{10}N_4O_2S_2$.

Storage Sulphamethizole should be protected from light.

Preparation
Sulphamethizole Tablets

Action and use Antibacterial.

Sulphamethoxazole ☆

H₂N—⟨benzene⟩—SO₂·NH—⟨isoxazole⟩—Me

C₁₀H₁₁N₃O₃S   253.3   723-46-6

Sulphamethoxazole is N^1-(5-methylisoxazol-3-yl)sulphanilamide. It contains not less than 99.0 per cent and not more than 101.0 per cent of $C_{10}H_{11}N_3O_3S$, calculated with reference to the dried substance.

Characteristics A white or almost white, crystalline powder; odourless or almost odourless.

Solubility Practically insoluble in *water*; soluble in 50 parts of *ethanol (96%)* and in 3 parts of *acetone*; slightly soluble in *chloroform* and in *ether*. It dissolves in dilute solutions of *sodium hydroxide*.

Identification *Test A may be omitted if tests B, C and D are carried out. Tests B and C may be omitted if tests A and D are carried out.*
A. The *infra-red absorption spectrum*, Appendix II A, is concordant with the spectrum of *sulfamethoxazole EPCRS*.
B. The *light absorption*, Appendix II B, in the range 210 to 330 nm of a 0.001% w/v solution in 1M *sodium hydroxide* exhibits a maximum at 257 nm and a minimum at 224 nm. The A(1%, 1 cm) at 257 nm is 640 to 690.
C. Dissolve 20 mg in 0.5 ml of 2M *hydrochloric acid* and add 1 ml of *water*. The resulting solution yields the *reaction* characteristic of primary aromatic amines, Appendix VI, producing an orange-red precipitate.
D. *Melting point*, 169° to 172°, Appendix V A, Method I.

Acidity Heat a mixture of 1.25 g of the finely powdered substance and 25 ml of *carbon dioxide-free water* to 70° for 5 minutes, cool rapidly and filter. The pH of the filtrate is 4.0 to 5.0, Appendix V L.

Colour of solution A solution of 1.0 g in 10 ml of 2M *sodium hydroxide* is not more intensely coloured than *reference solution BY₅*, Appendix IV B, Method II.

Heavy metals 1.0 g complies with *limit test C for heavy metals*, Appendix VII (20 ppm). Use 2 ml of *lead standard solution (10 ppm Pb)* to prepare the standard.

Related substances Carry out the method for *thin-layer chromatography*, Appendix III A, using *silica gel HF254* as the coating substance and a mixture of 50 volumes of *1,4-dioxan*, 40 volumes of *nitromethane*, 5 volumes of *water* and 3 volumes of 5M *ammonia* as the mobile phase. Apply separately to the chromatoplate 5 µl of each of two solutions of the substance being examined in a mixture of 1 volume of 13.5M *ammonia* and 49 volumes of *methanol* containing (1) 2.0% w/v and (2) 0.0050% w/v. After removal of the plate, dry it at 100° to 105°, examine under *ultra-violet light (254 nm)* and then reveal the spots by *Method I*. When examined under ultra-violet light and after spraying, any *secondary spot* in the chromatogram obtained with solution (1) is not more intense than the spot in the chromatogram obtained with solution (2).

Loss on drying When dried to constant weight at 100° to 105°, loses not more than 0.5% of its weight. Use 1 g.

Sulphated ash Not more than 0.1%, Appendix IX A, Method II. Use 1 g.

Assay Dissolve 0.5 g in 50 ml of *acetone* and carry out Method II for *non-aqueous titration*, Appendix VIII A, using 0.1M *tetrabutylammonium hydroxide VS* as titrant and a 0.3% w/v solution of *thymol blue* in *methanol* as indicator. Each ml of 0.1M *tetrabutylammonium hydroxide VS* is equivalent to 0.02533 g of $C_{10}H_{11}N_3O_3S$.

Storage Sulphamethoxazole should be kept in a well-closed container and protected from light.

Preparations
Co-trimoxazole Oral Suspension
Paediatric Co-trimoxazole Oral Suspension
Co-trimoxazole Intravenous Infusion
Co-trimoxazole Tablets
Dispersible Co-trimoxazole Tablets
Paediatric Co-trimoxazole Tablets

Action and use Antibacterial.

Sulphamethoxypyridazine

H₂N—⟨benzene⟩—SO₂·NH—⟨pyridazine N=N⟩—OMe

C₁₁H₁₂N₄O₃S   280.3   80-35-3

Sulphamethoxypyridazine is N^1-(6-methoxy-pyridazin-3-yl)sulphanilamide. It contains not less than 99.0 per cent and not more than 101.0 per cent of $C_{11}H_{12}N_4O_3S$, calculated with reference to the dried substance.

Characteristics A white or yellowish-white, crystalline powder; odourless or almost odourless.

Solubility Very slightly soluble in *water*; sparingly soluble in *ethanol (96%)*; soluble in 25 parts of *acetone*. It dissolves in dilute mineral acids and in aqueous solutions of the alkali hydroxides.

Identification A. The *infra-red absorption spectrum*, Appendix II A, is concordant with the *reference spectrum* of sulphamethoxypyridazine. If the spectra are not concordant, dissolve the substance in the minimum volume of hot *ethanol (96%)*, add an equal volume of *2,2,4-trimethylpentane*, evaporate to dryness on a water-bath and prepare a new spectrum of the residue. Avoid excessive grinding in the preparation of the disc.
B. Yields the *reaction* characteristic of primary aromatic amines, Appendix VI, producing a bright orange-red precipitate.

Acidity Heat 1 g with 50 ml of *carbon dioxide-free water* at about 70° for 5 minutes, cool quickly to 20° and filter. 25 ml of the filtrate requires not more than 0.35 ml of 0.1M *sodium hydroxide VS* for titration to pH 7.0, Appendix V L.

Melting point 180° to 183°, Appendix V A.

Clarity and colour of solution A solution containing 1.0 g in a mixture of 10 ml of 1M *sodium hydroxide* and 15 ml of *water* is *clear*, Appendix IV A, and not more intensely coloured than *reference solution BY₄*, Appendix IV B, Method I.

Heavy metals 1.0 g complies with *limit test C for heavy metals*, Appendix VII (20 ppm). Use 2 ml of *lead standard solution (10 ppm Pb)* to prepare the standard.

Related substances Complies with test A for *related substances in sulphonamides*, Appendix III A.

Loss on drying When dried to constant weight at 100° to 105°, loses not more than 0.5% of its weight. Use 1 g.

Sulphated ash Not more than 0.1%, Appendix IX A.

Assay Dissolve 0.5 g in a mixture of 75 ml of *water* and 10 ml of *hydrochloric acid* and carry out the method for *amperometric titration*, Appendix VIII B. Each ml of 0.1M *sodium nitrite VS* is equivalent to 0.02803 g of $C_{11}H_{12}N_4O_3S$.

Storage Sulphamethoxypyridazine should be protected from light.

Preparation
Sulphamethoxypyridazine Tablets

Action and use Antibacterial.

Sulphapyridine

H_2N—⟨O⟩—$SO_2 \cdot NH$—⟨O⟩
                                    N

$C_{11}H_{11}N_3O_2S$ 249.3   *144-83-2*

Sulphapyridine is N^1-2-pyridylsulphanilamide. It contains not less than 99.0 per cent and not more than 101.0 per cent of $C_{11}H_{11}N_3O_2S$, calculated with reference to the dried substance.

Characteristics A white or yellowish-white, crystalline powder; odourless or almost odourless.

Solubility Very slightly soluble in *water*; slightly soluble in *ethanol (96%)*; sparingly soluble in *acetone*. It dissolves in dilute mineral acids and in aqueous solutions of alkali hydroxides.

Identification A. The *infra-red absorption spectrum*, Appendix II A, is concordant with the *reference spectrum* of sulphapyridine. If the spectra are not concordant, dissolve 0.1 g in the minimum volume of 1M *sodium hydroxide* and neutralise to *litmus paper* with 1M *hydrochloric acid*. Filter, wash the precipitate with *water*, dry at 100° to 105° and prepare a new spectrum of the residue.
B. Heat 10 mg in a dry tube. A brown colour is produced, yellow fumes are evolved and the odour of sulphur dioxide is detectable.
C. Yields the *reaction* characteristic of primary aromatic amines, Appendix VI, producing an orange-red precipitate which darkens on standing.

Acidity Heat 1 g with 50 ml of *carbon dioxide-free water* at about 70° for 5 minutes, cool quickly to 20° and filter. 25 ml of the filtrate requires not more than 0.1 ml of 0.1M *sodium hydroxide VS* for titration to pH 7.0, Appendix V L.

Melting point 191° to 193°, Appendix V A.

Clarity and colour of solution A 5.0% w/v solution in 2M *hydrochloric acid* is *clear*, Appendix IV A, and not more intensely coloured than *reference solution Y_5*, Appendix IV B, Method I.

Heavy metals 1.0 g complies with *limit test C for heavy metals*, Appendix VII (20 ppm). Use 2 ml of *lead standard solution (10 ppm Pb)* to prepare the standard.

Related substances Carry out the method for *thin-layer chromatography*, Appendix III A, using *silica gel G* as the coating substance and a mixture of 90 volumes of *acetone*, 15 volumes of *4-methylpentan-2-one* and 7.5 volumes of 13.5M *ammonia* as the mobile phase. Apply separately to the chromatoplate 10 µl of each of two solutions in a mixture of 1 volume of 13.5M *ammonia* and 9 volumes of *ethanol (96%)* containing (1) 1.0% w/v of the substance being examined and (2) 0.0050% w/v of *sulphanilamide*. After removal of the plate, dry it at 105° for 10 minutes and spray with a 0.1% w/v solution of *4-dimethylamino-benzaldehyde* in *ethanol (96%)* containing 1% v/v of *hydrochloric acid*. Any *secondary spot* in the chromatogram obtained with solution (1) is not more intense than the spot in the chromatogram obtained with solution (2).

Loss on drying When dried to constant weight at 105°, loses not more than 0.5% of its weight. Use 1 g.

Sulphated ash Not more than 0.1%, Appendix IX A.

Assay Dissolve 0.5 g in a mixture of 75 ml of *water* and 10 ml of *hydrochloric acid* and carry out the method for *amperometric titration*, Appendix VIII B. Each ml of 0.1M *sodium nitrite VS* is equivalent to 0.02493 g of $C_{11}H_{11}N_3O_2S$.

Storage Sulphapyridine should be protected from light.

Preparation
Sulphapyridine Tablets

Action and use Antibacterial.

Sulphathiazole

H_2N—⟨O⟩—$SO_2 \cdot NH$—⟨S⟩
                                    N

$C_9H_9N_3O_2S_2$ 255.3   *72-14-0*

Sulphathiazole is N^1-thiazol-2-ylsulphanilamide. It contains not less than 99.0 per cent and not more than 101.0 per cent of $C_9H_9N_3O_2S_2$, calculated with reference to the dried substance.

Characteristics A white or almost white, crystalline powder; odourless or almost odourless.

Solubility Very slightly soluble in *water*; slightly soluble in *ethanol (96%)*. It dissolves in dilute mineral acids and in aqueous solutions of alkali hydroxides and carbonates.

Identification A. The *infra-red absorption spectrum*, Appendix II A, is concordant with the *reference spectrum* of sulphathiazole.
B. Dissolve 10 mg in a mixture of 10 ml of *water* and 2 ml of 0.1M *sodium hydroxide* and add 0.5 ml of *copper sulphate solution*. A greyish-purple precipitate is produced.
C. Yields the *reaction* characteristic of primary aromatic amines, Appendix VI, producing an orange-red precipitate.

Acidity Heat 1.0 g with 50 ml of *carbon dioxide-free water* at 70° for 5 minutes, cool rapidly to 20° and filter. 25 ml of the filtrate requires not more than 0.1 ml of 0.1M *sodium hydroxide VS* for titration to pH 7.0, Appendix V L.

Melting point 200° to 203°, Appendix V A.

Heavy metals 1.0 g complies with *limit test C for heavy metals*, Appendix VII (20 ppm). Use 2 ml of *lead standard solution (10 ppm Pb)* to prepare the standard.

Related substances Complies with test A for *related substances in sulphonamides*, Appendix III A.

Loss on drying When dried to constant weight at 105°, loses not more than 0.5% of its weight. Use 1 g.

Sulphated ash Not more than 0.1%, Appendix IX A.

Assay Dissolve 0.5 g in a mixture of 75 ml of *water* and 10 ml of *hydrochloric acid* and carry out the method for *amperometric titration*, Appendix VIII B. Each ml of 0.1M *sodium nitrite VS* is equivalent to 0.02553 g of $C_9H_9N_3O_2S_2$.

Storage Sulphathiazole should be protected from light.

Preparation
Sulphathiazole Tablets

Action and use Antibacterial.

Sulphinpyrazone

$C_{23}H_{20}N_2O_3S$ 404.5   *57-96-5*

Sulphinpyrazone is 1,2-diphenyl-4-(2-phenyl-sulphinylethyl)pyrazolidine-3,5-dione. It contains not less than 99.0 per cent and not more than 101.0 per cent of $C_{23}H_{20}N_2O_3S$, calculated with reference to the dried substance.

Characteristics A white or almost white powder; odourless or almost odourless.

Solubility Practically insoluble in *water* and in *petroleum spirit*; soluble in 40 parts of *ethanol (96%)* and in 2 parts of *chloroform*; slightly soluble in *ether*.

Identification A. The *infra-red absorption spectrum*, Appendix II A, is concordant with the *reference spectrum* of sulphinpyrazone.
B. The *light absorption*, Appendix II B, in the range 230 to 350 nm of a 0.002% w/v solution in 0.01M *sodium hydroxide* exhibits a maximum only at 260 nm. The *absorbance* at 260 nm is about 1.1.
C. Dissolve 10 mg in 3 ml of *acetone* and add 0.05 ml of *iron(III) chloride test-solution* and 3 ml of *water*. A red colour is produced.

Melting point 131° to 135°, Appendix V A.

Solubility in acetone A 5.0% w/v solution in *acetone* is *clear*, Appendix IV A. The *absorbance* of a 4-cm layer at 420 nm is not more than 0.1, Appendix II B.

Solubility in 1M sodium hydroxide A 5.0% w/v solution in 1M *sodium hydroxide* is *clear*, Appendix IV A. The *absorbance* of a 4-cm layer at 420 nm is not more than 0.15, Appendix II B.

Heavy metals Dissolve the residue obtained in the test for Sulphated ash in 0.5 ml of *hydrochloric acid*, evaporate to dryness, dissolve the residue in 2 ml of *water*, neutralise to *phenolphthalein solution* with 1.25M *sodium hydroxide* and dilute to 15 ml with *water*. 12 ml of the resulting solution

complies with *limit test A for heavy metals*, Appendix VII (10 ppm). Use *lead standard solution (1 ppm Pb)* to prepare the standard.

Related substances Carry out the method for *thin-layer chromatography*, Appendix III A, using a silica gel F254 precoated chromatoplate (Merck silica gel 60 F254 plates are suitable) and a mixture of 80 volumes of *chloroform* and 20 volumes of *glacial acetic acid* as the mobile phase. Place the plate in a tank containing a beaker of *glacial acetic acid* and allow it to stand for 10 minutes. Heat the plate at 60° for 40 minutes, cool and pass a stream of carbon dioxide over the surface of the plate for 10 minutes. Apply separately to the plate, under an atmosphere of carbon dioxide, 5 µl of each of the following solutions in *acetone*. Solutions (1) and (2) contain 2.0% w/v and 0.0060% w/v respectively of the substance being examined. Solutions (3) and (4) contain 0.040% w/v and 0.020% w/v respectively of *1,2-diphenyl-4-(2-phenylsulphonylethyl)pyrazolidine-3,5-dione BPCRS*. Solutions (5) and (6) contain 0.040% w/v and 0.020% w/v respectively of *1,2-diphenyl-4-(2-phenylthioethyl)-pyrazolidine-3,5-dione BPCRS*.

After removal of the plate, allow it to dry in air and examine under *ultra-violet light (254 nm)*. The spots in the chromatograms obtained with solutions (3) and (5) and at least one of the spots in the chromatograms obtained with solutions (4) and (6) are more intense than any corresponding spots in the chromatogram obtained with solution (1) Any other *secondary spot* in the chromatogram obtained with solution (1) is not more intense than the spot in the chromatogram obtained with solution (2).

Loss on drying When dried to constant weight at 105°, loses not more than 0.5% of its weight. Use 1 g.

Sulphated ash Not more than 0.1%, Appendix IX A, Method II. Use 1.5 g.

Assay Dissolve 0.5 g in 25 ml of *acetone* and titrate with 0.1M *sodium hydroxide VS* using *bromothymol blue solution* as indicator. Each ml of 0.1M *sodium hydroxide VS* is equivalent to 0.04045 g of $C_{23}H_{20}N_2O_3S$.

Preparation
Sulphinpyrazone Tablets

Action and use Used in treatment of gout.

Sulphobromophthalein Sodium

$C_{20}H_8Br_4Na_2O_{10}S_2$ 838.0   *71-67-0*

Sulphobromophthalein Sodium is disodium 5,5'-(4,5,6,7-tetrabromo-3-oxo-(3*H*)-isobenzofuran-1-ylidene)bis(2-hydroxybenzenesulphonate). It contains not less than 36.0 per cent and not more than 39.0 per cent of Br and not less than 7.4 per cent and not more than 8.2 per cent of

S, both calculated with reference to the dried substance.

Characteristics A white, crystalline powder; odourless or almost odourless; hygroscopic.

Solubility Soluble in 12 parts of *water*; practically insoluble in *ethanol (96%)* and in *acetone*.

Identification A. *Absorbance* of a 0.0005% w/v solution in 0.05M *sodium hydroxide* at 580 nm, about 0.40, Appendix II B.

B. When moistened with *hydrochloric acid* and introduced on a platinum wire into a flame, imparts a yellow colour to the flame.

C. Mix 0.1 g with 0.5 g of *sodium carbonate*, ignite until thoroughly charred, cool, add 5 ml of hot *water*, heat for 5 minutes on a water-bath and filter. The filtrate yields the *reactions* characteristic of bromides, Appendix VI.

Colour and completeness of solution 0.20 g dissolves completely in 10 ml of *water* yielding a solution that is *colourless*, Appendix IV B, Method I.

Calcium Ignite 5 g in a platinum dish until free from carbon, cool, add 1 ml of *hydrochloric acid* and 10 ml of *water*, heat on a water-bath for 5 minutes, add 1 g of *ammonium sulphate* and 4 ml of 5M *ammonia* and heat for a further 5 minutes. Transfer the contents of the dish to a flask using 50 ml of *water*, add 20 ml of 13.5M *ammonia*, dilute to 100 ml with *water*, add 0.3 ml of *sodium sulphide solution*, 1 ml of *potassium cyanide solution* and 74 ml of *absolute ethanol* and titrate with 0.01M *disodium edetate VS* using 0.1 g of *methyl thymol blue mixture* as indicator and titrating to a faint grey colour. Not more than 6.25 ml of 0.01M *disodium edetate VS* is required.

Halide ions To 5 ml of a 1.0% w/v solution add 1 ml of 2M *nitric acid* and 1 ml of *silver nitrate solution*. Not more than a slight opalescence is produced.

Sulphate To 10 ml of a 0.2% w/v solution add 0.25 ml of 2M *hydrochloric acid*, boil and add 1 ml of *barium chloride solution*. The hot solution remains clear for 2 minutes but on cooling crystals of the barium salt of sulphobromo-phthalein may be produced.

Loss on drying When dried to constant weight at 105°, loses not more than 5.0% of its weight. Use 1 g.

Assay *For Br* Carry out the method for *oxygen-flask combustion*, Appendix VIII C, using 0.2 g, a 1000-ml glass-stoppered flask and a mixture of 10 ml of 0.1M *sodium hydroxide*, 0.5 ml of *hydrogen peroxide solution (100 vol)* and 10 ml of *water* as the absorbing liquid. When the process is complete, boil the solution for 5 minutes, cool, acidify with 2M *nitric acid*, add 20 ml of 0.1M *silver nitrate VS*, shake and titrate the excess of silver nitrate with 0.1M *ammonium thiocyanate VS* using *ammonium iron(III) sulphate solution* as indicator. Each ml of 0.1M *silver nitrate VS* is equivalent to 0.007991 g of Br.

For S Carry out Method II for sulphur described under *oxygen-flask combustion*, Appendix VIII C, using 0.2 g, a 1000-ml glass-stoppered flask and a mixture of 30 ml of *water* and 0.5 ml of *hydrogen peroxide solution (100 vol)* as the absorbing liquid. When the process is complete, add 2 ml of *hydrochloric acid*, dilute to 250 ml with *water*, heat to boiling and slowly add 10 ml of *barium chloride solution*. Heat on a water-bath for 1 hour, filter, wash the precipitate with *water*, dry and ignite at about 600° until, after further ignition, two successive weighings do not differ by more than 0.2%. Each g of residue is equivalent to 0.1374 g of S.

Storage Sulphobromophthalein Sodium should be stored in a well-closed container.

Action and use Dye used in tests of hepatic function.

Sulphuric Acid

H_2SO_4 98.07   7664-93-9

Sulphuric Acid contains not less than 95.0 per cent w/w and not more than 100.5 per cent w/w of H_2SO_4.

Characteristics A colourless liquid of oily consistence; corrosive; evolves much heat when added to water.

Identification A. It is strongly acidic even when freely diluted with *water*.

B. Carefully add 1 ml to 10 ml of *water*. The resulting solution yields the *reactions* characteristic of sulphates, Appendix VI.

Weight per ml About 1.84 g, Appendix V G.

Arsenic Dilute 0.5 g to 25 ml with *water*. The resulting solution complies with the *limit test for arsenic*, Appendix VII (2 ppm).

Iron 0.25 g complies with the *limit test for iron*, Appendix VII (40 ppm).

Lead Not more than 10 ppm when determined by the following procedure and using the following solutions. For solution (1) use 4.0 g of the substance being examined. For solution (2) mix 2.0 g with 2 ml of *lead standard solution (10 ppm Pb)*. Make solutions (1) and (2) alkaline with 5M *ammonia* and to each add 1 ml of *potassium cyanide solution PbT*. The solutions should be not more than faintly opalescent. If the colours of the solutions differ, equalise by the addition of about 0.2 ml of a highly diluted solution of burnt sugar or other non-reactive substance. Dilute each solution to 50 ml with *water*, add 0.1 ml of a 10% w/v solution of *sodium sulphide* to each and mix thoroughly. The colour produced in solution (1) is not more intense than that produced in solution (2) when viewed against a white background.

Chloride Carefully add 5.0 g to 50 ml of *water*, neutralise to *litmus paper* with 5M *ammonia* and dilute to 100 ml with *water*. 15 ml of the resulting solution complies with the *limit test for chlorides*, Appendix VII (70 ppm).

Nitrate Carefully add 5.0 ml to a mixture of 5 ml of *water* and 0.5 ml of *indigo carmine solution* and allow to stand for 1 minute. The colour of the solution is not discharged.

Oxidisable substances Carefully add 5.0 ml to 20 ml of *water*, cool, add 0.1 ml of 0.02M *potassium permanganate* and allow to stand for 5 minutes. The colour of the solution is not discharged.

Non-volatile matter Evaporate 10 g by heating gently. The residue, when ignited to constant weight, weighs not more than 1.0 mg.

Assay Carefully add 2 g to 40 ml of *water* and titrate with 1M *sodium hydroxide VS* using *methyl orange solution* as indicator. Each ml of 1M *sodium hydroxide VS* is equivalent to 0.04904 g of H_2SO_4.

Storage Sulphuric Acid should be kept in a well-closed container.

Preparation
Dilute Sulphuric Acid

Dilute Sulphuric Acid

Dilute Sulphuric Acid contains 9.5 per cent to 10.5 per cent w/w of H_2SO_4. It is prepared by adding 104 g of Sulphuric Acid to 896 g of Purified Water with constant stirring and cooling.

Weight per ml 1.062 g to 1.072 g, Appendix V G.

Assay To 10 g add 40 ml of *water* and titrate with 1M *sodium hydroxide VS* using *methyl orange solution* as indicator. Each ml of 1M *sodium hydroxide VS* is equivalent to 0.04904 g of H_2SO_4.

Sulthiame

$C_{10}H_{14}N_2O_4S_2$ 290.4   *61-56-3*

Sulthiame is 4-(tetrahydro-2*H*-1,2-thiazin-2-yl)-benzenesulphonamide *S,S*-dioxide. It contains not less than 98.0 per cent and not more than 100.5 per cent of $C_{10}H_{14}N_2O_4S_2$, calculated with reference to the dried substance.

Characteristics A white, crystalline powder; odourless or almost odourless.

Solubility Very slightly soluble in *water*; slightly soluble in *ethanol (96%)*, in *chloroform* and in *ether*.

Identification A. The *infra-red absorption spectrum*, Appendix II A, is concordant with the *reference spectrum* of sulthiame.

B. The *light absorption*, Appendix II B, in the range 220 to 350 nm of a 0.002% w/v solution in *methanol* exhibits a maximum only at 246 nm. The *absorbance* at 246 nm is about 0.80.

C. Mix 0.5 g with 0.5 g of *benzhydrol*, 0.5 g of *toluene-p-sulphonic acid* and 5 ml of *glacial acetic acid* and heat for 30 minutes under a reflux condenser in a water-bath. Pour the hot solution into 25 ml of hot *water* and shake vigorously for 30 minutes. Filter the cooled mixture and wash the filter with 10 ml of *water*. The *melting point* of the precipitate, after recrystallisation from 50 ml of *ethanol (96%)* and drying at a pressure not exceeding 2 kPa, is about 190°, Appendix V A. Mix the residue with an equal quantity of the substance being examined; the *melting point* is reduced by not less than 10°.

Melting point 185° to 188°, Appendix V A.

Heavy metals Dissolve 2.0 g in 7 ml of 5M *sodium hydroxide* and dilute to 20 ml with *water*. 12 ml of the resulting solution complies with *limit test A for heavy metals*, Appendix VII (20 ppm). Use *lead standard solution (2 ppm Pb)* to prepare the standard.

Related substances A. Carry out the method for *thin-layer chromatography*, Appendix III A, using a 0.5-mm layer of *silica gel HF254* as the coating substance and a mixture of 80 volumes of *1,2-dichloroethane* and 20 volumes of *absolute ethanol* as the mobile phase. Apply separately to the chromatoplate 20 μl of each of two solutions in *acetone*

containing (1) 5.0% w/v of the substance being examined and (2) 0.010% w/v of *sulphanilamide*. After removal of the plate, allow it to dry in air and examine under *ultra-violet light (254 nm)*. Any *secondary spot* in the chromatogram obtained with solution (1) is not more intense than the spot in the chromatogram obtained with solution (2).

B. Complies with test A using a mixture of 90 volumes of *ethyl acetate*, 10 volumes of *absolute ethanol* and 2 volumes of 5M *ammonia* as the mobile phase.

Loss on drying When dried to constant weight at 105°, loses not more than 0.5% of its weight. Use 1 g.

Sulphated ash Not more than 0.1%, Appendix IX A.

Assay Dissolve 0.5 g in 70 ml of *dimethylformamide* and carry out Method II for *non-aqueous titration*, Appendix VIII A, using 0.1M *tetrabutylammonium hydroxide VS* as titrant and determining the end-point potentiometrically. Each ml of 0.1M *tetrabutylammonium hydroxide VS* is equivalent to 0.02904 g of $C_{10}H_{14}N_2O_4S_2$.

Preparation

Sulthiame Tablets

Action and use Anticonvulsant.

In some countries the material described in this monograph may be known as Sultiame.

Suxamethonium Bromide

Succinylcholine Bromide

$C_{14}H_{30}Br_2N_2O_4$ 450.3   *55-94-7 (dihydrate)*

Suxamethonium Bromide is 2,2'-succinyldioxy-bis(ethyltrimethylammonium) dibromide. It contains not less than 99.0 per cent and not more than 101.0 per cent of $C_{14}H_{30}Br_2N_2O_4$, calculated with reference to the dried substance.

Characteristics A white or creamy-white powder; odourless or almost odourless; hygroscopic.

Solubility Soluble in 0.3 part of *water* and in 5 parts of *ethanol (96%)*; practically insoluble in *chloroform* and in *ether*.

Identification A. Dissolve 0.1 g in 10 ml of *water* and add 10 ml of 1M *sulphuric acid* and 30 ml of a 1% w/v solution of *ammonium reineckate*; a pink precipitate is produced. Allow to stand for 30 minutes, filter and wash with *water*, with *ethanol (96%)* and with *ether*. The *melting point* of the residue, after drying at 80°, is about 180°, Appendix V A.

B. Yields the *reactions* characteristic of bromides, Appendix VI.

C. *Melting point*, about 225°, Appendix V A.

Acidity Dissolve 1.0 g in 10 ml of *carbon dioxide-free water* and add 0.1 ml of *bromothymol blue solution* and 0.05 ml of 0.1M *hydrochloric acid*; the solution is yellow. Immediately add 0.35 ml of 0.1M *sodium hydroxide*; a blue colour is produced.

Related substances Carry out the method for *thin-layer chromatography*, Appendix III A, using *cellulose* as the coating substance and as the mobile phase the freshly prepared upper layer, which may be cloudy, obtained by shaking together for 10 minutes 50 volumes of *butan-1-ol*, 40 volumes of *water* and 10 volumes of *anhydrous formic acid*. Apply separately to the chromatoplate 5 μl of each of four solutions in *methanol (60%)* containing (1) 4.0% w/v of the substance being examined, (2) 0.040% w/v of *choline iodide* and (3) and (4) 0.040% w/v and 0.020% w/v respectively of *2-(3-carboxypropionoxy)ethyltrimethyl-ammonium bromide BPCRS*. After removal of the plate, allow it to dry in air and spray with *dilute potassium iodobismuthate solution*. In the chromatogram obtained with solution (1) any spot corresponding to choline is not more intense than the spot in the chromatogram obtained with solution (2), any other *secondary spot* is not more intense than the spot in the chromatogram obtained with solution (3) and not more than one such spot is more intense than the spot in the chromatogram obtained with solution (4).

Loss on drying When dried to constant weight at 105°, loses not more than 2.0% of its weight. Use 1 g.

Sulphated ash Not more than 0.1%, Appendix IX A.

Assay Carry out Method I for *non-aqueous titration*, Appendix VIII A, using 0.5 g and *crystal violet solution* as indicator. Each ml of 0.1M *perchloric acid VS* is equivalent to 0.02251 g of $C_{14}H_{30}Br_2N_2O_4$.

Storage Suxamethonium Bromide should be protected from light.

Preparation
Suxamethonium Bromide Injection

Action and use Skeletal muscle relaxant.

Suxamethonium Chloride ☆

CO·OCH₂·CH₂·ṄMe₂
|
(CH₂)₂   2Cl⁻
|
CO·OCH₂·CH₂·ṄMe₂

$C_{14}H_{30}Cl_2N_2O_4,2H_2O$ 397.3   *6101-15-1*

Suxamethonium Chloride is 2,2′-succinyldioxy-bis(ethyltrimethylammonium) dichloride dihydrate. It contains not less than 98.0 per cent and not more than of 101.0 per cent of $C_{14}H_{30}Cl_2N_2O_4$, calculated with reference to the anhydrous substance.

Characteristics A white or almost white, crystalline powder; almost odourless; hygroscopic. The undried substance melts at about 160°.

Solubility Soluble in 1 part of *water*; slightly soluble in *ethanol (96%)*; practically insoluble in *chloroform* and in *ether*.

Identification *Test A may be omitted if tests B, C and D are carried out. Tests B and C may be omitted if tests A and D are carried out.*

A. The *infra-red absorption spectrum*, Appendix II A, is concordant with the spectrum of *suxamethonium chloride EPCRS*.

B. Dissolve 25 mg in 1 ml of *water*, add 0.1 ml of a 1% w/v solution of *cobalt(II) chloride* and 0.1 ml of a 5% w/v solution of *potassium hexacyanoferrate(II)*. A green colour is produced.

C. To 10 ml of a 0.5% w/v solution add 10 ml of 1M *sulphuric acid* and 30 ml of a 1% w/v solution of *ammonium reineckate*; a pink precipitate is produced. Allow to stand for 30 minutes, filter and wash with *water*, then with *ethanol (96%)* and finally with *ether*. The *melting point* of the residue after drying at 80° is 180° to 185°, Appendix V A, Method I.

D. 20 mg yields *reaction A* characteristic of chlorides, Appendix VI.

Acidity pH of a 0.5% w/v solution, 4.0 to 5.0, Appendix V L.

Clarity and colour of solution A 5.0% w/v solution in *carbon dioxide-free water* is *clear*, Appendix IV A. 4 ml of the solution diluted to 10 ml with *water* is *colourless*, Appendix IV B, Method II.

Choline chloride Carry out the method for *thin-layer chromatography*, Appendix III A, using *microcrystalline cellulose* as the coating substance and as the mobile phase the upper layer obtained by shaking together for 10 minutes and then allowing to separate 50 volumes of *butan-1-ol*, 40 volumes of *water* and 10 volumes of *anhydrous formic acid*. Apply separately to the chromato-plate 5 μl of each of two solutions in *methanol* containing (1) 4.0% w/v of the substance being examined and (2) 4.0% w/v of *suxamethonium chloride EPCRS* and 0.02% w/v of *choline chloride*. After removal of the plate, allow it to dry in air and spray with *acetic potassium iodobismuthate solution*. Any *secondary spot* in the chromatogram obtained with solution (1) is not more intense than the spot due to choline chloride in the chromatogram obtained with solution (2). The test is not valid unless the chromatogram obtained with solution (2) shows two clearly separated principal spots.

Sulphated ash Not more than 0.1%, Appendix IX A, Method II. Use 1 g.

Water 8.0 to 10.0% w/w, Appendix IX C. Use 0.3 g.

Assay Dissolve 0.15 g in 15 ml of *anhydrous glacial acetic acid*, add 15 ml of *acetic anhydride* and 10 ml of *mercury (II) acetate solution* and carry out Method I for *non-aqueous titration*, Appendix VIII A, using *crystal violet solution* as indicator. Each ml of 0.1M *perchloric acid VS* is equivalent to 0.01807 g of $C_{14}H_{30}Cl_2N_2O_4$.

Storage Suxamethonium Chloride should be kept in a well-closed container and protected from light.

Preparation
Suxamethonium Chloride Injection

Action and use Skeletal muscle relaxant.

Purified Talc ☆

14807-96-6

Purified Talc★ is a powdered, selected natural hydrated magnesium silicate. It may contain varying amounts of aluminium and iron in forms insoluble in 1M sulphuric acid. Purified Talc should be free from microscopic asbestos fibres.

Characteristics A light, homogeneous, white or almost white, unctuous powder; odourless.

Solubility Practically insoluble in *water* and in dilute solutions of acids or alkalis.

Identification A. When examined microscopically, shows irregular plates, the majority less than 50 μm in length, which are not notably stained by a 0.1% w/v solution of *methylene blue* in *ethanol (96%)*.

B. In a metal crucible melt 0.5 g with 1 g of *potassium nitrate* and 3 g of *anhydrous sodium carbonate*, add 20 ml of boiling *water*, mix and filter. Wash the residue remaining on the filter with 50 ml of *water*. Mix the residue with 0.5 ml of *hydrochloric acid* and 5 ml of *water* and filter. To the filtrate add 1 ml of 9M *ammonia* and 1 ml of 2M *ammonium chloride* and filter. To the filtrate add 1 ml of a 9% w/v solution of *disodium hydrogen orthophosphate*. A white, crystalline precipitate is produced.

C. Yields the *reaction* characteristic of silicates, Appendix VI. Use 0.1 g.

Acid-soluble matter IRON Not more than 250 ppm of Fe soluble in 1M *sulphuric acid* when determined by *atomic absorption spectrophotometry*, Appendix II D, using solution A prepared in the test for Calcium as the test solution and measuring at 248.3 nm using, if possible, a transmission band of 0.2 nm and an air—acetylene flame. For the reference solutions add 10 ml of a 1% w/v solution of *potassium chloride* and 40 ml of 1M *sulphuric acid* to suitable volumes of *iron standard solution (10 ppm Fe)* and dilute to 100 ml with *water*.

MAGNESIUM Not more than 0.4% of Mg soluble in 1M *sulphuric acid* when determined by *atomic absorption spectrophotometry*, Appendix II D. Prepare the test solution by adding 10 ml of a 1% w/v solution of *potassium chloride* to 5 ml of solution A and dilute to 100 ml with *water*. Measure at 285.2 nm using, if possible, a transmission band of 1 nm and an air—acetylene flame. For the reference solutions add 10 ml of a 1% w/v solution of *potassium chloride* to suitable volumes of *magnesium standard solution (10 ppm Mg)* and dilute to 100 ml with *water*.

Calcium Not more than 0.6% of Ca soluble in 1M *sulphuric acid*, using solution (1) as the test solution and not more than 500 ppm of Ca insoluble in 1M *sulphuric acid* using solution (2) as the test solution. Determine by *atomic absorption spectrophotometry*, Appendix II D, measuring at 422.7 nm using a transmission band, if possible, of 1 nm and using either a nitrous oxide—acetylene or an air—acetylene flame.

Suspend 0.25 g in 40 ml of 1M *sulphuric acid*, shake for 15 minutes, add 10 ml of a 1% w/v solution of *potassium chloride*, dilute to 100 ml with *water* and filter quantitatively through filter paper previously washed with hydrochloric acid and hydrofluoric acid (solution A). Wash the residue obtained in solution A with 10 ml of a 1% w/v solution of *potassium chloride* until the filtrate is free from chloride. Place the filter containing the insoluble residue in a platinum crucible and ignite to dark red until no traces of carbon remain. Add 2.5 ml of *sulphuric acid*, heat until white fumes of sulphur trioxide are evolved and allow to cool. Add cautiously 5 ml to 10 ml of *hydrofluoric acid* and evaporate without boiling until fumes of hydrofluoric acid are no longer evolved and white fumes of sulphur trioxide are evolved. Allow to cool completely, add cautiously 20 ml of *water*, mix, add 10 ml of a 1% w/v solution of *potassium chloride* and dilute to 100 ml with *water*. If the solution is opalescent or turbid, allow to stand until it becomes clear (solution B).

For solution (1) add 10 ml of a 1% w/v solution of *potassium chloride* to 20 ml of solution A and dilute to 100 ml with *water*. Prepare solution (2) in the same manner as solution (1) but use solution B in place of solution A. To prepare the reference solutions add 10 ml of a 1% w/v solution of *potassium chloride* and 8 ml of 1M *sulphuric acid* to suitable volumes of *calcium standard solution (10 ppm Ca)* and dilute to 100 ml with *water*.

Carbonate When preparing solution A in the test for Calcium, the addition of 1M *sulphuric acid* produces no effervescence.

Chloride Suspend 0.7 g in 10 ml of *water*, add 10 ml of 2M *nitric acid*, shake for 15 minutes and filter. 10 ml of the filtrate diluted to 15 ml with *water* complies with the *limit test for chlorides*, Appendix VII (140 ppm).

Readily carbonisable substances The residue obtained in the test for Loss on drying is not more than slightly yellow or grey.

Loss on drying When dried at 180° for 1 hour, loses not more than 1.0% of its weight. Use 1 g.

Preparation

Talc Dusting Powder

The title of the monograph in the European Pharmacopœia is Talc.

*In certain states party to the convention on the Elaboration of a European Pharmacopœia, Purified Talc may be required to comply with a limit for a total viable aerobic count of 10^2 micro-organisms per gram when determined by plate count, Appendix XVI B2.

Tamoxifen Citrate

C$_{26}$H$_{29}$NO,C$_6$H$_8$O$_7$ 563.6   *54965-24-1*

Tamoxifen Citrate is (Z)-2-[p-(1,2-diphenylbut-1-enyl)phenoxy]ethyldimethylamine citrate. It contains not less than 99.0 per cent and not more than 101.0 per cent of C$_{26}$H$_{29}$NO,C$_6$H$_8$O$_7$, calculated with reference to the dried substance.

Characteristics A white or almost white, crystalline powder.

Solubility Slightly soluble in *water* and in *acetone*; soluble in *methanol*.

Identification A. The *infra-red absorption spectrum*, Appendix II A, is concordant with the *reference spectrum* of tamoxifen citrate.

B. The *light absorption*, Appendix II B, in the range 220 to 350 nm of a 0.002% w/v solution in *methanol* exhibits two maxima, at 237 nm and 275 nm. The *absorbance* at 237 nm is about 0.7 and at 275 nm is about 0.4.

C. Carry out the method for *thin-layer chromatography*, Appendix III A, using *silica gel GF254* as the coating substance and a mixture of 90 volumes of *toluene* and 10 volumes of *triethylamine* as the mobile phase. Apply separately to the chromatoplate 5 μl of each of two solutions in *methanol* containing (1) 1% w/v of the substance being examined and (2) 1% w/v of *tamoxifen citrate BPCRS*. After removal of the plate, allow it to dry in air and examine under *ultra-violet light (254 nm)*. The principal spot in the chromatogram obtained with solution (1) corresponds to that in the chromatogram obtained with solution (2).

D. To 10 mg add 4 ml of *pyridine* and 2 ml of *acetic anhydride* and shake; a yellow colour is produced immediately. Heat on a water-bath for 2 minutes; a rose-pink to red colour is produced.

E-isomer and related substances Carry out the method for *high-performance liquid chromatography*, Appendix III D, using the following solutions. For solution (1) dissolve 25 mg of the substance being examined in a mixture of 12 volumes of *acetonitrile*, 5 volumes of *water* and 3 volumes of *tetrahydrofuran* and dilute to 10 ml with the same solvent mixture. Prepare solution (2) in the same manner but using 25 mg of *tamoxifen citrate impurity standard BPCRS* in place of the substance being examined. For solution (3) dilute 1 volume of solution (1) to 100 volumes with the same solvent mixture.

The chromatographic procedure may be carried out using (a) a stainless steel column (20 cm × 5 mm) packed with *stationary phase C* (5 μm) (Spherisorb ODS 1 is suitable), (b) a mixture of 300 volumes of *acetonitrile*, 125 volumes of *water*, 75 volumes of *tetrahydrofuran* and 2 volumes of 18M *ammonia* as the mobile phase with a flow rate of 1.5 ml per minute and (c) a detection wavelength of 240 nm.

In the chromatogram obtained with solution (2) a peak due to the *E*-isomer immediately follows the peak due to *Z*-tamoxifen. Adjust the sensitivity of the instrument so that the height of the peak due to *E*-tamoxifen is about 15% of full-scale deflection on the chart paper. Measure the height of the peak due to *E*-tamoxifen by dropping a perpendicular from the apex of the peak to a line drawn tangentially between the troughs on each side of the *E*-isomer peak or the trough between the *E*- and *Z*-isomer peaks and the baseline, whichever is appropriate.

The content of *E*-isomer in the substance being examined is not more than 1% when calculated using the declared content of *E*-isomer in *tamoxifen citrate impurity standard BPCRS*. The area of any *secondary peak* in the chromatogram obtained with solution (1), other than any peak due to the *E*-isomer, is not greater than half that of the peak due to tamoxifen in the chromatogram obtained with solution (3) and the sum of the areas of all such peaks is not greater than the peak due to tamoxifen in the chromatogram obtained with solution (3).

The test is not valid unless the height of the trough separating the peaks due to *E*- and *Z*-tamoxifen in the chromatogram obtained with solution (2) is less than 7% of full-scale deflection on the chart paper and the retention time of the main peak is not more than 30 minutes. The retention time decreases with increasing concentration of ammonia in the mobile phase.

Loss on drying When dried to constant weight at 105°, loses not more than 0.5% of its weight. Use 1 g.

Sulphated ash Not more than 0.2%, Appendix IX A.

Assay Dissolve 1 g in 150 ml of *anhydrous glacial acetic acid* and carry out Method I for *non-aqueous titration*, Appendix VIII A using *1-naphtholbenzein solution* as indicator. Each ml of 0.1M *perchloric acid VS* is equivalent to 0.05636 g of $C_{26}H_{29}NO,C_6H_8O_7$.

Preparation

Tamoxifen Tablets

Action and use Anti-oestrogen.

Tar

Tar is a bituminous liquid obtained from the wood of various trees of the family Pinaceae by destructive distillation and is known in commerce as Stockholm tar.

Characteristics Dark brown or nearly black, semi-liquid; denser than water; odour, characteristic and empyreumatic.

Solubility Soluble in *ethanol (90%)*, in *chloroform*, in *ether* and in fixed and volatile oils.

Identification Shake 1 g with 20 ml of *water* for 5 minutes. To 5 ml of the aqueous liquid, filtered if necessary with the aid of *kieselguhr*, add 0.15 ml of a 0.1% w/v solution of *iron(III) chloride hexahydrate*. A red colour is produced.

Acidity The aqueous liquid obtained by shaking 1 g with 20 ml of *water* for 5 minutes is acidic to *litmus paper*.

Coal tar Shake about 0.5 g vigorously with 10 ml of *petroleum spirit (boiling range, 40° to 60°)*. No fluorescence is produced.

Action and use Used in treatment of psoriasis.

Coal Tar

Coal Tar is a product obtained from bituminous coal by destructive distillation at about 1000°.

Characteristics A nearly black, viscous liquid; odour, strong, penetrating and characteristic. On exposure to air, the viscosity gradually increases. It burns in air with a luminous, sooty flame. It has a weight per ml of about 1.15 g.

Solubility Slightly soluble in *water*, partly soluble in *ethanol*, in *chloroform*, in *ether* and in volatile oils.

Identification A. A saturated solution is alkaline to *litmus solution*.

B. Carefully add 0.5 g to 10 ml of *petroleum spirit (boiling range, 40° to 60°)* and allow to stand for 30 minutes. When examined in daylight, the supernatant liquid has a blue fluorescence which becomes more intense when viewed under ultra-violet light (365 nm).

Ash Not more than 2.0%, Appendix XI J.

Preparations

Coal Tar Solution

Strong Coal Tar Solution

Coal Tar and Salicylic Acid Ointment

Zinc and Coal Tar Paste

Action and use Used in treatment of psoriasis.

Tartaric Acid ☆

CO₂H
|
HCOH
|
HOCH
|
CO₂H

C₄H₆O₆   150.1   87-69-4

Tartaric Acid is L-tartaric acid [(2R,3R)-2,3-dihydroxybutane-1,4-dioic acid]. It contains not less than 99.5 per cent and not more than 101.0 per cent of $C_4H_6O_6$, calculated with reference to the dried substance.

Characteristics Colourless crystals, or a white or almost white, crystalline powder.

Solubility Soluble in less than 1 part of *water* and in 2.5 parts of *ethanol (96%)*.

Identification A. A 10.0% w/v solution in *distilled water* (solution A) is strongly acidic.
B. Yields *reactions A and B* characteristic of tartrates, Appendix VI.

Clarity and colour of solution Solution A is *clear*, Appendix IV A, and not more intensely coloured than *reference solution Y₆*, Appendix IV B, Method I.

Specific optical rotation In a 20% w/v solution, +12.0° to +12.8°, Appendix V F.

Calcium To 5 ml of solution A add 10 ml of a 5.0% w/v solution of *sodium acetate* in *distilled water*. The resulting solution complies with the *limit test for calcium*, Appendix VII (200 ppm).

Heavy metals 2.0 g complies with *limit test C for heavy metals*, Appendix VII (10 ppm). Use 2 ml of *lead standard solution (10 ppm Pb)* to prepare the standard.

Chloride 5 ml of solution A diluted to 15 ml with *water* complies with the *limit test for chlorides*, Appendix VII (100 ppm).

Oxalate Dissolve 0.8 g in 4 ml of *water*, add 3 ml of *hydrochloric acid* and boil with 1 g of *granulated zinc* for 1 minute. Allow to stand for 2 minutes, decant the liquid into a test-tube containing 0.25 ml of a 1% w/v solution of *phenylhydrazine hydrochloride* and heat to boiling. Cool rapidly, transfer to a graduated cylinder, add an equal volume of *hydrochloric acid* and 0.25 ml of a 5% w/v solution of *potassium hexacyanoferrate(III)*, shake and allow to stand for 30 minutes. Any pink colour is not more intense than that produced by treating 4 ml of a 0.01% w/v solution of *oxalic acid* at the same time and in the same manner (350 ppm, calculated as anhydrous oxalic acid).

Sulphate 10 ml of solution A diluted to 15 ml with *distilled water* complies with the *limit test for sulphates*, Appendix VII (150 ppm).

Loss on drying When dried to constant weight at 100° to 105°, loses not more than 0.2% of its weight. Use 1 g.

Sulphated ash Not more than 0.1%, Appendix IX A, Method II. Use 1 g.

Assay Dissolve 0.65 g in 25 ml of *water* and titrate with 1M *sodium hydroxide VS* using 0.5 ml of *dilute phenolphthalein solution* as indicator. Each ml of 1M *sodium hydroxide VS* is equivalent to 0.07505 g of $C_4H_6O_6$.

Temazepam

C₁₆H₁₃ClN₂O₂   300.7   846-50-4

Temazepam is 7-chloro-1,3-dihydro-3-hydroxy-1-methyl-5-phenyl-1,4-benzodiazepin-2-one. It contains not less than 99.0 per cent and not more than 101.0 per cent of $C_{16}H_{13}ClN_2O_2$, calculated with reference to the dried substance.

Characteristics A white or almost white, crystalline powder; odourless or almost odourless.

Solubility Practically insoluble in *water*; sparingly soluble in *ethanol (96%)*; freely soluble in *chloroform*.

Identification A. The *infra-red absorption spectrum*, Appendix II A, is concordant with the *reference spectrum* of temazepam.
B. Protect the solutions from light and measure the absorbance immediately. The *light absorption*, Appendix II B, in the range 210 to 350 nm of a 0.0008% w/v solution in *ethanol (96%)* exhibits maxima at 230 and 315 nm and an inflection at 250 nm. A minor inflection may be observed at 275 nm. The *absorbance* at 230 nm is about 0.87.
C. *Melting point*, about 159°, Appendix V A.

Related substances Carry out in subdued light the method for *thin-layer chromatography*, Appendix III A, using a silica gel F254 precoated chromatoplate (Merck silica gel 60 F254 plates are suitable) and a mixture of 98 volumes of *chloroform* and 2 volumes of *methanol* as the mobile phase. Apply separately to the plate 5 μl of each of three freshly prepared solutions of the substance being examined in a mixture of equal volumes of *dichloroethane* and *methanol* containing (1) 4.0% w/v (2) 0.020% w/v and (3) 0.0080% w/v. After removal of the plate, allow it to dry in air and examine under *ultra-violet light (254 nm)*. Any *secondary spot* in the chromatogram obtained with solution (1) is not more intense than the spot in the chromatogram obtained with solution (2) and not more than one such spot is more intense than the spot in the chromatogram obtained with solution (3).

Loss on drying When dried at 70° at a pressure not exceeding 0.7 kPa for 4 hours, loses not more than 0.5% of its weight. Use 1 g.

Sulphated ash Not more than 0.1%, Appendix IX A, Method II. Use 1 g.

Assay Dissolve 0.25 g in 50 ml of *nitromethane* and carry out Method I for *non-aqueous titration*, Appendix VIII A, determining the end-point potentiometrically. Each ml of 0.1M *perchloric acid VS* is equivalent to 0.03007 g of $C_{16}H_{13}ClN_2O_2$.

Storage Temazepam should be kept in a well-closed container and protected from light.

Action and use Sedative and hypnotic.

Terbutaline Sulphate

$(C_{12}H_{19}NO_3)_2,H_2SO_4$ 548.6   *23031-32-5*

Terbutaline Sulphate is 2-(*tert*-butylamino)-1-(3,5-dihydroxyphenyl)ethanol sulphate. It contains not less than 98.0 per cent and not more than 101.0 per cent of $(C_{12}H_{19}NO_3)_2$, H_2SO_4 calculated with reference to the dried substance.

Characteristics A white or almost white, crystalline powder; odourless or almost odourless.

Solubility Soluble in 4 parts of *water*; slightly soluble in *ethanol (96%)*; practically insoluble in *chloroform* and in *ether*.

Identification A. The *infra-red absorption spectrum*, Appendix II A, is concordant with the *reference spectrum* of terbutaline sulphate. If the spectra are not concordant, dissolve the substance in the minimum volume of *methanol*, evaporate to dryness on a water-bath and prepare a new spectrum of the residue.
B. The *light absorption*, Appendix II B, in the range 230 to 350 nm of a 0.02% w/v solution in 0.1M *hydrochloric acid* exhibits two maxima, at 276 nm and 280 nm, which may be fused. The *absorbance* is about 1.4 at both 276 nm and 280 nm.
C. Yields the *reactions* characteristic of sulphates, Appendix VI.

Acidity Dissolve 0.2 g in 10 ml of *carbon dioxide-free water* and titrate with 0.01M *sodium hydroxide VS* using *methyl red solution* as indicator. Not more than 1.2 ml of 0.01M *sodium hydroxide VS* is required to change the colour of the solution to yellow.

Clarity of solution A 2.0% w/v solution is *clear*, Appendix IV A, Method II B.

Colour of solution *Absorbance* of a 4-cm layer of a 2.0% w/v solution at 400 nm, not more than 0.22, Appendix II B.

Heavy metals Mix 0.8 g with 0.3 g of *anhydrous sodium sulphate* and ignite without melting the sodium sulphate. Cool, add 1.5 ml of 2M *hydrochloric acid*, boil, add sufficient hot *water* to produce 20 ml, cool and filter. 12 ml of the resulting solution complies with *limit test A for heavy metals*, Appendix VII (25 ppm). Use *lead standard solution (1 ppm Pb)* to prepare the standard.

ω-*tert*-Butylamino-3,5-dihydroxyacetophenone *Absorbance* of a 2.0% w/v solution in 0.01M *hydrochloric acid* at 330 nm, not more than 0.50, Appendix II B.

Loss on drying When dried at 105° for 3 hours, loses not more than 0.5% of its weight. Use 1 g.

Assay Dissolve 0.4 g in a mixture of 60 ml of *anhydrous glacial acetic acid* and 60 ml of *acetonitrile* with the aid of heat and cool to room temperature. Carry out Method II for *non-aqueous titration*, Appendix VIII A, using 0.05M *perchloric acid VS* as titrant and *crystal violet solution* as indicator. Each ml of 0.05M *perchloric acid VS* is equivalent to 0.02743 g of $(C_{12}H_{19}NO_3)_2,H_2SO_4$.

Storage Terbutaline Sulphate should be kept in a well-closed container and protected from light.

Preparation
Terbutaline Tablets
Action and use Beta-adrenoceptor antagonist.

Terpineol

$C_{10}H_{18}O$ 154.3   *98-55-5*

Terpineol is a mixture of structural isomers in which α-terpineol predominates.

Characteristics A colourless, slightly viscous, liquid which may deposit crystals; odour, pleasant and characteristic.

Solubility Very slightly soluble in *water*; soluble in 2 parts of *ethanol (70%)*; soluble in *ether*.

Refractive index 1.4825 to 1.4855, Appendix V E.

Weight per ml 0.931 to 0.935 g, Appendix V G.

Low-boiling substances Not more than 4.0% v/v distils below 214°, Appendix V C.

Action and use Pharmaceutical aid.

Testosterone

$C_{19}H_{28}O_2$ 288.4   *58-22-0*

Testosterone is 17β-hydroxyandrost-4-en-3-one. It contains not less than 97.0 per cent and not more than 103.0 per cent of $C_{19}H_{28}O_2$, calculated with reference to the dried substance.

Characteristics A white, crystalline powder; odourless or almost odourless.

Solubility Practically insoluble in *water*; soluble in 5 parts of *ethanol (96%)*; slightly soluble in *ethyl oleate*.

Identification A. The *infra-red absorption spectrum*, Appendix II A, is concordant with the *reference spectrum* of testosterone.
B. Complies with the test for *identification of steroids*, Appendix III A, using *impregnating solvent II* and *mobile phase D*.
C. To 0.1 g in a stoppered tube add 3 ml of *anhydrous pyridine* and 0.6 ml of *acetic anhydride*. Heat on a water-bath for 3 hours, add *water* dropwise until crystals begin to form, then add slowly a further 15 ml of *water* and allow to stand until precipitation is complete. Filter using a sintered-glass crucible and wash with *water* until the washings are neutral to *methyl red solution*. Recrystallise from *ethanol (96%)*, adding a few drops of *water* if necessary to aid crystallisation, and dry at 105°. The *melting point* is about 140°, Appendix V A.

Melting point 152° to 156°, Appendix V A.

Specific optical rotation In a 1% w/v solution in *absolute ethanol*, +106° to +112°, Appendix V F.

Loss on drying When dried to constant weight at 105°, loses not more than 0.5% of its weight. Use 1 g.

Sulphated ash Not more than 0.1%, Appendix IX A.

Assay Dissolve 10 mg in sufficient *absolute ethanol* to produce 100 ml, dilute 5 ml to 50 ml with *absolute ethanol* and measure the *absorbance* of the resulting solution at the maximum at 240 nm, Appendix II B. Calculate the content of $C_{19}H_{28}O_2$ taking 560 as the value of A(1%, 1 cm) at the maximum at 240 nm.

Storage Testosterone should be protected from light.

Preparation
Testosterone Implants

Action and use Androgen; anabolic steroid.

Testosterone Decanoate

$C_{29}H_{46}O_3$ 442.7   *5721-91-5*

Testosterone Decanoate is 3-oxo-androst-4-en-17β-yl decanoate. It contains not less than 97.0 per cent and not more than 103.0 per cent of $C_{29}H_{46}O_3$, calculated with reference to the dried substance.

Characteristics White to creamy-white crystals or crystalline powder.

Solubility Practically insoluble in *water*; very soluble in *ethanol (96%)* and in *chloroform*.

Identification A. The *infra-red absorption spectrum*, Appendix II A, is concordant with the *reference spectrum* of testosterone decanoate.

B. Carry out the method for *thin-layer chromatography*, Appendix III A, using a chromatoplate precoated with silica gel F254 the surface of which has been modified with chemically-bonded octadecylsilyl groups (Whatman KC18F plates are suitable) and a mixture of 60 volumes of *propan-2-ol*, 40 volumes of *acetonitrile* and 20 volumes of *water* as the mobile phase. Apply separately to the plate 5 µl of each of three solutions in a mixture of 9 volumes of *chloroform* and 1 volume of *methanol* containing (1) 0.05% w/v of the substance being examined, (2) 0.05% w/v of *testosterone decanoate BPCRS* and (3) 0.05% w/v each of *testosterone decanoate BPCRS*, *testosterone enanthate BPCRS* and *testosterone isocaproate BPCRS*. After removal of the plate, allow it to dry in air until the odour of solvent is no longer detectable and heat at 100° for 10 minutes. Allow to cool and examine under *ultra-violet light (254 nm)*. The principal spot in the chromatogram obtained with solution (1) corresponds to that in the chromatogram obtained with solution (2). Spray the plate with *ethanolic sulphuric acid (20%)*, heat at 120° for 10 minutes and allow to cool. The principal spot in the chromatogram obtained with solution (1) is green and corresponds in position and size to the spot in the chromatogram obtained with solution (2). The test is not

valid unless the chromatogram obtained with solution (3) shows three distinct principal spots by both methods of visualisation.

C. To 25 mg add 2 ml of a 1% w/v solution of *potassium hydroxide* in *methanol*, heat under a reflux condenser for 1 hour, cool, add 10 ml of *water*, acidify to *litmus paper* with 2M *hydrochloric acid*, filter and wash the precipitate with a small volume of *water*. The *melting point* of the residue, after drying at 60° at a pressure not exceeding 0.7 kPa for 3 hours, is about 152°, Appendix V A.

D. *Melting point*, about 50°, Appendix V A, but the compound may occur in a form which melts at about 55°.

Free decanoic acid Dissolve 0.65 g in 10 ml of *ethanol (96%)*, previously neutralised to *bromothymol blue solution*, and titrate immediately with 0.01M *sodium hydroxide VS* using *bromothymol blue solution* as indicator. Not more than 0.6 ml of 0.01M *sodium hydroxide VS* is required to change the colour of the solution.

Related substances Carry out the method for *thin-layer chromatography*, Appendix III A, using *silica gel G* as the coating substance and a mixture of 80 volumes of *toluene* and 20 volumes of *ethyl acetate* as the mobile phase. Apply separately to the chromatoplate 5 µl of each of two solutions in a mixture of 9 volumes of *chloroform* and 1 volume of *methanol* containing (1) 2.0% w/v of the substance being examined and (2) 0.020% w/v of *testosterone*. After removal of the plate, allow it to dry in air until the odour of solvent is no longer detectable, heat at 110° for 10 minutes and spray the hot plate with *ethanolic sulphuric acid (10%)* and heat at 110° for a further 10 minutes. Any *secondary spot* in the chromatogram obtained with solution (1) is not more intense than the spot in the chromatogram obtained with solution (2).

Loss on drying When dried to constant weight over *phosphorus pentoxide* at a pressure not exceeding 0.7 kPa, loses not more than 0.5% of its weight. Use 1 g.

Assay Dissolve 10 mg in sufficient *absolute ethanol* to produce 100 ml, dilute 5 ml to 50 ml with *absolute ethanol* and measure the *absorbance* of the resulting solution at the maximum at 241 nm, Appendix II B. Calculate the content of $C_{29}H_{46}O_3$ taking 382 as the value of A(1%, 1 cm) at the maximum at 241 nm.

Storage Testosterone Decanoate should be kept in a well-closed container, protected from light and stored at a temperature not exceeding 15°.

Action and use Androgen; anabolic steroid.

Testosterone Enanthate

$C_{26}H_{40}O_3$ 400.6   *313-37-7*

Testosterone Enanthate is 3-oxo-androst-4-en-17β-yl heptanoate. It contains not less than 97.0 per cent and not more than 103.0 per cent of $C_{26}H_4O_3$, calculated with reference to the dried substance.

Characteristics A white to creamy-white, crystalline powder.

Solubility Practically insoluble in *water*; very soluble in *ether*; freely soluble in *fixed oils*.

Identification A. The *infra-red absorption spectrum*, Appendix II A, is concordant with the *reference spectrum* of testosterone enanthate.

B. Carry out the method for *thin-layer chromatography*, Appendix III A, using a chromatoplate precoated with silica gel F254 the surface of which has been modified with chemically-bonded octadecylsilyl groups (Whatman KC18F plates are suitable) and a mixture of 60 volumes of *propan-2-ol*, 40 volumes of *acetonitrile* and 20 volumes of *water* as the mobile phase. Apply separately to the plate 5 μl of each of three solutions in a mixture of 9 volumes of *chloroform* and 1 volume of *methanol* containing (1) 0.05% w/v of the substance being examined, (2) 0.05% w/v of *testosterone enanthate BPCRS* and (3) 0.05% w/v each of *testosterone decanoate BPCRS*, *testosterone enanthate BPCRS* and *testosterone isocaproate BPCRS*. After removal of the plate, allow it to dry in air until the odour of solvent is no longer detectable and heat at 100° for 10 minutes. Allow to cool and examine under *ultra-violet light (254 nm)*. The principal spot in the chromatogram obtained with solution (1) corresponds to that in the chromatogram obtained with solution (2). Spray the plate with *ethanolic sulphuric acid (20%)*, heat at 120° for 10 minutes and allow to cool. The principal spot in the chromatogram obtained with solution (1) is green and corresponds in position and size to the spot in the chromatogram obtained with solution (2). The test is not valid unless the chromatogram obtained with solution (3) shows three distinct principal spots by both methods of visualisation.

C. To 25 mg add 2 ml of a 1% w/v solution of *potassium hydroxide* in *methanol*, heat under a reflux condenser for 1 hour, cool, add 10 ml of *water*, make acidic to *litmus paper* with 2M *hydrochloric acid*, filter and wash the precipitate with a small volume of *water*. The *melting point* of the residue, after drying at 60° at a pressure not exceeding 0.7 kPa for 3 hours, is about 152°, Appendix V A.

D. *Melting point*, about 37°, Appendix V A.

Specific optical rotation In a 1% w/v solution in *1,4-dioxan*, +77° to +82°, Appendix V F.

Free heptanoic acid Dissolve 0.5 g in 10 ml of *ethanol (96%)*, previously neutralised to *bromothymol blue solution*, and titrate immediately with 0.01M *sodium hydroxide VS* using *bromothymol blue solution* as indicator. Not more than 0.6 ml of 0.01M *sodium hydroxide VS* is required to change the colour of the solution.

Related substances Carry out the method for *thin-layer chromatography*, Appendix III A, using *silica gel G* as the coating substance and a mixture of 80 volumes of *toluene* and 20 volumes of *ethyl acetate* as the mobile phase. Apply separately to the chromatoplate 5 μl of each of two solutions in a mixture of 9 volumes of *chloroform* and 1 volume of *methanol* containing (1) 2.0% w/v of the substance being examined and (2) 0.020% w/v of *testosterone*. After removal of the plate, allow it to dry in air until the odour of solvent is no longer detectable, heat at 110° for 10 minutes and spray the hot plate with *ethanolic sulphuric acid (10%)* and heat at 110° for a further 10 minutes. Any *secondary spot* in the chromatogram obtained with solution (1) is not more intense than the spot in the chromatogram obtained with solution (2).

Loss on drying When dried to constant weight over *phosphorus pentoxide* at a pressure not exceeding 0.7 kPa, loses not more than 0.5% of its weight. Use 1 g.

Assay Dissolve 10 mg in sufficient *absolute ethanol* to produce 100 ml, dilute 5 ml to 50 ml with *absolute ethanol* and measure the *absorbance* of the resulting solution at the maximum at 241 nm, Appendix II B. Calculate the content of $C_{26}H_{40}O_3$ taking 422 as the value of A(1%, 1 cm) at the maximum at about 241 nm.

Storage Testosterone Enanthate should be kept in a well-closed container, protected from light and stored at a temperature not exceeding 15°.

Action and use Androgen; anabolic steroid.

Testosterone Isocaproate

$C_{25}H_{38}O_3$ 386.6   *15262-86-9*

Testosterone Isocaproate is 3-oxo-androst-4-en-17β-yl 4-methylpentanoate. It contains not less than 97.0 per cent and not more than 103.0 per cent of $C_{25}H_{38}O_3$, calculated with reference to the dried substance.

Characteristics White to creamy-white crystals or crystalline powder.

Solubility Practically insoluble in *water*; very soluble in *ethanol (96%)* and in *chloroform*.

Identification A. The *infra-red absorption spectrum*, Appendix II A, is concordant with the *reference spectrum* of testosterone isocaproate.

B. Carry out the method for *thin-layer chromatography*, Appendix III A, using a chromatoplate precoated with silica gel F254 the surface of which has been modified with chemically-bonded octadecylsilyl groups (Whatman KC18F plates are suitable) and a mixture of 60 volumes of *propan-2-ol*, 40 volumes of *acetonitrile* and 20 volumes of *water* as the mobile phase. Apply separately to the plate 5 μl of each of three solutions in a mixture of 9 volumes of *chloroform* and 1 volume of *methanol* containing (1) 0.05% w/v of the substance being examined, (2) 0.05% w/v of *testosterone isocaporate BPCRS* and (3) 0.05% w/v each of *testosterone decanoate BPCRS*, *testosterone enanthate BPCRS* and *testosterone isocaproate BPCRS*. After removal of the plate, allow it to dry in air until the odour of solvent is no longer detectable and heat at 100° for 10 minutes. Allow to cool and examine under *ultra-violet light (254 nm)*. The principal spot in the chromatogram obtained with solution (1) corresponds to that in the chromatogram obtained with solution (2). Spray the plate with *ethanolic sulphuric acid (20%)*, heat at 120° for 10 minutes and allow to cool. The principal spot in the chromatogram obtained with solution (1) is green and corresponds in position and size to the spot in the chromatogram obtained with solution (2). The test is not valid unless the chromatogram obtained with solution (3) shows three distinct principal spots by both methods of visualisation.

C. To 25 mg add 2 ml of a 1% w/v solution of *potassium hydroxide* in *methanol*, heat under a reflux condenser for 1 hour, cool, add 10 ml of *water*, make acidic to *litmus paper* with 2M *hydrochloric acid*, filter and wash the precipitate with a small volume of *water*. The *melting point* of the residue, Appendix V A, after drying at 60° at a pressure not exceeding 0.7 kPa for 3 hours, is about 152°.

D. *Melting point*, about 80°, Appendix V A.

Specific optical rotation In a 1% w/v solution in *1,4-dioxan*, +79° to +83°, Appendix V F.

Related substances Carry out the method for *thin-layer chromatography*, Appendix III A, using *silica gel G* as the coating substance and a mixture of 80 volumes of *toluene* and 20 volumes of *ethyl acetate* as the mobile phase. Apply separately to the chromatoplate 5 μl of each of two solutions in a mixture of 9 volumes of *chloroform* and 1 volume of *methanol* containing (1) 2.0% w/v of the substance being examined and (2) 0.020% w/v of *testosterone*. After removal of the plate, allow it to dry in air until the odour of solvent is no longer detectable, heat at 110° for 10 minutes and spray the hot plate with *ethanolic sulphuric acid (10%)* and heat at 110° for a further 10 minutes. Any *secondary spot* in the chromatogram obtained with solution (1) is not more intense than the spot in the chromatogram obtained with solution (2).

Loss on drying When dried to constant weight over *phosphorus pentoxide* at a pressure not exceeding 0.7 kPa, loses not more than 0.5% of its weight. Use 1 g.

Assay Dissolve 10 mg in sufficient *absolute ethanol* to produce 100 ml, dilute 5 ml to 50 ml with *absolute ethanol* and measure the *absorbance* of the resulting solution at the maximum at 241 nm, Appendix II B. Calculate the content of $C_{25}H_{38}O_3$ taking 439 as the value of A(1%, 1 cm) at the maximum at 241 nm.

Storage Testosterone Isocaproate should be kept in a well-closed container, protected from light and stored at a temperature not exceeding 15°.

Action and use Androgen; anabolic steroid.

Testosterone Propionate ☆

$C_{22}H_{32}O_3$ 344.5   57-85-2

Testosterone Propionate is 3-oxo-androst-4-en-17β-yl propionate. It contains not less than 97.0 per cent and not more than 103.0 per cent of $C_{22}H_{32}O_3$, calculated with reference to the dried substance.

Characteristics A white or almost white powder or colourless crystals.

Solubility Practically insoluble in *water*; soluble in 6 parts of *ethanol* (96%) and in 4 parts of *acetone*; very soluble in *chloroform*; freely soluble in *methanol* and in fixed oils.

Identification *Test A may be omitted if tests B and C are carried out. Tests B and C may be omitted if test A is carried out.*

A. The *infra-red absorption spectrum*, Appendix II A, is concordant with the spectrum of *testosterone propionate EPCRS*.

B. Examine the chromatograms obtained in the test for Related substances under *ultra-violet light (254 nm)*. The principal spots in the chromatograms obtained with solutions (2) and (3) correspond to the principal spots in the chromatograms obtained with solutions (5) and (6) respectively. Spray the plate with *ethanolic sulphuric acid (20%)*, heat at 120° for 15 minutes and allow to cool. Examine in daylight and under *ultra-violet light (365 nm)*. The principal spots in the chromatograms obtained with solutions (2) and (3) are similar in colour in daylight, fluorescence under ultra-violet light (365 nm), position and size to the principal spots in the chromatograms obtained with solutions (5) and (6) respectively. The Rf values of the principal spots in the chromatograms obtained with solutions (2) and (5) are distinctly lower than those of the principal spots in the chromatograms obtained with solutions (3) and (6) respectively.

C. *Melting point*, 119° to 123°, Appendix V A, Method I.

Specific optical rotation In a 1% w/v solution in *absolute ethanol*, +83° to +90°, Appendix V F.

Related substances Carry out the method for *thin-layer chromatography*, Appendix III A, using as the coating substance a suitable silica gel containing a fluorescent indicator with an optimal intensity at 254 nm (Merck silica gel 60 F254 is suitable) and a mixture of 70 volumes of *butyl acetate*, 30 volumes of *petroleum spirit (boiling point, 60° to 80°)* and 1 volume of *anhydrous glacial acetic acid* as the mobile phase. Apply separately to the chromatoplate 5 μl of each of solutions (2), (3), (5) and (6) and 2 μl of each of solutions (1), (4), (7) and (8). Solution (1) contains 5.0% w/v of the substance being examined in *chloroform*. For solution (2) dissolve 50 mg of the substance being examined in 6 ml of *methanol* and add 2 ml of 1M *sodium hydroxide*; place a small funnel in the neck of the flask to act as a condenser and heat on a water-bath for 5 minutes; cool under running water, add 2.0 ml of 1M *hydrochloric acid* and dilute to 25 ml with *methanol*. Solutions (3) and (4) contain 0.2% w/v and 0.5% w/v respectively of the substance being examined in *chloroform*. Prepare solution (5) as for solution (2), but using 50 mg of *testosterone propionate EPCRS* in place of the substance being examined. Solution (6) contains 0.2% w/v of *testosterone propionate EPCRS* in *chloroform*. Solution (7) contains 0.1% w/v of *testosterone acetate EPCRS* in *chloroform*. For solution (8) add 1.0 ml of solution (1) to 5.0 ml of solution (7) and dilute to 15.0 ml with *chloroform*. After removal of the plate, allow it to dry in air and examine under *ultra-violet light (254 nm)*. Any spot corresponding to testosterone acetate in the chromatogram obtained with solution (1) is not more intense than the spot in the chromatogram obtained with solution (7). Any other *secondary spot* in the chromatogram obtained with solution (1) is not more intense than the spot in the chromatogram obtained with solution (4). The test is not valid unless the chromatogram obtained with solution (8) shows two clearly separated principal spots.

Loss on drying When dried at 100° to 105° for 2 hours, loses not more than 0.5% of its weight. Use 0.5 g.

Assay Dissolve 25 mg in sufficient *absolute ethanol* to produce 250 ml, dilute 10 ml to 100 ml with the same solvent and measure the *absorbance* of the resulting solution at the maximum at 241 nm, Appendix II B.

Calculate the content of $C_{22}H_{32}O_3$ taking 490 as the value of $A(1\%, 1 \text{ cm})$ at the maximum at 241 nm.

Storage Testosterone Propionate should be kept in a well-closed container and protected from light.

Preparation

Testosterone Propionate Injection

Action and use Androgen; anabolic steroid.

Tetrachloroethylene

Perchloroethylene

$Cl_2C{=}CCl_2$

C_2Cl_4 165.8   *127-18-4*

Tetrachloroethylene contains 0.01 per cent w/w of Thymol.

Characteristics A colourless, mobile liquid; odour, characteristic.

Solubility Practically insoluble in *water*; soluble in *ethanol (96%)*; miscible with *ether* and with oils.

Identification Transfer 5 ml to a stoppered cylinder, add 5 ml of *bromine water* and shake vigorously at intervals of 15 minutes for 1 hour. The aqueous layer is decolorised and a white turbidity is produced in the lower layer (distinction from chloroform and from carbon tetrachloride).

Acidity or alkalinity To 100 ml of *carbon dioxide-free water* in a stoppered flask add 0.15 ml of *bromocresol purple solution* and, if necessary, neutralise by the dropwise addition of 0.1M *sodium hydroxide VS* or 0.1M *hydrochloric acid VS*. Transfer 50 ml of the neutralised water to another stoppered flask, add 100 ml of the substance being examined and shake well. The aqueous layer is not more acidic than the neutralised water. If it is more alkaline, titrate the mixed liquids with 0.1M *hydrochloric acid VS*, added dropwise near the end-point and shaking after each addition, until the colour of the aqueous layer matches that of the neutralised water. Not more than 0.6 ml of 0.1M *hydrochloric acid VS* is required.

Distillation range Distils completely between 119° and 122°, not less than 95% v/v distilling within a range of 1.5°, Appendix V C.

Weight per ml 1.620 to 1.626 g, Appendix V G.

Chloride Shake 10 ml with 20 ml of *carbon dioxide-free water* for 3 minutes and allow to separate. Reserve 10 ml of the aqueous layer for the test for Free chlorine. To 5 ml of the aqueous layer add 5 ml of *water*, 0.05 ml of *nitric acid* and 0.2 ml of *silver nitrate solution*. The solution is *clear*, Appendix IV A.

Acetylenic compounds To 5 ml contained in a stoppered cylinder add 1 ml of *ammoniacal copper nitrate solution* and 5 ml of *absolute ethanol*, mix, add 0.1 g of *hydroxylamine hydrochloride*, shake gently and allow to stand in the dark for 15 minutes. No orange-red colour is produced.

Free chlorine To 10 ml of the aqueous layer reserved in the test for Chloride add 1 ml of a 5% w/v solution of *cadmium iodide* and 0.1 ml of *starch mucilage*. No blue colour is produced.

Phosgene Place 50 ml in a dry 350-ml bottle, suspend a strip of *phosgene test paper* vertically inside the bottle with the lower end about 1 cm above the surface of the liquid, insert the stopper and allow to stand in the dark for 16 hours. The test paper is not yellow.

Thymol Use three dry 25-ml stoppered cylinders. In cylinder (1) place 0.5 ml of the substance being examined, in cylinder (2) place 0.5 ml of a 0.0193% w/v solution of *thymol* in *carbon tetrachloride* and in cylinder (3) place 0.5 ml of a 0.01287% w/v solution of *thymol* in *carbon tetrachloride*. To each cylinder add 5 ml of *carbon tetrachloride* and 5.0 ml of *titanium dioxide solution*, shake vigorously for 30 seconds and allow to separate. The intensity of the yellowish-brown colour of the lower layer in cylinder (1) is between those of the corresponding layers in cylinders (2) and (3) (0.008 to 0.012% w/w of thymol).

Non-volatile matter When evaporated on a water-bath and dried at 105° for 2 hours, leaves not more than 0.002% w/v of residue.

Storage Tetrachloroethylene should be kept in a well-closed container and protected from light.

Action and use Anthelmintic.

Tetracosactrin

Ser—Tyr—Ser—Met—Glu—His—Phe—Arg—Trp—Gly—Lys—Pro—
Val—Gly—Lys—Lys—Arg—Arg—Pro—Val—Lys—Val—Tyr—Pro

$C_{136}H_{210}N_{40}O_{31}S$ 2933   *16960-16-0*

Tetracosactrin is a tetracosapeptide that increases the rate at which corticoid hormones are secreted by the adrenal gland. Its amino acid sequence is the same as that of the first twenty-four residues of human corticotrophin. It contains not less than 800 Units per mg, calculated with reference to the anhydrous and acetic acid-free substance. It is available in the acetate form.

Characteristics A white to yellow, amorphous powder.

Solubility Soluble in 70 parts of *water*.

Identification A. Stimulates the production of corticosterone by isolated rat adrenal cells when administered as directed in the Assay.

B. Dissolve 1 mg in 0.2 ml of a 1.54% w/v solution of *ammonium acetate* adjusted to pH 8.2 with 1M *ammonia*. Add 10 µl of a 0.2% w/v solution of *trypsin*, maintain the mixture at 37° to 38° for 40 minutes, heat in a water-bath for 3 minutes and add 5 µl of *glacial acetic acid*. Evaporate to dryness at 40° at a pressure not exceeding 2.7 kPa, dry the glassy residue at 40° for 1 hour and dissolve in 0.1 ml of *glacial acetic acid*. Freeze dry the solution, dissolve the residue in 0.1 ml of *water* and again freeze dry. Dry the final residue at 45° at a pressure not exceeding 2.7 kPa for 1 hour and dissolve in 50 µl of *water* [solution (1)]. At the same time, carry out the operation described above using 1 mg of *tetracosactrin BPCRS* [solution (2)].

Using electrophoresis and thin-layer chromatography, perform a two-dimensional separation on each of two chromatoplates (200 mm × 200 mm) coated with a thin layer of *microcrystalline cellulose* by the following procedures. Spray the plates with a buffer solution containing 0.2% v/v of *glacial acetic acid* and 0.2% v/v of *pyridine*. Adjust the filter paper tongues connecting the plate with the appropriate compartment of each trough to cover an area 1.5 cm wide at each end of the plates, close the tank and allow to stand for 30 minutes. Apply to the first plate, at a point about 2.5 cm from two adjacent edges, 4 µl of solution (1). Apply to the second plate, in a similar position, 4 µl of solution (2). Subject both plates to electrophoresis at 280 volts for 90 minutes. After removal of the plates, dry them in air for 30 minutes and in a current of air at 30° for a further 30 minutes. Carry out a second development on each plate, at right angles to the direction of electrophoresis, by ascending chromatography, using a mixture of 38 volumes of *butan-1-ol*, 30 volumes of *water*, 24 volumes of *pyridine* and 8 volumes of *glacial acetic acid* as the mobile phase. After removal of the plates, dry them in a current of air and spray with *cadmium and ninhydrin solution*. The principal spots in the chromatogram obtained with solution (1) correspond to those in the chromatogram obtained with solution (2). The overall position of the spots should be similar in each chromatogram but the intensity of the spots may vary.

Light absorption *Absorbance* of a 0.02% w/v solution in 0.1M *hydrochloric acid* at the maximum at 276 nm, 0.51 to 0.61, calculated with reference to the anhydrous and acetic acid-free substance, Appendix II B. The ratio of the *absorbance* at 276 nm to that at 248 nm is 2.4 to 2.9.

Specific optical rotation In a 1% w/v solution containing 1% v/v of *glacial acetic acid*, $-99°$ to $-109°$, Appendix V F, calculated with reference to the anhydrous and acetic acid-free substance.

Acetic acid 8 to 13% w/w when determined by the method for *gas chromatography*, Appendix III B, using solutions in *water* containing (1) 0.1% w/v of *glacial acetic acid* and 0.1% v/v of *1,4-dioxan* (internal standard), (2) 1.0% w/v of the substance being examined and (3) 1.0% w/v of the substance being examined and 0.1% v/v of the internal standard.

The chromatographic procedure may be carried out using a glass column (2 m × 2 mm) packed with porous polymer beads (100 to 120 mesh) (Porapak Q is suitable) and maintained at 150°.

Amino acids Carry out the method for *amino acid analysis*, Appendix III G, using 4.6 mg. Use 0.03% w/v of DL-*norleucine* (internal standard) and heat for 24 hours. Express the content of each amino acid in moles and calculate the relative proportions of the amino acids taking that for valine to be equivalent to 3. The values are within the following limits: lysine, 3.5 to 4.7; histidine, 0.9 to 1.1; arginine, 2.7 to 3.3; serine, 1.1 to 2.2; glutamic acid, 0.9 to 1.1; proline, 2.5 to 3.5; glycine, 1.8 to 2.2; methionine, 0.9 to 1.1; tyrosine, 1.7 to 2.2; phenylalanine, 0.9 to 1.1. Not more than traces of other amino acids are present in the hydrolysate.

Peptide Not less than 85.0% of the peptide $C_{136}H_{210}N_{40}O_{31}S$, calculated with reference to the anhydrous and acetic acid-free substance, when determined by the following method. Carry out the method for *high-performance liquid chromatography*, Appendix III D, using two solutions in *water* containing (1) 0.1% w/v of the substance being examined and (2) 0.1% w/v of *tetracosactrin BPCRS*.

The chromatographic procedure may be carried out using (a) a stainless steel column (20 cm × 4.6 mm) packed with *stationary phase C* (10 µm) (Nucleosil C18 is suitable), (b) a mixture of 365 ml of *acetonitrile*, 10 ml of *glacial acetic acid* and 10 g of *ammonium sulphate* diluted to 2000 ml with water as the mobile phase with a flow rate of 2 ml per minute and (c) a detection wavelength of 254 nm.

Calculate the content of the peptide $C_{136}H_{210}N_{40}O_{31}S$ using the declared content of $C_{136}H_{210}N_{40}O_{31}S$ in *tetracosactrin BPCRS*.

The result obtained is not valid unless the *resolution factor* between the peaks due to tetracosactrin and tetracosactrin sulphoxide in the chromatogram obtained with solution (2) in test A for Related peptides is not less than 7.

Related peptides A. *Tetracosactrin sulphoxide* Carry out the method for *high-performance liquid chromatography*, Appendix III D, using the following solutions. Solution (1) contains 0.1% w/v of the substance being examined in *water*. For solution (2) add 50 µl of a solution prepared by diluting 1 volume of *hydrogen peroxide solution (20 vol)* to 200 volumes with *water* to 1 ml of a 0.1% w/v solution of the substance being examined in a 1% v/v solution of *glacial acetic acid* and allow to stand for 2 hours.

The chromatographic conditions described in the test for Peptide may be used.

The chromatogram obtained with solution (2) exhibits a peak due to tetracosactrin corresponding to the principal peak in the chromatogram obtained with solution (1) and a peak with shorter retention time, due to tetracosactrin sulphoxide, of significantly greater area than the corresponding peak in the chromatogram obtained with solution (1). In the chromatogram obtained with solution (1) the relative amount of tetracosactrin sulphoxide, by *normalisation*, is not more than 4%.

B. *Other related peptides* Carry out the method for *thin-layer chromatography*, Appendix III A, using *cellulose* as the coating substance and a mixture of 42 volumes of *butan-1-ol*, 30 volumes of *water*, 24 volumes of *pyridine* and 4 volumes of *glacial acetic acid* as the mobile phase. Apply separately to the chromatoplate, as bands about 1 cm wide, 10 µl of each of three solutions of the substance being examined in 1M *acetic acid* containing (1) 0.20% w/v, (2) 0.010% w/v and (3) 0.0050% w/v. As a fourth band, about 1 cm wide, apply 10 µl of a solution prepared in the following manner. To 0.5 ml of a 0.20% w/v solution of the substance being examined in 1M *acetic acid* add 50 µl of a solution prepared by diluting 1 volume of *hydrogen peroxide solution (20 vol)* to 200 volumes with *water* and allow to stand for 2 hours [solution (4)].

After removal of the plate, dry it in a current of air, and spray with *cadmium and ninhydrin solution*. The chromatogram obtained with solution (4) exhibits a band corresponding in position to, but less intense than, the principal band in the chromatogram obtained with solution (1) and a prominent band of lower Rf value, attributable to tetracosactrin sulphoxide. In the chromatogram obtained with solution (1) any *secondary band* other than that corresponding to tetracosactin sulphoxide is not more intense than the band in the chromatogram obtained with solution (2) and not more than one such band is more intense than the band in the chromatogram obtained with solution (3).

Water 5 to 16% w/w, Appendix IX C. Use 0.8 mg.

Assay Carry out the *biological assay of tetracosactrin*, Appendix XIV C8. The estimated potency is not less than 80% and not more than 125% of the stated potency. The fiducial limits of error are not less than 64% and not more than 156% of the stated potency.

Storage Tetracosactrin should be kept under an atmosphere of nitrogen, protected from light and stored at a temperature of 2° to 8°.

Labelling The label states (1) the number of Units per mg; (2) the weight of the peptide in the container; (3) the date after which the material is not intended to be used; (4) the conditions under which it should be stored.

Preparations

Tetracosactrin Injection

Tetracosactrin Zinc Injection

Action and use Corticotrophic peptide.

In some countries the material described in this monograph may be known as Tetracosactide.

Tetracycline ☆

$C_{22}H_{24}N_2O_8$ 444.4   60-54-8

Tetracycline is (4S,4aS,5aS,6S,12aS)-4-dimethylamino-1,4,4a,5,5a,6,11,12a-octahydro-3,6,10,12,12a-pentahydroxy-6-methyl-1,11-dioxonaphthacene-2-carboxamide. It contains a variable quantity of water. The potency is not less than 1000 Units per mg, calculated with reference to the dried substance.

Characteristics A yellow, crystalline powder; odourless.

Solubility Very slightly soluble in *water*; soluble in *ethanol (96%)* and in *methanol*; sparingly soluble in *acetone*; slightly soluble in *chloroform*; practically insoluble in *ether*. It dissolves in dilute acid and alkaline solutions.

Identification A. Complies with the test for *identification of tetracyclines*, Appendix III A, using the following solutions. Solution (1) contains 0.05% w/v each of the substance being examined, *chlortetracycline hydrochloride EPCRS*, *demeclocycline hydrochloride EPCRS*, *doxycycline hyclate EPCRS* and *oxytetracycline hydrochloride EPCRS*. Solution (2) contains 0.05% w/v each of *chlortetracycline hydrochloride EPCRS*, *demeclocycline hydrochloride EPCRS*, *doxycycline hyclate EPCRS* and *oxytetracycline hydrochloride EPCRS*.

B. To 2 mg add 5 ml of *sulphuric acid*; a reddish-violet colour is produced. Add the solution to 2.5 ml of *water*; the colour changes to yellow.

C. Dissolve 10 mg in a mixture of 1 ml of 2M *nitric acid* and 5 ml of *water*, shake and add 1 ml of a 1.7% w/v solution of *silver nitrate*. Any opalescence produced is not more intense than that in a solution prepared in the same manner but omitting the substance being examined.

Acidity pH of a 1% w/v suspension, 3.5 to 6.0, Appendix V L.

Light absorption Dissolve 10 mg in 10 ml of 0.1M *hydrochloric acid* and dilute to 100 ml with *water*. To 10 ml of the resulting solution add 75 ml of *water*, 12 ml of 2M *sodium hydroxide* and sufficient *water* to produce 100 ml. The A(1%, 1 cm) at 380 nm, when determined exactly 6 minutes after the addition of the sodium hydroxide solution, is 390 to 420, Appendix II B.

Specific optical rotation In a 0.5% w/v solution in 0.1M *hydrochloric acid*, −260° to −280°, Appendix V F.

Heavy metals 0.5 g complies with *limit test C for heavy metals*, Appendix VII (50 ppm). Use 2.5 ml of *lead standard solution (10 ppm Pb)* to prepare the standard.

Light-absorbing impurities Dissolve 50 mg in 2.5 ml of 0.1M *hydrochloric acid* and dilute to 25 ml with *water*. The absorbance at 430 nm, measured within 1 hour of preparing the solution, is not more than 0.54, Appendix II B.

Related substances Carry out in subdued light the method for *thin-layer chromatography* using the mobile phase and the chromatoplate prepared as described under the test for *identification of tetracyclines*, Appendix III A, but using 0.1M *disodium edetate* previously adjusted to pH 7.0 by the addition of 2M *sodium hydroxide* in place of the citro-phosphate buffer. Apply separately to the plate 1 μl of each of seven solutions in 0.01M *methanolic hydrochloric acid* containing (1) 1% w/v of the substance being examined, (2) 0.25% w/v of the substance being examined, (3) 0.005% w/v of *4-epianhydrotetracycline hydrochloride EPCRS*, (4) 0.0125% w/v of *4-epitetracycline hydrochloride EPCRS*, (5) 0.005% w/v of *anhydrotetracycline hydrochloride EPCRS*, (6) 0.02% w/v of *chlortetracycline hydrochloride EPCRS* and (7) 0.01% w/v of *tetracycline hydrochloride EPCRS*, 0.005% w/v of *4-epi-anhydrotetracycline hydrochloride EPCRS*, 0.0125% w/v of *4-epitetracycline hydrochloride EPCRS*, 0.005% w/v of *anhydrotetracycline hydrochloride EPCRS* and 0.02% w/v of *chlortetracycline hydrochloride EPCRS*. Spray the plate very finely and evenly with a 5% w/v solution of *2,4,6-collidine*, freshly prepared at 5°, until traces of moisture appear (about 8 ml for a 200 mm × 200 mm plate) and if necessary allow to dry at room temperature before allowing the chromatography to proceed. After removal of the plate, allow it to dry in air, expose it to ammonia vapour and examine immediately under *ultra-violet light (365 nm)*; the lamp and the conditions of visualisation used in the test should be sufficient to reveal the spots due to the reference substances.

In the chromatogram obtained with solution (1) any spots corresponding to 4-epianhydrotetracycline hydrochloride, anhydrotetracycline hydrochloride and chlortetracycline hydrochloride are not more intense than the principal spots in the chromatograms obtained with solutions (3), (5) and (6) respectively. In the chromatogram obtained with solution (2) any spot corresponding to 4-epitetracycline hydrochloride is not more intense than the principal spot obtained with solution (4). The test is not valid unless the chromatogram obtained with solution (7) shows five clearly separated principal spots.

Loss on drying When dried to constant weight at 100° to 105°, loses not more than 13.0% of its weight. Use 1 g.

Sulphated ash Not more than 0.5%, Appendix IX A, Method II. Use 1 g.

Assay Carry out the *biological assay of antibiotics*, Appendix XIV A, using a solution of the substance being examined in 0.01M *hydrochloric acid*. The precision of the assay is such that the fiducial limits of error are not less than 95% and not more than 105% of the estimated potency.

Storage Tetracycline should be kept in a well-closed container and protected from light.

Labelling The label states (1) the date after which the material is not intended to be used; (2) the conditions under which it should be stored.

Preparation
Tetracycline Oral Suspension

Action and use Antibacterial.

Tetracycline Hydrochloride ☆

C₂₂H₂₄N₂O₈,HCl   480.9   *64-75-5*

Tetracycline Hydrochloride is (4*S*,4a*S*,5a*S*,6*S*, 12a*S*)-4-dimethylamino-1,4,4a,5,5a,6,11,12a-octahydro-3,6,10,12,12a-pentahydroxy-6-methyl-1,11-dioxonaphthacene-2-carboxamide hydrochloride. The potency is not less than 950 Units per mg, calculated with reference to the dried substance.

Characteristics A yellow, crystalline powder; odourless.

Solubility Soluble in 10 parts of *water* and in 100 parts of *ethanol (96%)*; practically insoluble in *acetone*, in *chloroform* and in *ether*. It dissolves in aqueous solutions of alkali hydroxides and carbonates. Solutions in *water* become turbid on standing due to the precipitation of tetracycline.

Identification A. Complies with the test for *identification of tetracyclines*, Appendix III A, using the following solutions. Solution (1) contains 0.05% w/v each of the substance being examined, *chlortetracycline hydrochloride EPCRS*, *demeclocycline hydrochloride EPCRS*, *doxycycline hyclate EPCRS* and *oxytetracycline hydrochloride EPCRS*. Solution (2) contains 0.05% w/v each of *chlortetracycline hydrochloride EPCRS*, *demeclocycline hydrochloride EPCRS*, *doxycycline hyclate EPCRS* and *oxytetracycline hydrochloride EPCRS*.
B. To 2 mg add 5 ml of *sulphuric acid*; a reddish-violet colour is produced. Add the solution to 2.5 ml of *water*; the colour changes to yellow.
C. Yields *reaction A* characteristic of chlorides, Appendix VI.

Acidity pH of a 1% w/v solution, 1.8 to 2.8, Appendix V L.

Light absorption Dissolve 10 mg in sufficient 0.01M *hydrochloric acid* to produce 100 ml. To 10 ml of the solution add 75 ml of *water*, 12 ml of 2M *sodium hydroxide* and sufficient *water* to produce 100 ml and mix immediately. The A(1%, 1 cm) at 380 nm, when determined exactly 6 minutes after the addition of the sodium hydroxide solution, is 360 to 390, Appendix II B.

Specific optical rotation In a 1% w/v solution in 0.1M *hydrochloric acid*, −240° to −255°, Appendix V F.

Heavy metals 0.5 g complies with *limit test C for heavy metals*, Appendix VII (50 ppm). Use 2.5 ml of *lead standard solution (10 ppm Pb)* to prepare the standard.

Light-absorbing impurities Dissolve 20 mg in sufficient 0.01M *hydrochloric acid* to produce 10 ml. The *absorbance* at 430 nm, when measured within 1 hour of preparing the solution, is not more than 0.50, Appendix II B.

Related substances Carry out in subdued light the method for *thin-layer chromatography* using the mobile phase and the chromatoplate prepared as described under

the test for *identification of tetracyclines*, Appendix III A, but using 0.1M *disodium edetate* previously adjusted to pH 7.0 by the addition of 2M *sodium hydroxide* in place of the citro-phosphate buffer. Apply separately to the plate 1 μl of each of seven solutions in 0.01M *methanolic hydrochloric acid* containing (1) 1% w/v of the substance being examined, (2) 0.25% w/v of the substance being examined, (3) 0.005% w/v of *4-epianhydrotetracycline hydrochloride EPCRS*, (4) 0.0125% w/v of *4-epitetracycline hydrochloride EPCRS*, (5) 0.005% w/v of *anhydrotetracycline hydrochloride EPCRS*, (6) 0.02% w/v of *chlortetracycline hydrochloride EPCRS* and (7) 0.01% w/v of *tetracycline hydrochloride EPCRS*, 0.005% w/v of *4-epi-anhydrotetracycline hydrochloride EPCRS*, 0.0125% w/v of *4-epitetracycline hydrochloride EPCRS*, 0.005% w/v of *anhydrotetracycline hydrochloride EPCRS* and 0.02% w/v of *chlortetracycline hydrochloride EPCRS*. Spray the plate very finely and evenly with a 5% w/v solution of *2,4,6-collidine*, freshly prepared at 5°, until traces of moisture appear (about 8 ml for a 200 mm × 200 mm plate) and if necessary allow to dry at room temperature before allowing the chromatography to proceed. After removal of the plate, allow it to dry in air, expose it to ammonia vapour and examine immediately under *ultra-violet light (365 nm)*; the lamp and the conditions of visualisation used in the test should be sufficient to reveal the spots due to the reference substances.

In the chromatogram obtained with solution (1) any spots corresponding to 4-epianhydrotetracycline hydrochloride, anhydrotetracycline hydrochloride and chlortetracycline hydrochloride are not more intense than the principal spots in the chromatograms obtained with solutions (3), (5) and (6), respectively. In the chromatogram obtained with solution (2) any spot corresponding to 4-epitetracycline hydrochloride is not more intense than the principal spot obtained with solution (4). The test is not valid unless the chromatogram obtained with solution (7) shows five clearly separated principal spots.

Loss on drying When dried over *phosphorus pentoxide* at 60° at a pressure not exceeding 0.7 kPa for 3 hours, loses not more than 2.0% of its weight. Use 1 g.

Sulphated ash Not more than 0.5%, Appendix IX A, Method II. Use 1 g.

Assay Carry out the *biological assay of antibiotics*, Appendix XIV A. The precision of the assay is such that the fiducial limits of error are not less than 95% and not more than 105% of the estimated potency.

Storage Tetracycline Hydrochloride should be kept in a well-closed container and protected from light. If the material is intended for use in the manufacture of a parenteral dosage form the container should be sterile, tamper-evident and sealed so as to exclude micro-organisms.

Labelling The label states (1) the date after which the material is not intended to be used; (2) the conditions under which it should be stored; (3) whether or not it is intended for use in the manufacture of a parenteral dosage form.

Preparations
Tetracycline Capsules
Tetracycline Intravenous Infusion
Tetracycline Tablets

Action and use Antibacterial.

Tetracycline Hydrochloride intended for use in the manufacture of a parenteral dosage form complies with the following additional requirements.

Pyrogens Complies with the *test for pyrogens*, Appendix XIV K. Use per kg of the rabbit's weight 1 ml of *water for injections* containing 5 mg per ml.

Sterility Complies with the *test for sterility*, Appendix XVI A.

Theobroma Oil

Cocoa Butter

Theobroma Oil is the solid fat obtained from the roasted seeds of *Theobroma cacao* L.

Characteristics A yellowish-white, solid fat; odour, slight, agreeable and resembling that of cocoa. Somewhat brittle.

Solubility Slightly soluble in *ethanol (96%)*; freely soluble in *chloroform*, in *ether* and in *petroleum spirit (boiling range, 40° to 60°)*.

Acid value Not more than 4.0, Appendix X B.

Iodine value 35 to 40 (*iodine monochloride method*), Appendix X E.

Melting point 31° to 34°, Appendix V A, Method IV.

Refractive index At 40°, 1.456 to 1.458, Appendix V E.

Saponification value 188 to 196, Appendix X G.

Storage Theobroma Oil should be stored at a temperature not exceeding 25°.

Action and use Suppository basis.

Theobromine ☆

$C_7H_8N_4O_2$ 180.2 *83-67-0*

Theobromine is 3,7-dimethylpurine-2,6($3H$,$1H$)-dione. It contains not less than 99.0 per cent and not more than 101.0 per cent of $C_7H_8N_4O_2$, calculated with reference to the dried substance.

Characteristics A white powder; odourless.

Solubility Very slightly soluble in *water*, in *ethanol (96%)* and in *chloroform*; practically insoluble in *ether*; slightly soluble in aqueous ammonia. It dissolves in dilute solutions of alkali hydroxides and in mineral acids.

Identification *Test A may be omitted if tests B and C are carried out. Test B may be omitted if tests A and C are carried out.*

A. The *infra-red absorption spectrum*, Appendix II A, is concordant with the spectrum of *theobromine EPCRS*.

B. Dissolve 20 mg in 2 ml of *6M ammonia* with gentle warming and cool. Add 2 ml of *0.1M silver nitrate*; the solution remains clear. Boil the solution for a few minutes; a white, crystalline precipitate is produced.

C. Yields the *reaction* characteristic of xanthines, Appendix VI.

Acidity To 0.4 g add 20 ml of *water*, heat to boiling for 1 minute, cool, filter and add 0.05 ml of *bromothymol blue*

solution. The solution is yellow or yellowish-green and not more than 0.2 ml of *0.01M sodium hydroxide VS* is required to change the colour to blue.

Heavy metals 1.0 g complies with *limit test C for heavy metals*, Appendix VII (20 ppm). Use 2 ml of *lead standard solution (10 ppm Pb)* to prepare the standard.

Related substances Carry out the method for *thin-layer chromatography*, Appendix III A, using *silica gel GF254* as the coating substance and a mixture of 40 volumes of *butan-1-ol*, 30 volumes of *acetone*, 30 volumes of *chloroform* and 10 volumes of *13.5M ammonia* as the mobile phase. Apply separately to the chromatoplate 10 μl of each of the following solutions. For solution (1) add 10 ml of a mixture of 6 volumes of *chloroform* and 4 volumes of *methanol* to 0.2 g of the finely powdered substance being examined, heat on a water-bath under a reflux condenser for 15 minutes, shaking occasionally, allow to cool and filter. Solution (2) contains 0.01% w/v of *theobromine EPCRS* in a mixture of 6 volumes of *chloroform* and 4 volumes of *methanol*. After removal of the plate, allow it to dry in air and examine under *ultra-violet light (254 nm)*. Any *secondary spot* in the chromatogram obtained with solution (1) is not more intense than the spot in the chromatogram obtained with solution (2).

Loss on drying When dried to constant weight at 100° to 105°, loses not more than 0.5% of its weight. Use 1 g.

Sulphated ash Not more than 0.1%, Appendix IX A, Method II. Use 1 g.

Assay Dissolve 0.15 g in 125 ml of boiling *water*, cool to about 55° and add 25 ml of *0.1M silver nitrate*. Titrate with *0.1M sodium hydroxide VS* using 1 ml of *dilute phenolphthalein solution* as indicator. Each ml of *0.1M sodium hydroxide VS* is equivalent to 0.01802 g of $C_7H_8N_4O_2$.

Theophylline ☆

$C_7H_8N_4O_2$ 180.2 *58-55-9*

Theophylline is 1,3-dimethylpurine-2,6($3H$,$1H$)-dione. It contains not less than 99.0 per cent and not more than 101.0 per cent of $C_7H_8N_4O_2$, calculated with reference to the dried substance.

Characteristics A white, crystalline powder; odourless.

Solubility Slightly soluble in *water* and in *chloroform*; soluble in 80 parts of *ethanol (96%)*; very slightly soluble in *ether*. It dissolves in solutions of alkali hydroxides, in aqueous ammonia and in mineral acids.

Identification *Test A may be omitted if tests B, C, D and E are carried out. Tests B and D may be omitted if tests A, C and E are carried out.*

A. The *infra-red absorption spectrum*, Appendix II A, is concordant with the spectrum of *theophylline EPCRS*.

B. Dissolve 10 mg in 10 ml of *water*, add 0.5 ml of a 5% w/v solution of *mercury(II) acetate* and allow to stand. A white, crystalline precipitate is produced.

C. Complies with the test for Loss on drying.
D. Yields the *reaction* characteristic of xanthines, Appendix VI.
E. The *melting point*, after drying at 100° to 105°, is 270° to 274°, Appendix V A, Method I.

Acidity Dissolve 0.5 g in *carbon dioxide-free water* with heating, allow to cool and dilute to 75 ml with the same solvent (solution A). To 50 ml of solution A add 0.1 ml of *methyl red solution*. The solution is red and not more than 1.0 ml of 0.01M *sodium hydroxide VS* is required to change the colour of the solution to yellow.

Clarity and colour of solution Solution A is *clear*, Appendix IV A, and *colourless*, Appendix IV B, Method II.

Heavy metals 1.0 g complies with *limit test C for heavy metals*, Appendix VII (20 ppm). Use 2 ml of *lead standard solution (10 ppm Pb)* to prepare the standard.

Related substances Carry out the method for *thin-layer chromatography*, Appendix III A, using *silica gel GF254* as the coating substance and a mixture of 40 volumes of *butan-1-ol*, 30 volumes of *acetone*, 30 volumes of *chloroform* and 10 volumes of 13.5M *ammonia* as the mobile phase. Apply separately to the chromatoplate 10 μl of each of two solutions of the substance being examined in a mixture of 6 volumes of *chloroform* and 4 volumes of *methanol* containing (1) 2% w/v and (2) 0.01% w/v. After removal of the plate, allow it to dry in air and examine under *ultra-violet light (254 nm)*. Any *secondary spot* in the chromatogram obtained with solution (1) is not more intense than the spot in the chromatogram obtained with solution (2).

Loss on drying When dried to constant weight at 100° to 105°, loses not more than 0.5% of its weight. Use 1 g.

Sulphated ash Not more than 0.1%, Appendix IX A, Method II. Use 1 g.

Assay Dissolve 0.15 g in 100 ml of *water*, add 20 ml of 0.1M *silver nitrate* and shake. Titrate with 0.1M *sodium hydroxide VS* until a blue colour is obtained using as indicator 1 ml of a solution prepared by dissolving 50 mg of *bromothymol blue* in a mixture of 4 ml of 0.02M *sodium hydroxide* and 20 ml of *ethanol (96%)* and diluting to 100 ml with *water*. Each ml of 0.1M *sodium hydroxide VS* is equivalent to 0.01802 g of $C_7H_8N_4O_2$.

Preparation
Aminophylline Injection

Action and use Xanthine bronchodilator.

Theophylline Hydrate ☆

$C_7H_8N_4O_2,H_2O$ 198.2   *5967-84-0*

Theophylline Hydrate is 1,3-dimethylpurine-2,6(3H,1H)-dione monohydrate. It contains not less than 99.0 per cent and not more than 101.0 per cent of $C_7H_8N_4O_2$, calculated with reference to the anhydrous substance.

Characteristics A white, crystalline powder; odourless.

Solubility Slightly soluble in *water* and in *chloroform*; soluble in 80 parts of *ethanol (96%)*; very slightly soluble in *ether*. It dissolves in solutions of alkali hydroxides, in aqueous ammonia and in mineral acids.

Identification *Test A may be omitted if tests B, C, D and E are carried out. Tests B and D may be omitted if tests A, C and E are carried out.*
A. Dry the substance being examined at 100° to 105°. The *infra-red absorption spectrum* of the residue, Appendix II A, is concordant with the spectrum of *theophylline EPCRS*.
B. Dissolve 10 mg in 10 ml of *water*, add 0.5 ml of a 5% w/v solution of *mercury(II) acetate* and allow to stand. A white, crystalline precipitate is produced.
C. Complies with the test for Water.
D. Yields the *reaction* characteristic of xanthines, Appendix VI.
E. The *melting point*, after drying at 100° to 105°, is 270° to 274°, Appendix V A, Method I.

Acidity; Clarity and colour of solution; Heavy metals; Related substances; Sulphated ash Complies with the requirements stated under Theophylline.

Water 8.0 to 9.5% w/w, Appendix IX C. Use 1 g.

Assay Carry out the Assay described under Theophylline but using 0.16 g.

Preparation
Aminophylline Injection

Action and use Xanthine bronchodilator.

The title of the monograph in the European Pharmacopœia is Theophylline Monohydrate.

Thiabendazole

$C_{10}H_7N_3S$ 201.3   *148-79-8*

Thiabendazole is 2-(thiazol-4-yl)benzimidazole. It contains not less than 98.0 per cent and not more than 101.0 per cent of $C_{10}H_7N_3S$, calculated with reference to the dried substance.

Characteristics A white to cream powder; odourless or almost odourless.

Solubility Practically insoluble in *water*; slightly soluble in *ethanol (96%)*, in *chloroform* and in *ether*. It dissolves in dilute mineral acids.

Identification A. The *infra-red absorption spectrum*, Appendix II A, is concordant with the *reference spectrum* of thiabendazole.
B. The *light absorption*, Appendix II B, in the range 230 to 350 nm of a 0.0008% w/v solution in 0.1M *hydrochloric acid* exhibits two maxima, at 243 nm and 302 nm. The *absorbance* at 243 nm is about 0.47 and at 302 nm is about 0.98.
C. Dissolve 5 mg in 5 ml of 0.1M *hydrochloric acid*, add 3 mg of p-*phenylenediamine dihydrochloride* and shake until dissolved. Add 0.1 g of *zinc powder*, mix, allow to stand for 2 minutes and add 10 ml of *ammonium iron(III) sulphate solution*. A deep blue or bluish-violet colour is produced.

Related substances Carry out the method for *thin-layer chromatography*, Appendix III A, using *silica gel GF254* as the coating substance and a mixture of 50 volumes of *toluene*, 20 volumes of *glacial acetic acid*, 8 volumes of *acetone* and 2 volumes of *water* as the mobile phase. Apply separately to the chromatoplate 10 µl of each of two solutions of the substance being examined in *methanol* containing (1) 1.0% w/v and (2) 0.015% w/v. After removal of the plate, allow it to dry in air and examine under *ultra-violet light (254 nm)*. Any *secondary spot* in the chromatogram obtained with solution (1) is not more intense than the spot in the chromatogram obtained with solution (2).

Loss on drying When dried to constant weight at 105°, loses not more than 0.5% of its weight. Use 1 g.

Sulphated ash Not more than 0.2%, Appendix IX A.

Assay Carry out Method I for *non-aqueous titration*, Appendix VIII A, using 0.16 g and *crystal violet solution* as indicator. Each ml of 0.1M *perchloric acid VS* is equivalent to 0.02013 g of $C_{10}H_7N_3S$.

Preparation
Thiabendazole Tablets

Action and use Anthelmintic.

In some countries the material described in this monograph may be known as Tiabendazole.

Thiamine Hydrochloride ☆

$C_{12}H_{17}ClN_4OS,HCl$ 337.3   *67-03-8*

Thiamine Hydrochloride is 3-[(4-amino-2-methylpyrimidin-5-yl)methyl]-5-(2-hydroxy-ethyl)-4-methylthiazolium chloride hydrochloride. It contains not less than 98.5 per cent and not more than 101.5 per cent of $C_{12}H_{17}ClN_4OS,HCl$, calculated with reference to the anhydrous substance.

Characteristics Colourless crystals or a white or almost white, crystalline powder; odour, faint and characteristic.

Solubility Soluble in 1 part of *water*, in 100 parts of *ethanol (96%)* and in 20 parts of *glycerol*; practically insoluble in *chloroform* and in *ether*.

Identification *Test A may be omitted if tests B and C are carried out. Test B may be omitted if tests A and C are carried out.*

A. The *infra-red absorption spectrum*, Appendix II A, is concordant with the spectrum of *thiamine hydrochloride EPCRS*. If the spectra are not concordant, dissolve the substances in *water*, evaporate the solutions to dryness and prepare new spectra of the residues.

B. Dissolve 20 mg in 10 ml of *water*, add 1 ml of 2M *acetic acid* and 1.6 ml of 1M *sodium hydroxide*, heat on a water-bath for 30 minutes and cool. Add 5 ml of 2M *sodium hydroxide*, 10 ml of a 5% w/v solution of *potassium hexacyanoferrate(III)* and 10 ml of *butan-1-ol* and shake vigorously for 2 minutes. The alcoholic layer exhibits an intense light blue fluorescence, particularly under ultra-violet light (365 nm). Repeat the test but adding 0.9 ml of 1M *sodium hydroxide* and 0.2 g of *sodium sulphite* in place of the 1.6 ml of 1M *sodium hydroxide*. Practically no fluorescence is produced.

C. Yields the *reactions* characteristic of chlorides, Appendix VI.

Acidity pH of a 2.5% w/v solution, 2.7 to 3.3, Appendix V L.

Clarity and colour of solution A 5.0% w/v solution is *clear*, Appendix IV A, and not more intensely coloured than *reference solution* Y_7 or GY_7, Appendix IV B, Method II.

Heavy metals A 10.0% w/v solution complies with *limit test A for heavy metals*, Appendix VII (20 ppm). Use *lead standard solution (2 ppm Pb)* to prepare the standard.

Nitrate To 0.4 ml of a 10.0% w/v solution add 1.6 ml of *water* and 2 ml of *sulphuric acid* and cool. Superimpose 2 ml of an 8.0% w/v solution of *iron(II) sulphate* in *carbon dioxide-free water* prepared immediately before use. No brown ring is produced at the junction of the two layers.

Sulphate 0.5 g complies with the *limit test for sulphates*, Appendix VII (300 ppm).

Sulphated ash Not more than 0.1%, Appendix IX A, Method II. Use 1 g.

Water Not more than 5.0% w/w, Appendix IX C. Use 0.4 g.

Assay Dissolve 0.15 g in 5 ml of *anhydrous formic acid*, add 65 ml of *anhydrous glacial acetic acid* and 10 ml of *mercury(II) acetate solution* and carry out Method I for *non-aqueous titration*, Appendix VIII A, determining the end-point potentiometrically. Each ml of 0.1M *perchloric acid VS* is equivalent to 0.01686 g of $C_{12}H_{17}ClN_4OS,HCl$.

Storage Thiamine Hydrochloride should be kept in a well-closed, non-metallic container and protected from light. Sterile solutions of pH 4.0 or less lose activity only very slowly. Neutral and alkaline solutions deteriorate rapidly, especially in contact with air.

Preparations
Thiamine Injection
Thiamine Tablets

Action and use Component of vitamin B.

Thiamine Nitrate ☆

$C_{12}H_{17}N_5O_4S$ 327.4   *532-43-4*

Thiamine Nitrate is 3-[4-amino-2-methyl-pyrimidin-5-yl]-5-(2-hydroxyethyl)-4-methyl-thiazolium nitrate. It contains not less than 98.0 per cent and not more than 102.0 per cent of $C_{12}H_{17}N_5O_4S$, calculated with reference to the dried substance.

Characteristics A white or almost white, crystalline powder or small, colourless crystals.

Solubility Sparingly soluble in *water*; freely soluble in boiling *water*; slightly soluble in *ethanol (96%)* and in *methanol*.

Identification *Test A may be omitted if tests B and C are carried out. Test B may be omitted if tests A and C are carried out.*

A. The *infra-red absorption spectrum*, Appendix II A, is concordant with the spectrum of *thiamine nitrate EPCRS*.

B. Dissolve 20 mg in 10 ml of *water*, add 1 ml of 2M *acetic acid* and 1.6 ml of 1M *sodium hydroxide*, heat on a water-bath for 30 minutes and allow to cool. Add 5 ml of 2M *sodium hydroxide*, 10 ml of a 5% w/v solution of *potassium hexacyanoferrate(III)* and 10 ml of *butan-1-ol* and shake vigorously for 2 minutes. The upper layer exhibits an intense light blue fluorescence under ultra-violet light (365 nm). Repeat the procedure using 0.9 ml of 1M *sodium hydroxide* and 0.2 g of *sodium sulphite* in place of the 1.6 ml of 1M *sodium hydroxide*; practically no fluorescence is produced.

C. 5 mg yields *reaction A* characteristic of nitrates, Appendix VI.

Acidity or alkalinity pH of a 2% w/v solution, 6.8 to 7.6, Appendix V L.

Clarity and colour of solution A 2.0% w/v solution in *carbon dioxide-free water* is *clear*, Appendix IV A, and not more intensely coloured than *reference solution Y₇*, Appendix IV B, Method II.

Heavy metals 1.0 g complies with *limit test D for heavy metals*, Appendix VII (20 ppm). Use 2 ml of *lead standard solution (10 ppm Pb)* to prepare the standard.

Chloride Dilute 8.3 ml of a 2.0% w/v solution in *carbon dioxide-free water* to 15 ml with *water*. The resulting solution complies with the *limit test for chlorides*, Appendix VII (300 ppm).

Loss on drying When dried to constant weight at 100° to 105°, loses not more than 1.0% of its weight. Use 1 g.

Sulphated ash Not more than 0.1%, Appendix IX A, Method II. Use 1 g.

Assay Dissolve 0.14 g in 5 ml of *anhydrous formic acid*, add 70 ml of *acetic anhydride* and carry out the method for *non-aqueous titration*, Appendix VIII A, determining the end-point potentiometrically. Repeat the operation without the substance being examined. The difference between the titrations represents the amount of perchloric acid required. Each ml of 0.1M *perchloric acid VS* is equivalent to 0.01637 g of $C_{12}H_{17}N_5O_4S$.

Storage Thiamine Nitrate should be kept in a well-closed, non-metallic container and protected from light.

Action and use Component of vitamin B.

Thiamphenicol ☆

MeSO₂—⟨benzene ring⟩—C—C—CH₂OH
(with OH H above, H NH·CO·CHCl₂ below)

$C_{12}H_{15}Cl_2NO_5S$ 356.2   *15318-45-3*

Thiamphenicol is 2,2-dichloro-*N*-[(αR,βR)-β-hydroxy-α-hydroxymethyl-4-methylsulphonyl-phenethyl]acetamide. It contains not less than 98.0 per cent and not more than 100.5 per cent of $C_{12}H_{15}Cl_2NO_5S$, calculated with reference to the dried substance.

Characteristics A fine, white to yellowish-white, crystalline powder or crystals; odourless. A solution in *absolute ethanol* is dextrorotatory; a solution in *dimethylformamide* is laevorotatory.

Solubility Slightly soluble in *water*, in *ether* and in *ethyl acetate*; sparingly soluble in *absolute ethanol* and in *acetone*; soluble in *methanol*; freely soluble in *acetonitrile* and in *dimethylformamide*; very soluble in *dimethylacetamide*.

Identification A. The *infra-red absorption spectrum*, Appendix II A, of the substance being examined, previously dried at 105° for 2 hours, examined as a potassium bromide disc, is concordant with the spectrum of a similar preparation of *thiamphenicol EPCRS*.

B. Carry out the method for *thin-layer chromatography*, Appendix III A, using *silica gel GF254* as the coating substance and a mixture of 97 volumes of *ethyl acetate* and 3 volumes of *methanol* as the mobile phase but allowing the solvent front to ascend 10 cm above the line of application. Apply separately to the chromatoplate 5 µl of each of two solutions in *methanol* containing (1) 1% w/v of the substance being examined and (2) 1% w/v of *thiamphenicol EPCRS*. After removal of the plate, allow it to dry in air and examine under *ultra-violet light (254 nm)*. The principal spot in the chromatogram obtained with solution (1) is similar in position and size to the spot in the chromatogram obtained with solution (2).

C. To 50 mg in a porcelain crucible add 0.5 g of *anhydrous sodium carbonate* and heat over an open flame for 10 minutes. Allow to cool, dissolve the residue in 5 ml of 2M *nitric acid* and filter. To 1 ml of the filtrate add 1 ml of *water*. The resulting solution yields *reaction A* characteristic of chlorides, Appendix VI.

Acidity or alkalinity Shake 0.1 g with 20 ml of *carbon dioxide-free water* and add 0.1 ml of *aqueous bromothymol blue solution*. Not more than 0.1 ml of either 0.02M *hydrochloric acid VS* or 0.02M *sodium hydroxide VS* is required to change the colour of the solution.

Light absorption The *light absorption*, Appendix II B, of a 0.020% w/v solution, prepared by heating at about 40°, in the range 240 to 300 nm exhibits two maxima, at 266 nm and 273 nm. The A(1%, 1 cm) at 266 nm is 25 to 28 and at 273 nm is 21.5 to 23.5. Dilute 1 volume of the solution to 20 volumes with *water*. The *light absorption* of the resulting solution in the range 200 to 240 nm exhibits a maximum only at 224 nm. The A(1%, 1 cm) at 224 nm is 370 to 400.

Melting point 163° to 167°, Appendix V A, Method I.

Specific optical rotation In a 5% w/v solution in *dimethylformamide*, −21° to −24°, Appendix V F.

Heavy metals 1.0 g complies with *limit test C for heavy metals*, Appendix VII (10 ppm). Use 1 ml of *lead standard solution (10 ppm Pb)* to prepare the standard.

Chloride Shake 0.50 g with 30 ml of *water* for 5 minutes and filter. 15 ml of the filtrate complies with the *limit test for chlorides*, Appendix VII (200 ppm).

Loss on drying When dried to constant weight at 100° to 105°, loses not more than 1.0% of its weight. Use 1 g.

Sulphated ash Not more than 0.1%, Appendix IX A, Method II. Use 2 g.

Assay Dissolve 0.3 g in 30 ml of *ethanol (96%)*, add 20 ml of a 50% w/v solution of *potassium hydroxide*, mix and heat under a reflux condenser for 4 hours. Cool, dilute with 100 ml of *water* and neutralise with 2M *nitric acid*. Add a further 5 ml of 2M *nitric acid* and titrate with 0.1M *silver nitrate VS* determining the end-point potentiometrically. Repeat the operation without the substance being examined. The difference between the titrations represents the amount of silver nitrate required. Each ml of 0.1M *silver nitrate VS* is equivalent to 0.01781 g of $C_{12}H_{15}Cl_2NO_5S$.

Storage Thiamphenicol should be kept in a well-closed container and protected from light and moisture.

Action and use Antibacterial.

Thioguanine

C₅H₅N₅S   167.2   *154-42-7*

Thioguanine is 2-aminopurine-6(1*H*)-thione. It contains not less than 98.0 per cent and not more than 101.0 per cent of $C_5H_5N_5S$, calculated with reference to the dried substance.

Characteristics A pale yellow, crystalline powder; odourless or almost odourless.

Solubility Practically insoluble in *water*, in *ethanol (96%)* and in *chloroform*. It dissolves in dilute solutions of alkali hydroxides.

Identification A. Heat a suitable quantity at 105° at a pressure not exceeding 0.7 kPa for 5 hours. The *infra-red absorption spectrum* of the residue, Appendix II A, is concordant with the *reference spectrum* of thioguanine.
B. The *light absorption*, Appendix II B, in the range 230 to 370 nm of a 0.001% w/v solution in 0.1M *hydrochloric acid* exhibits two maxima, at 258 nm and 348 nm. The *absorbance* at 348 nm is about 1.24.
C. Mix 10 mg with 10 mg of *sodium formate* in a test-tube and heat gently until melted. A gas is evolved which turns *lead acetate paper* black.

Phosphate To 0.5 g add 2 ml of 5M *sulphuric acid* and heat on a water-bath for 5 minutes. Add, dropwise, 5 ml of *nitric acid* and continue heating until a clear solution is obtained. Cool and add 10 ml of *water* and 0.75 ml of a solution prepared by dissolving 8.3 g of *ammonium molybdate* in 40 ml of *water* and adding 33 ml of 5M *sulphuric acid* and sufficient *water* to produce 100 ml. Add 1.0 ml of *aminohydroxynaphthalenesulphonic acid solution*, mix and dilute to 25 ml with *water*. Measure the *absorbance* of the resulting solution at 820 nm, Appendix II B, using in the reference cell a solution prepared in the same manner but omitting the substance being examined. The absorbance is not more than that obtained by treating 1.5 ml of *phosphate standard solution (100 ppm PO₄)* in the same manner, beginning at the words 'add 0.75 ml of a solution . . .'.

Free sulphur Dissolve 50 mg in 5 ml of 1M *sodium hydroxide*. The solution is *clear*, Appendix IV A.

Related substances Carry out the method for *thin-layer chromatography*, Appendix III A, using *silica gel GF254* as the coating substance and a mixture of 90 volumes of *methanol* and 15 volumes of 13.5M *ammonia* as the mobile phase. Apply separately to the chromatoplate 2 μl of solution (1) and 5 μl and 1 μl of solution (2). Solution (1) contains 1.0% w/v of the substance being examined in 0.1M *sodium hydroxide*. Solution (2) contains 0.010% w/v of *guanine* in the same solvent. After removal of the plate, allow it to dry in air and examine under *ultra-violet light (254 nm)*. Any spot corresponding to guanine in the chromatogram obtained with solution (1) is not more intense than the spot in the chromatogram obtained with 5 μl of solution (2). Any other *secondary spot* in the chromatogram obtained with solution (1) is not more

intense than the spot in the chromatogram obtained with 1 μl of solution (2).

Loss on drying When dried at 105° at a pressure not exceeding 0.7 kPa for 5 hours, loses not more than 1.0% of its weight. Use 1 g.

Assay Carry out Method I for *non-aqueous titration*, Appendix VIII A, using a solution prepared by dissolving 0.15 g in 15 ml of *anhydrous formic acid*, adding 50 ml of *butan-2-one* and determining the end-point potentiometrically. Each ml of 0.1M *perchloric acid VS* is equivalent to 0.01672 g of $C_5H_5N_5S$.

Storage Thioguanine should be kept in a well-closed container.

Preparation
Thioguanine Tablets

Action and use Cytotoxic.

In some countries the material described in this monograph may be known as Tioguanine.

Thiomersal
Thimerosal

C₉H₉HgNaO₂S   404.8   *54-64-8*

Thiomersal is the sodium salt of (2-carboxyphenylthio)ethylmercury. It contains not less than 98.0 per cent and not more than 100.5 per cent of $C_9H_9HgNaO_2S$, calculated with reference to the dried substance.

Characteristics A light, cream, crystalline powder; odour, slight and characteristic.

Solubility Soluble in 1 part of *water* and in 8 parts of *ethanol (96%)*; practically insoluble in *ether*.

Identification A. Dissolve 0.1 g in 10 ml of *water* and add 2 ml of *silver nitrate solution*. A white precipitate is produced.
B. Dissolve 0.5 g in 10 ml of *water* and add 2 ml of 2M *hydrochloric acid*. A pale yellow precipitate is produced which, after washing with *water* and drying over *phosphorus pentoxide* at a pressure not exceeding 0.7 kPa, has a *melting point* of about 110°, Appendix V A.

Acidity or alkalinity pH of a 1% w/v solution, 6.0 to 8.0, Appendix V L.

Mercuric salts Dissolve 0.1 g in 10 ml of *water* and add an equal volume of *ammonium sulphide solution*; a white precipitate is produced. Allow to stand for 30 minutes in the dark; no blackening occurs.

Ether-soluble matter Shake 0.5 g with 20 ml of *ether* for 10 minutes, filter and evaporate the filtrate to dryness. The residue, after drying over *phosphorus pentoxide* at a pressure not exceeding 0.7 kPa for 24 hours, weighs not more than 3 mg.

Loss on drying When dried over *phosphorus pentoxide* at a pressure not exceeding 0.7 kPa for 24 hours, loses not more than 0.5% of its weight. Use 1 g.

Assay Place 0.5 g in a 100-ml long-necked flask, add 5 ml of *sulphuric acid* and heat gently until charring occurs; continue to heat and add *hydrogen peroxide solution (100* vol), dropwise, until the mixture is colourless. Dilute with *water*, evaporate until slight fuming occurs, dilute to 10 ml with *water*, cool and titrate with 0.1M *ammonium thiocyanate VS* using *ammonium iron(III) sulphate solution* as indicator. Each ml of 0.1M *ammonium thiocyanate VS* is equivalent to 0.02024 g of $C_9H_9HgNaO_2S$.

Storage Thiomersal should be protected from light.

Action and use Antiseptic; antimicrobial preservative.

Thiopentone Sodium ☆

$C_{11}H_{17}N_2NaO_2S$ 264.3   *71-73-8*

Thiopentone Sodium is a mixture of sodium 5-ethyl-5-(1-methylbutyl)-2-thiobarbiturate and anhydrous sodium carbonate. It contains not less than 84.0 per cent and not more than 87.0 per cent of $C_{11}H_{18}N_2O_2S$ and not less than 10.2 per cent and not more than 11.2 per cent of Na, both calculated with reference to the dried substance.

Characteristics A yellowish-white powder; odour, faintly alliaceous; hygroscopic.

Solubility Soluble in 1.5 parts of *water;* practically insoluble in *ether*. It is partly soluble in *ethanol (96%)*.

Identification *Test A may be omitted if tests B, C, D and E are carried out. Tests B and D may be omitted if tests A, C and E are carried out.*

A. Acidify 10 ml of a 10% w/v solution in *carbon dioxide-free water* with 2M *hydrochloric acid*. The solution effervesces. Shake the solution with 20 ml of *ether*, separate the ether layer, wash with 10 ml of *water* and dry over *anhydrous sodium sulphate*. Filter, evaporate the filtrate to dryness and dry the residue at 100° to 105°. The *infra-red absorption spectrum* of the residue, Appendix II A, is concordant with the spectrum of *thiopental EPCRS*.

B. Complies with the test for *identification of barbiturates*, Appendix III A, but using the following solutions. Solution (1) contains 0.1% w/v of the substance being examined in *water*. For solution (2) dissolve 85 mg of *thiopental EPCRS* in 10 ml of 2M *sodium hydroxide* and dilute to 100 ml with *water*.

C. Determine the *melting point*, Appendix V A, Method I, of the residue obtained in test A and of a mixture of equal parts of the residue and *thiopental EPCRS*. The difference between the melting points, which are about 160°, is not greater than 2°.

D. Yields the *reaction* characteristic of non-nitrogen substituted barbiturates, Appendix VI.

E. Yields *reaction A* characteristic of sodium salts, Appendix VI.

Clarity and colour of solution A 10.0% w/v solution in *carbon dioxide-free water* is *clear*, Appendix IV A, and not more intensely coloured than *reference solution GY₃*, Appendix IV B, Method II.

Chloride To 5 ml of a 10.0% w/v solution in *carbon dioxide-free water* add 35 ml of *water* and 10 ml of 2M *nitric acid*. Shake successively with three 25-ml quantities of *ether*, discard the ether layers and heat the aqueous solution on a water-bath to remove any residual ether.

15 ml of the aqueous layer complies with the *limit test for chlorides*, Appendix VII (330 ppm).

Related substances Complies with the test for *related substances in barbiturates*, Apppendix III A, but using *water* as the solvent for solutions (1) and (2). Disregard any slight residue in solution (1). After removal of the chromatoplate, examine it under *ultra-violet light (254 nm)* but do not spray the plate with the diphenylcarbazone—mercury reagent.

Loss on drying When dried at 100° at a pressure of 1.5 to 2.5 kPa for 4 hours, loses not more than 2.5% of its weight. Use 0.5 g.

Assay *For Na* Dissolve 0.4 g in 30 ml of *water* and titrate with 0.1M *hydrochloric acid VS*, using 0.1 ml of *methyl red solution* as indicator, until the colour of solution changes to red. Boil gently for 2 minutes, cool and, if necessary, continue the titration with 0.1M *hydrochloric acid VS* until the red colour is restored. Each ml of 0.1M *hydrochloric acid VS* is equivalent to 0.002299 g of Na.

For $C_{11}H_{18}N_2O_2S$ Dissolve 0.15 g in 5 ml of *water*, add 2 ml of 1M *sulphuric acid* and extract with four 10-ml quantities of *chloroform*. Filter the combined chloroform extracts, evaporate the filtrate to dryness on a water-bath and dissolve the residue in 30 ml of *dimethylformamide* previously neutralised with 0.1M *lithium methoxide VS*. Titrate immediately with 0.1M *lithium methoxide VS*, using 0.1 ml of a 0.2% w/v solution of *thymol blue* in *methanol* as indicator, until a blue colour is obtained. Protect the solution from atmospheric carbon dioxide during the titration. Each ml of 0.1M *lithium methoxide VS* is equivalent to 0.02423 g of $C_{11}H_{18}N_2O_2S$.

Storage Thiopentone Sodium should be kept in an airtight container and protected from light.

Preparation
Thiopentone Injection

Action and use General anaesthetic.

The title of the monograph in the European Pharmacopœia is Thiopental Sodium and Sodium Carbonate.

Thioridazine Hydrochloride

$C_{21}H_{26}N_2S_2,HCl$ 407.0   *130-61-0*

Thioridazine Hydrochloride is 10-[2-(1-methyl-2-piperidyl)ethyl]-2-methylthiophenothiazine hydrochloride. It contains not less than 99.0 per cent and not more than 101.0 per cent of $C_{21}H_{26}N_2S_2,HCl$, calculated with reference to the dried substance.

Characteristics A white or cream, crystalline powder; odour, slight.

Solubility Soluble in 9 parts of *water*, in 10 parts of *ethanol (96%)* and in 1.5 parts of *chloroform*; almost insoluble in *ether*.

Identification A. The *infra-red absorption spectrum*, Appendix II A, is concordant with the *reference spectrum* of thioridazine hydrochloride.

B. The *light absorption*, Appendix II B, in the range 230 to 350 nm of a 0.0013% w/v solution in *ethanol (96%)* exhibits a maximum at 264 nm and a less well-defined maximum at 315 nm. The *absorbance* at 264 nm is about 1.22.

C. Dissolve 5 mg in 2 ml of *sulphuric acid* and allow to stand for 5 minutes. A blue colour is produced.

D. Yields the *reactions* characteristic of chlorides, Appendix VI.

Acidity pH of a 1% w/v solution, 4.2 to 5.2, Appendix V L.

Related substances Carry out in subdued light the method for *thin-layer chromatography*, Appendix III A, using a silica gel F254 precoated chromatoplate (Merck silica gel 60 F254 plates are suitable) and a mixture of 74 volumes of *chloroform*, 25 volumes of *propan-2-ol* and 1 volume of 13.5M *ammonia* as the mobile phase. Apply separately to the plate 5 μl of each of three solutions of the substance being examined in *chloroform* containing (1) 1.0% w/v, (2) 0.010% w/v and (3) 0.0050% w/v. After removal of the plate, allow it to dry in air and spray with a mixture of 10 volumes of *acetic potassium iodobismuthate solution*, 20 volumes of *glacial acetic acid* and 70 volumes of *water* and then with *hydrogen peroxide solution (10 vol)* and immediately cover the plate with a clear glass plate of the same size. Any *secondary spot* in the chromatogram obtained with solution (1) is not more intense than the spot in the chromatogram obtained with solution (2) and not more than one such spot is more intense than the spot in the chromatogram obtained with solution (3).

Loss on drying When dried to constant weight at 105°, loses not more than 0.5% of its weight. Use 1 g.

Sulphated ash Not more than 0.1%, Appendix IX A.

Assay Dissolve 0.6 g in 200 ml of *acetone*, add 5 ml of *mercury(II) acetate solution* and carry out Method I for *non-aqueous titration*, Appendix VIII A, determining the end-point potentiometrically. Each ml of 0.1M *perchloric acid VS* is equivalent to 0.04070 g of $C_{21}H_{26}N_2S_2,HCl$.

Storage Thioridazine Hydrochloride should be kept in a well-closed container and protected from light.

Preparation
Thioridazine Tablets

Action and use Antipsychotic.

Thiotepa

$C_6H_{12}N_3PS$ 189.2   *52-24-4*

Thiotepa is phosphorothioic tri(ethyleneamide). It contains not less than 97.0 per cent and not more than 102.0 per cent of $C_6H_{12}N_3PS$, calculated with reference to the anhydrous substance.

Characteristics Fine, white crystalline flakes; odourless or almost odourless.

Solubility Soluble in 8 parts of *water*, in 2 parts of *ethanol (96%)* and in 2 parts of *chloroform*.

Identification A. The *infra-red absorption spectrum*, Appendix II A, is concordant with the *reference spectrum* of thiotepa.

B. Burn 20 mg by the method for *oxygen-flask combustion*, Appendix VIII C, using 5 ml of 1.25M *sodium hydroxide* as the absorbing liquid. When the process is complete, dilute to 25 ml with *water*. To 5 ml of the resulting solution add 0.1 ml of *hydrogen peroxide solution (100 vol)* and 1 ml of 1M *hydrochloric acid*, mix and add 0.05 ml of *barium chloride solution*. The solution becomes turbid.

C. To 2 ml of the solution obtained in test B add 40 ml of *water* and 4 ml of *ammonium molybdate solution*, mix, add 0.1 g of L-ascorbic acid and boil for 1 minute. A blue colour is produced.

Melting point 52° to 57°, Appendix V A.

Clarity of solution A 2.0% w/v solution is *clear*, Appendix IV A.

Water Not more than 2.0% w/w, Appendix IX C. Use 1.2 g.

Assay Transfer 0.2 g to an iodine flask with the aid of 50 ml of a 20% w/v solution of *sodium thiosulphate* and titrate immediately with 0.1M *hydrochloric acid VS*, using 0.05 ml of *methyl orange solution* as indicator, until a faint red colour persists for 10 seconds. Stopper the flask, allow to stand for 30 minutes and titrate with 0.1M *sodium hydroxide VS* using *phenolphthalein solution* as indicator. Subtract the volume of 0.1M *sodium hydroxide VS* used from the volume of 0.1M *hydrochloric acid VS* used. Repeat the operation without the substance being examined. The difference between the titrations represents the amount of hydrochloric acid required. Each ml of 0.1M *hydrochloric acid VS* is equivalent to 0.006307 g of $C_6H_{12}N_3PS$.

Storage Thiotepa should be kept in a well-closed container and stored at a temperature of 2° to 8°. At higher temperatures it polymerises and becomes inactive.

Preparation
Thiotepa Injection

Action and use Cytotoxic.

Thymol

$C_{10}H_{14}O$ 150.2   *89-83-8*

Thymol is 2-isopropyl-5-methylphenol and may be obtained from natural oils or by synthesis. It contains not less than 99.0 per cent and not more than 101.0 per cent w/v of $C_{10}H_{14}O$.

Characteristics Colourless crystals; odour, pungent, aromatic and thyme-like.

Solubility Very slightly soluble in *water*; soluble in 0.3 part of *ethanol (96%)*, in 0.6 part of *chloroform* and in 0.7 part of *ether*.

Identification A. The *infra-red absorption spectrum*, Appendix II A, is concordant with the *reference spectrum* of

thymol. Melt a sufficient quantity, prepare a thin film between two sodium bromide plates previously warmed to 65° and record the spectrum immediately. The film must remain liquid during the production of the spectrum.
B. Heat 1 g in a test-tube in a water-bath with 5 ml of a 10% w/v solution of *sodium hydroxide*; a clear, colourless or pink solution is produced which darkens on standing and no oily drops separate. Add 0.15 ml of *chloroform* and agitate the mixture; a violet colour is produced.
C. Dissolve a small quantity in 1 ml of *glacial acetic acid* and add 0.15 ml of *sulphuric acid* and 0.05 ml of *nitric acid*. A green colour is produced.

Acidity or alkalinity Dissolve 0.4 g in 5 ml of *ethanol (96%)*, add 5 ml of freshly boiled and cooled *water* and 0.05 ml of *bromocresol purple solution*. Not more than 0.2 ml of either 0.01M *sodium hydroxide VS* or 0.01M *hydrochloric acid VS* is required to change the colour of the solution.

Freezing point Not below 49.3°, Appendix V B.

Related substances Carry out the method for *gas chromatography*, Appendix III B, using solutions in *chloroform* containing (1) 0.01% w/v of the substance being examined and 0.02% w/v of *4-chlorophenol* (internal standard), (2) 1.0% w/v of the substance being examined and (3) 1.0% w/v of the substance being examined and 0.02% w/v of the internal standard.

The chromatographic procedure may be carried out using a glass column (1.5 m × 4 mm) packed with *acid-washed, silanised diatomaceous support* (80 to 100 mesh) coated with 3% w/w of polyethylene glycol (Carbowax 20M is suitable) and maintained at 135°.

In the chromatogram obtained with solution (3) the ratio of the sum of the areas of any *secondary peaks* to the area of the peak due to the internal standard is not greater than half of the ratio of the area of the principal peak to that of the peak due to the internal standard in the chromatogram obtained with solution (1).

Non-volatile matter When heated in an open dish on a water-bath and dried at 105°, leaves not more than 0.05% of residue. Use 5 g.

Assay Dissolve 0.1 g in 5 ml of 1M *sodium hydroxide VS* in a glass-stoppered conical flask, add 20 ml of *water* and 20 ml of hot 6M *hydrochloric acid VS* and titrate immediately with 0.05M *bromine VS* to within 1 to 2 ml of the calculated end-point. Warm the solution to 70° to 80°, add 0.1 ml of *methyl orange solution* and continue the titration slowly, swirling vigorously after each addition, until the colour is discharged. Add alternately 0.05 ml of 0.05M *bromine VS* and 0.05 ml of *methyl orange solution* until the red colour disappears after the addition of the methyl orange. Each ml of 0.05M *bromine VS* is equivalent to 0.003755 g of $C_{10}H_{14}O$.

Storage Thymol should be kept in a well-closed container and protected from light.

Preparation
Compound Thymol Glycerin

Action and use Antimicrobial preservative; antiseptic.

Thymoxamine Hydrochloride

$C_{16}H_{25}NO_3,HCl$ 315.8   *964-52-3*

Thymoxamine Hydrochloride is 4-(2-dimethyl-aminoethoxy)-5-isopropyl-2-methylphenyl acetate hydrochloride. It contains not less than 99.0 per cent and not more than 101.0 per cent of $C_{16}H_{25}NO_3,HCl$, calculated with reference to the dried substance.

Characteristics A white, crystalline powder; odourless or almost odourless.

Solubility Soluble in 2.5 parts of *water*, in 11 parts of *ethanol (96%)* and in 3 parts of *chloroform*; practically insoluble in *ether* and in petroleum spirit.

Identification A. The *infra-red absorption spectrum*, Appendix II A, is concordant with the *reference spectrum* of thymoxamine hydrochloride.
B. Dilute 20 ml of a 0.03% w/v solution to 100 ml with *water* (solution 1). Dilute a further 20 ml of the same solution to 100 ml with 0.1M *sodium hydroxide* (solution 2). The ratio of the *absorbance* of solution (2) at 302 nm, measured 30 minutes after preparation, to the *absorbance* of solution (1) at 275 nm is about 1.7, Appendix II B.
C. Boil 10 mg with 3 ml of 2M *hydrochloric acid* for 15 minutes and cool. Add dropwise sufficient 5M *sodium hydroxide* to produce a turbidity and then slowly, with shaking, add just sufficient 2M *hydrochloric acid* to redissolve the precipitate and 1 ml of *iron(III) chloride test-solution*. The colour changes to greenish-yellow and a yellow, crystalline precipitate is produced.
D. Yields *reaction A* characteristic of chlorides, Appendix VI.
E. *Melting point*, about 212°, Appendix V A.

Acidity pH of a 5% w/v solution, 4.5 to 5.5, Appendix V L.

Related substances Carry out the method for *high-performance liquid chromatography*, Appendix III D, using solutions in the mobile phase containing (1) 0.010% w/v of *2-(6-hydroxythymoxy)ethyldimethylamine hydrochloride BPCRS*, 0.0050% w/v of *2-thymoxyethyldimethylamine hydrochloride BPCRS* and 0.020% w/v of *2-(6-chloro-thymoxy)ethyldimethylamine hydrochloride BPCRS* and (2) 2.0% w/v of the substance being examined.

The chromatographic procedure may be carried out using (a) a stainless steel column (30 cm × 3.9 mm) packed with *stationary phase C* (10 µm) (µBondapak C18 is suitable), (b) 0.005M *sodium hexanesulphonate* in a mixture of 315 volumes of *methanol*, 185 volumes of *water* and 2 volumes of *glacial acetic acid* as the mobile phase with a flow rate of 1.0 ml per minute and (c) a detection wavelength of 276 nm.

The peaks in the chromatogram obtained with solution (1) are due to (a) 2-(6-hydroxythymoxy)ethyldimethyl-amine hydrochloride, (b) 2-thymoxyethyldimethylamine hydrochloride and (c) 2-(6-chlorothymoxy)ethyldimethyl-amine hydrochloride in order of their elution. The areas of any peaks corresponding to (a), (b) and (c) in the chromatogram obtained with solution (2) are not greater than the areas of the corresponding peaks in the chromatogram obtained with solution (1).

Loss on drying When dried to constant weight at 105°, loses not more than 0.5% of its weight. Use 1 g.

Sulphated ash Not more than 0.1%, Appendix IX A.

Assay Carry out Method I for *non-aqueous titration*, Appendix VIII A, using 0.5 g and *1-naphtholbenzein solution* as indicator. Each ml of 0.1M *perchloric acid VS* is equivalent to 0.03158 g of $C_{16}H_{25}NO_3,HCl$.

Storage Thymoxamine Hydrochloride should be protected from light.

Preparation
Thymoxamine Tablets

Action and use Vasodilator.

In some countries the material described in this monograph may be known as Moxisylyte Hydrochloride.

Thyroxine Sodium ☆

$C_{15}H_{10}I_4NNaO_4,xH_2O$ 799 *(anhydrous)*
55-03-8 (anhydrous)

Thyroxine Sodium is sodium O^4-(4-hydroxy-3,5-di-iodophenyl)-3,5-di-iodo-L-tyrosinate and contains a variable quantity of water of crystallisation. It contains not less than 97.0 per cent and not more than 101.0 per cent of $C_{15}H_{10}I_4NNaO_4$, calculated with reference to the dried substance.

Characteristics An almost white or slightly brownish-yellow powder or a fine, slightly coloured, crystalline powder.

Solubility Very slightly soluble in *water*; slightly soluble in *ethanol (96%)*; practically insoluble in *chloroform* and in *ether*. It dissolves in aqueous solutions of the alkali hydroxides.

Identification A. The *light absorption*, Appendix II B, in the range 230 to 350 nm of a 0.01% w/v solution in 0.1M *sodium hydroxide* exhibits a maximum only at 325 nm. The A(1%, 1 cm) at 325 nm is 73 to 79.
B. In the test for Liothyronine, the principal spot in the chromatogram obtained with solution (1) is similar in position, colour and size to the spot in the chromatogram obtained with solution (2).
C. Complies with the test for Specific optical rotation.
D. Prepare the sulphated ash, Appendix IX C, Method II, using 0.2 g and dissolve the residue in 2 ml of *water*. The solution yields *reaction A* characteristic of sodium salts, Appendix VI.

Colour of solution Dissolve 0.50 g in 23 ml of a gently boiling mixture of 1 volume of 1M *hydrochloric acid* and 4 volumes of *ethanol (96%)*. Cool and dilute to 25 ml with the same mixture of solvents (solution A). The freshly prepared solution is not more intensely coloured than *reference solution BY₃*, Appendix IV B, Method II.

Specific optical rotation In solution A, +16.0° to +20.0°, Appendix V F.

Liothyronine Carry out the method for *thin-layer chromatography*, Appendix III A, using a slurry of 30 g of *silica gel H* in 60 ml of a 0.75% w/v solution of *soluble starch* to coat the chromatoplate. Do not heat the plate before use. Use a mixture of 55 volumes of *ethyl acetate*, 35 volumes of *propan-2-ol* and 20 volumes of 13.5M *ammonia* as the mobile phase. Apply separately to the plate 5 μl of each of the following solutions in a mixture of 5 volumes of 13.5M *ammonia* and 70 volumes of *methanol*. Solution (1) contains 1.0% w/v of the substance being examined. Solution (2) contains 1.0% w/v of *levothyroxine sodium EPCRS*. Solution (3) contains 0.01% w/v of *liothyronine EPCRS*. Solution (4) contains 1.0% w/v of the substance being examined and 0.01% w/v of *liothyronine EPCRS*.

After removal of the plate, allow it to dry in air and spray lightly with *iron(III) chloride—ferricyanide—arsenite solution*. Any spot corresponding to liothyronine in the chromatogram obtained with solution (1) is not more intense than the spot in the chromatogram obtained with solution (3). The test is not valid unless the chromatogram obtained with solution (4) shows two clearly separated principal spots.

Loss on drying When dried to constant weight at 100° to 105°, loses 6.0 to 12.0% of its weight. Use 0.1 g.

Assay Carry out the method for *oxygen-flask combustion*, Appendix VIII C, using 25 mg and 5 ml of 1M *sodium hydroxide* as the absorbing liquid. Rinse the neck of the flask with 10 ml of *water*, add 20 ml of *alkaline sodium hypobromite solution* and three or four glass beads and boil gently for 5 minutes. Add 170 ml of *water* and 5 g of *potassium hydrogen phthalate*, heat rapidly to boiling and boil for 1 minute after decolorisation of the solution. Check that the pH of the solution remains between 4 and 5 and, if necessary, add 0.5 g of *potassium hydrogen phthalate*. Check that the solution does not turn *starch iodide paper* blue and, if it does, heat again to boiling. Dry the inside of the neck of the flask with filter paper, cool in ice, add 20 ml of a 16.6% w/v solution of *potassium iodide* and 5 ml of 1M *sulphuric acid*, close the flask and allow to stand in the dark for 30 minutes. Titrate with 0.1M *sodium thiosulphate VS* using 1 ml of *starch solution*, added towards the end of the titration, as indicator. Repeat the operation without the substance being examined. The difference between the titrations represents the amount of sodium thiosulphate required. Each ml of 0.1M *sodium thiosulphate VS* is equivalent to 0.003329 g of $C_{15}H_{10}I_4NNaO_4$.

Storage Thyroxine Sodium should be kept in a well-closed container and protected from light.

Preparation
Thyroxine Tablets

Action and use Thyroid hormone.

The title of the monograph in the European Pharmacopœia is Levothyroxine Sodium.

Timolol Maleate

$C_{13}H_{24}N_4O_3S,C_4H_4O_4$ 432.5   *26921-17-5*

Timolol Maleate is (S)-1-*tert*-butylamino-3-(4-morpholino-1,2,5-thiadiazol-3-yloxy)propan-2-ol hydrogen maleate. It contains not less than 98.0 per cent and not more than 101.0 per cent of $C_{13}H_{24}N_4O_3S,C_4H_4O_4$, calculated with reference to the dried substance.

Characteristics A white or almost white powder; odourless or almost odourless.

Solubility Soluble in 15 parts of *water*, in 21 parts of *ethanol (96%)* and in 40 parts of *chloroform*; practically insoluble in *ether*.

Identification A. The *infra-red absorption spectrum*, Appendix II A, is concordant with the *reference spectrum* of timolol maleate.
B. The *light absorption*, Appendix II B, in the range 230 to 350 nm of a 0.0025% w/v solution in 0.05M *sulphuric acid* exhibits a maximum at 295 nm. The *absorbance* at 295 nm is about 0.52.
C. Dissolve 0.2 g in 3 ml of *water*, add 2 ml of 5M *sodium hydroxide* and shake with three 3-ml quantities of *ether*. Warm the aqueous layer in a water-bath for 10 minutes with 2 ml of *bromine water*, boil, cool and add 0.2 ml to a solution of 10 mg of *resorcinol* in 3 ml of *sulphuric acid*. A bluish-black colour is produced on heating for 15 minutes in a water-bath.

Acidity pH of a 2% w/v solution, 3.8 to 4.3, Appendix V L.

Clarity and colour of solution A 2.0% w/v solution is *clear*, Appendix IV A, and *colourless*, Appendix IV B, Method I.

Specific optical rotation In a 5% w/v solution in 1M *hydrochloric acid*, −11.7° to −12.5°, determined at 405 nm, Appendix V F.

Related substances Carry out the method for *thin-layer chromatography*, Appendix III A, using a precoated silica gel GF254 chromatoplate (Merck silica gel 60 GF254 plates are suitable) and a mixture of 80 volumes of *dichloromethane*, 20 volumes of *methanol* and 1 volume of 13.5M *ammonia* as the mobile phase. Apply separately to the plate 10 μl of each of three solutions of the substance being examined in *methanol* containing (1) 5.0% w/v, (2) 0.020% w/v and (3) 0.010% w/v. After removal of the plate, allow it to dry in air and examine under *ultra-violet light (254 nm)* and then expose to iodine vapour for 2 hours and examine in daylight. Using both methods of visulisation, any *secondary spot* in the chromatogram obtained with solution (1) is not more intense than the spot in the chromatogram obtained with solution (2) and not more than two such spots are more intense than the spot in the chromatogram obtained with solution (3).

Loss on drying When dried to constant weight at 100° to 105° at a pressure not exceeding 0.7 kPa, loses not more than 0.5% of its weight. Use 1 g.

Sulphated ash Not more than 0.1%, Appendix IX A.

Assay Carry out Method I for *non-aqueous titration*, Appendix VIII A, using 0.85 g and *1-naphtholbenzein*

solution as indicator. Each ml of 0.1M *perchloric acid VS* is equivalent to 0.04325 g of $C_{13}H_{24}N_4O_3S,C_4H_4O_4$.

Preparations
Timolol Eye Drops
Timolol Tablets

Action and use Beta-adrenoceptor antagonist.

Titanium Dioxide ☆

TiO_2 79.90   *13463-67-7*

Titanium Dioxide is titanium(IV) oxide. It contains not less than 98.0 per cent and not more than 100.5 per cent of TiO_2.

Characteristics A white or almost white powder; odourless.

Solubility Practically insoluble in *water* and in dilute mineral acids; slowly soluble in hot *sulphuric acid*.

Identification A. When strongly heated it becomes pale yellow; the colour is discharged on cooling.
B. To 5 ml of solution A obtained in the assay add 0.1 ml of *hydrogen peroxide solution (100 vol)*. An orange-red colour is produced.
C. To 5 ml of solution A add 0.5 g of *granulated zinc*. After 45 minutes a violet-blue colour is produced.

Clarity and colour of solution Solution A is not more opalescent than *reference suspension II*, Appendix IV A, and is *colourless*, Appendix IV B, Method II.

Acidity or alkalinity Shake 5 g with 50 ml of *carbon dioxide-free water* for 5 minutes and centrifuge or filter until a clear solution is obtained. To 10 ml of the solution add 0.1 ml of *bromothymol blue solution*. Not more than 1 ml of either 0.01M *hydrochloric acid VS* or 0.01M *sodium hydroxide VS* is required to change the colour of the solution.

Water-soluble matter Boil 10 g for 5 minutes with 150 ml of *water* containing 0.5 g of *ammonium sulphate*. Cool, dilute to 200 ml with *water* and filter until a clear solution is obtained. Evaporate 100 ml of the filtrate to dryness and ignite. The residue weighs not more than 25 mg (0.5%).

Antimony To 10.0 ml of solution A add 10 ml of *hydrochloric acid* and 10 ml of *water*. Cool to 20°, if necessary, and add 0.15 ml of *sodium nitrite solution*. After 5 minutes add 5 ml of a 1% w/v solution of *hydroxylamine hydrochloride*, mix, add 10 ml of a freshly prepared 0.01% w/v solution of *rhodamine B* and mix. Add 10 ml of *toluene*, shake vigorously for 1 minute and collect the toluene layer. Prepare a reference solution at the same time and in the same manner using a solution prepared by adding 10 ml of *hydrochloric acid* and 15 ml of a solution containing 0.5 g of *anhydrous sodium sulphate* and 2 ml of *sulphuric acid* to 5 ml of *antimony standard solution (1 ppm Sb)* in place of the solution of the substance being examined. Any pink colour in the toluene layer of the test solution is not more intense than that in the toluene layer of the reference solution (100 ppm).

Arsenic To 0.20 g in a 100-ml long-necked combustion flask add 2 g of *anhydrous sodium sulphate*, 7 ml of *sulphuric acid* and 5 ml of *nitric acid*. Heat gently until a clear solution is obtained (about 20 minutes), cool, add 10 ml of *water*, cool again and add 5 g of *hydrazine* *reducing mixture* and 10 ml of *hydrochloric acid*. Immediately attach an air condenser and distil into 15 ml of cooled *water* until a total volume of 30 ml is obtained. Rinse the condenser and dilute the combined distillate and rinsings to 40 ml with *water*. 20 ml of the solution complies with the *limit test for arsenic*, Appendix VII (5 ppm). Use a mixture of 0.5 ml of *arsenic standard solution (1 ppm As)* and 24.5 ml of *water* to prepare the standard.

Barium Shake 20.0 g for 1 minute with 30 ml of *hydrochloric acid*, add 100 ml of *distilled water* and boil. Filter while hot through a hardened filter paper until a clear filtrate is obtained. Wash the filter with 60 ml of *distilled water* and dilute the combined filtrate and washings to 200 ml with *distilled water*. To 10 ml of the solution add 1 ml of 1M *sulphuric acid*. After 30 minutes any opalescence is not more intense than that of a mixture of 10 ml of the test solution and 1 ml of *distilled water*.

Heavy metals Dilute 10.0 ml of the solution prepared in the test for Barium to 20 ml with *water*. 12 ml of the solution complies with *limit test A for heavy metals*, Appendix VII (20 ppm). Use *lead standard solution (1 ppm Pb)* to prepare the standard.

Iron To 8.0 ml of solution A add 4 ml of *water*, mix and add 0.05 ml of *bromine water*, allow to stand for 5 minutes, remove the excess of bromine with a current of air and add 3 ml of 1M *potassium thiocyanate*. Any colour in the solution is not more intense than that in a standard prepared at the same time and in the same manner using a mixture of 4 ml of *iron standard solution (2 ppm Fe)* and 8 ml of a 20% w/v solution of *sulphuric acid* (200 ppm).

Assay To 0.5 g add 5 g of *anhydrous sodium sulphate* and 10 ml of *water*, mix and add 10 ml of *sulphuric acid*. Boil gently in a long-necked combustion flask until clear (about 20 to 25 minutes), cool, add slowly 40 ml of cooled *sulphuric acid (25%)*, cool again and dilute with *water* to 100 ml (solution A). To 300 g of *granulated zinc* add 300 ml of a 2% w/v solution of *mercury(II) nitrate* and 2 ml of *nitric acid*, shake for 10 minutes and wash with *water*. Pack the amalgamated zinc into a glass tube (400 mm × 20 mm) fitted with a tap and a filter plate. Pass through the column 100 ml of 1M *sulphuric acid* followed by 100 ml of *water*, ensuring that the amalgam is covered with liquid throughout. Pass slowly through the column, at a rate of about 3 ml per minute, 200 ml of 0.5M *sulphuric acid* followed by 100 ml of *water*. Collect the combined eluates in a flask containing 50 ml of a 15% w/v solution of *ammonium iron(III) sulphate* in *sulphuric acid (25%)* and titrate immediately with 0.1M *ammonium cerium(IV) nitrate VS* using *ferroin sulphate solution* as indicator (n_1 ml). Pass slowly through the column 200 ml of 0.5M *sulphuric acid* followed by 20 ml of solution A, wash with 100 ml of 0.5M *sulphuric acid* followed by 100 ml of *water*. Collect the combined eluates in a flask containing 50 ml of a 15% w/v solution of *ammonium iron(III) sulphate* in *sulphuric acid (25%)* and titrate immediately with 0.1M *ammonium cerium(IV) nitrate VS* using *ferroin sulphate solution* as indicator (n_2 ml). Calculate the percentage content of TiO_2 from the expression $3.99(n_2 - n_1)/w$ where w is the weight, in g, of the substance being examined taken to prepare solution A.

Preparations

Titanium Dioxide Paste
Titanium Dioxide Elastic Adhesive Bandage

Action and use Protective and pharmaceutical aid.

Tobramycin

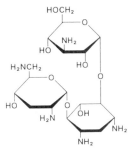

$C_{18}H_{37}N_5O_9$ 467.5   32986-56-4

Tobramycin is 6-*O*-(3-amino-3-deoxy-α-D-glucopyranosyl)-2-deoxy-4-*O*-(2,6-diamino-2,3,6-trideoxy-α-D-*ribo*-hexopyranosyl)-D-streptamine, an antimicrobial base produced by *Streptomyces tenebrarius* or by any other means. The potency is not less than 930 Units per mg, calculated with reference to the anhydrous substance.

Characteristics A white or almost white powder.

Solubility Soluble in 1.5 parts of *water*; very slightly soluble in *ethanol (96%)*; practically insoluble in *chloroform* and in *ether*.

Identification *Test A may be omitted if tests B and C are carried out. Tests B and C may be omitted if test A is carried out.*

A. The *nuclear magnetic resonance spectrum*, Appendix II C, of a 10% w/v solution in *deuterium oxide* is concordant with that of a similar solution of *tobramycin BPCRS*.

B. The *infra-red absorption spectrum*, Appendix II A, is concordant with the *reference spectrum* of tobramycin.

C. Carry out the method for *thin-layer chromatography*, Appendix III A, using a silica gel precoated chromatoplate (Merck silica gel 60 plates are suitable) and a mixture of 60 volumes of *methanol*, 40 volumes of 13.5M *ammonia* and 20 volumes of *chloroform* as the mobile phase. Apply separately to the plate 1 μl of each of the following solutions in *water*. Solution (1) contains 2% w/v of the substance being examined. Solution (2) contains 2% w/v of *tobramycin BPCRS*. Solution (3) is a mixture of equal volumes of solutions (1) and (2). After removal of the plate, allow it to dry in air, spray with a 1% w/v solution of *ninhydrin* in *butan-1-ol* and heat at 105° for 2 minutes. The principal red spot in the chromatogram obtained with solution (1) corresponds to that in the chromatogram obtained with solution (2). The principal red spot in the chromatogram obtained with solution (3) appears as a single compact spot.

Alkalinity pH of a 10% w/v solution, 9.0 to 11.0, Appendix V L.

Specific optical rotation In a 4% w/v solution, +138° to +148°, Appendix V F.

2-Methylpropan-1-ol Not more than 2.0% w/w when determined by the method for *gas chromatography*, Appendix III B, using solutions in *water* containing (1) 0.20% w/v of *2-methylpropan-1-ol* and 0.20% w/v of *propan-2-ol* (internal standard), (2) 10.0% w/v of the substance being examined and (3) 10.0% w/v of the substance being examined and 0.20% w/v of the internal standard.

The chromatographic procedure may be carried out using a glass column (1.5 m × 4 mm) packed with porous polymer beads (80 to 100 mesh) (Porapak Q is suitable) and maintained at 165°.

Calculate the percentage w/w of 2-methylpropan-1-ol.

Related substances Carry out the method for *thin-layer chromatography*, Appendix III A, using a silica gel precoated chromatoplate (Merck silica gel 60 plates are suitable) and a mixture of equal volumes of 13.5M *ammonia*, *butan-2-one* and *ethanol (96%)* as the mobile phase. Apply separately to the plate 1 µl of each of two solutions of the substance being examined in 0.01M *ammonia* containing (1) 4.0% w/v and (2) 0.080% w/v. After removal of the plate, allow it to dry in air, heat at 110° for 10 minutes and spray the hot plate with a solution prepared immediately before use by diluting *sodium hypochlorite solution* with *water* to contain 0.5% of available chlorine. Dry in a current of cold air until a sprayed area of the plate below the line of application gives at most a very faint blue colour with a drop of a 0.5% w/v solution of *potassium iodide* in *starch mucilage*; avoid prolonged exposure to cold air. Spray the plate with a 0.5% w/v solution of *potassium iodide* in *starch mucilage*. Any *secondary spot* in the chromatogram obtained with solution (1) is not more intense than the spot in the chromatogram obtained with solution (2).

Sulphated ash Not more than 0.3%, Appendix IX A.

Water Not more than 8.0% w/w, Appendix IX C. Use 0.3 g.

Assay Carry out the *biological assay of antibiotics*, Appendix XIV A. The precision of the assay is such that the fiducial limits of error are not less than 95% and not more than 105% of the estimated potency.

Storage Tobramycin should be kept in a well-closed container and stored at a temperature not exceeding 25°.

Labelling The label states (1) the number of Units per mg; (2) the date after which the material is not intended to be used; (3) the conditions under which it should be stored; (4) whether or not it is intended for use in the manufacture of a parenteral dosage form.

Preparation
Tobramycin Injection

Action and use Antibacterial.

Tobramycin intended for use in the manufacture of a parenteral dosage form complies with the following additional requirements.

Depressor substances Complies with the *test for depressor substances*, Appendix XIV M. Use per kg of the cat's weight 1 ml of a solution in *water* or *saline solution* containing 3 mg per ml.

Pyrogens Complies with the *test for pyrogens*, Appendix XIV K. Use per kg of the rabbit's weight 1 ml of a solution in *sodium chloride injection* containing 10 mg per ml.

Sterility When intended for use in the manufacture of a parenteral dosage form without further sterilisation, complies with the *test for sterility*, Appendix XVI A.

Alpha Tocopheryl Acetate ☆
α-Tocopheryl Acetate

$C_{31}H_{52}O_3$ 472.7   7695-91-2

Alpha Tocopheryl Acetate is *all-rac*-α-tocopherol acetate. It contains not less than 96.0 per cent and not more than 102.0 per cent of $C_{31}H_{52}O_3$.

Characteristics A clear, slightly greenish-yellow, viscous, oily liquid.

Solubility Practically insoluble in *water*; freely soluble in *absolute ethanol*, in *acetone*, in *chloroform*, in *ether* and in fixed oils; soluble in *ethanol (96%)*.

Identification *Test A may be omitted if tests B and C are carried out. Tests B and C may be omitted if test A is carried out.*

A. The *infra-red absorption spectrum*, Appendix II A, is concordant with the spectrum of α-*tocopherol acetate EPCRS*.

B. The *light absorption*, Appendix II B, in the range 230 to 350 nm of a 0.01% w/v solution in *absolute ethanol* exhibits a maximum only at 284 nm, a shoulder at 278 nm and a minimum only at 254 nm.

C. Carry out the method for *thin-layer chromatography*, Appendix III A, using *silica gel HF254* as the coating substance and a mixture of 80 volumes of *cyclohexane* and 20 volumes of *ether* as the mobile phase. Apply separately to the chromatoplate 10 µl of each of the following solutions. Solution (1) contains 0.5% w/v of the substance being examined in *cyclohexane*. For solution (2) dissolve 10 mg of the substance being examined in 2 ml of 5M *ethanolic sulphuric acid*, heat in a water-bath for 5 minutes, cool, add 2 ml of *water* and 2 ml of *cyclohexane* and shake for 1 minute; use the upper layer. Solution (3) contains 0.5% w/v of α-*tocopherol acetate EPCRS* in *cyclohexane*. Prepare solution (4) in the same manner as solution (2) but using 10 mg of α-*tocopherol acetate EPCRS* in place of the substance being examined.

After removal of the plate, allow it to dry in air and examine under *ultra-violet light (254 nm)*. The principal spot in the chromatogram obtained with solution (1) is similar in position and size to the principal spot in the chromatogram obtained with solution (3). There are two spots in each of the chromatograms obtained with solutions (2) and (4). The spots of higher Rf value are due to α-tocopherol acetate and correspond to the spot in the chromatogram obtained with solution (3). The spots of lower Rf value are due to α-tocopherol. Spray the plate with a mixture of 1 volume of *hydrochloric acid*, 4 volumes of a 0.25% w/v solution of *iron(III) chloride hexahydrate* in *ethanol (96%)* and 4 volumes of a 1% w/v solution of *1,10-phenanthroline hydrochloride* in *ethanol (96%)*. In the chromatograms obtained with solutions (2) and (4) the spot of lower Rf value (α-tocopherol) is orange.

Acid value Not more than 2.0, Appendix X B. Use 2 g.

Light absorption Dissolve 0.150 g in sufficient *absolute ethanol* to produce 100 ml. Dilute separately 10 ml to 100 ml (solution A) and 20 ml to 50 ml (solution B) with the same solvent. Measure the *absorbance* of solution A at the maximum at 284 nm and the *absorbance* of solution B at the minimum at 254 nm, Appendix II B. The A(1%, 1 cm) at 284 nm is 42.0 to 45.0 and the A(1%, 1 cm) at 254 nm is 7.0 to 9.0.

Free tocopherol Not more than 1.0% when determined by the following method. Dissolve 0.5 g in 100 ml of 0.25M *ethanolic sulphuric acid*, add 20 ml of *water* and 0.1 ml of a 0.25% w/v solution of *diphenylamine* in *sulphuric acid* and titrate with 0.01M *ammonium cerium(IV) nitrate VS* until a blue colour is produced that persists for at least 5 seconds. Repeat the operation without the substance being examined. The difference between the titrations represents the amount of ammonium cerium(IV) sulphate required. Each ml of 0.01M *ammonium cerium(IV) nitrate VS* is equivalent to 0.002154 g of tocopherol.

Heavy metals 0.5 g complies with *limit test D for heavy metals*, Appendix VII (20 ppm). Use 1 ml of *lead standard solution (10 ppm Pb)* to prepare the standard.

Sulphated ash Not more than 0.1%, Appendix IX A, Method II. Use 1 g.

Assay Carry out the method for *gas chromatography*, Appendix III B, using the following solutions. Dissolve 1 g of *dotriacontane* (internal standard) in sufficient *hexane* to produce 100 ml (solution A). For solution (1) dissolve 0.1 g of the substance being examined in 10 ml of solution A and dilute to 50 ml with *hexane*. For solution (2) dissolve 0.1 g of *α-tocopherol acetate EPCRS* in 10 ml of solution A and dilute to 50 ml with *hexane*. Solution (3) contains 0.2% w/v of the substance being examined in *hexane*.

The chromatographic procedure may be carried out using a silanised glass column (2 to 3 m × 2.2 to 4.0 mm) packed with *diatomaceous support* (125 to 150 mesh or 150 to 180 mesh) silanised with dimethyldichlorosilane (Chromosorb W/AW/DMCS 80-100 mesh is suitable) and coated with 1% to 5% w/w of methyl silicone gum; place a plug of silanised glass wool at each end of the column. Set the temperature of the column and the rate of flow of carrier gas at values such that the required resolution is achieved (a column temperature of 245° to 280° and a rate of flow of carrier gas of 25 to 90 ml per minute are suitable). Maintain the injection port and the detector at a constant temperature between 270° and 320°. Inject the solutions either directly on to the column or using a glass-lined injection port using an automatic injection device or other reproducible method.

Use an electronic integrator to measure the areas of the peaks. The *resolution factor* determined using the peaks due to the internal standard and α-tocopherol acetate in the chromatogram obtained with solution (2) should be greater than 1.4. Inject 1 μl of solution (2) repeatedly until the response factor as determined below is constant to within 2%.

Inject 1 μl of solution (3) and record the chromatogram using an attenuation such that the height of the peak corresponding to α-tocopherol acetate is greater than 50% of full-scale deflection on the chart paper; during the recording, change the attenuation so that any peak with the same retention time as that of the internal standard is recorded with a sensitivity at least eight times greater than that used for recording the alpha-tocopheryl acetate peak. If a peak with a height of at least 2% of full-scale deflection of the paper is recorded use for the final calculation the corrected peak area (*a*) if necessary, determined using the expression $a = D - (ia_1/fa_2)$, where

D is the area of the internal standard peak in the chromatogram with solution (1), *i* is the area of the interfering peak, a_1 is the area of the α-tocopherol acetate peak in the chromatogram obtained with solution (1), a_2 is the area of the α-tocopherol acetate peak in the chromatogram obtained with solution (3) and *f* is the factor by which the attenuation was changed.

After having verified the resolution factor of the column determine the response factor in the following manner. Inject 1 μl of solution (2) using an attenuation such that the height of the peak due to α-tocopherol acetate is greater than 50% of full-scale deflection on the chart paper. Measure the areas of the peaks corresponding to α-tocopherol acetate and the internal standard and calculate the response factor, *R*, as the ratio of the area of the internal standard peak to the area of the α-tocopherol acetate peak.

Inject 1 μl of solution (1) using the same attenuation and measure the areas of the peaks corresponding to the internal standard and α-tocopherol acetate. Calculate the percentage content of $C_{31}H_{52}O_3$ using the expression $a_1R \times 10^4/aw$ where *w* is the weight of the substance taken in mg.

Storage Alpha Tocopheryl Acetate should be kept in a well-closed container and protected from light.

Action and use Used in prevention and treatment of vitamin E deficiencies.

The title of the monograph in the European Pharmacopœia is α-Tocopherol Acetate.

Tolazamide

Me—⟨◯⟩—SO₂·NH·CO·NH—N⟨◯⟩

$C_{14}H_{21}N_3O_3S$ 311.4   *1156-19-0*

Tolazamide is 1-perhydroazepin-1-yl-3-*p*-tolyl-sulphonylurea. It contains not less than 98.0 per cent and not more than 101.0 per cent of $C_{14}H_{21}N_3O_3S$, calculated with reference to the dried substance.

Characteristics A white or almost white, crystalline powder; odourless or almost odourless.

Solubility Very slightly soluble in *water*; slightly soluble in *ethanol (96%)*; soluble in *acetone*; freely soluble in *chloroform*.

Identification A. The *infra-red absorption spectrum*, Appendix II A, is concordant with the *reference spectrum* of tolazamide.
B. The *light absorption*, Appendix II B, in the range 230 to 350 nm of a 0.04% w/v solution in *ethanol (96%)* exhibits maxima at 256, 263 and 275 nm and a shoulder at 268 nm. The *absorbance* at 256 nm is about 0.78, at 263 nm, about 0.83 and at 275 nm, about 0.62.
C. *Melting point*, about 165°, Appendix V A.

Heavy metals Moisten the residue obtained in the test for Sulphated ash with 1 ml of *hydrochloric acid*, evaporate to dryness and dissolve the residue in 20 ml of *water*. 12 ml of the resulting solution complies with *limit test A for heavy metals*, Appendix VII (20 ppm). Use *lead standard solution (1 ppm Pb)* to prepare the standard.

Related substances Carry out the method for *thin-layer chromatography*, Appendix III A, using *silica gel G* as the coating substance and a mixture of 200 volumes of *chloroform*, 100 volumes of *methanol*, 60 volumes of *cyclohexane* and 23 volumes of 13.5M *ammonia* as the mobile phase. Apply separately to the chromatoplate 10 µl of each of two solutions in *acetone* containing (1) 2.0% w/v of the substance being examined and (2) 0.010% w/v of *toluene*-p-*sulphonamide*. After removal of the plate, dry it in a current of cold air, heat at 110° for 10 minutes, place the hot plate in a tank of chlorine gas prepared by the addition of *hydrochloric acid* to a 5% w/v solution of *potassium permanganate* contained in a beaker placed in the tank and allow to stand for 2 minutes. Dry it in a current of cold air until an area of the plate below the line of application gives at most a very faint blue colour with a 0.5% w/v solution of *potassium iodide* in *starch mucilage*; avoid prolonged exposure to cold air. Spray the plate with a 0.5% w/v solution of *potassium iodide* in *starch mucilage*. Any *secondary spot* in the chromatogram obtained with solution (1) is not more intense than the spot in the chromatogram obtained with solution (2).

Loss on drying When dried to constant weight at 60° at a pressure not exceeding 0.7 kPa, loses not more than 0.5% of its weight. Use 1 g.

Sulphated ash Not more than 0.2%, Appendix IX A. Use 1.0 g.

Assay Dissolve 0.5 g in 20 ml of *butan-2-one* with the aid of gentle heat. Allow to cool, add 30 ml of *ethanol (96%)* and titrate with 0.1M *sodium hydroxide VS* using *phenolphthalein solution* as indicator. Each ml of 0.1M *sodium hydroxide VS* is equivalent to 0.03114 g of $C_{14}H_{21}N_3O_3S$.

Storage Tolazamide should be kept in a well-closed container.

Preparation
Tolazamide Tablets

Action and use Hypoglycaemic.

Tolbutamide ☆

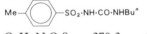

$C_{12}H_{18}N_2O_3S$ 270.3   *64-77-7*

Tolbutamide is 1-butyl-3-tosylurea. It contains not less than 99.0 per cent and not more than 101.0 per cent of $C_{12}H_{18}N_2O_3S$, calculated with reference to the dried substance.

Characteristics A white, crystalline powder; almost odourless.

Solubility Practically insoluble in *water*; soluble in 10 parts of *ethanol (96%)*; soluble in *acetone* and in *chloroform*; slightly soluble in *ether*. It dissolves in dilute aqueous solutions of alkali hydroxides.

Identification *Test A may be omitted if tests B, C and D are carried out. Tests B and C may be omitted if tests A and D are carried out.*

A. The *infra-red absorption spectrum*, Appendix II A, is concordant with the spectrum of *tolbutamide EPCRS*.

B. Dissolve 25 mg in sufficient *methanol* to produce 100 ml. The *light absorption* of the resulting solution,

Appendix II B, in the range 245 to 300 nm exhibits maxima at 258, 263 and 275 nm and a shoulder at 268 nm. Dilute the solution with sufficient *methanol* to produce a 0.001% w/v solution. The *light absorption* in the range 220 to 235 nm exhibits a maximum only at 228 nm. The A(1%, 1 cm) at the maximum at 228 nm is 480 to 520.

C. Boil 0.2 g under a reflux condenser for 30 minutes with 8 ml of 5M *sulphuric acid* and allow to cool. The *melting point* of the resulting crystals, after recrystallisation from hot *water* and drying at 100° to 105°, is 135° to 140°, Appendix V A, Method I.

D. *Melting point*, 128° to 131°, Appendix V A, Method I.

Acidity To 2 g add 50 ml of *carbon dioxide-free water*, heat at 70° for 5 minutes, cool rapidly and filter. The pH of the filtrate is 4.5 to 5.5, Appendix V L.

Clarity and colour of solution A 2.0% w/v solution in 1M *sodium hydroxide* is *clear*, Appendix IV A, and *colourless*, Appendix IV B, Method II.

Heavy metals Dissolve 1.0 g in 20 ml of a mixture of 15 volumes of *water* and 85 volumes of *acetone*. 12 ml of the resulting solution complies with *limit test B for heavy metals*, Appendix VII (20 ppm). Use the solution obtained by diluting 1 ml of *lead standard solution (100 ppm Pb)* to 100 ml with a mixture of 15 volumes of *water* and 85 volumes of *acetone* to prepare the standard.

Related substances Carry out the method for *thin-layer chromatography*, Appendix III A, using *silica gel G* as the coating substance and a mixture of 90 volumes of *chloroform*, 8 volumes of *methanol* and 2 volumes of *anhydrous formic acid* as the mobile phase. Apply separately to the chromatoplate 5 µl of each of solutions (1) and (2) and 10 µl of solution (3). Solution (1) contains 5% w/v of the substance being examined in *acetone*. Solution (2) contains 0.015% w/v of *toluene*-p-*sulphonamide* in *acetone*. Solution (3) is a mixture of equal volumes of solutions (1) and (2). After removal of the plate, dry it in a current of warm air and heat at 110° for 10 minutes. While still hot, place the plate in a chromatographic tank with an evaporating dish containing a 5% w/v solution of *potassium permanganate*, add an equal volume of *hydrochloric acid* and close the tank. Leave the plate in the tank for 2 minutes, then place it in a current of cold air until the excess of chlorine is removed and an area of coating below the line of application gives only a very faint blue colour with *potassium iodide and starch solution*; avoid prolonged exposure to cold air. Spray the plate with *potassium iodide and starch solution* and allow to stand for 5 minutes. Any *secondary spot* in the chromatogram obtained with solution (1) is not more intense than the spot in the chromatogram obtained with solution (2). The test is not valid unless the chromatogram obtained with solution (3) shows two clearly separated spots.

Loss on drying When dried to constant weight at 100° to 105°, loses not more than 0.5% of its weight. Use 1 g.

Sulphated ash Not more than 0.1%, Appendix IX A, Method II. Use 1 g.

Assay Dissolve 0.25 g in a mixture of 40 ml of *ethanol (96%)* and 20 ml of *water* and titrate with 0.1M *sodium hydroxide VS* using 1 ml of *dilute phenolphthalein solution* as indicator. Each ml of 0.1M *sodium hydroxide VS* is equivalent to 0.02703 g of $C_{12}H_{18}N_2O_3S$.

Storage Tolbutamide should be kept in a well-closed container.

Preparation
Tolbutamide Tablets
Action and use Hypoglycaemic.

Tolnaftate

C$_{19}$H$_{17}$NOS   307.4   *2398-96-1*

Tolnaftate is *O*-2-naphthyl *N*-methyl-*m*-tolyl-thiocarbamate. It contains not less than 97.0 per cent and not more than 103.0 per cent of C$_{19}$H$_{17}$NOS, calculated with reference to the dried substance.

Characteristics A white to creamy-white powder; odourless or almost odourless.

Solubility Practically insoluble in *water*; very slightly soluble in *ethanol (96%)*; soluble in 9 parts of *acetone*, in 3 parts of *chloroform* and in 55 parts of *ether*.

Identification A. The *infra-red absorption spectrum*, Appendix II A, is concordant with the *reference spectrum* of tolnaftate.

B. The *light absorption*, Appendix II B, in the range 230 to 350 nm of a 0.001% w/v solution in *methanol* exhibits a maximum only at 257 nm. The *absorbance* at 257 nm is about 0.71.

C. Carry out the method for *thin-layer chromatography*, Appendix III A, using *silica gel GF254* as the coating substance and *toluene* as the mobile phase. Apply separately to the chromatoplate 10 μl of each of two solutions in a mixture of equal volumes of *toluene* and *ethanol (96%)* containing (1) 0.1% w/v of the substance being examined and (2) 0.1% w/v of *tolnaftate BPCRS*. After removal of the plate, allow it to dry in air and examine under *ultra-violet light (254 nm)*. The principal spot in the chromatogram obtained with solution (1) corresponds to that in the chromatogram obtained with solution (2).

Melting point 109° to 112°, Appendix V A.

Loss on drying When dried at 60° at a pressure not exceeding 0.7 kPa for 3 hours, loses not more than 0.5% of its weight. Use 1 g.

Sulphated ash Not more than 0.1%, Appendix IX A.

Assay Dissolve 0.1 g in sufficient *methanol* to produce 250 ml, dilute 2 ml to 100 ml with *methanol* and measure the *absorbance* of the resulting solution at the maximum at 257 nm, Appendix II B. Calculate the content of C$_{19}$H$_{17}$NOS taking 708 as the value of A(1%, 1 cm) at the maximum at 257 nm.

Action and use Antifungal.

Tragacanth ☆

Tragacanth is the air-hardened gummy exudate, flowing naturally or obtained by incision, from the trunk and branches of *Astragalus gummifer* Labillardière and certain other species of *Astragalus* grown in Western Asia.

Characteristics Odourless; almost tasteless. On the addition of about 10 times its weight of *water*, it forms a mucilaginous gel.

Macroscopical Occurs as thin, flattened ribbons, about 30 mm long, 10 mm wide and up to 1 mm in thickness, more or less curved, marked on the surface by fine longitudinal striae and concentric transverse ridges; white, translucent, horny; fracture, short. Occurs also as thicker, less brittle pieces, pale yellow to white and more opaque.

Microscopical When powdered, it shows in the gummy mass numerous stratified cellular membranes which turn violet on the addition of *iodinated zinc chloride solution*. The mass includes starch granules, isolated or in small groups, rounded or occasionally deformed, diameter 4 to 10 μm, occasionally up to 20 μm, with a central hilum, visible in polarised light.

Identification A. Carry out the method for *thin-layer chromatography*, Appendix III A, using a slurry of *kieselguhr G* in a 1.6% w/v solution of *sodium dihydrogen orthophosphate* to coat the chromatoplate and a mixture of 50 volumes of *acetone*, 40 volumes of *butan-1-ol* and 10 volumes of a 1.6% w/v solution of *sodium dihydrogen orthophosphate* as the mobile phase, but allowing the mobile phase to ascend 10 cm above the line of application. Apply separately to the plate, as bands 20 mm long and not more than 3 mm wide, 10 μl of each of the following solutions. For solution (1) add to 1 g, in powder, 25 ml of a mixture of 4 volumes of *sulphuric acid* and 96 volumes of *water* and heat under a reflux condenser in a water-bath for 90 minutes; cool, neutralise 10 ml with 3 g of *barium carbonate*, shake for 90 minutes, filter, add 9 ml of *methanol* to 1 ml of the filtrate, centrifuge and use the supernatant liquid. For solution (2) dissolve 10 mg of *L-arabinose*, 10 mg of *L-fucose*, 10 mg of *D-galactose* and 10 mg of *D-xylose* in 1 ml of *water* and add sufficient *methanol* to produce 10 ml.

After removal of the plate, dry it in a current of warm air for a few minutes and develop again using the same mobile phase but allowing the solvent front to ascend 15 cm from the line of application. After removal of the plate, dry it at 110° for 10 minutes, spray with *aminohippuric acid reagent*, using 10 ml for a plate 200 mm × 200 mm in size, and dry it at 110° for 10 minutes. In the chromatogram obtained with solution (2) four clearly separated coloured bands are seen which, in order of increasing Rf value, are due to galactose (yellowish-brown), arabinose (reddish-brown), xylose (red) and fucose (yellow). The chromatogram obtained with solution (1) shows four coloured bands corresponding to those in the chromatogram obtained with solution (2); in addition a faint yellowish band is seen at the solvent front and a yellow band is seen between the bands corresponding to galactose and arabinose. No red band is seen near the solvent front (methylcellulose).

B. Moisten 0.5 g, in powder, with 1 ml of *ethanol (96%)* and add gradually, with shaking, 50 ml of *water* until a homogeneous mucilage is produced. To 5 ml of the mucilage add 5 ml of *water* and 2 ml of a 4.73% w/v solution of *barium hydroxide*; a slightly flocculent precipitate is produced. Heat on a water-bath for 10 minutes; an intense yellow colour is produced.

C. Heat a mixture of 4 ml of a 0.5% w/v dispersion in *water* and 0.5 ml of *hydrochloric acid* on a water-bath for 30 minutes, add 3 ml of 10M *sodium hydroxide* and 6 ml of *modified potassium cupri-tartrate solution* and heat on a water-bath. A reddish-brown precipitate is produced.

Flow time Not less than 10 seconds, or not less than 50 seconds if the substance is to be used for the preparation of emulsions, when determined by the following method. To 1.0 g, in *No. 125* to *No. 250 powder*, in a 1000-ml round-bottomed glass-stoppered flask add 8 ml of *ethanol (96%)* and disperse the suspension on the inner surface of the flask by shaking, taking care not to wet the stopper. Add 72 ml of *water* in one portion, close the flask, shake vigorously for 3 minutes, allow to stand for 24 hours and again shake vigorously for 3 minutes. Eliminate air bubbles by reducing the pressure above the mucilage for 5 minutes and transfer the mucilage to a 50-ml cylinder. Dip into the mucilage a glass tube (200 mm × 6.0 mm) graduated at 20 mm and 120 mm from the lower end; the tube must not be rinsed with surface-active substances. Close the tube with a finger when the mucilage reaches the upper mark, withdraw the closed tube, remove the finger and measure with a stop-watch the time needed for the meniscus to reach the lower graduation. Repeat the operation a further three times and determine the average value of the last three determinations.

Acacia and other soluble gums Disperse 50 mg, in *No. 355 powder*, in 20 ml of *carbon dioxide-free water* and add 10 ml of *lead(II) acetate solution*; a flocculent precipitate is produced. Centrifuge and add 10 ml of *lead subacetate solution* to the clear supernatant liquid; the solution may become slightly cloudy but no precipitate is produced.

Foreign matter To 2 g, in *No. 355 powder*, in a 250-ml round-bottomed flask add 95 ml of *methanol*, swirl to moisten the powder and add 60 ml of *7M hydrochloric acid*. Add a few glass beads about 4 mm in diameter and heat under a reflux condenser in a water-bath for 3 hours, shaking occasionally. Remove the glass beads and filter the hot suspension under reduced pressure through a sintered-glass crucible (BS porosity No. 1). Rinse the flask with a small quantity of *water*, passing the rinsings through the filter. Wash the residue on the filter with 40 ml of *methanol* and dry to constant weight at 110°. The residue weighs not more than 20 mg (1.0%).

Sterculia A. Shake 2 g, in *No. 355 powder*, with 10 ml of *ethanol (60%)* in a 10-ml stoppered cylinder, graduated in 0.1 ml intervals. Any gel produced occupies not more than 1.5 ml.
B. Shake 1 g, in *No. 355 powder*, with 100 ml of *water* and titrate with *0.01M sodium hydroxide VS* using *methyl red solution* as indicator. Not more than 5.0 ml of *0.01M sodium hydroxide VS* is required to change the colour of the solution.

Ash Not more than 4.0%, Appendix XI J, Method II. Use 1 g, in powder.

Microbial contamination* 1.0 g is free from *Escherichia coli* and 10.0 g is free from Salmonellae, Appendix XVI B1.

Storage Tragacanth should be kept in a well-closed container.

Labelling The label states whether the material is suitable for use in the preparation of emulsions.

*In certain states party to the Convention on the Elaboration of a European Pharmacopœia, Tragacanth may be required to comply with a limit for a total viable aerobic count of 10^4 micro-organisms per gram, determined by plate count, Appendix XVI B2.

Powdered Tragacanth

Powdered Tragacanth is Tragacanth in powder.

Characteristics White or almost white; in colourless, angular, microscopic fragments which, when treated with *water*, increase in size and finally disappear; odourless or almost odourless. Diagnostic structures: exhibits numerous, stratified cellular membranes which turn violet on the addition of *iodinated zinc chloride solution*; starch granules, isolated or in small groups, rounded or occasionally deformed, diameter 4 to 10 μm, occasionally up to 20 μm, with central hilum visible in polarised light.

Identification Complies with the tests described under Tragacanth.

Apparent viscosity Introduce 0.88 g, accurately weighed, into a dry 500-ml conical flask and add 5 ml of *ethanol (96%)*. Ensure that the gum is completely wetted and evenly dispersed over the inner surface of the flask, add 195 ml of *water* as quickly as possible and shake. Allow to stand for 1 hour, swirling frequently. Attach a reflux condenser to the flask and immerse in vigorously boiling water so that the surface of the water is about 2.5 cm above the surface of the mucilage. Continue heating for 1 hour, gently swirling at intervals of 15 minutes without removing the flask from the water. Remove the flask from the water, stopper, allow to stand for 2 hours, shaking frequently, and allow to stand for 24 hours. Determine the efflux time, at 20°, of 50 ml using a Redwood No. 1 viscometer. Multiply the mean of six readings by $27/x$ where x is the efflux time, in seconds, at 20° of 50 ml of *water* determined in the same instrument. The corrected efflux time is not less than 100 seconds.

Acacia and other soluble gums; Foreign matter; Sterculia; Ash Complies with the requirements stated under Tragacanth.

Microbial contamination 1.0 g is free from *Escherichia coli* and 10.0 g is free from Salmonellae, Appendix XVI B1.

Storage Powdered Tragacanth should be kept in a well-closed container.

Labelling The label states whether the material is suitable for use in the preparation of emulsions.

Tranexamic Acid

$C_8H_{15}NO_2$ 157.2   *1197-18-8*

Tranexamic Acid is *trans*-4-aminomethylcyclo-hexanecarboxylic acid. It contains not less than 99.0 per cent and not more than 101.0 per cent of $C_8H_{15}NO_2$, calculated with reference to the dried substance.

Characteristics A white, crystalline powder; odourless or almost odourless.

Solubility Freely soluble in *water* and in *glacial acetic acid*; practically insoluble in *ethanol (96%)* and in *ether*.

Identification A. The *infra-red absorption spectrum*, Appendix II A, is concordant with the *reference spectrum* of tranexamic acid.

B. To 1 ml of a 1% w/v solution add 1 ml of a 0.2% w/v solution of *ninhydrin* in *ethanol (96%)* and heat on a water-bath for 2 minutes. A dark bluish-violet colour is produced.

C. Dissolve 0.2 g in 10 ml of 5M *sodium hydroxide*, add 0.2 ml of *benzoyl chloride* and shake vigorously for 10 minutes. Acidify to pH 4 with 2M *hydrochloric acid*, filter, wash the residue with 5 ml of *ether* and dry at 50° at a pressure of 2 kPa. The *melting point* of the residue is about 186°, Appendix V A.

Acidity or alkalinity pH of a 5% w/v solution, 6.5 to 7.5, Appendix V L.

Bromide Add 1 ml of a 5.0% w/v solution dropwise to 2 ml of *peroxymonosulphuric acid reagent* in a stoppered tube, mix well, allow to stand for 3 minutes at room temperature and then cool in ice for 1 minute. Add dropwise 1 ml of a 0.006% w/v solution of *magenta*. Three minutes after the first drop of the magenta solution has been added add 10 ml of *benzyl alcohol*, shake vigorously, centrifuge and measure the *absorbance* of the alcohol layer at the maximum at 570 nm, Appendix II B, using *benzyl alcohol* in the reference cell. The *absorbance* is not more than that obtained by repeating the procedure using 1 ml of a 0.005% w/v solution of *potassium bromide* in place of the solution of the substance being examined.

Heavy metals 12 ml of a 5.0% w/v solution complies with *limit test A for heavy metals*, Appendix VII (20 ppm). Use *lead standard solution (1 ppm Pb)* to prepare the standard.

Iminodi-acid Carry out the method for *thin-layer chromatography*, Appendix III A, using *silica gel G* as the coating substance and a mixture of 80 volumes of *butan-1-ol*, 20 volumes of *glacial acetic acid* and 20 volumes of *water* as the mobile phase. Apply separately to the chromatoplate 2 µl of each of two solutions in *water* containing (1) 10.0% w/v of the substance being examined and (2) 0.10% w/v of trans-trans-*4,4'-iminodimethylene-di(cyclohexanecarboxylic acid)* BPCRS. After removal of the plate, allow it to dry in air, spray with a 0.25% w/v solution of *ninhydrin* in a mixture of equal volumes of *methanol* and *pyridine* and heat at 130° for 15 minutes. Any spot corresponding to the iminodi-acid in the chromatogram obtained with solution (1) is not more intense than the spot in the chromatogram obtained with solution (2).

Cis-**isomer** Carry out the method for *high-performance liquid chromatography*, Appendix III D, using the following solutions. For solution (1) dilute 1 volume of solution (2) to 200 volumes with *ethanol-free chloroform*. For solution (2) dissolve 20 mg of the substance being examined in 1 ml of 0.1M *boric acid*, add 4 ml of a 10% w/v solution of *4-fluoro-3-nitrobenzotrifluoride* in *dimethyl sulphoxide* and shake for 10 minutes. Add 50 ml of 0.1M *hydrochloric acid* and extract with two 10-ml quantities of *chloroform*. Evaporate the chloroform extract to dryness and dissolve the residue in 2 ml of *ethanol-free chloroform*.

The chromatographic procedure may be carried out using (a) a stainless steel column (30 cm × 4 mm) packed with *stationary phase A* (10 µm) (µPorasil is suitable), (b) a mixture of 120 volumes of *hexane*, 80 volumes of *ethanol-free chloroform* and 1 volume of *glacial acetic acid* as the mobile phase with a flow rate of 2 ml per minute and (c) a detection wavelength of 420 nm.

In the chromatogram obtained with solution (2) the area of any peak eluting immediately before the principal peak

is not greater than the area of the principal peak in the chromatogram obtained with solution (1).

Loss on drying When dried to constant weight at 105°, loses not more than 1% of its weight. Use 1 g.

Sulphated ash Not more than 0.1%, Appendix IX A.

Assay Carry out Method I for *non-aqueous titration*, Appendix VIII A, using 0.25 g and *crystal violet solution* as indicator. Each ml of 0.1M *perchloric acid VS* is equivalent to 0.01572 g of $C_8H_{15}NO_2$.

Preparations
Tranexamic Acid Injection
Tranexamic Acid Tablets

Action and use Antifibrinolytic; haemostatic.

Tranylcypromine Sulphate

$(C_9H_{11}N)_2,H_2SO_4$ 364.5   *13492-01-8*

Tranylcypromine Sulphate is *trans*-2-phenylcyclo-propylamine sulphate. It contains not less than 98.0 per cent and not more than 101.0 per cent of $(C_9H_{11}N)_2,H_2SO_4$, calculated with reference to the dried substance.

Characteristics A white or almost white, crystalline powder; odourless or with a faint odour similar to that of cinnamaldehyde.

Solubility Soluble in 20 parts of *water*; very slightly soluble in *ethanol (96%)* and in *ether*; insoluble in *chloroform*.

Identification A. The *infra-red absorption spectrum*, Appendix II A, is concordant with the *reference spectrum* of tranylcypromine sulphate.

B. The *light absorption*, Appendix II B, in the range 230 to 350 nm of a 0.05% w/v solution in 0.1M *sulphuric acid* exhibits three maxima, at 258, 264 and 271 nm. The *absorbance* at 258 nm is about 0.72, at 264 nm, about 0.81 and at 271 nm, about 0.58.

C. Suspend 5 mg in 0.5 ml of *ethanol (96%)* and add 5 mg of *ninhydrin*. A purple colour is produced within 15 minutes.

D. Yields the *reactions* characteristic of sulphates, Appendix VI.

Related substances Dissolve 10 mg of *4-chloroaniline* (internal standard) in sufficient 0.1M *hydrochloric acid* to produce 20 ml (solution A). Carry out the method for *gas chromatography*, Appendix III B, using the following solutions. For solution (1) add 5 ml of 1M *sodium hydroxide* to 1 ml of solution A, extract with 10 ml of *dichloromethane*, add 1 ml of *trifluoroacetic anhydride* to the dichloromethane extract and allow to stand for 10 minutes. Evaporate the solution at a pressure of 2 kPa using a rotary evaporator and a water-bath at 20° and dissolve the residue in 2 ml of *dichloromethane*. For solution (2) dissolve 0.1 g of the substance being examined in 5 ml of *water*, add 1 ml of 5M *sodium hydroxide* and continue as for solution (1), beginning at the words 'extract with . . .'. For solution (3) dissolve 0.1 g of the substance being examined in 5 ml of *water*, add 1 ml of solution A and 1 ml of 5M *sodium hydroxide* and continue as for solution (1), beginning at the words 'extract with . . .'.

The chromatographic procedure may be carried out using a glass column (1.5 m × 4 mm) packed with *acid-washed, silanised diatomaceous support* (100 to 120 mesh) coated with 3% w/w of cyanopropylmethylphenyl methyl silicone fluid (OV-225 is suitable) and maintained at 170°.

In the chromatogram obtained with solution (3) the area of any *secondary peak* is not greater than that of the peak due to the trifluoracetyl derivative of 4-chloroaniline.

Loss on drying When dried to constant weight at 105°, loses not more than 0.5% of its weight. Use 1 g.

Sulphated ash Not more than 0.1%, Appendix IX A.

Assay Carry out Method I for *non-aqueous titration*, Appendix VIII A, using 0.3 g and determining the end-point potentiometrically. Each ml of 0.1M *perchloric acid VS* is equivalent to 0.03645 g of $(C_9H_{11}N)_2,H_2SO_4$.

Storage Tranylcypromine Sulphate should be kept in a well-closed container.

Preparation
Tranylcypromine Tablets

Action and use Monoamine oxidase inhibitor.

Tretinoin

Me Me   Me   Me
                              CO₂H

$C_{20}H_{28}O_2$ 300.4   *302-79-4*

Tretinoin is 15-apo-β-caroten-15-oic acid. It contains not less than 97.0 per cent and not more than 103.0 per cent of $C_{20}H_{28}O_2$, calculated with reference to the dried substance.

Characteristics A yellow to light orange, crystalline powder. It is very sensitive to light and oxygen.

Solubility Insoluble in *water*; slightly soluble in *ethanol (96%)* and in *chloroform*; soluble in *ether*.

Identification A. The *infra-red absorption spectrum*, Appendix II A, is concordant with the *reference spectrum* of tretinoin.
B. The *light absorption*, Appendix II B, in the range 300 to 450 nm of a 0.0005% w/v solution in a 0.0085% v/v solution of *hydrochloric acid* in *propan-2-ol* exhibits a maximum only at 353 nm. The *absorbance* at 353 nm is about 0.76.

Related substances Carry out in subdued light the method for *high-performance liquid chromatography*, Appendix III D, using three freshly prepared solutions in *methanol* containing (1) 0.0010% w/v of the substance being examined, (2) 0.20% w/v of the substance being examined and (3) 0.0040% w/v of *isotretinoin BPCRS*.

The chromatographic procedure may be carried out using (a) a stainless steel column (20 cm × 4.6 mm) packed with *stationary phase C* (10 μm) (Spherisorb ODS 1 is suitable), (b) as the mobile phase a solution containing 0.5% v/v of *glacial acetic acid* in a mixture of *methanol* and *water* adjusted to give a retention time for tretinoin of about 15 minutes (a mixture of 77 volumes of *methanol* and 23 volumes of *water* is usually suitable) and (c) a detection wavelength of 353 nm.

In the chromatogram obtained with solution (2) the area of any peak corresponding to isotretinoin is not greater than the area of the peak in the chromatogram obtained with solution (3) and the sum of the areas of any other *secondary peaks* is not greater than the area of the principal peak in the chromatogram obtained with solution (1). Adjust the sensitivity of the instrument to give a recorder response of about 70% of full-scale deflection for the principal peak in the chromatogram obtained with solution (1). The method is not valid unless the *column efficiency* is not less than 10,000 theoretical plates per metre determined using this peak.

Loss on drying When dried at 105° for 3 hours, loses not more than 0.5% of its weight. Use 1 g.

Sulphated ash Not more than 0.1%, Appendix IX A.

Assay Dissolve 0.5 g in 75 ml of *dimethylformamide* and carry out in subdued light Method II for *non-aqueous titration*, Appendix VIII A, using 0.1M *tetrabutylammonium hydroxide VS* as titrant and *thymolphthalein solution* as indicator. Each ml of 0.1M *tetrabutylammonium hydroxide VS* is equivalent to 0.03004 g of $C_{20}H_{28}O_2$.

Storage Tretinoin should be kept in a well-closed container, protected from light and stored at a temperature not exceeding −15°.

Preparations
Tretinoin Gel
Tretinoin Solution

Action and use Used in treatment of acne.

Triamcinolone

                    CH₂OH
        HO   Me   CO
                        --OH
        Me   H
                        ''OH
          F   H
    O

$C_{21}H_{27}FO_6$ 394.4   *124-94-7*

Triamcinolone is 9α-fluoro-11β,16α,17α,21-tetrahydroxypregna-1,4-diene-3,20-dione. It contains not less than 97.0 per cent and not more than 103.0 per cent of $C_{21}H_{27}FO_6$, calculated with reference to the dried substance.

Characteristics A white or almost white, crystalline powder; slightly hygroscopic.

Solubility Slightly soluble in *water*; soluble in 40 parts of *ethanol (96%)*; very slightly soluble in *chloroform* and in *ether*.

Identification A. The *infra-red absorption spectrum*, Appendix II A, is concordant with the *reference spectrum* of triamcinolone. If the spectra are not concordant dissolve a sufficient quantity in the minimum volume of *methanol*, evaporate to dryness, dry the residue at 60° at a pressure not exceeding 0.7 kPa and prepare a new spectrum of the residue.
B. The *light absorption*, Appendix II B, in the range 230 to 350 nm of a 0.002% w/v solution in *methanol* exhibits a maximum only at 238 nm. The *absorbance* at 238 nm is about 0.78.
C. Dissolve 1 mg in 6 ml of *ethanol (96%)*, add 5 ml of a 1% w/v solution of *butylated hydroxytoluene* in *ethanol*

(96%) and 5 ml of 1M *sodium hydroxide* and heat on a water-bath under a reflux condenser for 20 minutes. A pinkish-lavender colour is produced.

Specific optical rotation In a 1% w/v solution in *dimethylformamide*, +65° to +72°, Appendix V F.

Related substances Carry out the method for *high-performance liquid chromatography*, Appendix III D, using three solutions of the substance being examined in *methanol* containing (1) 0.0010% w/v, (2) 0.0040% w/v and (3) 0.10% w/v.

The chromatographic procedure may be carried out using (a) a stainless steel column (20 cm × 4 mm) packed with *stationary phase C* (5 μm) (Hypersil ODS is suitable), (b) as the mobile phase a mixture of *methanol* and *water*, adjusted so that the retention time of triamcinolone is about 5 minutes (a mixture of equal volumes of *methanol* and *water* is usually suitable) with a flow rate of 2 ml per minute and (c) a detection wavelength of 238 nm.

For solution (3) allow the chromatography to proceed for four times the retention time of the triamcinolone peak. The area of any *secondary peak* in the chromatogram obtained with solution (3) is not greater than twice the area of the principal peak in the chromatogram obtained with solution (1) and not more than one such peak has an area greater than that of the principal peak in the chromatogram obtained with solution (1). The sum of the areas of any such peaks is not greater than the area of the principal peak in the chromatogram obtained with solution (2). The test is not valid unless the *column efficiency*, determined using the principal peak in the chromatogram obtained with solution (2), is 10,000 theoretical plates per metre or more.

Loss on drying When dried at 60° at a pressure not exceeding 0.7 kPa for 3 hours, loses not more than 2.0% of its weight. Use 1 g.

Sulphated ash Not more than 0.2%, Appendix IX A.

Assay Dissolve 25 mg in sufficient *ethanol* (96%) to produce 100 ml. Dilute 2 ml to 50 ml with *ethanol* (96%) and measure the *absorbance* of the resulting solution at the maximum at 238 nm, Appendix II B. Calculate the content of $C_{21}H_{27}FO_6$ taking 380 as the value of A(1%, 1 cm) at the maximum at 238 nm.

Storage Triamcinolone should be kept in a well-closed container.

Preparation
Triamcinolone Tablets

Action and use Corticosteroid.

Triamcinolone Acetonide ☆

$C_{24}H_{31}FO_6$ 434.5   76-25-5

Triamcinolone Acetonide is 9α-fluoro-11β,21-dihydroxy-16α,17α-isopropylidenedioxypregna-1,4-diene-3,20-dione. It contains not less than 96.0 per cent and not more than 104.0 per cent of $C_{24}H_{31}FO_6$, calculated with reference to the dried substance.

Characteristics A white or almost white, crystalline powder.

Solubility Practically insoluble in *water*; sparingly soluble in *ethanol* (96%) and in *chloroform*; very slightly soluble in *ether*.

Identification *Test A may be omitted if tests B, C and D are carried out. Tests C and D may be omitted if tests A and B are carried out.*

A. The *infra-red absorption spectrum*, Appendix II A, is concordant with the spectrum of *triamcinolone acetonide EPCRS*. If the spectra are not concordant, dissolve the substances separately in the minimum volume of *methanol*, evaporate to dryness on a water-bath and prepare new spectra of the residues.

B. Complies with the test for *identification of steroids*, Appendix III A, using *impregnating solvent I* and *mobile phase H* and applying 5 μl of each solution.

C. Complies with the test for *identification of steroids*, Appendix III A, using the conditions specified in test B and the following solutions. For solution (1) dissolve 10 mg of the substance being examined in 1.5 ml of *glacial acetic acid* in a separating funnel, add 0.5 ml of a 2% w/v solution of *chromium trioxide* and allow to stand for 30 minutes. Add 5 ml of water and 2 ml of *dichloromethane*, shake vigorously for 2 minutes, allow to separate and use the lower layer. Prepare solution (2) in the same manner as solution (1) but using 10 mg of *triamcinolone acetonide EPCRS* in place of the substance being examined.

D. Heat 0.5 ml of *chromic—sulphuric acid mixture* in a small test-tube in a naked flame until white fumes appear in the upper part of the tube; the solution wets the sides of the tube readily and there is no greasiness. Add 2 mg of the substance being examined and again heat in a naked flame until white fumes appear; the solution does not wet the sides of the tube and does not pour easily from the tube.

Light absorption Dissolve 10 mg in sufficient *ethanol* (96%) to produce 100 ml and dilute 10 ml to 100 ml with *ethanol* (96%). The *light absorption* of the resulting solution, Appendix II B, in the range 225 to 320 nm exhibits a maximum at 239 nm. The A(1%, 1 cm) at the maximum at 239 nm is 340 to 370.

Specific optical rotation In a 1% w/v solution in *1,4-dioxan*, +100° to +107°, Appendix V F.

Related substances Carry out the method for *thin-layer chromatography*, Appendix III A, using *silica gel GF254* as the coating substance and a mixture of 77 volumes of *dichloromethane*, 15 volumes of *ether*, 8 volumes of *methanol* and 1.2 volumes of *water* as the mobile phase. Apply separately to the chromatoplate 5 µl of each of three solutions of the substance being examined in *chloroform* containing (1) 1.0% w/v, (2) 0.020% w/v and (3) 0.010% w/v. After removal of the plate, allow it to dry in air and examine under *ultra-violet light (254 nm)*. Any *secondary spot* in the chromatogram obtained with solution (1) is not more intense than the spot in the chromatogram obtained with solution (2) and not more than one such spot is more intense than the spot in the chromatogram obtained with solution (3).

Loss on drying When dried at 100° to 105° for 3 hours, loses not more than 2.0% of its weight. Use 0.5 g.

Assay Carry out the *tetrazolium assay of steroids*, Appendix VIII P, and calculate the content of $C_{24}H_{31}FO_6$ from the *absorbance* obtained by repeating the operation using *triamcinolone acetonide EPCRS* in place of the substance being examined.

Storage Triamcinolone Acetonide should be kept in a well-closed container and protected from light.

Preparations
Triamcinolone Cream
Triamcinolone Ointment
Triamcinolone Dental Paste

Action and use Corticosteroid.

Triamterene ☆

$C_{12}H_{11}N_7$ 253.3   *396-01-0*

Triamterene is 2,4,7-triamino-6-phenyl-pteridine. It contains not less than 99.0 per cent and not more than 101.0 per cent of $C_{12}H_{11}N_7$, calculated with reference to the dried substance.

Characteristics A yellow, crystalline powder; odourless.

Solubility Very slightly soluble in *water*, in *ethanol (96%)* and in *chloroform*; practically insoluble in *ether*.

Identification A. The *light absorption*, Appendix II B, in the range 255 to 380 nm of a 0.001% w/v solution in a mixture of 1 volume of 1M *hydrochloric acid* and 9 volumes of *ethanol (96%)* exhibits two maxima, at 262 nm and 360 nm, and a shoulder at 285 nm.
B. A 0.1% w/v solution in *anhydrous formic acid*, when examined under ultra-violet light (365 nm), exhibits an intense blue fluorescence. Solutions in other acids also exhibit a blue fluorescence.

Acidity Boil 1 g with 20 ml of *water* for 5 minutes, cool, filter and wash the filter with three 10-ml quantities of *water*. Combine the filtrate and washings and add 0.3 ml of *dilute phenolphthalein solution*. Not more than 1.5 ml of 0.01M *sodium hydroxide VS* is required to change the colour of the solution.

5-Nitroso-2,4,6-triaminopyrimidine Carry out the method for *thin-layer chromatography*, Appendix III A, using *silica*

gel HF254 as the coating substance. Apply separately to the chromatoplate, as bands 1.5 cm long, two applications of 10 µl of each of two freshly prepared solutions in *anhydrous formic acid* containing (1) 4.0% w/v of the substance being examined and (2) 0.0040% w/v of *5-nitroso-2,4,6-triaminopyrimidine EPCRS*, drying the band in a current of air after each application. Develop over a path of 5 cm using *ether* as the mobile phase, remove the plate, allow it to dry in air and develop over a path of 10 cm using as the mobile phase a 0.05% w/v solution of *fluorescein sodium* in a mixture of 80 volumes of *ethyl acetate*, 10 volumes of *glacial acetic acid* and 10 volumes of *methanol*. After removal of the plate, dry it in a current of air, expose to ammonia vapour for a few seconds and examine under *ultra-violet light (254 nm and 365 nm)*. Any band corresponding to 5-nitroso-2,4,6-triaminopyrimidine in the chromatogram obtained with solution (1) is not more intense than the band in the chromatogram obtained with solution (2).

Related substances Carry out the method for *thin-layer chromatography*, Appendix III A, using *silica gel G* as the coating substance and a mixture of 90 volumes of *ethyl acetate*, 10 volumes of 18M *ammonia* and 10 volumes of *methanol* as the mobile phase. Apply separately to the chromatoplate 5 µl of each of the following solutions. For solution (1) dissolve 0.10 g in 20 ml of *dimethyl sulphoxide* and dilute 2 ml of the resulting solution to 50 ml with *methanol*. For solution (2) dilute 1 volume of solution (1) to 200 volumes with *methanol*. After removal of the plate, allow it to dry in air until the odour of solvent is no longer detectable and examine under *ultra-violet light (365 nm)*. Any *secondary spot* in the chromatogram obtained with solution (1) is not more intense than the spot in the chromatogram obtained with solution (2).

Loss on drying When dried to constant weight at 100° to 105°, loses not more than 1.0% of its weight. Use 1 g.

Sulphated ash Not more than 0.1%, Appendix IX A, Method II. Use 1 g.

Assay Dissolve 0.15 g in 5 ml of *anhydrous formic acid*, add 100 ml of *anhydrous glacial acetic acid* and carry out Method I for *non-aqueous titration*, Appendix VIII A, determining the end-point potentiometrically. Each ml of 0.1M *perchloric acid VS* is equivalent to 0.02533 g of $C_{12}H_{11}N_7$.

Storage Triamterene should be kept in a well-closed container and protected from light.

Preparation
Triamterene Capsules

Action and use Diuretic.

Trichlorofluoromethane
Propellant 11

CCl_3F 137.4   *75-69-4*

Trichlorofluoromethane is a gas above 24°. For convenience in use it is compressed in metal cylinders.

Characteristics A colourless, non-flammable gas; odour, faintly ethereal. The liquid form has a weight per ml of about 1.61 g at −35° and about 1.50 g at 15°.

Solubility In the liquid state, immiscible with *water*; miscible with *absolute ethanol*.

Identification It boils at about 23.7°.

Acidity Not more than 2 ppm, calculated as HCl, when determined by the following method. Transfer 200 ml of *water* previously neutralised to *bromocresol purple solution* to a gas-washing bottle fitted with a sintered-glass distribution tube, pass 200 g of the gas being examined through the water and titrate with 0.02M *sodium hydroxide VS* using *bromocresol purple solution* as indicator. Each ml of 0.02M *sodium hydroxide VS* is equivalent to 0.000729 g of HCl.

Distillation range 0.3°, Appendix V C, Method II, using a water-bath at 54° and correcting the temperatures by ±0.263° per kPa.

Chloride Mix 5 ml with 5 ml of *methanol* and add 0.2 ml of a saturated solution of *silver nitrate* in *methanol*. The solution is *clear*, Appendix IV A.

High-boiling matter Not more than 0.01% v/v when determined by the following method. Allow the boiling tube containing the remaining 15 ml of liquid from the determination of Distillation range to stand in a water-bath at 54° for 30 minutes and measure the volume.

Water Not more than 0.001% w/w, Appendix IX C, Method I C.

Storage Trichlorofluoromethane should be kept compressed in a metal cylinder and stored at a temperature of 8° to 15°.

Action and use Aerosol propellant.

Triclofos Sodium

$$CCl_3 \cdot CH_2 \cdot O\overset{\displaystyle O}{\underset{\displaystyle OH}{\overset{\|}{P}}}{-}ONa$$

$C_2H_3Cl_3NaO_4P$ 251.4   7246-20-0

Triclofos Sodium is sodium 2,2,2-trichloroethyl hydrogen orthophosphate. It contains not less than 41.3 per cent and not more than 43.2 per cent of Cl and not less than 97.0 per cent and not more than 102.0 per cent of $C_2H_3Cl_3NaO_4P$, both calculated with reference to the dried substance.

Characteristics A white or almost white powder; odourless or almost odourless; hygroscopic.

Solubility Soluble in 2 parts of *water*; slightly soluble in *ethanol* (96%); practically insoluble in *ether*.

Identification A. Heat 50 mg with 1 ml of a 50% v/v solution of *sulphuric acid* and 1 ml of a 5% w/v solution of *potassium permanganate* in a water-bath for 5 minutes. Add 7 ml of *water* and decolorise the solution with 1 ml of a 5% w/v solution of *oxalic acid*. To 1 ml add 1 ml of *pyridine* and 1 ml of 5M *sodium hydroxide* and heat in a water-bath for 1 minute, stirring continuously. A pink colour is produced in the pyridine layer.

B. Dissolve 0.1 g in 5 ml of *water* and add 2 ml of *silver nitrate solution*. A white precipitate is produced which is soluble in 5M *ammonia* and in 2M *nitric acid*.

C. Yields the *reactions* characteristic of sodium salts, Appendix VI.

D. Heat 0.1 g with 1 g of *anhydrous sodium carbonate* to a dull red heat and maintain for 10 minutes, cool, extract the residue with *water* and filter. The filtrate yields the *reactions* characteristic of chlorides and of phosphates, Appendix VI.

Acidity pH of a 2% w/v solution, 3.0 to 4.5, Appendix V L.

Clarity of solution A 2.0% w/v solution is *clear*, Appendix IV A.

Heavy metals A 10.0% w/v solution complies with *limit test A for heavy metals*, Appendix VII (20 ppm). Use *lead standard solution* (2 ppm Pb) to prepare the standard.

Chloride Dissolve 0.1 g in 50 ml of *water*. 15 ml of the solution complies with the *limit test for chlorides*, Appendix VII (0.175%).

Phosphate Not more than 1.0%, calculated as PO_4^{3-}, when determined by the following method. Dissolve 25 mg in 10 ml of *water*, add 4 ml of 1M *sulphuric acid*, 1 ml of a 10% w/v solution of *ammonium molybdate* and 2 ml of *methylaminophenol—sulphite solution* and allow to stand for 15 minutes. Add sufficient *water* to produce 25 ml, allow to stand for a further 15 minutes and measure the *absorbance* of a 4-cm layer of the resulting solution at 730 nm, Appendix II B. Calculate the content of phosphate from a calibration curve prepared by treating suitable volumes of a 0.00143% w/v solution of *potassium dihydrogen orthophosphate* in the same manner.

Loss on drying When dried at 100° at a pressure not exceeding 0.7 kPa for 3 hours, loses not more than 5.0% of its weight. Use 1 g.

Assay *For Cl* Mix 0.25 g with 1 g of *anhydrous sodium carbonate* in a nickel crucible about 3 cm in diameter, fill the crucible completely with *anhydrous sodium carbonate* and invert into a nickel crucible about 4 cm in diameter; cover the smaller crucible with *anhydrous sodium carbonate*, well pressed down, using about 25 g of *anhydrous sodium carbonate* in all. Heat for 30 minutes at a dull red heat, cool, transfer to a 400-ml beaker, add 150 ml of *water* and boil gently for 10 minutes. Filter through absorbent cotton into a 600-ml beaker, washing the residue thoroughly with hot *water*, until about 400 ml of filtrate has been collected. Cool, cautiously add *nitric acid* until the solution is neutral to *litmus paper* and add 3 ml of *nitric acid* in excess. Add 50 ml of 0.1M *silver nitrate VS*, allow to stand until precipitation is complete, filter, wash the precipitate with *water* and titrate the combined filtrate and washings with 0.1M *ammonium thiocyanate VS* using *ammonium iron(III) sulphate solution* as indicator. Each ml of 0.1M *silver nitrate VS* is equivalent to 0.003545 g of Cl.

For $C_2H_3Cl_3NaO_4P$ Heat 0.2 g in a long-necked flask with 2 ml of *sulphuric acid* and 2.5 ml of *nitric acid* until brown fumes cease to be evolved, cool, add 1 ml of *nitric acid* and heat again. Continue adding *nitric acid* and heating until brown fumes are no longer evolved and the solution is colourless when cold. Heat until dense, white fumes are evolved, cool, transfer the solution to a flask with the aid of 150 ml of *water*, add 50 ml of *citric—molybdic acid solution* and heat slowly to boiling. Swirling the flask continuously, add 25 ml of *quinoline solution* at first dropwise and then in a steady stream, heat on a water-bath for 5 minutes and cool. Filter, wash the precipitate with *water* until free from acid, transfer the precipitate to a flask with the aid of 100 ml of *water*, add 50 ml of 0.5M *sodium hydroxide VS* and shake until dissolved. Titrate the excess of alkali with 0.5M *hydrochloric acid VS* using *phenolphthalein—thymol blue* *solution* as indicator. Each ml of 0.5M *sodium hydroxide VS* is equivalent to 0.004835 g of $C_2H_3Cl_3NaO_4P$. Correct the result for the content of phosphate, as determined by the test described above; each g of PO_4^{3-} is equivalent to 2.65 g of $C_2H_3Cl_3NaO_4P$.

Storage Triclofos Sodium should be kept in a well-closed container.

Preparation
Triclofos Oral Solution

Action and use Sedative and hypnotic.

Triethanolamine

Triethanolamine is a variable mixture of bases consisting mainly of 2,2′,2′′-nitrilotriethanol $(HOCH_2.CH_2)_3N$, together with 2,2′-iminobis-ethanol and smaller amounts of 2-amino-ethanol. It contains not less than 80.0 per cent of nitrilotriethanol, $C_6H_{15}NO_3$.

Characteristics A clear, colourless or pale yellow liquid; odourless or almost odourless; hygroscopic.

Solubility Miscible with *water* and with *ethanol (96%)*; slightly soluble in *ether*.

Identification A. A 10% w/v solution in 2M *hydrochloric acid* produces a copious precipitate with *phosphotungstic acid solution*, a slight precipitate with *iodine solution* and no precipitate with *potassium mercuri-iodide solution* or *chloroplatinic acid solution*.
B. Mix 1 ml with 1 ml of *water* and neutralise to *litmus paper* with *hydrochloric acid*. A crystalline precipitate is produced which, after washing with *ethanol (96%)* and drying, has a *melting point* of about 178°, Appendix V A.
C. A 10% w/v solution is strongly alkaline to *litmus solution*.

Refractive index 1.482 to 1.485, Appendix V E.

Weight per ml 1.120 to 1.130 g, Appendix V G.

Related substances Carry out the method for *gas chromatography*, Appendix III B, using the following solutions. Solution (1) contains 2.0% w/v of each of *ethanolamine, diethanolamine* and *triethanolamine* in *methanol*. Solution (2) is the substance being examined.

The chromatographic procedure may be carried out using a glass column (1.5 m × 4 mm) packed with porous polymer beads (Tenax-GC, 60 to 80 mesh, is suitable), at a temperature rising at a rate of 8° per minute from 120° to 290° and maintaining this temperature for 15 minutes. In order to ensure a consistent response it may be necessary to saturate the column prior to analysis by making repeated injections of the substance being examined.

In the chromatogram obtained with solution (2) the area of any peak corresponding to ethanolamine does not exceed 3.0%, the area of any peak corresponding to diethanolamine does not exceed 12.0% and the sum of the areas of any other *secondary peaks* does not exceed 5.0%, by *normalisation*.

Total bases Mix 3 g with 20 ml of *water* and titrate with 1M *hydrochloric acid VS* using *methyl red solution* as indicator. 19.9 ml to 22.1 ml of 1M *hydrochloric acid VS* is required.

Sulphated ash Not more than 0.1%, Appendix IX A.

Assay Mix 0.5 g with 5 ml of 2M *hydrochloric acid* and evaporate to dryness on a water-bath. Stir the residue with 5 ml of *propan-2-ol*, transfer to a tared sintered-glass crucible and wash the dish and residue with three 5-ml quantities of *propan-2-ol*, thoroughly drying the residue in the crucible by suction after each washing. Dry the residue to constant weight at 105° and add a correction of 0.2 mg for each ml of *propan-2-ol* used. Each g is equivalent to 0.8035 g of $C_6H_{15}NO_3$.

Storage Triethanolamine should be kept in a well-closed container.

Trifluoperazine Hydrochloride ☆

$C_{21}H_{24}F_3N_3S,2HCl$ 480.4   *440-17-5*

Trifluoperazine Hydrochloride is 10-[3-(4-methylpiperazin-1-yl)propyl]-2-trifluoromethyl-phenothiazine dihydrochloride. It contains not less than 99.0 per cent and not more than 101.0 per cent of $C_{21}H_{24}F_3N_3S,2HCl$, calculated with reference to the dried substance.

Characteristics A white to pale yellow, crystalline powder; odourless or almost odourless; slightly hygroscopic. It melts at about 242° with decomposition.

Solubility Soluble in 2 parts of *water*; soluble in *ethanol (96%)*; slightly soluble in *chloroform*; practically insoluble in *ether*.

Identification A. Carry out the following procedure in subdued light. The *light absorption*, Appendix II B, in the range 280 to 350 nm of a 0.01% w/v solution in 0.1M *hydrochloric acid* measured immediately after preparation exhibits a maximum only at 305 nm. Dilute 5 ml to 100 ml with 0.1M *hydrochloric acid*. The *light absorption* of the resulting solution in the range 230 to 280 nm exhibits a maximum only at 255 nm. The A(1%, 1 cm) at 255 nm is about 650.
B. Complies with the test for *identification of phenothiazines*, Appendix III A, using as solution (2) a 0.2% w/v solution of *trifluoperazine hydrochloride EPCRS* in *chloroform*.
C. Dissolve 0.5 mg in 1 ml of *water*, add 0.1 ml of *bromine water* and shake for 1 minute. Add dropwise 1 ml of *sulphuric acid*, shaking vigorously. A red colour is produced.
D. To 0.25 g add 5 ml of *water* and 2 ml of 2M *sodium hydroxide* and shake vigorously with 20 ml of *ether*. Wash the ether layer with 5 ml of *water*, add 0.15 g of *maleic acid* and evaporate the ether. The *melting point* of the residue, after recrystallisation from 30 ml of *ethanol (96%)* and drying, is about 192°, Appendix V A, Method I.
E. To 5 ml of a 1% w/v solution add 2 ml of *nitric acid*. A dark red colour is produced which becomes pale yellow. The yellow solution yields *reaction A* characteristic of chlorides, Appendix VI.

Acidity pH of a 10% w/v solution, 1.6 to 2.5, Appendix V L.

Related substances Complies with the test for *related substances in phenothiazines*, Appendix III A, using *mobile phase A*.

Loss on drying When dried to constant weight at 100° to 105°, loses not more than 1.5% of its weight. Use 1 g.

Sulphated ash Not more than 0.1%, Appendix IX A, Method II. Use 1 g.

Assay Dissolve 0.3 g in 50 ml of *anhydrous glacial acetic acid*, add 10 ml of *mercury(II) acetate solution* and carry out Method I for *non-aqueous titration*, Appendix VIII A, determining the end-point potentiometrically. Each ml of 0.1M *perchloric acid VS* is equivalent to 0.02402 g of $C_{21}H_{24}F_3N_3S,2HCl$.

Storage Trifluoperazine Hydrochloride should be kept in a well-closed container and protected from light.

Preparation
Trifluoperazine Tablets

Action and use Antipsychotic.

Trimeprazine Tartrate

$$\left[\begin{array}{c}CH_2 \cdot CHMe \cdot CH_2 \cdot NMe_2\end{array}\right]_2 \quad \begin{array}{c}OH\\CH \cdot CO_2H\\CH \cdot CO_2H\\OH\end{array}$$

$(C_{18}H_{22}N_2S)_2,C_4H_6O_6$ 747.0   *4330-99-8*

Trimeprazine Tartrate is dimethyl[2-methyl-3-(phenothiazin-10-yl)propyl]amine tartrate. It contains not less than 99.0 per cent and not more than 101.0 per cent of $(C_{18}H_{22}N_2S)_2$, $C_4H_6O_6$, calculated with reference to the dried substance.

Characteristics A white or slightly cream powder; odourless or almost odourless. It darkens on exposure to light.

Solubility Soluble in 4 parts of *water*, in 30 parts of *ethanol (96%)* and in 4 parts of *chloroform*; very slightly soluble in *ether*.

Identification A. Dissolve 0.1 g in 10 ml of *water* and add 2 ml of 1M *sodium hydroxide*. Extract with 25 ml of *ether*, wash the extract with 5 ml of *water*, dry over *anhydrous sodium sulphate*, evaporate to dryness and dissolve the residue in 1 ml of *chloroform*. The *infra-red absorption spectrum* of the resulting solution, Appendix II A, is concordant with the *reference spectrum* of trimeprazine.
B. The *light absorption*, Appendix II B, in the range 230 to 350 nm of a 0.0008% w/v solution in a mixture of 1 volume of 5M *ammonia* and 99 volumes of *methanol* exhibits a maximum at 255 nm and a less well-defined maximum at 301 nm. The *absorbance* at 255 nm is about 0.70.
C. To 1 mg add 0.05 ml of a mixture of equal volumes of *formaldehyde solution* and *sulphuric acid*. A purple colour is produced.
D. Dissolve 0.5 g in 5 ml of *water*, add 1.5 ml of 5M *sodium hydroxide* and extract with two 10-ml quantities of *ether*. To 2 ml of the aqueous layer add 6M *acetic acid* until it is acidic to *litmus paper* and add 1 ml of *ammonium metavanadate solution*. An orange-red colour is produced.

Acidity pH of a 2% w/v solution, 5.0 to 6.5, Appendix V L.

Melting point 159° to 163°, Appendix V A.

Related substances Complies with the test for *related substances in phenothiazines*, Appendix III A, using *mobile phase A*.

Loss on drying When dried to constant weight at 100° at a pressure not exceeding 0.7 kPa, loses not more than 0.5% of its weight. Use 1 g.

Sulphated ash Not more than 0.1%, Appendix IX A.

Assay Carry out Method I for *non-aqueous titration*, Appendix VIII A, using 1 g and *crystal violet solution* as indicator. Each ml of 0.1M *perchloric acid VS* is equivalent to 0.03735 g of $(C_{18}H_{22}N_2S)_2,C_4H_6O_6$.

Storage Trimeprazine Tartrate should be protected from light.

Preparation
Paediatric Trimeprazine Oral Solution
Strong Paediatric Trimeprazine Oral Solution
Trimeprazine Tablets

Action and use Histamine H_1-receptor antagonist; sedative.

In some countries the material described in this monograph may be known as Alimemazine Tartrate.

Trimethoprim ☆

$C_{14}H_{18}N_4O_3$ 290.3   *738-70-5*

Trimethoprim is 5-(3,4,5-trimethoxybenzyl)-pyrimidine-2,4-diamine. It contains not less than 98.5 per cent and not more than 101.0 per cent of $C_{14}H_{18}N_4O_3$, calculated with reference to the dried substance.

Characteristics A white or yellowish-white powder; odourless or almost odourless.

Solubility Very slightly soluble in *water*; slightly soluble in *ethanol (96%)*; soluble in 55 parts of *chloroform*; practically insoluble in *ether*.

Identification *Test A may be omitted if tests B, C and D are carried out. Tests B and C may be omitted if tests A and D are carried out.*
A. The *infra-red absorption spectrum*, Appendix II A, is concordant with the spectrum of *trimethoprim EPCRS*.
B. The *light absorption*, Appendix II B, in the range 230 to 350 nm of a 0.002% w/v solution in 0.1M *sodium hydroxide* exhibits a maximum only at 287 nm. The A(1%, 1 cm) at 287 nm is about 245.
C. Dissolve 25 mg in 5 ml of 0.005M *sulphuric acid*, with heating if necessary, and add 2 ml of a 1.6% w/v solution of *potassium permanganate* in 0.1M *sodium hydroxide*. Heat to boiling and to the hot solution add 0.4 ml of *formaldehyde solution*. Mix, add 1 ml of 0.5M *sulphuric*

acid, mix and heat to boiling. Cool and filter. Add 2 ml of *chloroform* to the filtrate and shake vigorously. The chloroform layer exhibits a green fluorescence when examined under ultra-violet light (365 nm).

D. *Melting point*, 199° to 203°, Appendix V A, Method I.

Colour of solution A 5% w/v solution in a mixture of 10 volumes of *chloroform*, 9 volumes of *methanol* and 2 volumes of *water* is not more intensely coloured than *reference solution BY₇*, Appendix IV B, Method II.

Heavy metals 2.0 g complies with *limit test C for heavy metals*, Appendix VII (20 ppm). Use 4 ml of *lead standard solution (10 ppm Pb)* to prepare the standard.

Related substances Carry out the method for *thin-layer chromatography*, Appendix III A, using *silica gel GF254* as the coating substance and a mixture of 85 volumes of *ethyl acetate*, 10 volumes of *methanol*, 5 volumes of *water* and 2 volumes of *anhydrous formic acid* as the mobile phase but carrying out the chromatography using an unsaturated tank and allowing the solvent front to ascend 17 cm above the line of application. Apply separately to the chromatoplate 5 μl of each of two solutions of the substance being examined in a mixture of 10 volumes of *chloroform*, 9 volumes of *methanol* and 2 volumes of *water* containing (1) 4% w/v and (2) 0.008% w/v. After removal of the plate, allow it to dry in a current of cold air for 5 minutes and examine under *ultra-violet light (254 nm)*. Place the plate in a closed tank containing chlorine that has been produced by mixing 2 volumes of a 1.5% w/v solution of *potassium permanganate*, 1 volume of 7M *hydrochloric acid* and 1 volume of *water* in a container placed at the bottom of the tank and allow to stand for 20 minutes. Remove the plate from the tank and remove the chlorine in a current of cold air until an area below the line of application does not give a blue colour on the addition of one drop of *potassium iodide and starch solution*. Spray the plate with *potassium iodide and starch solution* and examine in daylight. Any *secondary spot* in the chromatogram obtained with solution (1), before or after the treatment with chlorine, is not more intense than the spot in the chromatogram obtained with solution (2).

Loss on drying When dried to constant weight at 100° to 105°, loses not more than 1.0% of its weight. Use 1 g.

Sulphated ash Not more than 0.1%, Appendix IX A, Method II. Use 1 g.

Assay Dissolve 0.25 g in 50 ml of *anhydrous glacial acetic acid* and carry out Method I for *non-aqueous titration*, Appendix VIII A, determining the end-point potentiometrically. Each ml of 0.1M *perchloric acid VS* is equivalent to 0.02903 g of $C_{14}H_{18}N_4O_3$.

Preparations

Co-trimoxazole Oral Suspension
Paediatric Co-trimoxazole Oral Suspension
Co-trimoxazole Injection
Co-trimoxazole Tablets
Dispersible Co-trimoxazole Tablets
Paediatric Co-trimoxazole Tablets

Action and use Antibacterial.

Trimipramine Maleate ☆

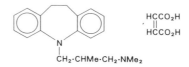

$C_{20}H_{26}N_2,C_4H_4O_4$ 410.5   *521-78-8*

Trimipramine Maleate is 3-(10,11-dihydro-5*H*-dibenz[*b,f*]azepin-5-yl)-2-methylpropyl-dimethylamine hydrogen maleate. It contains not less than 98.0 per cent and not more than 101.0 per cent of $C_{20}H_{26}N_2,C_4H_4O_4$, calculated with reference to the dried substance.

Characteristics A white or almost white, crystalline powder.

Solubility Slightly soluble in *water* and in *ethanol (96%)*; freely soluble in *chloroform*; practically insoluble in *ether*.

Identification Test A may be omitted if tests B, C, D and E are carried out. Tests B, C and D may be omitted if tests A and E are carried out.

A. The *infra-red absorption spectrum*, Appendix II A, is concordant with the spectrum of *trimipramine maleate EPCRS*.

B. The *light absorption*, Appendix II B, in the range 230 to 350 nm of a 0.002% w/v solution in 0.01M *hydrochloric acid* exhibits a maximum at 250 nm and a shoulder at 270 nm. The A(1%, 1 cm) at 250 nm is 205 to 235.

C. In the test for Related substances, the principal spot in the chromatogram obtained with solution (2) is similar in position, colour and size to that in the chromatogram obtained with solution (3).

D. Carry out the method for *thin-layer chromatography*, Appendix III A, using *silica gel GF254* as the coating substance and a mixture of 90 volumes of *di-isopropyl ether*, 7 volumes of *anhydrous formic acid* and 3 volumes of *water* as the mobile phase but allowing the solvent front to ascend 12 cm above the line of application. Apply separately to the chromatoplate as 10-mm bands 5 μl of each of two solutions in *methanol* containing (1) 2% w/v of the substance being examined and (2) 0.56% w/v of *maleic acid*. After removal of the plate, dry it in a current of air for a few minutes and then at 120° for 10 minutes and examine under *ultra-violet light (254 nm)*. The chromatogram obtained with solution (1) shows a band on the line of application and another band which is similar in position and size to the principal band in the chromatogram obtained with solution (2).

E. *Melting point*, 140° to 144°, Appendix V A, Method I.

Colour of solution A 10.0% w/v solution in *chloroform* is not more intensely coloured than *reference solution BY₅*, Appendix IV B, Method II.

Heavy metals 2.0 g complies with *limit test C for heavy metals*, Appendix VII (20 ppm). Use 4 ml of *lead standard solution (10 ppm Pb)* to prepare the standard.

Related substances Carry out the method for *thin-layer chromatography*, Appendix III A, using *silica gel G* as the coating substance and a mixture of 90 volumes of *toluene*, 10 volumes of *ethanol* and 0.7 volume of 13.5M *ammonia* as the mobile phase. Apply separately to the chromatoplate 5 μl of each of six solutions prepared immediately before use in *methanol* containing (1) 5% w/v of the substance being examined, (2) 0.25% w/v of the substance being examined, (3) 0.25% w/v of *trimipramine maleate EPCRS*, (4) 0.025% w/v of *trimipramine maleate EPCRS*, (5) 0.010% w/v of *trimipramine maleate EPCRS* and (6) 0.025% w/v of *iminodibenzyl*. After removal of the plate, allow it to dry in air for 15 minutes and spray with a 0.5% w/v solution of *potassium dichromate* in *sulphuric acid (20%)*. Examine the plate immediately. Any spot corresponding to iminodibenzyl in the chromatogram obtained with solution (1) is not more intense than the spot in the chromatogram obtained with solution (6). Any other *secondary spot* is not more intense than the spot in the chromatogram obtained with solution (4) and not more than three such spots are more intense than the spot in the chromatogram obtained with solution (5). Disregard any spot on the line of application.

Loss on drying When dried to constant weight at 100° to 105°, loses not more than 0.5% of its weight. Use 1 g.

Sulphated ash Not more than 0.1%, Appendix IX A, Method II. Use 1 g.

Assay Dissolve 0.35 g in 50 ml of *anhydrous glacial acetic acid* and carry out Method I for *non-aqueous titration*, Appendix VIII A, determining the end-point potentiometrically. Each ml of 0.1M *perchloric acid VS* is equivalent to 0.04105 g of $C_{20}H_{26}N_2,C_4H_4O_4$.

Storage Trimipramine Maleate should be kept in a well-closed container and protected from light.

Preparation
Trimipramine Tablets

Action and use Antidepressant.

Triprolidine Hydrochloride

$C_{19}H_{22}N_2,HCl,H_2O$ 332.9   *6138-79-0*

Triprolidine Hydrochloride is (*E*)-2-(3-pyrrolidin-1-yl-1-*p*-tolylprop-1-enyl)pyridine hydrochloride monohydrate. It contains not less than 98.5 per cent and not more than 101.0 per cent of $C_{19}H_{22}N_2,HCl$, calculated with reference to the anhydrous substance.

Characteristics A white, crystalline powder; odourless or almost odourless.

Solubility Soluble in 2 parts of *water*, in 1.5 parts of *ethanol (96%)* and in less than 1 part of *chloroform*; practically insoluble in *ether*.

Identification A. The *infra-red absorption spectrum*, Appendix II A, is concordant with the *reference spectrum* of triprolidine hydrochloride.

B. The *light absorption*, Appendix II B, in the range 240 to 350 nm of a 0.004% w/v solution in 0.05M *sulphuric acid* exhibits a maximum only at 290 nm. The *absorbance* at 290 nm is about 1.2.

C. The *light absorption*, Appendix II B, in the range 220 to 350 nm of a 0.002% w/v solution exhibits two maxima, at 230 nm and 276 nm. The *absorbance* at 230 nm is about 0.99 and at 276 nm is about 0.49.

D. Dissolve 0.1 g in 2 ml of 2M *hydrochloric acid* and add 0.5 ml of *potassium mercuri-iodide solution*. A pale yellow precipitate is produced.

E. Yields *reaction A* characteristic of chlorides, Appendix VI.

Related substances Carry out the method for *thin-layer chromatography*, Appendix III A, using a silica gel F254 precoated chromatoplate (Merck silica gel 60 F254 plates are suitable) and a mixture of equal volumes of *butan-2-one* and *dimethylformamide* as the mobile phase. Apply separately to the plate 5 μl of each of three solutions in *methanol* containing (1) 1.0% w/v of the substance being examined, (2) 0.020% w/v of *Z-triprolidine BPCRS* and (3) 0.010% w/v of the substance being examined. After removal of the plate, allow it to dry in air and examine under *ultra-violet light (254 nm)*. In the chromatogram obtained with solution (1) any spot corresponding to Z-triprolidine is not more intense than the spot in the chromatogram obtained with solution (2) and any other *secondary spot* is not more intense than the spot in the chromatogram obtained with solution (3).

Sulphated ash Not more than 0.1%, Appendix IX A.

Water 4.5 to 6.0% w/w, Appendix IX C. Use 0.4 g.

Assay Carry out Method I for *non-aqueous titration*, Appendix VIII A, using 0.25 g dissolved in a mixture of 50 ml of *anhydrous glacial acetic acid* and 0.5 ml of *acetic anhydride* and *crystal violet solution* as indicator. Each ml of 0.1M *perchloric acid VS* is equivalent to 0.01574 g of $C_{19}H_{22}N_2,HCl$.

Preparation
Triprolidine Tablets

Action and use Histamine H₁-receptor antagonist.

Tropicamide

$C_{17}H_{20}N_2O_2$ 284.4   *1508-75-4*

Tropicamide is *N*-ethyl-*N*-(4-pyridylmethyl)-tropamide. It contains not less than 99.0 per cent and not more than 101.0 per cent of $C_{17}H_{20}N_2O_2$, calculated with reference to the dried substance.

Characteristics A white or almost white, crystalline powder; odourless or almost odourless.

Solubility Slightly soluble in *water*; soluble in 3.5 parts of *ethanol (96%)* and in 2 parts of *chloroform*.

Identification A. The *infra-red absorption spectrum*, Appendix II A, is concordant with the *reference spectrum* of tropicamide.

B. The *light absorption*, Appendix II B, in the range 230 to 350 nm of a 0.005% w/v solution in 0.1M *hydrochloric acid* exhibits a maximum only at 254 nm. The *absorbance* at 254 nm is about 0.9.

C. Dissolve 5 mg in 3 ml of a mixture of 9 ml of *acetic anhydride*, 1 ml of 6M *acetic acid* and 0.1 g of *citric acid* and heat on a water-bath for 5 to 10 minutes. A reddish-yellow colour is produced.

Melting point 95° to 98°, Appendix V A.

Related substances Carry out the method for *thin-layer chromatography*, Appendix III A, using *silica gel GF254* as the coating substance and a mixture of 190 volumes of *chloroform*, 10 volumes of *methanol* and 1 volume of 13.5M *ammonia* as the mobile phase. Apply separately to the chromatoplate 20 μl of each of three solutions of the substance being examined in *chloroform* containing (1) 1.0% w/v, (2) 0.0050% w/v and (3) 0.0020% w/v. After removal of the plate, allow it to dry in air and examine under *ultra-violet light (254 nm)*. Any *secondary spot* in the chromatogram obtained with solution (1) is not more intense than the spot in the chromatogram obtained with solution (2) and not more than one such spot is more intense than the spot in the chromatogram obtained with solution (3).

Loss on drying When dried at 80° at a pressure not exceeding 0.7 kPa for 4 hours, loses not more than 0.5% of its weight. Use 1 g.

Sulphated ash Not more than 0.1%, Appendix IX A.

Assay Carry out Method I for *non-aqueous titration*, Appendix VIII A, using 0.5 g and *1-naphtholbenzein solution* as indicator. Each ml of 0.1M *perchloric acid VS* is equivalent to 0.02844 g of $C_{17}H_{20}N_2O_2$.

Preparation
Tropicamide Eye Drops

Action and use Mydriatic; cycloplegic.

Troxidone ☆

$C_6H_9NO_3$ 143.1   *127-48-0*

Troxidone is 3,5,5-trimethyloxazolidine-2,4-dione. It contains not less than 98.0 per cent and not more than 102.0 per cent of $C_6H_9NO_3$, calculated with reference to the dried substance.

Characteristics Colourless or almost colourless crystals; odour, slightly camphoraceous.

Solubility Soluble in 13 parts of *water*; very soluble in *ethanol (96%)*, in *chloroform* and in *ether*.

Identification *Test A may be omitted if tests B, C and D are carried out. Tests B, C and D may be omitted if test A is carried out.*
A. The *infra-red absorption spectrum*, Appendix II A, is concordant with the spectrum of *trimethadione EPCRS*. Examine the substances as discs prepared from a dispersion of 3 mg in 0.4 g of *potassium bromide IR*.
B. To 2 ml of a 5% w/v solution in *carbon dioxide-free water* add 1 ml of a 4.73% w/v solution of *barium hydroxide*. A white precipitate is immediately produced which dissolves on the addition of 1 ml of 2M *hydrochloric acid*.
C. Dissolve 0.3 g in a mixture of 5 ml of *ethanolic potassium hydroxide solution* and 5 ml of *ethanol (96%)* and allow to stand for 10 minutes. Add 0.05 ml of a 1.0% w/v solution of *phenolphthalein* in *ethanol (96%)* and carefully add *hydrochloric acid* until the solution is neutral.

Evaporate to dryness on a water-bath, shake the residue with four 5-ml quantities of *ether*, filter the combined ether extracts and evaporate to dryness. The *melting point* of the dried residue, after recrystallisation from 5 ml of *toluene*, is about 80°, Appendix V A, Method I.
D. *Melting point* of the undried substance, 45° to 47°, Appendix V A, Method I.

Acidity or alkalinity To 10 ml of a 5% w/v solution in *carbon dioxide-free water* add 0.1 ml of *methyl red solution*. Not more than 0.1 ml of 0.01M *hydrochloric acid VS* or 0.01M *sodium hydroxide VS* is required to change the colour of the solution.

Clarity and colour of solution A 5.0% w/v solution in *carbon dioxide-free water* is *clear*, Appendix IV A, and *colourless*, Appendix IV B, Method II.

Heavy metals A 5.0% w/v solution in *carbon dioxide-free water* complies with *limit test A for heavy metals*, Appendix VII (20 ppm). Use *lead standard solution (1 ppm Pb)* to prepare the standard.

Loss on drying When dried over *self-indicating silica gel* for 6 hours, loses not more than 0.5% of its weight. Use 1 g.

Sulphated ash Not more than 0.1%, Appendix IX A, Method II. Use 1 g.

Assay Dissolve 0.125 g of *decan-1-ol* (internal standard) in sufficient *absolute ethanol* to produce 25 ml (solution A). Carry out the method for *gas chromatography*, Appendix III B, using the following solutions. For solution (1) dissolve 0.1 g of the substance being examined in sufficient of solution A to produce 10 ml. For solution (2) dissolve 0.1 g of *trimethadione EPCRS* in sufficient of solution A to produce 10 ml.

The chromatographic procedure may be carried out using a stainless steel column (0.75 m × 3 mm) packed with porous polymer beads (120 to 150 mesh) (Chromosorb 101 is suitable) and maintained at 210° with an inlet port temperature of 240° and a detector temperature of 270° and using an injection volume of 1 μl.

Calculate the content of $C_6H_9NO_3$ using the declared content of $C_6H_9NO_3$ in *trimethadione EPCRS*.

Storage Troxidone should be kept in a well-closed container and protected from light.

Action and use Anticonvulsant.

The title of the monograph in the European Pharmacopœia is Trimethadione.

Tubocurarine Chloride ☆

$C_{37}H_{41}ClN_2O_6,HCl,5H_2O$ 772   *6989-98-6*

Tubocurarine Chloride is 7′,12′-dihydroxy-6,6′-dimethoxy-2,2′,2′-trimethyltubocuraranium chloride hydrochloride pentahydrate. It contains not less than 98.0 per cent and not more than 102.0 per cent of $C_{37}H_{41}ClN_2O_6,HCl$, calculated with reference to the anhydrous substance.

Characteristics A white to slightly yellowish, crystalline powder. It melts at about 270°, with decomposition.

Solubility Soluble in 20 parts of *water* and in 30 parts of *ethanol (96%)*; practically insoluble in *acetone*, in *chloroform* and in *ether*. It dissolves in aqueous solutions of alkali hydroxides.

Identification *Test A may be omitted if tests B, C, D, E and F are carried out. Tests B, C, D and F may be omitted if tests A and E are carried out.*

A. The *infra-red absorption spectrum*, Appendix II A, is concordant with the spectrum of *tubocurarine chloride EPCRS*.

B. The *light absorption*, Appendix II B, in the range 230 to 350 nm of a 0.005% w/v solution exhibits a maximum at 280 nm and a minimum at 255 nm. The A(1%, 1 cm) at the maximum at 280 nm is 113 to 123.

C. To 1 ml of a 2.5% w/v solution add 0.2 ml of a 1.3% w/v solution of *iron(III) chloride hexahydrate* and heat on a water-bath for 1 minute; a green colour is produced. Treat 1 ml of *water* in the same manner; a brown colour is produced.

D. To 1 ml of a 1.0% w/v solution in *carbon dioxide-free water* add 1 ml of *mercury—nitric acid solution*. A red colour is produced slowly.

E. Yields *reaction A* characteristic of chlorides, Appendix VI.

F. Yields the *reactions* characteristic of alkaloids, Appendix VI.

Acidity pH of a 1% w/v solution, 4.0 to 6.0, Appendix V L.

Clarity and colour of solution A 1.0% w/v solution in *carbon dioxide-free water* is *clear*, Appendix IV A, and not more intensely coloured than *reference solution Y_6*, Appendix IV B, Method II.

Specific optical rotation +210° to +222°, Appendix V F, determined in a solution prepared by dissolving 0.25 g in sufficient *carbon dioxide-free water* to produce 25 ml and allowing to stand for 3 hours.

Chloroform-soluble substances Dissolve 0.25 g in 150 ml of *water*. Add 5 ml of a saturated solution of *sodium hydrogen carbonate* and extract with three 20-ml quantities of *chloroform*. Wash the combined chloroform extracts with 10 ml of *water*, filter the chloroform solution and wash the filter with two 5-ml quantities of *chloroform*. Evaporate the combined filtrate and washings on a water-bath and dry the residue at 100° to 105° for 1 hour. The dried residue weighs not more than 5 mg. It does not dissolve in 10 ml of *water* but dissolves on the addition of 1 ml of 2M *hydrochloric acid*.

Related substances Carry out the method for *thin-layer chromatography*, Appendix III A, using *silica gel G* as the coating substance and as the mobile phase the lower layer of a mixture of equal volumes of *chloroform*, *methanol* and a 12.5% w/v solution of *trichloroacetic acid* in a non-saturated tank. Apply separately to the chromatoplate 5 µl of each of three solutions of the substance being examined in *water* containing (1) 2.5% w/v, (2) 0.0375% w/v and (3) 0.01875% w/v. After removal of the plate, allow it to dry in a current of cold air and spray with a mixture of 1 volume of a freshly prepared 5% w/v solution of *potassium hexacyanoferrate(III)*, 1 volume of *water* and 2 volumes of a 10.5% w/v solution of *iron(III) chloride hexahydrate*,

prepared immediately before use. Any *secondary spot* in the chromatogram obtained with solution (1) is not more intense than the spot in the chromatogram obtained with solution (2) and not more than one such spot is more intense than the spot in the chromatogram obtained with solution (3).

Sulphated ash Not more than 0.25%, Appendix IX A, Method II. Use 0.2 g.

Water 9.0 to 12.0% w/w, Appendix IX C. Use 0.3 g.

Assay Dissolve 25 mg in sufficient *water* to produce 500 ml and measure the *absorbance* of the resulting solution at the maximum at 280 nm, Appendix II B. Calculate the content of $C_{37}H_{41}ClN_2O_6,HCl$ from the *absorbance* obtained by repeating the operation using 25 mg of *tubocurarine chloride EPCRS* in place of the substance being examined and from the declared content of $C_{37}H_{41}ClN_2O_6,HCl$ in *tubocurarine chloride EPCRS*.

Storage Tubocurarine Chloride should be kept in an airtight container.

Preparation
Tubocurarine Injection

Action and use Skeletal muscle relaxant.

Turpentine Oil

Turpentine Oil is obtained by distillation from the oleoresin obtained from various species of *Pinus* and rectified.

Characteristics A clear, bright, colourless liquid, visibly free from water; odour, characteristic.

Refractive index 1.467 to 1.477, Appendix V E.

Solubility in ethanol Soluble, at 20°, in 7 volumes of *ethanol (90%)* and in 3 volumes of *ethanol (96%)*, Appendix X M.

Weight per ml 0.855 to 0.868 g, Appendix V G.

Residue on evaporation Not more than 0.5% when determined by the method for *residue on evaporation of volatile oils*, Appendix X M. Use 2 g and heat for 4 hours.

Storage Turpentine Oil should be kept in a well-filled, well-closed container, protected from light and stored at a temperature not exceeding 25°.

Preparations
Turpentine Liniment
White Liniment

Action and use Rubefacient.

Undecenoic Acid ☆

CH₂=CH·(CH₂)₈·CO₂H

$C_{11}H_{20}O_2$ 184.3   *112-38-9*

Undecenoic Acid consists mainly of undec-10-enoic acid. It contains not less than 97.0 per cent and not more than 102.0 per cent of $C_{11}H_{20}O_2$.

Characteristics A white or very pale yellow, crystalline mass or a colourless or pale yellow liquid; odour, characteristic.

Solubility Practically insoluble in *water*, freely soluble in *ethanol (96%)*, in *chloroform*, in *ether*, in fixed oils and in volatile oils.

Identification A. Dissolve 0.1 g in a mixture of 2 ml of 1M *sulphuric acid* and 5 ml of *glacial acetic acid* and add dropwise 0.25 ml of *potassium permanganate solution*. The colour of the permanganate solution is discharged.

B. Boil 2 g under a reflux condenser with 2 ml of recently distilled *aniline* for 10 minutes, cool, add 30 ml of *ether* and extract with three 20-ml quantities of 2M *hydrochloric acid* and then with 20 ml of *water*. Evaporate the organic layer to dryness. The *melting point* of the residue, after recrystallising twice from *ethanol (70%)* and drying over *phosphorus pentoxide* at a pressure of 1.5 to 2.5 kPa for 3 hours, is 66° to 68°, Appendix V A, Method I.

C. *Freezing point*, 21° to 24°, Appendix V B.

D. *Refractive index*, at 25°, 1.447 to 1.450, Appendix V E.

Peroxide value Not more than 10, Appendix X F.

Degree of unsaturation Dissolve 85 mg in a mixture of 5 ml of 2M *hydrochloric acid* and 30 ml of *glacial acetic acid* and titrate with 0.05M *bromine VS* using 0.05 ml of *ethoxychrysoidine hydrochloride solution* as indicator. The volume of 0.05M *bromine VS* required to discharge the red colour is 8.9 to 9.4 ml.

Fixed and mineral oils Boil 1.0 g with 25 ml of *water* and 5 ml of *sodium carbonate solution* for 3 minutes. The hot solution is not more opalescent than *reference suspension II*, Appendix IV A.

Water-soluble acids Shake 1 g with 20 ml of *water* at 35° to 45° for 2 minutes, cool and filter the aqueous layer through a moistened filter. To 10 ml of the filtrate add 0.05 ml of *dilute phenolphthalein solution*. Not more than 0.1 ml of 0.1M *sodium hydroxide VS* is required to change the colour of the solution.

Sulphated ash Not more than 0.1%, Appendix IX A, Method II. Use 0.5 g.

Assay Dissolve 0.75 g in 10 ml of *ethanol (96%)* and titrate with 0.5M *sodium hydroxide VS* using 0.1 ml of *dilute phenolphthalein solution* as indicator. Each ml of 0.5M *sodium hydroxide VS* is equivalent to 0.09214 g of $C_{11}H_{20}O_2$.

Storage Undecenoic Acid should be kept in a well-closed, non-metallic container, protected from light and stored at a temperature of 8° to 15°.

The title of the monograph in the European Pharmacopœia is Undecylenic Acid.

Urea

$H_2N \cdot CO \cdot NH_2$

CH_4N_2O 60.06   *37-13-6*

Urea is the diamide of carbonic acid. It contains not less than 99.5 per cent and not more than 100.5 per cent of CH_4N_2O.

Characteristics Colourless, transparent, prismatic crystals; odourless or almost odourless; slightly hygroscopic.

Solubility Soluble in 1 part of *water*, in 12 parts of *ethanol (96%)* and in 1.5 parts of boiling *ethanol (96%)*; practically insoluble in *chloroform* and in *ether*.

Identification A. Carry out the method for *thin-layer chromatography*, Appendix III A, using a silica gel precoated chromatoplate (Merck silica gel 60 plates are suitable) and a mixture of 99 volumes of *absolute ethanol* and 1 volume of 13.5M *ammonia* as the mobile phase. Apply separately to the plate 10 µl of each of the following solutions. For solution (1) dissolve 50 mg of the substance being examined in 1 ml of *water* and add 4 ml of *acetone*. For solution (2) dissolve 50 mg of *urea* in 1 ml of *water* and add 4 ml of *acetone*. After removal of the plate, allow it to dry in air and spray with a solution containing 0.5% w/v of *4-dimethylaminobenzaldehyde* and 0.5% v/v of *sulphuric acid* in *absolute ethanol*. The principal spot in the chromatogram obtained with solution (1) corresponds to that in the chromatogram obtained with solution (2).

B. Heat 0.5 g in a test-tube; it liquefies and ammonia is evolved. Continue heating until the liquid becomes turbid, cool, dissolve in a mixture of 10 ml of *water* and 0.5 ml of 5M *sodium hydroxide* and add 0.05 ml of *copper sulphate solution*. A reddish-violet colour is produced.

C. Dissolve 20 mg in 5 ml of *water*, add 5 ml of *urease-active meal* and allow to stand for 30 minutes in a stoppered flask at 37°. Heat the resulting solution in a water-bath. A vapour is produced which turns moist *litmus paper* blue.

Melting point 132° to 134°, Appendix V A.

Heavy metals Dissolve 1.0 g in 20 ml of *water* and add 5 ml of 0.1M *hydrochloric acid*, dilute to 40 ml with *water*, add 10 ml of *hydrogen sulphide solution* and allow to stand for 5 minutes. The colour of the solution is not more intense than that produced by treating 2 ml of *lead standard solution (10 ppm Pb)* in the same manner (20 ppm).

Chloride 0.70 g complies with the *limit test for chlorides*, Appendix VII (70 ppm).

Sulphate 1.5 g complies with the *limit test for sulphates*, Appendix VII (100 ppm).

Ethanol-insoluble matter Dissolve 5 g in 50 ml of warm *ethanol (96%)*, filter through a tared filter, wash the filter with 20 ml of warm *ethanol (96%)* and dry at 105° for 1 hour. The residue weighs not more than 2 mg.

Sulphated ash Not more than 0.1%, Appendix IX A.

Assay Transfer 0.17 g to a 300-ml long-necked flask, add 2 ml of a 3% w/v solution of *copper(II) sulphate* and 8 ml of *sulphuric acid* and heat gently until copious fumes of sulphur trioxide are evolved. Continue heating for 15 minutes, cool, carefully add 100 ml of *water* and 0.2 g of *granulated zinc* and connect the flask to an ammonia-distillation apparatus the delivery tube of which reaches just below the surface of 50 ml of 0.2M *hydrochloric acid VS*. Heat the flask until the air contained in it has been replaced by steam, slowly add 75 ml of 5M *sodium hydroxide* and distil the ammonia. Titrate the excess of acid with 0.2M *sodium hydroxide VS* using *methyl red solution* as indicator. Repeat the operation without the substance being examined. The difference between the titrations represents the amount of ammonia evolved. Each ml of 0.2M *hydrochloric acid VS* is equivalent to 0.006006 g of CH_4N_2O.

Preparation
Urea Cream

Action and use Keratolytic.

Valerian ☆

Valerian consists of the subterranean organs, carefully dried at a temperature below 40°, of *Valeriana officinalis* L. *s.l.*, including the rhizome, root and stolon.

Characteristics Odour, characteristic, penetrating, resembling that of valeric acid and camphor; taste, somewhat sweet at first, then spicy and slightly bitter.

Macroscopical Rhizome, yellowish-grey to pale greyish-brown, obconical to cylindrical, up to 5 cm long and up to 3 cm in diameter, base elongated or compressed, covered by and merging with numerous roots; apex usually bearing a cup-shaped scar from aerial parts, stem bases rarely present in longitudinal section, pith exhibiting a central cavity traversed by septa. Roots, numerous, almost cylindrical and of the same colour as the rhizome, 1 to 3 mm in diameter and occasionally more than 10 cm long; a few filiform, fragile secondary roots; fracture, short. Stolon, pale yellowish-grey, showing prominent nodes separated by longitudinally striated internodes, each 2 to 5 cm long; fracture, fibrous.

Microscopical Root, in transverse section, shows small, suberised, epidermal cells some with root hairs, exodermis of one or occasionally two layers of larger, suberised secretory cells often containing droplets of volatile oil; outer cortex of two to four layers of resin-containing cells with thin or collenchymatous, sometimes suberised, walls; inner cortex of numerous layers of polygonal to rounded cells filled with starch. Starch granules simple or compound; simple granules rounded, 5 to 15 μm in diameter, sometimes showing a cleft or stellate hilum; compound granules with two to six components, up to 20 μm in diameter. Endodermis consisting of a single layer of suberised, tangentially elongated cells. Pericycle continuous, starch-filled; parenchyma surrounding the phloem zone; cambium frequently indistinct; vascular bundles forming an interrupted ring surrounding the starch-filled cells. Rhizome, in transverse section, different from the root, its structure being complicated by the presence of numerous vascular bundles from root and stolon; epidermis and exodermis partially replaced by poorly developed periderm; central pith, wide, including cavities of various sizes, the larger ones being separated by plates of partially sclerified tissue.

Identification A. Carry out the method for *thin-layer chromatography*, Appendix III A, using *silica gel G* as the coating substance and a mixture of 70 volumes of *hexane* and 30 volumes of *ethyl acetate* as the mobile phase. Apply separately to the chromatoplate as bands (20 mm × 3 mm) 10 μl of each of the following solutions. For solution (1) add 5 ml of *dichloromethane* to 0.2 g of the freshly powdered material, allow to stand for 5 minutes, shaking several times, and filter, washing the filter with 2 ml of *dichloromethane*. Heat the combined filtrate and washings in a water-bath for the minimum time required to remove the solvent and dissolve the residue in 0.2 ml of *methanol*. For solution (2) dissolve 10 mg of *4-aminoazobenzene* and 2 mg of *sudan red G* in sufficient *methanol* to produce 10 ml. Develop the plate twice, each time allowing the solvent front to ascend 10 cm above the line of application. After removal of the plate, spray with *anisaldehyde solution*, using 10 ml for a plate 200 mm × 200 mm in size, and examine while heating to 100° to 105° for 5 minutes. The chromatogram obtained with

solution (1) shows in the middle part, at an Rf value between those of the pink and orange bands in the chromatogram obtained with solution (2) (sudan red G and aminoazobenzene respectively), a deep violet band (valerenic acid) and sometimes at a higher Rf value a greyish-brown band (valtrate and isovaltrate), a faint violet band (acetoxyvalerenic acid) with an Rf value lower than that of the band due to aminoazobenzene and grey bands situated between the band due to valerenic acid and the line of application. In the upper part of the chromatogram there are a number of violet bands of variable intensity; any violet band immediately above the line of application is, at most, very faint.

B. To the remainder of solution (1) used in test A add 3 ml of a mixture of equal volumes of 6M *acetic acid* and 7M *hydrochloric acid* and shake. A blue colour is produced within 15 minutes.

Extractable matter Not less than 15.0% when determined by the following method. Mix 2 g in *No. 250 powder* with a mixture of 12 g of *ethanol (96%)* and 8 g of *water* and allow to stand for 2 hours, shaking frequently. Filter, evaporate 5 g of the filtrate to dryness on a water-bath and dry the residue at 100° to 105°.

Volatile oil Not less than 0.5% v/w when determined by the method for *volatile oil in drugs*, Appendix XI E, using 25 g, in freshly prepared *No. 500 powder*. Use a 1000-ml flask, 300 ml of *water* as the distillation liquid and 0.50 ml of *xylene* in the graduated tube and distil at a rate of 3 to 4 ml per minute for 4 hours.

Acid-insoluble ash Not more than 7.0%, Appendix XI K, Method II.

Sulphated ash Not more than 15.0%, Appendix IX A, Method II. Use 1 g, in powder.

Storage Valerian should be kept in a well-closed container and protected from light.

Action and use Sedative.

The title of the monograph in the European Pharmacopœia is Valerian Root.

Powdered Valerian

Powdered Valerian is Valerian in powder.

Characteristics Light brown. Diagnostic structures: numerous fragments of parenchyma composed of rounded or elongated cells containing starch granules; occasional cells filled with light brown resin; rectangular sclereids with pitted walls, 5 to 15 μm thick; xylem vessels isolated or in small groups, 10 to 50 μm in diameter; root hairs and fragments of cork also present.

Identification; Extractable matter; Acid-insoluble ash; Sulphated ash Complies with the requirements stated under Valerian.

Storage Powdered Valerian should be kept in a well-closed container and protected from light.

Action and use Sedative.

Vancomycin Hydrochloride

$C_{66}H_{75}Cl_2N_9O_{24}$,HCl   1485   *1404-93-9*

Vancomycin Hydrochloride is the hydrochloride of (1*S*,2*R*,18*R*,19*R*,22*S*,25*R*,28*R*,40*S*)-50-[2-*O*-(3-amino-2,3,6-trideoxy-3*C*-methyl-α-L-lyxo-pyranosyl)-β-D-glucopyranosyloxy]-22-carbamoylmethyl-5,15-dichloro-2,18,32,35,37-pentahydroxy-19-(*N*²-methyl-D-leucylamino)-20,23,26,42,44-pentaoxo-7,13-dioxa-21,24,27,41,43-penta-azaoctacyclo-[26.14.2.2³,⁶.2¹⁴,¹⁷.1⁸,¹².1²⁹,³³.0¹⁰,²⁵.0³⁴,³⁹]pentaconta-3,5,8,10,12(50),14,16,29,31,33(49),34,36,38,45,47-pentadecaene-40-carboxylic acid, an antibiotic produced by certain strains of *Streptomyces orientalis* or by any other means. The potency is not less than 900 Units per mg, calculated with reference to the anhydrous substance.

Characteristics A light brown powder; very hygroscopic.

Solubility Soluble in 10 parts of *water*; slightly soluble in *ethanol (96%)* and in *ether*; practically insoluble in *chloroform*.

Identification A. Carry out the method for *descending paper chromatography*, Appendix III E, using a mixture of 40 volumes of *2-methylbutan-2-ol*, 40 volumes of *water* and 20 volumes of *acetone* as the saturating solvent and as the mobile phase. Apply separately to the paper suitable volumes of solutions in *water* of the substance being examined and of the Standard Preparation of vancomycin containing 3 Units and develop for 16 hours. Place the dried paper on nutrient agar medium previously inoculated with *Bacillus subtilis* (NCTC 8236). After 30 minutes remove the paper and maintain the agar plate at 37° overnight. Clear zones of inhibition are produced at corresponding positions on the two chromatograms.
B. Dissolve 0.2 g in 5 ml of *water*, add 1 ml of *hydrochloric acid* and heat in a water-bath for 10 minutes. Dissolve the precipitate in the minimum volume of 5M *sodium hydroxide* and add dropwise to the boiling solution 2.5 ml of *potassium cupri-tartrate solution*; a copious red precipitate is produced. Repeat the test omitting the addition of 5M *sodium hydroxide*; only a slight red precipitate is produced.

C. Yields the *reactions* characteristic of chlorides, Appendix VI.

Acidity pH of a 5% w/v solution, 2.8 to 4.5, Appendix V L.

Completeness of solution 0.10 g dissolves completely in 1 ml of *water*.

Sulphated ash Not more than 1.0%, Appendix IX A.

Water Not more than 4.5% w/w, Appendix IX C. Use 0.5 g.

Assay Carry out the *biological assay of antibiotics*, Appendix XIV A. The precision of the assay is such that the fiducial limits of error are not less than 95% and not more than 105% of the estimated potency.

Storage Vancomycin Hydrochloride intended for use in the manufacture of a parenteral dosage form should be kept in a sterile container, sealed so as to exclude micro-organisms.

Labelling The label states (1) the number of Units per mg; (2) the date after which the material is not intended to be used; (3) the conditions under which it should be stored; (4) whether or not it is intended for use in the manufacture of a parenteral dosage form.

Preparation
Vancomycin Injection

Action and use Antibacterial.

Vancomycin Hydrochloride intended for use in the manufacture of a parenteral dosage form complies with the following additional requirements.

Abnormal toxicity Complies with the *test for abnormal toxicity*, Appendix XIV L. Use a quantity containing 2000 Units.

Pyrogens Complies with the *test for pyrogens*, Appendix XIV K. Use per kg of the rabbit's weight 1 ml of *water for injections* containing 10,000 Units per ml.

Sterility When intended for use in the manufacture of a parenteral dosage form without further sterilisation, complies with the *test for sterility*, Appendix XVI A.

Vanillin

$C_8H_8O_3$ 152.1   *121-33-5*

Vanillin is 4-hydroxy-3-methoxybenzaldehyde and may be obtained from *Vanilla planifolia* Andrews or other species of *Vanilla* or prepared synthetically.

Solubility Soluble in 100 parts of *water* and in 20 parts of *glycerol*; soluble in *ethanol (96%)* and in fixed and volatile oils. It dissolves in aqueous solutions of alkali hydroxides.

Characteristics White or cream, crystalline needles or powder; odour, characteristic of vanilla.

Identification A. To 1 ml of a saturated solution in *water* add 1 ml of *lead acetate solution*. A white precipitate is produced which is soluble in hot *water*; on cooling it separates as flakes.

B. To 10 ml of a saturated solution in *water* add 0.2 ml of *iron(III) chloride test-solution*; a blue colour is produced. Heat at 80° for 3 minutes; the solution becomes brown. Cool; a white or almost white precipitate is produced.

Melting point 81° to 83°, Appendix V A.

Sulphated ash Not more than 0.1%, Appendix IX A.

Storage Vanillin should be kept in a well-closed container and protected from light.

Action and use Flavour.

Verapamil Hydrochloride

$C_{27}H_{38}N_2O_4,HCl$ 491.1   *152-11-4*

Verapamil Hydrochloride is 5-[*N*-(3,4-dimethoxyphenethyl)methylamino]-2-(3,4-dimethoxyphenyl)-2-isopropylvaleronitrile hydrochloride. It contains not less than 99.0 per cent and not more than 101.0 per cent of $C_{27}H_{38}N_2O_4,HCl$, calculated with reference to the dried substance.

Characteristics A white or almost white, crystalline powder; odourless or almost odourless.

Solubility Soluble in 20 parts of *water*; sparingly soluble in *ethanol (96%)*; freely soluble in *chloroform*.

Identification A. The *infra-red absorption spectrum*, Appendix II A, is concordant with the *reference spectrum* of verapamil hydrochloride.
B. To 2 ml of a 1% w/v solution add 0.2 ml of a 5% w/v solution of *mercury(II) chloride*. A white precipitate is produced.
C. To 2 ml of a 1% w/v solution add 0.5 ml of 3M *sulphuric acid* and 0.2 ml of *potassium permanganate solution*. A violet precipitate is produced which quickly dissolves to produce a very pale yellow solution.
D. Yields *reaction B* characteristic of chlorides, Appendix VI.

Acidity pH of a 5% w/v solution, 4.5 to 6.5, Appendix V L.

Clarity and colour of solution 10 ml of a 5.0% w/v solution is *clear*, Appendix IV A, and *colourless*, Appendix IV B, Method II.

Light absorption *Absorbance* of a 0.002% w/v solution in 0.01M *hydrochloric acid* at the maximum at 229 nm, 0.61 to 0.64, and at the maximum at 278 nm, 0.23 to 0.24, Appendix II B.

Melting point 141° to 144°, Appendix V A.

Readily carbonisable substances Dissolve 0.1 g in 5 ml of *sulphuric acid*. After 5 minutes the solution is clear and not more intensely coloured than *reference solution BY₄*, Appendix IV B, Method II.

Related substances A. Carry out the method for *thin-layer chromatography*, Appendix III A, using a silica gel precoated chromatoplate (Merck silica gel 60 plates are suitable) and a mixture of 85 volumes of *cyclohexane* and 15 volumes of *diethylamine* as the mobile phase. Apply separately to the plate 10 μl of each of three solutions of

the substance being examined in *chloroform* containing (1) 5.0% w/v, (2) 0.0050% w/v and (3) 0.0025% w/v. Dry the plate for 10 minutes at room temperature and repeat the development. After removal of the plate, heat at 110° for 1 hour, allow to cool, spray with a solution prepared by dissolving 5 g of *iron(III) chloride hexahydrate* and 2 g of *iodine* in a mixture of 50 ml of *acetone* and 50 ml of a 20% w/v solution of *tartaric acid*, applying a total of 15 to 20 ml of the reagent, and examine immediately. Any *secondary spot* in the chromatogram obtained with solution (1) is not more intense than the spot in the chromatogram obtained with solution (2) and not more than three such spots are more intense than the spot in the chromatogram obtained with solution (3). Disregard any spot on the line of application.
B. Carry out test A but use a mixture of 70 volumes of *toluene*, 20 volumes of *methanol*, 5 volumes of *acetone* and 5 volumes of *glacial acetic acid* as the mobile phase.

Loss on drying When dried to constant weight at 105°, loses not more than 0.5% of its weight. Use 1 g.

Sulphated ash Not more than 0.1%, Appendix IX A.

Assay Carry out Method I for *non-aqueous titration*, Appendix VIII A, using 0.5 g, 10 ml of *mercury(II) acetate solution* and *1-naphtholbenzein solution* as indicator. Each ml of 0.1M *perchloric acid VS* is equivalent to 0.04911 g of $C_{27}H_{38}N_2O_4,HCl$.

Storage Verapamil Hydrochloride should be kept in a well-closed container and protected from light.

Preparations
Verapamil Injection
Verapamil Tablets

Action and use Anti-arrhythmic.

Vinblastine Sulphate

$C_{46}H_{58}N_4O_9,H_2SO_4$ 909.1   *143-67-9*

Vinblastine Sulphate is the sulphate of an alkaloid, vincaleukoblastine, occurring in *Vinca rosea* L. It contains not less than 96.0 per cent and not more than 101.0 per cent of vinblastine sulphate, $C_{46}H_{58}N_4O_9,H_2SO_4$, calculated with reference to the dried substance.

Characteristics A white to slightly yellow, amorphous or crystalline powder; very hygroscopic.

Solubility Soluble in 10 parts of *water*; very slightly soluble in *ethanol (96%)*; soluble in 50 parts of *chloroform*; practically insoluble in *ether*.

Identification A. In the test for Related alkaloids the principal spot in the chromatogram obtained with solution (1) corresponds to that in the chromatogram obtained with solution (3).

B. To 1 mg add 0.2 ml of a freshly prepared 1% w/v solution of *vanillin* in *hydrochloric acid*. A pink colour is produced in about 1 minute (distinction from vincristine sulphate).

C. Mix 0.5 mg with 5 mg of *4-dimethylaminobenzaldehyde* and 0.2 ml of *glacial acetic acid* and add 0.2 ml of *sulphuric acid*; a reddish-brown colour is produced. Add 1 ml of *glacial acetic acid*; the colour changes to pink.

D. Yields the *reactions* characteristic of sulphates, Appendix VI.

Acidity pH of a 0.15% w/v solution, 3.5 to 5.0, Appendix V L.

Clarity of solution A 0.30% w/v solution is *clear*, Appendix IV A.

Specific optical rotation In a 2% w/v solution in *methanol*, $-28°$ to $-35°$, Appendix V F.

Related alkaloids Carry out the method for *thin-layer chromatography*, Appendix III A, using *silica gel GF254* as the coating substance and a mixture of 80 volumes of *toluene*, 40 volumes of *chloroform* and 6 volumes of *diethylamine* as the mobile phase. Apply separately to the chromatoplate 5 µl of each of three solutions in *methanol* containing (1) 1.0% w/v of the substance being examined, (2) 0.020% w/v of *vincristine sulphate BPCRS* and (3) 1.0% w/v of *vinblastine sulphate BPCRS*. After removal of the plate, allow it to dry in air and examine under *ultraviolet light (254 nm)*. Any *secondary spot* in the chromatogram obtained with solution (1) is not more intense than the spot in the chromatogram obtained with solution (2).

Loss on drying When dried at 60° at a pressure not exceeding 0.7 kPa for 16 hours, loses not more than 17.0% of its weight.

Assay Dissolve 10 mg in sufficient *methanol* to produce 500 ml and measure the *absorbance* of the resulting solution at the maximum at 267 nm, Appendix II B. Calculate the content of $C_{46}H_{58}N_4O_9,H_2SO_4$ taking 185 as the value of A(1%, 1 cm) at the maximum at 267 nm.

Storage Vinblastine Sulphate should be kept in a well-closed container, protected from light and stored at a temperature of 2° to 8°.

Preparation
Vinblastine Injection

Action and use Cytotoxic.

Vincristine Sulphate

$C_{46}H_{56}N_4O_{10},H_2SO_4$ 923.1   *2068-78-2*

Vincristine Sulphate is the sulphate of an alkaloid, 22-oxovincaleukoblastine, occurring in *Vinca rosea* L. It contains not less than 90.0 per cent and not more than 105.0 per cent of vincristine sulphate, $C_{46}H_{56}N_4O_{10},H_2SO_4$, calculated with reference to the dried substance.

Characteristics A white to slightly yellow, amorphous or crystalline powder; very hygroscopic.

Solubility Soluble in 2 parts of *water*; slightly soluble in *ethanol* (96%); soluble in 30 parts of *chloroform*; practically insoluble in *ether*.

Identification A. In the test for Related alkaloids the principal spot in the chromatogram obtained with solution (1) corresponds to that in the chromatogram obtained with solution (3).

B. To 1 mg add 0.2 ml of a freshly prepared 1% w/v solution of *vanillin* in *hydrochloric acid*. An orange colour is produced in about 1 minute (distinction from vinblastine sulphate).

C. Mix 0.5 mg with 5 mg of *4-dimethylaminobenzaldehyde* and 0.2 ml of *glacial acetic acid* and add 0.2 ml of *sulphuric acid*; a reddish-brown colour is produced. Add 1 ml of *glacial acetic acid*; the colour changes to pink.

D. Yields the *reactions* characteristic of sulphates, Appendix VI.

Acidity pH of a 0.1% w/v solution, 3.5 to 4.5, Appendix V L.

Related alkaloids Carry out the method for *thin-layer chromatography*, Appendix III A, using *silica gel HF254* as the coating substance and a mixture of 80 volumes of *toluene*, 40 volumes of *chloroform* and 6 volumes of *diethylamine* as the mobile phase. Apply separately to the chromatoplate 5 µl of each of three solutions in *methanol* containing (1) 1.0% w/v of the substance being examined, (2) 0.020% w/v of *vinblastine sulphate BPCRS* and (3) 1.0% w/v of *vincristine sulphate BPCRS*. After removal of the plate, allow it to dry in air and examine under *ultraviolet light (254 nm)*. Any *secondary spot* in the chromatogram obtained with solution (1) is not more intense than the spot in the chromatogram obtained with solution (2).

Loss on drying When dried at 40° at a pressure not exceeding 0.7 kPa for 16 hours, loses not more than 12.0% of its weight.

Assay Dissolve 10 mg in sufficient *methanol* to produce 500 ml and measure the *absorbance* of the resulting solution at the maximum at 297 nm, Appendix II B.

Calculate the content of $C_{46}H_{56}N_4O_{10},H_2SO_4$ taking 177 as the value of A(1%, 1 cm) at the maximum at 297 nm.

Storage Vincristine Sulphate should be kept in a well-closed container, protected from light and stored at a temperature of 2° to 8°.

Preparation
Vincristine Injection

Action and use Cytotoxic.

Vinyl Ether

$(H_2C{=}CH)_2O$

C_4H_6O 70.09   *109-93-3*

Vinyl Ether is divinyl ether to which has been added about 4 per cent of absolute ethanol and not more than 0.01 per cent w/v of 1-naphthyl(phenyl)amine or other suitable stabiliser.

Characteristics A clear, colourless, flammable liquid, often with a purplish fluorescence; odour, characteristic.

Solubility Soluble in 100 parts of *water*; miscible with *ethanol (96%)*, with *chloroform* and with *ether*.

Identification A. Warm 2 ml with 2 ml of 1M *sulphuric acid*. Acetaldehyde, recognisable by its odour, is evolved.
B. Shake 2 ml with 2 ml of *bromine water*. The colour is immediately discharged.

Acidity or alkalinity Shake 5 ml with 2 ml of *water* for 2 minutes. The aqueous layer is neutral to *litmus solution*.

Distillation range None distils below 28° and not more than 5% v/v distils above 31°, Appendix V C.

Weight per ml 0.770 to 0.778 g, Appendix V G.

Aldehyde Shake vigorously 5 ml for 3 minutes in a stoppered cylinder with 1 ml of a solution of 0.1 g of *phloroglucinol* in a mixture of 10 ml of 5M *sodium hydroxide* and 15 ml of *water*. The colour of the aqueous layer, when examined against a white background, is not more intense than that produced by repeating the test using 5 ml of *toluene* in place of the substance being examined.

Chlorinated compounds Mix 25 ml with 20 ml of *amyl alcohol* in a flask fitted with a reflux condenser and add 2 g of *sodium* in small pieces. Heat on a water-bath until evolution of hydrogen ceases, boil gently until all the sodium has dissolved and continue the heating for a further 20 minutes. Cool, add 25 ml of *water*, 15 ml of *nitric acid*, 1 ml of *dibutyl phthalate* and 10 ml of 0.02M *silver nitrate VS*, shake well and titrate the excess of silver nitrate with 0.02M *ammonium thiocyanate VS* using *ammonium iron(III) sulphate solution* as indicator. Repeat the operation without the substance being examined. The difference between the titrations does not exceed 4 ml.

Foreign odour Pour 10 ml in successive portions on to clean filter paper and allow to evaporate spontaneously. No foreign odour is detectable at any stage of the evaporation.

Peroxides Add 3.0 ml of the substance being examined to 5.0 ml of a freshly prepared 0.3% w/v solution of N,N-diethyl-p-phenylenediamine sulphate in a mixture of 9 volumes of *methanol* and 1 volume of *water*, mix and allow to stand in the dark for 5 minutes. No pink or red colour is produced.

Non-volatile matter When evaporated spontaneously and dried at 105°, leaves not more than 0.01% w/v of residue.

Storage Vinyl Ether should be kept in a well-closed container of not more than 200-ml capacity, protected from light and stored at a temperature of 8° to 15°. It should be used within 48 hours of first opening the container.

Action and use General anaesthetic.

Vitamin A Ester Concentrate (Natural)

Vitamin A Ester Concentrate (Natural) consists of a natural ester or a mixture of natural esters of retinol or of a solution of the ester or mixture of esters in Arachis Oil or other suitable vegetable oil. It contains in 1 g not less than 485,000 Units of vitamin A and not less than 97.0 per cent of the number of Units of vitamin A stated on the label. It may contain a suitable antioxidant or mixture of antioxidants.

Characteristics A yellow oil or a mixture of oil and crystalline material which yields a homogeneous yellow oil on warming; odour, faint.

Solubility Practically insoluble in *water*; soluble or partly soluble in *ethanol (96%)*; miscible with *chloroform*, with *ether* and with *petroleum spirit*.

Identification A. Dissolve a quantity containing 10 Units in a mixture of 100 parts of *absolute ethanol* and 1 part of *hydrochloric acid*. The *light absorption* of the solution immediately after preparation, Appendix II B, exhibits a single maximum at 326 nm. Heat the solution in a water-bath for 30 seconds and cool rapidly. The *light absorption* in the range 300 to 400 nm exhibits a low maximum or inflection at 332 nm and sharp maxima at 348, 367 and 389 nm.
B. Dissolve a quantity containing 30 Units in 1 ml of *chloroform* and add 10 ml of *antimony trichloride solution*. A transient bright blue colour is produced immediately.

Acid value Not more than 2.0, Appendix X B.

Peroxide value Place 1 g in a boiling-tube (20 cm × 2.5 cm) and dissolve in 20 ml of a mixture of 2 volumes of *glacial acetic acid* and 1 volume of *ethanol-free chloroform*. Add 1 g of finely powdered *potassium iodide* and pass a rapid stream of *oxygen-free nitrogen* through the mixture for 1 minute. Stopper the tube loosely, partly immerse in boiling water for 30 seconds and then in water at 80° for 2 minutes, tighten the stopper and cool rapidly. Transfer the contents to a flask containing 25 ml of a freshly prepared 1% w/v solution of *potassium iodide*, rinse the tube with a further 25 ml of the potassium iodide solution, shake the combined solution and rinsings and titrate with 0.01M *sodium thiosulphate VS*. Repeat the procedure without the concentrate. The difference between the titrations does not exceed 1.4 ml.

Retinol Carry out the method for *descending paper chromatography*, Appendix III E, using a mixture of 70 volumes of *1,4-dioxan*, 15 volumes of *methanol* and 15 volumes of *water* containing 1% w/v of *butylated hydroxyanisole* in the bottom of the tank and as the mobile phase. Saturate the paper with a 10% w/v solution of *liquid paraffin* in *petroleum spirit (boiling range, 40° to 60°)*

and dry without the aid of heat. Apply separately to the impregnated paper 5 µl and 10 µl of each of two freshly prepared solutions in *petroleum spirit (boiling range, 40° to 60°)* containing (1) sufficient of the concentrate to yield a solution containing 16,150 to 17,850 Units per ml and (2) 0.01% w/v of retinol. Solution (2) may be prepared in the following manner. Saponify a portion of the concentrate by the method described under the *assay of vitamin A, other vitamin A*, Appendix VIII K, and adjust the volume of the solution of the extracted retinol to contain about 340 Units per ml.

Develop until the solvent front approaches the bottom of the paper. Examine the dried paper under ultra-violet light (365 nm). The fluorescence of any spot corresponding to retinol in the chromatograms obtained with solution (1) is not more intense than that of the spots in the corresponding chromatogram obtained with solution (2).

Assay Carry out the *assay of vitamin A*, Appendix VIII K.

Storage Vitamin A Ester Concentrate (Natural) should be kept in an airtight container, protected from light and stored at a temperature of 8° to 15°. Once the container has been opened its contents should be used as soon as possible; any part of the contents not used at once should be protected by an atmosphere of an inert gas.

Labelling The label states (1) the number of Units of vitamin A in 1 g; (2) the name and proportion of any added stabilising agents; (3) the method of restoring the solution if partial crystallisation has occurred.

In some countries the material described in this monograph may be known as Retinol Ester Concentrate (Natural).

Synthetic Vitamin A Concentrate (Oily Form) ☆

Synthetic Vitamin A Concentrate (Oily Form) consists of an ester or a mixture of esters of retinol (the acetate, propionate or palmitate) prepared by synthesis. It may be diluted with a suitable vegetable oil. It contains in 1 g not less than 500,000 Units of Vitamin A and not less than 95.0 per cent and not more than 110.0 per cent of the number of Units of Vitamin A stated on the label. It may contain suitable stabilising agents such as antioxidants.

Characteristics A yellow to brownish-yellow, oily liquid; odour, faint and characteristic.

Solubility Practically insoluble in *water*; soluble or partly soluble in *absolute ethanol*; miscible with organic solvents. Partial crystallisation may occur in highly concentrated solutions.

Identification A. The *light absorption*, Appendix II B, of a solution in *propan-2-ol UV* containing 10 to 15 Units per ml exhibits a maximum at 325 to 327 nm.
B. Carry out the method for *thin-layer chromatography*, Appendix III A, using *silica gel G* as the coating substance and a mixture of 80 volumes of *cyclohexane* and 20 volumes of *ether* as the mobile phase. Apply separately to the chromatoplate 2 µl of each of four solutions in *cyclohexane* containing about 5 Units per µl of (1) the

substance being examined, (2) *retinyl acetate EPCRS*, (3) *retinyl propionate EPCRS* and (4) *retinyl palmitate EPCRS*. Develop the chromatogram immediately without evaporating the solvent. After removal of the plate, allow it to dry in air and spray with *antimony trichloride solution*. The principal spot or spots in the chromatogram obtained with solution (1) corresponds to one or more of the spots in the chromatograms obtained with solutions (2), (3) or (4).
C. Dissolve a quantity containing 10 to 15 Units in 1 ml of *chloroform* and add 5 ml of *antimony trichloride solution*. A transient bright blue colour is produced immediately.

Acid value Not more than 2.0, Appendix X B. Use 2 g.

Peroxides Add 0.30 g to 25.0 ml of a mixture of 4 volumes of *methanol* and 6 volumes of *toluene* (solution A). Mix in a test-tube, in the following order, 0.3 ml of a 1.8% w/v solution of *ammonium thiocyanate*, 10.0 ml of *methanol*, 0.3 ml of *acid iron(II) sulphate solution* and 15.0 ml of *toluene* and add 1.0 ml of solution A. The colour produced after 5 minutes is not more intense than that obtained in a solution prepared at the same time and in the same manner but using a solution prepared in the following manner in place of solution A. Add 1.0 ml of a 27.0% w/v solution of *iron(III) chloride hexahydrate* to 99 ml of a mixture of 4 volumes of *methanol* and 6 volumes of *toluene* and dilute 2.0 ml to 100 ml with the same solvent mixture.

Assay Carry out the *assay of vitamin A*, Appendix VIII K, Method I.

Storage Synthetic Vitamin A Concentrate (Oily Form) should be kept in an airtight container, protected from light and stored at a temperature of 8° to 15°. Once the container has been opened its contents should be used as soon as possible; any part of the contents not used at once should be protected by an atmosphere of an inert gas.

Labelling The label states (1) the number of Units of vitamin A in 1 g; (2) the name and proportion of any added stabilising agents; (3) the method of restoring the solution if partial crystallisation has occurred; (4) the name of the ester or esters.

In some countries the material described in this monograph may be known as Synthetic Retinol Concentrate (Oily Form).

Synthetic Vitamin A Concentrate (Powder Form) ☆

Synthetic Vitamin A Concentrate (Powder Form) consists of an ester or a mixture of esters of retinol (the acetate, propionate or palmitate) prepared by synthesis and dispersed in a matrix of gelatin, acacia or other suitable material. It contains in 1 g not less than 250,000 Units of Vitamin A activity and not less than 95.0 per cent and not more than 115.0 per cent of the number of Units of Vitamin A stated on the label. It may contain suitable stabilising agents such as antioxidants.

Characteristics A yellowish powder usually in the form of particles of almost uniform size.

Solubility Depending on the formulation, may be practically insoluble in *water*, swell or form an emulsion.

Identification To a quantity containing 50,000 Units add 1.5 ml of 2M *ammonia* previously heated to 60° and heat in a water-bath at 60°, shaking occasionally. After 10 minutes add 40 ml of *ethanol (96%)*, dilute to 200 ml with *ether* and shake. Allow to stand for a few minutes and use the supernatant liquid (solution A) for the following tests.

Certain batches do not react sufficiently during the course of the above treatment. For these batches the volume of solution A used in the tests should be increased. The increase may be as much as tenfold.

A. The *light absorption*, Appendix II B, of a solution prepared by diluting 5 ml of solution A to 100 ml with *propan-2-ol UV* exhibits a maximum at 325 to 327 nm.

B. Complies with test B for Identification described under Synthetic Vitamin A Concentrate (Oily Form) using as solution (1) a solution prepared by evaporating 10 ml of solution A to dryness in a stream of nitrogen and dissolving the residue in 0.5 ml of *cyclohexane*.

C. Dilute 2 ml of solution A to 50 ml with n-*pentane* and evaporate 1 ml of the solution to dryness in a stream of nitrogen. Dissolve the residue in 1 ml of *chloroform* and add 5 ml of *antimony trichloride solution*. A transient bright blue colour is produced immediately.

Related substances and degradation products Using the relative absorbances obtained in the Assay, the ratio A_{300}/A_{325} is not more than 0.612 and the sum of the ratios A_{300}/A_{325} and A_{350}/A_{325} is not more than 1.054, where A_{300}, A_{325} and A_{350} are the absorbances measured at 300, 325 and 350 nm respectively.

Assay Carry out the *assay of vitamin A*, Appendix VIII K, Method I B, using *propan-2-ol UV* in the reference cell and taking 0.612 as the maximum value of the ratio A_{300}/A_{325}.

Storage Synthetic Vitamin A Concentrate (Powder Form) should be kept in an airtight container, protected from light and stored at a temperature of 8° to 15°. Once the container has been opened its contents should be used as soon as possible; any part of the contents not used at once should be protected by an atmosphere of an inert gas.

Labelling The label states (1) the number of Units of vitamin A in 1 g; (2) the name of the ester or esters; (3) the name of the principal excipient or excipients used; (4) the name of any added stabiliser.

In some countries the material described in this monograph may be known as Synthetic Retinol Concentrate (Powder Form).

Synthetic Vitamin A Concentrate (Water-dispersible Form) ☆

Synthetic Vitamin A Concentrate (Water-dispersible Form) consists of an ester or a mixture of esters of retinol (the acetate, propionate or palmitate) prepared by synthesis to which suitable solubilisers have been added. It contains in 1 g not less than 100,000 Units of Vitamin A and not less than 95.0 per cent and not more than 115.0 per cent of the number of Units of Vitamin A stated on the label. It may contain suitable stabilising agents such as antimicrobial preservatives and antioxidants.

Characteristics A yellow or yellowish liquid of variable opalescence and viscosity; odour, characteristic. Highly concentrated solutions may become cloudy at low temperatures or take the form of a gel at room temperature.

Identification To a quantity containing about 10,000 Units add 5 ml of *water* and mix until a homogeneous dispersion is obtained. Add 5 ml of *ethanol (96%)* and 20 ml of n-*pentane* and shake vigorously for 30 seconds. Allow to stand for a few minutes and use the supernatant liquid (solution A) for the following tests.

A. Dilute solution A with sufficient *propan-2-ol UV* so that the *absorbance* at the wavelength of maximum absorption is between 0.3 and 0.7, Appendix II B. The solution exhibits a maximum at 325 to 327 nm.

B. Complies with test B for Identification described under Synthetic Vitamin A Concentrate (Oily Form) using as solution (1) a solution prepared by evaporating 10 ml of solution A to dryness in a stream of nitrogen and dissolving the residue in 0.5 ml of *cyclohexane*.

C. Evaporate 0.1 ml of solution A to dryness in a stream of nitrogen, dissolve the residue in 1 ml of *chloroform* and add 5 ml of *antimony trichloride solution*. A transient bright blue colour is produced immediately.

Water miscibility Mix 1 g with 10 ml of *water* previously heated to 50° and allow to cool to 20°. Immediately after cooling a uniform, slightly opalescent and slightly yellow dispersion is obtained.

Related substances and degradation products Using the relative absorbances obtained in the Assay, the ratio A_{300}/A_{325} is not more than 0.618 and the sum of the ratios A_{300}/A_{325} and A_{350}/A_{325} is not more than 1.060, where A_{300}, A_{325} and A_{350} are the absorbances measured at 300, 325 and 350 nm respectively.

Assay Carry out the *assay of vitamin A*, Appendix VIII K, Method I B, using *propan-2-ol UV* in the reference cell and taking 0.618 as the maximum value of the ratio A_{300}/A_{325}.

Storage Synthetic Vitamin A Concentrate (Water-dispersible Form) should be kept in an airtight container, protected from light and stored at the temperature stated on the label. Once the container has been opened, its contents should be used as soon as possible; any part of the contents not used at once should be protected by an atmosphere of an inert gas.

Labelling The label states (1) the number of Units of vitamin A in 1 g; (2) the name of the ester or esters; (3) the name of the principal solubiliser or solubilisers used; (4) the name of any added stabiliser; (5) the temperature at which it should be stored.

In some countries the material described in this monograph may be known as Synthetic Retinol Concentrate (Water-dispersible Form).

Warfarin Sodium

C₁₉H₁₅NaO₄   330.3   *129-06-6*

Warfarin Sodium is the sodium derivative of 4-hydroxy-3-(3-oxo-1-phenylbutyl)coumarin or the clathrate of this substance with propan-2-ol. It contains not less than 98.0 per cent and not more than 102.0 per cent of C₁₉H₁₅NaO₄, calculated with reference to the anhydrous substance or the anhydrous, propan-2-ol-free substance.

Characteristics A white, crystalline powder; odourless or almost odourless.

Solubility Soluble in less than 1 part of *water* and in less than 1 part of *ethanol (96%)*; slightly soluble in *chloroform* and in *ether*.

Identification A. Dissolve 0.1 g in 10 ml of *water*, acidify with 1M *hydrochloric acid*, filter, wash the precipitate with *water* and dry the residue at 105°. The *infra-red absorption spectrum* of the residue, Appendix II A, is concordant with the *reference spectrum* of warfarin.

B. Dissolve 0.1 g in 25 ml of *water*, add 0.1 ml of 2M *hydrochloric acid* and filter. The *melting point* of the precipitate, after washing with *water* and drying at 105°, is about 162°, Appendix V A.

C. Dissolve 1 g in 10 ml of *water*, add 5 ml of *nitric acid* and filter. To the filtrate add 2 ml of 0.0167M *potassium dichromate* and shake for 5 minutes. A light greenish-blue colour is produced with the clathrate.

D. The filtrate obtained in test B yields the *reactions* characteristic of sodium salts, Appendix VI.

Alkalinity pH of a 1% w/v solution, 7.2 to 8.3, Appendix V L.

Clarity of solution A 5.0% w/v solution is not more opalescent than *reference suspension II* and a 2.0% w/v solution in *acetone* is *clear*, Appendix IV A.

Colour of solution *Absorbance* of a 4-cm layer of a 2.0% w/v solution in *acetone* at 460 nm, not more than 0.12, Appendix II B.

Phenolic ketones *Absorbance* of a 12.5% w/v solution in 1.25M *sodium hydroxide* at 385 nm, measured within 15 minutes of preparing the solution, not more than 0.3, Appendix II B.

Propan-2-ol In the clathrate, 4.3 to 8.3% w/w when determined by the method for *gas chromatography*, Appendix III B, using solutions in *water* containing (1) 0.50% v/v of *propan-2-ol* and 0.50% v/v of *propan-1-ol* (internal standard), (2) 5.0% w/v of the substance being examined and (3) 5.0% w/v of the substance being examined and 0.50% v/v of the internal standard.

The chromatographic procedure may be carried out using (a) a column (1.5 m × 5 mm) packed with *diatomaceous support* (100 to 120 mesh) coated with 10% w/w of polyethylene glycol 1500 and maintained at 70°.

Calculate the percentage w/w of propan-2-ol, taking 0.785 g as its weight per ml.

Related substances Carry out the method for *thin-layer chromatography*, Appendix III A, using *silica gel GF254* as the coating substance and a mixture of 50 volumes of *chloroform*, 50 volumes of *cyclohexane* and 20 volumes of *glacial acetic acid* as the mobile phase. Apply separately to the chromatoplate 20 µl of each of two solutions of the substance being examined in *acetone* containing (1) 2.0% w/v and (2) 0.0020% w/v. After removal of the plate, allow it to dry in air and examine immediately under *ultra-violet light (254 nm)*. Any *secondary spot* in the chromatogram obtained with solution (1) is not more intense than the spot in the chromatogram obtained with solution (2).

Water Not more than 2.0% w/w, Appendix IX C. Use 1.2 g.

Assay Dissolve 0.1 g in sufficient 0.01M *sodium hydroxide* to produce 100 ml, dilute 10 ml to 100 ml with 0.01M *sodium hydroxide* and dilute 20 ml of the solution to 100 ml with 0.01M *sodium hydroxide*. Measure the *absorbance* of the resulting solution at the maximum at 308 nm, Appendix II B. Calculate the content of C₁₉H₁₅NaO₄ taking 431 as the value of A(1%, 1 cm) at the maximum at 308 nm.

Storage Warfarin Sodium should be kept in a well-closed container and protected from light.

Preparation
Warfarin Tablets

Action and use Anticoagulant.

Purified Water ☆

H₂O   18.02   *7732-18-5*

Purified Water is prepared by distillation, by means of ion exchange or by any other appropriate method, from suitable potable water.

Characteristics A clear, colourless liquid; odourless and tasteless.

Acidity or alkalinity To 10.0 ml, freshly boiled and cooled in a borosilicate glass flask, add 0.05 ml of *methyl red solution*; the resulting solution is not red. To 10.0 ml add 0.1 ml of *bromothymol blue solution*; the resulting solution is not blue.

Ammonium To 20.0 ml add 1 ml of *alkaline potassium mercuri-iodide reagent* and allow to stand for 5 minutes. When viewed vertically the solution is not more intensely coloured than a solution prepared at the same time by adding 1 ml of *alkaline potassium mercuri-iodide solution* to a mixture of 4 ml of *ammonium standard solution (1 ppm NH₄)* and 16 ml of *ammonia-free water* (0.2 ppm).

Calcium and magnesium To 100 ml add 2 ml of *ammonia buffer pH 10.0*, 50 mg of *mordant black 11 mixture* and 0.5 ml of 0.01M *disodium edetate*. A pure blue colour is produced.

Heavy metals In a glass evaporating dish evaporate 150.0 ml to 15 ml on a water-bath. 12 ml of the resulting solution complies with *limit test A for heavy metals*, Appendix VII (0.1 ppm). Use *lead standard solution (1 ppm Pb)* to prepare the standard.

Chloride To 10.0 ml add 1 ml of 2M *nitric acid* and 0.2 ml of 0.1M *silver nitrate*. The appearance of the solution does not change within 15 minutes.

Nitrate To 5.0 ml in a test-tube immersed in ice add 0.4 ml of a 10% w/v solution of *potassium chloride*, 0.1 ml of *diphenylamine solution* and, dropwise with shaking, 5 ml of *sulphuric acid*. Transfer the tube to a water-bath at 50° and allow to stand for 15 minutes. Any blue colour in the solution is not more intense than that in a solution prepared at the same time and in the same manner using a mixture of 4.5 ml of *nitrate-free water* and 0.5 ml of *nitrate standard solution (2 ppm NO₃)* (0.2 ppm).

Sulphate To 10.0 ml add 0.1 ml of 2M *hydrochloric acid* and 0.1 ml of 0.25M *barium chloride*. The solution shows no change in appearance for at least 1 hour.

Oxidisable substances To 100 ml add 10 ml of 1M *sulphuric acid* and 0.1 ml of 0.02M *potassium permanganate VS* and boil for 5 minutes. The pink colour is not completely discharged.

Non-volatile matter When evaporated to dryness on a water-bath and dried at 100° to 105°, leaves not more than 0.001% of residue. Use 100 ml.

Storage Purified Water should be kept in a well-closed container of a material that does not alter the properties of the water.

When Distilled Water is prescribed or demanded, Purified Water shall be dispensed or supplied.

Injections are made with Water for Injections; Purified Water is unsuitable for this purpose.

Water for Injections ☆

H₂O   18.02   *7732-18-5*

Water for Injections is sterilised, distilled water free from pyrogens. It is obtained by distilling potable water, Purified Water or distilled water from a neutral glass, quartz or suitable metal still fitted with an efficient device for preventing the entrainment of droplets; the first portion of the distillate is discarded and the remainder is collected in suitable containers, previously rinsed with freshly distilled water obtained under the same conditions from the apparatus, and closed so as to avoid contamination.

Water for Injections is distributed in suitable containers complying with the requirements stated under Containers for Water for Injections, Appendix XIX C, which are sealed and sterilised by *Heating in an Autoclave* under conditions that ensure that, whenever tested, the water will comply with the Test for Pyrogens, Appendix XIV K. Each container contains a sufficient quantity of Water for Injections to permit the nominal volume to be withdrawn.

Water for Injections complies with the tests prescribed under Purified Water with the following modifications and additional tests.

Acidity or alkalinity To 20 ml add 0.05 ml of *phenol red solution*. Not more than 0.1 ml of 0.01M *sodium hydroxide*

VS or 0.15 ml of 0.01M *hydrochloric acid VS* is required to change the colour of the solution.

Clarity and colour When examined under optimal conditions of visibility, it is clear, colourless and practically free from suspended particles.

Chloride When the volume in the final container is 100 ml or less, 15.0 ml complies with the *limit test for chlorides*, Appendix VII (0.5 ppm). Use a mixture of 1.5 ml of *chloride standard solution (5 ppm Cl)* and 13.5 ml of *water* to prepare the standard.

Oxidisable substances Boil 100 ml with 10 ml of 1M *sulphuric acid*, add 0.2 ml of 0.02M *potassium permanganate* and boil for 5 minutes. The pink colour is not completely discharged.

Non-volatile matter When evaporated on a water-bath and dried at 100° to 105°, the residue from Water for Injections in containers of not more than 10 ml does not exceed 0.004% and in containers of more than 10 ml does not exceed 0.003%. Use 100 ml.

Pyrogens When the volume in the final container is 15 ml or more, or if the container is labelled 'apyrogenic', carry out the *test for pyrogens*, Appendix XIV K. Use the water from a number of final containers representative of the batch and use per kg of the rabbit's weight 10 ml of the water, rendered isotonic by the addition of pyrogen-free *sodium chloride*.

Sterility Complies with the *test for sterility*, Appendix XVI A.

Wool Alcohols
Wool Wax Alcohols

Wool Alcohols may be prepared by saponification of the grease of the wool of sheep and separation of the fraction containing cholesterol and other alcohols. It contains not less than 30.0 per cent of cholesterol and not less than 500 and not more than 1000 parts per million of Butylated Hydroxytoluene.

Characteristics A golden brown solid, somewhat brittle when cold but becoming plastic when warm; odour, faint and characteristic. Fracture, smooth and shiny.

Solubility Practically insoluble in *water*; slightly soluble in *ethanol (96%)*; soluble in 25 parts of boiling *absolute ethanol*; freely soluble in *chloroform*, in *ether* and in *petroleum spirit (boiling range, 40° to 60°)*.

Identification Dissolve 0.5 g in 5 ml of *chloroform* and add 1 ml of *acetic anhydride* and 0.1 ml of *sulphuric acid*. A green colour is produced.

Acid value Not more than 2.0, Appendix X B.

Melting point Not lower than 58°, Appendix V A, Method V.

Copper Heat 5.0 g over a small flame until charred, ignite the residue at about 550° and dissolve the ash in 5 ml of *hydrochloric acid* with the aid of heat. Cool, dilute with *water*, make alkaline with 13.5M *ammonia*, boil to remove the excess of ammonia, add a few drops of *bromine water*, boil again and filter. To the filtrate add 1 ml of *sodium diethyldithiocarbamate solution*, 0.2 ml of 5M *ammonia* and sufficient *water* to produce 50 ml. Any colour produced is not more intense than that produced by adding 1 ml of *sodium diethyldithiocarbamate solution* and 0.2 ml of 5M *ammonia* to 2.5 ml of *copper standard solution (10 ppm Cu)* and diluting to 50 ml with *water* (5 ppm).

Soap; Mineral acid Boil 10 g with 100 ml of *water* for 5 minutes, stirring frequently. Remove the source of heat and add 0.5 ml of *phenolphthalein solution* while stirring; no pink colour is produced. Add 0.5 ml of *methyl orange solution* while stirring; no red colour is produced.

Saponification value Not more than 12, Appendix X G. Use 5 g and boil with the 0.5M ethanolic potassium hydroxide for 4 hours.

Butylated hydroxytoluene Carry out the method for *gas chromatography*, Appendix III B, using three solutions in *carbon disulphide* containing (1) 0.0050% w/v each of *butylated hydroxytoluene* and *methyl n-decanoate* (internal standard), (2) 5.0% w/v of the substance being examined and (3) 5.0% w/v of the substance being examined and 0.0050% w/v of the internal standard.

The chromatographic procedure may be carried out using a column (1.5 m × 4 mm) packed with *silanised diatomaceous support* (100 to 120 mesh) coated with 10% w/w of silicone gum rubber (methyl) (SE-30 is suitable), maintained at 150° and used in conjunction with a pre-column containing silanised glass wool.

In the chromatogram obtained with solution (3) the ratio of the area of the peak corresponding to butylated hydroxytoluene to the area of the peak due to the internal standard is not greater than the corresponding ratio in the chromatogram obtained with solution (1).

Loss on drying When dried at 105° for 1 hour, loses not more than 0.5% of its weight. Use 1 g.

Sulphated ash Not more than 0.15%, Appendix IX A.

Assay Melt 20 g on a water-bath, mix thoroughly and allow to cool. Dissolve 1 g in 25 ml of warm *ethanol (90%)*, filter while still warm through a sintered-glass filter (BS porosity No. 2) and wash the residue with 50 ml of warm *ethanol (90%)*. Cool the combined filtrate and washings and add sufficient *ethanol (90%)* to produce 100 ml. To 10 ml of the resulting solution add 40 ml of a 0.5% w/v solution of *digitonin* in *ethanol (90%)*, warm to 60° and allow to stand for 18 hours. Filter through a sintered-glass filter (BS porosity No. 2) with the aid of gentle suction, wash the residue with successive 15-ml quantities of *ethanol (90%)*, *acetone* and hot *carbon tetrachloride* and dry to constant weight at 105°. Each g of residue is equivalent to 0.239 g of cholesterol.

Storage Wool Alcohols should be kept in a well-closed container, protected from light and stored at a temperature not exceeding 25°.

Preparation
Wool Alcohols Ointment

Wool Fat ☆
Anhydrous Lanolin

Wool Fat is a purified anhydrous waxy material obtained from the wool of sheep. It may contain not more than 200 parts per million of Butylated Hydroxytoluene.

Characteristics A pale yellow substance with the consistency of an ointment; odour, characteristic. Melted wool fat is a clear or almost clear, yellow liquid.

Solubility Practically insoluble in *water*; slightly soluble in boiling *ethanol (96%)*; soluble in *chloroform* and in *ether*. A solution in *petroleum spirit (boiling range, 50° to 70°)* is opalescent.

Identification A. To a solution of 0.5 g in 5 ml of *chloroform* add 1 ml of *acetic anhydride* and 0.1 ml of *sulphuric acid*. An emerald-green colour is produced.
B. To a solution of 50 mg in 5 ml of *chloroform* add 5 ml of *sulphuric acid* and shake. A red colour is produced and a strong green fluorescence appears in the lower layer.

Acid value Not more than 1.0, Appendix X B. Use 5 g dissolved in 25 ml of the prescribed mixture of solvents.

Melting point 38° to 44°, Appendix V A, Method III, Test B. To fill the metal cup, melt the substance being examined on a water-bath, cool to about 50°, pour into the cup and allow to stand for 24 hours at 15° to 20°.

Peroxide value Not more than 20, Appendix X F.

Saponification value 90 to 105, Appendix X G, Method II. Boil with the 0.5M ethanolic potassium hydroxide for 4 hours.

Water absorption capacity Weigh 10 g into a mortar. Add *water* in quantities of 0.2 to 0.5 ml from a burette and stir vigorously, incorporating all the water before proceeding to the next addition. The end-point is reached when visible droplets remain that cannot be incorporated. Not less than 20 ml of *water* is absorbed.

Water-soluble acidic or alkaline substances Shake vigorously 5 g, previously melted on a water-bath, for 2 minutes with 75 ml of *water* previously heated to 90° to 95°. Allow to cool to ambient temperature and filter through filter paper previously washed with *water*. To 60 ml of the filtrate, which may not be clear, add 0.25 ml of *bromothymol blue solution*. Not more than 0.2 ml of 0.02M *hydrochloric acid VS* or 0.15 ml of 0.02M *sodium hydroxide VS* is required to change the colour of the solution.

Water-soluble oxidisable substances To 10 ml of the filtrate obtained in the test for Water-soluble acidic or alkaline substances add 1 ml of 1M *sulphuric acid* and 0.1 ml of 0.02M *potassium permanganate VS*. The solution is not completely decolorised within 10 minutes.

Chloride Boil 1.0 g with 20 ml of *ethanol (90%)* under a reflux condenser for 5 minutes, cool, add 40 ml of *water* and 0.5 ml of *nitric acid* and filter. To the filtrate add 0.15 ml of a 1% w/v solution of *silver nitrate in ethanol (90%)*. Any turbidity produced is not greater than that produced by adding 0.15 ml of a 1% w/v solution of *silver nitrate in ethanol (90%)* to a mixture of 0.2 ml of 0.02M *hydrochloric acid VS*, 20 ml of *ethanol (90%)*, 40 ml of *water* and 0.5 ml of *nitric acid*. Examine the liquids after 5 minutes (150 ppm).

Paraffins Prepare an alumina column (23 cm × 2 cm) by adding a slurry of *anhydrous aluminium oxide* and *petroleum spirit (boiling range, 40° to 60°)* to a glass tube fitted with a tap and containing the petroleum spirit. Allow to settle and reduce the depth of the solvent above the column to about 4 cm; the tap and absorbent cotton plugs should be free from grease. Dissolve 3 g of the substance being examined in 50 ml of warm *petroleum spirit (boiling range, 40° to 60°)*, cool, pass the solution through the column at a rate of 3 ml per minute and wash with 250 ml of the petroleum spirit. Distil the combined eluate and washings to low bulk, evaporate to dryness on a water-bath and heat the residue at 105° for periods of 10 minutes until the difference between two successive weighings is not greater than 1 mg. The residue weighs not more than 30 mg.

Butylated hydroxytoluene Carry out the method for *gas chromatography*, Appendix III B, using three solutions in *carbon disulphide* containing (1) 0.0020% w/v each of *butylated hydroxytoluene* and *methyl* n-*decanoate* (internal standard), (2) 10.0% w/v of the substance being examined and (3) 10.0% w/v of the substance being examined and 0.0020% w/v of the internal standard.

The chromatographic procedure may be carried out using a column (1.5 m × 4 mm) packed with *silanised diatomaceous support* (80 to 100 mesh) (Diatomite CQ is suitable) coated with 10% w/w of silicone gum rubber (methyl) (SE-30 is suitable), maintained at 150° and used in conjunction with a pre-column containing silanised glass wool.

In the chromatogram obtained with solution (3) the ratio of the area of the peak corresponding to butylated hydroxytoluene to the area of the peak due to the internal standard is not greater than the corresponding ratio in the chromatogram obtained with solution (1) (200 ppm).

Loss on drying When dried at 100° to 105° for 1 hour, loses not more than 0.5% of its weight. Use 1 g.

Sulphated ash Not more than 0.15%, Appendix IX A, Method II. Ignite 5 g and use the residue to determine the sulphated ash.

Storage Wool Fat should be kept in a well-closed container and stored at a temperature not exceeding 25°.

Labelling The label states the proportion of any butylated hydroxytoluene present.

Preparation
Hydrous Wool Fat

Hydrous Wool Fat ☆
Lanolin

Hydrous Wool Fat is a mixture of 75 per cent w/w of Wool Fat and 25 per cent w/w of Purified Water. It is obtained by the gradual addition of Purified Water to melted Wool Fat with continuous stirring. It may contain not more than 150 parts per million of Butylated Hydroxytoluene.

Characteristics A pale yellow substance with the consistency of an ointment; odour, faint and characteristic.

Identification Complies with the tests for Identification described under Wool Fat.

Acid value Not more than 0.8, Appendix X B. Use 5 g dissolved in 25 ml of the prescribed mixture of solvents.

Melting point 38° to 44°, Appendix V A, Method III, Test B, when determined on the residue obtained in the test for Non-volatile matter. To fill the metal cup, melt the residue on a water-bath, cool to about 50°, pour into the cup and allow to stand for 24 hours at 15° to 20°.

Peroxide value Not more than 15, Appendix X F.

Saponification value 67 to 79, Appendix X G, Method II. Boil with the 0.5M ethanolic potassium hydroxide for 4 hours.

Water absorption capacity Complies with the test described under Wool Fat. Use 10 g of the residue obtained in the test for Non-volatile matter.

Water-soluble acidic or alkaline substances Shake vigorously 6.7 g previously melted on a water-bath for 2 minutes with 75 ml of *water* previously heated to 90° to 95°. Allow to cool and filter through filter paper previously washed with *water*. To 60 ml of the filtrate, which may not be clear, add 0.25 ml of *bromothymol blue solution*. Not more than 0.2 ml of 0.02M *hydrochloric acid VS* or 0.15 ml of 0.02M *sodium hydroxide VS* is required to change the colour of the solution.

Water-soluble oxidisable substances Complies with the test described under Wool Fat. Use 10 ml of the filtrate obtained in the test for Water-soluble acidic or alkaline substances.

Chloride Carry out the test described under Wool Fat. Use 1.3 g (115 ppm).

Paraffins Complies with the test described under Wool Fat. Use 3 g of the residue obtained in the test for Non-volatile matter.

Butylated hydroxytoluene Carry out the test described under Wool Fat using in solutions (2) and (3) 10.0% w/v of the residue obtained in the test for Non-volatile matter (150 ppm).

Non-volatile matter When heated to constant weight on a water-bath, stirring occasionally with a glass rod, leaves 72.5% to 77.5% of residue. Use 30 g.

Sulphated ash Not more than 0.1%, Appendix IX A, Method II. Ignite 5 g and use the residue to determine the sulphated ash.

Storage Hydrous Wool Fat should be kept in a well-closed container and stored at a temperature not exceeding 25°.

Labelling The label states the proportion of any butylated hydroxytoluene present.

Xylometazoline Hydrochloride

$C_{16}H_{24}N_2,HCl$ 280.8   *1218-35-5*

Xylometazoline Hydrochloride is 2-(4-*tert*-butyl-2,6-dimethylbenzyl)-2-imidazoline hydrochloride. It contains not less than 99.0 per cent and not more than 101.0 per cent of $C_{16}H_{24}N_2$, HCl, calculated with reference to the dried substance.

Characteristics A white or almost white, crystalline powder; odourless or almost odourless.

Solubility Soluble in 12 parts of *water*, in 4 parts of *ethanol (96%)* and in 25 parts of *chloroform*; practically insoluble in *ether*.

Identification A. The *infra-red absorption spectrum*, Appendix II A, is concordant with the *reference spectrum* of xylometazoline hydrochloride.

B. The *light absorption*, Appendix II B, in the range 250 to 350 nm of a 0.1% w/v solution in 0.1M *hydrochloric acid* exhibits a minimum at 257 nm, a maximum at 265 nm and two inflections, at 270 nm and 275 nm. The *absorbance* at 265 nm is about 1.0.

C. To 1 ml of a 0.05% w/v solution add 0.2 ml of a 5% w/v solution of *sodium nitroprusside* and 0.1 ml of 5M *sodium hydroxide* and allow to stand for 10 minutes. Add 2 ml of *sodium hydrogen carbonate solution*. A violet colour is produced.

D. Yields *reaction A* characteristic of chlorides, Appendix VI.

Acidity pH of a 5% w/v solution, 5.0 to 6.6, Appendix V L.

Iron Moisten the residue obtained in the test for Sulphated ash with 5 ml of *hydrochloric acid*, evaporate to dryness and dissolve the residue in sufficient *water* to produce 50 ml. 10 ml of the resulting solution complies with the *limit test for iron*, Appendix VII (50 ppm).

Sulphate 0.75 g complies with the *limit test for sulphates*, Appendix VII (200 ppm).

***N*-(2-Aminoethyl)-4-*tert*-butyl-2,6-xylylacetamide** Carry out the method for *thin-layer chromatography*, Appendix III A, using *silica gel HF254* as the coating substance and a mixture of 200 volumes of *methanol* and 3 volumes of 13.5M *ammonia* as the mobile phase. Apply separately to the chromatoplate 5 μl of each of two solutions in *methanol* containing (1) 2.0% w/v of the substance being examined and (2) 0.010% w/v of N-(*2-aminoethyl*)-*4*-tert-*butyl*-*2,6*-*xylylacetamide BPCRS*. After removal of the plate, allow it to dry in air and spray with a solution containing 0.3 g of *ninhydrin* in a mixture of 100 ml of *butan-1-ol* and 3 ml of *glacial acetic acid*. Heat at 100° for 10 minutes, allow to cool and spray with *dilute potassium iodobismuthate solution*. Any spot corresponding to *N*-(2-aminoethyl)-4-*tert*-butyl-2,6-xylylacetamide in the chromatogram obtained with solution (1) is not more intense than the spot in the chromatogram obtained with solution (2).

Loss on drying When dried to constant weight at 105°, loses not more than 0.5% of its weight. Use 1 g.

Sulphated ash Not more than 0.1%, Appendix IX A. Use 1.0 g.

Assay Carry out Method I for *non-aqueous titration*, Appendix VIII A, using 0.5 g and *1-naphtholbenzein solution* as indicator. Each ml of 0.1M *perchloric acid VS* is equivalent to 0.02808 g of $C_{16}H_{24}N_2,HCl$.

Storage Xylometazoline Hydrochloride should be kept in a well-closed container and protected from light.

Preparation
Xylometazoline Nasal Drops

Action and use Sympathomimetic amine.

Xylose

D–Xylose

$C_5H_{10}O_5$ 150.1   58-86-6

Characteristics Colourless needles or a white, crystalline powder; odourless or almost odourless.

Solubility Soluble in less than 1 part of *water*; soluble in hot *ethanol* (96%).

Identification A. Carry out the method for *thin-layer chromatography*, Appendix III A, using a suspension of *silica gel G* in a 0.3% w/v solution of *sodium acetate* as the coating substance. Spread the suspension to form a uniform layer 0.5 mm thick. Use as the mobile phase a mixture of 70 volumes of *glacial acetic acid*, 60 volumes of *chloroform* and 10 volumes of *water*. Apply separately to the chromatoplate 2 μl of each of three solutions containing (1) 5.0% w/v of the substance being examined, (2) 5.0% w/v of *D–xylose* and (3) a mixture of equal volumes of solutions (1) and (2). Develop the plate in a continuous elution tank for about 4 hours. After removal of the plate, dry it in a current of warm air, spray with a solution in *acetone* containing 1% w/v of *diphenylamine*, 1% v/v of *aniline* and 1% v/v of *orthophosphoric acid* and heat for 10 minutes at 130°. The principal spot in the chromatogram obtained with solution (1) corresponds to that in the chromatogram obtained with solution (2). The principal spot in the chromatogram obtained with solution (3) appears as a single, compact spot.

B. When heated with *potassium cupri-tartrate solution* it produces a copious precipitate of copper(I) oxide.

Acidity Dissolve 5 g in 50 ml of *carbon dioxide-free water*. Not more than 0.2 ml of 0.1M *sodium hydroxide VS* is required to neutralise the solution using *phenolphthalein solution* as indicator.

Clarity and colour of solution A 10.0% w/v solution in *carbon dioxide-free water* is *clear*, Appendix IV A, and *colourless*, Appendix IV B, Method I.

Specific optical rotation In a 10% w/v solution containing 0.4% v/v of 5M *ammonia*, +18.5° to +19.5°, Appendix V F.

Heavy metals Dissolve 1.0 g in 20 ml of *water*. 12 ml of the resulting solution complies with *limit test A for heavy metals*, Appendix VII (20 ppm). Use *lead standard solution (1 ppm Pb)* to prepare the standard.

Chloride Dissolve 0.50 g in 50 ml of *water*. 15 ml of the resulting solution complies with the *limit test for chlorides*, Appendix VII (330 ppm).

Loss on drying When dried to constant weight at 100° at a pressure not exceeding 0.7 kPa, loses not more than 0.5% of its weight. Use 1 g.

Sulphated ash Not more than 0.1%, Appendix IX A.

Action and use For investigation of intestinal absorption.

Zinc Chloride ☆

ZnCl₂   136.3   7646-85-7

Zinc Chloride contains not less than 95.0 per cent and not more than 100.5 per cent of ZnCl₂.

Characteristics A white, crystalline powder or cast white sticks; odourless; deliquescent.

Solubility Very soluble in *water*; freely soluble in *ethanol* (96%) and in *glycerol*.

Identification A. To 2.0 g add 38 ml of *carbon dioxide-free water* prepared from *distilled water*, add 2M *hydrochloric acid* dropwise until solution is complete and dilute to 40 ml with *carbon dioxide-free water* prepared from *distilled water* (solution A). 5 ml of solution A yields the *reaction* characteristic of zinc salts, Appendix VI.

B. A 5% w/v solution in 2M *nitric acid* yields *reaction A* characteristic of chlorides, Appendix VI.

Acidity pH of a solution prepared by dissolving 1 g in 9 ml of *carbon dioxide-free water*, disregarding any slight turbidity, 4.6 to 5.5, Appendix V L.

Aluminium, calcium, magnesium, heavy metals and iron To 8 ml of solution A add 2 ml of 13.5M *ammonia* and shake; the solution is *clear*, Appendix IV A, and *colourless*, Appendix IV B, Method II. Add 1 ml of a 9% w/v solution of *disodium hydrogen orthophosphate*; the resulting solution remains clear for at least 5 minutes. Add 0.2 ml of *sodium sulphide solution*; a white precipitate is produced and the supernatant liquid remains colourless.

Ammonium 0.5 ml of solution A diluted to 15 ml with *water* complies with the *limit test for ammonium*, Appendix VII (400 ppm).

Oxychloride Dissolve 1.5 g in 1.5 ml of *carbon dioxide-free water*; the solution is not more opalescent than *reference suspension II*, Appendix IV A. Add 7.5 ml of *ethanol (96%)*; the solution may become cloudy within 10 minutes, but becomes clear on the addition of 0.2 ml of 2M *hydrochloric acid*.

Sulphate 5 ml of solution A diluted to 15 ml with *distilled water* complies with the *limit test for sulphates*, Appendix VII (200 ppm). Use 5 ml of *sulphate standard solution (10 ppm SO₄)* diluted to 15 ml with *distilled water* as the standard solution.

Assay Carry out the *complexometric titration of zinc*, Appendix VIII D, using 0.25 g dissolved in 5 ml of 2M *acetic acid*. Each ml of 0.1M *disodium edetate VS* is equivalent to 0.01363 g of $ZnCl_2$.

Storage Zinc Chloride should be kept in a well-closed, non-metallic container.

Zinc Oxide ☆

ZnO   81.4   *1341-13-2*

Zinc Oxide contains not less than 99.0 per cent and not more than 100.5 per cent of ZnO, calculated with reference to the substance ignited at 500°.

Characteristics A soft, white or faintly yellowish-white, amorphous powder, free from grittiness; odourless.

Solubility Practically insoluble in *water* and in *ethanol (96%)*. It dissolves in dilute mineral acids.

Identification A. Becomes yellow when strongly heated. The yellow colour disappears on cooling.
B. Dissolve 0.1 g in 1.5 ml of 2M *hydrochloric acid* and dilute to 5 ml with *water*. The resulting solution yields the *reaction* characteristic of zinc salts, Appendix VI.

Alkalinity Mix 1.0 g with 10 ml of boiling *water*, add 0.1 ml of *dilute phenolphthalein solution* and filter. If the filtrate is red, not more than 0.3 ml of 0.1M *hydrochloric acid VS* is required to discharge the colour.

Arsenic 0.2 g complies with the *limit test for arsenic*, Appendix VII (5 ppm).

Cadmium Not more than 10 ppm of Cd when determined by *atomic absorption spectrophotometry*, Appendix II D, Method II, measuring at 228.8 nm and using either an air—acetylene or an air—propane flame. Dissolve 2 g of the substance being examined in 14 ml of a mixture of equal volumes of *water* and *cadmium- and lead-free nitric acid*, boil for 1 minute, cool and dilute to 100 ml with

water. Use *cadmium solution ASp*, suitably diluted with a 3.5% v/v solution of *cadmium- and lead-free nitric acid*, for the standard solution.

Iron Dissolve 50 mg in 1 ml of 2M *hydrochloric acid* and dilute to 10 ml with *water*. The resulting solution complies with the *limit test for iron*, Appendix VII (200 ppm). Use 0.5 ml of *mercaptoacetic acid* in the test.

Lead Not more than 50 ppm of Pb when determined by *atomic absorption spectrophotometry*, Appendix II D, Method II, measuring at 283.3 nm or 217 nm using an air—acetylene flame. Dissolve 5 g of the substance being examined in 24 ml of a mixture of equal volumes of *water* and *cadmium- and lead-free nitric acid*, boil for 1 minute, cool and dilute to 100 ml with *water*. Use *lead solution ASp* suitably diluted with a 3.5% v/v solution of *cadmium- and lead-free nitric acid*, for the standard solution.

Carbonate and acid-insoluble substances Dissolve 1.0 g in 15 ml of 2M *hydrochloric acid*. No effervescence is produced and the solution is not more opalescent than *reference suspension II*, Appendix IV A, and is *colourless*, Appendix IV B, Method II.

Loss on ignition When ignited at 500°, loses not more than 1.0% of its weight.

Assay Carry out the *complexometric titration of zinc*, Appendix VIII D, using a solution of 0.15 g in 10 ml of 2M *acetic acid*. Each ml of 0.1M *disodium edetate VS* is equivalent to 0.00814 g of ZnO.

Preparations
Zinc Cream
Zinc Ointment
Zinc and Castor Oil Ointment
Zinc and Salicylic Acid Paste
Zinc and Coal Tar Paste
Compound Zinc Paste

Action and use Mild astringent.

Zinc Stearate ☆

$(C_{17}H_{35}CO_2)_2Zn$ 632.0   *557-05-1*

Zinc Stearate consists mainly of zinc stearate but may contain variable proportions of zinc palmitate, $(C_{15}H_{31}CO_2)_2Zn$, and zinc oleate, $(C_{17}H_{33}CO_2)_2Zn$. It contains not less than 10.0 per cent and not more than 12.0 per cent of Zn.

Characteristics A light, white, amorphous powder, free from gritty particles; odour, faint and characteristic.

Solubility Practically insoluble in *water*, in *ethanol (96%)* and in *ether*.

Identification A. To 5.0 g add 50 ml of *ether* and 40 ml of a 7.5% v/v solution of *cadmium- and lead-free nitric acid* in *distilled water* and heat under a reflux condenser until dissolution is complete. Allow to cool, separate the aqueous layer and shake the ether layer with two 4-ml quantities of *distilled water*. Combine the washings with the aqueous layer and reserve for test B. Evaporate the ether layer to dryness and dry the residue at 105°. The *freezing point* of the residue is not lower than 53°, Appendix V B.
B. Wash the aqueous extracts reserved in test A with 15 ml of *ether*, separate and heat the aqueous layer on a

water-bath until the odour of ether is no longer detectable. Allow to cool and dilute to 50 ml with *water* (solution A). Neutralise 5 ml of the solution to *litmus paper* with 10M *sodium hydroxide*. The resulting solution yields the *reactions* characteristic of zinc salts, Appendix VI.

Acidity or alkalinity Shake 1 g with 5 ml of *ethanol (96%)* and add 20 ml of *carbon dioxide-free water* and 0.1 ml of *phenol red solution*. Not more than 0.3 ml of 0.1M *hydrochloric acid VS* or 0.1 ml of 0.1M *sodium hydroxide VS* is required to change the colour of the solution.

Colour of solution Solution A is not more intensely coloured than *reference solution* Y_6, Appendix IV B, Method II.

Acid value of the fatty acids 195 to 210, Appendix X B, when determined on 0.2 g of the residue obtained in test A for Identification. Use 25 ml of the prescribed mixture of solvents.

Clarity and colour of solution of the fatty acids Dissolve 0.5 g of the dried residue obtained in test A for Identification in 10 ml of *chloroform*. The solution is *clear*, Appendix IV A, and not more intensely coloured than *reference solution* Y_5, Appendix IV B, Method II.

Cadmium Not more than 5 ppm of Cd when determined by *atomic absorption spectrophotometry*, Appendix II D, Method II, using as the test solution 20 ml of solution A diluted to 50 ml with a 3.5% v/v solution of *cadmium- and lead-free nitric acid* and measuring at 228.8 nm using either an air—acetylene or an air—propane flame. Use *cadmium solution ASp*, diluted if necessary with a 3.5% v/v *cadmium- and lead-free nitric acid*, for the standard solution.

Lead Not more than 25 ppm of Pb when determined by *atomic absorption spectrophotometry*, Appendix II D, Method II, using solution A, measuring at 283.3 or 217 nm and using an air—acetylene flame. Use *lead solution ASp*, diluted if necessary with a 3.5% v/v solution of *cadmium- and lead-free nitric acid*, for the standard solution.

Chloride 2 ml of solution A diluted to 15 ml with *water* complies with the *limit test for chlorides*, Appendix VII (250 ppm).

Sulphate Dilute 1 ml of solution A to 50 ml with *water*. 12.5 ml of the resulting solution diluted to 15 ml with *water* complies with the *limit test for sulphates*, Appendix VII (0.6%).

Assay Boil 1 g with 50 ml of 2M *acetic acid* for at least 10 minutes or until the layer of fatty acids is clear, adding *water* if necessary to maintain the original volume. Cool, filter and wash the filter and the flask with *water* until the washings are no longer acidic to *litmus paper*. Combine the filtrate and washings and carry out the *complexometric titration of zinc*, Appendix VIII D. Each ml of 0.1M *disodium edetate VS* is equivalent to 0.00654 g of Zn.

Action and use Pharmaceutical aid.

Zinc Sulphate ☆

ZnSO$_4$,7H$_2$O   287.5   *7733-02-0*

Zinc Sulphate contains not less than 99.0 per cent and not more than 104.0 per cent of ZnSO$_4$,7H$_2$O.

Characteristics Colourless, transparent crystals or a white, crystalline powder; odourless; efflorescent.

Solubility Very soluble in *water*; practically insoluble in *ethanol (96%)*.

Identification A 5.0% w/v solution in *carbon dioxide-free water* (solution A) yields the *reactions* characteristic of zinc salts and of sulphates, Appendix VI.

Acidity pH of solution A, 4.4 to 5.6, Appendix V L.

Clarity and colour of solution Solution A is *clear*, Appendix IV A, and *colourless*, Appendix IV B, Method II.

Iron 2 ml of solution A diluted to 10 ml with *water* complies with the *limit test for iron*, Appendix VII (100 ppm). Use 0.5 ml of *mercaptoacetic acid* in the test.

Chloride 3.3 ml of solution A diluted to 15 ml with *water* complies with the *limit test for chlorides*, Appendix VII (300 ppm).

Assay Carry out the *complexometric titration of zinc*, Appendix VIII D, using 0.5 g dissolved in 5 ml of 2M *acetic acid*. Each ml of 0.1M *disodium edetate VS* is equivalent to 0.02875 g of ZnSO$_4$,7H$_2$O.

Storage Zinc Sulphate should be kept in a well-closed, non-metallic container.

Preparations
Zinc Sulphate Eye Drops
Zinc Sulphate Lotion

Action and use Astringent.

Zinc Undecenoate ☆

[CH$_2$=CH·(CH$_2$)$_8$·CO$_2$]$_2$Zn

C$_{22}$H$_{38}$O$_4$Zn   431.9   *557-08-4*

Zinc Undecenoate is zinc di(undec-10-enoate). It contains not less than 98.0 per cent and not more than 102.0 per cent of C$_{22}$H$_{38}$O$_4$Zn, calculated with reference to the dried substance.

Characteristics A white or almost white, fine powder. It melts at 116° to 121° but may leave a slight solid residue.

Solubility Practically insoluble in *water*, in *ethanol (96%)* and in *ether*.

Identification A. Dissolve 0.1 g in a mixture of 2 ml of 1M *sulphuric acid* and 5 ml of *glacial acetic acid* and add, dropwise, 0.25 ml of *potassium permanganate solution*. The permanganate solution is decolorised.
B. To 2.5 g add 10 ml of *water* and 10 ml of 1M *sulphuric acid* and extract with two 10-ml quantities of *ether*. Reserve the aqueous layer for test C. Wash the combined ether extracts with *water* and evaporate the ether. To the residue add 2 ml of recently distilled *aniline* and boil under a reflux condenser for 10 minutes, cool and add 30 ml of *ether*; extract with three 20-ml quantities of 2M *hydrochloric acid* and then with 20 ml of *water*. Evaporate the organic layer to dryness on a water-bath. The *melting point* of the residue, after recrystallising twice from *ethanol (70%)* and drying at a pressure of 2 kPa for 3 hours, is 66° to 68°, Appendix V A, Method I.
C. A mixture of 1 ml of the aqueous layer reserved in test B and 4 ml of *water* yields the *reaction* characteristic of zinc salts, Appendix VI.

Alkalinity Mix 1.0 g with 5 ml of *ethanol (96%)* and 0.5 ml of *phenol red solution* and add 50 ml of *carbon* *dioxide-free water*. No reddish colour is produced immediately.

Alkali and alkaline-earth metals To 1.0 g add 25 ml of *water* and 5 ml of *hydrochloric acid*, heat to boiling and filter whilst hot. Wash the filter and the residue with 25 ml of hot *water*, combine the filtrate and washings and add 13.5M *ammonia* until the solution is alkaline. Add 7.5 ml of a 4% w/v solution of *thioacetamide* and warm on a water-bath for 30 minutes. Filter, wash the precipitate with two 10-ml quantities of *water*, combine the filtrate and washings and evaporate to dryness on a water-bath. The residue, after ignition, weighs not more than 20 mg (2%).

Sulphate To 0.10 g add 10 ml of *distilled water* and 2 ml of 2M *hydrochloric acid*. Cool, filter and dilute the filtrate to 15 ml with *distilled water*. The resulting solution complies with the *limit test for sulphates*, Appendix VII (500 ppm). Use a mixture of 5 ml of *sulphate standard solution (10 ppm SO₄)* and 10 ml of *water* as the standard solution.

Degree of unsaturation Dissolve 0.10 g in a mixture of 5 ml of 2M *hydrochloric acid* and 30 ml of *glacial acetic acid* and titrate with 0.05M *bromine VS* using 0.05 ml of *ethoxychrysoidine hydrochloride solution*, added towards the end of the titration, as indicator. Not less than 9.1 ml and not more than 9.4 ml of 0.05M *bromine VS* is required to discharge the red colour.

Loss on drying When dried at 100° to 105°, loses not more than 1.5% of its weight. Use 0.5 g.

Assay To 0.35 g add 25 ml of 2M *acetic acid*, heat to boiling and carry out the *complexometric titration of zinc*, Appendix VIII D. Each ml of 0.1M *disodium edetate VS* is equivalent to 0.04319 g of $C_{22}H_{38}O_4Zn$.

Storage Zinc Undecenoate should be kept in a well-closed container and protected from light.

Action and use Used topically in the treatment of fungal infections.

The title of the monograph in the European Pharmacopœia is Zinc Undecylenate.

Infra-red Reference Spectra

Preparation of Infra-red Reference Spectra

All spectra presented in this section were recorded on a Perkin-Elmer model 682 infra-red spectrophotometer using a twofold reduction for both abscissa and ordinate scales.

Pressed discs, 13 mm in diameter, were prepared using potassium bromide or potassium chloride. Liquid paraffin mulls and thin films were prepared between potassium bromide plates and solution spectra were prepared using cells with potassium bromide windows. Solution spectra were recorded against a solvent reference and all other spectra were recorded against air.

As stated in Appendix II A, for solution spectra the regions of the spectrum within which the solvent shows strong absorption should be disregarded. Solvent 'cut-offs' in the reference spectra are recorded as horizontal straight lines.

The spectra for polyurethane (form A) and polyurethane (form B) were obtained by the multiple internal reflectance technique, using a Perkin-Elmer high-performance multiple internal reflectance accessory and a 45° KRS-5 (thallium bromide/iodide) internal reflecting plate.

Polystyrene

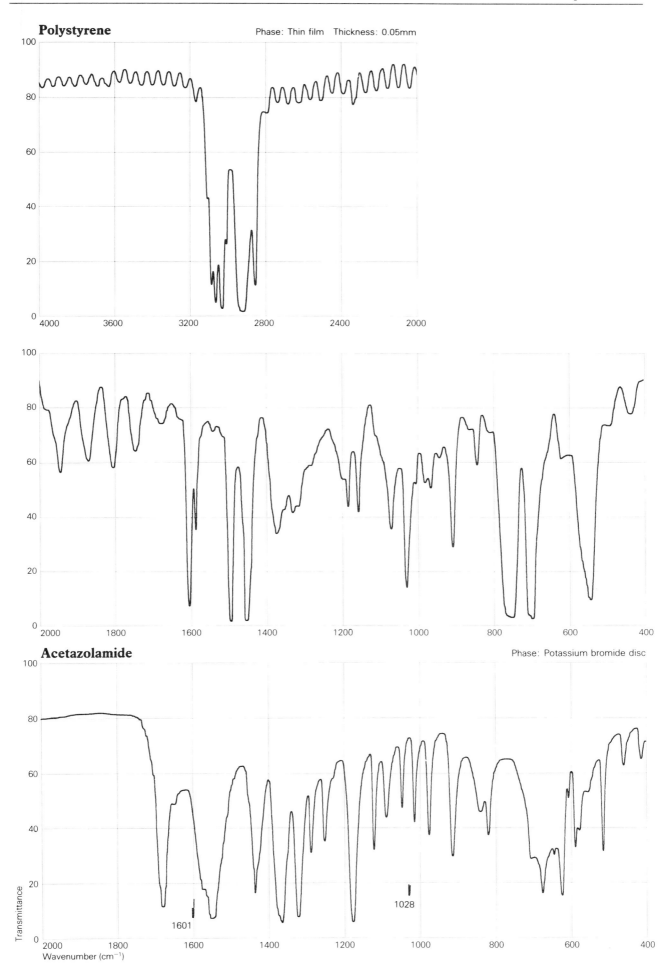

Phase: Thin film   Thickness: 0.05mm

Acetazolamide

Phase: Potassium bromide disc

1601

1028

Transmittance

Wavenumber (cm^{-1})

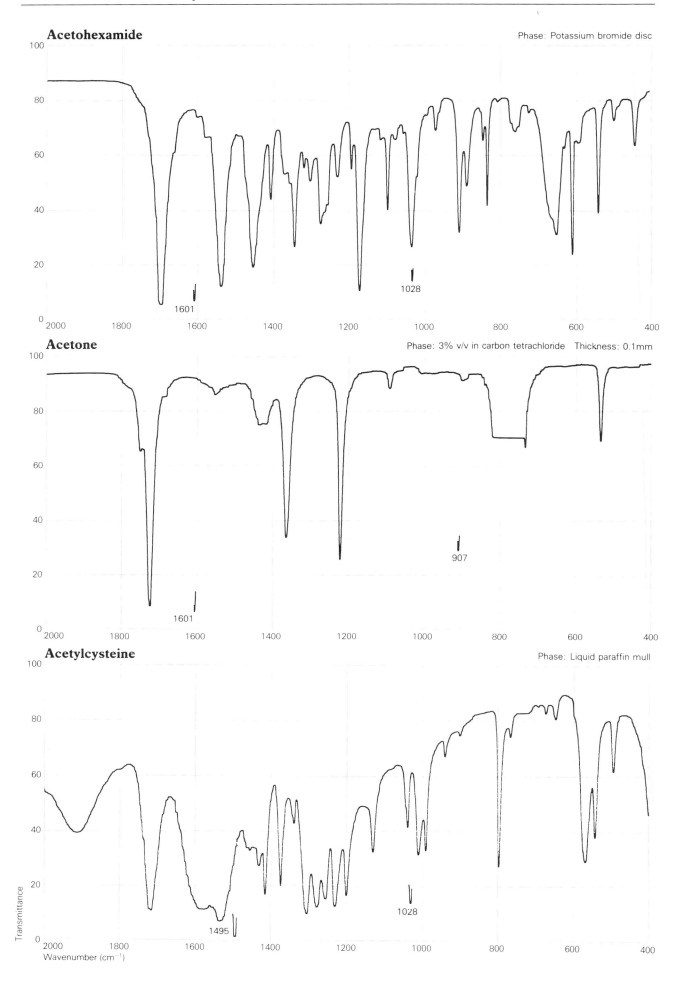

Acetohexamide   Phase: Potassium bromide disc

1601

1028

Acetone   Phase: 3% v/v in carbon tetrachloride   Thickness: 0.1mm

1601

907

Acetylcysteine   Phase: Liquid paraffin mull

1495

1028

Transmittance

Wavenumber (cm⁻¹)

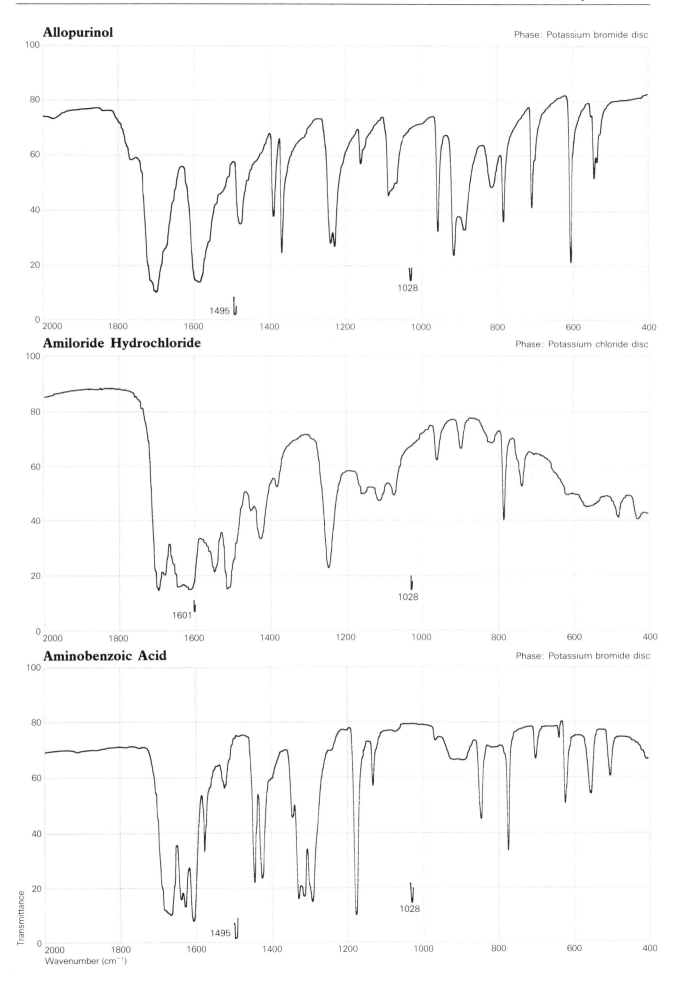

Allopurinol

Phase: Potassium bromide disc

1495

1028

Amiloride Hydrochloride

Phase: Potassium chloride disc

1601

1028

Aminobenzoic Acid

Phase: Potassium bromide disc

1495

1028

Transmittance

Wavenumber (cm⁻¹)

Aminocaproic Acid

Phase: Potassium bromide disc

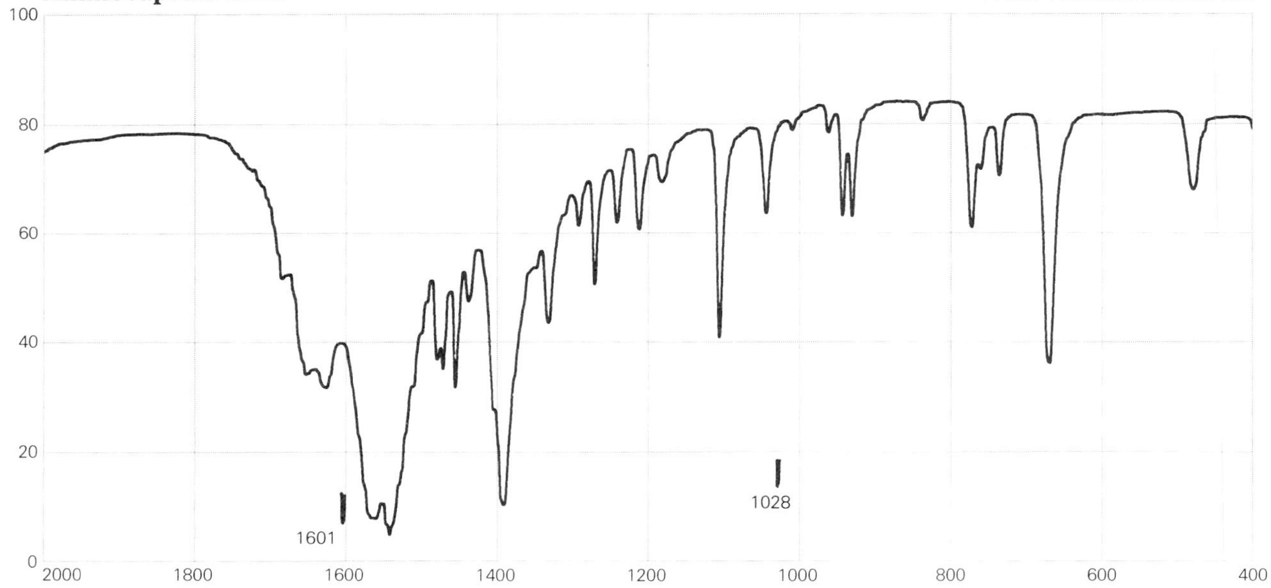

1601

1028

Amitriptyline

Phase: Thin film

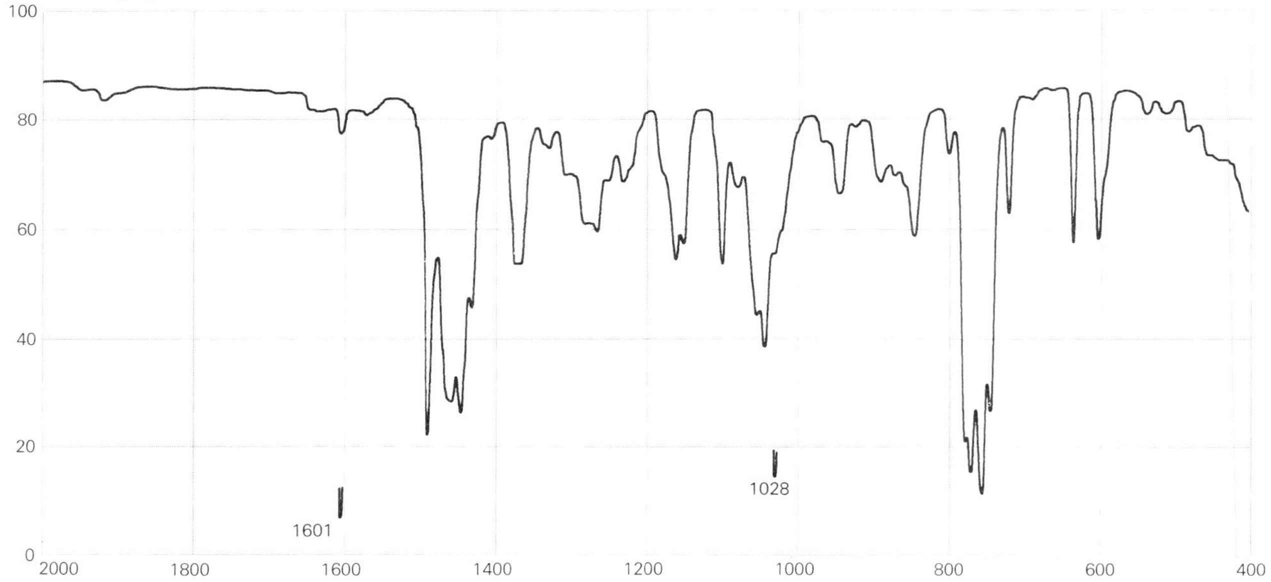

1601

1028

Amodiaquine

Phase: 5% w/v solution in chloroform   Thickness: 0.1mm

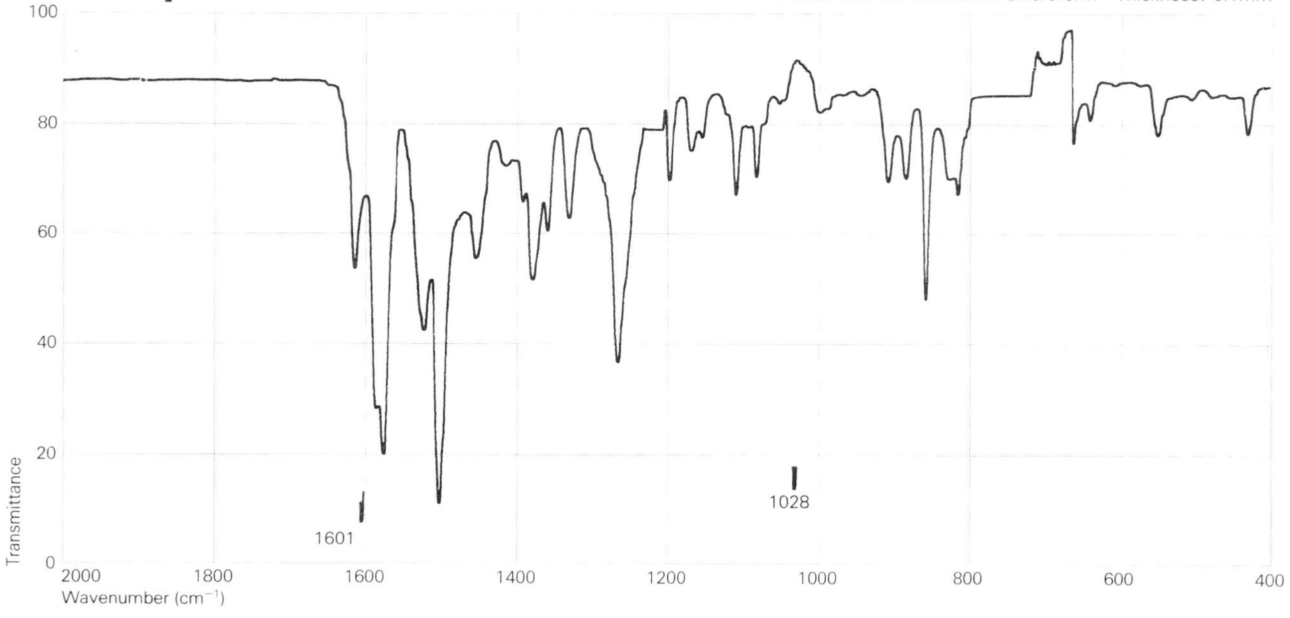

1601

1028

Transmittance

Wavenumber (cm⁻¹)

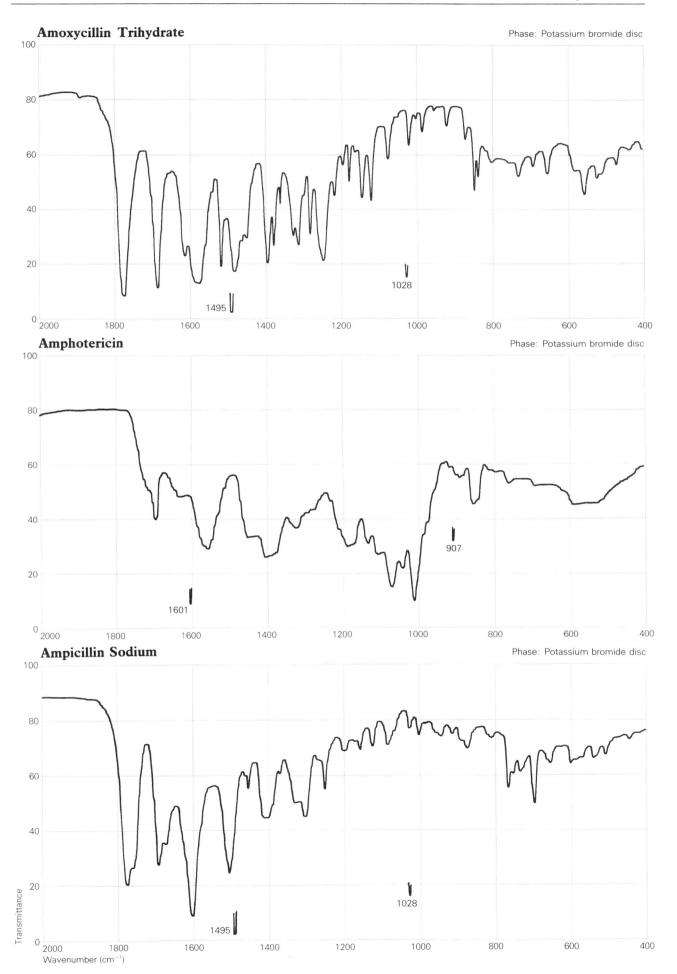

Amoxycillin Trihydrate   Phase: Potassium bromide disc

1495

1028

Amphotericin   Phase: Potassium bromide disc

1601

907

Ampicillin Sodium   Phase: Potassium bromide disc

1495

1028

Transmittance

Wavenumber (cm⁻¹)

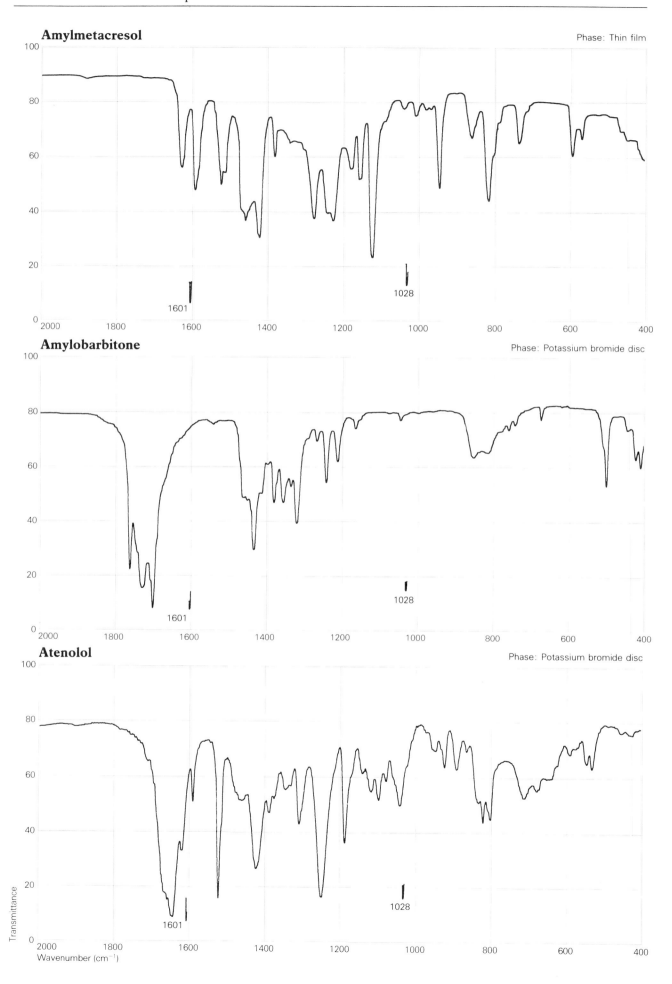

Amylmetacresol   Phase: Thin film

Amylobarbitone   Phase: Potassium bromide disc

Atenolol   Phase: Potassium bromide disc

Baclofen

Phase: Potassium bromide disc

Beclamide

Phase: Potassium bromide disc

Beclomethasone Dipropionate

Phase: 5% w/v solution in chloroform   Thickness: 0.1mm

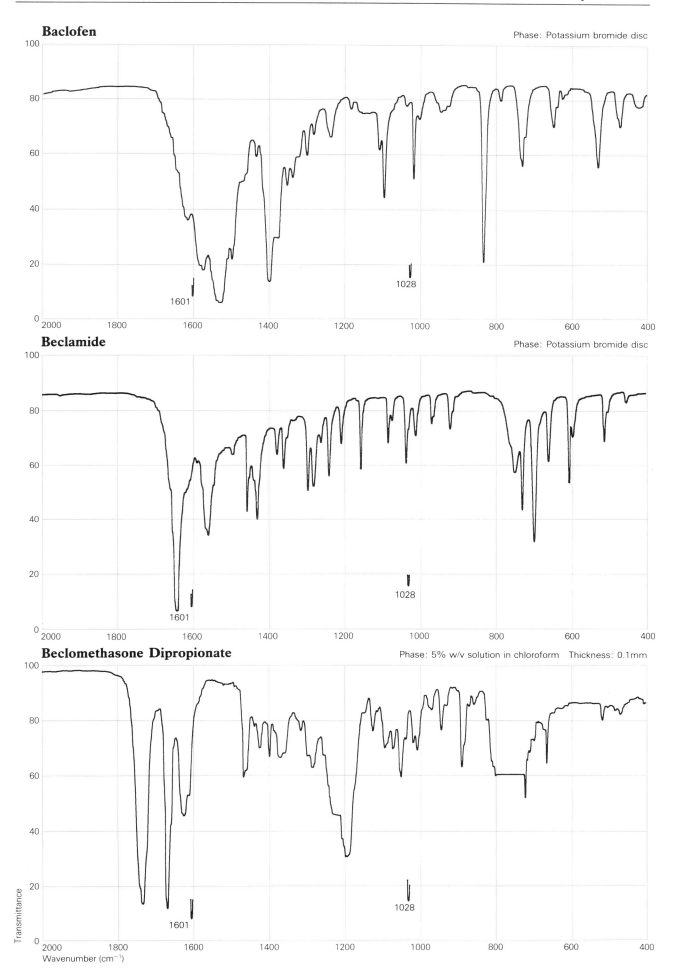

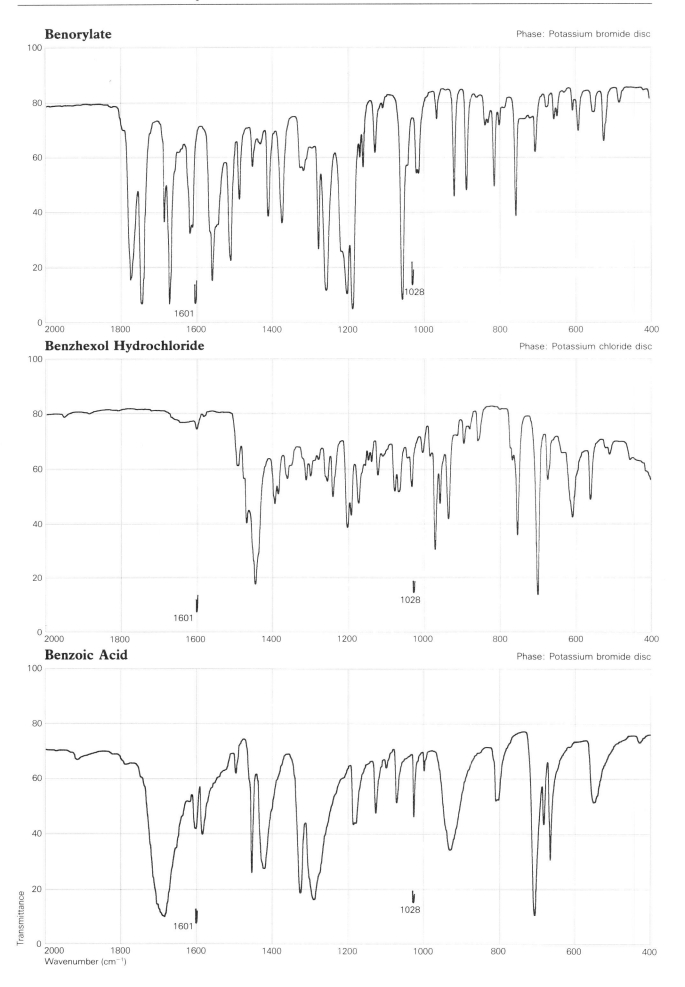

Benorylate Phase: Potassium bromide disc

1601
1028

Benzhexol Hydrochloride Phase: Potassium chloride disc

1601
1028

Benzoic Acid Phase: Potassium bromide disc

1601
1028

Transmittance

Wavenumber (cm⁻¹)

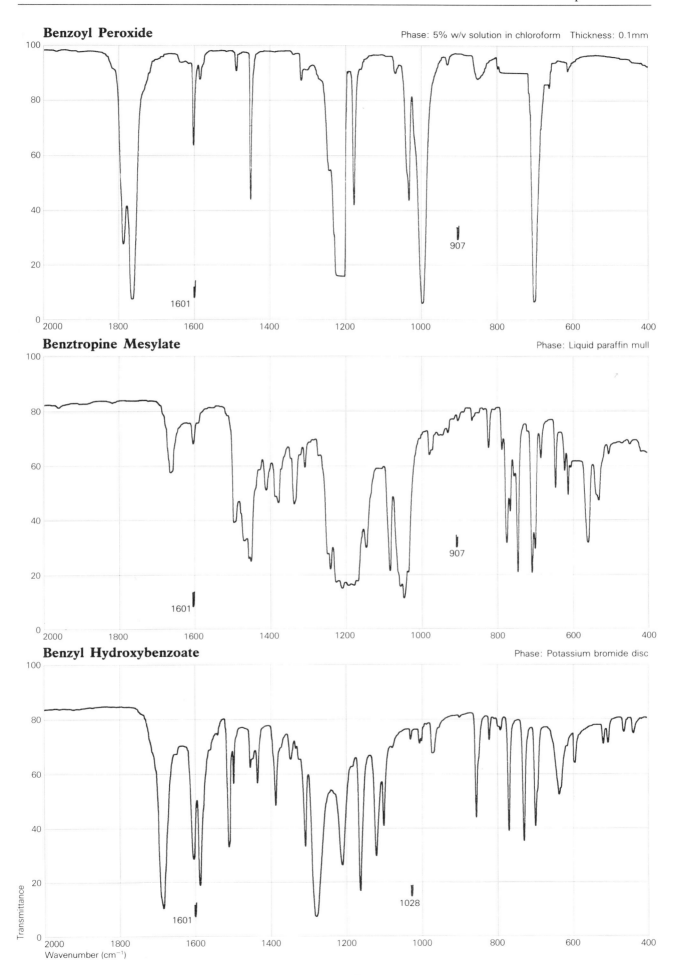

Benzoyl Peroxide   Phase: 5% w/v solution in chloroform   Thickness: 0.1mm

907

1601

Benztropine Mesylate   Phase: Liquid paraffin mull

907

1601

Benzyl Hydroxybenzoate   Phase: Potassium bromide disc

1601

1028

Transmittance

Wavenumber (cm⁻¹)

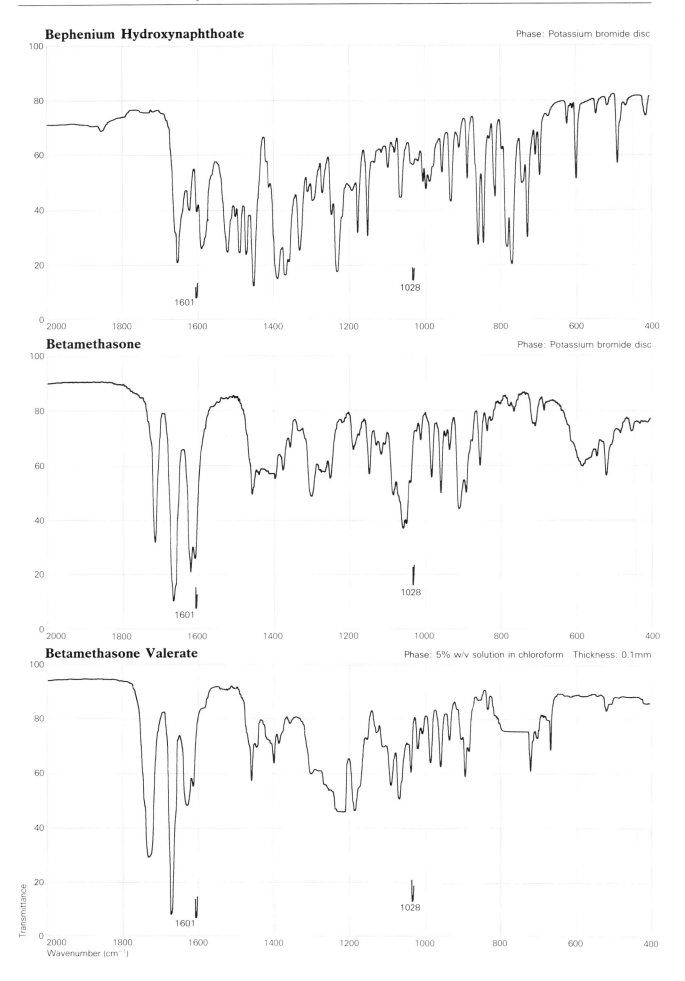

Bephenium Hydroxynaphthoate

Phase: Potassium bromide disc

1601

1028

Betamethasone

Phase: Potassium bromide disc

1601

1028

Betamethasone Valerate

Phase: 5% w/v solution in chloroform   Thickness: 0.1mm

1601

1028

Transmittance

Wavenumber (cm⁻¹)

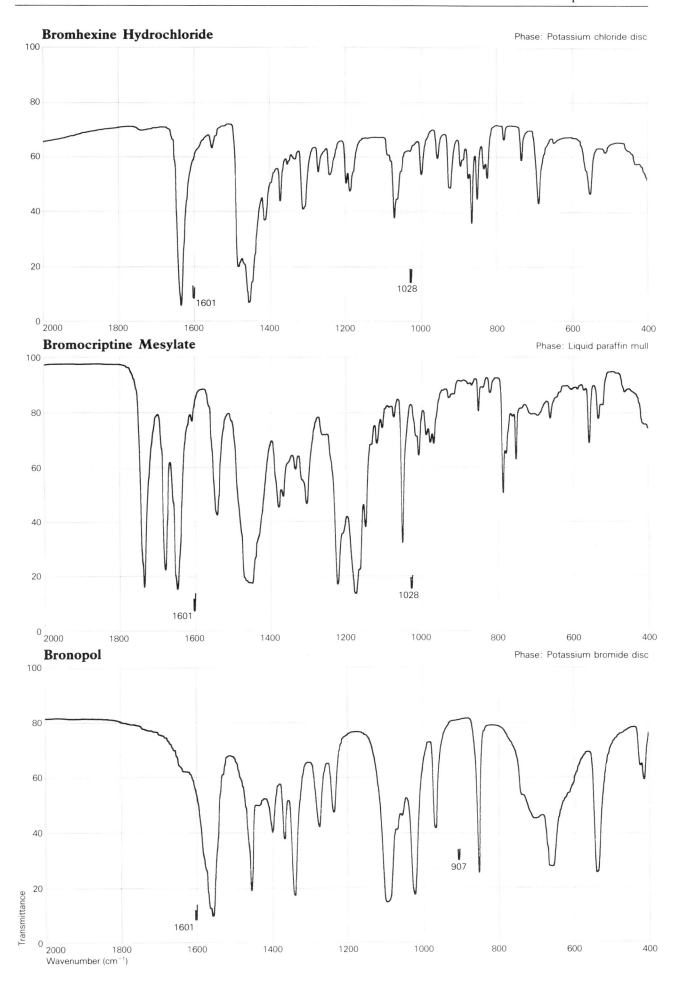

Bromhexine Hydrochloride   Phase: Potassium chloride disc

1601
1028

Bromocriptine Mesylate   Phase: Liquid paraffin mull

1601
1028

Bronopol   Phase: Potassium bromide disc

907
1601

Transmittance

Wavenumber (cm⁻¹)

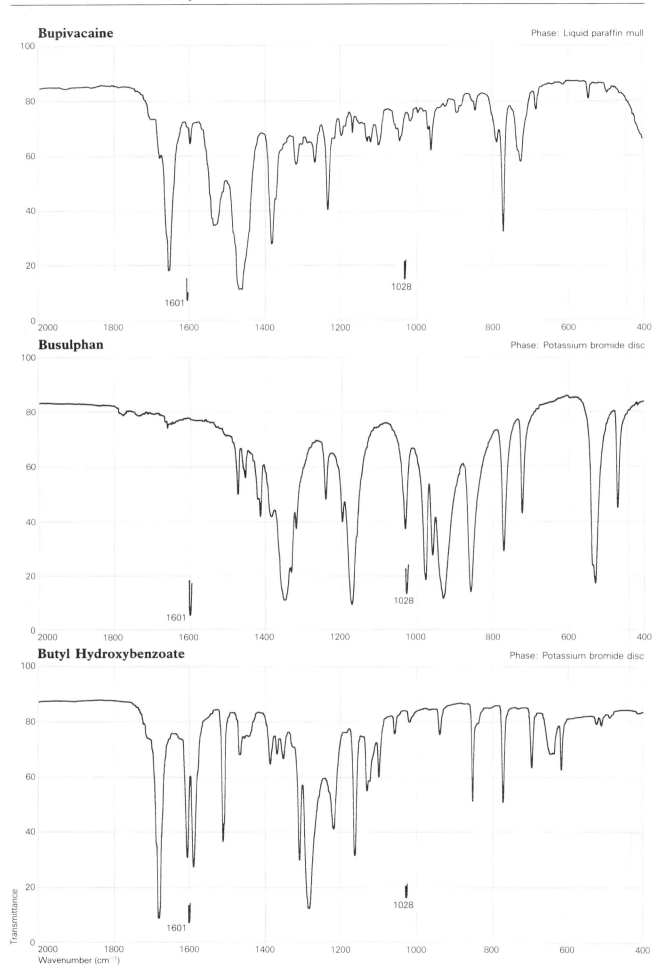

Bupivacaine

Phase: Liquid paraffin mull

Busulphan

Phase: Potassium bromide disc

Butyl Hydroxybenzoate

Phase: Potassium bromide disc

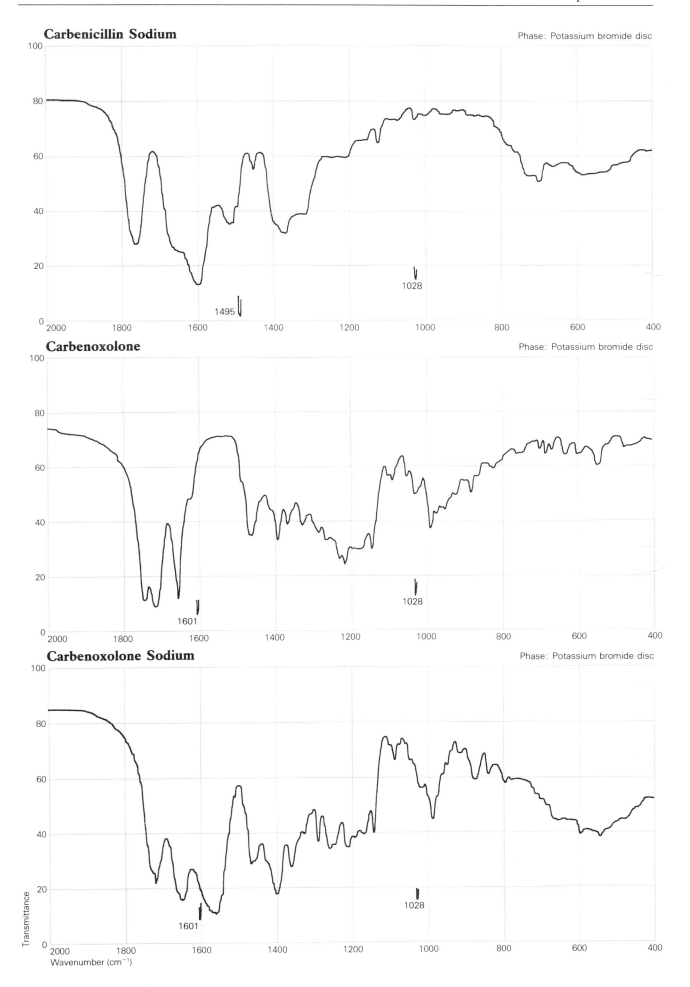

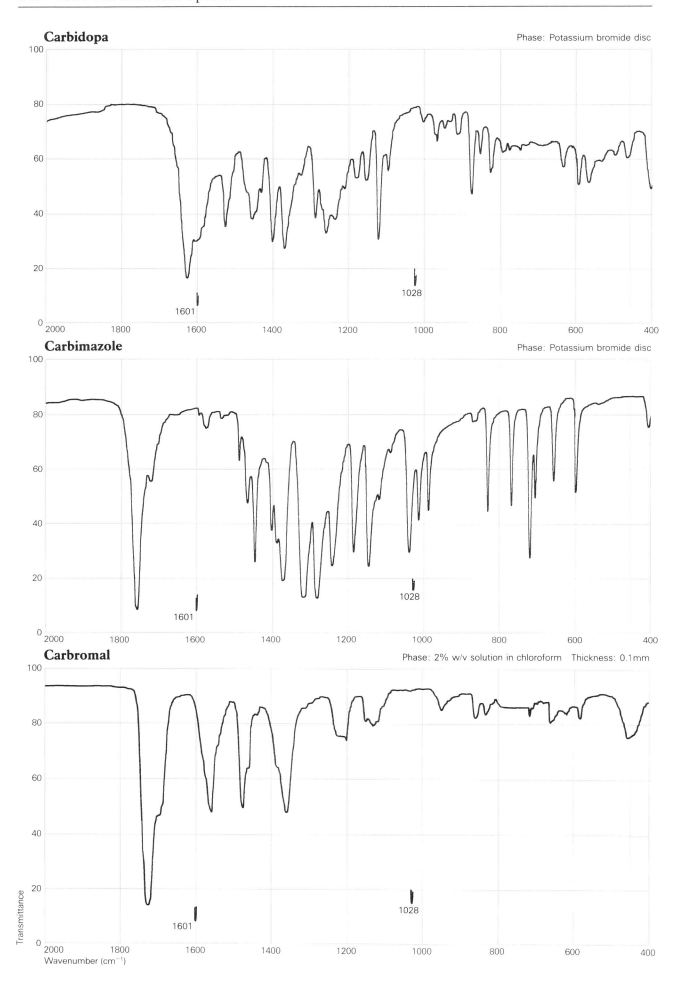

Carbidopa   Phase: Potassium bromide disc

1601
1028

Carbimazole   Phase: Potassium bromide disc

1601
1028

Carbromal   Phase: 2% w/v solution in chloroform   Thickness: 0.1mm

1601
1028

Transmittance

Wavenumber (cm⁻¹)

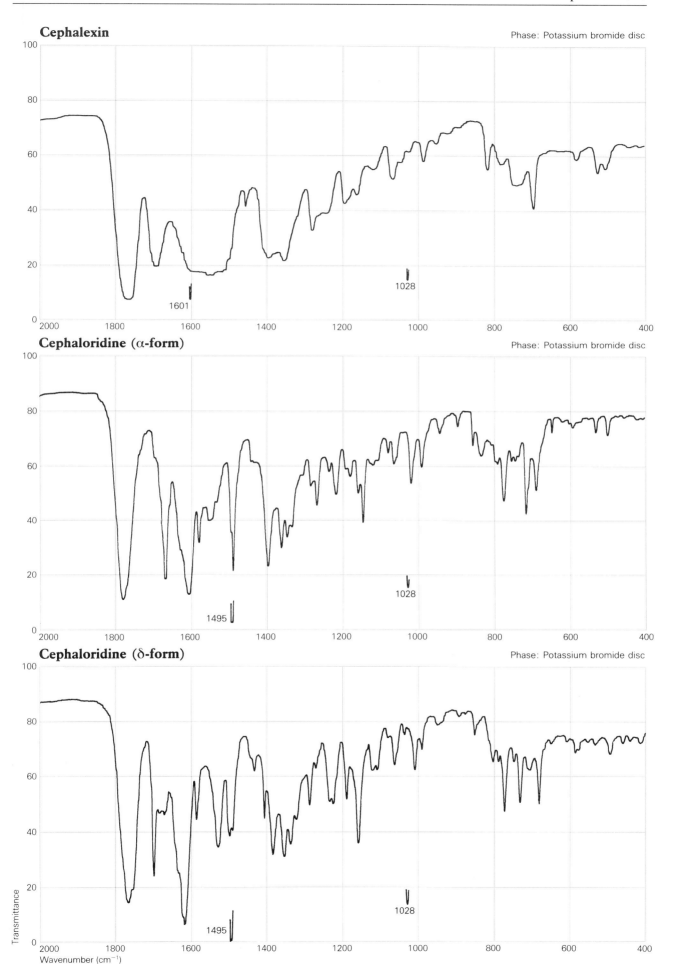

Cephalexin

Phase: Potassium bromide disc

1601
1028

Cephaloridine (α-form)

Phase: Potassium bromide disc

1495
1028

Cephaloridine (δ-form)

Phase: Potassium bromide disc

1495
1028

Transmittance

Wavenumber (cm⁻¹)

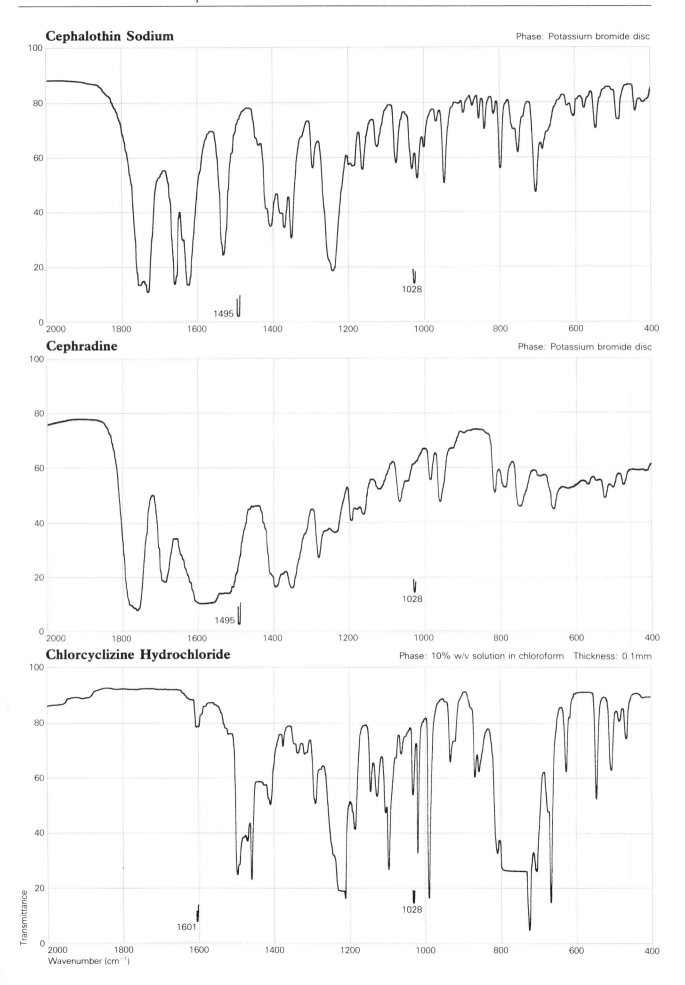

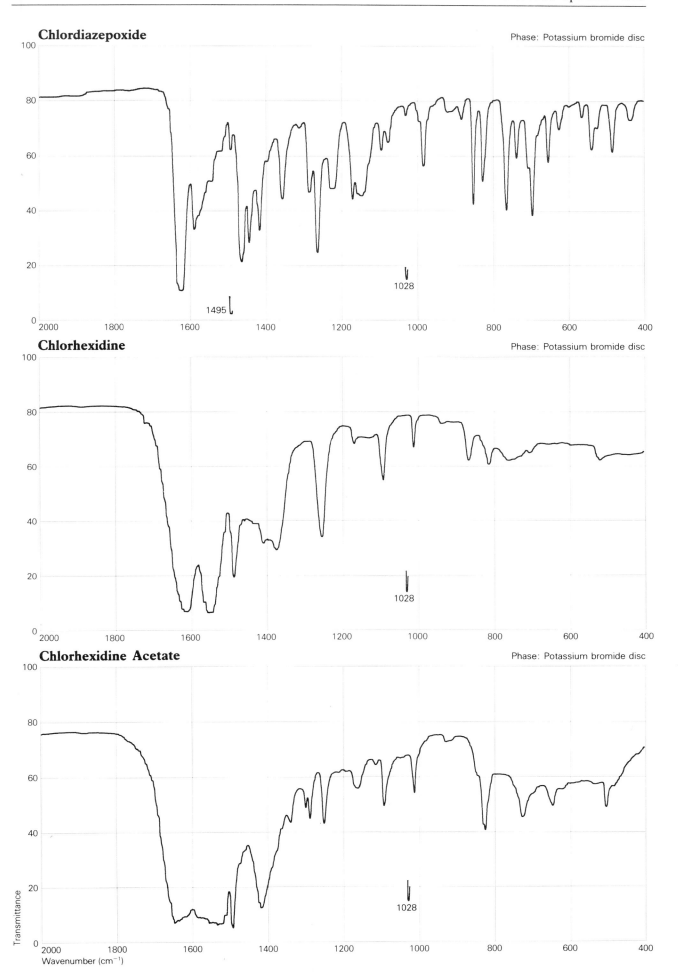

Chlordiazepoxide

Phase: Potassium bromide disc

1495

1028

Chlorhexidine

Phase: Potassium bromide disc

1028

Chlorhexidine Acetate

Phase: Potassium bromide disc

1028

Transmittance

Wavenumber (cm⁻¹)

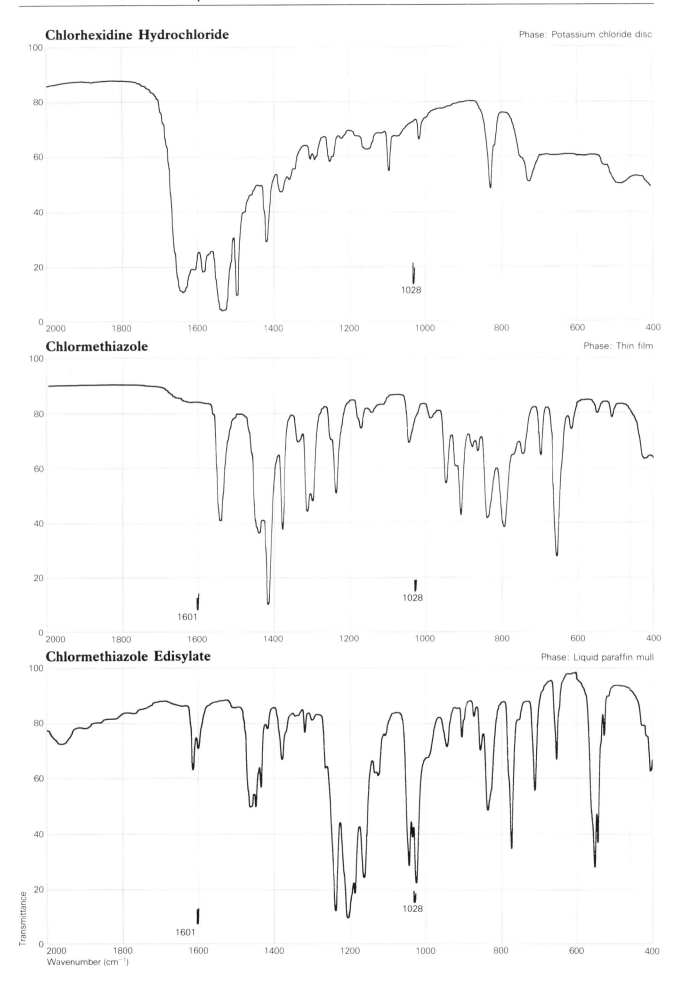

Chlorhexidine Hydrochloride

Phase: Potassium chloride disc

1028

Chlormethiazole

Phase: Thin film

1601

1028

Chlormethiazole Edisylate

Phase: Liquid paraffin mull

1601

1028

Transmittance

Wavenumber (cm⁻¹)

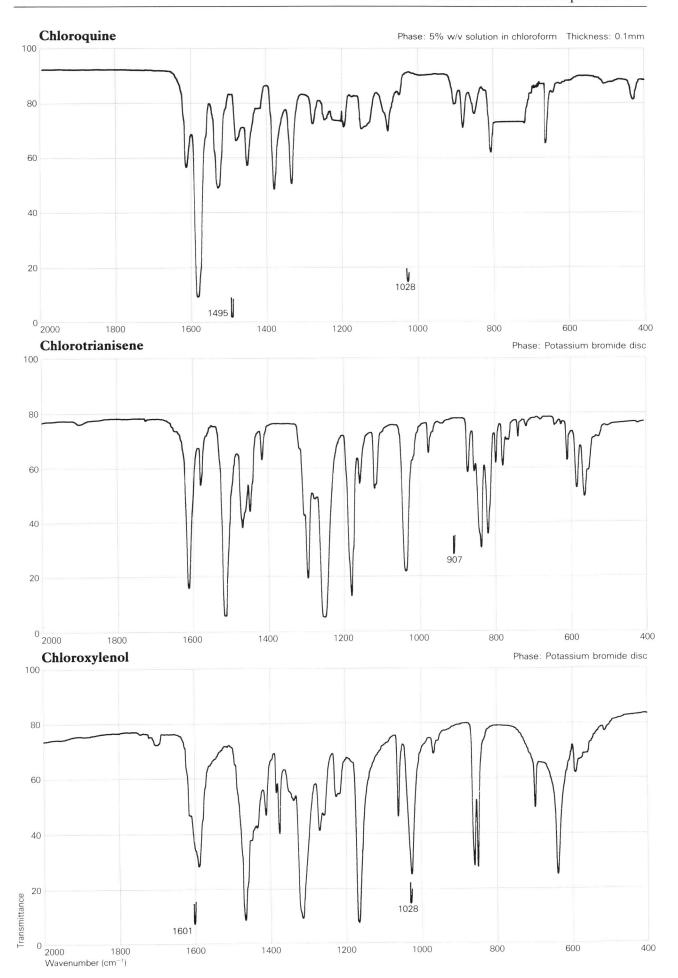

Chloroquine   Phase: 5% w/v solution in chloroform   Thickness: 0.1mm

1495

1028

Chlorotrianisene   Phase: Potassium bromide disc

907

Chloroxylenol   Phase: Potassium bromide disc

1601

1028

Transmittance

Wavenumber (cm⁻¹)

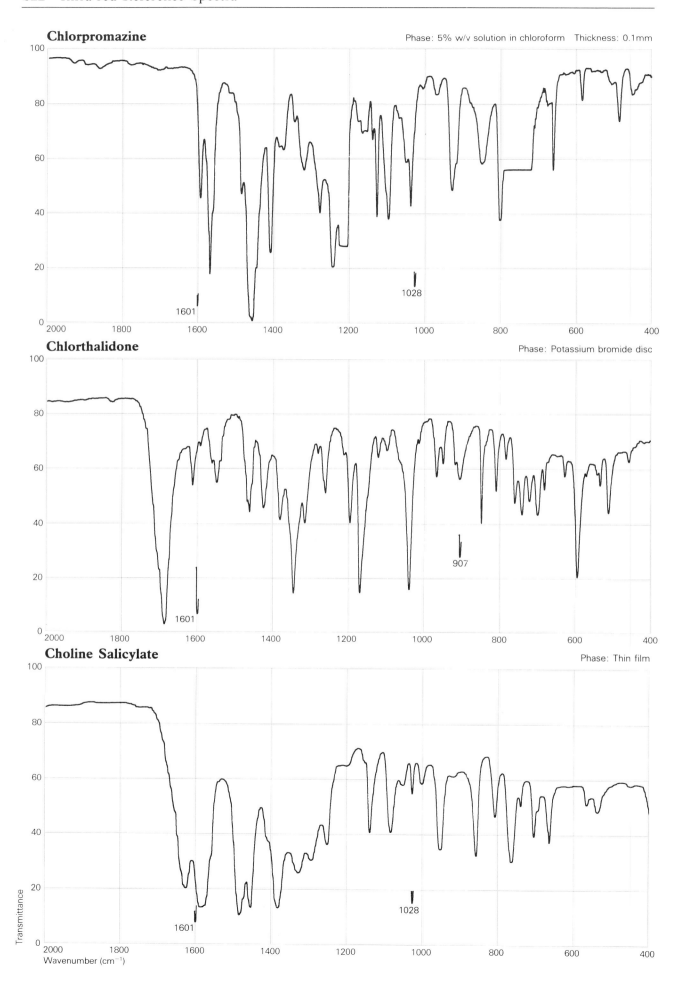

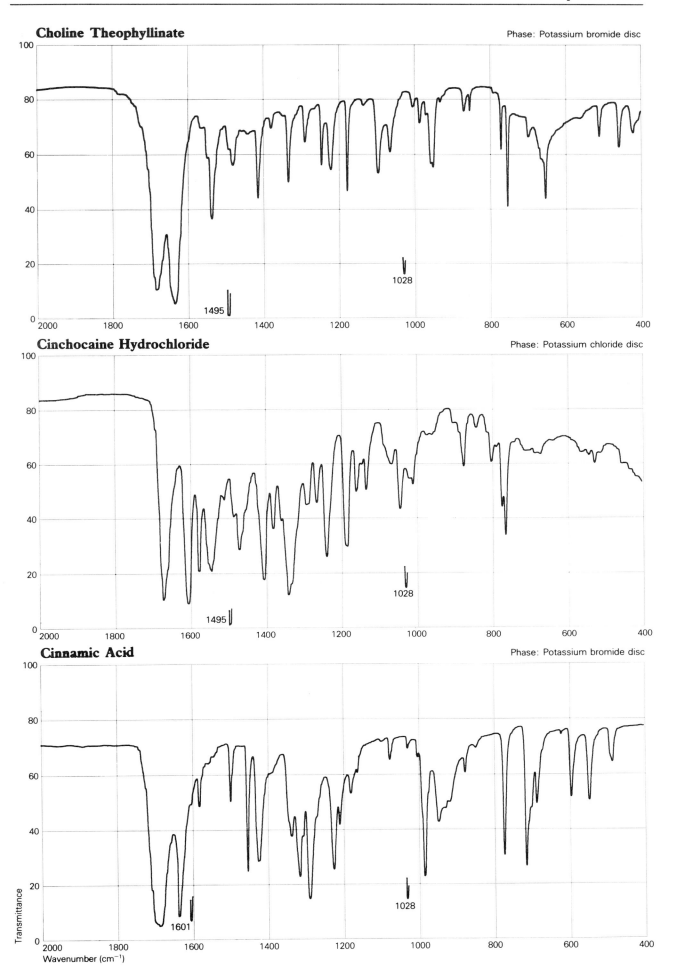

Choline Theophyllinate

Phase: Potassium bromide disc

1495
1028

Cinchocaine Hydrochloride

Phase: Potassium chloride disc

1495
1028

Cinnamic Acid

Phase: Potassium bromide disc

1601
1028

Transmittance

Wavenumber (cm⁻¹)

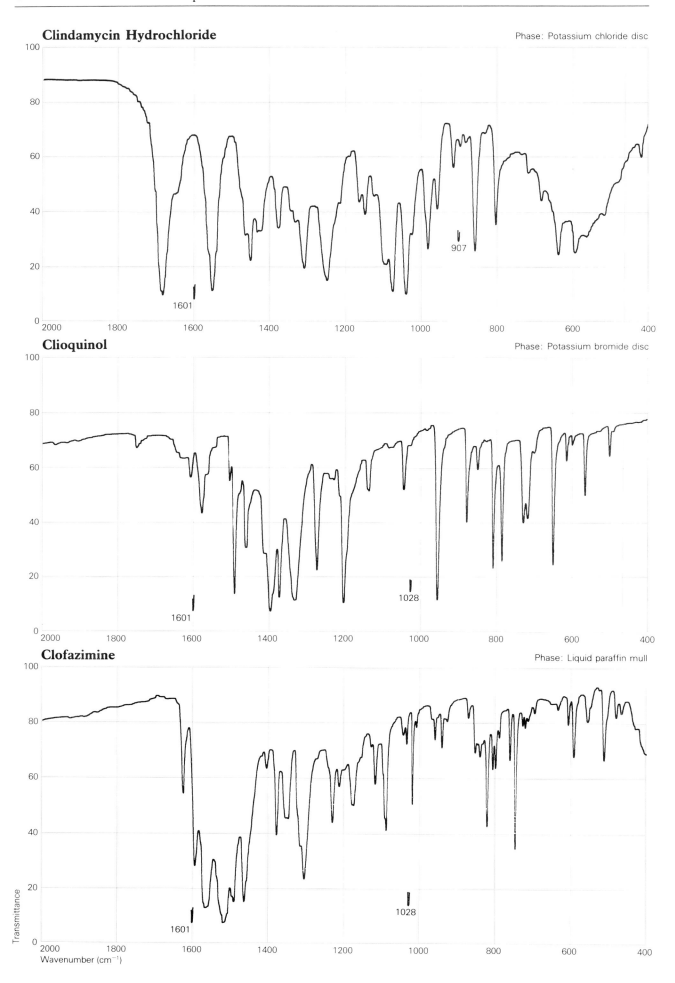

Clindamycin Hydrochloride

Phase: Potassium chloride disc

1601

907

Clioquinol

Phase: Potassium bromide disc

1601

1028

Clofazimine

Phase: Liquid paraffin mull

1601

1028

Transmittance

Wavenumber (cm⁻¹)

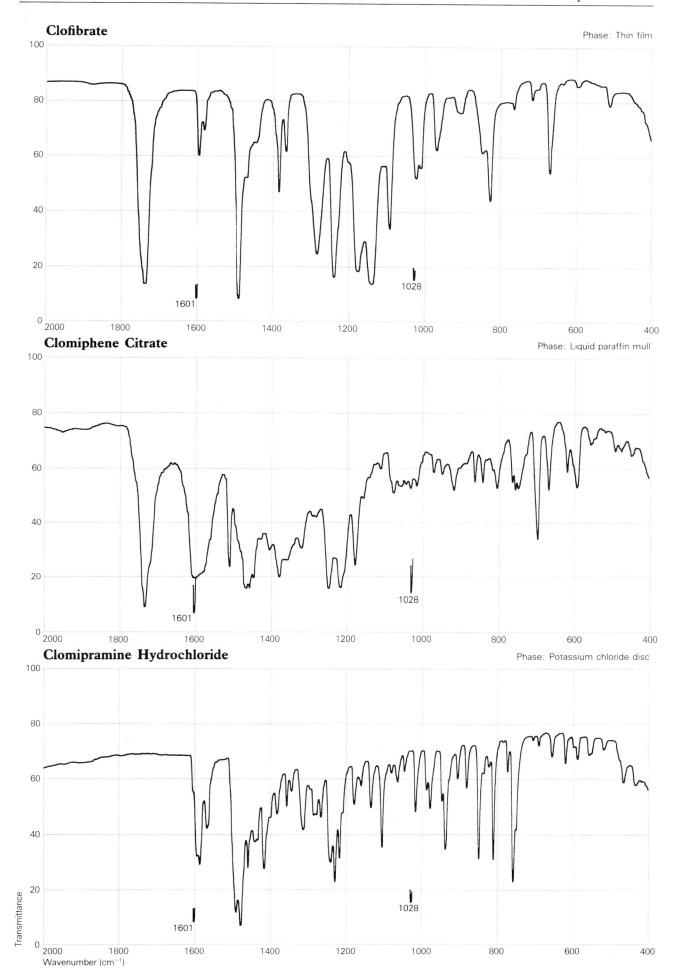

Clofibrate
Phase: Thin film

1601

1028

Clomiphene Citrate
Phase: Liquid paraffin mull

1601

1028

Clomipramine Hydrochloride
Phase: Potassium chloride disc

1601

1028

Transmittance

Wavenumber (cm⁻¹)

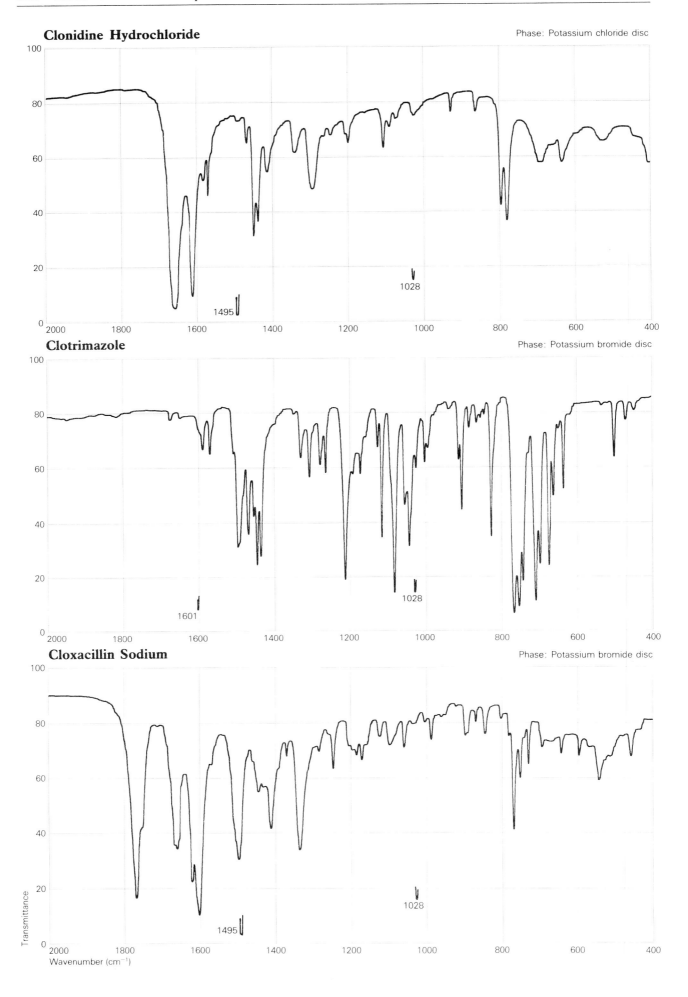

Clonidine Hydrochloride Phase: Potassium chloride disc

Clotrimazole Phase: Potassium bromide disc

Cloxacillin Sodium Phase: Potassium bromide disc

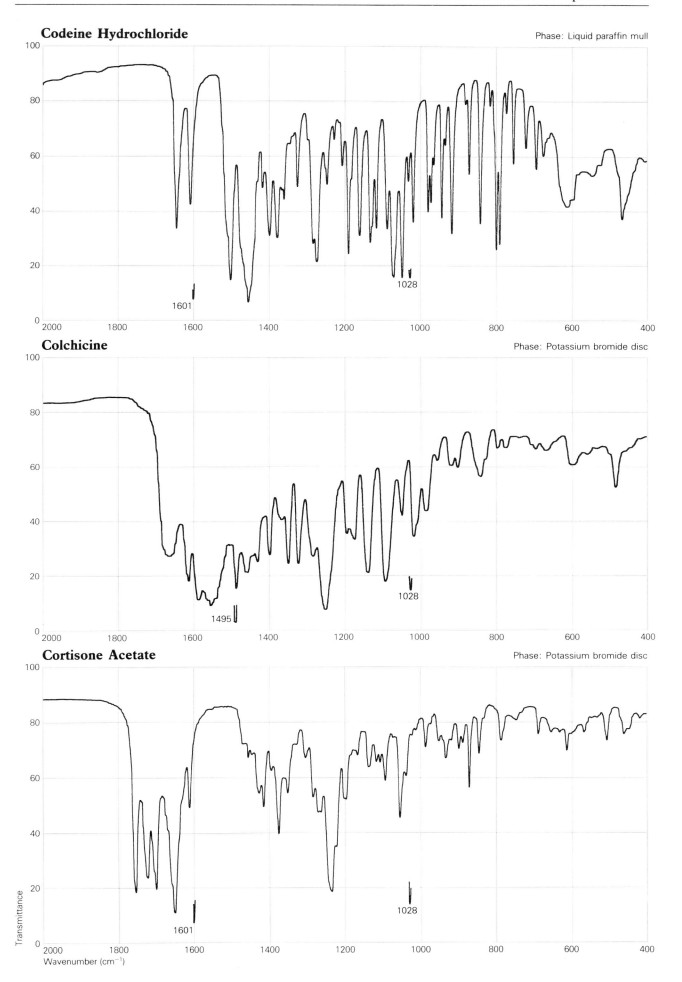

Codeine Hydrochloride

Phase: Liquid paraffin mull

1601

1028

Colchicine

Phase: Potassium bromide disc

1495

1028

Cortisone Acetate

Phase: Potassium bromide disc

Transmittance

1601

1028

Wavenumber (cm⁻¹)

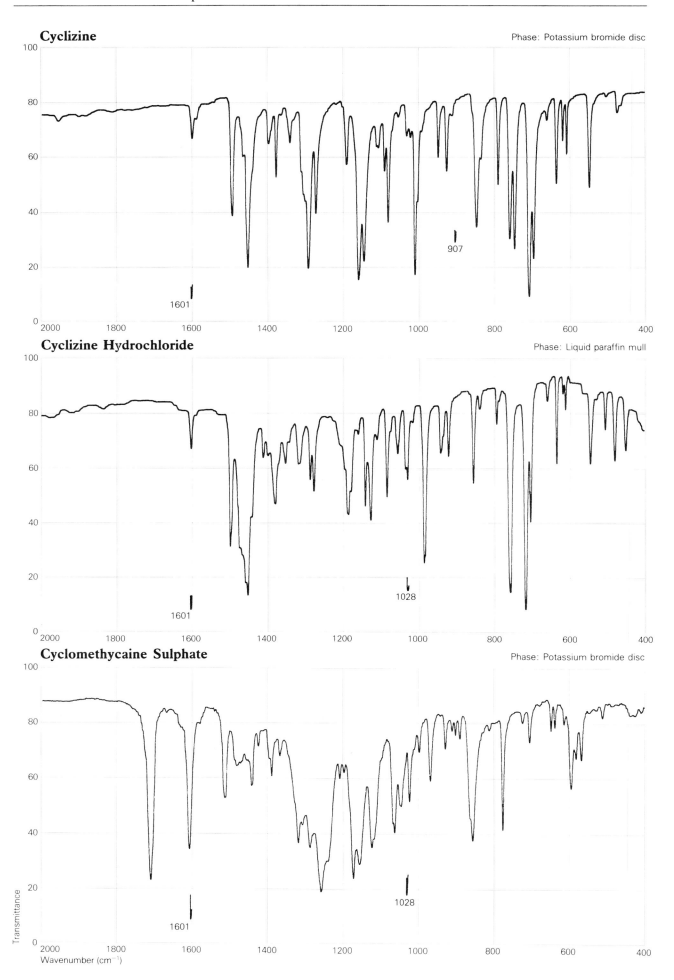

Cyclizine   Phase: Potassium bromide disc

1601
907

Cyclizine Hydrochloride   Phase: Liquid paraffin mull

1601
1028

Cyclomethycaine Sulphate   Phase: Potassium bromide disc

1601
1028

Transmittance

Wavenumber (cm⁻¹)

Cyclopenthiazide

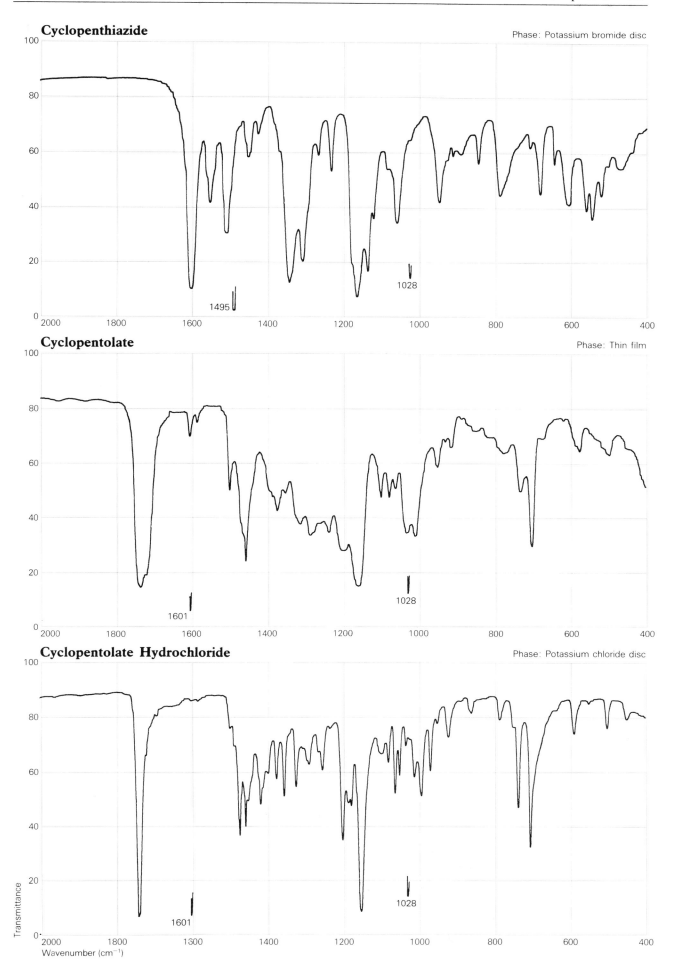

Phase: Potassium bromide disc

Cyclopentolate

Phase: Thin film

Cyclopentolate Hydrochloride

Phase: Potassium chloride disc

Cyclophosphamide

Phase: 10% w/v solution in chloroform   Thickness: 0.1mm

Cyproheptadine

Phase: Potassium bromide disc

Cytarabine

Phase: Potassium bromide disc

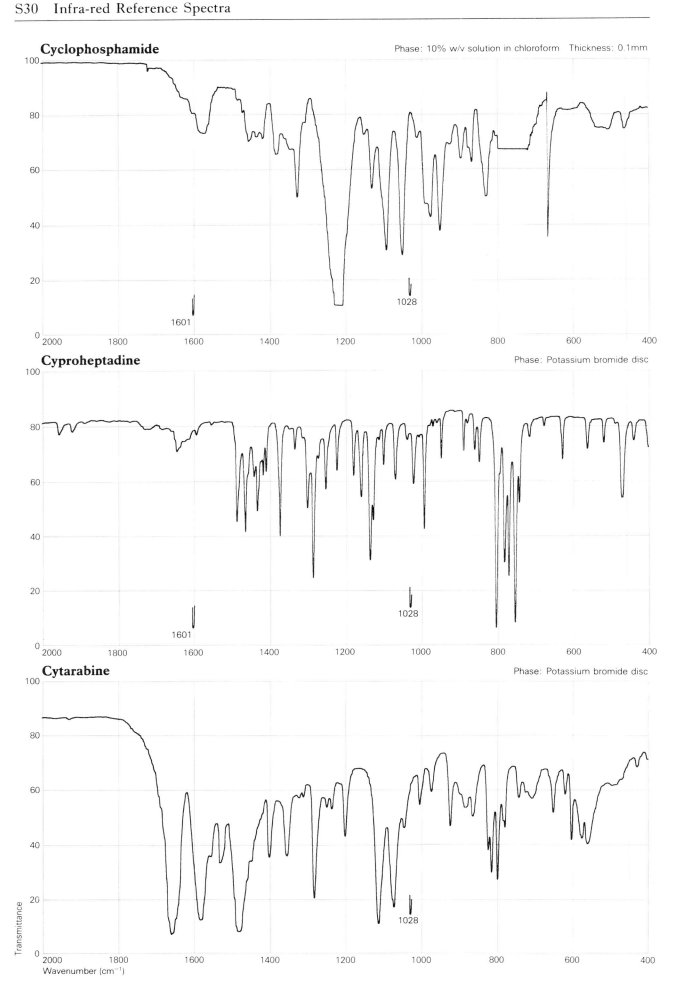

Transmittance

Wavenumber (cm⁻¹)

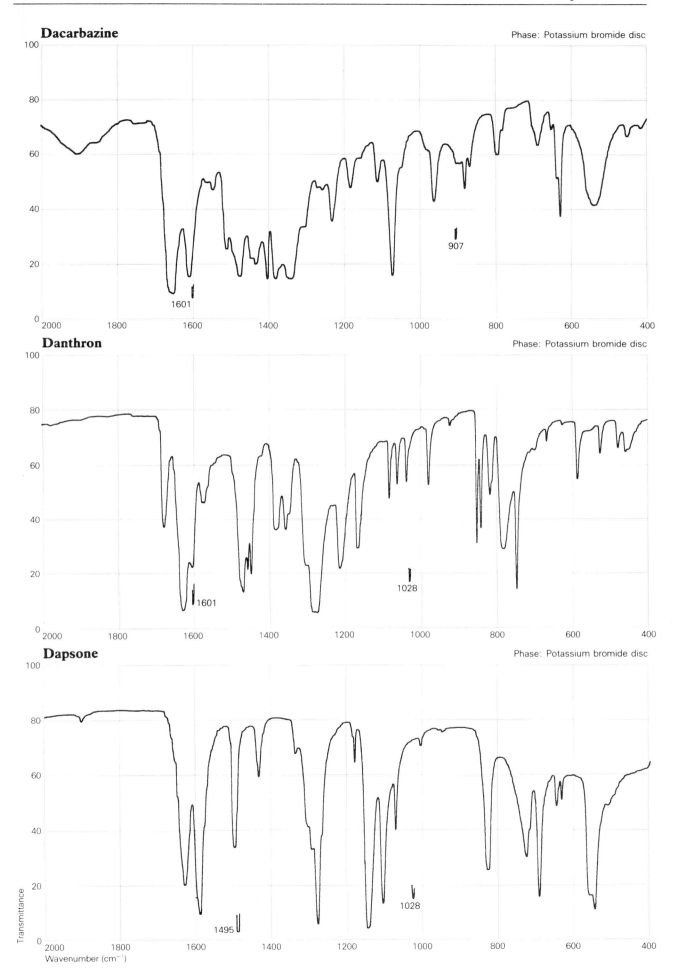

Dacarbazine

Phase: Potassium bromide disc

907

1601

Danthron

Phase: Potassium bromide disc

1601

1028

Dapsone

Phase: Potassium bromide disc

1495

1028

Transmittance

Wavenumber (cm⁻¹)

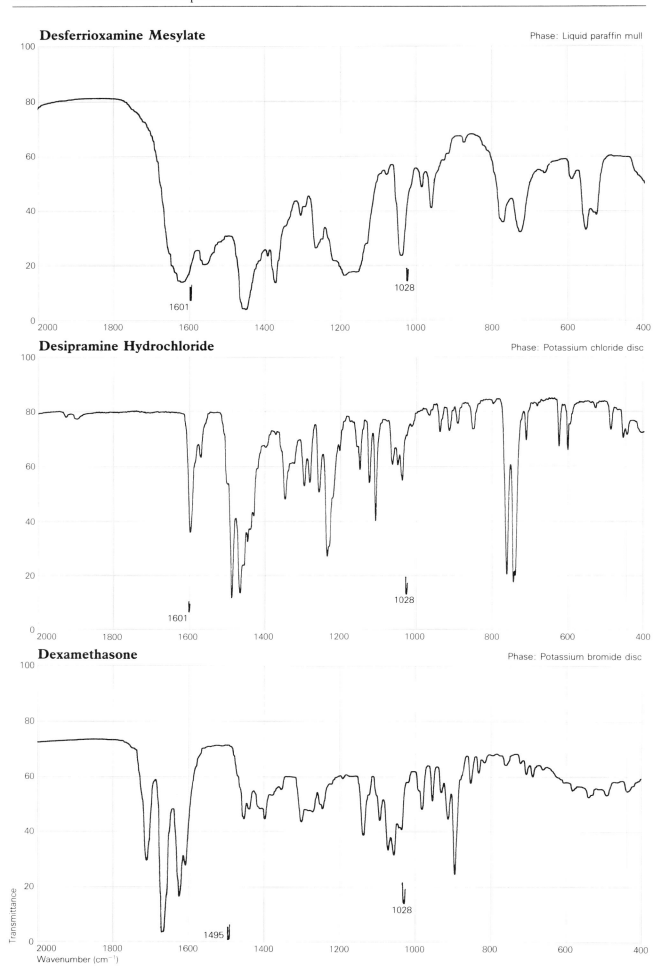

Desferrioxamine Mesylate

Phase: Liquid paraffin mull

Desipramine Hydrochloride

Phase: Potassium chloride disc

Dexamethasone

Phase: Potassium bromide disc

Dextromoramide

Phase: Potassium bromide disc

Dextropropoxyphene Hydrochloride

Phase: 10% w/v solution in chloroform   Thickness: 0.1mm

Dextropropoxyphene Napsylate

Phase: Liquid paraffin mull

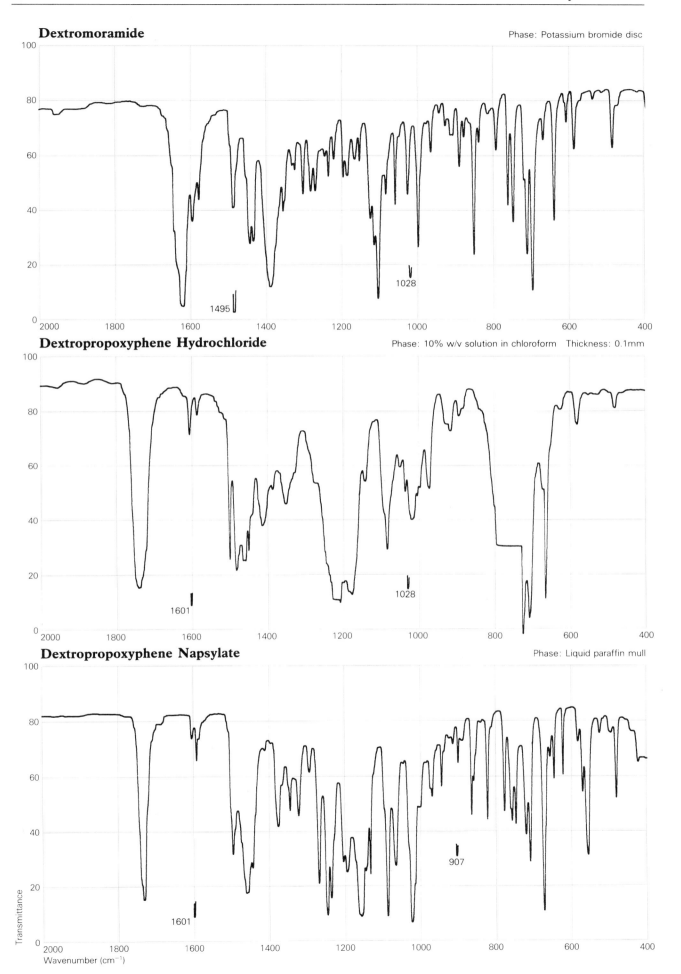

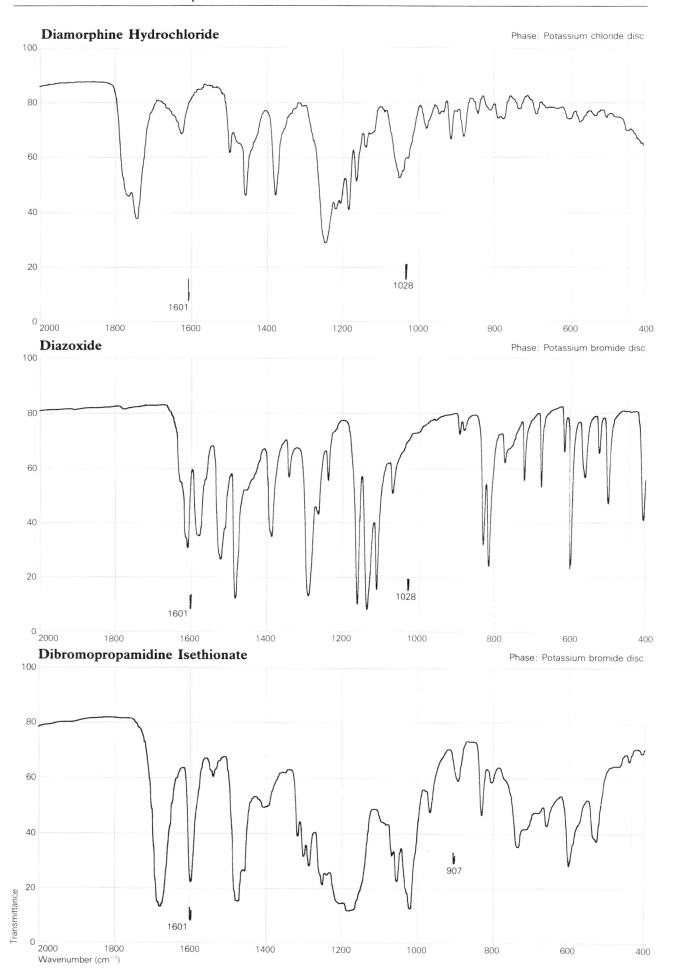

Diamorphine Hydrochloride

Phase: Potassium chloride disc

1601

1028

Diazoxide

Phase: Potassium bromide disc

1601

1028

Dibromopropamidine Isethionate

Phase: Potassium bromide disc

1601

907

Transmittance

Wavenumber (cm⁻¹)

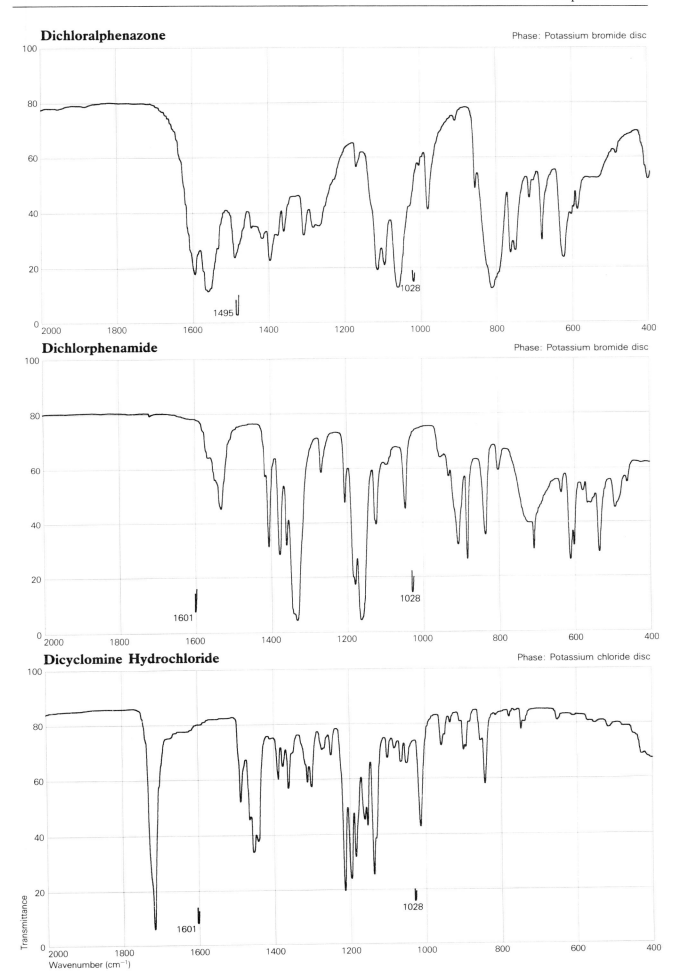

Dichloralphenazone   Phase: Potassium bromide disc

Dichlorphenamide   Phase: Potassium bromide disc

Dicyclomine Hydrochloride   Phase: Potassium chloride disc

Wavenumber (cm⁻¹)

Transmittance

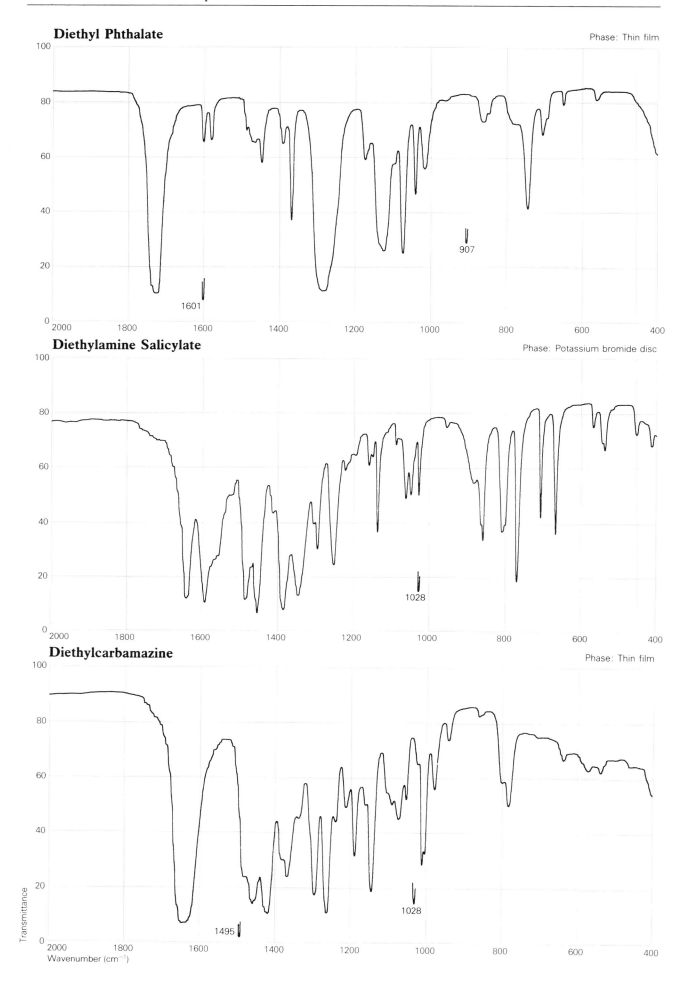

Diethyl Phthalate Phase: Thin film

Diethylamine Salicylate Phase: Potassium bromide disc

Diethylcarbamazine Phase: Thin film

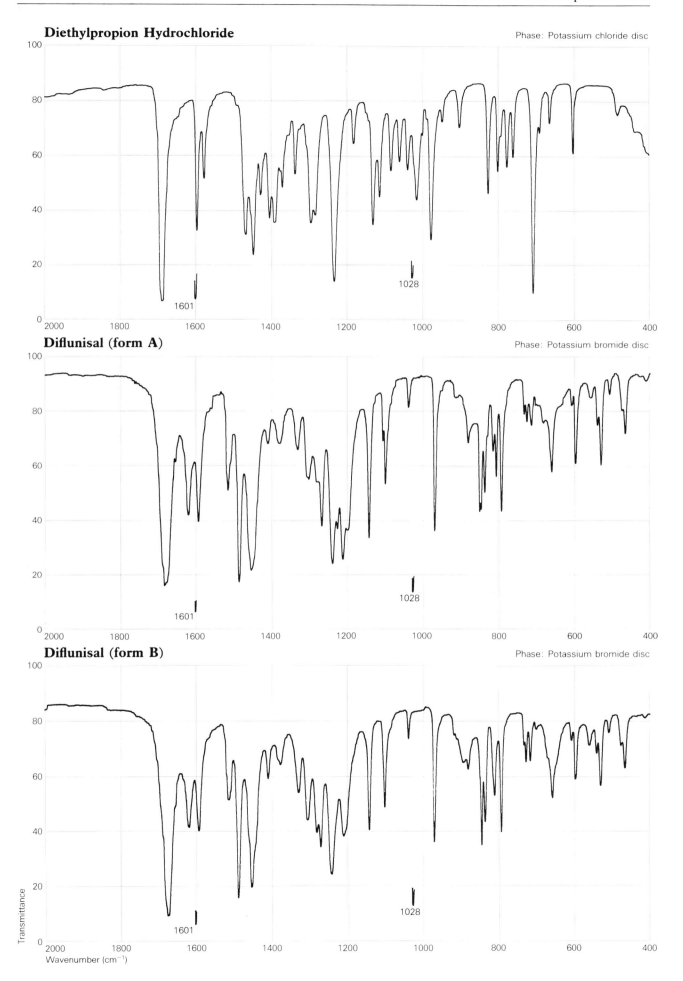

Diethylpropion Hydrochloride

Phase: Potassium chloride disc

1601

1028

Diflunisal (form A)

Phase: Potassium bromide disc

1601

1028

Diflunisal (form B)

Phase: Potassium bromide disc

1601

1028

Transmittance

Wavenumber (cm⁻¹)

Dihydroergotamine Mesylate

Phase: Liquid paraffin mull

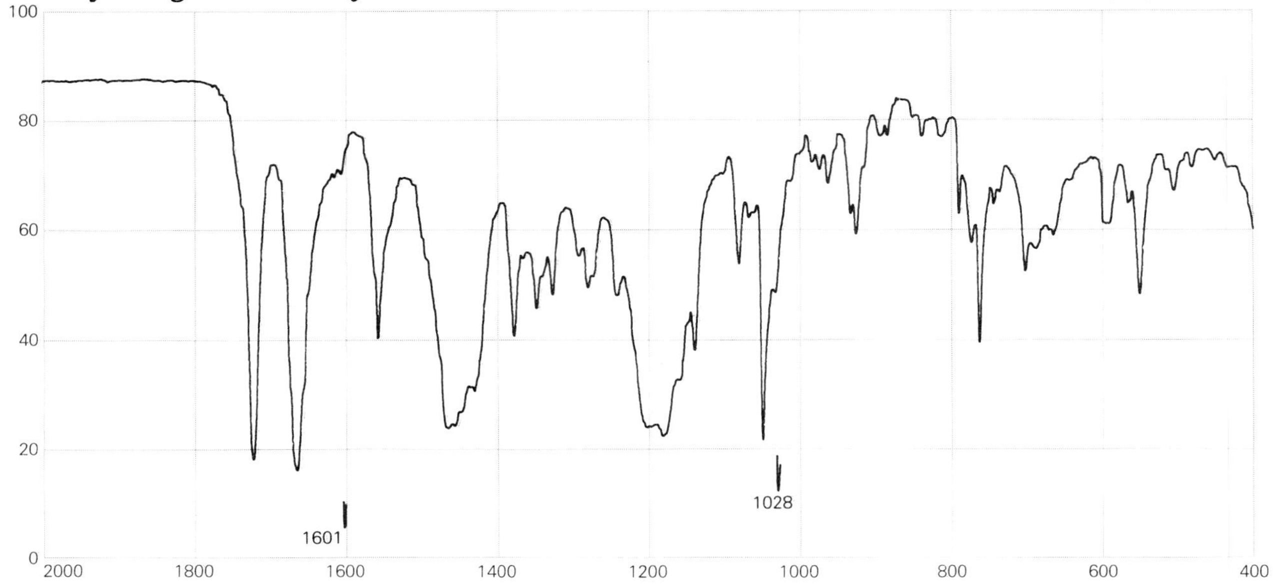

1601

1028

Diloxanide Furoate

Phase: Potassium bromide disc

1601

1028

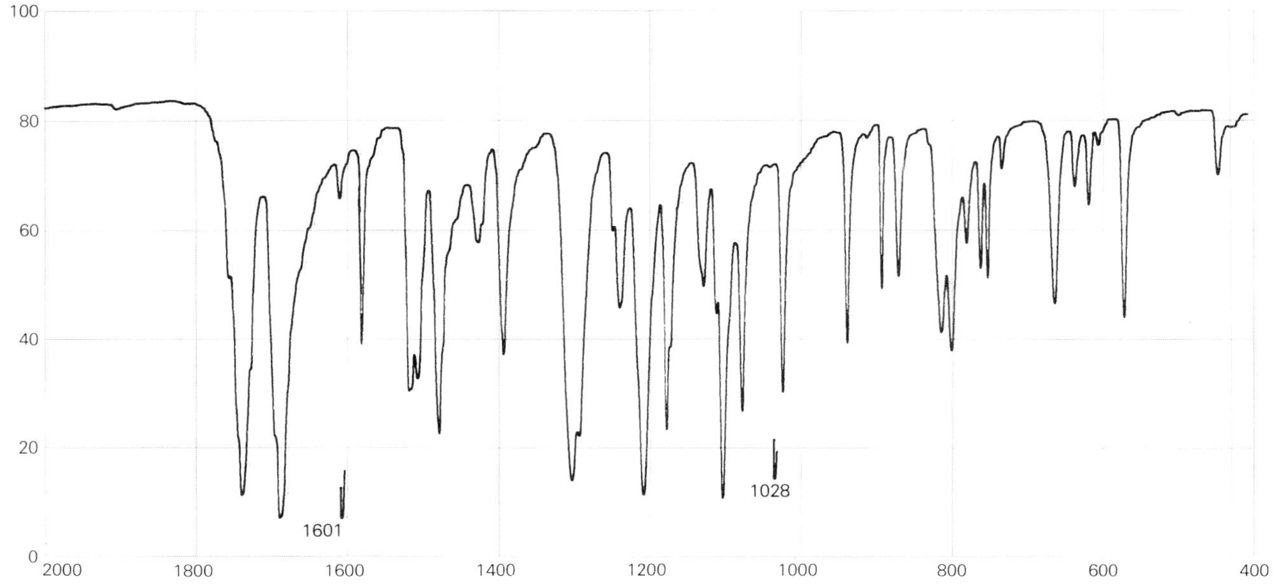

Dimenhydrinate

Phase: Potassium bromide disc

Transmittance

1495

1028

Wavenumber (cm⁻¹)

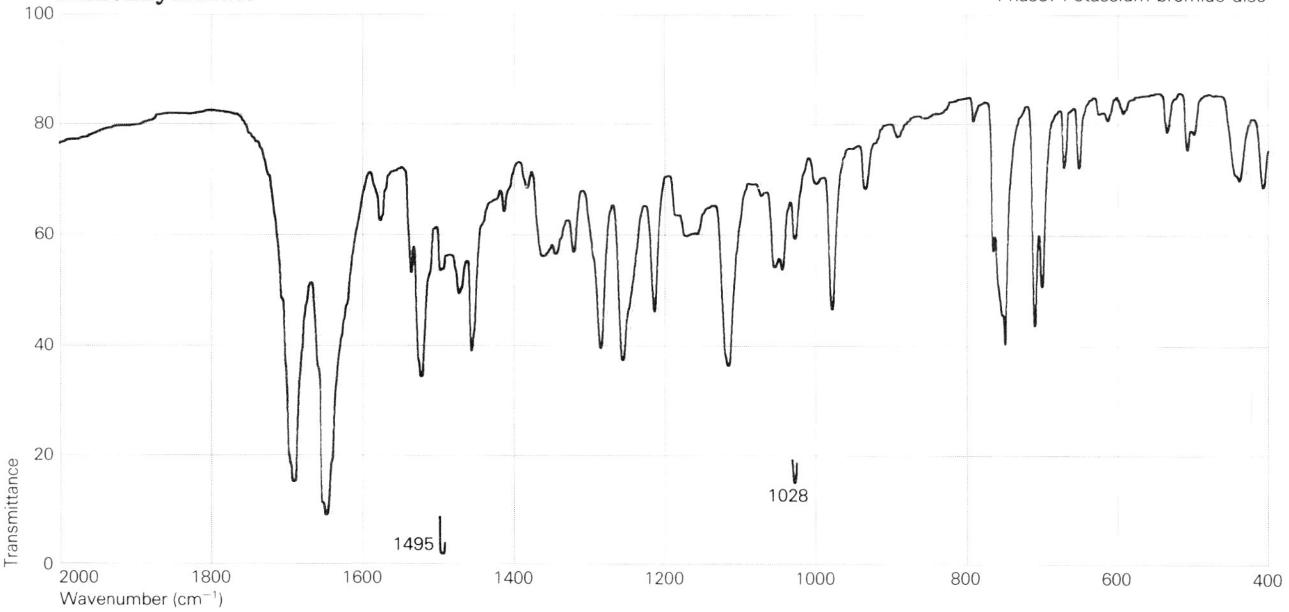

Dimethyl Phthalate

Diphenhydramine

Diphenoxylate Hydrochloride

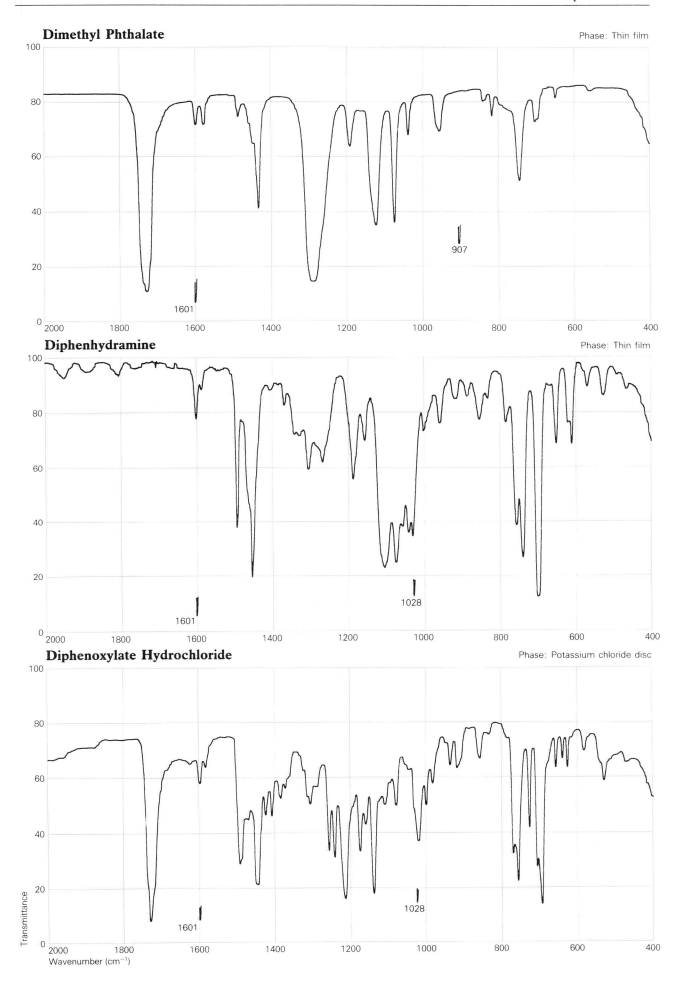

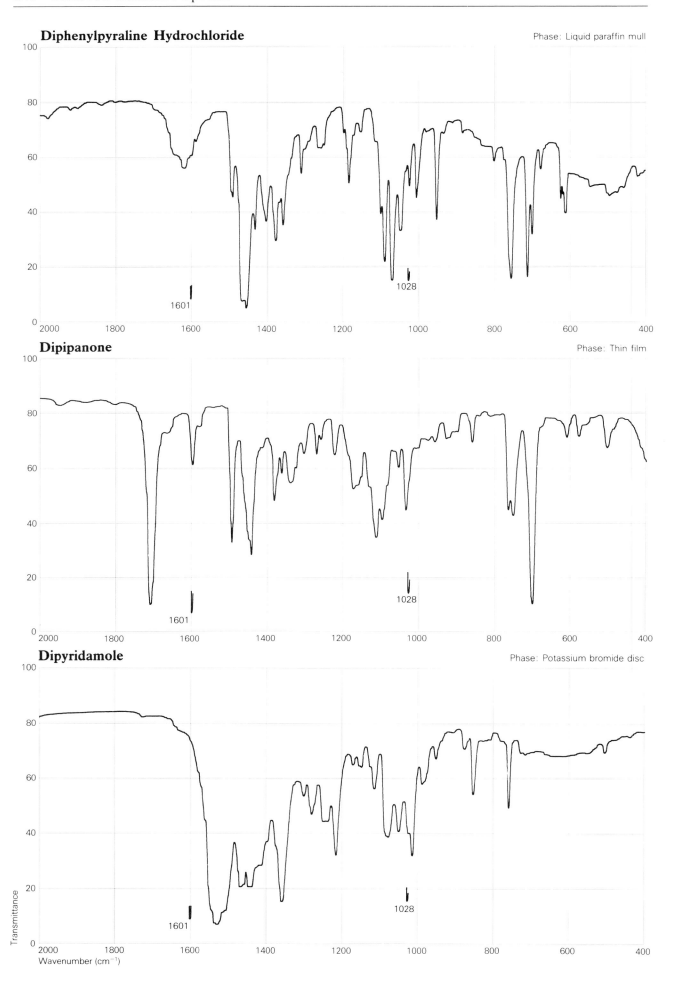

Diphenylpyraline Hydrochloride   Phase: Liquid paraffin mull

1601
1028

Dipipanone   Phase: Thin film

1601
1028

Dipyridamole   Phase: Potassium bromide disc

1601
1028

Transmittance

Wavenumber (cm⁻¹)

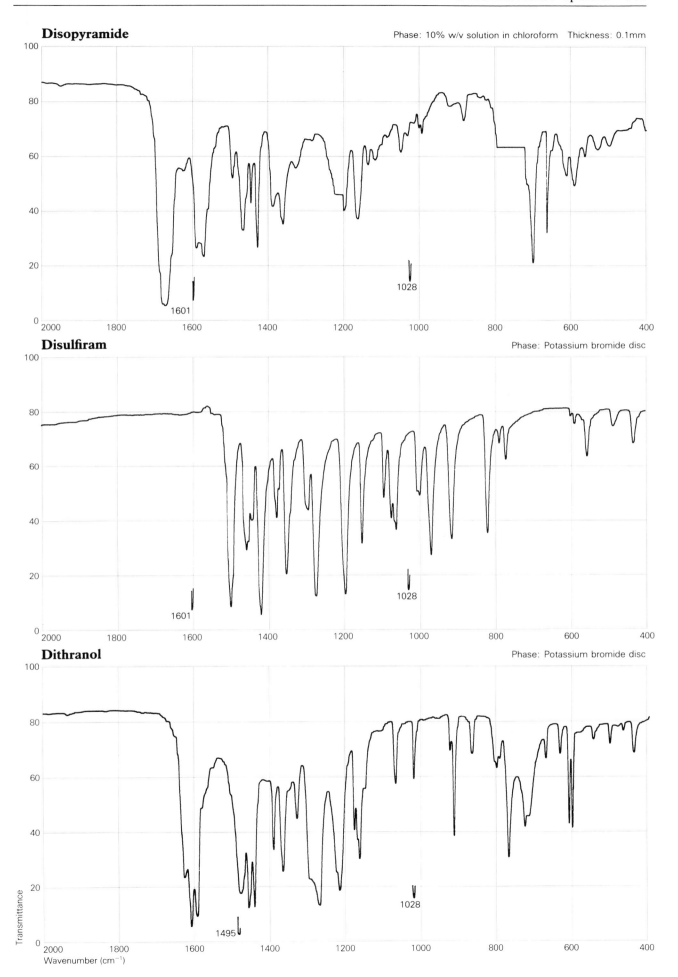

Disopyramide

Phase: 10% w/v solution in chloroform Thickness: 0.1mm

1601

1028

Disulfiram

Phase: Potassium bromide disc

1601

1028

Dithranol

Phase: Potassium bromide disc

1495

1028

Transmittance

Wavenumber (cm⁻¹)

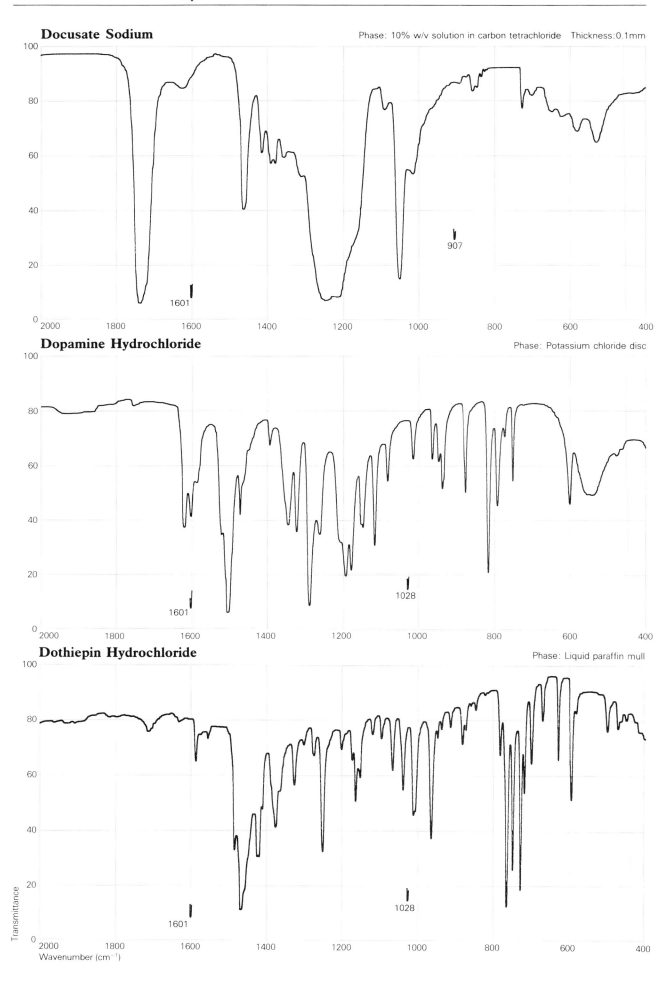

Docusate Sodium   Phase: 10% w/v solution in carbon tetrachloride   Thickness:0.1mm

907

1601

Dopamine Hydrochloride   Phase: Potassium chloride disc

1601

1028

Dothiepin Hydrochloride   Phase: Liquid paraffin mull

1601

1028

Transmittance

Wavenumber (cm⁻¹)

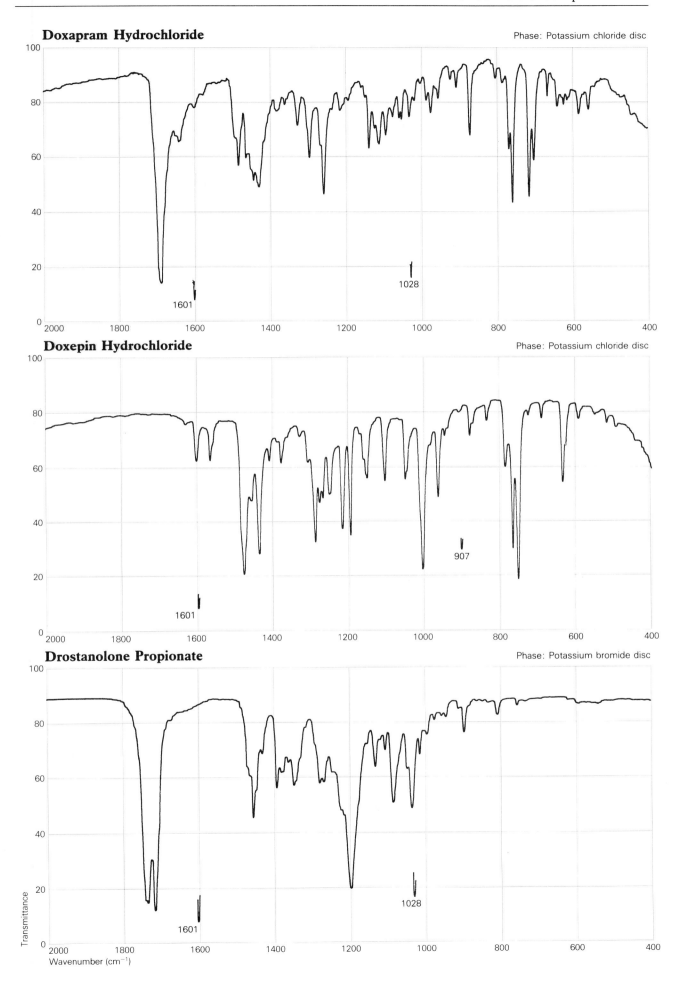

Doxapram Hydrochloride   Phase: Potassium chloride disc

1601
1028

Doxepin Hydrochloride   Phase: Potassium chloride disc

1601
907

Drostanolone Propionate   Phase: Potassium bromide disc

Transmittance

1601
1028

Wavenumber (cm⁻¹)

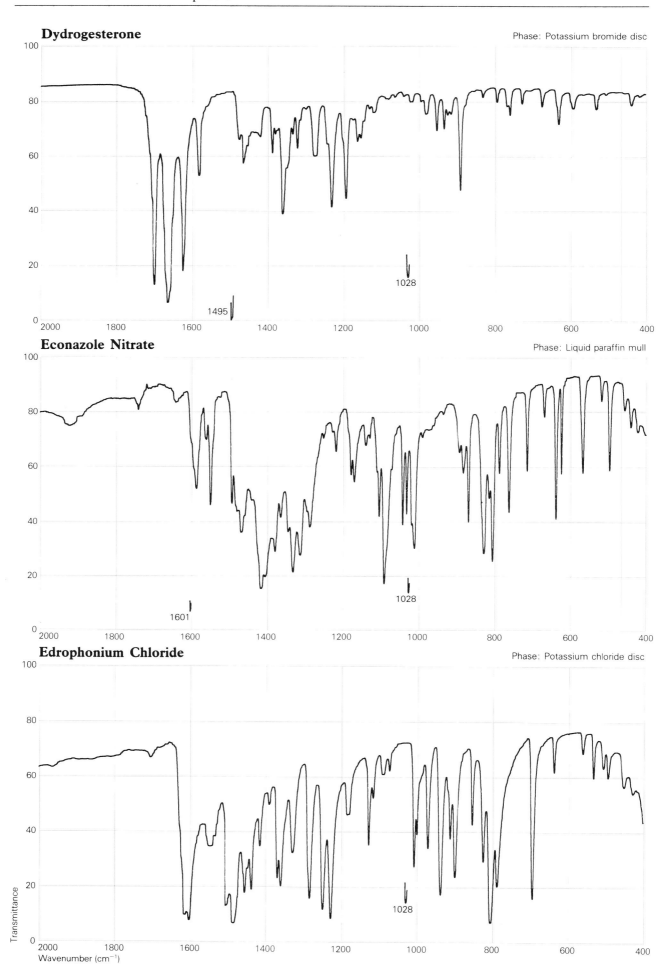

Dydrogesterone

Phase: Potassium bromide disc

1495

1028

Econazole Nitrate

Phase: Liquid paraffin mull

1601

1028

Edrophonium Chloride

Phase: Potassium chloride disc

1028

Transmittance

Wavenumber (cm⁻¹)

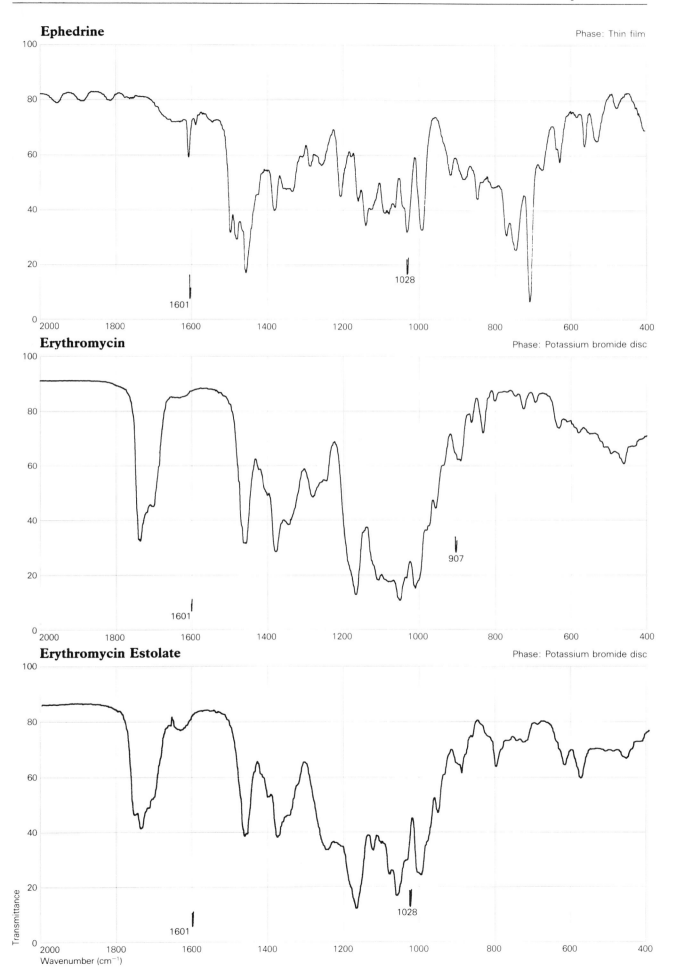

Ephedrine

Phase: Thin film

1601
1028

Erythromycin

Phase: Potassium bromide disc

907
1601

Erythromycin Estolate

Phase: Potassium bromide disc

1601
1028

Transmittance

Wavenumber (cm⁻¹)

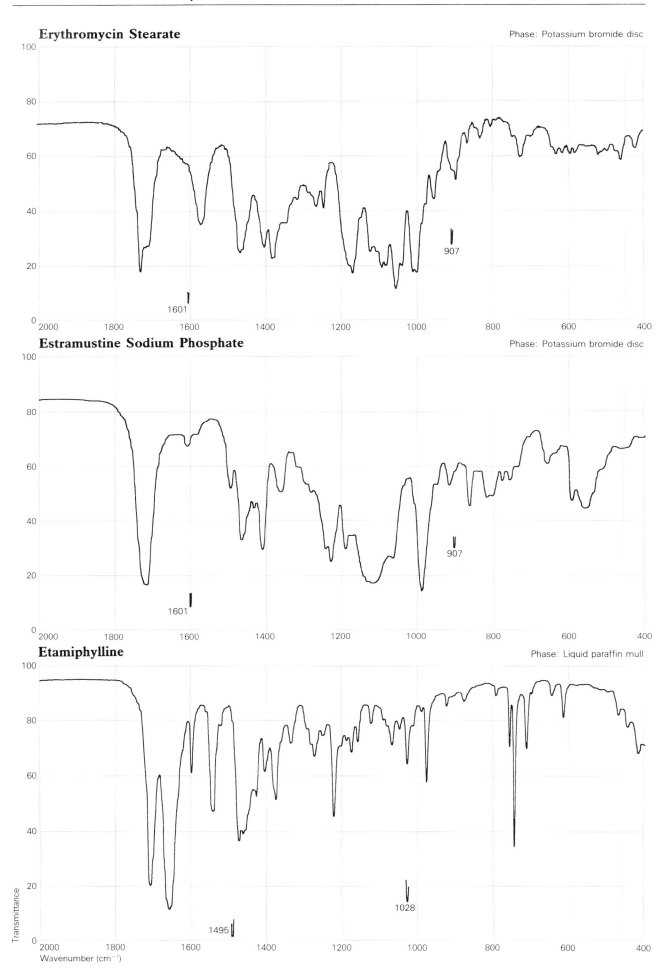

Erythromycin Stearate   Phase: Potassium bromide disc

Estramustine Sodium Phosphate   Phase: Potassium bromide disc

Etamiphylline   Phase: Liquid paraffin mull

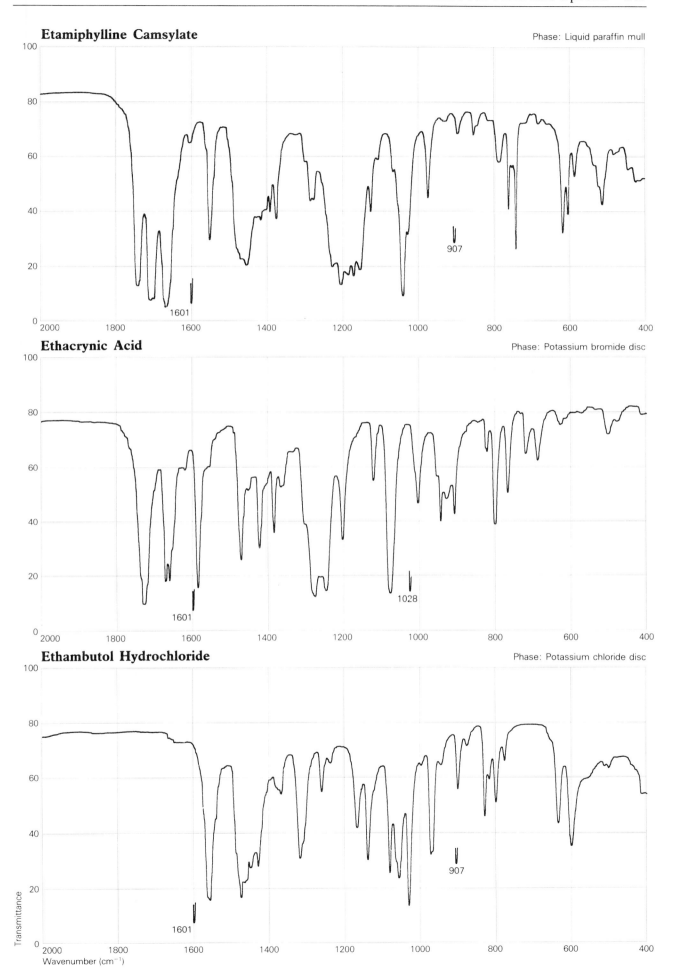

Etamiphylline Camsylate   Phase: Liquid paraffin mull

1601

907

Ethacrynic Acid   Phase: Potassium bromide disc

1601

1028

Ethambutol Hydrochloride   Phase: Potassium chloride disc

1601

907

Transmittance

Wavenumber (cm⁻¹)

Ethamivan   Phase: Potassium bromide disc

Ethosuximide   Phase: Thin film

Ethyl Cinnamate   Phase: Thin film

Wavenumber (cm⁻¹)

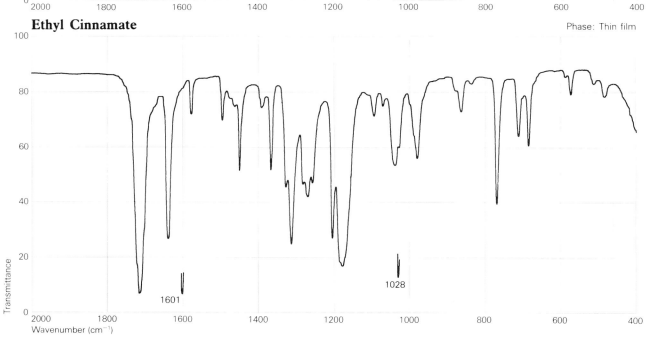

Ethyl Hydroxybenzoate

Phase: Potassium bromide disc

Ethylenediamine

Phase: Thin film

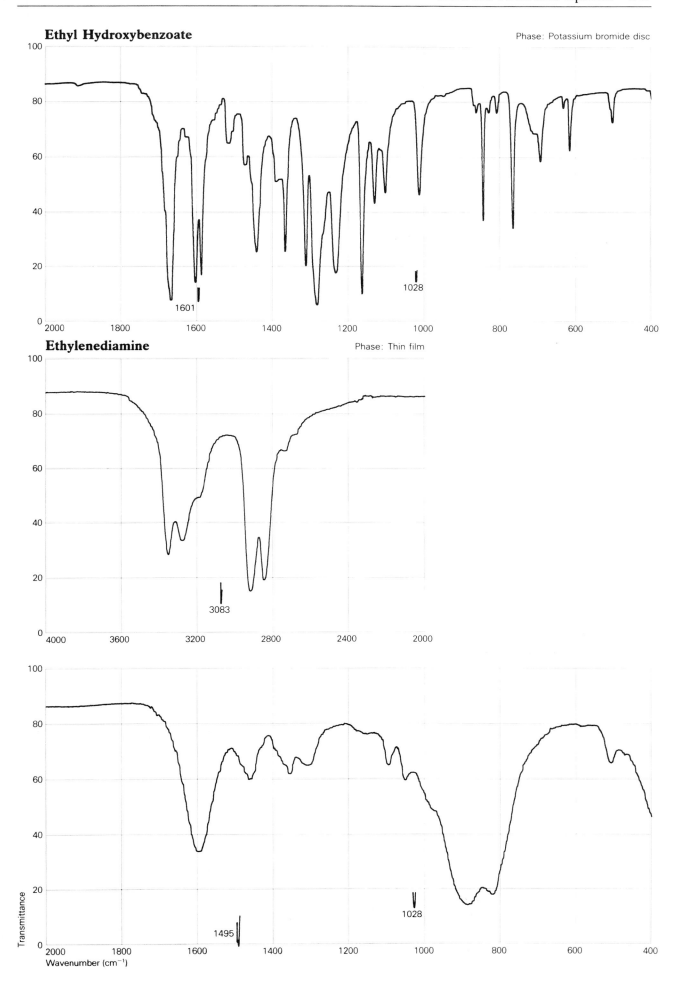

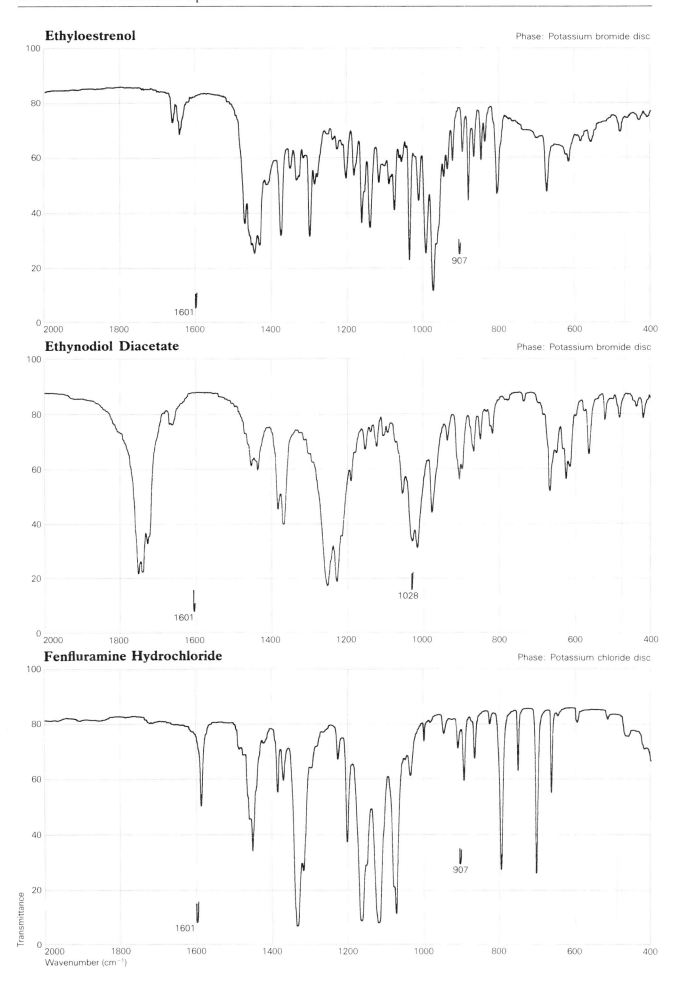

Fenoprofen

Phase: Thin film

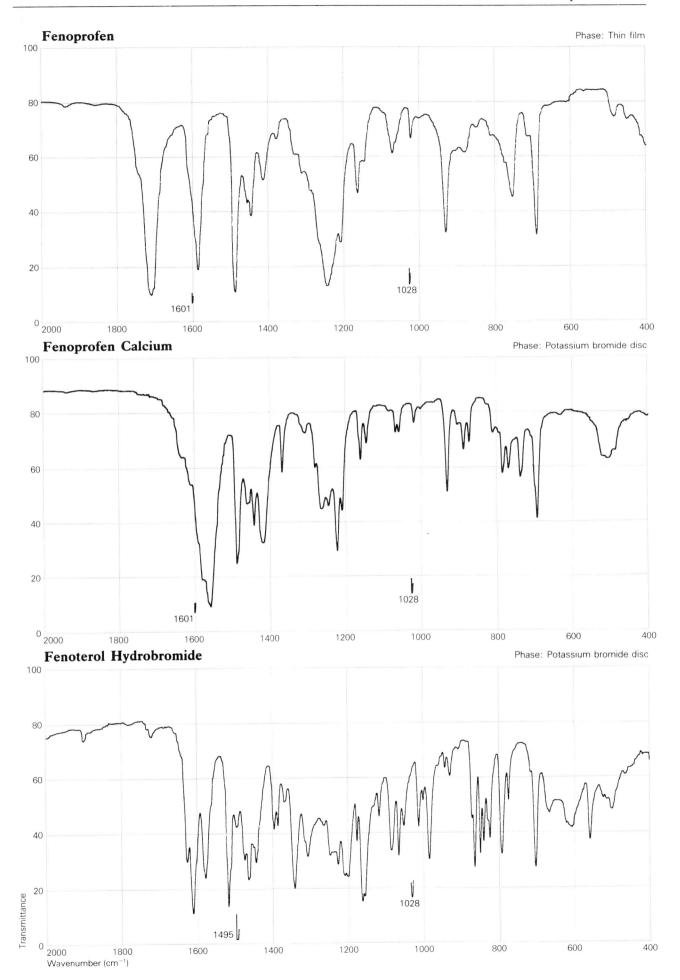

Fenoprofen Calcium

Phase: Potassium bromide disc

Fenoterol Hydrobromide

Phase: Potassium bromide disc

Transmittance

Wavenumber (cm⁻¹)

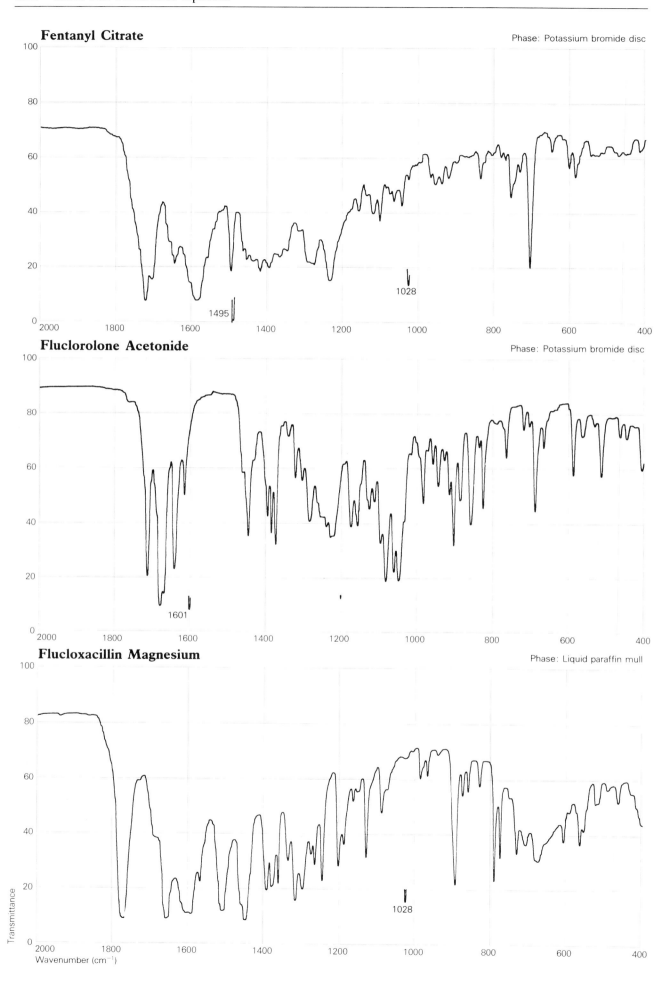

Fentanyl Citrate

Phase: Potassium bromide disc

1495

1028

Fluclorolone Acetonide

Phase: Potassium bromide disc

1601

Flucloxacillin Magnesium

Phase: Liquid paraffin mull

1028

Transmittance

Wavenumber (cm⁻¹)

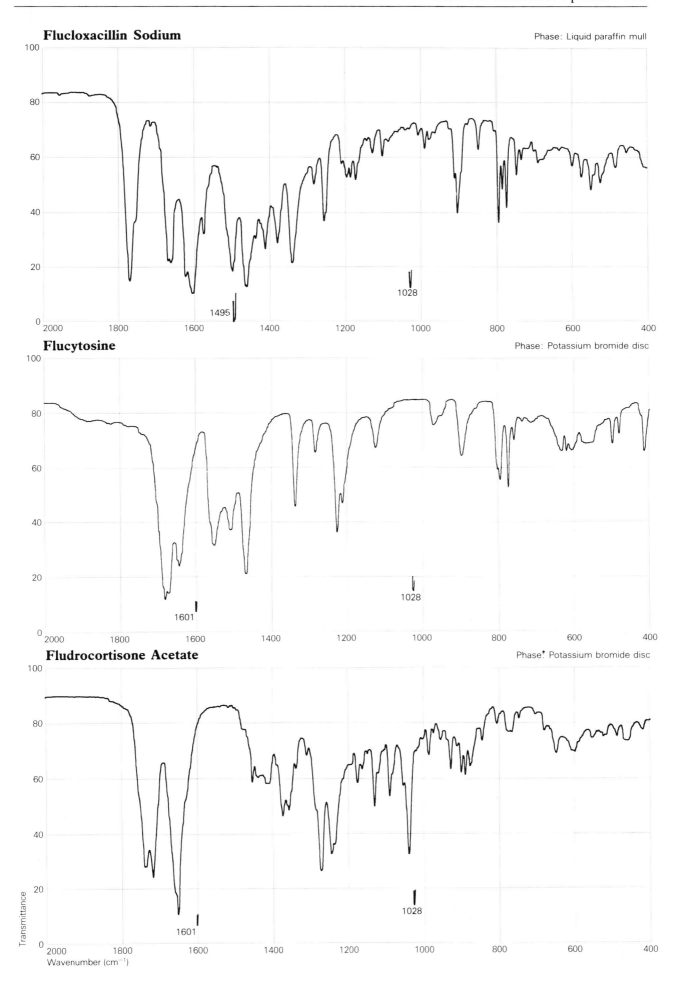

Flucloxacillin Sodium

Phase: Liquid paraffin mull

1495

1028

Flucytosine

Phase: Potassium bromide disc

1601

1028

Fludrocortisone Acetate

Phase: Potassium bromide disc

1601

1028

Transmittance

Wavenumber (cm⁻¹)

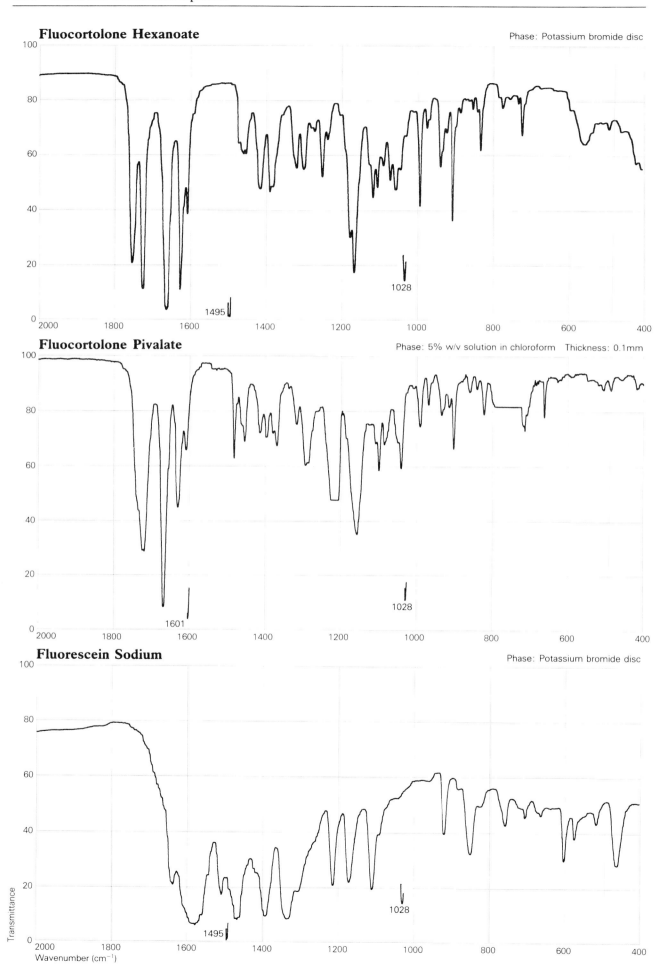

Fluocortolone Hexanoate   Phase: Potassium bromide disc

Fluocortolone Pivalate   Phase: 5% w/v solution in chloroform   Thickness: 0.1mm

Fluorescein Sodium   Phase: Potassium bromide disc

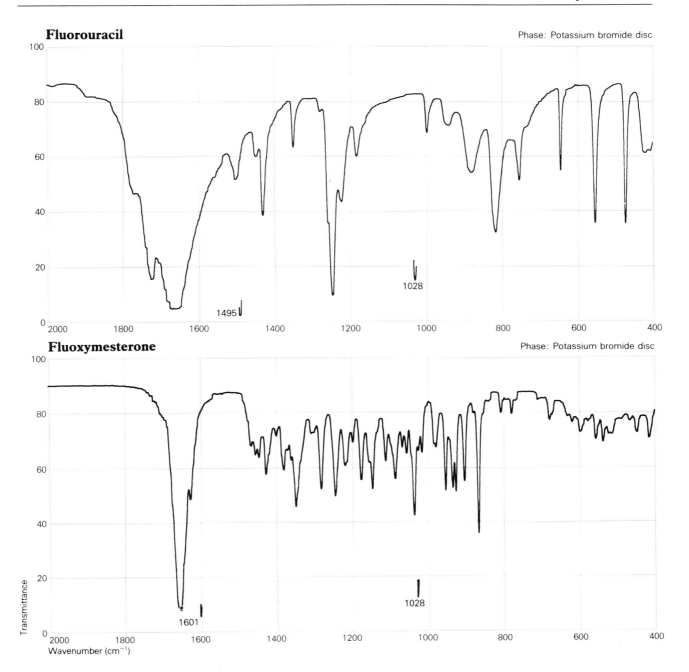

Fluorouracil

Phase: Potassium bromide disc

1495

1028

Fluoxymesterone

Phase: Potassium bromide disc

1601

1028

Transmittance

Wavenumber (cm⁻¹)

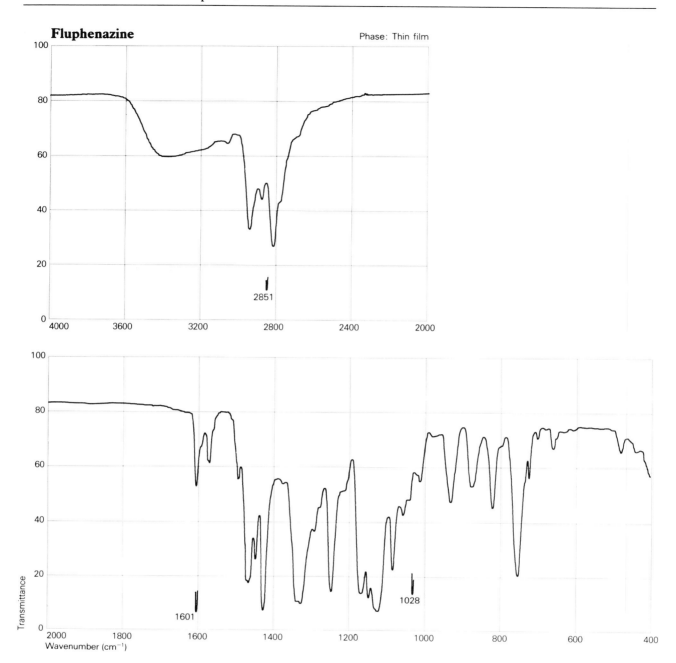

Fluphenazine Decanoate

Phase: 8% w/v solution in chloroform   Thickness: 0.1mm

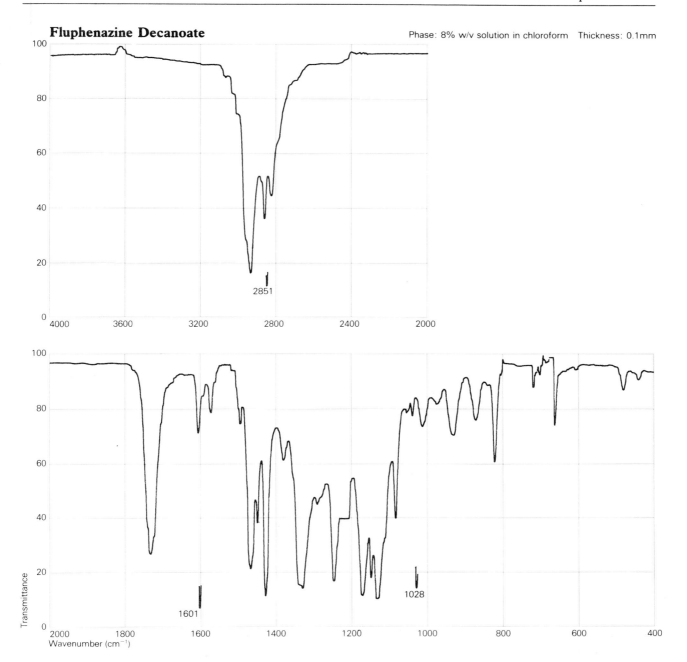

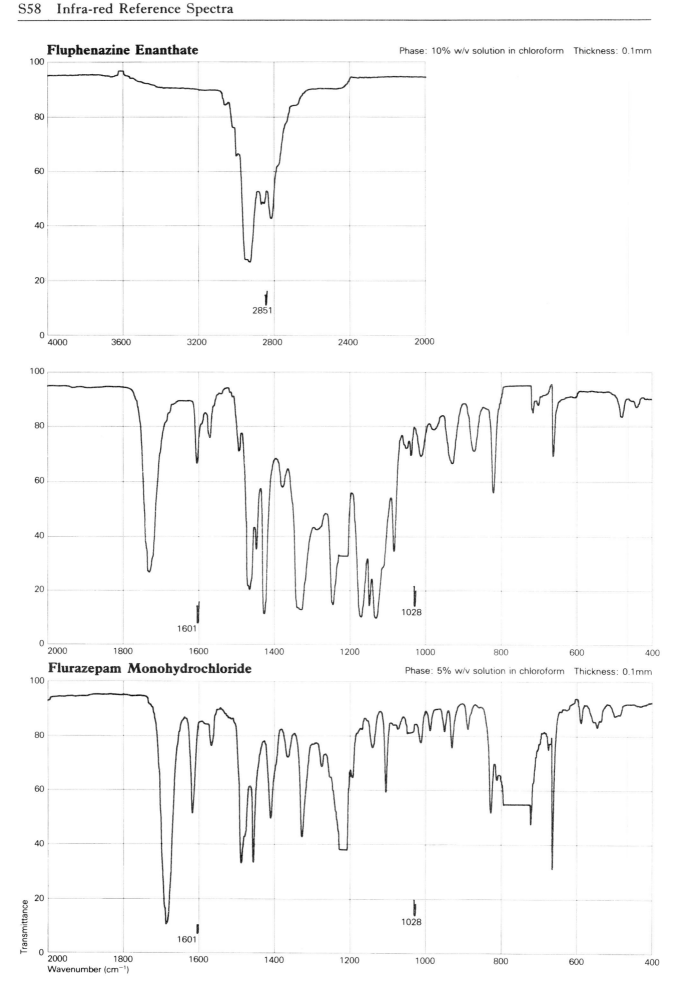

Fluphenazine Enanthate

Phase: 10% w/v solution in chloroform   Thickness: 0.1mm

2851

1601

1028

Flurazepam Monohydrochloride

Phase: 5% w/v solution in chloroform   Thickness: 0.1mm

1601

1028

Transmittance

Wavenumber (cm⁻¹)

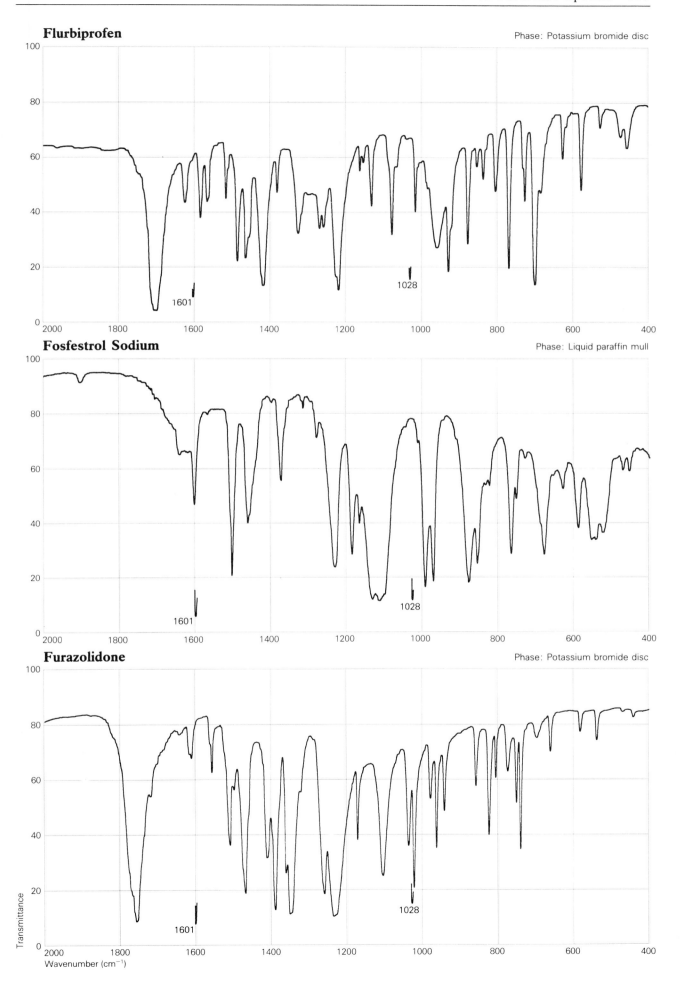

Flurbiprofen   Phase: Potassium bromide disc

1601
1028

Fosfestrol Sodium   Phase: Liquid paraffin mull

1601
1028

Furazolidone   Phase: Potassium bromide disc

1601
1028

Transmittance

Wavenumber (cm⁻¹)

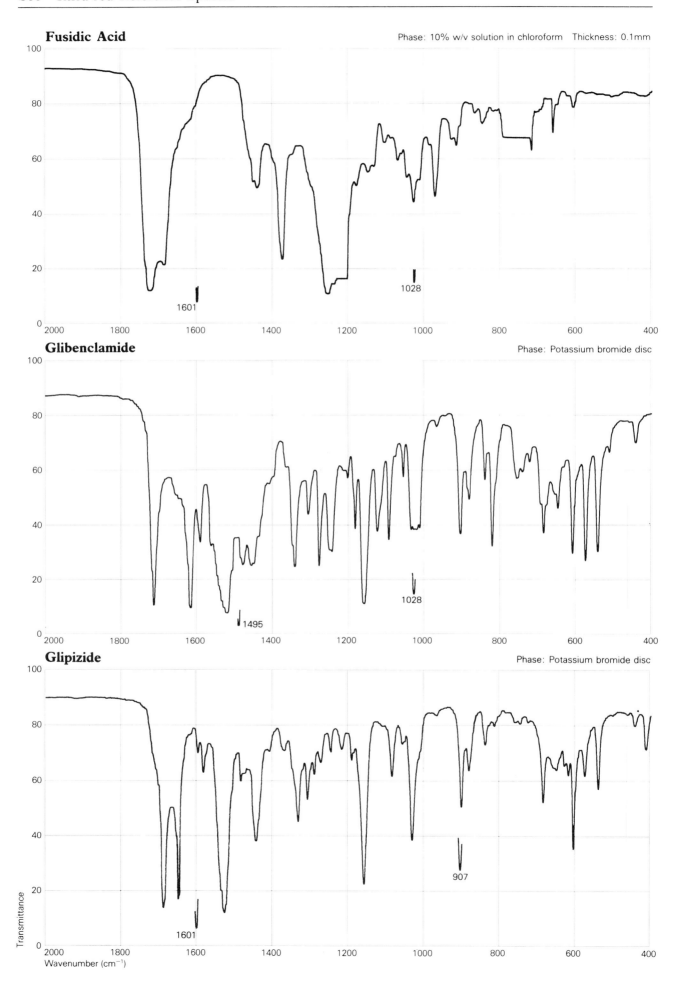

Fusidic Acid

Phase: 10% w/v solution in chloroform   Thickness: 0.1mm

1601

1028

Glibenclamide

Phase: Potassium bromide disc

1495

1028

Glipizide

Phase: Potassium bromide disc

1601

907

Transmittance

Wavenumber (cm⁻¹)

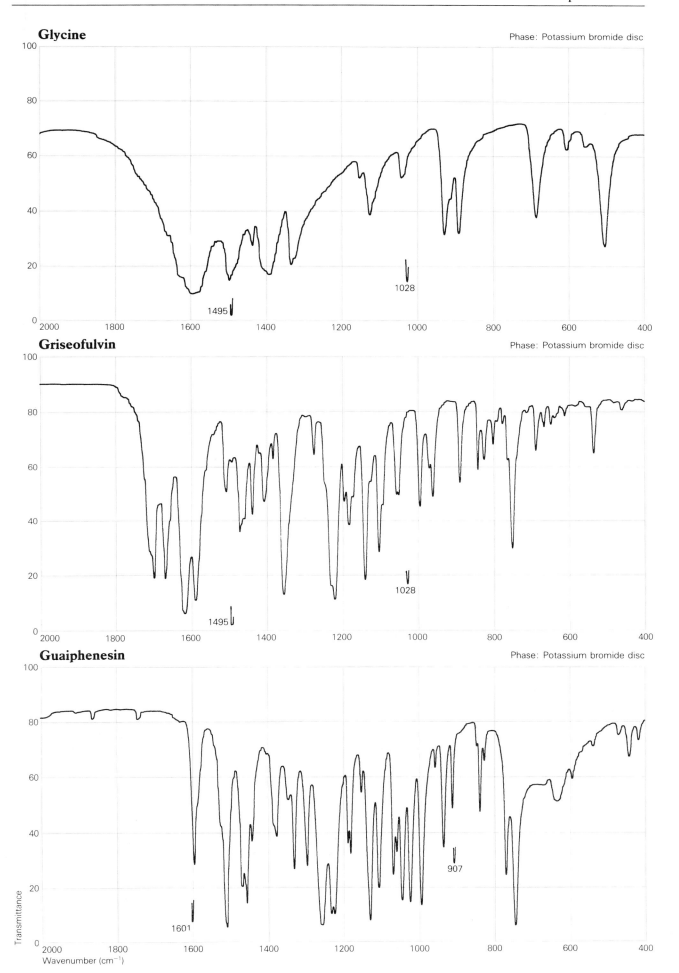

Glycine   Phase: Potassium bromide disc

Griseofulvin   Phase: Potassium bromide disc

Guaiphenesin   Phase: Potassium bromide disc

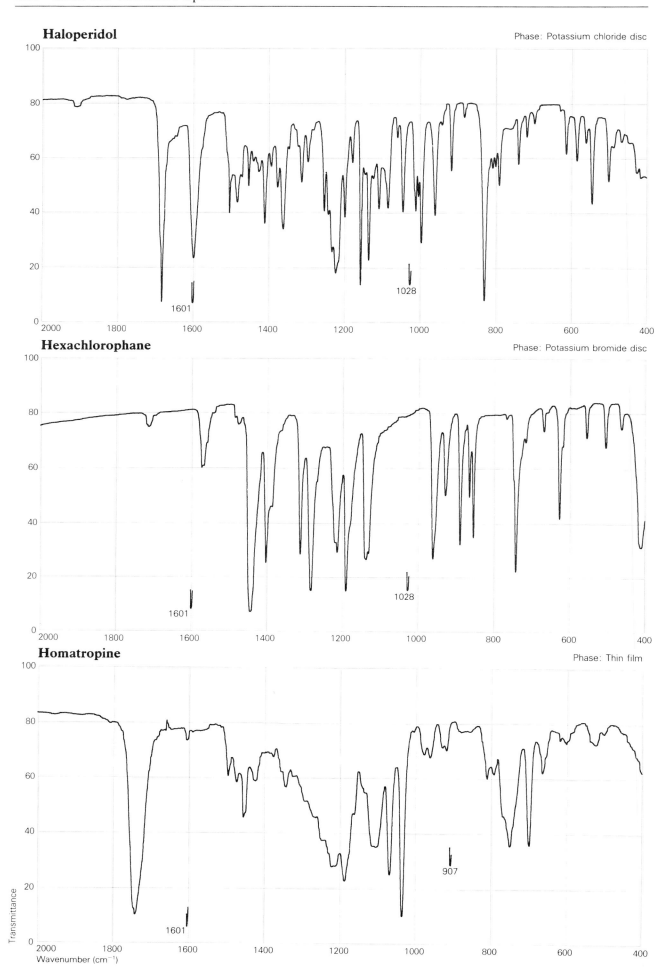

Haloperidol

Phase: Potassium chloride disc

Hexachlorophane

Phase: Potassium bromide disc

Homatropine

Phase: Thin film

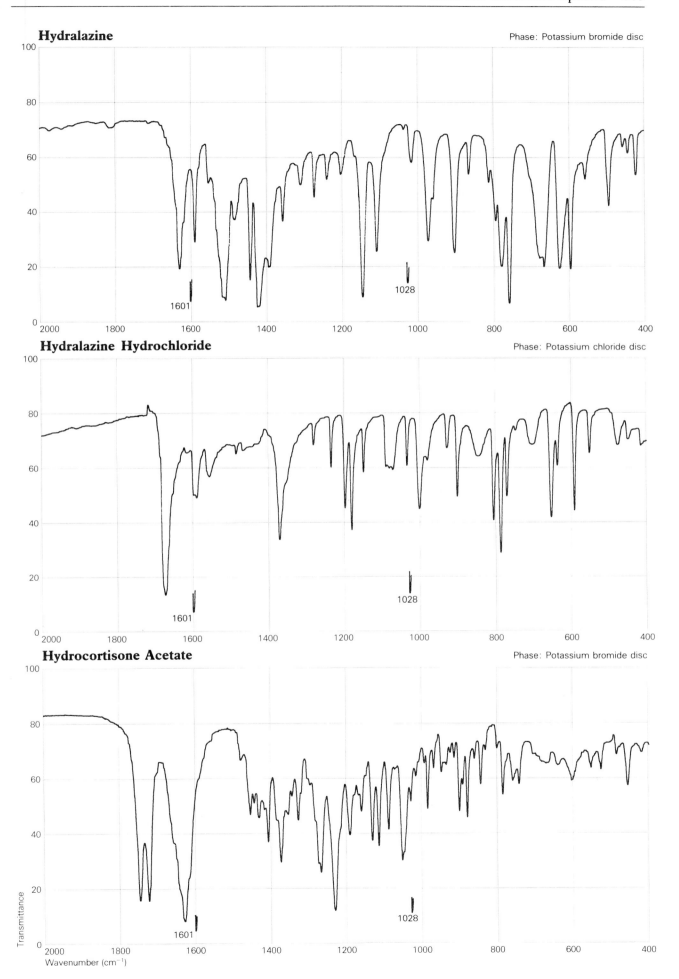

Hydralazine   Phase: Potassium bromide disc

Hydralazine Hydrochloride   Phase: Potassium chloride disc

Hydrocortisone Acetate   Phase: Potassium bromide disc

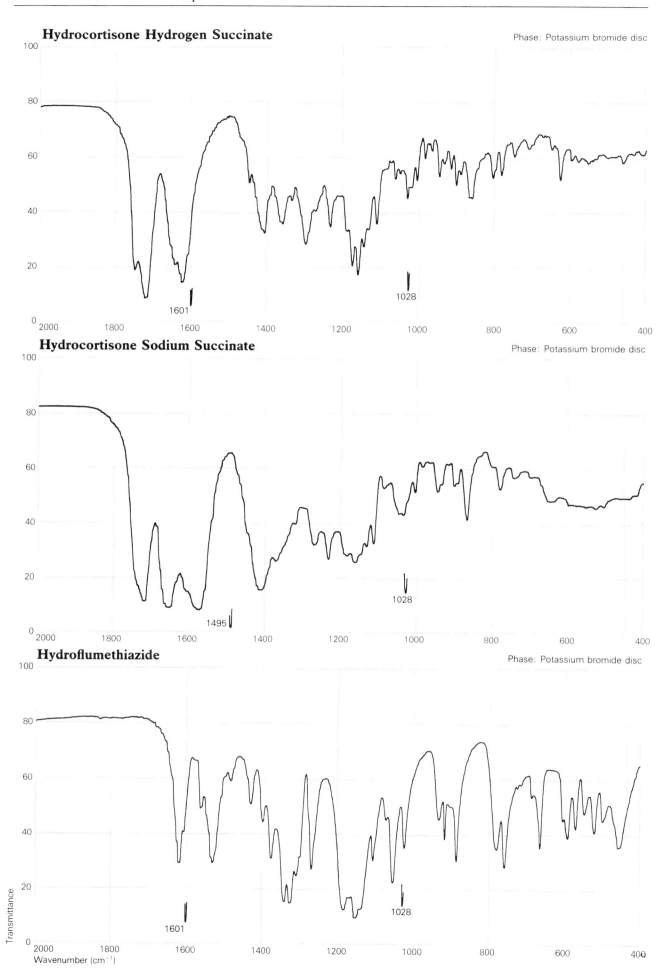

Hydrocortisone Hydrogen Succinate

Phase: Potassium bromide disc

1601

1028

Hydrocortisone Sodium Succinate

Phase: Potassium bromide disc

1028

1495

Hydroflumethiazide

Phase: Potassium bromide disc

1601

1028

Transmittance

Wavenumber (cm⁻¹)

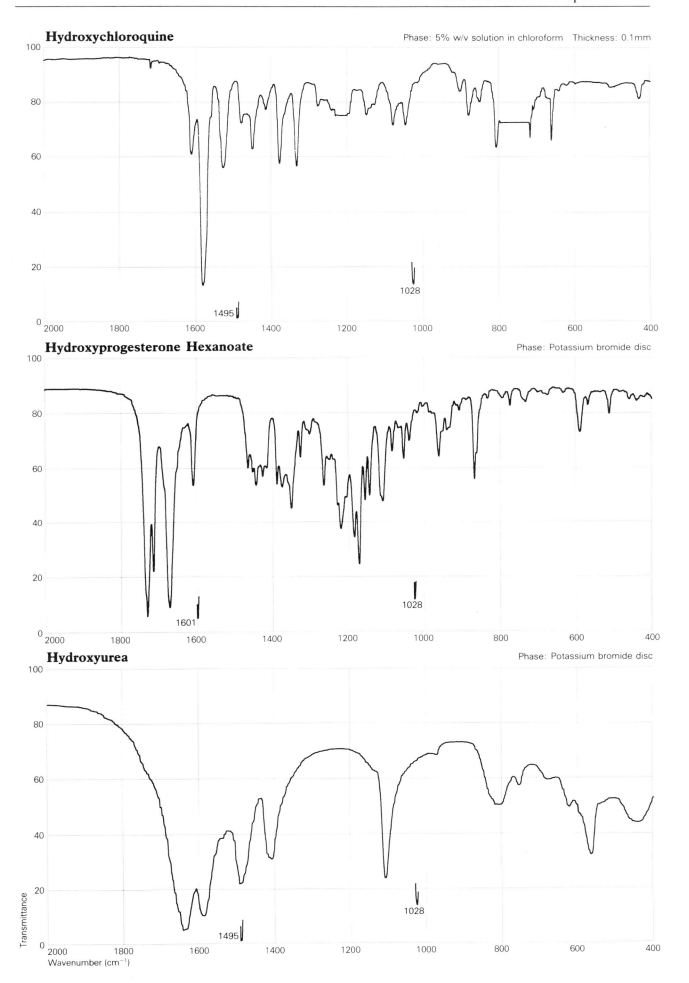

Hydroxychloroquine Phase: 5% w/v solution in chloroform Thickness: 0.1mm

1495

1028

Hydroxyprogesterone Hexanoate Phase: Potassium bromide disc

1601

1028

Hydroxyurea Phase: Potassium bromide disc

1495

1028

Transmittance

Wavenumber (cm⁻¹)

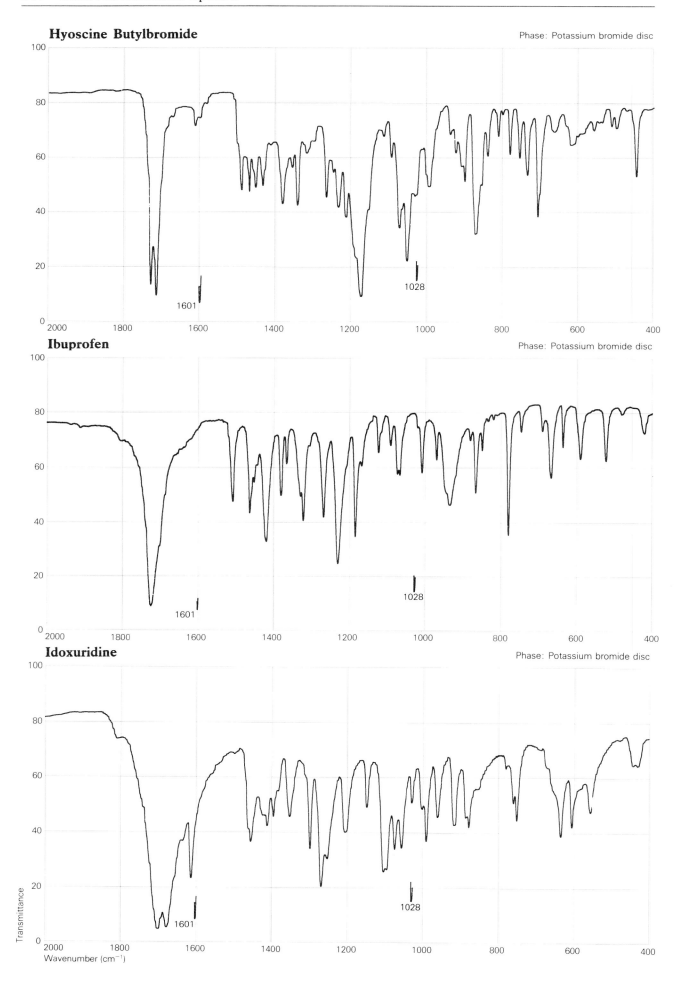

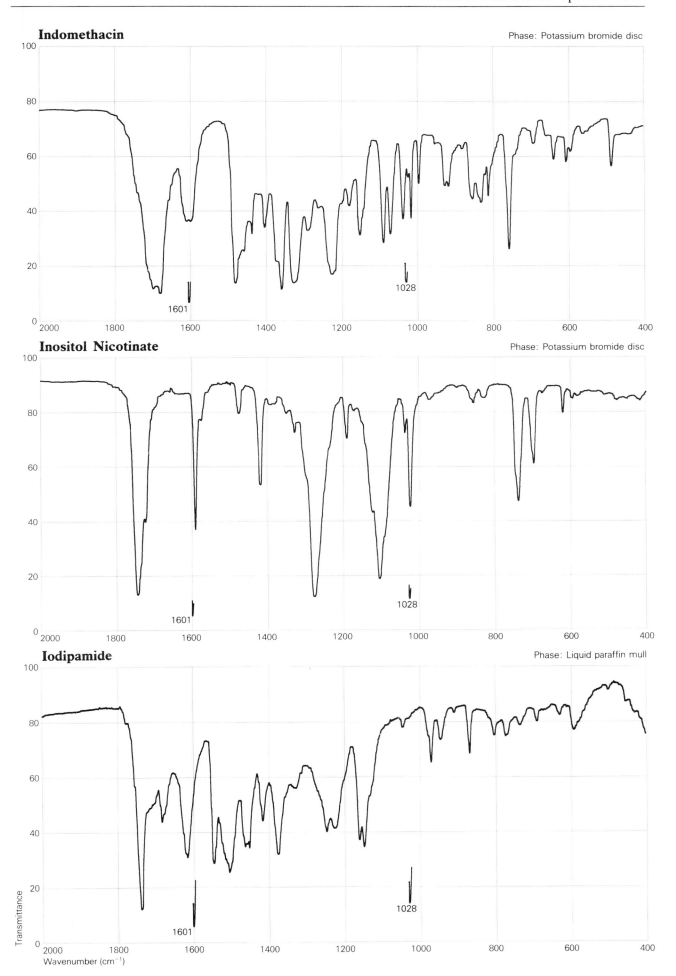

Indomethacin

Phase: Potassium bromide disc

1601
1028

Inositol Nicotinate

Phase: Potassium bromide disc

1601
1028

Iodipamide

Phase: Liquid paraffin mull

1601
1028

Transmittance

Wavenumber (cm⁻¹)

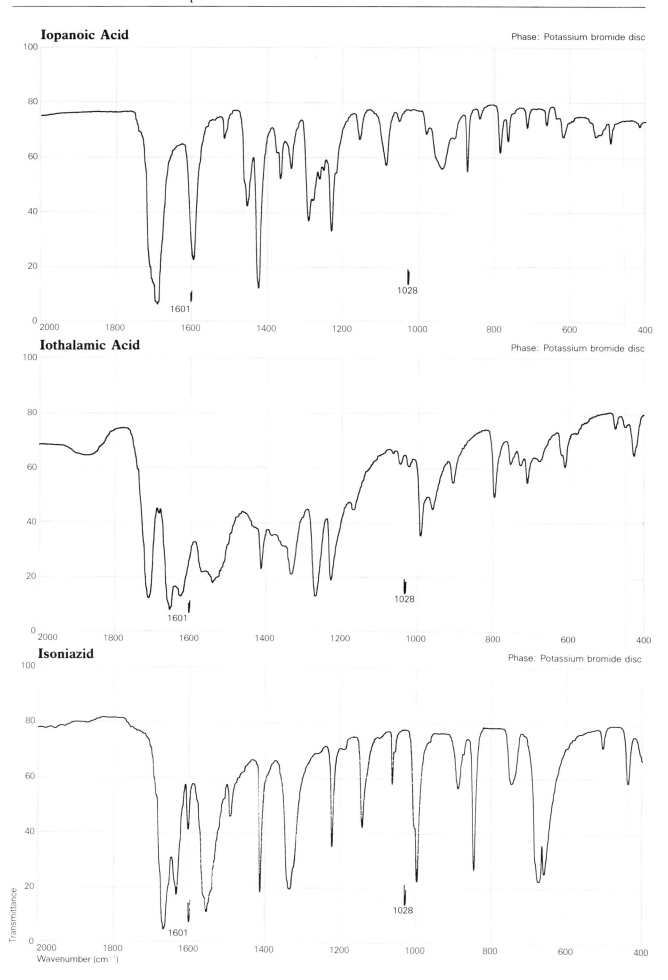

Iopanoic Acid
Phase: Potassium bromide disc

1601
1028

Iothalamic Acid
Phase: Potassium bromide disc

1601
1028

Isoniazid
Phase: Potassium bromide disc

1601
1028

Transmittance
Wavenumber (cm⁻¹)

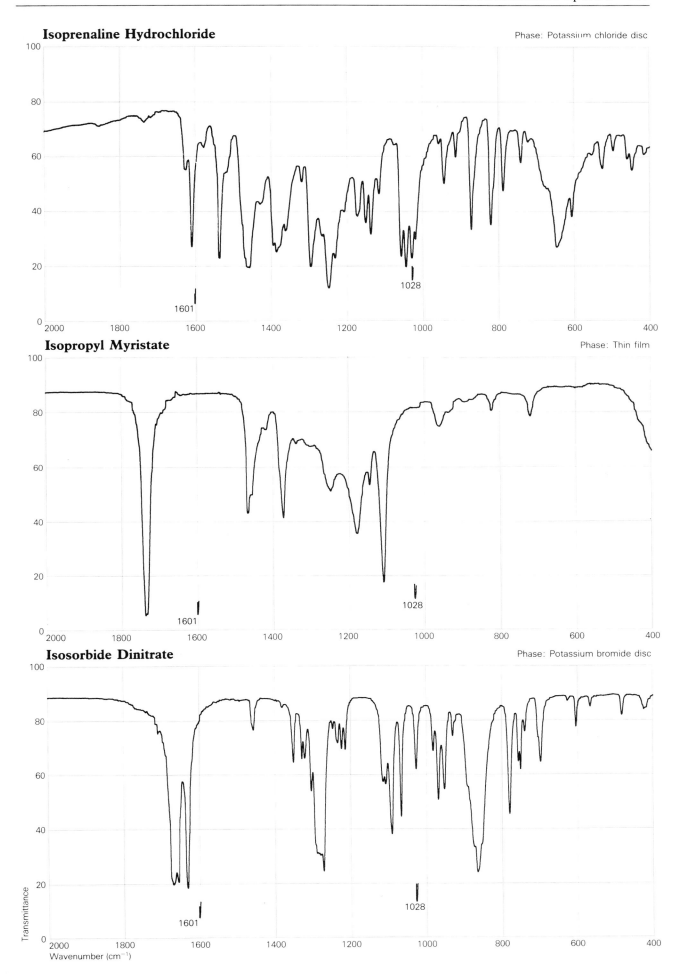

Isoprenaline Hydrochloride

Phase: Potassium chloride disc

1601

1028

Isopropyl Myristate

Phase: Thin film

1601

1028

Isosorbide Dinitrate

Phase: Potassium bromide disc

1601

1028

Transmittance

Wavenumber (cm⁻¹)

Isoxsuprine Hydrochloride

Phase: Potassium chloride disc

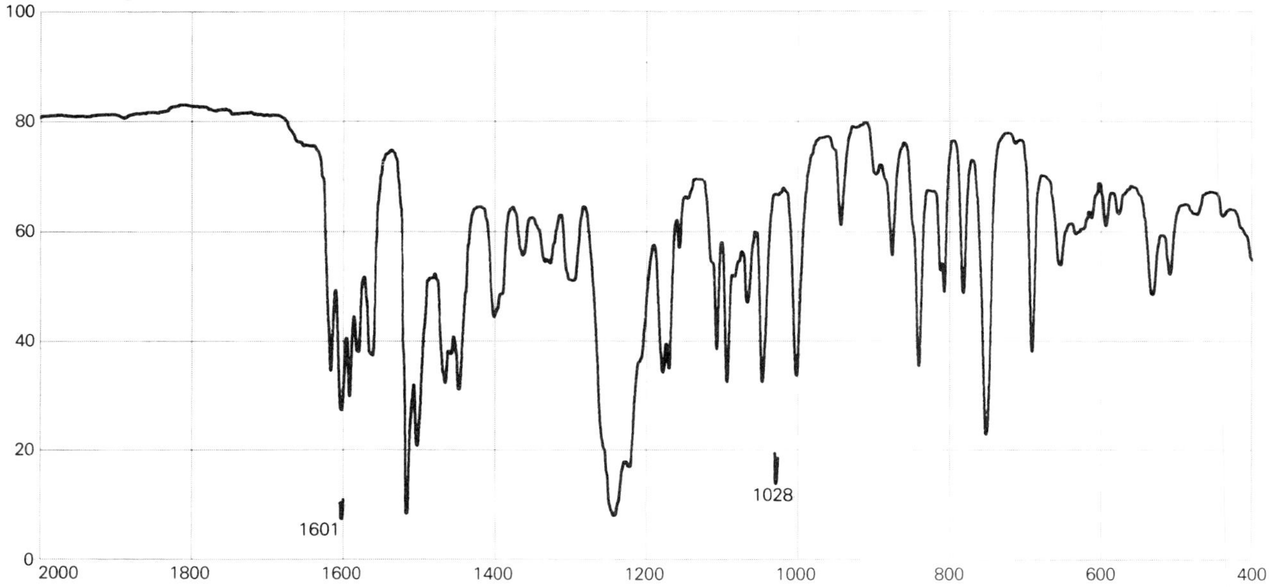

1601
1028

Ketoprofen

Phase: Potassium bromide disc

1601
1028

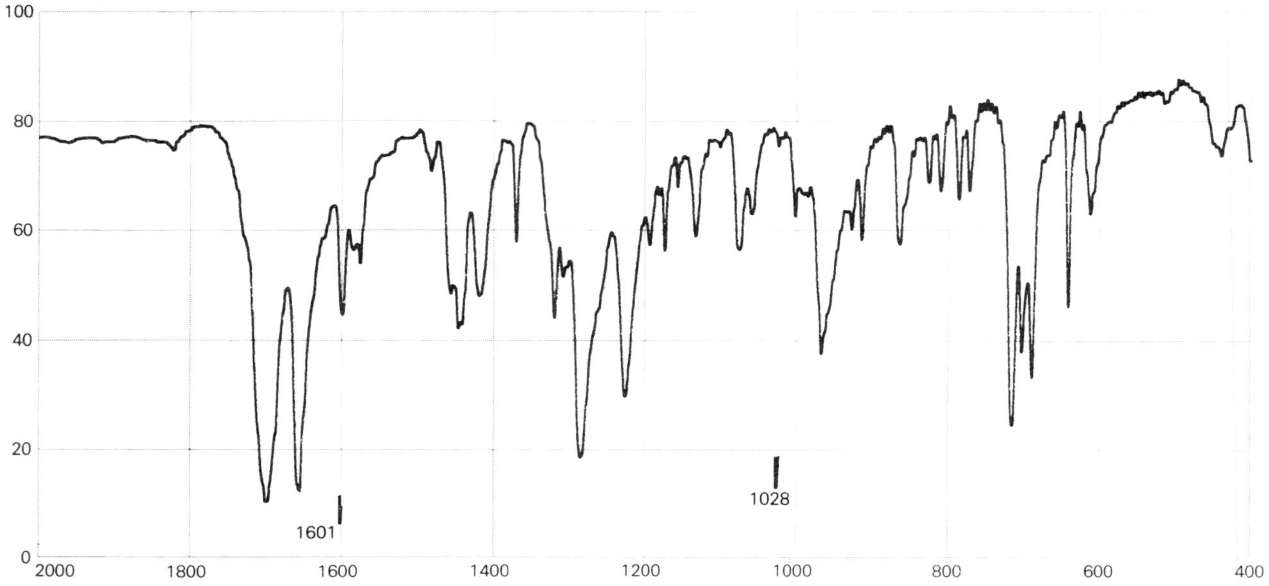

Labetalol

Phase: Potassium bromide disc

1601
1028

Transmittance

Wavenumber (cm^{-1})

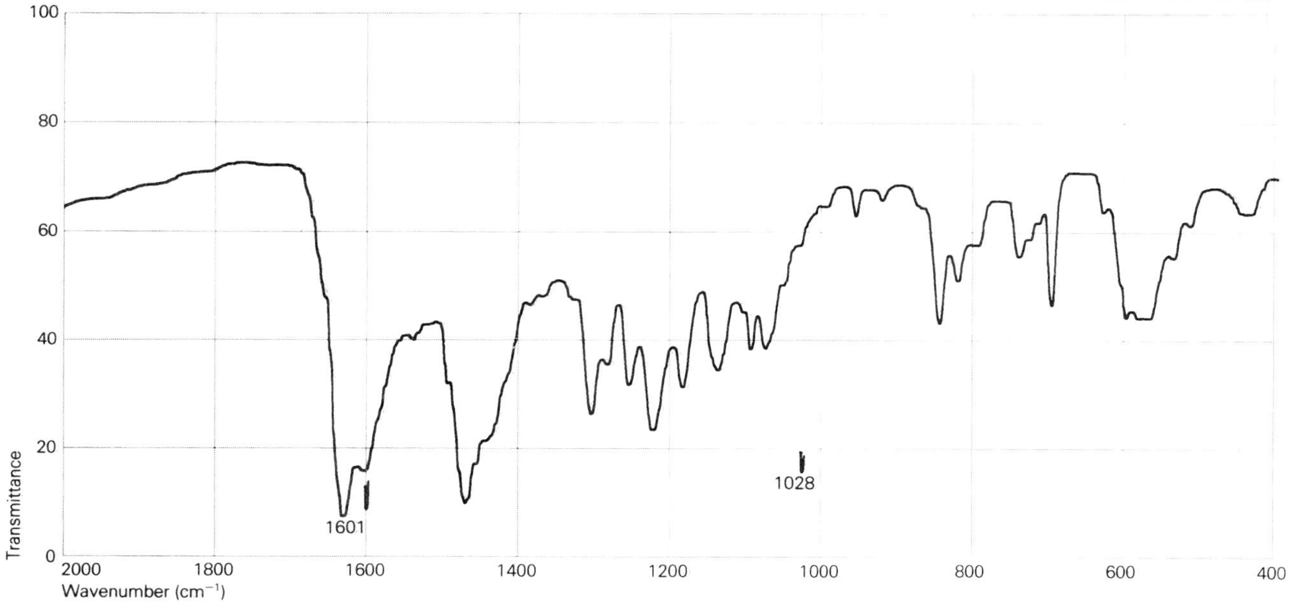

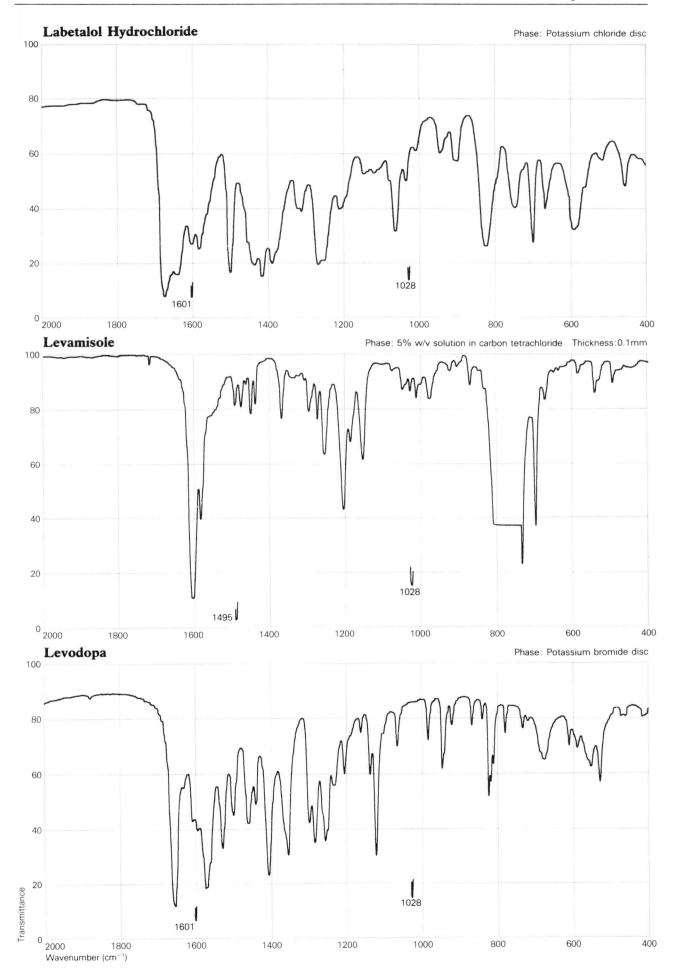

Labetalol Hydrochloride   Phase: Potassium chloride disc

1601
1028

Levamisole   Phase: 5% w/v solution in carbon tetrachloride   Thickness: 0.1mm

1495
1028

Levodopa   Phase: Potassium bromide disc

1601
1028

Transmittance

Wavenumber (cm⁻¹)

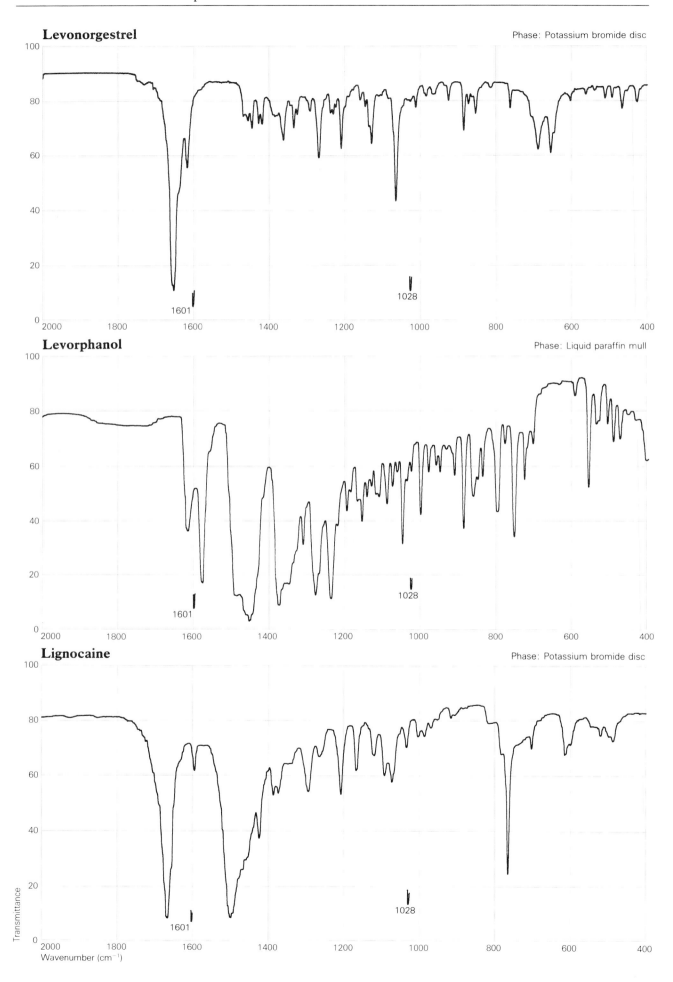

Levonorgestrel Phase: Potassium bromide disc

1601
1028

Levorphanol Phase: Liquid paraffin mull

1601
1028

Lignocaine Phase: Potassium bromide disc

1601
1028

Transmittance

Wavenumber (cm⁻¹)

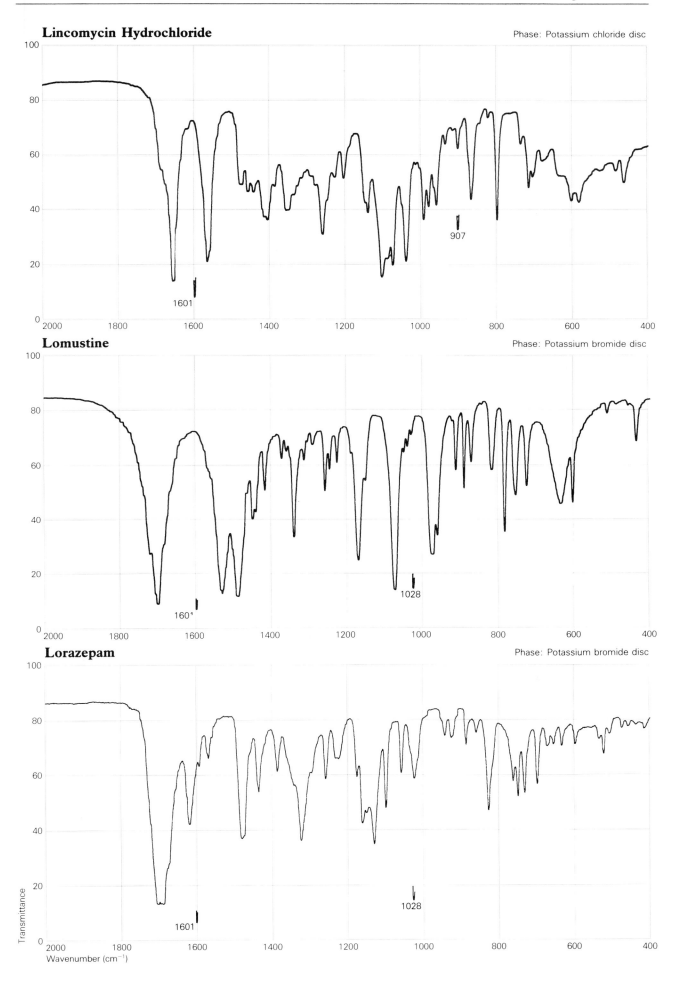

Lincomycin Hydrochloride

Phase: Potassium chloride disc

907

1601

Lomustine

Phase: Potassium bromide disc

1028

160'

Lorazepam

Phase: Potassium bromide disc

1028

1601

Transmittance

Wavenumber (cm⁻¹)

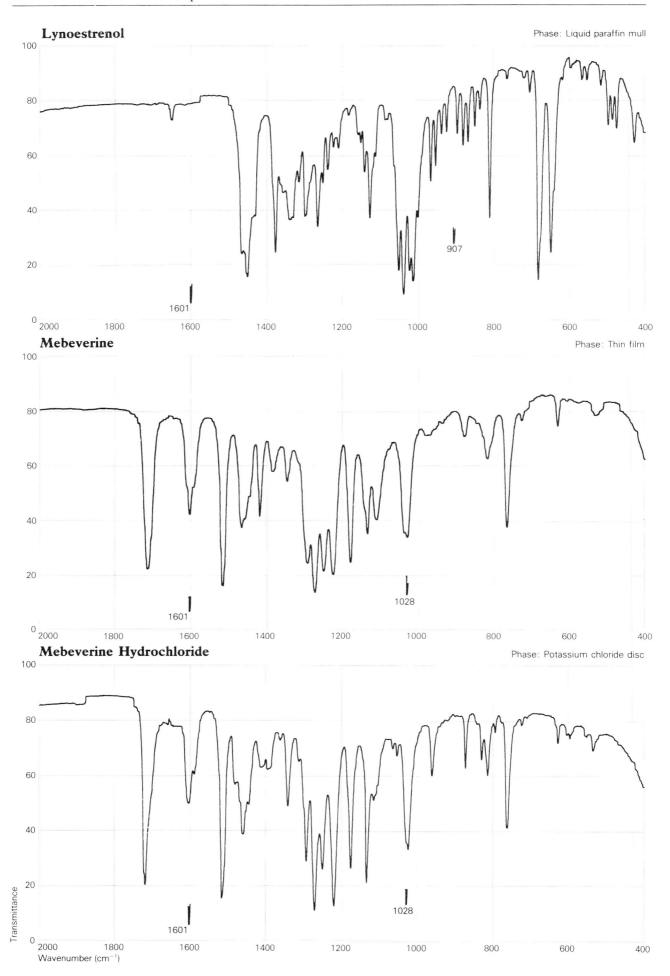

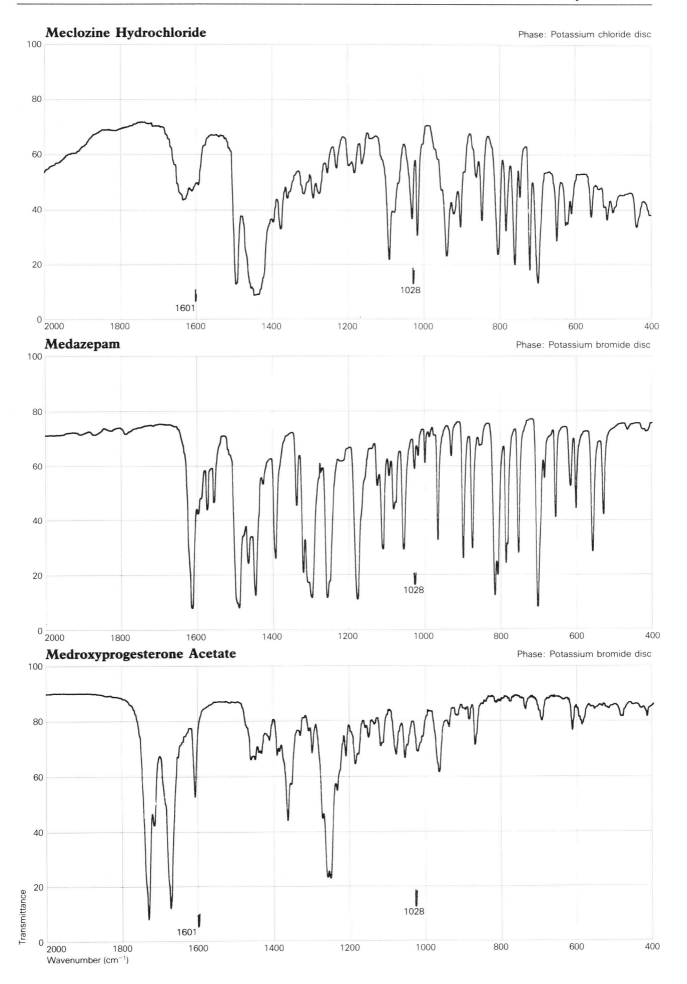

Meclozine Hydrochloride   Phase: Potassium chloride disc

1601
1028

Medazepam   Phase: Potassium bromide disc

1028

Medroxyprogesterone Acetate   Phase: Potassium bromide disc

1601
1028

Transmittance
Wavenumber (cm⁻¹)

Mefenamic Acid

Phase: Liquid paraffin mull

Megestrol Acetate

Phase: Potassium bromide disc

Menadiol Sodium Diphosphate

Phase: Potassium bromide disc

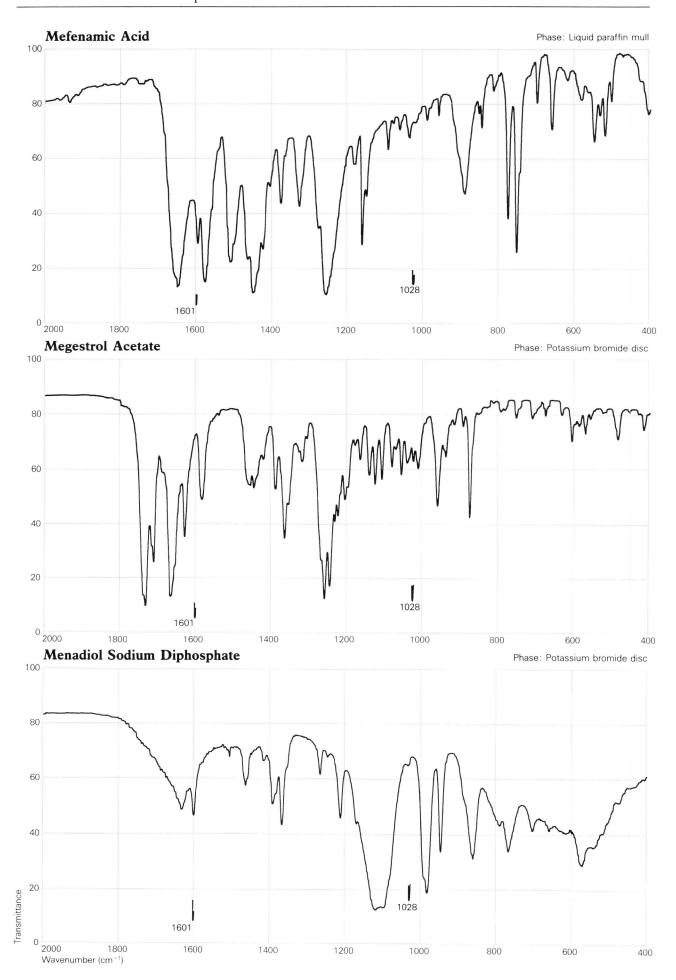

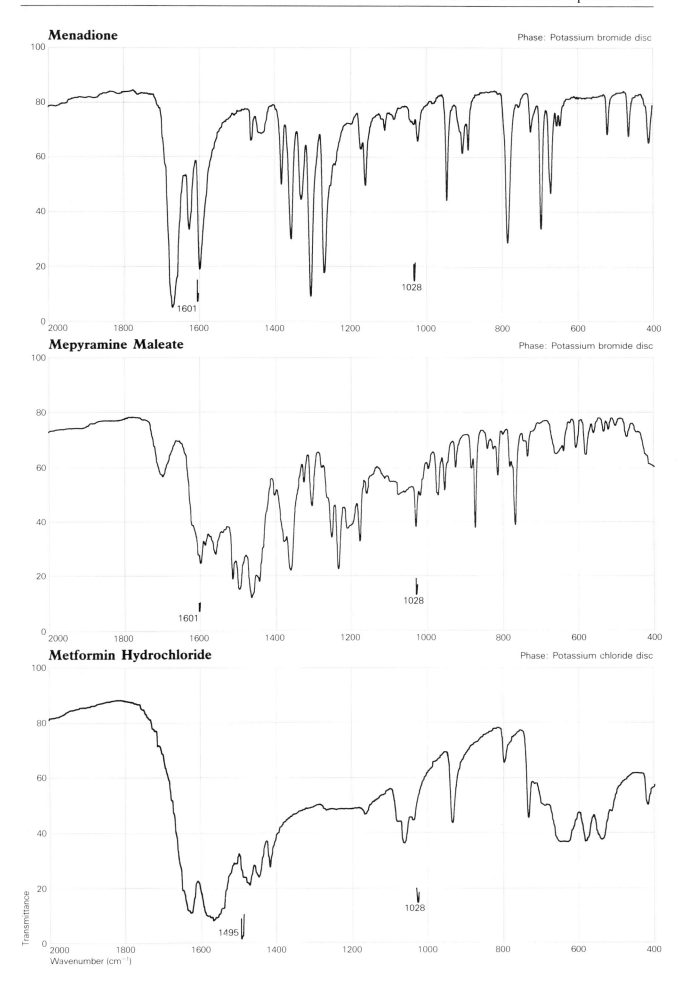

Menadione

Phase: Potassium bromide disc

1601
1028

Mepyramine Maleate

Phase: Potassium bromide disc

1601
1028

Metformin Hydrochloride

Phase: Potassium chloride disc

1495
1028

Transmittance

Wavenumber (cm⁻¹)

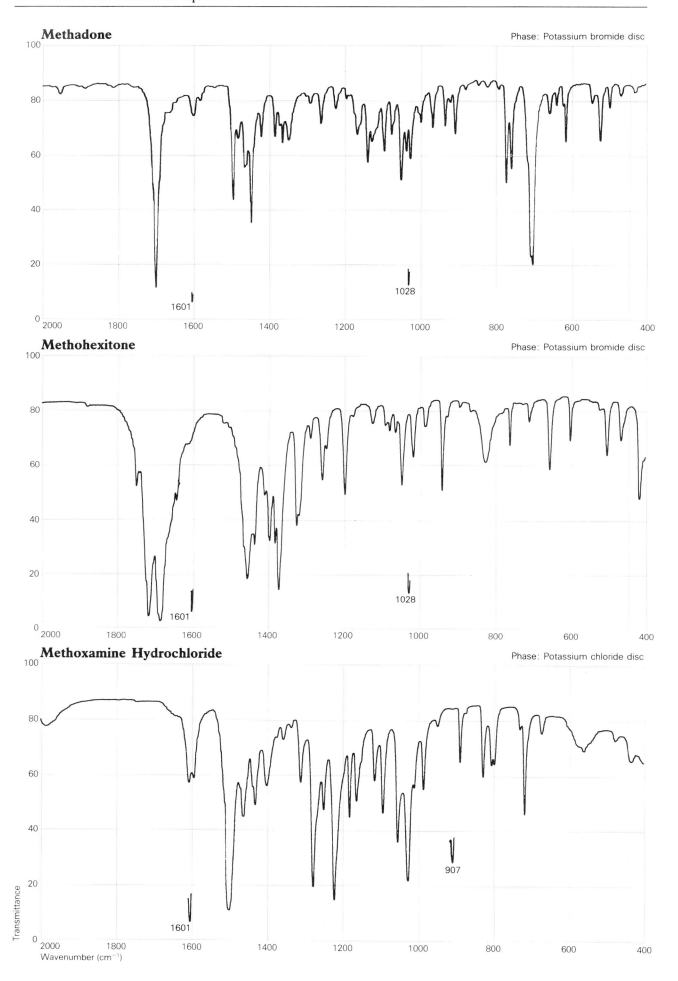

Methadone

Phase: Potassium bromide disc

Methohexitone

Phase: Potassium bromide disc

Methoxamine Hydrochloride

Phase: Potassium chloride disc

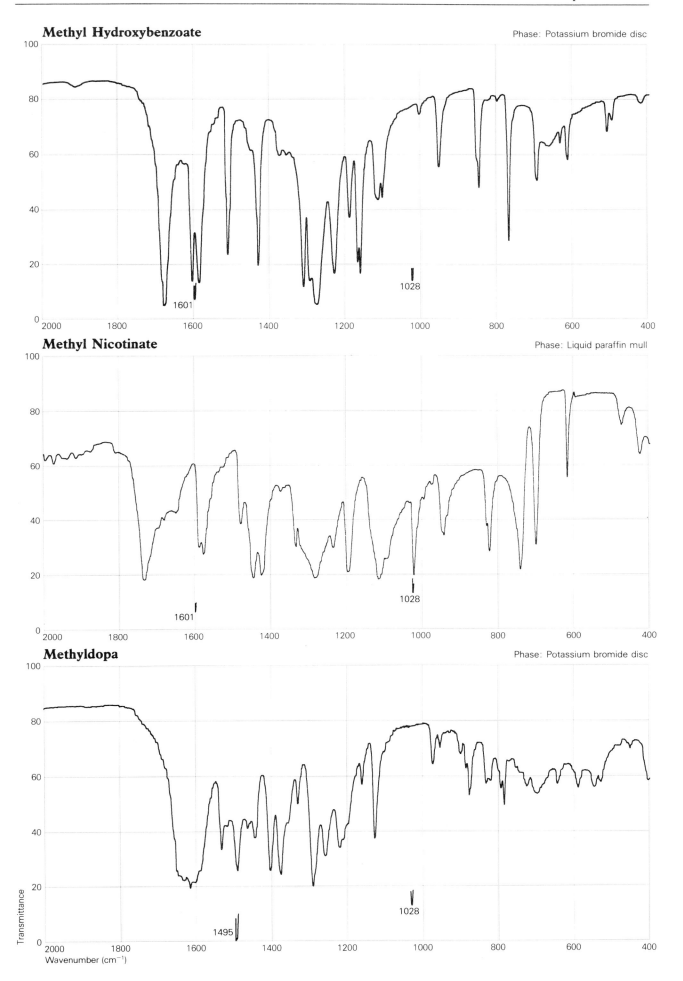

Methyl Hydroxybenzoate

Phase: Potassium bromide disc

1601
1028

Methyl Nicotinate

Phase: Liquid paraffin mull

1601
1028

Methyldopa

Phase: Potassium bromide disc

1495
1028

Transmittance

Wavenumber (cm⁻¹)

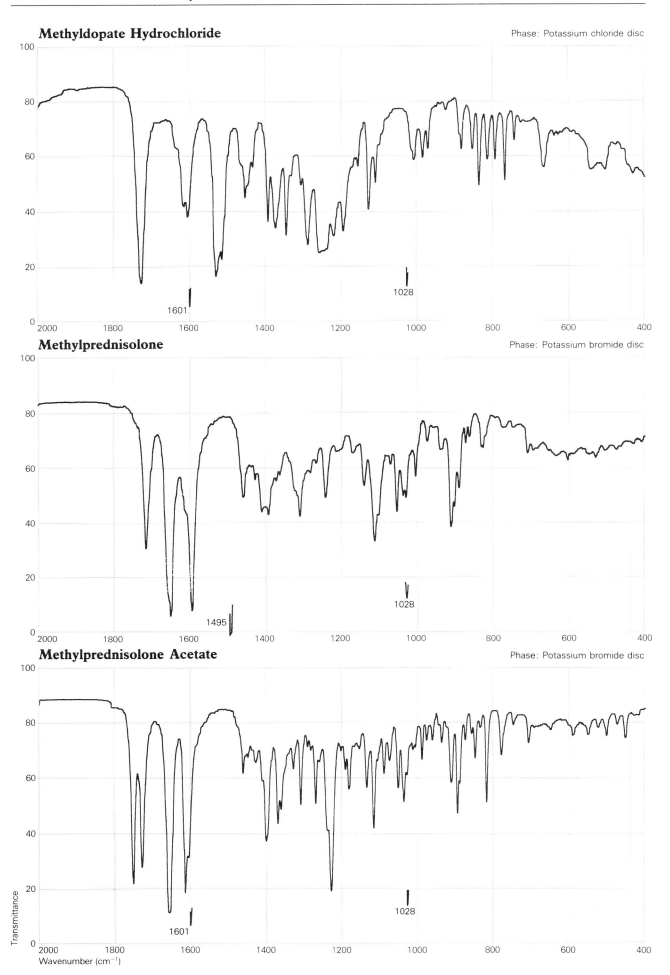

Methyldopate Hydrochloride Phase: Potassium chloride disc

1601

1028

Methylprednisolone Phase: Potassium bromide disc

1495

1028

Methylprednisolone Acetate Phase: Potassium bromide disc

1601

1028

Transmittance

Wavenumber (cm⁻¹)

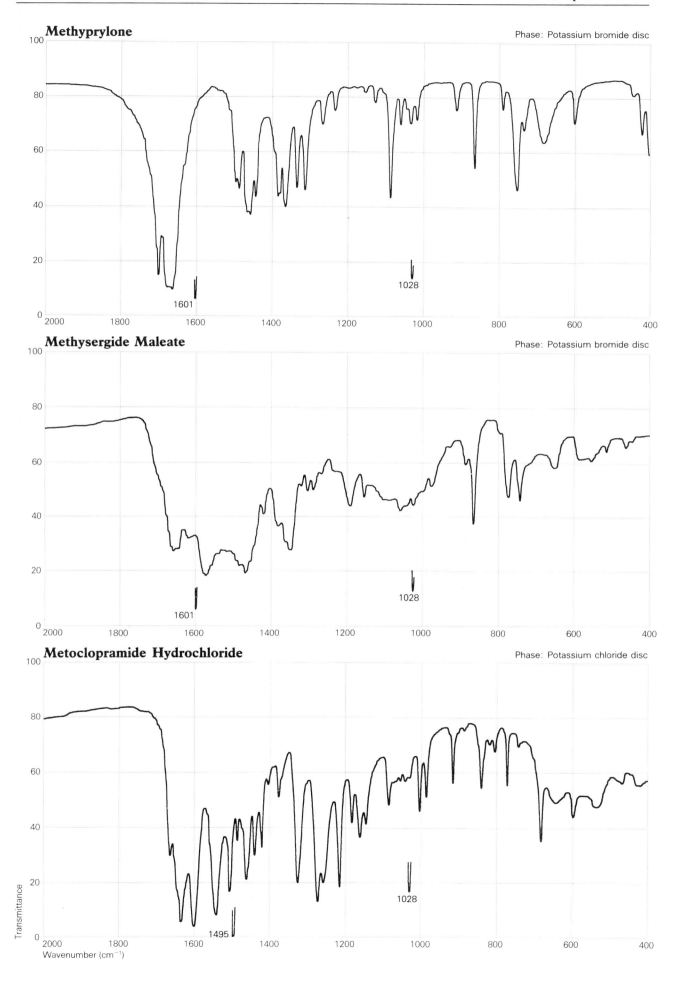

Methyprylone   Phase: Potassium bromide disc

1601

1028

Methysergide Maleate   Phase: Potassium bromide disc

1601

1028

Metoclopramide Hydrochloride   Phase: Potassium chloride disc

1495

1028

Transmittance

Wavenumber (cm⁻¹)

Metronidazole   Phase: Potassium bromide disc

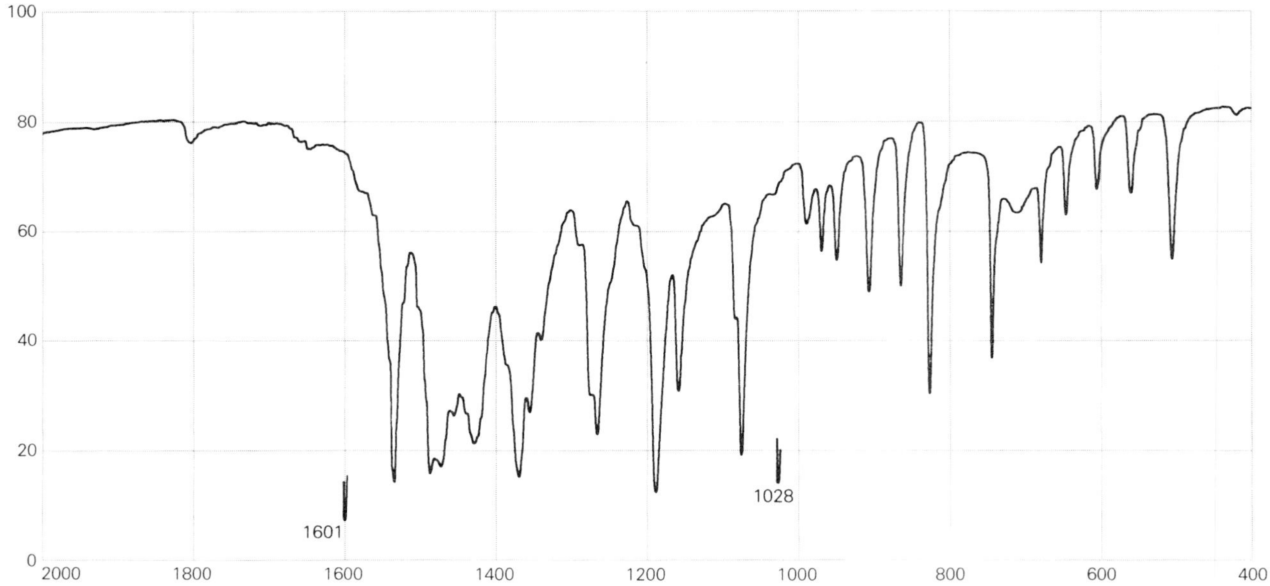

1601

1028

Metyrapone (1)   Phase: Liquid paraffin mull

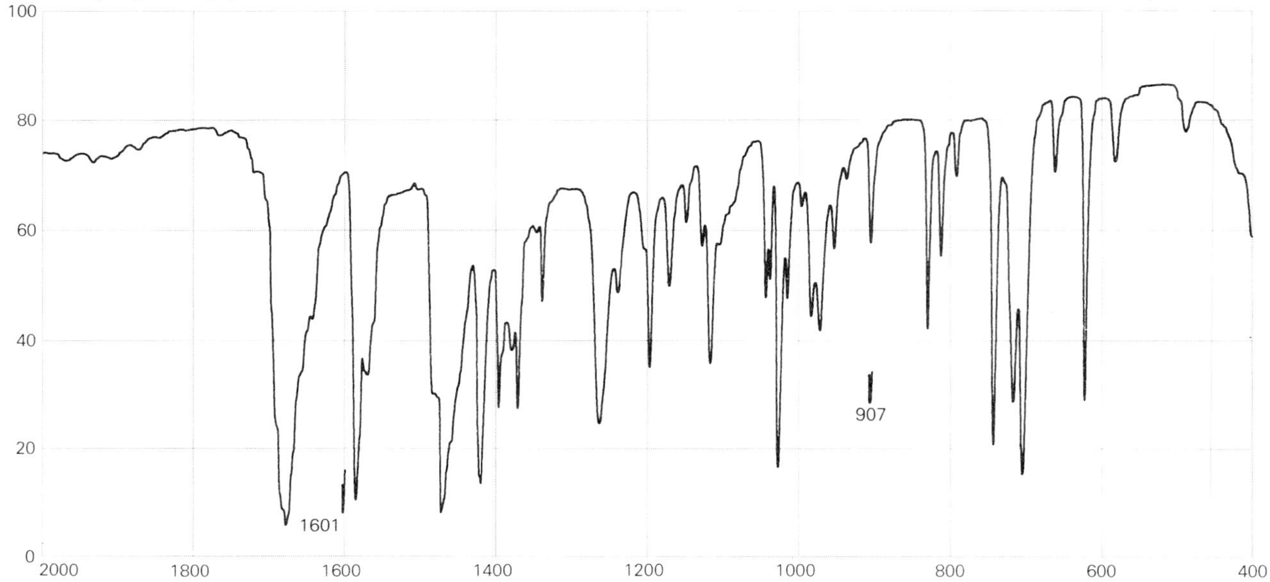

1601

907

Metyrapone (2)   Phase: 50% w/v solution in macrogol 400   Thickness: Thin film

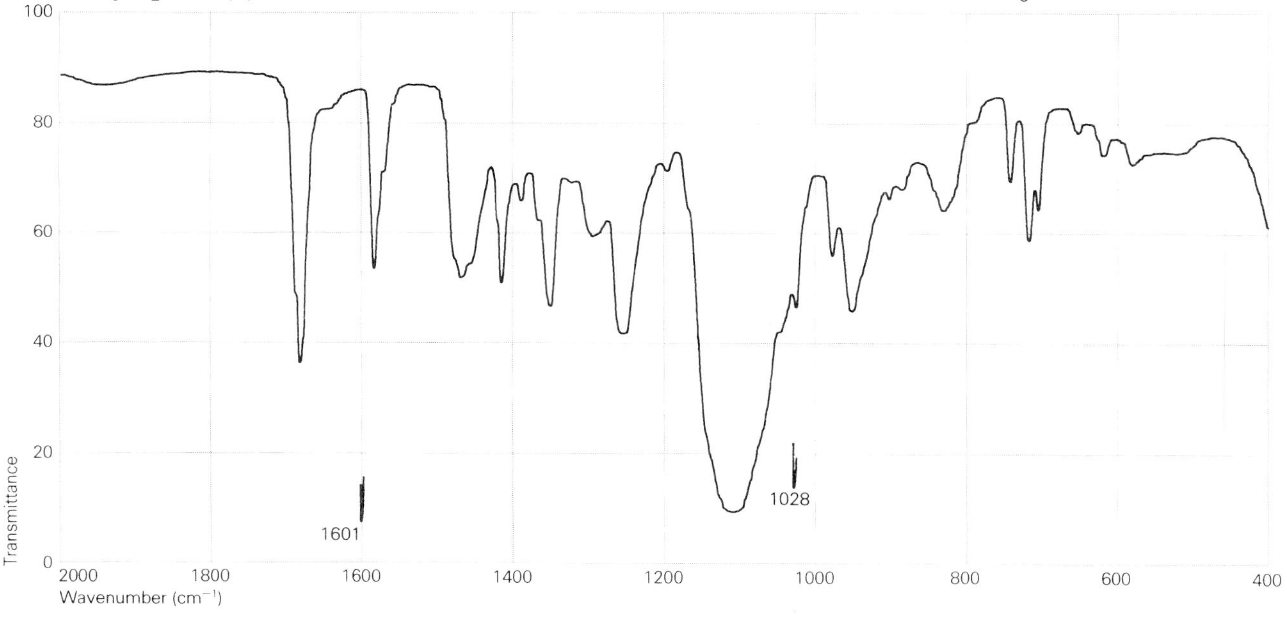

1601

1028

Transmittance

Wavenumber (cm⁻¹)

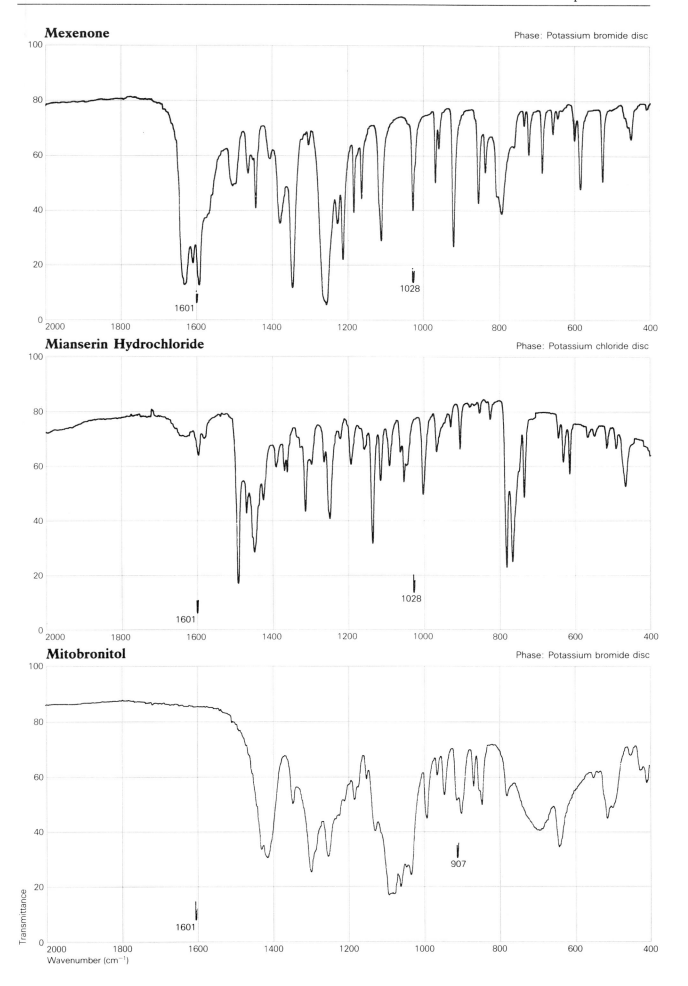

Mexenone   Phase: Potassium bromide disc

1601

1028

Mianserin Hydrochloride   Phase: Potassium chloride disc

1601

1028

Mitobronitol   Phase: Potassium bromide disc

907

1601

Transmittance

Wavenumber (cm⁻¹)

Nalidixic Acid

Phase: Potassium bromide disc

Nandrolone Decanoate

Phase: 10% w/v solution in chloroform   Thickness: 0.1mm

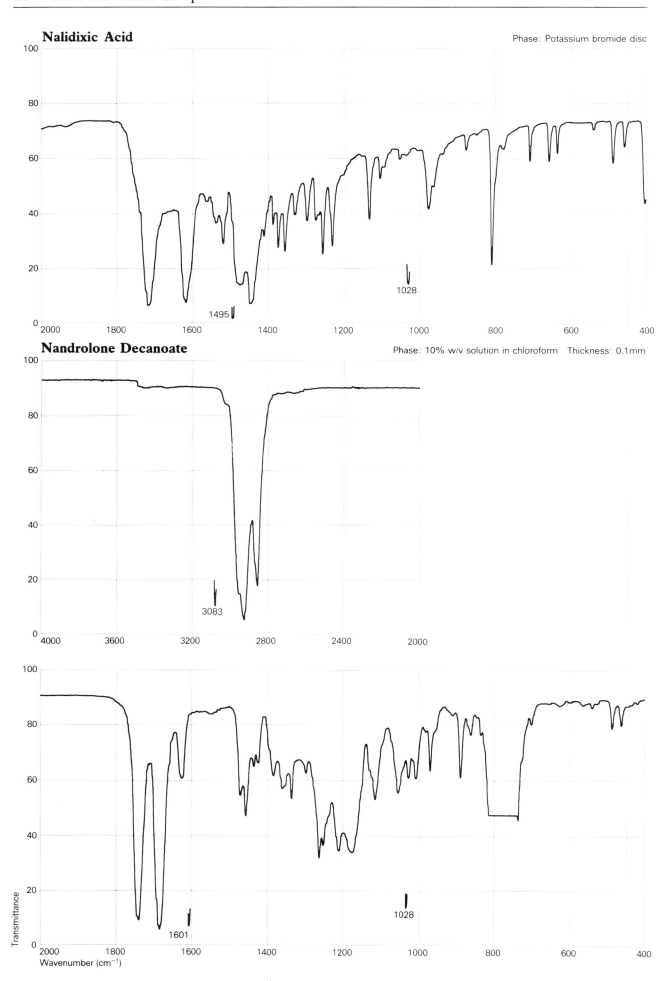

Nandrolone Phenylpropionate

Phase: 5% w/v solution in chloroform   Thickness: 0.1mm

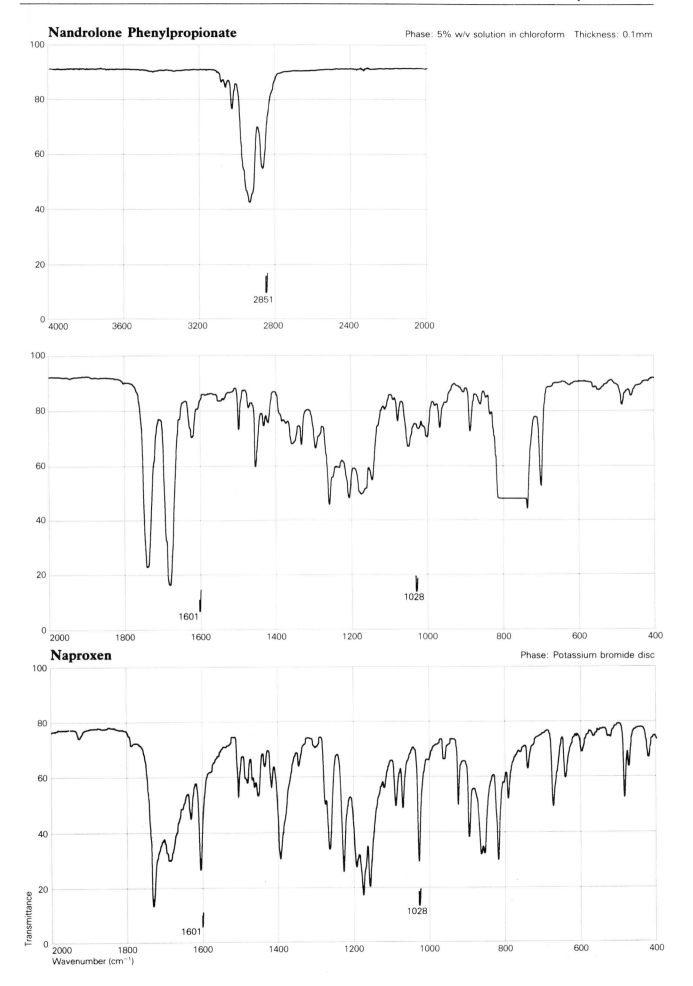

Naproxen

Phase: Potassium bromide disc

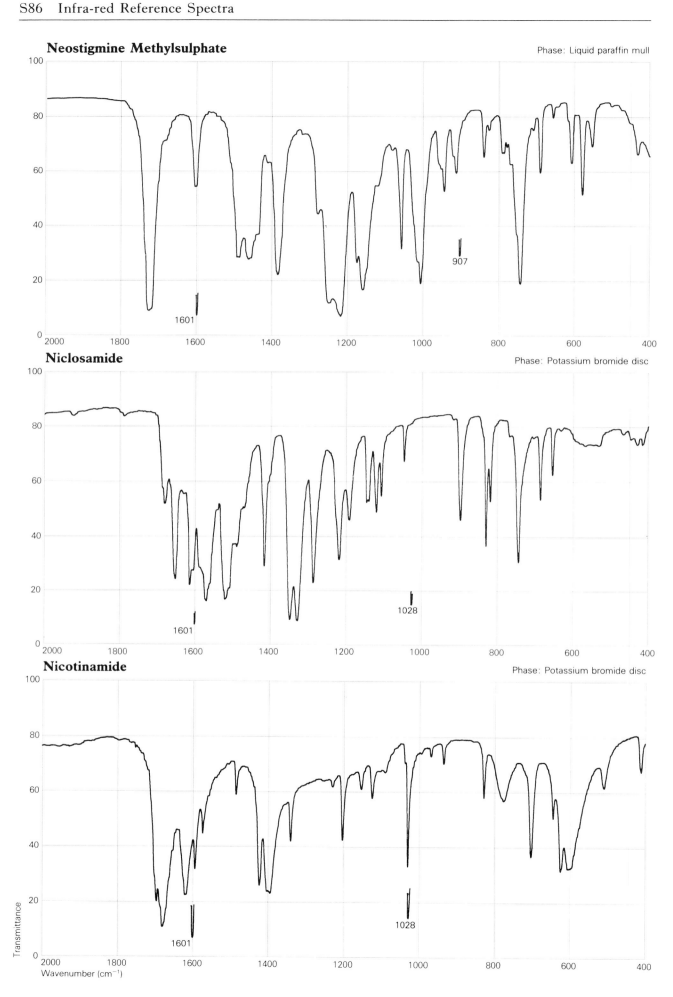

Neostigmine Methylsulphate

Phase: Liquid paraffin mull

1601

907

Niclosamide

Phase: Potassium bromide disc

1601

1028

Nicotinamide

Phase: Potassium bromide disc

1601

1028

Transmittance

Wavenumber (cm⁻¹)

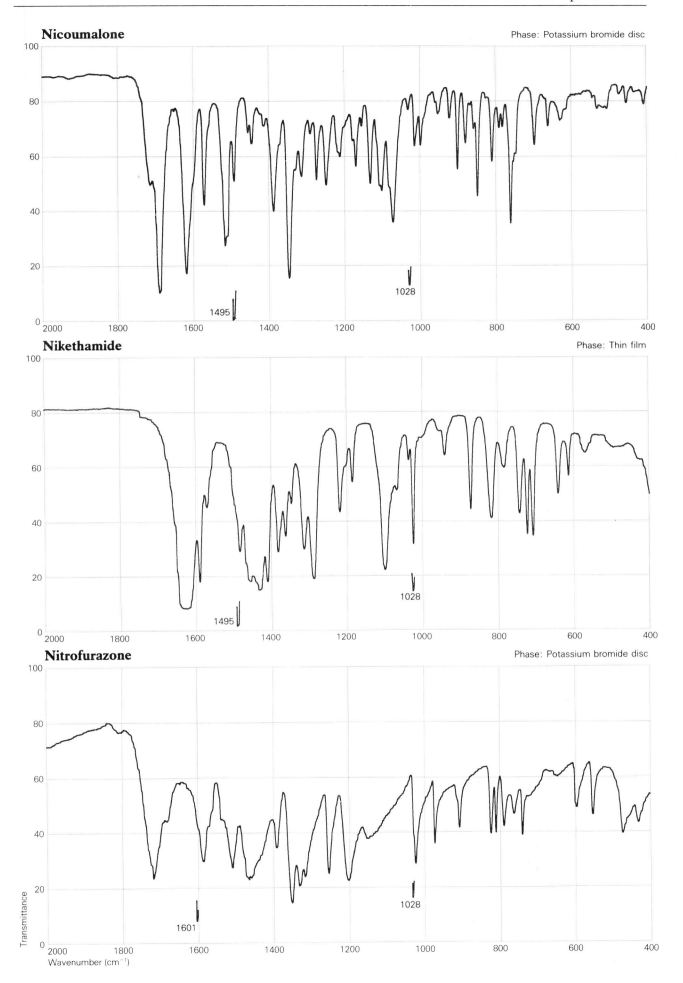

Nicoumalone   Phase: Potassium bromide disc

1495

1028

Nikethamide   Phase: Thin film

1495

1028

Nitrofurazone   Phase: Potassium bromide disc

1601

1028

Transmittance

Wavenumber (cm⁻¹)

Norethisterone Acetate

Phase: 5% w/v solution in chloroform   Thickness: 0.1mm

Nortriptyline

Phase: Thin film

Noscapine

Phase: Potassium bromide disc

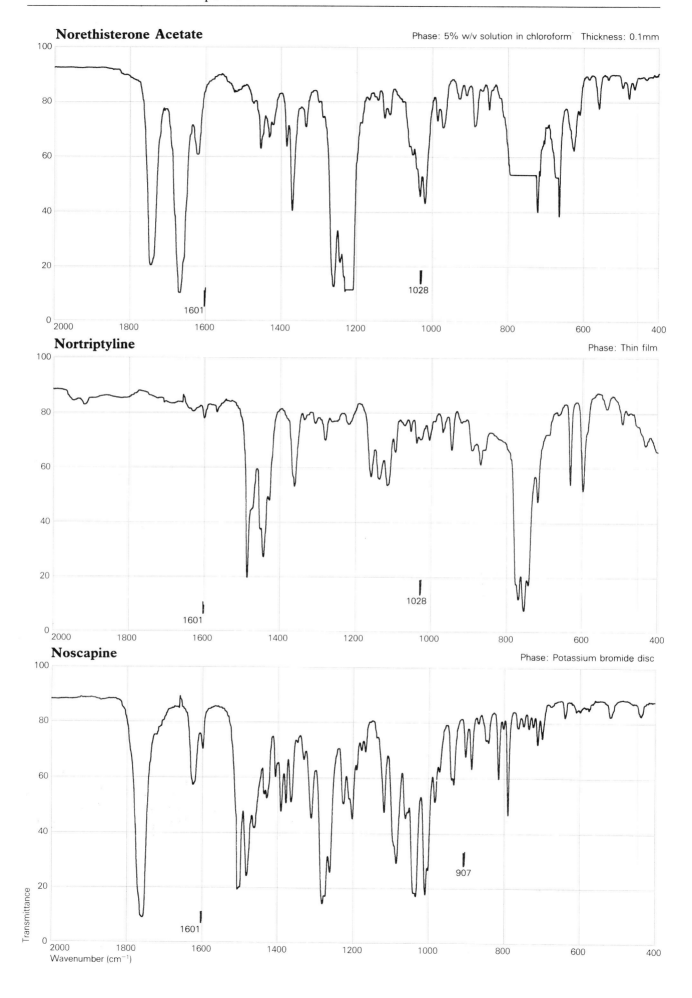

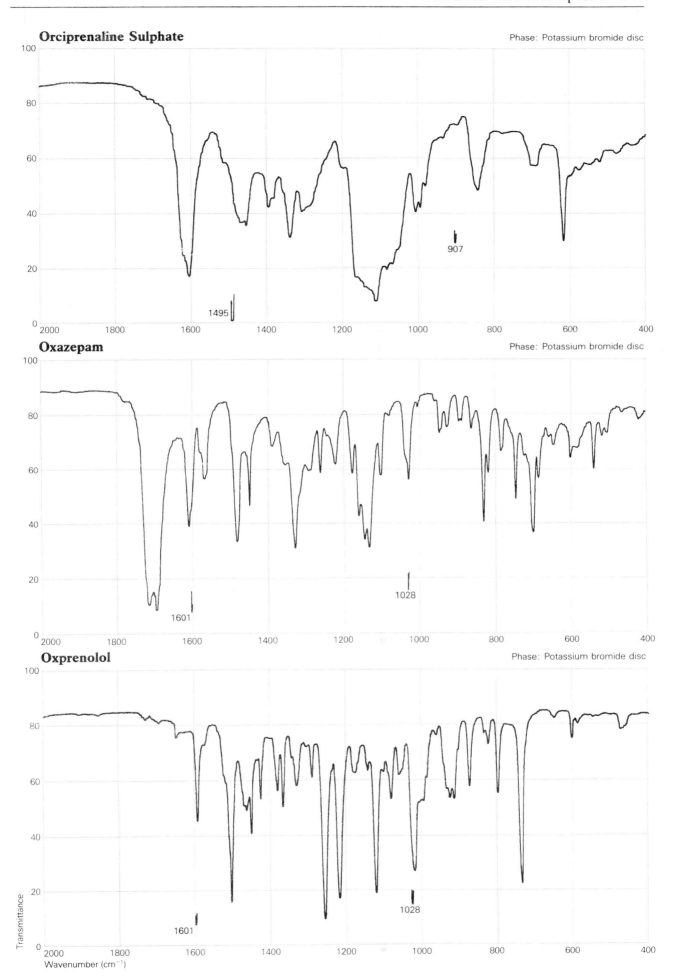

Orciprenaline Sulphate   Phase: Potassium bromide disc

1495

907

Oxazepam   Phase: Potassium bromide disc

1601

1028

Oxprenolol   Phase: Potassium bromide disc

1601

1028

Transmittance

Wavenumber (cm⁻¹)

Oxprenolol Hydrochloride

Phase: Potassium chloride disc

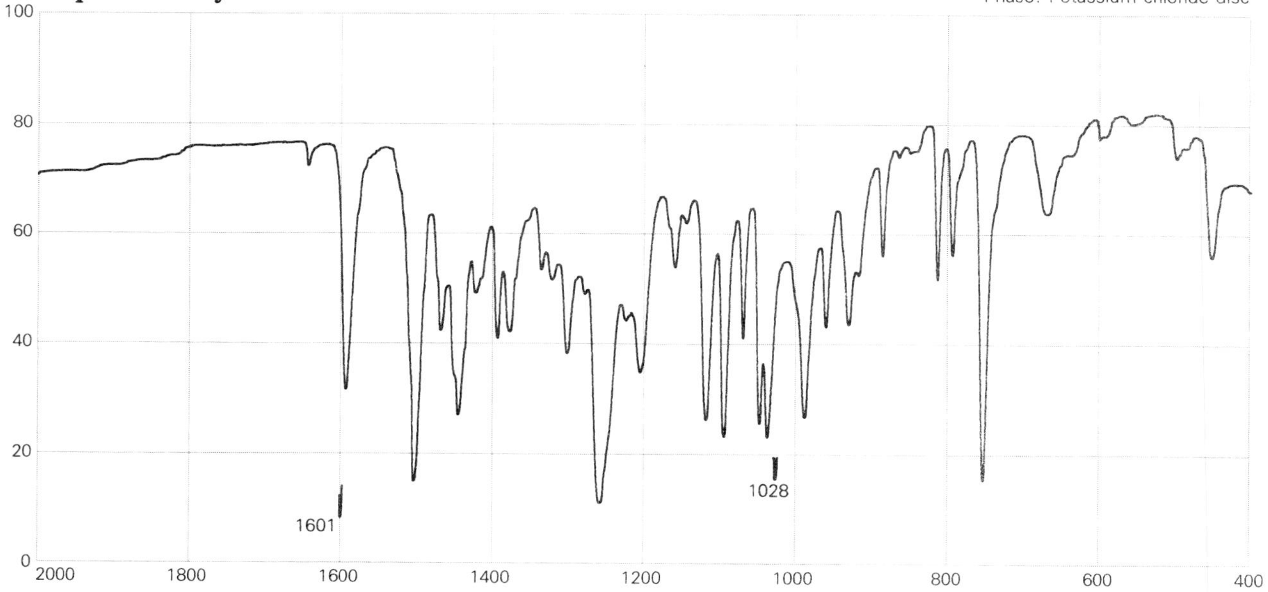

1601
1028

Oxymethalone

Phase: Potassium bromide disc

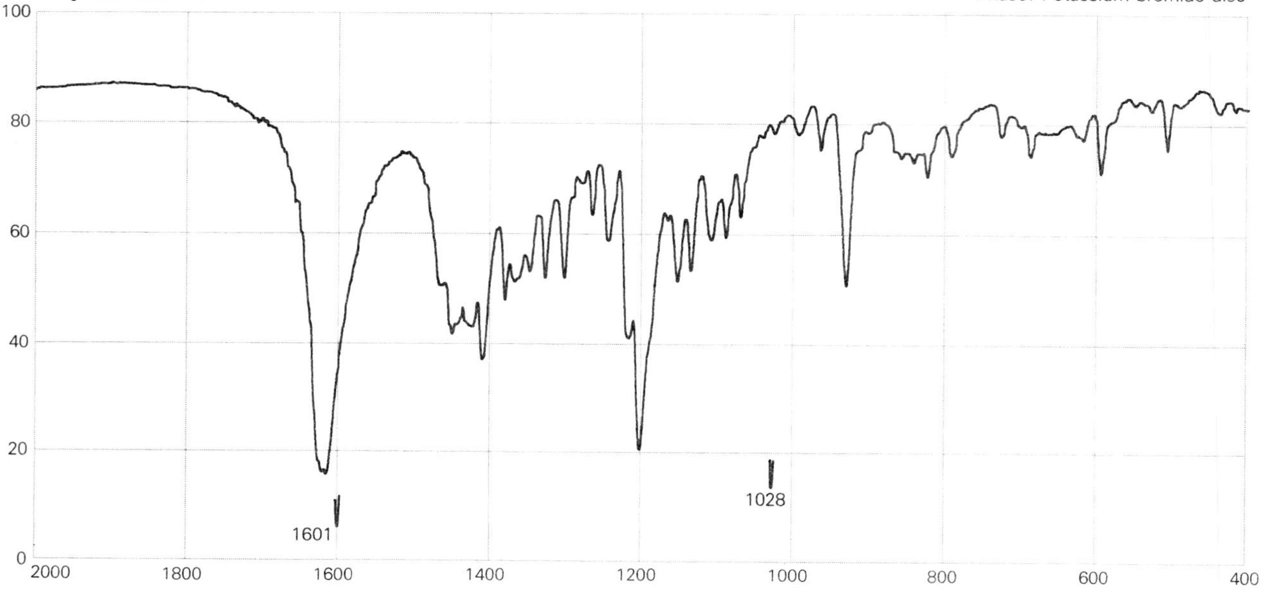

1601
1028

Oxyphenbutazone

Phase: 5% w/v solution in dichloromethane   Thickness: 0.1mm

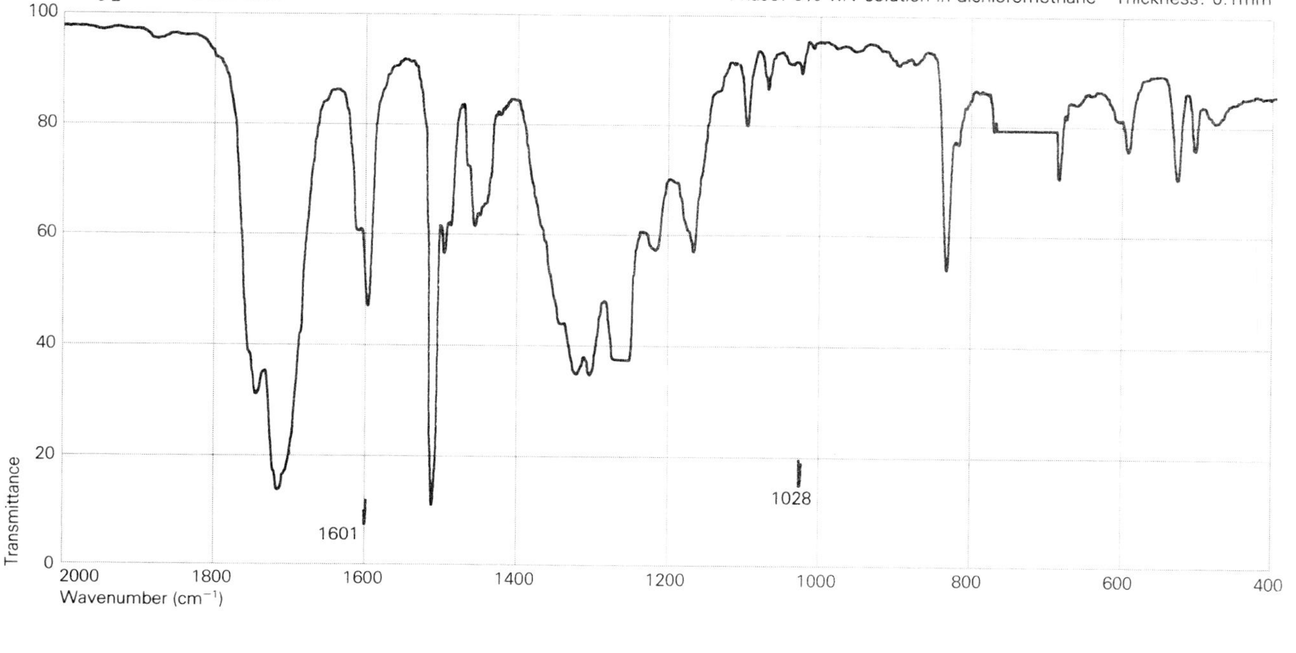

1601
1028

Transmittance

Wavenumber (cm⁻¹)

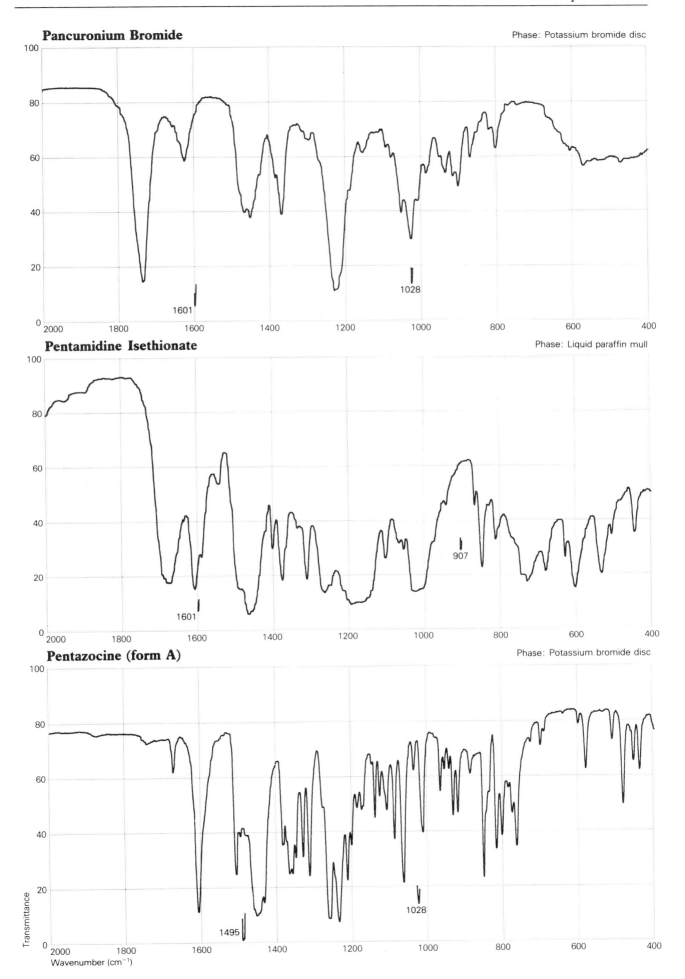

Pancuronium Bromide

Phase: Potassium bromide disc

1601
1028

Pentamidine Isethionate

Phase: Liquid paraffin mull

1601
907

Pentazocine (form A)

Phase: Potassium bromide disc

1495
1028

Transmittance

Wavenumber (cm⁻¹)

Pentazocine (form B)

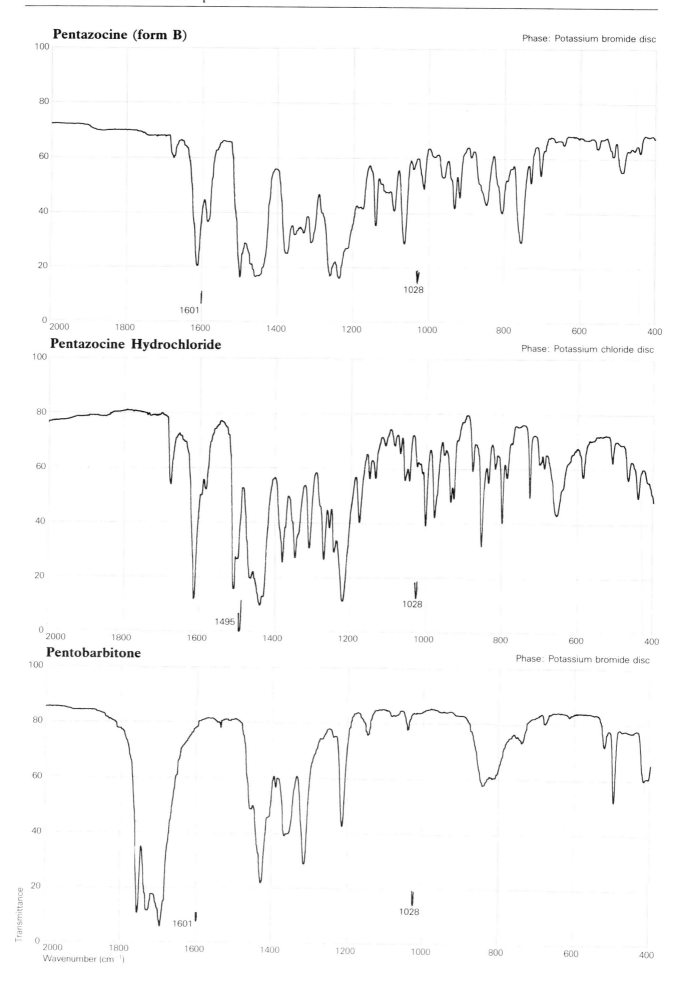

Phase: Potassium bromide disc

Pentazocine Hydrochloride

Phase: Potassium chloride disc

Pentobarbitone

Phase: Potassium bromide disc

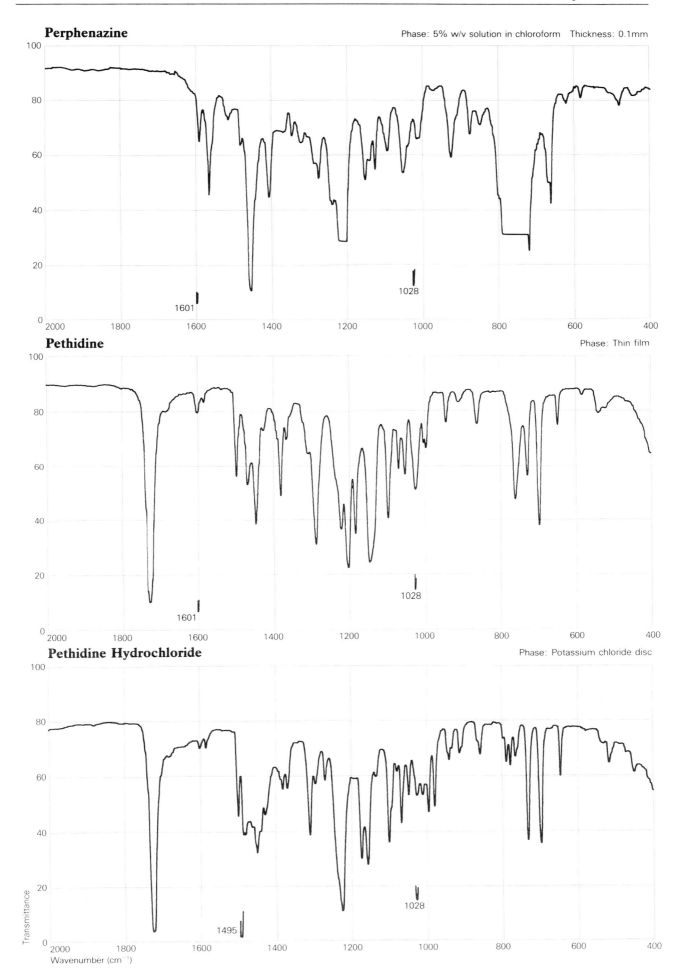

Perphenazine

Phase: 5% w/v solution in chloroform   Thickness: 0.1mm

1601
1028

Pethidine

Phase: Thin film

1601
1028

Pethidine Hydrochloride

Phase: Potassium chloride disc

1495
1028

Transmittance

Wavenumber (cm⁻¹)

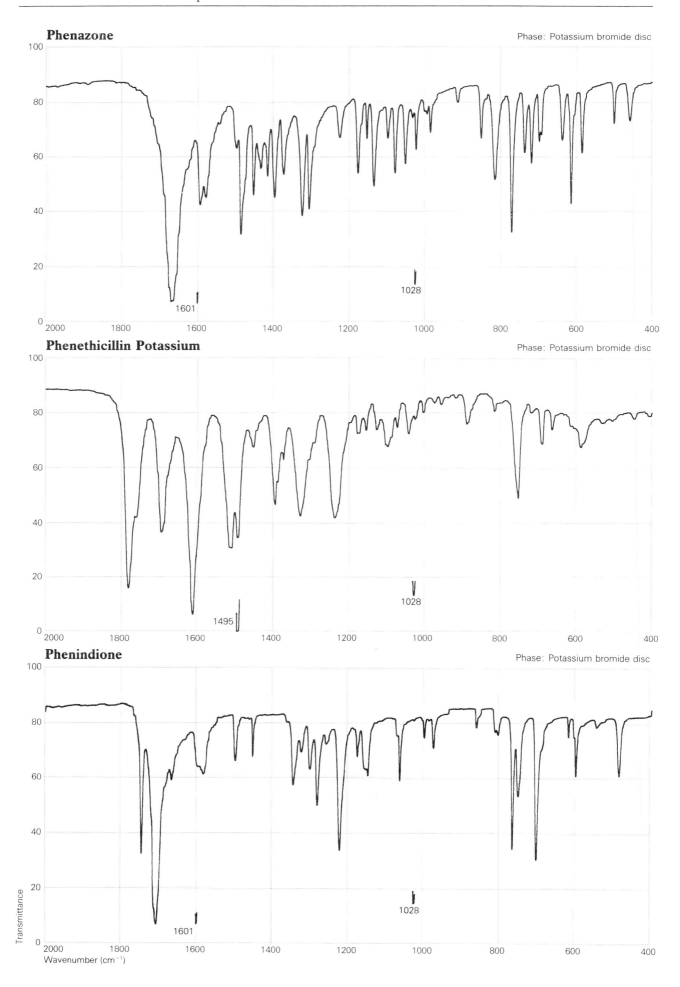

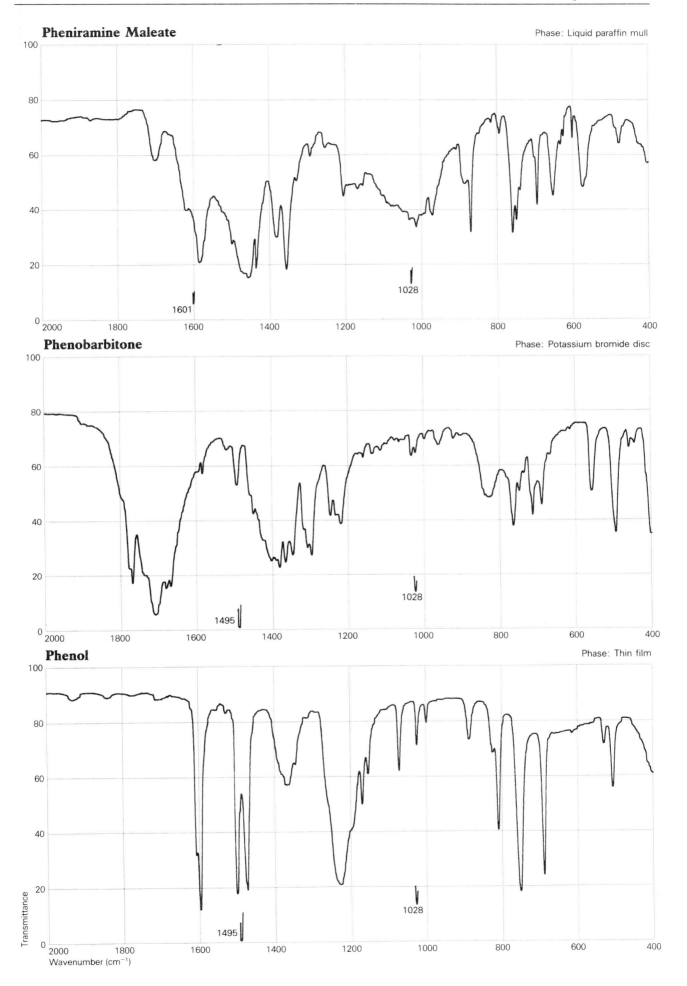

Pheniramine Maleate

Phase: Liquid paraffin mull

1601

1028

Phenobarbitone

Phase: Potassium bromide disc

1495

1028

Phenol

Phase: Thin film

1495

1028

Transmittance

Wavenumber (cm⁻¹)

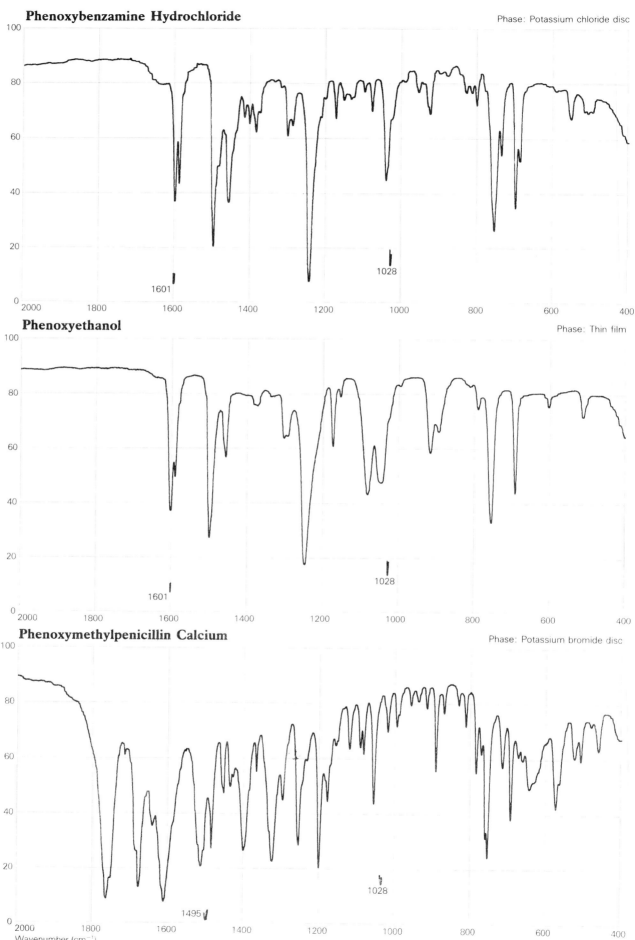

Phenoxybenzamine Hydrochloride   Phase: Potassium chloride disc

1601
1028

Phenoxyethanol   Phase: Thin film

1601
1028

Phenoxymethylpenicillin Calcium   Phase: Potassium bromide disc

1028
1495

Transmittance

Wavenumber (cm⁻¹)

Phentolamine Mesylate

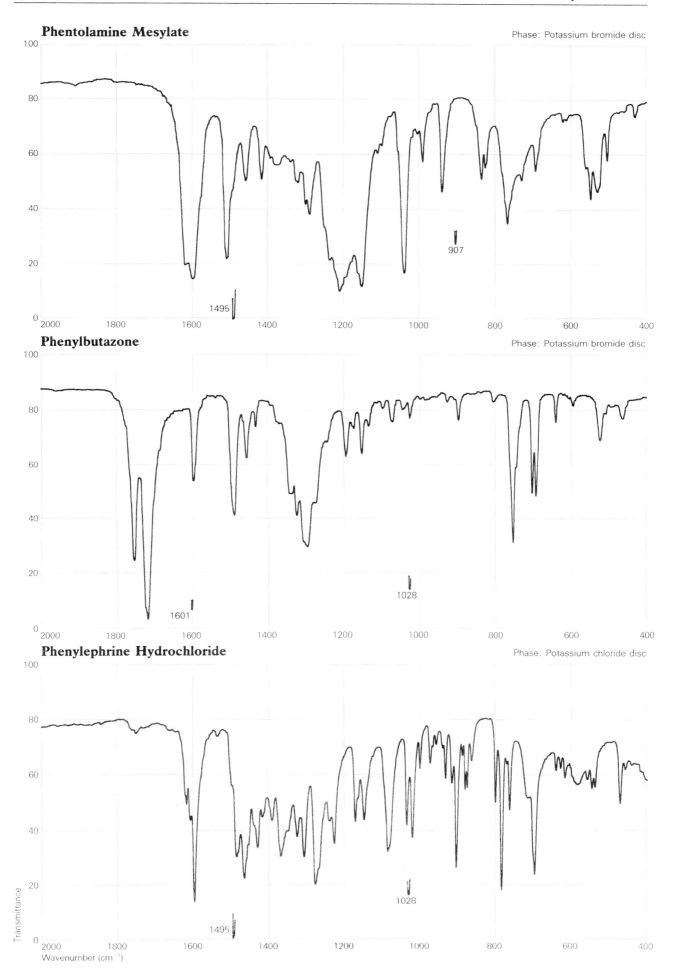

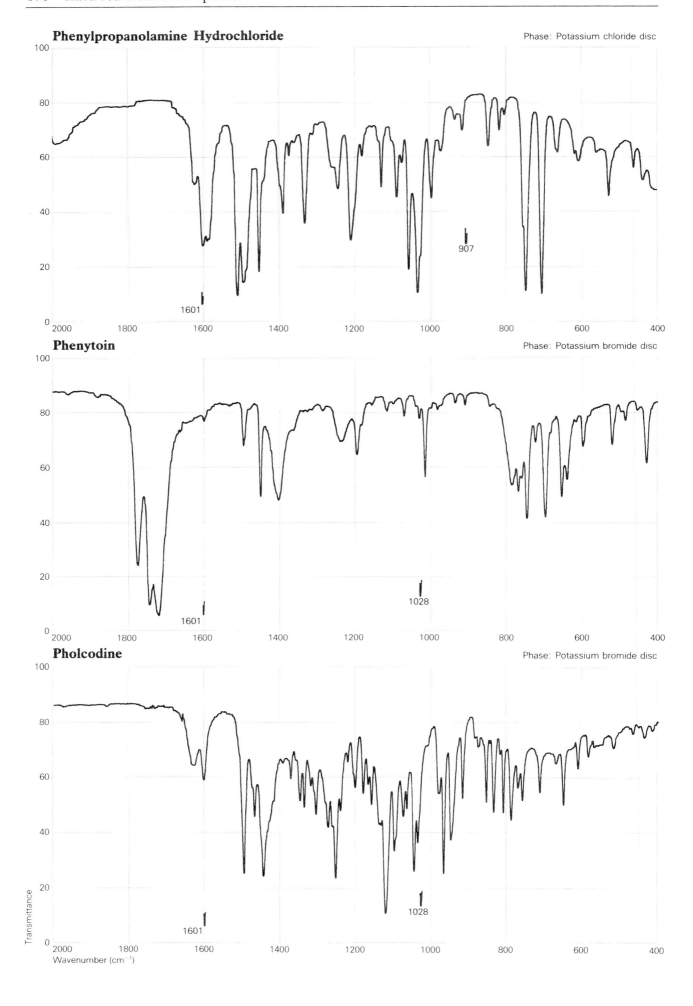

Phenylpropanolamine Hydrochloride   Phase: Potassium chloride disc

Phenytoin   Phase: Potassium bromide disc

Pholcodine   Phase: Potassium bromide disc

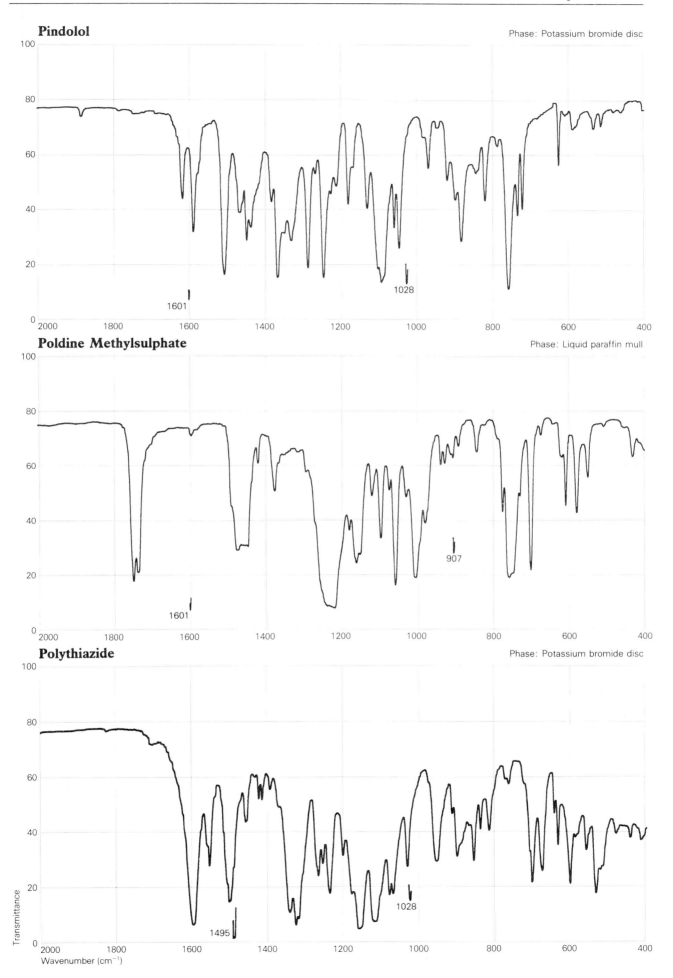

Pindolol   Phase: Potassium bromide disc

1601

1028

Poldine Methylsulphate   Phase: Liquid paraffin mull

1601

907

Polythiazide   Phase: Potassium bromide disc

Transmittance

Wavenumber (cm⁻¹)

1495

1028

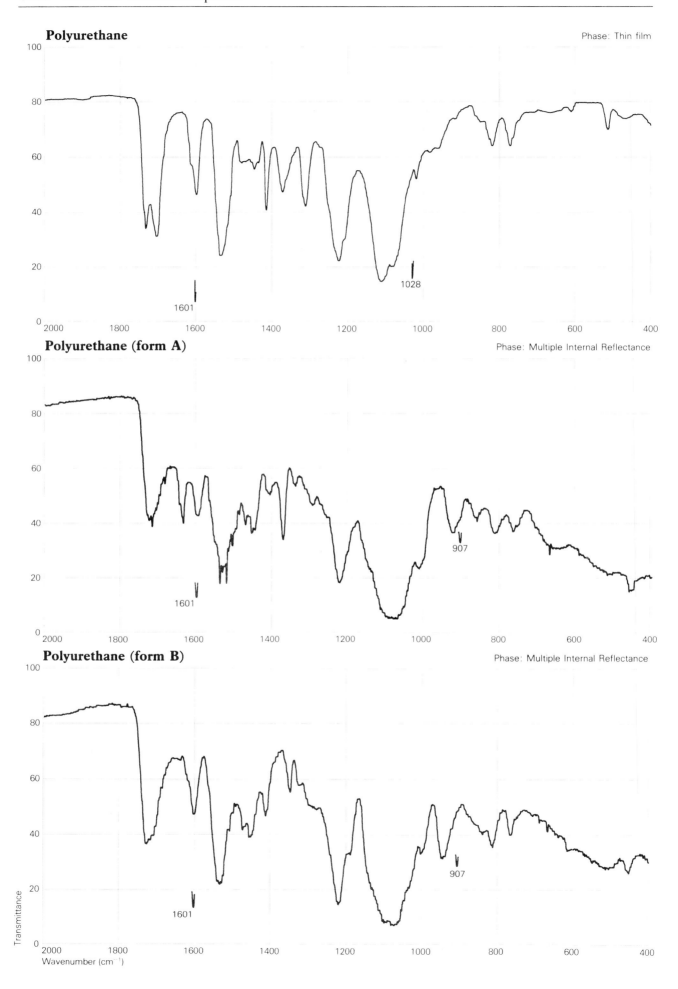

Polyurethane   Phase: Thin film

1601

1028

Polyurethane (form A)   Phase: Multiple Internal Reflectance

1601

907

Polyurethane (form B)   Phase: Multiple Internal Reflectance

1601

907

Transmittance

Wavenumber (cm⁻¹)

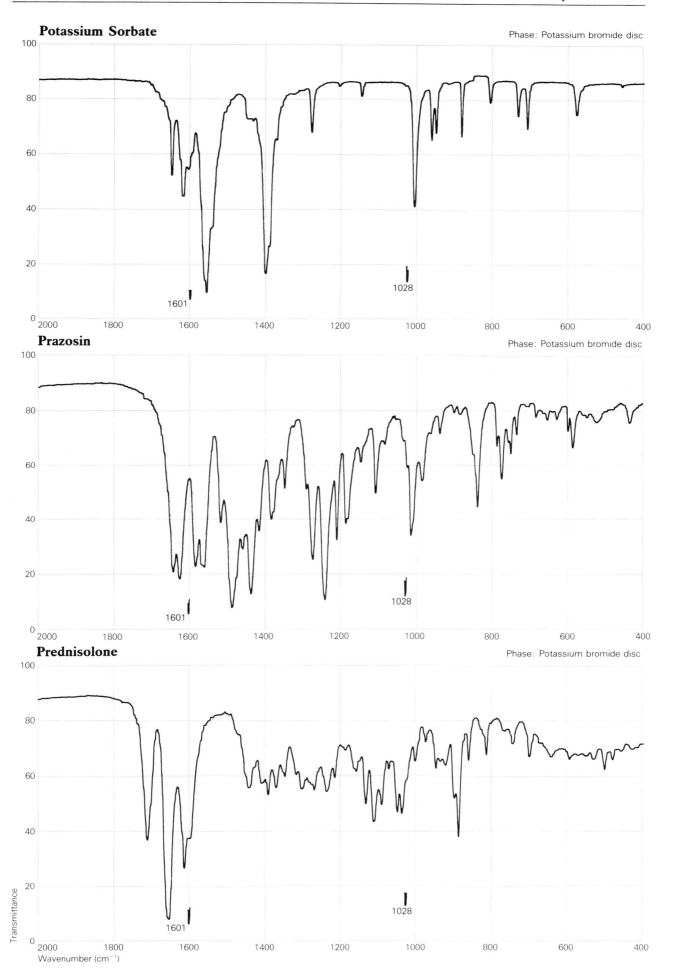

Potassium Sorbate   Phase: Potassium bromide disc

1601
1028

Prazosin   Phase: Potassium bromide disc

1601
1028

Prednisolone   Phase: Potassium bromide disc

1601
1028

Transmittance

Wavenumber (cm⁻¹)

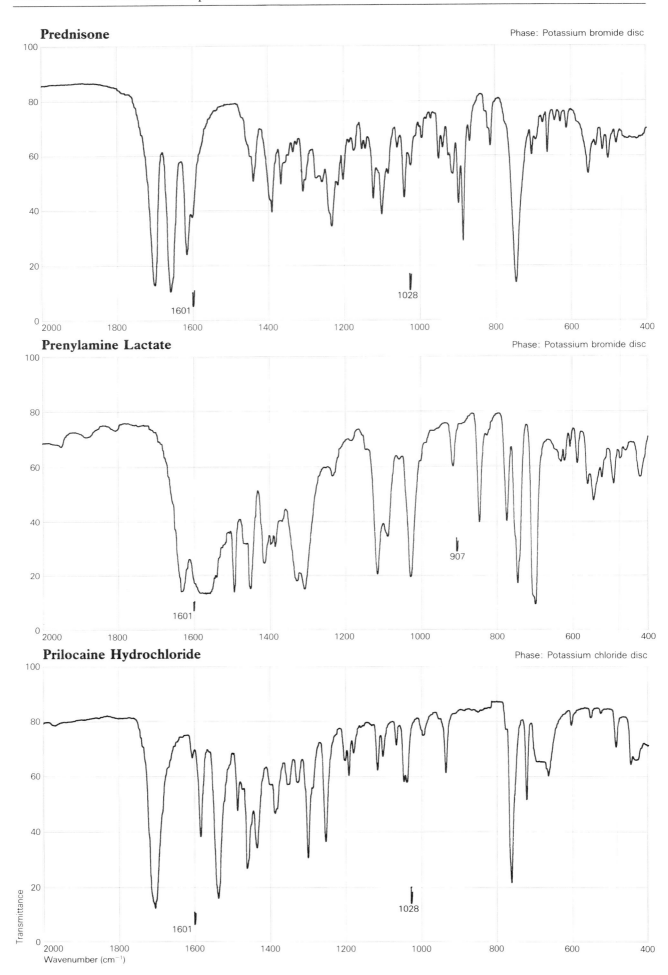

Prednisone   Phase: Potassium bromide disc

1601

1028

Prenylamine Lactate   Phase: Potassium bromide disc

1601

907

Prilocaine Hydrochloride   Phase: Potassium chloride disc

1601

1028

Transmittance

Wavenumber (cm⁻¹)

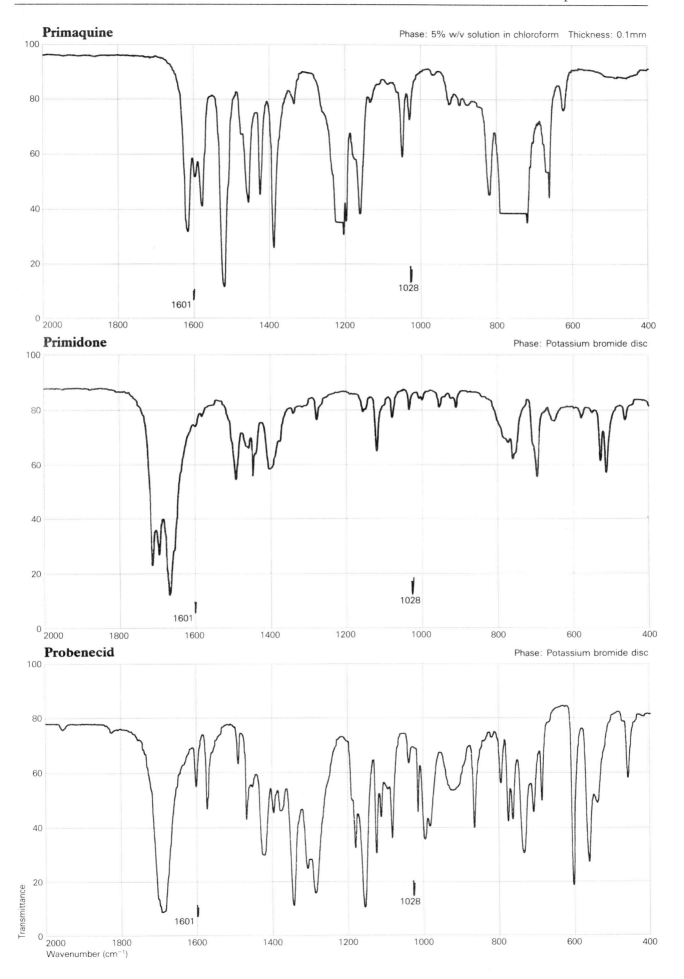

Primaquine

Phase: 5% w/v solution in chloroform   Thickness: 0.1mm

1601

1028

Primidone

Phase: Potassium bromide disc

1601

1028

Probenecid

Phase: Potassium bromide disc

1601

1028

Transmittance

Wavenumber (cm⁻¹)

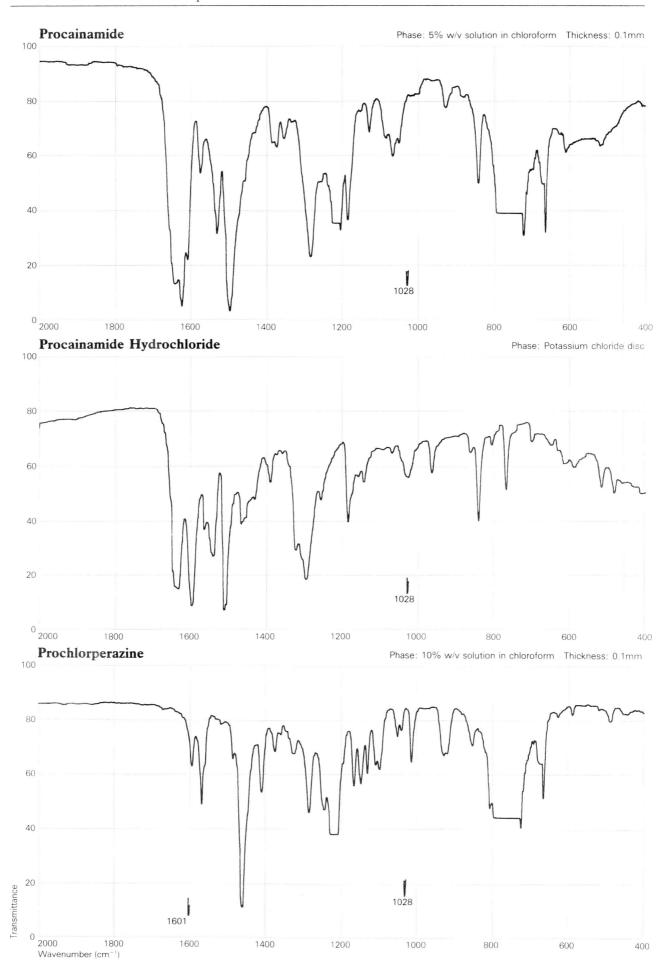

Procainamide

Phase: 5% w/v solution in chloroform   Thickness: 0.1mm

1028

Procainamide Hydrochloride

Phase: Potassium chloride disc

1028

Prochlorperazine

Phase: 10% w/v solution in chloroform   Thickness: 0.1mm

1601

1028

Transmittance

Wavenumber (cm⁻¹)

Prochlorperazine Mesylate

Phase: Liquid paraffin mull

Procyclidine Hydrochloride

Phase: Potassium chloride disc

Progesterone

Phase: Potassium bromide disc

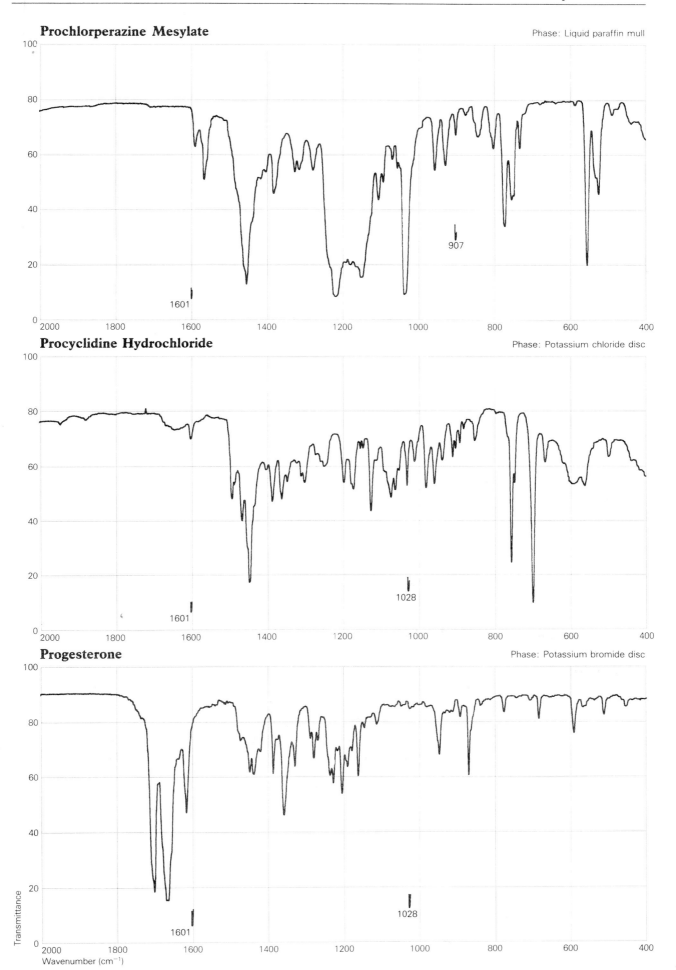

Transmittance

Wavenumber (cm⁻¹)

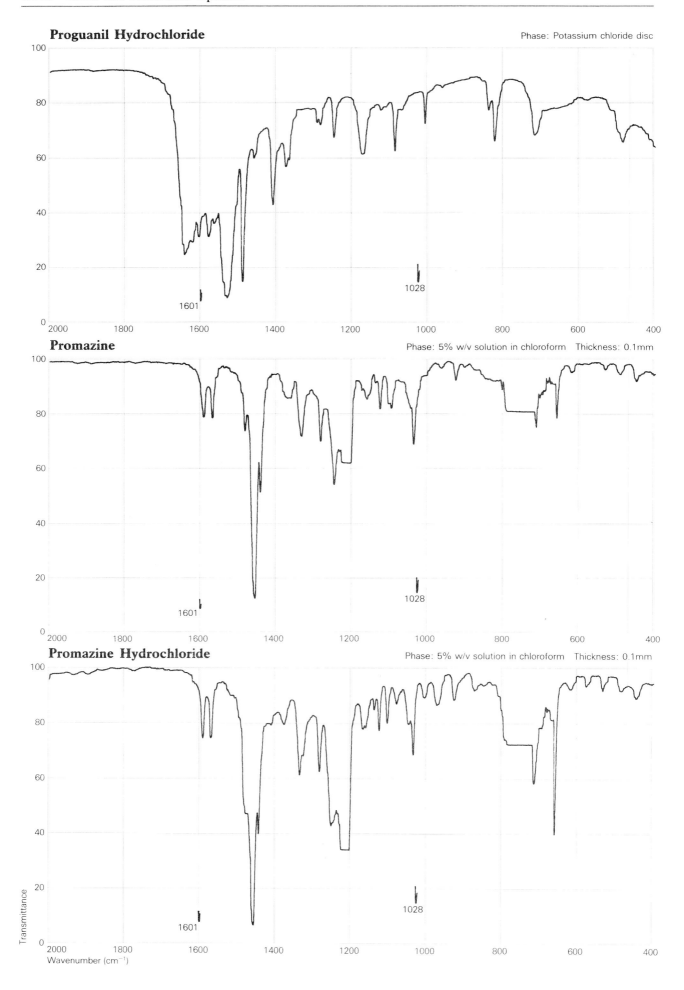

Proguanil Hydrochloride Phase: Potassium chloride disc

Promazine Phase: 5% w/v solution in chloroform   Thickness: 0.1mm

Promazine Hydrochloride Phase: 5% w/v solution in chloroform   Thickness: 0.1mm

Transmittance

Wavenumber (cm⁻¹)

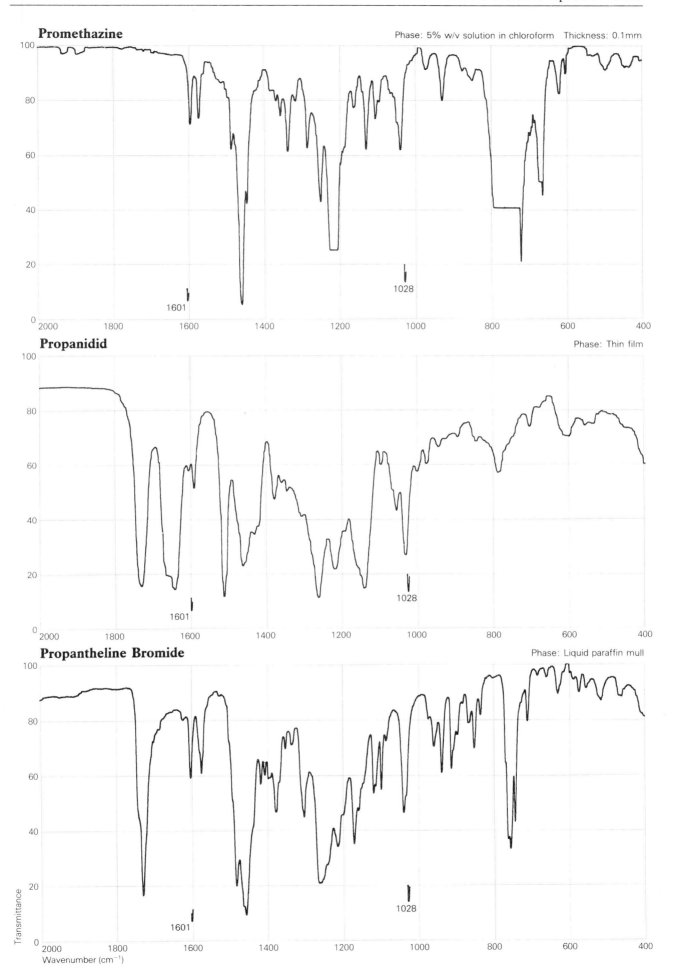

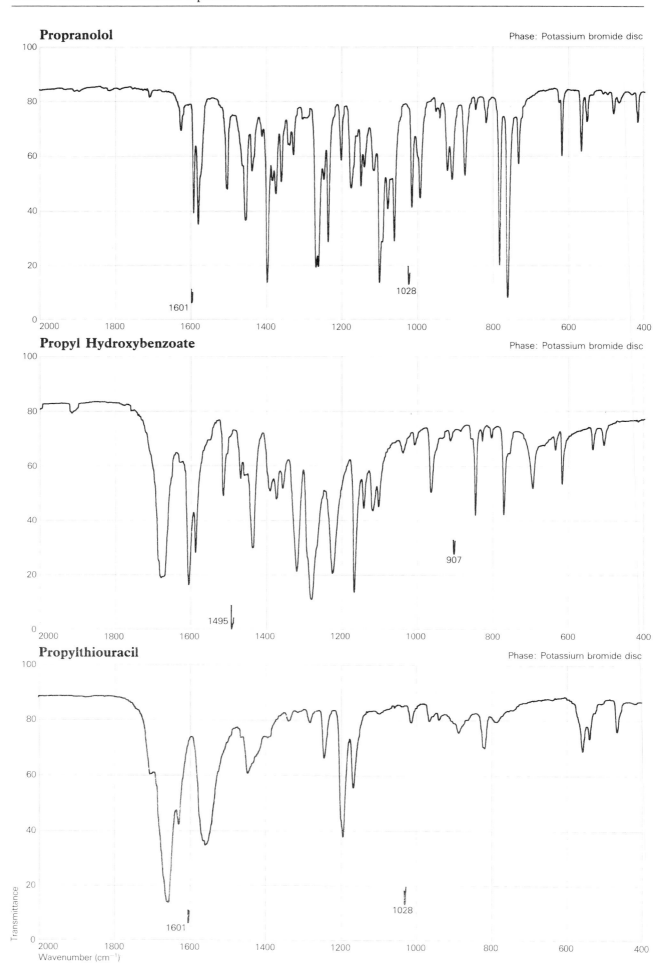

Propranolol

Phase: Potassium bromide disc

1601
1028

Propyl Hydroxybenzoate

Phase: Potassium bromide disc

1495
907

Propylthiouracil

Phase: Potassium bromide disc

1601
1028

Transmittance

Wavenumber (cm⁻¹)

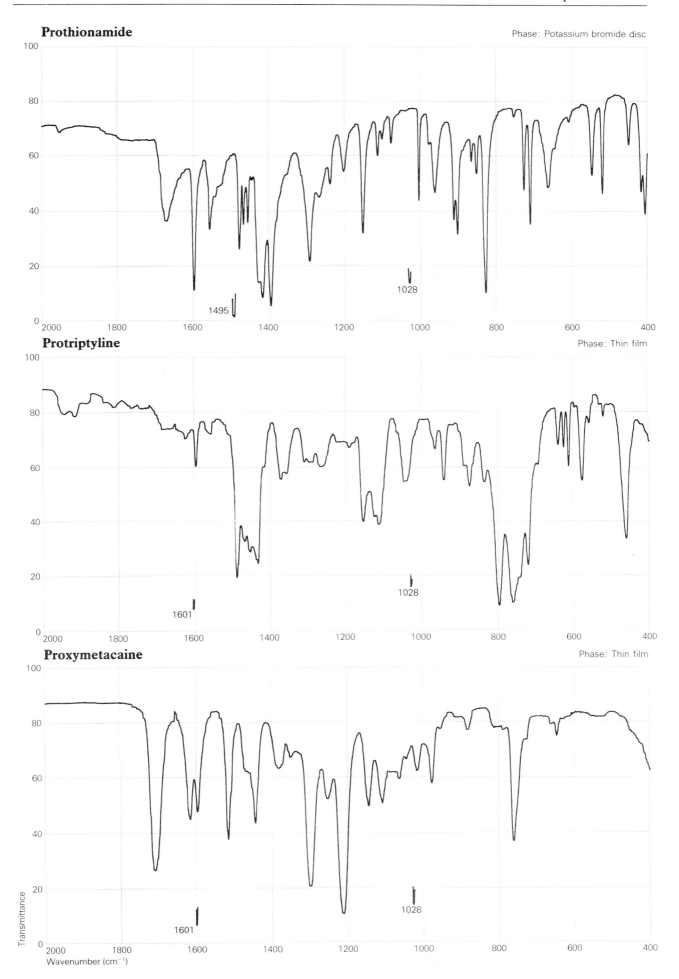

Prothionamide   Phase: Potassium bromide disc

1495

1028

Protriptyline   Phase: Thin film

1601

1028

Proxymetacaine   Phase: Thin film

1601

1028

Transmittance

Wavenumber (cm⁻¹)

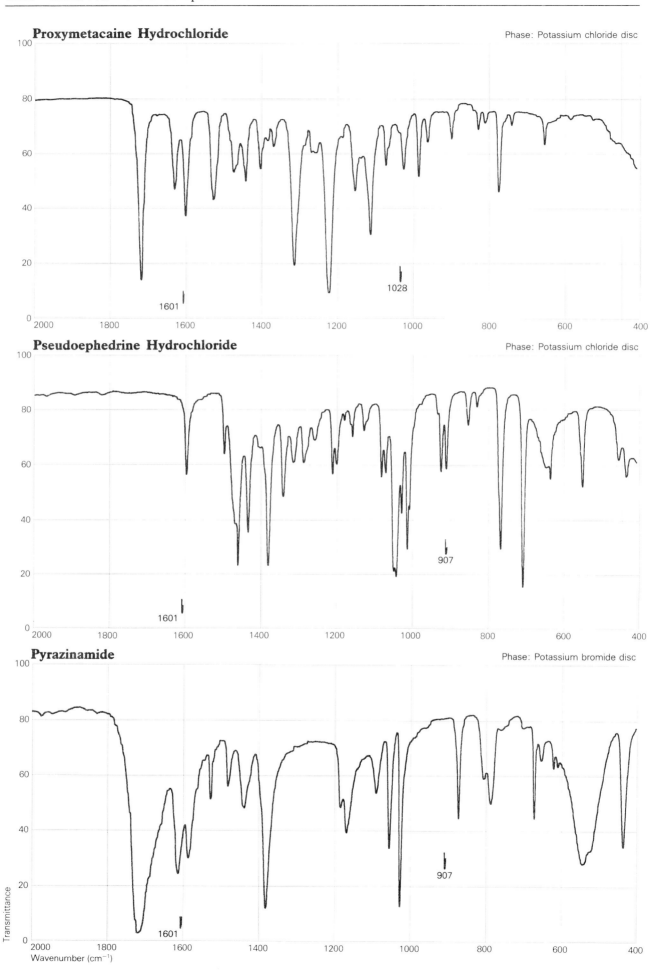

Proxymetacaine Hydrochloride

Phase: Potassium chloride disc

1601

1028

Pseudoephedrine Hydrochloride

Phase: Potassium chloride disc

1601

907

Pyrazinamide

Phase: Potassium bromide disc

1601

907

Transmittance

Wavenumber (cm⁻¹)

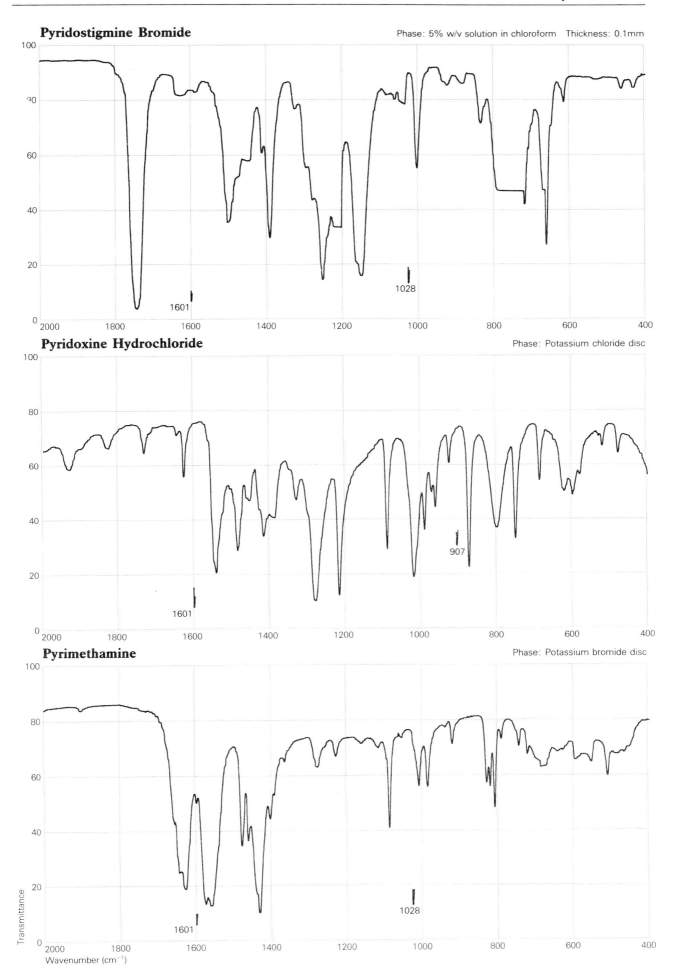

Pyridostigmine Bromide

Phase: 5% w/v solution in chloroform   Thickness: 0.1mm

1601
1028

Pyridoxine Hydrochloride

Phase: Potassium chloride disc

1601
907

Pyrimethamine

Phase: Potassium bromide disc

1601
1028

Transmittance

Wavenumber (cm⁻¹)

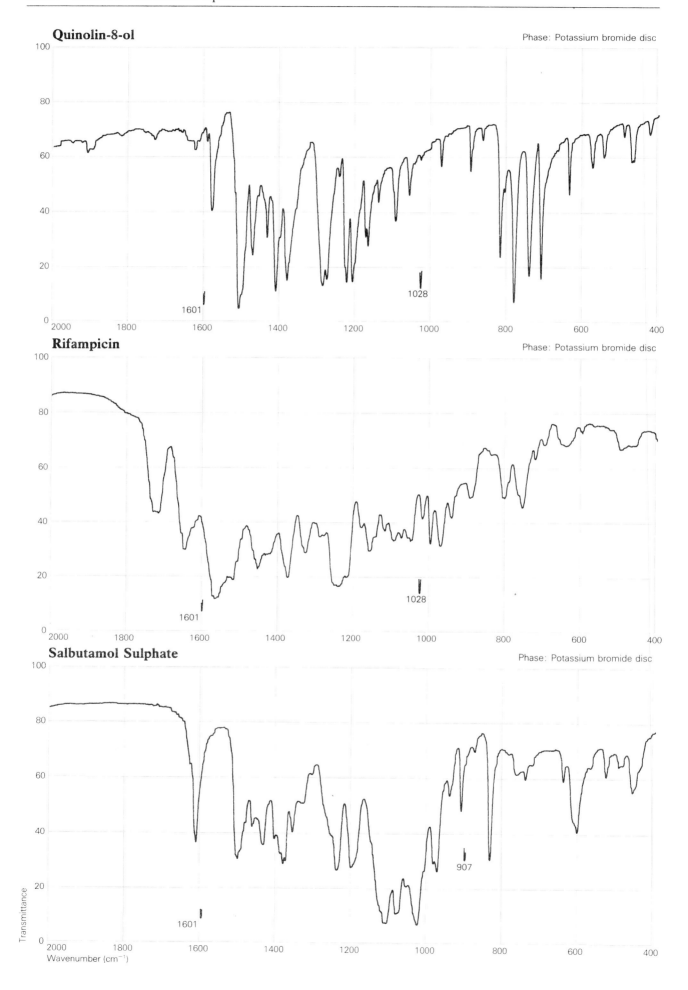

Quinolin-8-ol   Phase: Potassium bromide disc

Rifampicin   Phase: Potassium bromide disc

Salbutamol Sulphate   Phase: Potassium bromide disc

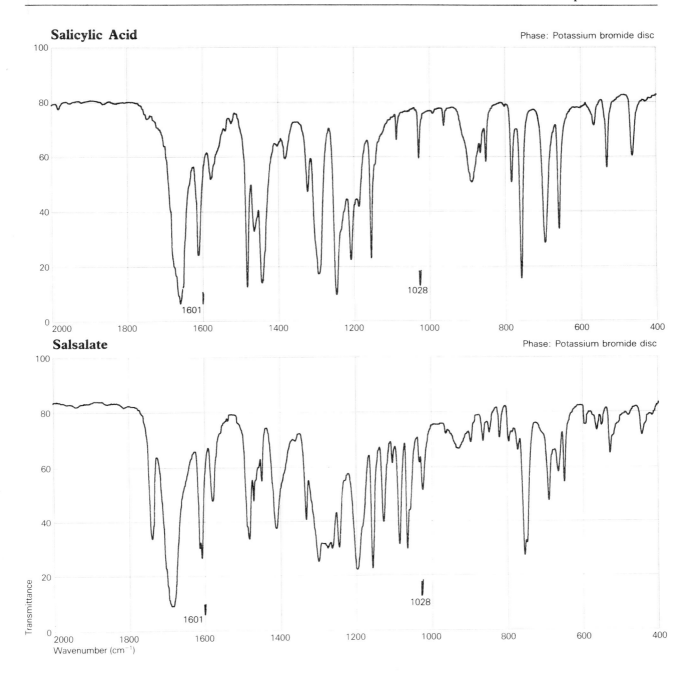

Salicylic Acid

Phase: Potassium bromide disc

1601

1028

Salsalate

Phase: Potassium bromide disc

1601

1028

Transmittance

Wavenumber (cm⁻¹)

Silicone Elastomer Base

Phase: Thin film

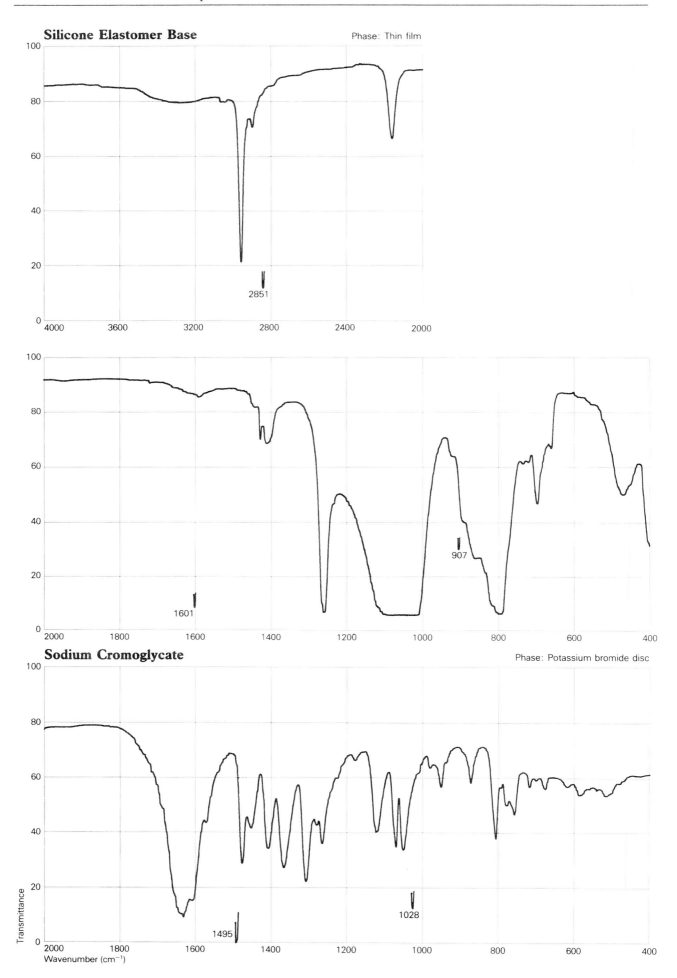

2851

1601

907

Sodium Cromoglycate

Phase: Potassium bromide disc

1495

1028

Transmittance

Wavenumber (cm⁻¹)

Sodium Diatrizoate

Phase: Potassium bromide disc

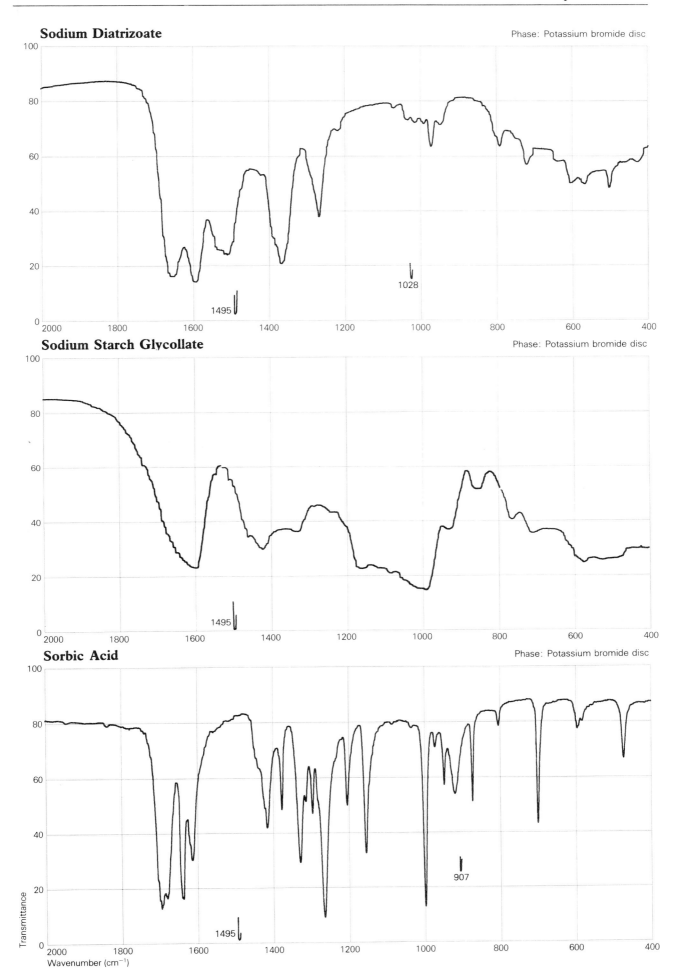

1495

1028

Sodium Starch Glycollate

Phase: Potassium bromide disc

1495

Sorbic Acid

Phase: Potassium bromide disc

907

1495

Transmittance

Wavenumber (cm⁻¹)

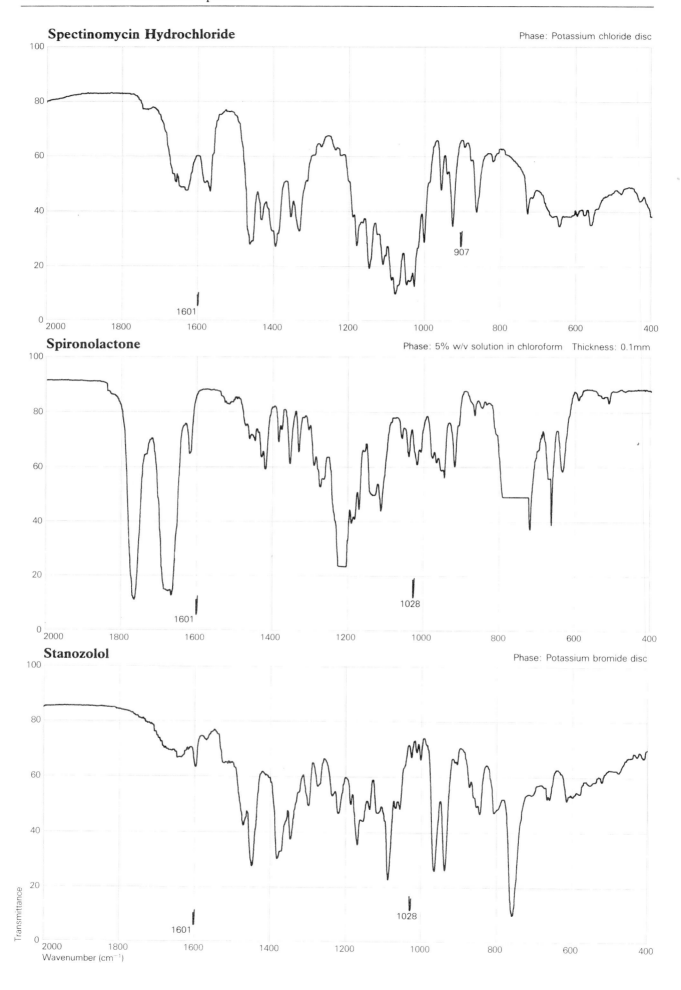

Spectinomycin Hydrochloride

Phase: Potassium chloride disc

1601
907

Spironolactone

Phase: 5% w/v solution in chloroform   Thickness: 0.1mm

1601
1028

Stanozolol

Phase: Potassium bromide disc

Transmittance

1601
1028

Wavenumber (cm⁻¹)

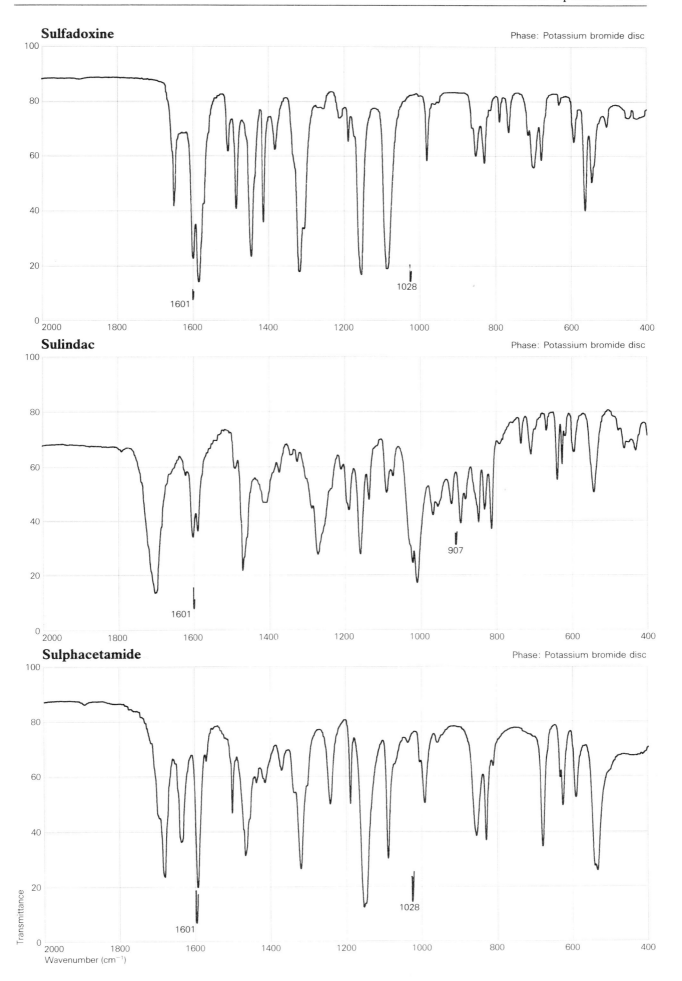

Sulfadoxine

Phase: Potassium bromide disc

1601
1028

Sulindac

Phase: Potassium bromide disc

1601
907

Sulphacetamide

Phase: Potassium bromide disc

1601
1028

Transmittance

Wavenumber (cm⁻¹)

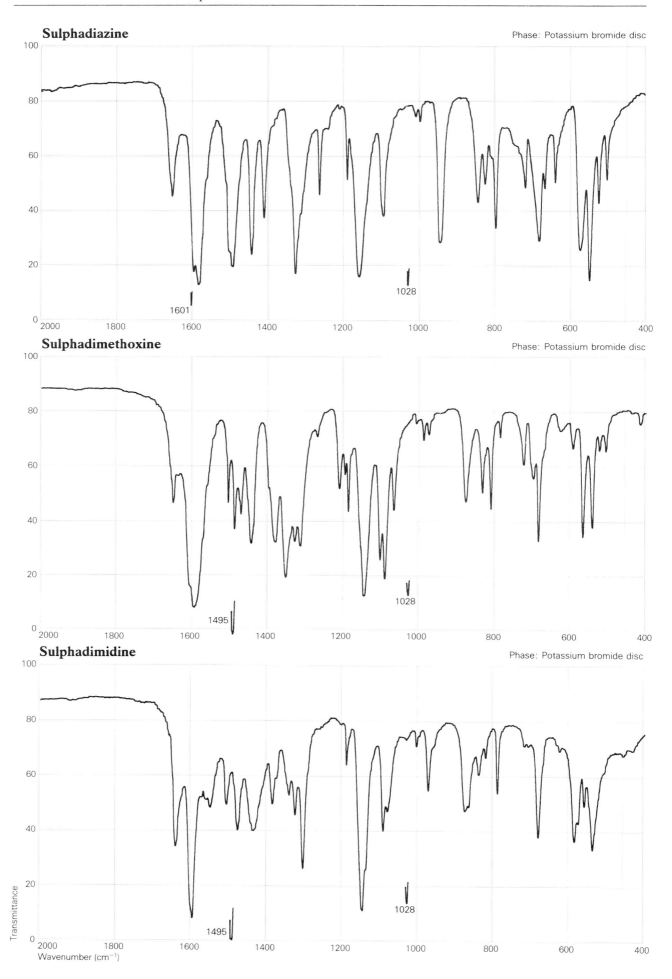

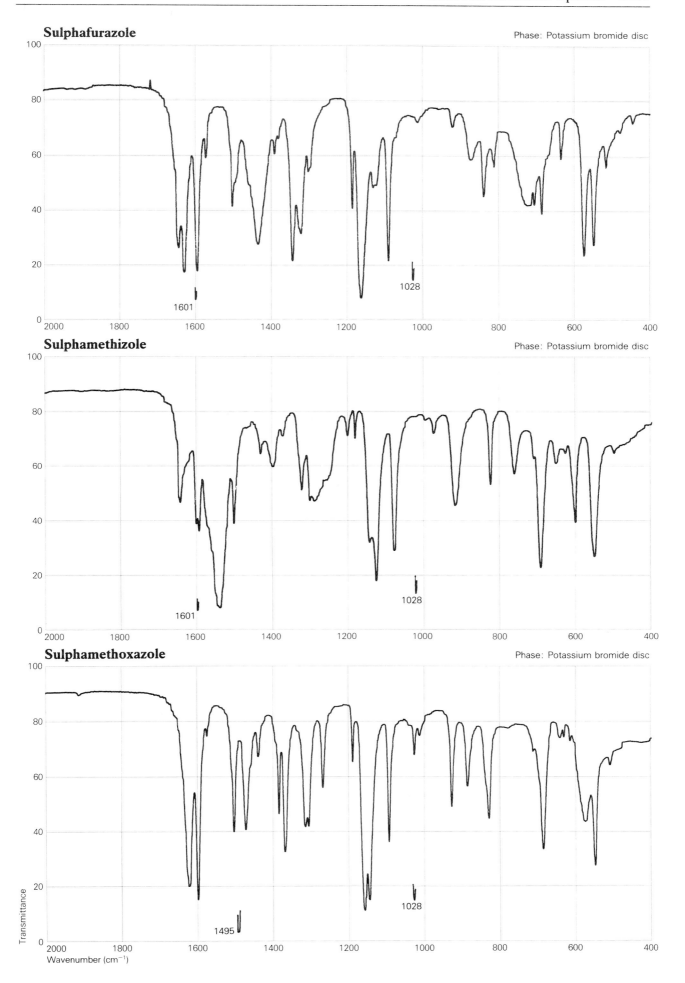

Sulphafurazole   Phase: Potassium bromide disc

1601

1028

Sulphamethizole   Phase: Potassium bromide disc

1601

1028

Sulphamethoxazole   Phase: Potassium bromide disc

1495

1028

Transmittance

Wavenumber (cm⁻¹)

Sulphamethoxypyridazine

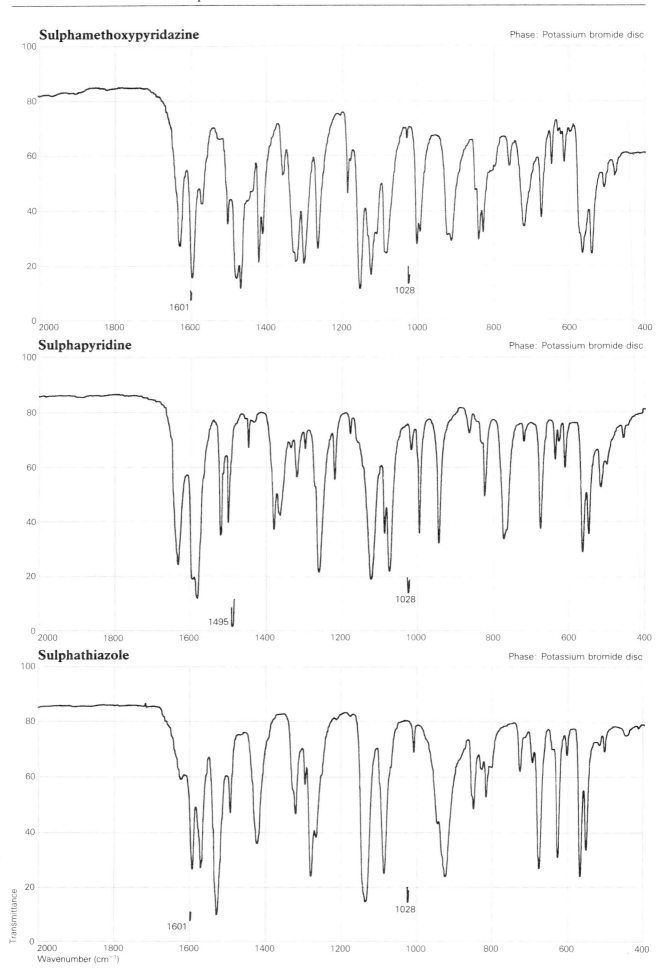

Phase: Potassium bromide disc

1601
1028

Sulphapyridine

Phase: Potassium bromide disc

1495
1028

Sulphathiazole

Phase: Potassium bromide disc

1601
1028

Transmittance

Wavenumber (cm⁻¹)

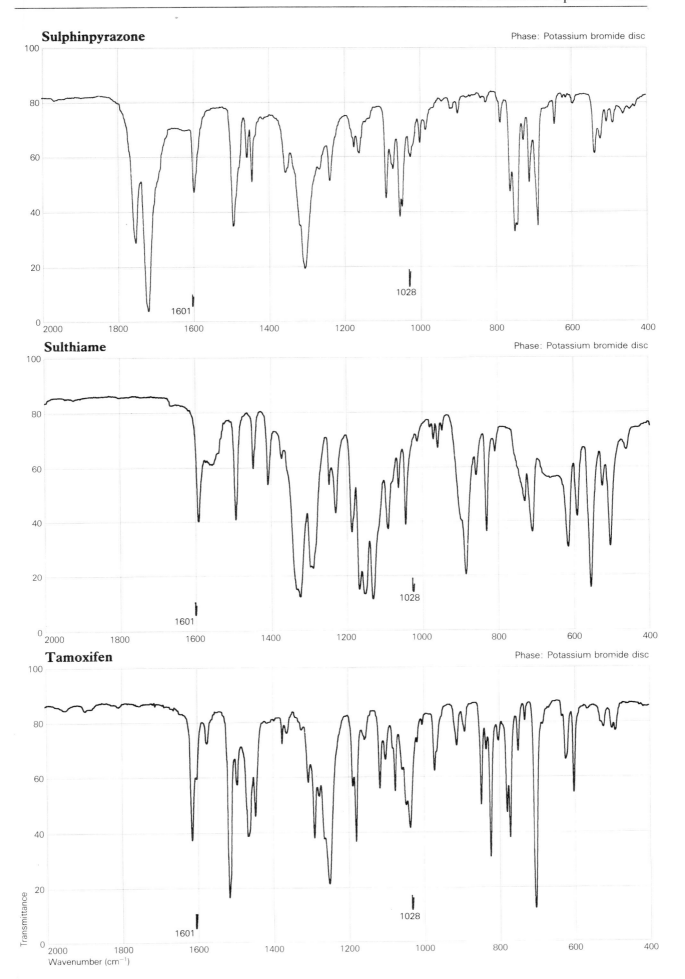

Sulphinpyrazone

Phase: Potassium bromide disc

1601

1028

Sulthiame

Phase: Potassium bromide disc

1601

1028

Tamoxifen

Phase: Potassium bromide disc

Transmittance

Wavenumber (cm⁻¹)

1601

1028

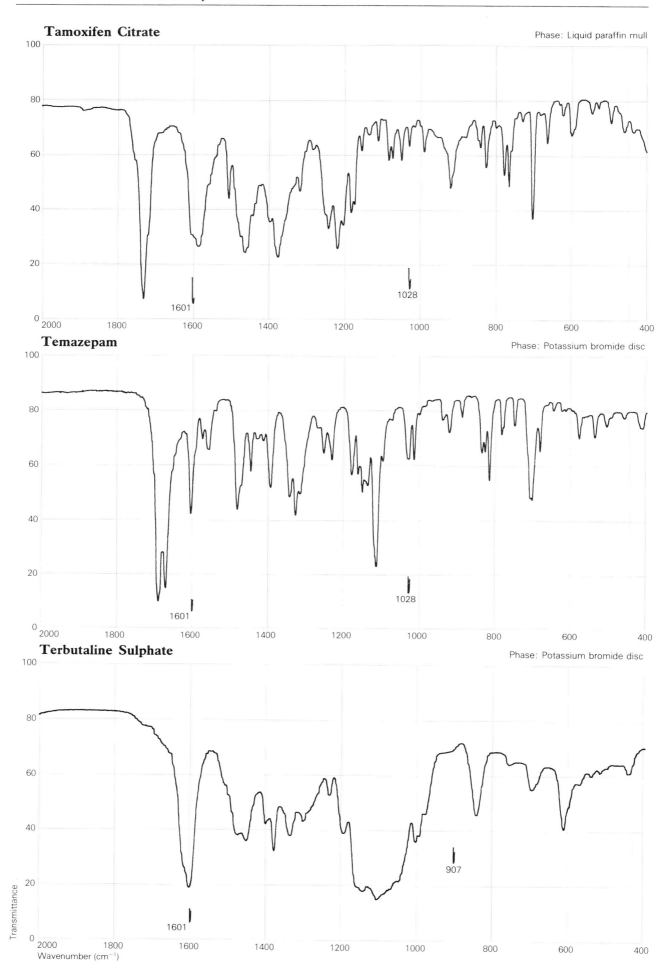

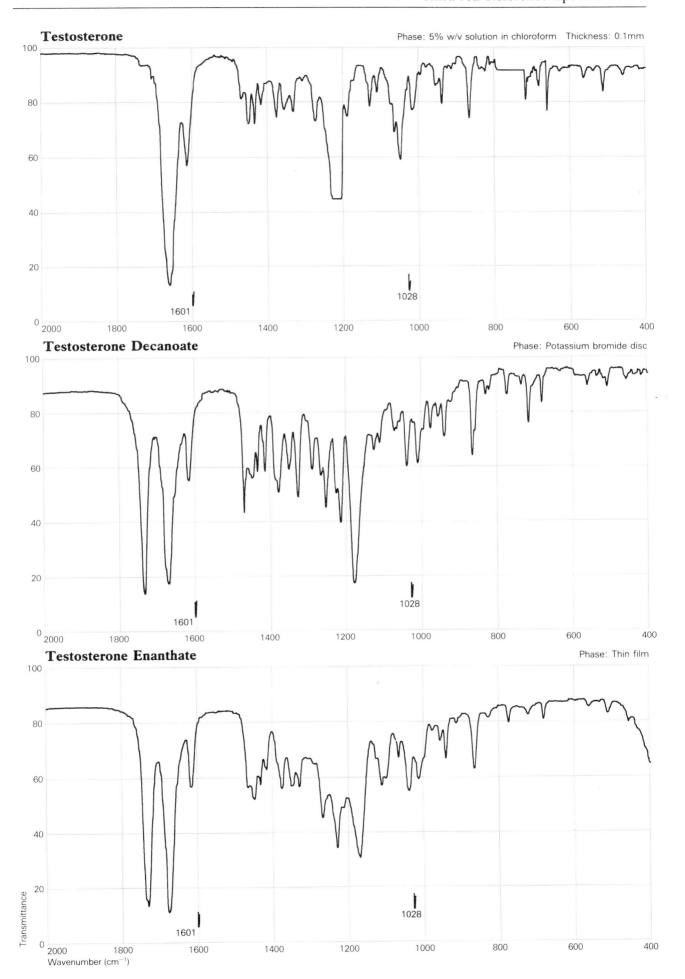

Testosterone

Phase: 5% w/v solution in chloroform   Thickness: 0.1mm

1601

1028

Testosterone Decanoate

Phase: Potassium bromide disc

1601

1028

Testosterone Enanthate

Phase: Thin film

1601

1028

Transmittance

Wavenumber (cm⁻¹)

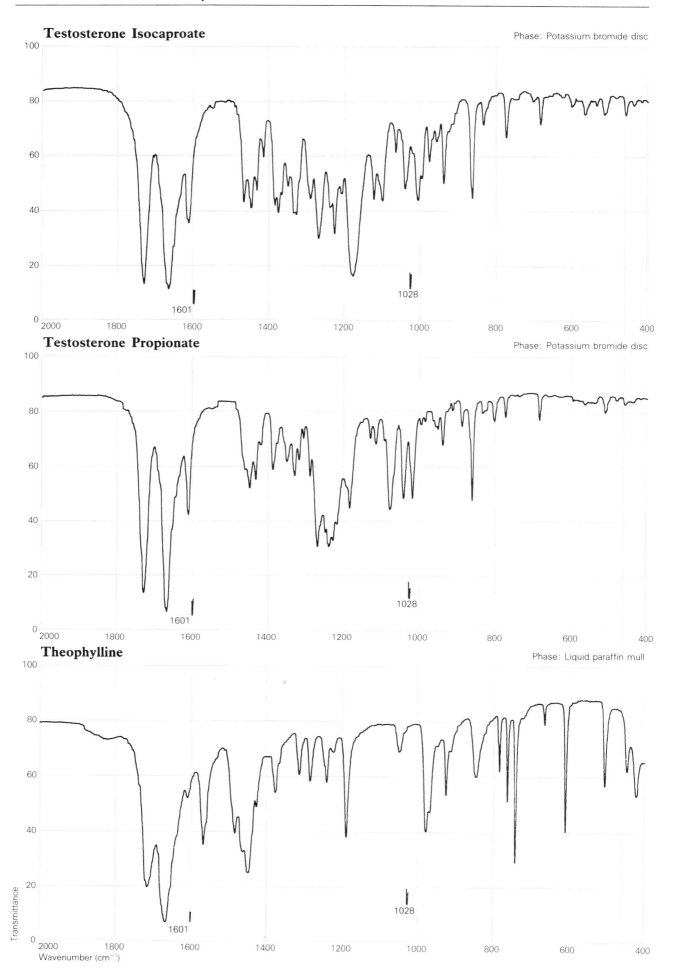

Testosterone Isocaproate

Phase: Potassium bromide disc

1601

1028

Testosterone Propionate

Phase: Potassium bromide disc

1601

1028

Theophylline

Phase: Liquid paraffin mull

1601

1028

Transmittance

Wavenumber (cm⁻¹)

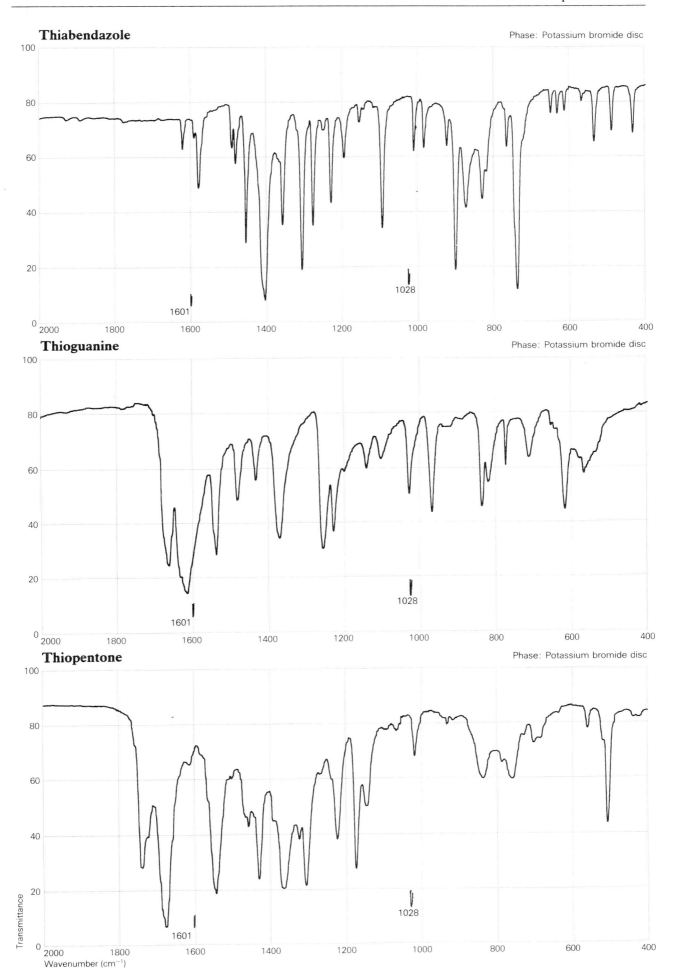

Thiabendazole

Phase: Potassium bromide disc

1601

1028

Thioguanine

Phase: Potassium bromide disc

1601

1028

Thiopentone

Phase: Potassium bromide disc

1601

1028

Transmittance

Wavenumber (cm⁻¹)

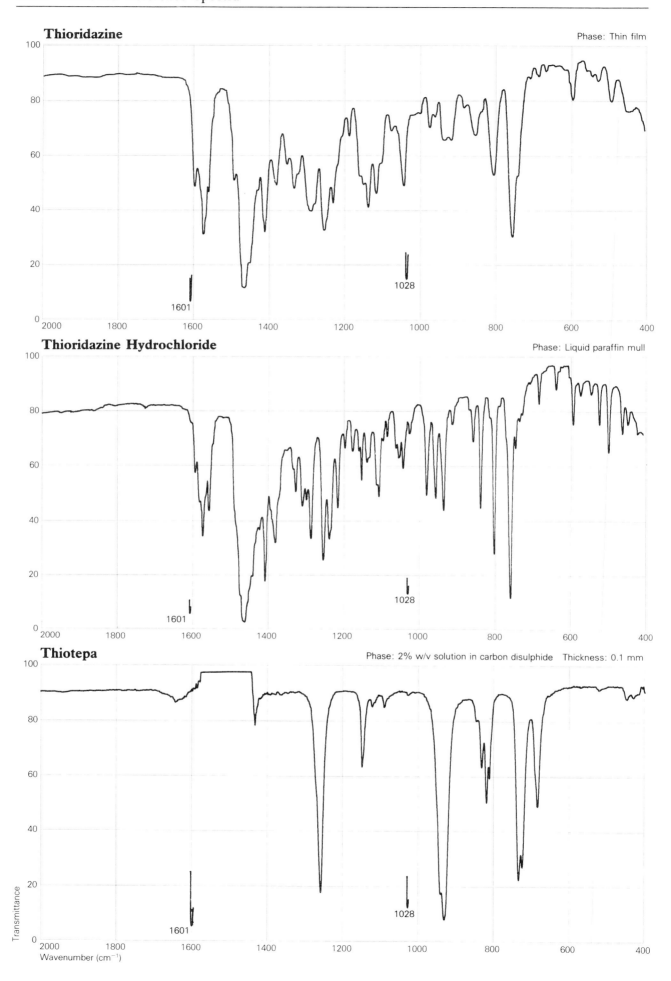

Thioridazine
Phase: Thin film

Thioridazine Hydrochloride
Phase: Liquid paraffin mull

Thiotepa
Phase: 2% w/v solution in carbon disulphide   Thickness: 0.1 mm

Transmittance

Wavenumber (cm⁻¹)

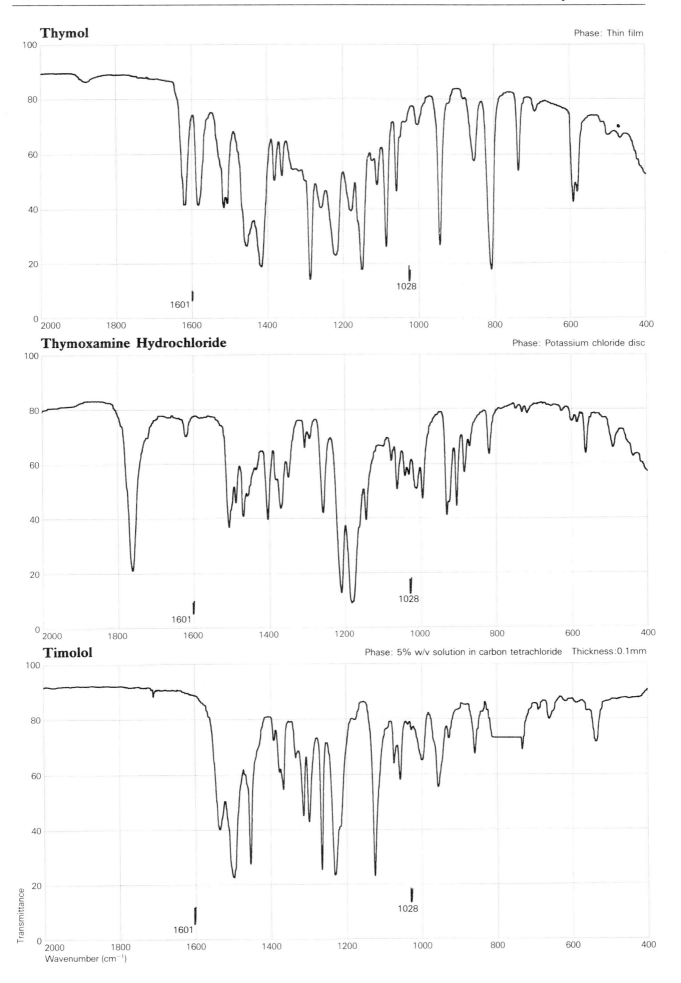

Thymol   Phase: Thin film

1601
1028

Thymoxamine Hydrochloride   Phase: Potassium chloride disc

1601
1028

Timolol   Phase: 5% w/v solution in carbon tetrachloride   Thickness:0.1mm

1601
1028

Transmittance

Wavenumber (cm⁻¹)

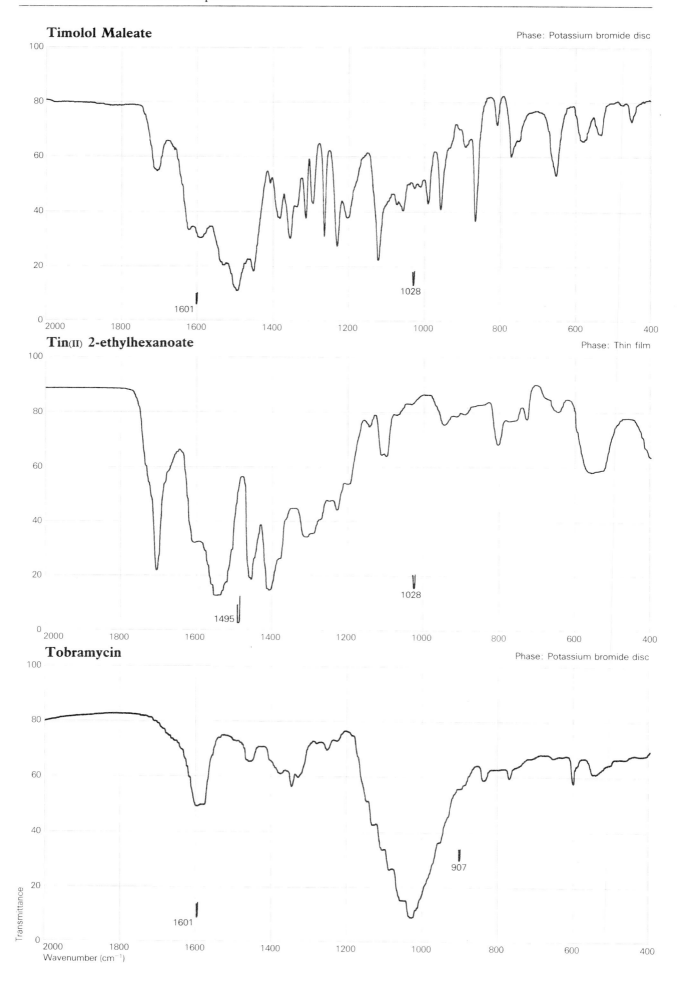

Timolol Maleate

Phase: Potassium bromide disc

1601

1028

Tin(II) 2-ethylhexanoate

Phase: Thin film

1495

1028

Tobramycin

Phase: Potassium bromide disc

907

1601

Transmittance

Wavenumber (cm⁻¹)

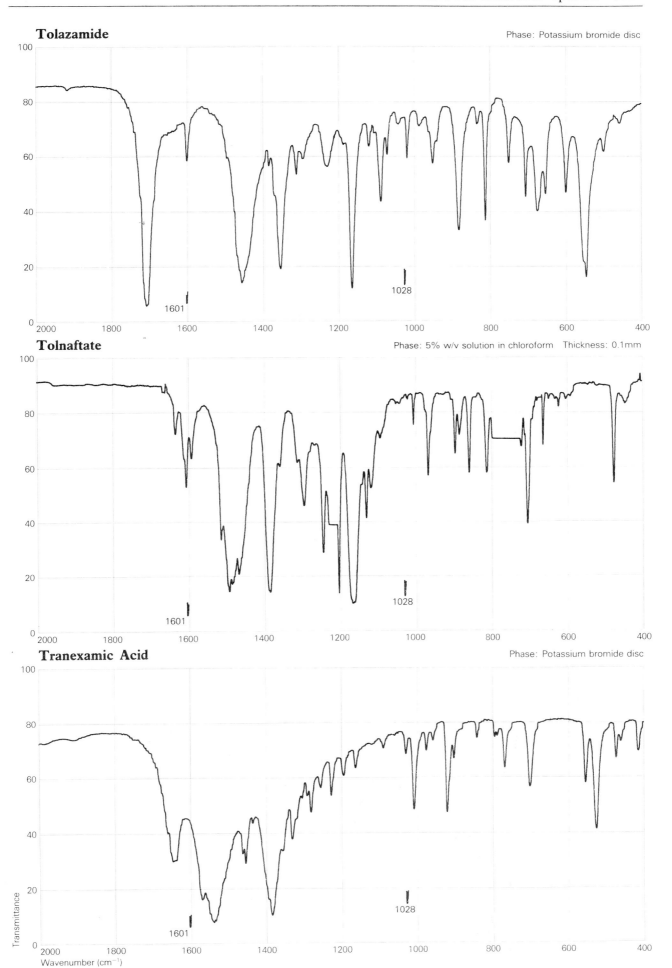

Tolazamide   Phase: Potassium bromide disc

Tolnaftate   Phase: 5% w/v solution in chloroform   Thickness: 0.1mm

Tranexamic Acid   Phase: Potassium bromide disc

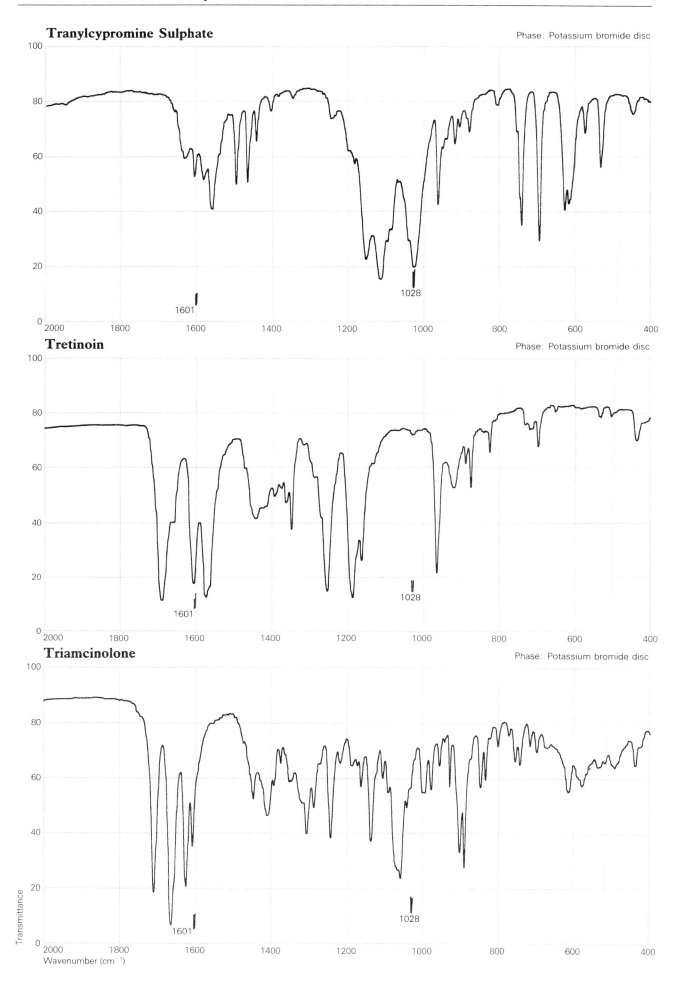

Tranylcypromine Sulphate

Phase: Potassium bromide disc

1601
1028

Tretinoin

Phase: Potassium bromide disc

1601
1028

Triamcinolone

Phase: Potassium bromide disc

1601
1028

Transmittance

Wavenumber (cm⁻¹)

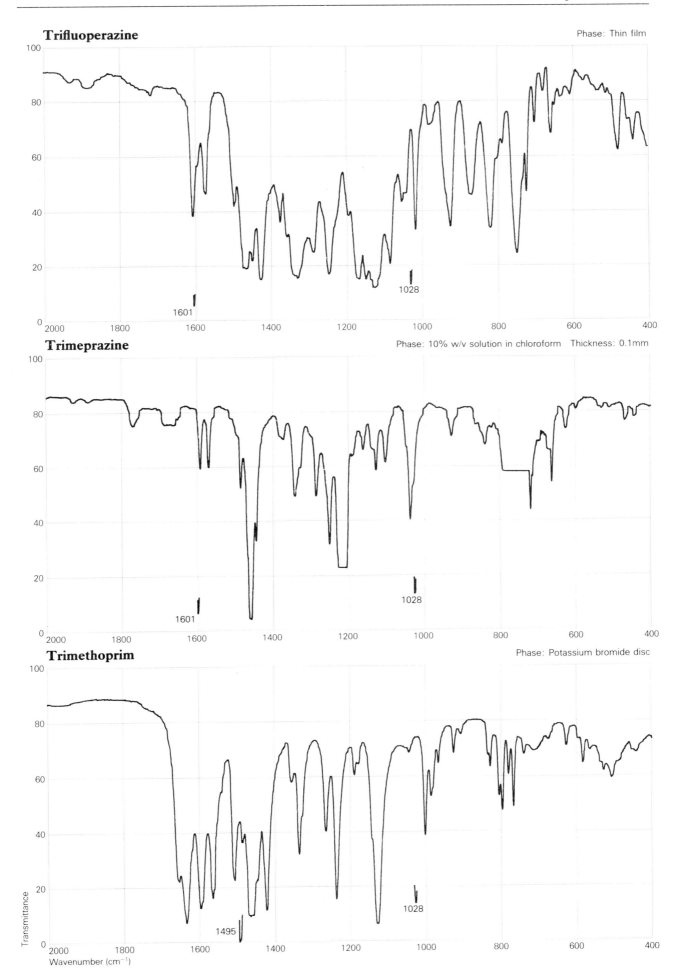

Trifluoperazine

Phase: Thin film

1601

1028

Trimeprazine

Phase: 10% w/v solution in chloroform   Thickness: 0.1mm

1601

1028

Trimethoprim

Phase: Potassium bromide disc

1495

1028

Transmittance

Wavenumber (cm⁻¹)

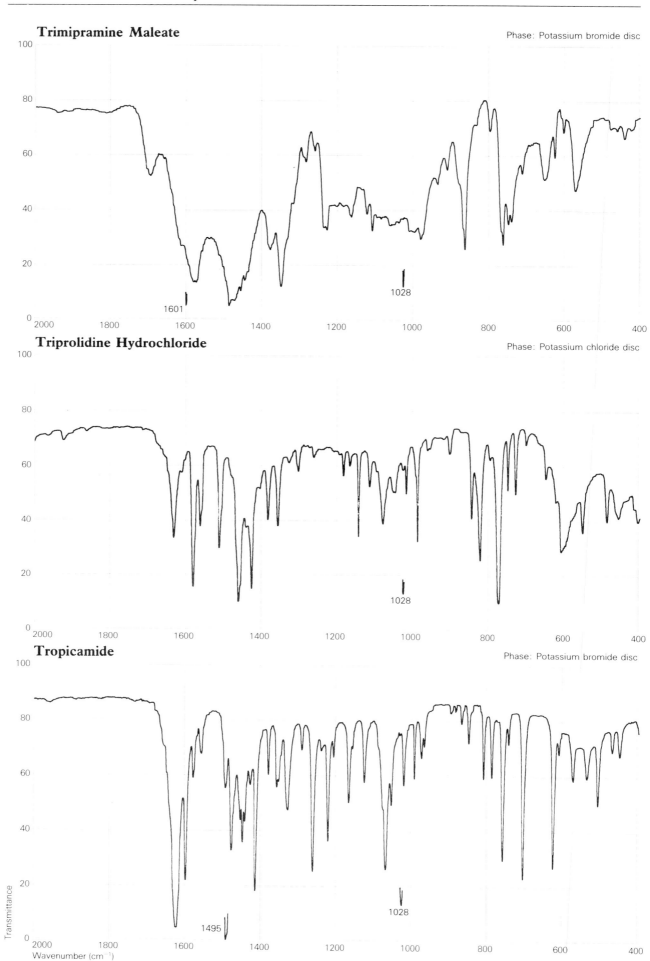

Trimipramine Maleate

Phase: Potassium bromide disc

1601

1028

Triprolidine Hydrochloride

Phase: Potassium chloride disc

1028

Tropicamide

Phase: Potassium bromide disc

1495

1028

Transmittance

Wavenumber (cm⁻¹)